Translational Medicine

Translational Medicine
Optimizing Preclinical Safety Evaluation
of Biopharmaceuticals

Edited by
Joy A. Cavagnaro and Mary Ellen Cosenza

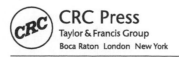

CRC Press
Taylor & Francis Group
Boca Raton London New York

CRC Press is an imprint of the
Taylor & Francis Group, an **Informa** business

First edition published 2022
by CRC Press
6000 Broken Sound Parkway NW, Suite 300, Boca Raton, FL 33487-2742

and by CRC Press
2 Park Square, Milton Park, Abingdon, Oxon, OX14 4RN

ISBN: 978-0-367-64427-7 (hbk)
ISBN: 978-0-367-64445-1 (pbk)
ISBN: 978-1-003-12454-2 (ebk)

DOI: 10.1201/9781003124542

Typeset in Times
by codeMantra

Contents

Part I   Principles

Part II   Practices

Part III   Product Attributes

Part IV   Practical Applications

Preface

The book *Preclinical Safety Evaluation of Biopharmaceuticals: A Science-Based Approach to Facilitating Clinical Trials*, ed. JA Cavagnaro, John Wiley & Sons, was published in 2008 over a decade ago. At the time, there were few comprehensive toxicology textbooks that focused on biotherapeutics, and it quickly became the premier reference and has remained the seminal book for biologics and advanced therapies to this day (so much so it is often referred to as the "BioBible"). The theme of the book was based upon experiences with the implementation of the "case-by-case" approach to preclinical safety evaluation: an approach which was accepted internationally in 1997 as guidance for the preclinical safety evaluation of biotechnology-derived products (ICH S6). The "case-by-case" approach is rational, flexible, innovative, science-, question-, and experiential-based, and targeted, taking into consideration a product's attributes. While most of the content of the "BioBible" is still relevant, experiences over the last decade have provided an opportunity to both revisit and expand the scope by providing relevance and application for the novel therapeutic modalities that have successfully advanced into clinical trials since 2008.

The goal of this book is to provide scientists responsible for the translation of novel biopharmaceuticals into clinical trials with a better understanding of how to navigate the obstacles that keep innovative medical research discoveries from becoming new therapies or even making it to clinical trials. The scope of products includes protein-based therapeutics, modified proteins, oligonucleotide-based therapies, monoclonal antibodies, antibody–drug conjugates, gene and cell-based therapies, gene-modified cell-based therapies, combination products, and therapeutic vaccines. Our intent is to provide examples and best practices that illustrate how to efficiently leverage discovery research for various modalities and how to implement science-based, rational, efficient, and predictive preclinical development programs to inform clinical efficacy and safety.

This book is divided into four areas of focus.

Part I Principles (Chapter 1–Chapter 5): This section addresses the "case-by-case" approach as influenced by product attributes and distinguishes characteristics between small and large molecules including oligos, cellular therapies, and gene-based therapies. Other topics include considerations for initial first-in-human (FIH) population/clinical POC (proof of concept) (normal subjects vs. index population; patient-specific therapies); dose extrapolation and support for dose regimens; considerations on how relevant species are defined; challenges of a development pathway where no animal toxicology studies are available; strategic planning; global regulatory expectations; and health authority interactions.

Part II Practices (Chapter 6–Chapter 18): This section describes how the principles in the first section are applied in the conduct of drug development including CMC (chemistry, manufacturing and controls), comparative toxicology testing, and unique routes of administration; and CRO selection, due diligence, and specific assessments such as immunogenicity, off-target binding assessments, immunotoxicity testing, and reproductive, developmental, and juvenile toxicity testing. Also, in this section biosimilars and combination products are discussed. IND best practices and pitfalls are also illustrated.

Part III Product Attributes (Chapter 19–Chapter 27): The objective of each of these chapters is to highlight the different preclinical approaches for various therapeutic modalities, i.e., "case-by-case", based on product attributes. These chapters cover peptides and therapeutic proteins, monoclonal antibodies, complex molecules such as ADCs, vaccines, oligonucleotides, cell and gene therapies, and gene-editing technologies. Rare diseases are also discussed. Each topic area discusses "What-Why-When-How" highlighting different considerations based upon product attributes.

Part IV Practical Applications (Chapter 28–Chapter 31): This section provides examples of implementation, "best practices", across specific therapeutic areas: oncology, immune-mediated diseases, infectious diseases, and neurodegenerative diseases.

-Joy A. Cavagnaro and Mary Ellen Cosenza

Acknowledgments

The editors would like to acknowledge all the chapter authors and colleagues who have embraced the case-by-case approach and shared their experiences for successful navigation of the "Valley of Death".

Thanks to all the scientists we have worked with globally over the years, including those from academia, industry, and health authorities. Maintaining active dialogues between and among the various groups has been key to the successful translation of novel biopharmaceuticals.

Special thanks to Shannon Shoup, our project manager extraordinaire, who was essential for completion of this book. She helped us to cross the finish line, never losing her persistence, her patience, or her pleasant disposition.

Extra special thanks to our families, both the Cavagnaro-Lewis and DeCiutiis-Cosenza clans. The answer to your most frequent question over these past few years—"Are you done yet?"—is: Yes, we are done!

Editors

Joy A. Cavagnaro, PhD, DABT, ATS, RAC, FRAPS, is the President of Access BIO where she consults on science-based preclinical development strategies for novel drug, biologics, and device combinations. She received her PhD in Biochemistry from the University of North Carolina at Chapel Hill. Her career spans academia, the CRO and biotechnology industries, and government. During her tenure at CBER/FDA, she was appointed to the SBRS and served as FDA's safety topic lead and rapporteur for "ICH S6". She was the first to advocate the "case-by-case" rational science-based approach to preclinical safety evaluation. In 2011, she received SOT's Biotechnology Specialty Section First Career Achievement Award, and in 2019, she received the Society's Arnold J. Lehman Award recognizing individuals who have made significant contributions to risk assessment and/or the regulation of chemical agents, including pharmaceuticals. She is Founder and past Chair of the leadership committee of BioSafe, an expert preclinical science committee within BIO. She is a past Chair of the Clinical and Regulatory Affairs Committee and Translational Science & Product Development Committee of the American Society of Gene & Cell Therapy. She served as President of the National Capital Area Chapter of Society of Toxicology and Chairman of the Board of Directors for Regulatory Affairs Professional Society. She was a member of the National Toxicology Program Scientific Advisory Committee on Alternative Toxicological Methods and is an advisor and member of the Grants Working Group of the California Institute for Regenerative Medicine. She serves on multiple scientific advisory boards (SABs) and consults and lectures internationally on translation and risk assessment of novel therapies. She is a past chair of CRRI, an independent investigational review board, and is currently a member of Advarra IRB. She has co-authored numerous white papers, articles, and book chapters related to various aspects of preclinical safety assessment. The book she edited, *Preclinical Safety Evaluation of Biopharmaceuticals: A Science-Based Approach to Facilitating Clinical Trials*, published by John Wiley & Sons, NJ, 2008, is commonly referred to as the "BioBible".

Mary Ellen Cosenza, PhD, DABT, ATS, ERT, RAC, is a regulatory consultant with over 30 years of senior leadership experience in the biopharmaceutical industry in the USA, Europe, and emerging markets. Before becoming a consultant, she served as the Executive Director, U.S. Regulatory Affairs, at Amgen, Inc. During her 20-year tenure at Amgen, she led the International Emerging Markets Regulatory Department and served as an Executive Director of Global Regulatory Affairs and Safety. In addition to her leadership roles in Regulatory Affairs, she also served as the Senior Director of Toxicology at Amgen. Prior to joining Amgen, she served as a Principal Scientist for the Medical Research Division of American Cyanamid Company (now Pfizer). Mary Ellen is a founding member of BIO's BioSafe Preclinical Safety Expert Group. She was also a member of an Expert Working Group, operating under the auspices of the International Conference on Harmonization (ICH) for ICH M3(R2). She has been awarded the ACT Mildred Christian Women's Leadership in Toxicology Award (2019) and SOT's Biotechnology Specialty Section Career Achievement Award (2015). Mary Ellen is a Diplomat of the American Board of Toxicology, a Fellow of the Academy of Toxicological Sciences, and a member of the Society of Toxicology (SOT), Drug Information Association (DIA), and Regulatory Affairs Professional Society (RAPS) and holds Regulatory Affairs Certification for both the U.S. and EU. Mary Ellen has been an active member of the American College of Toxicology (ACT) and has served as a member of the ACT Education Committee, as Councilor, and as Treasurer and President of the College. She is currently the Treasurer of the International Union of Toxicology (IUTOX). She is also an adjunct assistant professor at the University of Southern California where she teaches graduate-level courses in toxicology and regulation of biologics. Mary Ellen received her PhD in Toxicology from St. John's University, New York, and her MS in Regulatory Science from the University of Southern California, Los Angeles.

Contributors

D. Blanset
Boehringer Ingelheim
Ridgefield, Connecticut

Christopher J. Bowman
Worldwide Research, Development and Medical
Pfizer, Inc.
Groton, Connecticut

Ed Branson
PharmaDirections, Inc.
Cary, North Carolina

Frank R. Brennan
Preclinical Safety (PCS)
Novartis Institute of BioMedical Research
United Kingdom

Florence G. Burleson
Burleson Research Technologies, Inc.
Morrisville, North Carolina

Gary R. Burleson
Burleson Research Technologies, Inc.
Morrisville, North Carolina

Stefanie C.M. Burleson
Burleson Research Technologies, Inc.
Morrisville, North Carolina

Joy A. Cavagnaro
Access BIO, LC
Boyce, Virginia

C.W. Chen
Tox and Text Solutions, LLC
Anaheim, California

Simon Chivers
Integrated Biologix GmbH
Basel, Switzerland

Anu Connor
Novartis
Basel, Switzerland

Mary Ellen Cosenza
MEC Regulatory & Toxicology Consulting, LLC
Thousand Oaks, California

Cathaline den Besten
ProQR Therapeutics BV
Leiden, Netherlands

Maggie Dempster
GlaxoSmithKline
Middlesex, United Kingdom

M. Di Piazza
F. Hoffmann-La Roche AG
Basel, Switzerland

Benjamin J. Doranz
Integral Molecular
Philadelphia, Pennsylvania

C. E. Ellis
Division of Pharmacology/Toxicology for Infectious Diseases
(DPT-ID)
CDER, US-FDA
Silver Spring, Maryland

Hadi Falahatpisheh
AbbVie Inc.
Lake Bluff, Illinois

Ellen G. Feigal
NDA Partners LLC
Santa Rosa Valley, California

Gregory L. Finch
Independent Toxicologist
Waterford, Connecticut

Stephanie F. Greene
Trovare Preclinical Consulting, LLC
Consulting Toxicologist
Ventura, California

Magali Guffroy
AbbVie Inc.
Lake Bluff, Illinois

Helen G. Haggerty
Nonclinical Safety
Janssen
Beerse, Belgium

Melanie T. Hartsough
Hartsough Nonclinical Consulting LLC
Derwood, Maryland

Scott P. Henry
Ionis Pharmaceuticals, Inc.
Carlsbad, California

Jonathan Heyen
Drug Safety Research and Development
Pfizer, Inc.
Groton, Connecticut

D. N. Hovland, Jr.
Eledon Pharmaceuticals, Inc.
Irvine, California

Cris Kamperschroer
Early Phase Development Solutions
Labcorp
Saranac Lake, New York

A. Kimzey
Biopharmaceutical/Pharmaceutical Practice
ToxStrategies, Inc.
Katy, Texas

Sheri D. Klas
Klas Act Consulting, LLC
Bozeman, Montana

Janice Lansita
Toxicology Consultant
ToxAlliance LLC
Kennett Square, Pennsylvania

Michael W. Leach
Drug Safety Research and Development
Pfizer, Inc.
Groton, Connecticut

Anthony J. Lee
Seagen Inc.
Bothell, Washington

Arthur A. Levin
Avidity Biosciences
La Jolla, California

Lise I. Loberg
AbbVie Inc.
Lake Bluff, Illinois

Timothy MacLachlan
Preclinical Safety
Novartis Institutes for Biomedical Research
Basel, Switzerland

Andrew McDougal
Division of Transplant and Ophthalmology Products (DTOP)
Office of Antimicrobial Products (OAP), Office of New
    Drugs (OND)
Center for Drug Evaluation and Research (CDER)
U.S. Food and Drug Administration (FDA)
Silver Spring, Maryland

K. McKeever
Translational Sciences
Ultragenyx Pharmaceutical
Novato, California

Sara McKenzie
PharmaDirections, Inc.
Cary, North Carolina

K. Mease
Biopharmaceutical/Pharmaceutical Practice
ToxStrategies, Inc.
Katy, Texas

Kathleen Meyer-Tamaki
Nonclinical Development
Sangamo Therapeutics, Inc.
Brisbane, California

P. Mookherjee
Toxicology Department
Global Blood Therapeutics, Inc.
South San Francisco, California

B. Mounho-Zamora
Biopharmaceutical/Pharmaceutical Practice
ToxStrategies, Inc.
Katy, Texas

Eunice Musvasva
F. Hoffmann-La Roche AG
Basel, Switzerland

Janet Nokleby
Consultant
Moorpark, California

Diana M. Norden
Integral Molecular
Philadelphia, Pennsylvania

Deborah L. Novicki
DL Novicki Toxicology Consulting LLC
Marlborough, Massachusetts

Colin Phipps
AbbVie Inc.
Lake Bluff, Illinois

Rafael Ponce
Shape Therapeutics
Seattle, Washington

Sherry L. Ralston
AbbVie Inc.
Lake Bluff, Illinois

Stanley A. Roberts
SAR Safety Assessment
San Diego, California

Melissa M. Schutten
Genentech, Inc.
South San Francisco, California

B. B. Smith
Toxicology
Vir Biotechnology
San Francisco, California

Jane Sohn
Pharmacology/Toxicology Team Lead
Office of Nonprescription Drugs (ONPD)
Office of New Drugs (OND)
Center for Drug Evaluation and Research (CDER)
U.S. Food and Drug Administration (FDA)
Silver Spring, Maryland

Nicola J. Stagg
Genentech, Inc.
South San Francisco, California

John T. Sullivan
Regulatory, Safety, Clinical Pharmacology and Drug
    Development Consulting
Thousand Oaks, California

Steven J. Swanson
Steven J Swanson Consulting, LLC
Moorpark, California

Marque Todd
Renaissance Consulting
San Diego, California

Jay Tibbitts
Surrozen Inc.
South San Francisco, California

Gerhard F. Weinbauer
LabCorp Early Development Services GmbH
Münster, Germany

Shawna L. Weis
Vice President, Toxicology, Constellation Pharmaceuticals
Cambridge, Massachusetts

M. Wood
Biopharmaceutical/Pharmaceutical Practice
ToxStrategies, Inc.
Katy, Texas

Patricia D. Williams
Chief Executive Officer
IND Directions, LLC
Annandale, New Jersey

Part I

Principles

1

Case-by-Case Approach: A Historical Perspective

Joy A. Cavagnaro
Access BIO, LC

CONTENTS

1.1 Translational Imperative

Bringing safe new medicines to market is critical not only from a medical and economic perspective but also from a societal point of view. The speed at which drug development is expected to take place in order to achieve this goal is challenging not only for small start-up companies but also for large well-resourced companies. These expectations have not been higher than those created by the recent COVID-19 pandemic. The practical challenges to accelerating clinical development of novel therapies and "getting it right the first time" include managing the inevitable delays. Such delays can range from issues including unavailability of sufficient test article, analytical methods, reagents, relevant animal models, a clinical plan, to lack of reproducibility of the data, lack of experienced staff or alignment of the management team, or lack of understanding of the regulatory pathway. Regulatory authorities are expected to meet the challenge by providing the necessary guidance documents to ensure quality, safety, and efficacy and by conducting rapid review of the information. "Fast track" drug development in the US and priority regulatory review designations ex-US, however, are not defined by a "faster read" of an investigational new drug application by regulatory authorities. While FDA will provide more meetings and feedback/guidance, more importantly sponsors will need to ensure that sufficient resources are in place to be able to realize development efficiencies to ensure that the "right" decisions are made sooner in the development process not only to facilitate development but also to help manage potential risks (Cavagnaro 2001).

Accelerated development plans expect first-in-human (FIH) studies to provide data that are sufficient not only to identify potential development-limiting adverse events, but also to establish proof of concept, ideally in the patient population. Thus, the paradigm of a Phase I study in healthy volunteers to assess safety, Phase II study(ies) dose ranging in patients to confirm safety, determine clinical activity, and define an optimal dose, and Phase III well-controlled studies to confirm safety in efficacy has shifted for novel therapies, many of which are now targeting rare diseases. There is a high expectation that safety and efficacy can be determined by conducting Phase I (in patients) and Phase II/III studies and in some cases a single Phase I/II study. As such, the quality of the manufactured product and the quality of the preclinical data are critical components to support accelerated clinical timelines.

1.2 Role of Preclinical Development

The purpose of preclinical, pre-the-clinical, development is to support clinical decision-making. In order to facilitate clinical development, it is important to define risk and benefit in the most reasonable and appropriate way. Preclinical studies are the foundation for the initial ongoing assessment of potential risks and as such should be designed to realize their maximal value. The primary objective of preclinical safety evaluation is to provide data that clinical investigators can use to better predict adverse effects in study subjects and to help design clinical studies that will minimize their occurrence. The same information will also help to guide research toward new, less toxic drugs and, if harmful effects cannot be entirely avoided, to suggest means to lessen or alleviate the potential adverse reactions. Early in clinical development, preclinical studies are designed to support the recommendation of an initial safe starting dose and dose escalation scheme, identify potential target organ(s) of toxicity, determine reversibility of effects, and identify a specific risk to subjects. During development, studies are designed to support broader subject enrollment and longer study durations, as well as, if needed, to answer specific questions with respect to the mechanism of toxicity.

DOI: 10.1201/9781003124542-2

1.3 Improving the Science of Predicting Toxicity

In 1987, Professor Gerhard Zbinden challenged toxicologists to "refrain from following the beaten track of routine toxicology testing." In November 2005, this same message was echoed by the Preclinical Toxicology Working Group of the Academy of Medical Sciences in the Safe Medicines Report which concluded that "the challenge is to change the present culture of thinking about regulatory toxicology and replace it with the concept of science-driven toxicology" (Cavagnaro 2002).

Various initiatives have occurred over the past two decades to improve the science of predicting toxicity and improve extrapolation to humans. These include the encouragement and application of innovative designs, greater emphasis on mechanistic studies, greater understandings in PK/PD modeling approaches, and validation and acceptance of new in vitro models including organoid cultures. Other innovations include the utilization of in vivo humanized animal models and animals that mimic human disease for assessing safety in addition to efficacy, the incorporation of noninvasive and minimally invasive technologies, and the use of non-cellular and cell-based simulation models to enhance predictions.

Importantly, as preclinical translational scientists, we are humbled by our understandings that despite our best efforts to maximize the designs of our preclinical study designs and programs to improve predictive value, their inherent limitations mean that therapies may be ineffective in humans or more importantly unanticipated adverse events may occur in clinical trials. In some cases, these results have been explained by differences in sensitivity between normal and diseased states.

1.4 Development and Implementation of the Case-by-Case Approach

As previously stated, the case-by-case approach is not consistent with traditional practices, but this does not mean it is a minimalist approach. However, because it is not a prescriptive approach, it is less easy to predict that studies performed will be acceptable to regulatory authorities, which has been a key challenge to acceptance and implementation. The approach is, however, consistent with traditional principles. It is science-based, question-based, data-driven, and practical. Studies are designed to obtain maximum information with judicious animal use where limitations are identified. It is flexible, based on knowledge base, and innovative, as new models to answer new questions are ongoing activities.

The principles of safety evaluation remain the same as conventional pharmaceuticals including developing sufficient data for recommending a safe starting dose, dose escalations, and dose regimens; discerning the mechanism of toxicity if unexpected toxicity is demonstrated; identifying parameters to monitor in the clinic for potential toxicities and duration of follow-up; providing rationale for a specific patient population; determining potential unacceptable toxicities in certain patient populations; predicting potential adverse interactions with concomitant therapies; and providing a preliminary risk/benefit assessment. Examples of preclinical findings that can influence the design of early and subsequent clinical development strategies include difficult-to-monitor target organ effects, narrow therapeutic indexes, enhanced toxicity in the animal model of disease or with increased study durations, unanticipated cross-reactivity, similar toxicities across species, and delayed toxicities including those that may result in infection or tumors.

The successful implementation of a product-specific science-based, "case-by-case" approach requires individuals with a broad knowledge of toxicological processes and the ability to integrate data from molecular biology, pharmacology, physiology, pharmacokinetics, and pathology. This knowledge is gained through experience and/or training. However, as developers continue to innovate, there will often be no precedence. Sponsors are ultimately responsible for providing the data and scientific justification to support each case, "telling the story." Importantly, early and more frequent dialogue with regulatory authorities throughout development may be needed to ensure acceptability. Additionally, the clinical enterprise extends to clinical investigators as well as members on ethical review committees. Ultimately, we must have sufficient information to communicate to subjects to allow them to make informed decisions to enroll in trials with novel therapeutic agents.

1.5 Future Applications

The explicit intent of the initial ICH S6 guidance was primarily to recommend a basic framework for the preclinical safety evaluation of biotechnology-derived pharmaceuticals. At the time, the scope of applicable products included products derived from characterized cells through the use of a variety of expression systems including bacteria, yeast, insect, plant, and mammalian cells. The intended indications included in vivo diagnostic, therapeutic, or prophylactic uses. The active substances included proteins and peptides, their derivatives, and products of which they were components; they could be derived from cell cultures or produced using recombinant deoxyribonucleic acid (DNA) technology, including production by transgenic plants and animals. Examples included but were not limited to cytokines, plasminogen activators, recombinant plasma factors, growth factors, fusion proteins, enzymes, receptors, hormones, and monoclonal antibodies (mAbs). Although not formerly incorporated in the scope, it was acknowledged that the principles outlined in the guidance may also be applicable to recombinant DNA protein vaccines, chemically synthesized peptides, plasma-derived products, endogenous proteins extracted from human tissue, and oligonucleotide (ODN) drugs. At the time, the document excluded antibiotics, allergenic extracts, heparin, vitamins, cellular blood components, conventional bacterial or viral vaccines, DNA vaccines, and cellular and gene therapies. Current guidance has since extended the case-by-case approach to the preclinical safety evaluation of investigational cellular and gene therapy products (US FDA 2012).

The relevance for the case-by-case approach based upon product attributes is highlighted not only across but within product classes. All mAbs have not been created equal. Differences have included but are not limited to whole molecules or fragments (nanobodies, diabodies, triabodies, tetrabodies); different isotypes and modifications to Fc regions; use of different cell substrates for production including transgenic animals and plants; murine, chimeric, humanized, fully humanized versions; constructs have been monospecific, bispecific, and even trispecific; naked or conjugated with toxins or chemicals; uniquely species specific; functions include agonist or agonist activities; catalytic antibodies; targets can be endogenous or exogenous; and there have been variations of antibodies and Fc fusion molecules including peptibodies. Despite these important differences in product attributes, all have successfully advanced into clinic trials utilizing the case-by-case approach.

As previously discussed with flexibility to design toxicology studies using a science-based approach, the lack of a consensus approach could lead to variability in acceptance by regulatory authorities. ODN drugs are regulated as small molecules because they are chemically synthesized although they have attributes of both small and large molecules (Schubert et al. 2012). This dual characterization is why they were considered in the initial ICH S6 guidance. Of note, over a decade ago the ODN community challenged a potential third characterization by petitioning that synthetic RNA and DNA ODNs be exempt from the definition as a gene therapy requiring additional public review, arguing lack of transmission via the germ line or integration into the host genome. Discussions are currently ongoing in the community as to how to better predict regulatory acceptance by either generating a new guidance or tailoring the existing M3(R2) guidance based on a recent ODN therapeutics survey sponsored by EFPIA which was first presented at the Oligonucleotide-based Therapeutics Conference in October 2019. There were 22 respondents to the survey. The various types of ODNs considered included ssRNAaseH, ss splicing, ss immunostim, ss other, ss siRNA, ds siRNAs, ds other, and aptamers similar to the diversity within mAbs. Over half of the respondents acknowledged regulatory acceptance of innovative or "leaner packages," and approximately half considered that ICH S6 might be relevant. Should the community decide a new guidance is needed, principally to ensure consistency of acceptance among regulatory authorities, the cautionary note was that it not be prescriptive as to not unnecessarily limit the quickly advancing field.

The biotech field has and will continue to innovate not only new product classes but also the types of products within a product class. The confidence to innovate is both science-based and experiential-based. The development of novel therapies means that at times there will be no precedence. Moreover, we have to be humbled and accept the fact that there will likely be limitations in our preclinical assessments and predictions for clinical efficacy and safety, even if programs are optimally designed. This will continue to be true for therapies in development with unique species specify where the only relevant specie for the intended clinical product is "human" including those cases where preclinical species lack the human ortholog or paralog; in cases when only surrogates can be used; and in cases where animal models are lacking. Successful arguments for comparability will continue to be made not only when surrogates are used but also when manufacturing changes are made to the clinical product over the course of clinical development. Justification will be needed to support the definition a relevant species and animal models of disease. The unexpected demand of non-human primates caused by the pandemic has resulted in a global shortage, further emphasizing the importance of their use only if relevant and in optimizing study designs to ensure judicious use. The use of patient cells should further improve our extrapolations in addition to the increased acceptance of the use of animal models of disease to assess both safety and efficacy. This is especially true in cases where the subjects in the FIH study are patients and where disease models are more sensitive to toxicity which should improve extrapolations for safety. Assessment and interpretation of immunogenicity data and translation to humans will continue to be the most challenging areas of extrapolation, impacting the determination of no observed adverse effect levels (NOAELs), especially problematic when adverse antibody-mediated findings are observed at the lowest dose level or only at the lowest dose level. Optimization of methods to better assess and interpret consequences and relevance of off-target or unintended target effects will continue to be important for a variety of modalities spanning mAbs, ONs, and gene-based technologies, including gene-editing. The speed at which drug development is expected to take place is only increasing. While we may be able to capitalize on learnings from acceleration opportunities enacted to address the COVID pandemic, realization of development efficiencies is only ensured if the "right" decisions are made sooner in the development process. An understating of basic ("M") components for accelerating translation of novel modalities into the clinic can be useful for projecting both efficient and realistic development timelines: Medical (unmet need); bioMarkers (safety and/or efficacy endpoints); Models (availability/relevance); Materials (quality); Methods (feasibility); Manufacturing (capacity); Multiple disciplines (collaboration); huManpower (experienced); Milestones (achievable); Management (aligned); and Money (much more).

REFERENCES

Cavagnaro, J. 2001. Pre-clinical development strategies for new medicines: Are the correct questions being asked? *Regulatory Affairs Journal* 12: 3–4.

Cavagnaro, J. 2002. Preclinical safety evaluation of biotechnology-derived pharmaceuticals. *Nature Reviews Drug Discovery* 1: 469–475.

FDA Guidance for Industry Preclinical Assessment of Investigational Cell and Gene Products. 2013. https://www.fda.gov/media/87564/download

ICHS6 and ICHS6(R1) Preclinical Safety Evaluation of Biotechnology-derived Pharmaceuticals. 1997, 2011. https://www.fda.gov/regulatory-information/search-fda-guidance-documents/s6r1-preclinical-safety-evaluation-biotechnology-derived-pharmaceuticals

Schubert, D., Levin, A., Kornbrust, D., Berman, C.L., Cavagnaro, J., Henry, S., Sequin, R., Ferrari, N., and Shrewsbury, S.B. 2012. Oligonucleotide Safety Working Group (OSWG). *Nucleic Acid Therapeutics* 22: 211–212.

2

Selection of Relevant Animal Models/Species

D. Blanset
Boehringer Ingelheim

M. Di Piazza and E. Musvasva
F. Hoffmann-La Roche AG

CONTENTS

2.1 Introduction

The preclinical safety evaluation program for a pharmaceutical is designed to provide information on the potential toxicities of the pharmaceutical, the reversibility of any toxicity, the potential safety parameters for clinical monitoring, and the safe starting dose and dose escalation scheme for the initial clinical trial. For chemically synthesized pharmaceuticals, toxicities are often "off-target" (i.e., not related to the desired pharmacological effect) and related to interactions of the chemical with non-target molecules or to the effects of reactive compounds that are formed during metabolism. Due to the possibility of

DOI: 10.1201/9781003124542-3

the generating reactive metabolites, species selection for small molecules is driven primarily by similarities in the metabolite profiles predicted by *in vitro* assays. In contrast, as biopharmaceutical products generally exhibit high specificity for the intended target, the toxicities for these compounds are primarily related to the mechanism of action or to immune responses to the biopharmaceutical. Therefore, in order to appropriately assess potential adverse effects of biopharmaceuticals, it is important to perform the toxicology studies in animal models which exhibit the intended pharmacology after exposure. This allows for the identification of adverse or exaggerated pharmacological effects and is consistent with ICH S6(R1), the international guideline that describes the preclinical development of biotechnology-derived pharmaceuticals. The scope of this guidance includes biopharmaceuticals produced in cells, such as recombinant peptides, proteins, and monoclonal antibodies. While the scope excludes certain biopharmaceuticals such as cellular blood components, cell therapies, and gene therapies, the principles of animal model selection for these types of products are similar to those described in ICH S6(R1). In this guidance, a relevant species is defined as "one in which the test material is pharmacologically active" and it indicates that several factors such as sequence homology, target binding, and functional activity should be considered when selecting relevant species. In addition to these factors, species differences in target expression patterns, target biology, and immune system function can also affect the translation of the preclinical data to humans. Moreover, differences in anatomy can affect species selection for certain routes of administration such as intravitreal or intracochlear. For example, the use of at least one pigmented species is recommended for products administered via intravitreal injection to address potential differences in toxicity and distribution due to melanin binding (Short 2008). These studies are often performed in non-human primates due to the structural similarity to the human eye (e.g., presence of a macula). Finally, there may be situations where it is not possible to identify a relevant species, and the preclinical safety profiling is limited to an *in vitro* assessment (e.g., target structure or biology is unique to humans or to the disease state).

ICH S6(R1) indicates that toxicology studies to support the initial clinical trial should, where possible, be conducted in two relevant species, one rodent and one non-rodent species. However, the guidance clearly states that "toxicology studies in non-relevant species are discouraged and may be misleading" and indicates that a toxicology program in only one species may be appropriate under certain circumstances. This chapter will discuss various experimental approaches to select relevant animal models for safety assessments of biopharmaceuticals. The use of traditional toxicology species and alternative models such as animal models of disease and genetically modified animals will also be discussed.

2.2 Experimental Approaches for Species Selection

There are several methodologies available to assess the relevance of a potential animal model for safety assessments. These methods are used to generate information on target tissue distribution, sequence homology, binding, and functional activity/potency. Generally, several of these methods are applied and an evidence-based approach is taken to determine the relevance of the animal species. While the entire data set should be included in the evaluation, the most compelling evidence of species relevance is generated from *in vivo* models or *ex vivo*/*in vitro* tissue or cell assays. Data derived from analysis of isolated molecules (e.g., binding affinity) are less convincing and are primarily used in screening assays to select species for further testing in *in vitro*/*ex vivo* functional assays and *in vivo* pharmacology studies.

2.2.1 Target Distribution

A comparison of the cellular/tissue distribution of the target between the toxicology species and humans aids in the selection of a relevant species. The degree of similarity between the expression patterns is important as pharmacological effects on cells that express the target but are not implicated in the disease process can lead to clinically relevant toxicities. For example, cetuximab has been approved for the treatment of head and neck cancer and colorectal cancer (FDA 2004). This monoclonal antibody targets epidermal growth factor receptor (EGFR), which is expressed on a variety of malignant tissues, as well as on epithelial cells in normal tissues such as the skin, tongue, and salivary glands. As cetuximab demonstrated binding to cynomolgus monkey EGFR and the expression pattern of EGFR is similar to that of humans, cynomolgus monkeys were considered to be a relevant species for toxicity testing. During the toxicology studies, severe hematologic and dermatologic toxicities were observed in cynomolgus monkeys and were considered predictive of the dose-limiting toxicities observed in patients (FDA 2004).

If the cellular/tissue distribution is different between the species, this can limit the ability to use a species for toxicity evaluations or the translatability of the findings. For example, alemtuzumab binds to CD52 in humans, macaques, and baboons. However, the expression of CD52 varies between the species, with expression on erythrocytes in baboons, rhesus monkeys, and some cynomolgus monkeys, but not in humans (Hale et al. 1983). As this expression increases the risk of vascular hemolysis and hemolytic anemia, the most relevant model for toxicology studies would be cynomolgus monkeys that do not express CD52 on erythrocytes. CD33, a myeloid differentiation antigen, is another example of a target that is not expressed on the same cell types/tissues across species. CD33 is expressed on the cell surface of leukocytes of the myeloid lineage and with high frequency on malignant cells in acute myeloid leukemia, chronic myeloid leukemia, and myelodysplastic syndrome (Laszlo et al. 2014). Several CD33 targeting approaches have been tested in clinical trials, including monoclonal antibodies and antibody conjugates (Laszlo et al. 2014). However, CD33 expression patterns on leukocytes of the myeloid lineage differ between humans and mice. In humans, expression is seen on monocytes, whereas in mice, expression is primarily on granulocytes (Brinkman-Van der Linden et al. 2003). Therefore, biopharmaceuticals intended to deplete CD33+ cells will deplete different cell types in humans and in mice.

Target expression and distribution information may be obtained from the scientific literature and from public and commercial databases such the National Center for Biotechnology Information (NCBI, https://www.ncbi.nlm.nih.gov/), BioGPS (www.biogps.org), the Human Protein Atlas (www.proteinatlas.org), and Proteomics Database (www.proteomicsdb.org). NCBI provides access to databases containing extensive biomedical and genomic information and provides information on gene function and tissue messenger ribonucleic acid (mRNA) expression. Target expression can also be evaluated through a number of molecular methods, such as reverse transcription polymerase chain reaction (RT-PCR), in situ hybridization (ISH), Northern blots, Western blots, and immunohistochemistry. Techniques such as RT-PCR, ISH, and northern blots provide information on mRNA expression in tissues; however, they do not provide information on protein expression. If there are significant differences in mRNA expression between the species or differences in the regulation of mRNA translation are to be expected, it is useful to evaluate protein expression through techniques such as immunohistochemistry to determine if the mRNA expression translates to protein expression. Figure 2.1 provides an example of the type of data that can be generated by RT-PCR.

2.2.2 Target Biology

In addition to understanding target distribution, it is also important to determine if the target biology in the selected animal species is similar to humans. If the target is well characterized, this information may be available from the scientific literature and from public databases. As a starting point, the NCBI gene database provides a synopsis of gene information. For novel targets that are not well described in the scientific literature, comparative *in vitro* pharmacology assays using animal and human cells/tissues can be used to determine if the target biology is similar between the species. The greater the similarity in target biology between the species, the higher the likelihood that the species will be predictive of the pharmacological effects of the biopharmaceutical in humans.

When assessing target biology for immunomodulatory molecules, it is also important to evaluate interspecies differences in the mechanisms regulating activation and kinetics of immune responses. For example, human T cells have stronger proliferative responses upon activation via the T-cell receptor compared to other nonhuman primate (NHPs). This may be related to a loss in inhibitory CD33-related Siglec expression that down-regulates cellular activation pathways (Nguyen et al. 2006). As humans have a stronger proliferative response, toxicology studies may underestimate the effects of immunostimulatory molecules targeting T cells in humans.

The importance of having a clear understanding of the target expression and biology is exemplified by the results of the first-in-man Phase I clinical trial of the anti-CD28 agonistic antibody TGN1412. In this trial, six healthy volunteers became critically ill within 12–16 hours after the initial infusion from a systemic inflammatory immune response to TGN1412 (Suntharalingam et al. 2006). The clinical starting dose for this trial was justified by a toxicology study in cynomolgus monkeys. In this study, doses of up to 50 mg/kg/week were well tolerated with no signs of immune stimulation

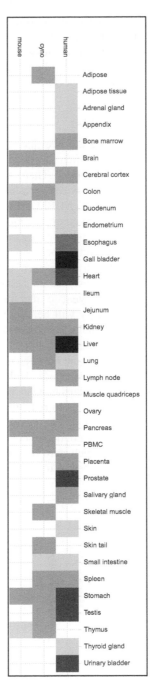

FIGURE 2.1 Comparative RNA expression data for thymic stromal lymphopoietin (TSLP) in human, cynomolgus monkey, and mouse tissues. The values represented in the heatmap are median reads per kilobase of transcript per million mapped reads (RPKM) per tissue and are expressed as relative values versus average expression across all tissues. Low-to-high expression is shown by light-to-dark colors on the heatmap. Tissues where data were not available were left blank.

(TeGenero 2005) even though the intended pharmacological effect involved superactivation of T cells. Subsequent research has suggested that the cytokine storm in the healthy volunteers was likely related to activation of CD4+ effector memory T cells (Eastwood et al. 2010). As CD4+ effector memory T cells from cynomolgus and rhesus macaques do not express CD28 (Pitcher et al. 2002, Moniuszko et al. 2004), Eastwood et al. have hypothesized that this difference in CD28 expression may explain the species differences in responses to TGN1412 (Eastwood et al. 2010). This underscores the importance of exercising caution when translating toxicology data to first-in-human starting doses if the intended pharmacological effects are not seen in the toxicology species.

2.2.3 Sequence Homology

An initial step in assessing the relevance of a species for a specific biopharmaceutical often involves determining the sequence homology of the target. There are several public and commercial bioinformatics resources available to obtain information on sequences (e.g., NCBI UniGene), and there are BLAST functions available to compare sequences. In general, the higher the degree of sequence homology in the extracellular domain between queried animal species and the human protein, the more likely the biopharmaceutical will bind to the target. In addition, the more conserved the homology is between multiple species on the phylogenetic tree, the higher the likelihood that the target biology will be conserved. Figure 2.2 illustrates the sequence homology for IL36R between several species. For this protein, the similarity between humans and cynomolgus monkeys is 95% and between humans and rats is 63%, indicating that the biopharmaceutical is more likely to bind to the analogous cynomolgus monkey protein than the rat protein. However, it is important to remember that the use of sequence identity/similarity to determine relevance has limitations as it does not take into account the secondary and tertiary structure of the protein, which may be critical for binding. While the overall similarity between species may be high, the

similarity at the binding sites may not be sufficient to allow for interaction between the protein and the biopharmaceutical, and higher activity may be demonstrated in species with less homology due to conserved amino acids in the binding sites. For these reasons, it is recommended to conduct binding assays in support of the protein sequence homology investigation. If the protein sequence similarity is low among all species and humans, it is recommended to perform functional *in vitro* assays in addition to binding assays to determine if there is biological activity in a species.

2.2.4 Binding Assays

For protein-based therapeutics, there are several technologies available to assess binding of the biotherapeutic to its intended target. Surface plasmon resonance (SPR) technology is the most commonly used as it can provide quantitative data on binding affinity and on kinetics. Figure 2.3 shows the binding kinetics of a monoclonal antibody to a human protein and the analogous cynomolgus monkey and rat proteins which were generated using SPR. In this example, the antibody bound to the human and cynomolgus monkey proteins with similar affinity; however, it did not bind to the rat protein. In general, if the binding affinity between the animal and human proteins is within 10x, the biopharmaceutical is more likely to exhibit appropriate pharmacological activity in the species. However, biopharmaceuticals with >10x differences in binding affinities can still be pharmacologically relevant. Therefore, if there are no species with binding affinities within 10×, consideration should be given to further assessing the relevance of

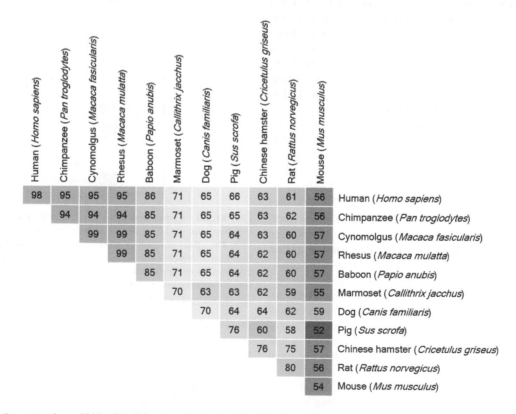

FIGURE 2.2 Percent amino acid identity of the extracellular domain of IL36R across species. Protein sequences were obtained from NCBI, and sequence alignment was performed using MUltiple Sequence Comparison by Log-Expectation (MUSCLE).

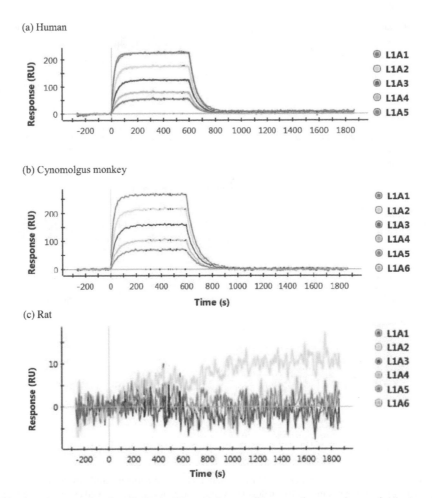

FIGURE 2.3 Binding kinetics of a monoclonal antibody (mAb) to (a) human, (b) cynomolgus monkey, and (c) rat protein using SPR (ProteOn XPR36). The mAb was captured on the surface of a sensorchip, and the protein was flowed over the mAb at increasing concentrations up to 100 nM. Sensorgrams were fit globally to 1:1 Langmuir binding to provide on-rate (ka), off-rate (kd), and affinity (KD). The KDs were 35 nM for the human antigen and 28 nM for the cynomolgus monkey antigen. The antibody did not bind to the rat protein.

the species using *in vitro* and *in vivo* pharmacological assays. For example, as illustrated in Figure 2.4, SPR was utilized to assess the relative binding affinities of a monoclonal antibody to the human antigen and to the analogous antigen in several potential toxicology species. In this example, the antibody binds to the human antigen with single-digit pM binding; however, it exhibits weak binding to cynomolgus monkey antigen and does not bind to the other species. As there were no species with binding affinities within 10× of the human, *in vitro* assessments of the pharmacological activity were performed with cynomolgus monkey cells to determine if the weak binding translated into biological activity.

There are several other technologies (e.g., flow cytometry, electrochemiluminescence (ECL), enzyme-linked immunosorbent assay (ELISA)) that can be used to assess binding of the biopharmaceutical to the intended target although not all of these technologies can provide quantitative data that can be used for cross-species comparison. In these assays, the strongest data are derived from assays using primary cells; however, cells transfected to express the target proteins or isolated proteins can also be used. When performing these assays, appropriate positive and negative controls for both the target and the biopharmaceutical should be included to evaluate nonspecific

binding. Figures 2.5 and 2.6 illustrate the use of flow cytometry to evaluate binding of a monoclonal antibody to a target.

2.2.5 Functional Activity

While binding of the biopharmaceutical to the target provides evidence of the relevance of the animal model, in some cases, binding to the target does not necessarily result in an appropriate biological effect. Functional *in vitro* and *ex vivo* assays can be used to determine if a biotherapeutic demonstrates appropriate biological activity in the species and for comparing the activity to that in a human system. There are many methods for assessing the biological activity of a biopharmaceutical, and appropriate assays should be developed specifically for the product based on the modality and mode of action. The following sections describe common methodologies that have been used to establish the biological activity of biopharmaceuticals.

2.2.5.1 Cellular Assays

The cellular assays developed for the *in vitro* pharmacological profiling of candidate molecules during drug discovery can be used as a basis for the development of cellular assays

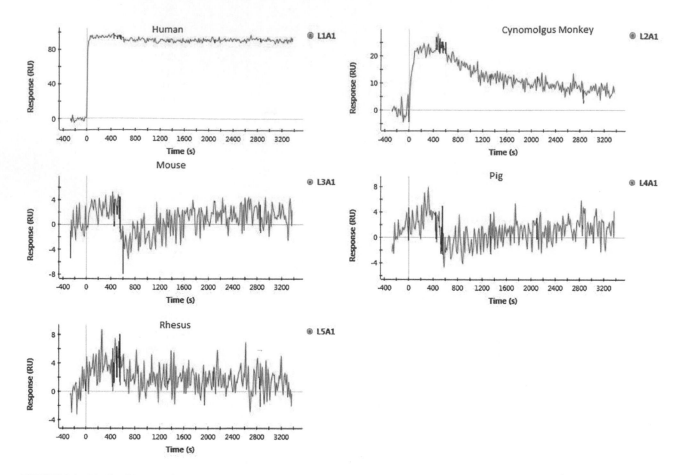

FIGURE 2.4 Binding kinetics of a monoclonal antibody (mAb) to human and animal antigens. SPR (ProteOn) was used to determine the binding affinities of a mAb to the target human protein and the analogous cynomolgus monkey, rhesus monkey, mouse, and pig proteins. The mAb was captured on the surface of a sensorchip, and the antigen was flowed over the mAb at a concentration of 500 nM. Sensorgrams were fit globally to 1:1 Langmuir binding to provide on-rate (ka), off-rate (kd), and affinity (KD). As shown in the sensorgrams, the mAb bound to human antigen. No binding was observed to mouse, pig, and rhesus monkey antigen at the highest tested concentration of 500 nM, whereas weak binding to cynomolgus monkey antigen was observed. Local fitting of the two observed binding curves revealed single-digit pM binding to the human antigen in comparison with 2 nM binding to the cynomolgus monkey antigen.

(bioassays) to compare the biological effects of a biopharmaceutical across species. Depending on the mechanism of action, these assays usually involve the measurement of either cellular proliferation, cytotoxicity, or signaling cascades. When developing these assays, endpoints that are directly related to the proposed mechanism of action of the biopharmaceutical are preferred. Assays using primary cells that physiologically express the target are also preferred as they are more closely related to the *in vivo* setting. However, culturing certain primary cell types may be challenging (e.g., neurons), and the disruption of the 3D architecture in the monolayer culture may alter the proliferative status of the cells and/or the target biochemical pathway(s). Therefore, assays that use tumor cell lines expressing the target or immortalized cell lines transfected with the target can also be used. In addition to cellular assays, developments are being made in *in vitro* testing systems such as 3D tissue models and organ-on-chips. These complex systems allow for the evaluation of the interaction of multiple cell types in a more appropriate architectural connection and may be useful to address specific hypotheses.

For antagonistic monoclonal antibodies, the most basic cellular assays evaluate the ability of the monoclonal antibody to block binding of the ligand(s) to its receptor. For example, Figure 2.7 shows human or cynomolgus monkey PD-1 that was transfected into CHO cells. The cells were incubated with either the human or cynomolgus monkey ligands (PD-L1 and PD-L2) and an anti-human PD-1 monoclonal antibody to compare the inhibition of ligand binding. In this assay, the monoclonal antibody effectively inhibited ligand binding in both species with comparable IC90 values. Cellular assays can also be developed to measure the ability of the antagonistic antibody to inhibit a biological effect of ligand binding. Figures 2.8 and 2.9 illustrate the use of such an assay to demonstrate the activity of an anti-granulocyte–macrophage colony-stimulating factor (GM-CSF) antibody against both human and cynomolgus monkey GM-CSF. First, the ability of recombinant human or cynomolgus monkey GM-CSF to induce CD11 stimulation in human granulocytes was demonstrated (Figure 2.8). The assay was then used to demonstrate that the antibody was capable of inhibiting both human and cynomolgus monkey GM-CSF-induced CD11 expression (Figure 2.9).

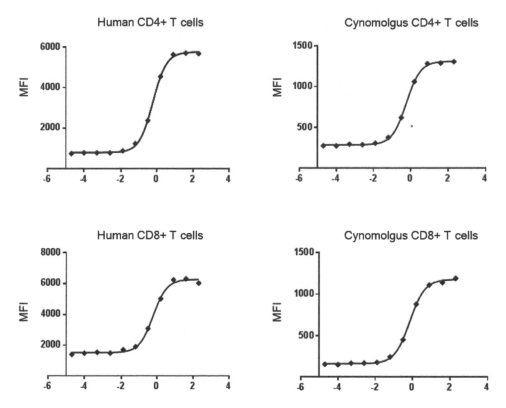

FIGURE 2.5 Binding of a monoclonal antibody to CD4+ and CD8+ T cells. Peripheral blood mononuclear cells (PBMCs) from three human subjects and three cynomolgus monkeys were stimulated with anti-CD3 and anti-CD28 antibodies and analyzed for binding of antibody to CD4+ and CD8+ T cells. The average EC50s for human CD4+ and CD8+ T-cell binding were 0.54 and 0.58 nM, respectively. The average EC50s for cynomolgus monkey CD4 and CD8 T cells were 0.46 and 0.58 nM, respectively.

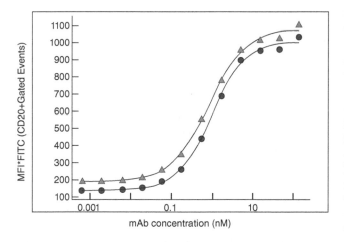

FIGURE 2.6 Binding of a monoclonal antibody to CD20+ cells. Increasing concentrations of antibody were incubated with human or cynomolgus monkey PBMCs. Binding was measured by flow cytometry, which indicated similar binding to human (▲) and cynomolgus monkey (●) CD20+ cells.

Assays that measure cellular signaling cascades can also be used to evaluate the relative potency of a biopharmaceutical in a toxicology species and humans. These assays typically measure the activation of kinases or other transcription factors or the release of chemokines or cytokines. Figure 2.10 depicts the biological activity of a monoclonal antibody directed toward a cell surface receptor in cynomolgus monkey and human dermal fibroblasts. Incubation of the ligand for the receptor with dermal fibroblasts induces NFkB activation, and the antagonism of this receptor with the monoclonal antibody should block this activation. In this experiment, dose-dependent reduction in NFkB activation in human dermal fibroblast was seen. In contrast, the monoclonal antibody demonstrated very weak activity in cynomolgus monkey dermal fibroblasts as demonstrated by the shape of the dose–response curve and incomplete inhibition of NFkB activation. For this monoclonal antibody, there was also a 2,000× difference in binding affinity to the cynomolgus monkey receptor compared to the human receptor. Therefore, the data indicate that cynomolgus monkeys are not a relevant species for toxicology studies as there are no indications that the model is capable of demonstrating potentially adverse consequences of target modulation. For this program, toxicology studies were conducted with a surrogate antibody in mice to support clinical development.

For biopharmaceuticals intended to induce cytotoxicity, there are several assay formats that can be used to assess the activity. Antibody-dependent cell-mediated cytotoxicity (ADCC) or complement-dependent cytotoxicity (CDC) assays are commonly used to assess the relative activity of cytotoxic monoclonal antibodies and have been used for products such as ocrelizumab and SGN-40 (FDA 2016, Kelley et al. 2006). In these assays, primary cells or cells transfected with the target are typically incubated with various concentrations of the biopharmaceutical and effector cells. Cytotoxicity is then measured by luminescence or absorbance. Cellular cytotoxicity assays can also be developed for other mechanisms of action involving cell killing. For example, for blinatumomab,

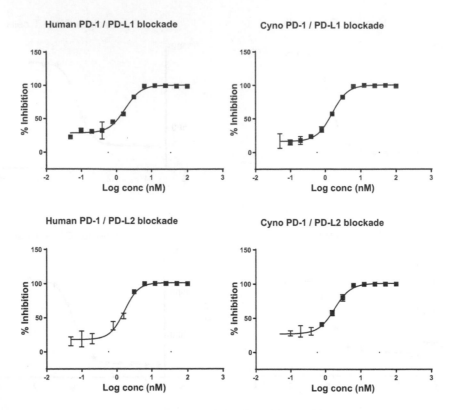

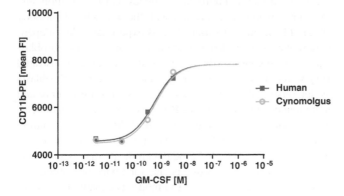

FIGURE 2.7 Inhibition of ligand binding in CHO cells stably transfected with either human PD-1 or cynomolgus monkey PD-1. In this assay, CHO cells were incubated with ligand (PD-L1 – top panel; PD-L2 – bottom panel) and an anti-human PD-1 monoclonal antibody at varying concentrations. The monoclonal antibody potently blocks binding of human PD-L1 and human PD-L2 to cell-associated human PD-1 with an average IC90 of 4.14 and 3.98 nM, respectively. Binding of cynomolgus PD-L1 and PD-L2 to cynomolgus PD-1-expressing cells was inhibited by the monoclonal antibody with an average IC90 of 5.61 nM and 7.54 nM.

FIGURE 2.8 Human whole blood was incubated with increasing concentrations of recombinant human GM-CSF or cynomolgus monkey GM-CSF. CD11b on primary granulocytes was quantified by flow cytometry using an anti-CD11b antibody. Recombinant human and cynomolgus monkey GM-CSF were equally potent at inducing stimulation of CD11b on human primary granulocytes.

a bispecific T-cell engager directed toward CD19-expressing cells, cytotoxicity assays involving the incubation of a CD19-expressing cell line, human T cells, and blinatumomab were developed to assess the *in vitro* activity (FDA 2014).

2.2.5.2 Ex Vivo Biological Effect

An additional method of assessing species relevance is through the demonstration of an *ex vivo* effect after the *in vivo* administration of a biopharmaceutical. These methods generally use

cellular assays similar to those used to demonstrate *in vitro* activity with slight modifications to test the activity in cells obtained from animals after exposure to the biopharmaceutical.

2.2.5.3 Gene Expression Profiling

Transcript profiling can be used to evaluate the effects of a biopharmaceutical on gene expression. In these assays, mRNA profiles are examined in tissues obtained from animals after exposure to the biopharmaceutical or in primary or transformed cells incubated with the biopharmaceutical. If gene expression profiles related to target modulation in humans have been described in the literature, the data from the assays in the animal species can be compared to the expression patterns in the scientific literature to determine if the gene expression profiles are similar between the species and humans (healthy subjects/patients). If little is known regarding the downstream effects of modulating the target, the data from treated human and animal tissues/cells can be compared to untreated samples to determine expression patterns. The function of genes that are up- or down-regulated after exposure to the biopharmaceutical can then be evaluated to determine if they are known to be involved in the pathway of interest or if they are known to affect pathways with similar biological functions. Comparison of the profiles from the potential toxicology species and humans can provide support for the relevance of the species if similar up-regulation and down-regulation patterns are observed. The expression patterns should also be evaluated to determine if there are pathways that are affected in one

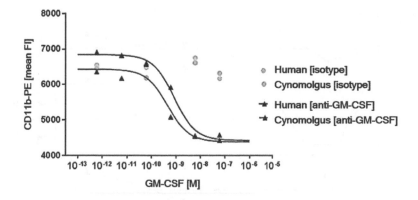

FIGURE 2.9 Whole blood was incubated with 3 nM of either recombinant human GM-CSF or cynomolgus monkey GM-CSF, followed by increasing amounts of isotype antibody or anti-human GM-CSF antibody. GM-CSF-induced CD11b expression on primary granulocytes was quantified by flow cytometry using an anti-CD11b antibody. GM-CSF-induced CD11b expression was inhibited by the addition of anti-GM-CSF antibody, demonstrating that the antibody is capable of neutralizing both human and cynomolgus monkey GM-CSF.

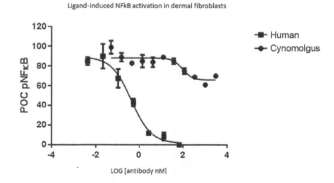

FIGURE 2.10 Primary human and cynomolgus monkey dermal fibroblasts were incubated with a ligand that induces NFkB activation. Co-incubation with an antagonistic monoclonal antibody directed toward the receptor for the ligand potently blocked NFkB activation in the primary human dermal fibroblasts with a near-complete inhibition at the highest concentration. In contrast, the antibody demonstrated very weak activity in cynomolgus monkey dermal fibroblasts. Data were fit using a four-parameter logistic curve.

species but not in others as this may indicate that the target has different functions across the species which could result in toxicity findings that are not relevant to the clinical situation.

2.2.5.4 In Vivo Pharmacodynamics

Demonstrating a pharmacological effect of the biopharmaceutical in an animal species provides the strongest evidence that a species is relevant for safety assessments. This could include activity in a relevant animal model of disease or a change in a pharmacodynamic marker in an animal model of disease or normal animal. A wide variety of endpoints have been used as pharmacodynamic markers including receptor internalization, changes in cell numbers or the concentration of the target in blood or tissue samples, and changes in downstream markers expected to be affected by target modulation. For targets with well-described biology, the effects of target modulation in humans may be known, and appropriate animal models of disease or pharmacodynamic markers may be available from the scientific literature. For less well-described pathways, the demonstration of the intended effect of the biopharmaceutical in the animal model under consideration can provide support

for the species relevance. Similarly, the lack of an effect in an appropriate model on a pharmacodynamic marker, even in the presence of positive binding and *in vitro* potency data, should be a cause for concern as it may indicate differences in target biology in the species or a lack of knowledge regarding target biology and/or the mechanism of action.

The strongest markers of biological activity are those that are directly related to the mechanism of action and the intended effect of the pharmaceutical. Some of these markers can easily be incorporated into pharmacology or toxicology studies as standard methods used to assess toxicity can also be used to demonstrate pharmacological activity. For example, the effects of a therapy intended to induce cytotoxicity of B cells can be measured by flow cytometry (Figure 2.11), which is routinely included in toxicology studies. Flow cytometry or immunohistochemical methods can also be used to examine cell populations in tissues obtained at necropsy (Figure 2.12). Other techniques for pharmacodynamic marker testing may require method development. For example, T-cell-dependent antigen response (TDAR) assays are routinely used to assess immunosuppression in toxicology species (ICH S8); however, only recently have these assays been adapted to assess the immunostimulatory effects of newly developed immuno-oncology drugs (Ferency et al. 2016, Satterwhite et al. 2016).

In addition to contributing to the selection of a relevant species, the evaluation of biomarkers can assist in providing information on the relationship between exposure and pharmacological activity/adverse effects (therapeutic window) if pharmacology and toxicology are evaluated in the same species. For example, anti-CD25 monoclonal antibodies (e.g., basiliximab and daclizumab) have been studied in non-human primate models of renal, lung, and islet allografts, autoimmune uveitis, and collagen-induced arthritis, and the use of these models could allow for estimations of the therapeutic window (Hausen et al. 2000, Wijkstrom et al. 2004, Guex-Crosier et al. 1997, Brok et al. 2001, Montgomery et al. 2002). Finally, if properly identified, quantified, and validated for clinical translatability, safety biomarkers used in nonclinical studies have the potential to be implemented in clinical trials to inform on dose escalation, to support planning of risk mitigation strategies, and to monitor onset of adverse events (Sasseville et al., 2013).

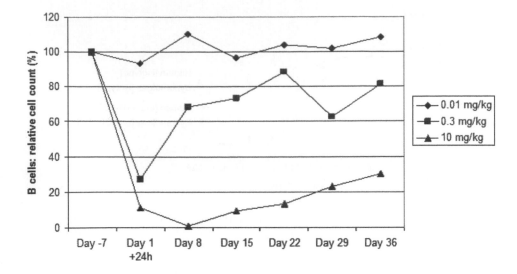

FIGURE 2.11 B-cell counts (percentage of Day −7 values) after a single intravenous administration of 0.01, 0.3, or 10 mg/kg of a monoclonal antibody to cynomolgus monkeys on Day 1.

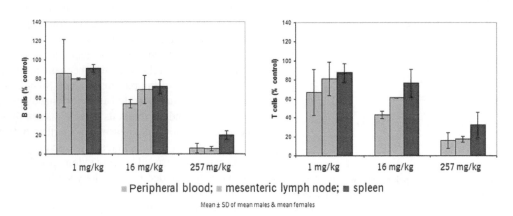

FIGURE 2.12 Relative B- and T-cell counts (% of control mean values) in mice after 5 weekly intravenous doses of a monoclonal antibody at 0, 1, 16, and 257 mg/kg.

2.3 Animal Models

2.3.1 Traditional Toxicology Species

Commonly used toxicology species should be initially considered when selecting nonclinical models for general toxicology testing with a focus on one non-rodent and one rodent candidate species. Species selection strategy should take into account the pharmacologic relevance of the species, practicality of use, the availability of historical control data, and the 3R principles of Replacement, Refinement, and Reduction of animal use in research. In some cases, the use of the most appropriate animal model based on pharmacological activity or target biology may be challenged by practical factors such as availability of reagents for specialized endpoints, availability of the model, the ability to collect appropriate endpoints, and the ability to use the desired clinical route of administration. When multiple non-rodent species are acceptable for use, the lowest order species should be used.

2.3.1.1 Rodents

Rats and mice are the most commonly used rodent species for nonclinical testing. Their use for biopharmaceuticals has been limited by the species specificity of many products, target biology divergence to humans, and immunogenicity. However, if pharmacologically relevant, rodents should be used for the initial safety assessments to allow for first-in-human clinical trials. If the toxicity profile in the rodent species is similar to that of the non-rodent species and administration is not limited by immunogenicity, it may be possible to justify the use of the rodent species as the only species for chronic toxicology studies as per ICH S6(R1).

When considering the use of rodents for reproductive and developmental toxicology evaluations, species differences in gestational biology and embryo–fetal exposure should be considered. In rodents, the period of organogenesis is a larger proportion of the gestational period compared to humans. In addition, there are differences in placentation between species, which can result in differences in embryo–fetal exposures including significant differences in placental transport of Fc-containing biotherapeutics across rats and humans with higher exposures in rats during early gestation (Bowman et al. 2013). This could translate into an overestimation of human risk due to differences in exposure during organogenesis.

2.3.1.2 Hamsters

Hamsters have also been used in toxicology studies and can be a more appropriate species than rats and mice in specific situations. Syrian hamsters were used for assessment of the GM-CSF-expressing oncolytic adenovirus, ONCOS-102, as this species is permissive for adenovirus replication while rat and mouse strains commonly used for toxicity testing are not (Kuryk et al. 2017, Ginsberg et al. 1991, Thomas et al. 2003, Toth et al. 2007).

2.3.1.3 Rabbits

Rabbits are not commonly used for general toxicity testing; however, they are standardly used for reproductive and developmental toxicity testing of small molecules based on the large litter size, large historical database, and established experience with this model. For biotherapeutics, the use of the rabbit is often limited by robust anti-therapeutic antibody response coupled with the frequently low sequence homology to the human target that reduces the likelihood of pharmacological relevance. Additionally, gestational biology in rabbits differs to humans and non-human primates in that the period of organogenesis comprises a larger portion of the gestational period than in non-human primates and in humans. Finally, placentation is different between rabbits and humans, which could result in differences in placental transfer. As with the rat, these factors could translate into greater exposure during organogenesis and, consequently, potential overestimation of toxicity compared to humans.

2.3.1.4 Dogs

While dogs are commonly used as a large animal species for toxicity testing of small-molecule drugs, the use of dogs for assessment of most proteins and monoclonal antibodies has been limited by a lack of pharmacological relevance, the development of immune responses against the exogenous protein and, until recently, the lack of reagents to evaluate immune responses. However, the dog has been used for toxicity assessment of small proteins and peptides, such as insulin analogues and erythropoiesis-stimulating agents (Heidel and Page 2010; Andrews et al. 2014).

2.3.1.5 Non-human Primates

Due to the phylogenic relationship to humans, similarity of biology, and availability of reagents for specialized endpoints, cynomolgus macaques became a preferred non-rodent animal species for toxicity assessments of early biotherapeutics, particularly for monoclonal antibodies. Cynomolgus monkeys continue to be a commonly used non-human primate species for toxicity assessments of biopharmaceuticals; however, consideration should be given to using a lower order species whenever possible. Rhesus monkeys have also been used for toxicity assessments of biopharmaceuticals such as HIV vaccines (Sui et al. 2013). However, the use of rhesus monkeys does present some technical challenges, primarily in reproductive and developmental toxicity evaluations as they are seasonal breeders. Although cynomolgus and rhesus monkeys are closely related, there are some genetic differences between the species, such as the previously mentioned differences in the expression of CD52 (Hale et al. 1983). Therefore, the relevance of these species should be evaluated on a case-by-case basis.

Marmosets can also be considered for use in safety assessments of biopharmaceuticals. This species has been used for toxicity assessments of small-molecule pharmaceuticals such as oseltamivir phosphate and mitomycin C (Orsi et al. 2011) and for at least one monoclonal antibody (FDA 2009). Although the use of marmosets has been limited, there are historical databases available in some toxicology laboratories. In addition, established animal models of disease for neurology, immunology, and infectious diseases applications (Hart et al. 2012, Jagessar et al. 2012) provide opportunities to use marmosets to address specific safety-related questions.

Chimpanzees are a protected species and their use in medical research is banned in several countries; therefore, toxicology studies are not conducted in this species. If a biotherapeutic does not demonstrate appropriate biology in commonly used toxicology species, approaches such as surrogate molecules or transgenic animals should be utilized instead of considering chimpanzees.

2.3.1.6 Other Species

In keeping with the principles of the respective guidelines for biotechnology-derived products, certain biotherapeutics may require the use of alternative species in addition or *in lieu* of the species described above. The type of product, route of administration, and similarity of organ physiology can be key aspects impacting the need for alternative animal models. For example, due to the similarity in lung physiology, sheep may be appropriate for evaluating inhaled biotherapeutics, while pigs may be appropriate for evaluating cardiovascular products due to similarities in the cardiovascular system. Alternative species should be considered as needed based on the specific development needs.

2.3.2 Animal Models of Disease

Although toxicology studies are typically conducted in healthy animals, there are situations where the use of animal models of disease can add value to the safety assessment. These include the following:

1. identification of hazards specific to disease conditions or when healthy animals lack the target
2. investigation of mechanisms of toxicities in patients that were not detected in healthy animals

3. evaluation of pharmacological effects occurring under normal physiologic conditions that may not be relevant in the disease state

4. evaluation of therapeutic windows in the animal model

The safety assessment package for recombinant human acid sphingomyelinase (rhASM) illustrates how animal models of disease can be useful in identifying hazards specific to disease conditions. rhASM has been evaluated as an enzyme replacement therapy for Niemann–Pick disease types A and B. In this disease, sphingomyelin accumulates in lysosomes due to acid sphingomyelinase deficiency. Standard toxicology studies were conducted in healthy rats, mice, and dogs, and no toxicities were detected (Murray et al. 2015). However, when rhASM was administered to acid sphingomyelinase knockout mice (ASMKO), severe toxicities were noted at dose levels lower than the no-observed-adverse-effect level (NOAEL) in healthy animals. Further investigation in the ASMKO mice suggested that the toxicities were related to the breakdown of sphingomyelin into toxic metabolites. As the healthy animals did not have high tissue levels of sphingomyelin, these toxicities could not be detected in the standard toxicology studies. As the efficacy of rhASM was also assessed in the ASMKO mice, the therapeutic window could also be established in the model. Finally, the model was used to investigate different dosing regimens, leading to an understanding that the toxicity could be reduced by intra-animal dose escalation (i.e., administering lower doses prior to escalating to higher doses within the same animal).

Animal models of disease can also be used to investigate toxicities occurring in patients that were not detected in healthy animals. For example, pancreatitis has been reported following administration of GLP-1 agonists in patients with type 2 diabetes and obesity. As the risk of pancreatitis is already elevated in these diseases, animal models of disease were used to assess if the administration of GLP-1 agonists induced or potentiated pancreatitis (Tatarkiewicz et al. 2010). Normal and diabetic rats were treated with exenatide (a GLP-1 agonist), pancreatitis was chemically induced, and biomarkers of pancreatitis were evaluated. In these studies, administration of exenatide did not induce or potentiate pancreatitis.

In cases where the animal model of disease provides evidence of a relationship between the biotherapeutic and the adverse clinical effect(s), the model may also be useful to evaluate if the adverse effect can be managed by altering either the product or the dosing regimen or by implementing clinical management practices.

Animal models of disease can also be utilized to determine if toxic effects seen in healthy animals are relevant to patients or if they are only occurring because of disruption of normal homeostasis. In many cases, this can be determined based on existing scientific knowledge. However, there may be effects where the relationship is not clear and can be further delineated using animal models of disease. This approach was utilized to determine if the development of peripheral neuropathy in healthy animals treated with insulin was related to intermittent hypoglycemia. Through the use of diabetic rats, it was determined that treatment with insulin only resulted in neuropathy when serum glucose fell below 50 mg/dL (Tabata 2000, Ozaki et al. 2010). Therefore, the neuropathy should be preventable in the clinical setting by maintaining serum glucose levels within the normal range.

While animal models of disease can be useful in safety assessments, and in some cases may be the most appropriate model, there are several limitations to these models and it is important to carefully consider the advantages and disadvantages of these models before implementing their use in safety assessments (Table 2.1). Animal models of disease are best utilized to address specific therapeutic modalities such as cell and gene therapies or hypotheses that cannot be adequately assessed in standard toxicology studies. The decision to use an animal model of disease in safety assessment should be based on the model characteristics and the ability of the model to address the safety questions. The ideal animal model of disease is a model where the disease arises from the same physiological mechanisms, has a similar progression, and includes all of the characteristics of the human disease, such as clinical signs and symptoms, laboratory changes, biomarkers of disease, and organ pathology. The intra-model and inter-model consistency should also be considered to determine if the model will allow for adequate consistency within a study and reproducibility across studies. Some animal models of disease have been well characterized with extensive documentation in the scientific

TABLE 2.1

Animal Models

Model	Advantages	Disadvantages
Traditional Tox species	Evaluates the clinical candidate Large historical database	May not identify effects that occur only in the disease condition
Animal models of disease	May mimic effects in disease condition May allow assessment of therapeutic window in the model May assist in understanding the pathogenesis of toxicity findings May aid in the development of biomarkers	Confounding effects of disease Poor analogy to disease may result in irrelevant effects May only represent one aspect of the disease Lack of historical data May be short-term models, which preclude the evaluation of long-term effects
Genetically modified animals	Can assess the effects of targeting the pathway May allow for assessment of the clinical candidate	May need to genotype all animals prior to study initiation May have limited animal availability Genetic manipulation may affect other endpoints Lack of historical control data
Surrogate molecules	Can assess the effects of targeting the pathway	Surrogate may not accurately reflect the pharmacology of the clinical product Different production process, impurities, and/or formulation

literature. However, other models may need to be characterized through natural history studies and other assays to assess the ability of the model to provide useful safety information.

The use of animal models of disease for safety assessment is also limited by confounding effects of the underlying disease. A thorough understanding of the range of clinical signs and pathological changes arising from the disease is needed to determine if toxicities arising from the administration of the biotherapeutic can be distinguished from background lesions. For example, animal models of inhalational anthrax were used to study the efficacy of raxibacumab when administered after signs of infection (e.g., toxemia) (FDA 2012). As anthrax infection results in acute inflammation and necrosis in multiple tissues, it can be very difficult to detect toxic effects of potential treatments against the background of multiple pathological changes. During the development of raxibacumab, there appeared to be a greater central nervous system (CNS) inflammatory response in non-surviving animals treated with raxibacumab compared to non-surviving animals treated with placebo (FDA 2012). As inflammation of the CNS is commonly found in animals infected with anthrax, it is difficult to determine if this apparent difference was a result of chance or was treatment related. However, additional animal models of inhalational anthrax were conducted with the inclusion of pathology evaluations. As CNS toxicities were not noted in surviving animals treated with raxibacumab, a positive risk–benefit analysis was achieved.

2.3.3 Non-traditional Approaches

The increasing complexity of modalities to treat disease has resulted in the development of products with no pharmacological activity in common toxicology species such that the conduct of traditional *in vivo* toxicology studies with the clinical candidate is not possible. Human-restricted pharmacological activity does not preclude the development and licensing of a new therapeutic, although it makes the development process more challenging and often results in the need to proceed more cautiously in the clinic with lower starting doses and conservative dose escalation schemes. The lack of appropriate animal models also limits the ability to investigate adverse clinical effects. In the absence of standard toxicology studies, non-traditional approaches to safety assessment can be applied to generate an assessment of the potential safety issues that could arise with the clinical product and to establish a starting dose for the initial clinical trial. These approaches can include the use of surrogate molecules, genetically modified animals, and/or well-designed *in vitro* pharmacological assessments.

2.3.3.1 Surrogate Molecules

In cases where a therapeutic is highly human specific such that it precludes the use of standard animal models for toxicity testing, a surrogate molecule that modulates the target in a similar manner as the clinical product can be used to assess the potential for adverse effects. As per the ICH S6(R1) guideline, surrogate molecules "can be used for hazard detection and understanding the potential for adverse effects due to exaggerated pharmacology, but are generally not useful for quantitative risk assessment." Therefore, while the use of a surrogate molecule can provide useful information regarding target modulation, this approach will not provide information on safety margins for adverse effects. This approach will need to be combined with appropriate *in vitro* pharmacology assays to determine an appropriate clinical starting dose and dose escalation scheme.

When using a surrogate approach for safety testing, the chosen molecule should have the same mechanism of action as the clinical candidate and be thoroughly characterized to assess the degree of similarity to the clinical candidate. These evaluations should include assessments of the mechanism of action, pharmacologic activity, *in vitro* potency, and *in vivo* pharmacodynamics. The assessment should also include assays specific for the modality such as binding affinity for monoclonal antibodies. Examples of products that were successfully developed using a surrogate approach include efalizumab (anti-CD11a antibody) and infliximab (anti-TNFα antibody). As these products exhibited human and chimpanzee specific reactivity, mouse surrogate antibodies were used in general toxicology and reproductive toxicology studies to support clinical trials (Clarke et al. 2004, EMEA 2005, Treacy 2000). More recently, a mouse surrogate antibody was used to support development of an anti-IL36R antibody (Ganesan et al. 2017) as the clinical candidate did not demonstrate adequate activity in common toxicology species based on binding and potency in functional assays. Extensive characterization of the mouse surrogate antibody was undertaken and included epitope mapping and *in vitro* and *in vivo* pharmacological evaluations to demonstrate functional similarity between the clinical candidate and the surrogate. Surrogate molecules have also been used to address specific safety questions. During the development of denosumab, an anti-RANKL monoclonal antibody that prevents the development of osteoclasts, an osteoprotegerin-Fc surrogate molecule was included as part of the safety assessment to evaluate potential effects on growth plates (FDA 2010).

2.3.3.2 Genetically Modified Animals

Information regarding the consequences of target modulation can also be obtained from genetically modified animals. There are several different types of genetically modified animals including knockout models that lack specific gene(s), transgenic animals that are designed to overexpress the target, and transgenic animals that express the human target. Usually, these models involve genetic manipulation at the single-cell embryonic stage resulting in a permanent genetic change. However, conditional tissue-specific or temporal models can also be developed and are particularly useful when a permanent genetic modification results in embryolethality. Knockout models that do not express the target can be useful to evaluate the consequences of target deficiency or inhibition. The generation of viable animals with no apparent adverse effects on physiology provides supportive evidence that inhibiting the target is unlikely to result in severe adverse effects in humans. However, the generation of animals with a defined phenotype can provide information on the types of effects that may result from target modulation in humans. For example, genetic deficiency of the immune-modulating target CTLA4 or PD-1 results in phenotypes that indicate the potential for immune-mediated adverse effects (Waterhouse et al. 1995, Okazaki and Honjo 2006). This is consistent with the primary adverse effects of marketed products that antagonize these pathways (Keytruda®, Opdivo®; Hodi et al. 2010).

For biotherapeutics that do not demonstrate activity in common toxicology species, it may be possible to use a transgenic animal model expressing the human target for safety assessments. However, when inserting a human gene into an animal species, it is essential to determine if the human gene product interacts with the relevant animal proteins resulting in appropriate biology. If the gene product does not result in appropriate downstream signaling, the usefulness of the model for safety assessment is limited. This approach was successfully used for keliximab, a monoclonal antibody directed toward human CD4 (Bugelski et al. 2000). As keliximab did not exhibit pharmacological activity in common toxicology species, a transgenic mouse model expressing human CD4 was utilized for the toxicology assessment, including reproductive and developmental toxicology assessments.

When using genetically modified animal models to evaluate the potential effects of target modulation, it is important to fully characterize the model to determine the relevance to the human safety assessment. These evaluations should include assessment of the gene expression, function, and regulation, and of the gene product expression, distribution, and function. Other factors that can affect the ability of these models to provide relevant data for safety assessment include phenotypic instability, inappropriate feedback controls, and unintentional modification of other genes. Finally, in models where the genetic modification is present from conception, the model may not reflect the effects of target modulation in humans as compensatory mechanisms may influence the development of the relevant pathways resulting in effects that are different from those resulting from temporary modulation of the pathway after development.

2.3.3.3 Preclinical Safety Assessment in the Absence of an Appropriate Animal Model for Toxicology Studies

When the specificity of the biotherapeutic precludes the use of all animal models to conduct toxicology studies, the nonclinical safety assessment relies on a scientific understanding of the potential implication of modulating the target, the possible toxicities related to the treatment modality (e.g., immunological responses to the product), and the conduct of *in vitro* assays to address specific questions. This situation may arise when there is a human-specific target and/or epitope, when the target is only present in the disease state, or when the treatment modality precludes assessment in animals. For example, approaches such as T-cell receptor mimic antibodies (TCRm) that target specific tumor antigens in the context of major histocompatibility complex (MHC) molecules cannot be assessed in conventional nonclinical species where the MHCs are dissimilar to humans and the tumor antigen is not expressed, not processed, or not presented in a manner comparable to the therapeutic principle in humans. In these cases, the preclinical safety assessment is based primarily on *in vitro* target expression and specificity evaluations to provide information on which cells/tissues are likely to be targeted by the therapy and on *in vitro* functional assays that elucidate the mechanism of action. Additionally, for individualized cell-based therapies such as chimeric antigen receptor (CAR) T cells where patient-derived T cells are genetically engineered to express a specific antigen receptor in an HLA-independent manner, the usefulness of *in vivo* models is limited. In these cases, *in vivo* toxicology studies in NSG mice or other immunodeficient models may be requested by health authorities; however, dose extrapolation from these studies is not possible, and these models do not properly educate about biodistribution and off-target toxicities.

2.4 Special Considerations for Specific Modalities

2.4.1 Peptides and Protein-Based Therapeutics

For peptides and protein-based therapeutics including monoclonal antibodies, the selection of toxicology species is generally based on a stepwise assessment of the sequence homology, target binding, *in vitro/ex vivo* activity, and *in vivo* pharmacological activity. See Chapter 19 for further discussion. For peptides, signaling proteins, and agonistic monoclonal antibodies, it is important to demonstrate that the biotherapeutic binds to the target(s) resulting in appropriate downstream signaling and biological responses. For antagonistic products, it is important to demonstrate that the product binds to the appropriate target(s), blocks binding of the ligand(s), and prevents downstream signaling and biological responses. Generally, *in vitro/ex vivo* cellular assays are utilized to demonstrate that the product elicits appropriate biological reactions and to compare the potency between the animal species and humans. *In vivo* pharmacodynamic markers should also be used if applicable to demonstrate activity in the toxicology species. For example, administration of recombinant human GM-CSF results in an increase in mature granulocytes in rhesus monkeys (Mayer et al. 1987) which can be used as a pharmacodynamic marker. However, it is not always possible to measure *in vivo* pharmacological activity in healthy animals as the target may not be expressed or not expressed in sufficient quantities to elicit a biological effect after administration of the biotherapeutic. For example, the administration of an antagonistic monoclonal antibody targeting GM-CSF alpha receptor did not result in any effects on hematologic parameters in healthy cynomolgus monkeys (Ryan et al. 2014). When pharmacodynamic markers are not available, the relevance of the species should be based on a comparison of the *in vitro/ex vivo* potency between the animal species and humans, preferably in a cell-based assay using primary cells.

When selecting toxicology species for monoclonal antibodies, the activity of the Fc region of the monoclonal antibody should also be considered. This is especially important for monoclonal antibodies intended to elicit effector functions such as phagocytosis, cytotoxicity, release of inflammatory mediators, and antigen presentation. If the intended mechanism of action involves effector functions, it is important to review the functionality/potency of the specific class of the human immunoglobulin in the proposed toxicology species.

For example, human IgG1 has been shown to be less potent than cynomolgus monkey IgG1 in eliciting effector functions upon binding to cynomolgus monkey FcγR (Jacobsen et al. 2011). In addition, there are differences in the expression of Fc receptors between species. In humans, CD16a is expressed on monocytes, macrophages, and natural killer cells, while CD16b is expressed on neutrophils and eosinophils (Kimberly et al. 2002). However, in rhesus and cynomolgus monkeys, CD16 expression is limited to natural killer cells and monocytes (Rogers et al. 2006). Therefore, if Fc interactions are involved in the mechanism of action, the potential impact of these differences in activity and expression of the Fc receptor should be considered during the safety evaluations.

2.4.2 Complex Antibody-Based Molecular Formats (ADCs, Bispecifics, Trispecifics)

The species selection for complex, antibody-based molecular formats such as bispecific antibodies follows the same paradigm as that of monoclonal antibodies. For formats that target more than one antigen, the binding and potency of each component should be determined and compared to those of the human antigens. If the multi-specific biopharmaceutical does not demonstrate activity toward one of the targets, the species would not be considered to be relevant. For example, the bispecific T-cell engager blinatumomab does not bind to CD3 from common toxicology species. Therefore, exposure to blinatumomab would not be expected to result in appropriate pharmacology (i.e., T-cell-mediated cytotoxicity of CD19-expressing cells). For this product, the safety assessment was based on the pharmacology data and toxicity assessments with a surrogate molecule (FDA 2014).

For antibody–drug conjugates (ADCs), species selection is based primarily on the pharmacological activity of the monoclonal antibody. However, if the monoclonal antibody demonstrates relevant activity in more than one species, species selection can be further refined based on the characteristics of the conjugated molecule. For example, if a chemotherapy agent is conjugated to the antibody, species selection can be refined based on the similarity of the metabolite profiles or known species sensitivities to the chemotherapy. See Chapter 22 for further discussion of these complex molecules.

2.4.3 Preventative and Therapeutic Vaccines

Vaccines represent a heterogeneous group of therapies including live attenuated preventative vaccines, inactivated vaccines, DNA and RNA vaccines, and autologous and allogeneic cell-based vaccines. Prophylactic vaccines intended to protect an individual from future infections are the most commonly encountered and widely used vaccines and typically consist of live attenuated or inactivated pathogen. The selection of an animal model for toxicology studies is primarily based on the ability of the animal species to mount an immune response to the antigen and adjuvant (if present) similar to the expected response in humans. For live attenuated vaccines, the infectivity of the pathogen in the toxicology species should also be considered (Forster 2012).

Safety assessments for prophylactic vaccines are generally conducted in a single species, with rodents and rabbits as the most commonly used species. However, a wide variety of species have been used for safety assessments of vaccines including mice, rats, rabbits, and pigs (EMA 2011, FDA 2015, Dincer et al. 2006, Hwa et al. 2013, Sheets et al. 2006). Ferrets have also been used to evaluate the influenza vaccines based on susceptibility to influenza virus, pathogenesis, and similarity of airway anatomy to humans (Belser et al. 2011, Zitzow et al. 2002). The safety of vaccines for viral, bacterial, and parasitic diseases such as tuberculosis, dengue fever, pertussis, Ebola, and human immunodeficiency virus (Qiu et al. 2009, Rivera-Hernandez et al. 2014, Sui et al. 2013) has been evaluated in non-human primates. In the case of HIV studies, the Indian rhesus macaque has been widely used based on appropriate viremia compared to the cynomolgus monkey or rhesus monkey of Chinese origin (Reimann et al. 2005).

Recently, there has been increased interest in the development of therapeutic vaccines for oncology indications, including approaches using autologous and allogeneic cells, dendritic cells, viral vectors, DNA/RNA, and proteins/peptides (Guo et al. 2013). As with prophylactic vaccines, the selection of species for toxicity testing of therapeutic vaccines is based on an assessment of the immune response to the vaccine. For autologous or dendritic cell-based vaccines, it may not be possible to use standard toxicology species due to the human-restricted specificity of these vaccines and due to immune responses to the human cells. In such cases, nonstandard approaches such as the use of humanized or syngeneic models should be assessed to determine if these strategies will add value to the safety assessment by addressing specific safety concerns. See Chapter 23 for more information on vaccines.

2.4.4 Oligonucleotide-Based Therapeutics

As toxicities arising from oligonucleotide therapeutics can be related to hybridization with the complementary sequence or can arise from mechanisms unrelated to hybridization, toxicology studies are generally conducted in rodent and non-rodent species with the clinical candidate regardless of the ability to hybridize with the analogous sequence in the toxicology species. However, it is still important to assess the ability of the oligonucleotide to hybridize with the analogous sequence and to produce pharmacological effects in the selected species to determine if hybridization-dependent toxicities can be detected in the species. If the oligonucleotide does not produce relevant *in vitro* or *in vivo* pharmacological activity in at least one toxicology species, species-specific surrogates are often synthesized and included in the toxicology program to assess hybridization-dependent toxicities. Chapter 24 further discusses this class of modalities.

2.4.5 Gene Therapies and Oncolytic Viruses

The field of gene therapy is comprised of several methodologies intended to modify the expression of normal genes or correct functionality of abnormal genes for the treatment or prevention of a variety of human diseases. Gene therapy products include plasmid DNA, viral and non-viral vectors, genetically modified viruses, and genetically modified cells. Although oncolytic viruses (OVs), which naturally or through genetic engineering preferentially infect and kill cancer cells, are a separate modality, the principles of species selection for gene therapies utilizing viral vectors apply. In addition, OVs may be genetically engineered to carry additional therapeutic gene(s) to increase anti-tumoral responses, and as such are considered by health authorities as gene therapy products. Therefore, species selection for OVs will also be discussed in this section.

As toxicities with these alternative therapeutic modalities can be associated with the delivery system, the transgene expression vector, and the gene product, all of these factors should be considered when selecting an appropriate species for safety assessments. Consideration should also be given to collection of toxicity endpoints in the animal model of disease used for the proof-of-concept studies as these models may allow for identification of hazards specific to the disease condition. In general, safety assessment in one species is generally acceptable, with rodents as the preferred species if they satisfy all the key requirements: comparability to human physiology and anatomy, pharmacological responsiveness and immune tolerance to the transgene, feasibility of using the planned clinical delivery device, and (for viral vectors) similar permissiveness and susceptibility to infection. If rodents do not fulfill all of the requirements, a non-rodent species is accepted either as single species or in support to the rodent studies. For example, if the clinical delivery method cannot be used in rodents due to differences in physiology, the impact of the clinical delivery method on the vector spread and transduction pattern could be evaluated in a small study in non-rodent species to supplement toxicology studies in rodents (e.g., pigs and sheep for cardiovascular and respiratory indications, respectively).

The functional relevance of the gene product is an important consideration in the species selection process. This can be assessed as described previously using a stepwise evaluation of the sequence homology, target binding, *in vitro/ex vivo* activity, and *in vivo* pharmacological activity. Gene function can be assessed *in vitro* by measuring restoration of activity in cells where the therapeutic gene is defective or has been removed, or by acquisition of activity in cells that physiologically do not express the therapeutic gene. If the gene product is not pharmacologically active in toxicology species, genetically modified animals expressing the human target of the gene product or a surrogate molecule comprised of the clinical viral vector with the murine version of the therapeutic gene can be considered to address specific safety concerns.

For gene therapies utilizing viral vectors and OVs, the selection of the toxicology species should consider the similarity in viral tropism, infectivity, and pathology between the animal species and humans. For example, mice, rats, and non-human primates were reported to be equally valuable to test antiviral immune responses against adenovirus and adenoviral vectors as these viruses induce comparable innate and adaptive immune responses across the three species (Muruve 2004). However, as not all strains of mice and rats support adenovirus replication, these species are not ideal to test the risk of viral replication or the impact of secondary infection-related immune responses. For rhabdoviruses such as Maraba virus pseudotyped with lymphocytic choriomeningitis virus (LCMV), rats and cynomolgus monkeys are preferred over mice as different innate immune responses are observed in the mouse, and mice do not recapitulate the early appearance of neutralizing antibodies against the virus as seen in humans (Evgin et al. 2016). Importantly, impactful differences can exist even within a species: C57BL/6 and BALB/c mice are biased respectively toward Th1 and Th2 CD4+ T-cell-dependent innate immune responses, and therefore, the choice of mouse strain should consider the type of innate response elicited by the viral vector (Schulte et al. 2008).

Lastly, it is important to consider the possibility of gender-related differences in biodistribution, as was observed for AAV2 injected in the salivary glands of BALB/c mice (Voutetakis et al. 2007). If gender-related differences are seen, it is crucial to assess the relevance in relation to species selection and to translation to the clinical setting, especially if employing gender restriction within the toxicology studies. Chapter 26 further discusses gene-based therapies.

2.4.6 Cell-Based Therapeutics and CAR T Cells

For cell-based therapies, the selection of a relevant animal model for safety assessment may be complicated by several factors including (1) immune responses to the cells that result in rejection, (2) differences in intended behavior of the cells in normal versus disease target tissues, (3) the ability to access the anatomic site to administer the cells, and (4) the ability to deliver a relevant dose.

For many products, the use of a single toxicology species (i.e., rodents) may be acceptable to address the major safety risks generally associated with cell therapies such as long-term stability, tumorigenesis, unwanted tissue formation, and increased immunogenicity at immune-privileged sites. To address differences in cell behavior in disease tissues versus healthy tissues, it may be advantageous to incorporate the use of relevant animal models of disease into the safety assessment. For therapies that result in immune rejection in immunocompetent animals, it can be useful to use immunosuppressed animals to contextualize safety outcomes and kinetics. This can be accomplished by the use of low-dose immunosuppressive agents such as cyclosporine or by using genetically modified animals such as severe combined immunodeficiency (SCID) mice. These approaches were utilized in the development of a cell-based therapy composed of human regulatory macrophages (Broichhausen et al. 2014). For this program, Non-obese diabetic SCID Gamma (NSG™) mice were used to evaluate the tissue distribution and survival of the cells and NMRI nude mice were used in toxicology studies. An interesting alternative is represented by humanized mice, whose use may progressively increase in the future with the perfection of human cell transplantation techniques. However, while humanized mice can overcome the issue of host-versus-graft rejection and can allow combined safety and efficacy assessment for some cellular products, these models still present limitations such as immature and/or partial differentiation of hematopoietic cell lineages, and deferred partial reconstitution of the mouse immune system.

Similarly to gene therapy products, the use of a non-rodent species (e.g., pigs, sheep, dogs, and non-human primates) may be preferred for the testing of certain cell therapy products due to closer physiology, comparable organ/tissue morphology, the ability to mimic the clinical route of administration, and the ability to use the clinical device for administration. Chapter 25 has further information on this product class.

2.4.7 Gene Editing Technologies

Therapeutic genome editing technology enables direct correction of genetic mutations in target pathological tissues by use of programmable nucleases such as zinc finger nucleases (ZFNs), transcription activator-like effector nucleases (TALENs), and the clustered regularly interspaced short palindromic repeat-associated nuclease Cas9 (CRISPR/Cas9). Modifications are achieved either by direct administration *in vivo* of viral or non-viral delivery vectors or by genetic manipulation of cells *ex vivo*, and therefore, these products can be considered respectively as gene and cell therapies with regard to recommendations for species selection. In addition to those recommendations, the differences in the genome between humans and animals must be considered when selecting the appropriate animal model or species.

In particular, for *in vivo* delivery, the selected animal species should be suitable for assessing both the vector and the genome editing components.

2.5 Conclusion

The selection of appropriate animal models for toxicity assessments is based on a strong understanding of the intended target as well as the specific mode of action and format of the biotherapeutic. A stepwise testing strategy (Figure 2.13) should be implemented which allows for screening of animal species and progresses to in-depth assessment of specific species that demonstrate the potential for pharmacological relevance in the screening assays. A wide variety of methods can be implemented to screen and more thoroughly interrogate species relevance, and development of assays based on the specific target/modality is generally required. In addition, non-traditional models such as animal models of disease or transgenic animals should be included in the assessment where appropriate. The selection of relevant animal models based on demonstration of appropriate pharmacological activity will lead to stronger nonclinical safety assessments and reduce the risks of improper translation of animal data to the clinical setting.

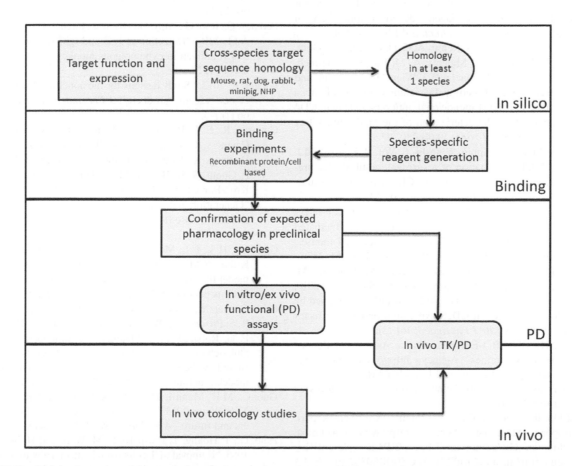

FIGURE 2.13 High-level overview of the process for selection of relevant animal models for nonclinical safety studies. PD: pharmacodynamics; TK: toxicokinetics.

REFERENCES

Andrews, D.A., Pyrah, I.T., Boren, B.M., Tannehill-Gregg, S.H., and R.M. Lightfoot-Dunn. 2014. "High hematocrit resulting from administration of erythropoiesis-stimulating agents is not fully predictive of mortality or toxicities in preclinical species." *Toxicol Pathol* 42 (3):510–23.

Belser, J. A., J. M. Katz, and T. M. Tumpey. 2011. "The ferret as a model organism to study influenza A virus infection." *Dis Model Mech* 4 (5):575–9.

Bowman, C. J., W. J. Breslin, A. V. Connor, P. L. Martin, G. J. Moffat, L. Sivaraman, M. B. Tornesi, and S. Chivers. 2013. "Placental transfer of Fc-containing biopharmaceuticals across species, an industry survey analysis." *Birth Defects Res B Dev Reprod Toxicol* 98 (6):459–85.

Brinkman-Van der Linden, E. C., T. Angata, S. A. Reynolds, L. D. Powell, S. M. Hedrick, and A. Varki. 2003. "CD33/Siglec-3 binding specificity, expression pattern, and consequences of gene deletion in mice." *Mol Cell Biol* 23 (12):4199–206.

Broichhausen, C., P. Riquelme, N. Ahrens, A. K. Wege, G. E. Koehl, H. J. Schlitt, B. Banas, F. Fandrich, E. K. Geissler, and J. A. Hutchinson. 2014. "In question: the scientific value of preclinical safety pharmacology and toxicology studies with cell-based therapies." *Mol Ther Methods Clin Dev* 1:14026.

Brok, H. P., J. M. Tekoppele, J. Hakimi, J. A. Kerwin, E. M. Nijenhuis, C. W. De Groot, R. E. Bontrop, and B. A. Hart. 2001. "Prophylactic and therapeutic effects of a humanized monoclonal antibody against the IL-2 receptor (DACLIZUMAB) on collagen-induced arthritis (CIA) in rhesus monkeys." *Clin Exp Immunol* 124 (1):134–41.

Bugelski, P. J., D. J. Herzyk, S. Rehm, A. G. Harmsen, E. V. Gore, D. M. Williams, B. E. Maleeff, A. M. Badger, A. Truneh, S. R. O'Brien, R. A. Macia, P. J. Wier, D. G. Morgan, and T. K. Hart. 2000. "Preclinical development of keliximab, a Primatized anti-CD4 monoclonal antibody, in human CD4 transgenic mice: characterization of the model and safety studies." *Hum Exp Toxicol* 19 (4):230–43.

Clarke, J., W. Leach, S. Pippig, A. Joshi, B. Wu, R. House, and J. Beyer. 2004. "Evaluation of a surrogate antibody for preclinical safety testing of an anti-CD11a monoclonal antibody." *Regul Toxicol Pharmacol* 40 (3):219–26.

Dincer, Z, Jones S, and R Haworth. 2006. "Preclinical safety assessment of a DNA vaccine using particle-mediated epidermal delivery in domestic pig, minipig and mouse." *Experimental and Toxicologic Pathology* 57 (5):351–357.

Eastwood, D., L. Findlay, S. Poole, C. Bird, M. Wadhwa, M. Moore, C. Burns, R. Thorpe, and R. Stebbings. 2010. "Monoclonal antibody TGN1412 trial failure explained by species differences in CD28 expression on CD4+ effector memory T-cells." *Br J Pharmacol* 161 (3):512–26.

EMA 2011. HBVAXPRO European Public Assessment Report. European Medicines Agency http://www.ema.europa.eu/docs/en_GB/document_library/EPAR_-_Scientific_Discussion/human/000373/WC500046812.pdf (accessed November 14, 2017).

EMEA 2005. Remicade®. European Public Assessment Report. European Medicines Agency. http://www.ema.europa.eu/docs/en_GB/document_library/EPAR_-_Scientific_Discussion/human/000240/WC500050885.pdf.EMA (accessed October 27, 2017).

Evgin, L., Ilkow, C.S., Bourgeois-Daigneault, M.-C., et al. 2016. "Complement inhibition enables tumor delivery of LCMV glycoprotein pseudotyped viruses in the presence of antiviral antibodies." *Molecular Therapy Oncolytics* 3:16027.

FDA 2004. Cetuximab Pharmacology Toxicology Review. https://www.accessdata.fda.gov/drugsatfda_docs/bla/2004/125084_erbitux_toc.cfm (accessed November 5, 2017).

FDA 2009. Ilaris® Pharmacology Review. https://www.accessdata.fda.gov/drugsatfda_docs/nda/2009/125319s000TOC.cfm (accessed November 5, 2017).

FDA 2010. Prolia® Pharmacology Review. https://www.accessdata.fda.gov/drugsatfda_docs/nda/2010/125320s0000TOC.cfm (accessed November 14, 2017.

FDA 2012. Raxibacumab: Pharmacology Review. https://www.accessdata.fda.gov/drugsatfda_docs/nda/2012/125349Orig1s000PharmR.pdf (accessed September 15, 2017).

FDA 2014. Blincyto® Pharmacology Review. https://www.accessdata.fda.gov/drugsatfda_docs/nda/2014/125557Orig1s000PharmR.pdf (accessed September 06, 2017).

FDA 2015. Gardasil® Approval History. https://www.fda.gov/BiologicsBloodVaccines/Vaccines/ApprovedProducts/UCM094042 (accessed November 05, 2017).

FDA 2016. Ocrelizumab Pharmacology Review. https://www.accessdata.fda.gov/drugsatfda_docs/nda/2017/761053Orig1s000TOC.cfm (accessed November 06, 2017).

Ferency, G., Rao, G., Amy, O., Olsen, J., Puchalski, J., and Frantz, A.M. 2016. "Detection of IgG and IgM responses to hepatitis B antigen in cynomolgous monkey." *The Toxicologist* 150 (1):1927.

Forster, R. 2012. "Study designs for the nonclinical safety testing of new vaccine products." *J Pharmacol Toxicol Methods* 66 (1):1–7.

Ganesan, R., E. L. Raymond, D. Mennerich, J. R. Woska, Jr., G. Caviness, C. Grimaldi, J. Ahlberg, R. Perez, S. Roberts, D. Yang, K. Jerath, K. Truncali, L. Frego, E. Sepulveda, P. Gupta, S. E. Brown, M. D. Howell, K. A. Canada, R. Kroe-Barrett, J. S. Fine, S. Singh, and M. L. Mbow. 2017. "Generation and functional characterization of anti-human and anti-mouse IL-36R antagonist monoclonal antibodies." *MAbs*:1–12.

Ginsberg, H.S., L.L. Moldawer, P.B. Sehgal, M. Redington, P.L. Kilian, R.M. Chanock, and G.A. Prince. 1991. "A mouse model for investigating the molecular pathogenesis of adenovirus pneumonia." *Proc Natl Acad Sci* 88 (5):1651–5.

Guex-Crosier, Y., J. Raber, C. C. Chan, M. S. Kriete, J. Benichou, R. S. Pilson, J. A. Kerwin, T. A. Waldmann, J. Hakimi, and F. G. Roberge. 1997. "Humanized antibodies against the alpha-chain of the IL-2 receptor and against the beta-chain shared by the IL-2 and IL-15 receptors in a monkey uveitis model of autoimmune diseases." *J Immunol* 158 (1):452–8.

Guo, C., M.H. Manjili, J.R. Subjeck, D. Sarkar, P.B. Fisher, and X.-Y. Wang. 2013. "Therapeutic cancer vaccines: past, present and future." *Adv Cancer Res* 119: 421–475.

Hale, G., T. Hoang, T. Prospero, S. M. Watt, and H. Waldmann. 1983. "Removal of T cells from bone marrow for transplantation. Comparison of rat monoclonal anti-lymphocyte antibodies of different isotypes." *Mol Biol Med* 1 (3):305–19.

Hart, B. A., D. H. Abbott, K. Nakamura, and E. Fuchs. 2012. "The marmoset monkey: a multi-purpose preclinical and translational model of human biology and disease." *Drug Discov Today* 17 (21–22):1160–5.

Hausen, B., J. Gummert, G. J. Berry, U. Christians, N. Serkova, T. Ikonen, L. Hook, F. Legay, W. Schuler, M. H. Schreier, and R. E. Morris. 2000. "Prevention of acute allograft rejection in nonhuman primate lung transplant recipients: induction with chimeric anti-interleukin-2 receptor monoclonal antibody improves the tolerability and potentiates the immuno-suppressive activity of a regimen using low doses of both microemulsion cyclosporine and 40-O-(2-hydroxyethyl)-rapamycin." *Transplantation* 69 (4):488–96.

Heidel, S.M., and T.J. Page. 2010. "Current practices in the preclinical safety assessment of peptides." In *Preclinical Safety Evaluation of Biopharmaceuticals: A Science-Based Approach to Facilitating Clinical Trials*, 499–515. Pharmaceutical Sciences Encyclopedia. John Wiley & Sons, Inc. ISBN: 9780470571224

DOI: 10.1002/9780470571224.

Hodi, F. S., S. J. O'Day, D. F. McDermott, R. W. Weber, J. A. Sosman, J. B. Haanen, R. Gonzalez, C. Robert, D. Schadendorf, J. C. Hassel, W. Akerley, A. J. van den Eertwegh, J. Lutzky, P. Lorigan, J. M. Vaubel, G. P. Linette, D. Hogg, C. H. Ottensmeier, C. Lebbe, C. Peschel, I. Quirt, J. I. Clark, J. D. Wolchok, J. S. Weber, J. Tian, M. J. Yellin, G. M. Nichol, A. Hoos, and W. J. Urba. 2010. "Improved survival with ipilimumab in patients with metastatic melanoma." *N Engl J Med* 363 (8):711–23.

Hwa, S. H., Y. A. Lee, J. N. Brewoo, C. D. Partidos, J. E. Osorio, and J. D. Santangelo. 2013. "Preclinical evaluation of the immunogenicity and safety of an inactivated enterovirus 71 candidate vaccine." *PLoS Negl Trop Dis* 7 (11):e2538.

ICH Guidance S6(R1). Preclinical safety evaluation of biotechnology-derived pharmaceuticals.

ICH Guidance S8. Immunotoxicity studies for human pharmaceuticals.

Jacobsen, F. W., R. Padaki, A. E. Morris, T. L. Aldrich, R. J. Armitage, M. J. Allen, J. C. Lavallee, and T. Arora. 2011. "Molecular and functional characterization of cynomolgus monkey IgG subclasses." *J Immunol* 186 (1):341–9.

Jagessar, S. A., N. Heijmans, L. Oh, J. Bauer, E. L. Blezer, J. D. Laman, T. S. Migone, M. N. Devalaraja, and B. A. Hart. 2012. "Antibodies against human BLyS and APRIL attenuate EAE development in marmoset monkeys." *J Neuroimmune Pharmacol* 7 (3):557–70.

Kelley, S. K., T. Gelzleichter, D. Xie, W. P. Lee, W. C. Darbonne, F. Qureshi, K. Kissler, E. Oflazoglu, and I. S. Grewal. 2006. "Preclinical pharmacokinetics, pharmacodynamics, and activity of a humanized anti-CD40 antibody (SGN-40) in rodents and non-human primates." *Br J Pharmacol* 148 (8):1116–23.

Keytruda®. Prescribing Information. https://www.merck.com/product/usa/pi_circulars/k/keytruda/keytruda_pi.pdf (accessed November 14, 2017).

Kimberly, R. P., J. Wu, A. W. Gibson, K. Su, H. Qin, X. Li, and J. C. Edberg. 2002. "Diversity and duplicity: human FCgamma receptors in host defense and autoimmunity." *Immunol Res* 26 (1–3):177–89.

Kuryk, L., L. Vassilev, T. Ranki, A. Hemminki, A. Karioja-Kallio, O. Levalampi, A. Vuolanto, V. Cerullo, and S. Pesonen. 2017. "Toxicological and bio-distribution profile of a GM-CSF-expressing, double-targeted, chimeric oncolytic adenovirus ONCOS-102- Support for clinical studies on advanced cancer treatment." *PLoS One* 12 (8):e0182715.

Laszlo, G. S., E. H. Estey, and R. B. Walter. 2014. "The past and future of CD33 as therapeutic target in acute myeloid leukemia." *Blood Rev* 28 (4):143–53.

Mayer, P., C. Lam, H. Obenaus, E. Liehl, and J. Besemer. 1987. "Recombinant human GM-CSF induces leukocytosis and activates peripheral blood polymorphonuclear neutrophils in nonhuman primates." *Blood* 70 (1):206–13.

Moniuszko, M., T. Fry, W. P. Tsai, M. Morre, B. Assouline, P. Cortez, M. G. Lewis, S. Cairns, C. Mackall, and G. Franchini. 2004. "Recombinant interleukin-7 induces proliferation of naive macaque CD4+ and CD8+ T cells in vivo." *J Virol* 78 (18):9740–9.

Montgomery, S. P., S. R. Mog, H. Xu, D. K. Tadaki, B. Hirshberg, J. D. Berning, J. Leconte, D. M. Harlan, D. Hale, and A. D. Kirk. 2002. "Efficacy and toxicity of a protocol using sirolimus, tacrolimus and daclizumab in a nonhuman primate renal allotransplant model." *Am J Transplant* 2 (4):381–5.

Murray, J. M., A. M. Thompson, A. Vitsky, M. Hawes, W. L. Chuang, J. Pacheco, S. Wilson, J. M. McPherson, B. L. Thurberg, K. P. Karey, and L. Andrews. 2015. "Nonclinical safety assessment of recombinant human acid sphingomyelinase (rhASM) for the treatment of acid sphingomyelinase deficiency: the utility of animal models of disease in the toxicological evaluation of potential therapeutics." *Mol Genet Metab* 114 (2):217–25.

Muruve, D. A. 2004. "The innate immune response to adenovirus vectors." *Hum Gene Ther* 15 (12):1157–66.

Nguyen, D. H., N. Hurtado-Ziola, P. Gagneux, and A. Varki. 2006. "Loss of Siglec expression on T lymphocytes during human evolution." *Proc Natl Acad Sci U S A* 103 (20):7765–70.

Okazaki, T., and T. Honjo. 2006. "The PD-1-PD-L pathway in immunological tolerance." *Trends Immunol* 27 (4):195–201.

Opdivo®. Prescribing Information. https://packageinserts.bms.com/pi/pi_opdivo.pdf (accessed November 4, 2017).

Orsi, A., D. Rees, I. Andreini, S. Venturella, S. Cinelli, and G. Oberto. 2011. "Overview of the marmoset as a model in nonclinical development of pharmaceutical products." *Regul Toxicol Pharmacol* 59 (1):19–27.

Ozaki, K., T. Sano, N. Tsuji, T. Matsuura, and I. Narama. 2010. "Insulin-induced hypoglycemic peripheral motor neuropathy in spontaneously diabetic WBN/Kob rats." *Comp Med* 60 (4):282–7.

Pitcher, C. J., S. I. Hagen, J. M. Walker, R. Lum, B. L. Mitchell, V. C. Maino, M. K. Axthelm, and L. J. Picker. 2002. "Development and homeostasis of T cell memory in rhesus macaque." *J Immunol* 168 (1):29–43.

Qiu, X., L. Fernando, J. B. Alimonti, P. L. Melito, F. Feldmann, D. Dick, U. Stroher, H. Feldmann, and S. M. Jones. 2009. "Mucosal immunization of cynomolgus macaques with the VSVDeltaG/ZEBOVGP vaccine stimulates strong ebola GP-specific immune responses." *PLoS One* 4 (5):e5547.

Reimann, K. A., R. A. Parker, M. S. Seaman, K. Beaudry, M. Beddall, L. Peterson, K. C. Williams, R. S. Veazey, D. C. Montefiori, J. R. Mascola, G. J. Nabel, and N. L. Letvin. 2005. "Pathogenicity of simian-human immunodeficiency virus SHIV-89.6P and SIVmac is attenuated in cynomolgus macaques and associated with early T-lymphocyte responses." *J Virol* 79 (14):8878–85.

Rivera-Hernandez, T., D. G. Carnathan, P. M. Moyle, I. Toth, N. P. West, P. R. Young, G. Silvestri, and M. J. Walker. 2014. "The contribution of non-human primate models to the development of human vaccines." *Discov Med* 18 (101):313–22.

Rogers, K. A., F. Scinicariello, and R. Attanasio. 2006. "IgG Fc receptor III homologues in nonhuman primate species: genetic characterization and ligand interactions." *J Immunol* 177 (6):3848–56.

Ryan, P.C., Sleeman, M.A., Rebelatto, M., Wang, B., Lu, H., Chen, X., et al. 2014. "Nonclinical safety of mavrilimumab, an anti-GMCSF receptor alpha monoclonal antibody, in cynomolgus monkeys: relevance for human safety. *Toxicol Appl Pharmacol* 279:230–9.

Sasseville, VG, Mansfield, KG, and Brees, DJ. 2013. "Safety biomarkers in preclinical development: translational potential." *Vet Pathol* 51(1):281–91.

Satterwhite, C.M., R.W. Comba, A. Oldendorp, and R. Prell. 2016. "Investigation of KLH (Keyhole Limpet Hemocyanin) antigen dose response in male and female cynomolgus monkeys to establish an optimal response to study immune enhancement." *The Toxicologist* 150 (1): 222.

Schulte, S., Sukhova, G., Libby, P. 2008. "Genetically programmed biases in Th1 and Th2 immune responses modulate atherogenesis." *Am J Pathol* 172 (6): 1500–8.

Sheets, R. L., J. Stein, T. S. Manetz, C. Andrews, R. Bailer, J. Rathmann, and P. L. Gomez. 2006. "Toxicological safety evaluation of DNA plasmid vaccines against HIV-1, ebola, severe acute respiratory syndrome, or west nile virus is similar despite differing plasmid backbones or gene-inserts." *Toxicol Sci* 91 (2):620–30.

Short, B. G. 2008. "Safety evaluation of ocular drug delivery formulations: techniques and practical considerations." *Toxicol Pathol* 36 (1):49–62.

Sui, Y., S. Gordon, G. Franchini, and J.A. Berzofsky. 2013. "Nonhuman primate models for HIV/AIDS vaccine development." *Cur Prot Immunol/edited by John E. Coligan... [et al.]* 102: 12.14.1–12.14.30.

Suntharalingam, G., M. R. Perry, S. Ward, S. J. Brett, A. Castello-Cortes, M. D. Brunner, and N. Panoskaltsis. 2006. "Cytokine storm in a phase 1 trial of the anti-CD28 monoclonal antibody TGN1412." *N Engl J Med* 355 (10):1018–28.

Tabata, H. 2000. "Peripheral neuropathy in B6C3F1 mice and SD rats induced by chronic intermittent insulin hypoglycemia." *Drug Chem Toxicol* 23 (3):485–96.

Tatarkiewicz, K., P. A. Smith, E. J. Sablan, C. J. Polizzi, D. E. Aumann, C. Villescaz, D. M. Hargrove, B. R. Gedulin, M. G. Lu, L. Adams, T. Whisenant, D. Roy, and D. G. Parkes. 2010. "Exenatide does not evoke pancreatitis and attenuates chemically induced pancreatitis in normal and diabetic rodents." *Am J Physiol Endocrinol Metab* 299 (6):E1076–86.

TeGenero. 2005. "Investigator's Brochure. TGN1412 humanized agonistic anti-CD28 monoclonal antibody. Edition 1.1." http://www.circare.org/foia5/tgn1412investigatorbrochure.pdf (accessed September 06, 2017).

Thomas, C. E., A. Ehrhardt, and M. A. Kay. 2003. "Progress and problems with the use of viral vectors for gene therapy." *Nat Rev Genet* 4 (5):346–58.

Thomas, M. A., J. F. Spencer, M. C. La Regina, D. Dhar, A. E. Tollefson, K. Toth, and W. S. Wold. 2006. "Syrian hamster as a permissive immunocompetent animal model for the study of oncolytic adenovirus vectors." *Cancer Res* 66 (3):1270–6.

Toth, K., J. F. Spencer, and W. S. Wold. 2007. "Immunocompetent, semi-permissive cotton rat tumor model for the evaluation of oncolytic adenoviruses." *Methods Mol Med* 130:157–68.

Treacy, G. 2000. "Using an analogous monoclonal antibody to evaluate the reproductive and chronic toxicity potential for a humanized anti-TNFalpha monoclonal antibody." *Hum Exp Toxicol* 19 (4):226–8.

Voutetakis, A., Zheng, C., Wang, J., Goldsmith, C.M., Afione, S., Chiorini, J.A., et al. 2007. Gender differences in serotype 2 adeno-associated virus biodistribution after administration to rodent salivary glands. *Hum Gene Ther.* 18(11):1109–18.

Waterhouse, P., J. M. Penninger, E. Timms, A. Wakeham, A. Shahinian, K. P. Lee, C. B. Thompson, H. Griesser, and T. W. Mak. 1995. "Lymphoproliferative disorders with early lethality in mice deficient in Ctla-4." *Science* 270 (5238):985–8.

Wijkstrom, M., N. S. Kenyon, N. Kirchhof, N. M. Kenyon, C. Mullon, P. Lake, S. Cottens, C. Ricordi, and B. J. Hering. 2004. "Islet allograft survival in nonhuman primates immunosuppressed with basiliximab, RAD, and FTY720." *Transplantation* 77 (6):827–35.

Zitzow, L. A., T. Rowe, T. Morken, W. J. Shieh, S. Zaki, and J. M. Katz. 2002. "Pathogenesis of avian influenza A (H5N1) viruses in ferrets." *J Virol* 76 (9):4420–9.

3

Dose Extrapolation to Humans for Novel Biologics

John T. Sullivan
Regulatory, Safety, Clinical Pharmacology and Drug Development Consulting

CONTENTS

3.1 Introduction

The overriding consideration in selection of doses administered to humans is safety for the subjects. Related to this is the nature of toxicity observed in nonclinical species or that anticipated to occur in humans, what the margin between toxicity and presumptive efficacy is likely to be, and what type of subjects will be selected (healthy vs those with disease of interest). The secondary considerations include a practical dose and schedule, confidence in planned extrapolations from animals to human exposure, and experience of the investigator(s). This chapter will begin with a discussion of nonclinical studies needed to proceed to human studies. The reasoning behind selection of the initial study population will be explored, and this will be followed by a discussion of the methods used to select an initial dose for administration to humans. Overall safety of first-in-human (FIH) trials will be discussed, including an elaboration on how and where to conduct an initial FIH study, designs, and appropriate dose escalation principles for FIH and early-phase trials of novel biologics. This discussion will include methods of FIH dose selection, for example, minimum anticipated biological effect level (MABEL), pharmacologically active dose (PAD), no-adverse-effect level (NOAEL), and highest non-severely toxic dose (HNSTD). Finally, there will be a brief discussion of regulatory issues in human trials.

3.2 Background

Before a potential therapeutic is administered to humans for the first time, a series of assessments are generally required and these usually include target liability (the target planned for interdiction is reviewed for potential risks (target liability) based on both known and theoretical concerns), in vitro studies, pharmacology, and Good Laboratory Practice (GLP) toxicology trials in order to ensure that it is reasonably safe to administer a novel biologic to humans. The more novel the target, the more uncertainty there is with respect to safety. A well-studied biological class such as tumor necrosis factor (TNF) sequestering agents will have safety liabilities identified in humans after many years of marketing exposure. For example, serious and opportunistic infections associated with TNF modulators were not typically identified either in animal studies or in human clinical trials at the time of marketing and not included in early labels. This is most likely related to the uncommonness of these infections and the fact that there is a given background rate in the various disease indications.

DOI: 10.1201/9781003124542-4

3.3 Key Considerations

For a completely novel target, theoretical concerns only may or may not be identified. Drug targets can be studied by profiling techniques. "Toxicogenomics is defined as the application of genomic technologies (for example, genetics, genome sequence analysis, gene expression profiling, proteomics, metabolomics, and related approaches) to study the adverse effects of environmental and pharmaceutical chemicals on human health and the environment" (Communicating Toxicogenomics Information to Nonexperts: A Workshop Summary. The National Academies Press US 2005). Toxicogenomics combines toxicology with genomics. It evaluates in organisms' tissues and cells various expression patterns. The purpose is to assess phenotypic responses in cells, tissues, or organisms. Different chemical compounds may produce similar gene expression profiles. For example, the expression profiles of chemically different compounds from the peroxisome proliferator class produce similar gene expression but distinct from those of phenobarbital, which results in similar histopathologic hepatic findings (Hamadeh et al. 2002). System-level understanding of molecular patterns can be important for understanding chemically induced toxicity risks. Microarray data, for example, may be instructive. An understanding of mechanism of action is also important for understanding toxicity that is likely to occur in humans. While this primarily applies to small-molecule therapeutics, it can apply to novel compounds such as antibody–drug conjugates (which have small-molecule components) but not typically to biologics since they have highly specific targets. The mechanism of action is generally understood for a biologic, and toxicity usually relates to exaggerated pharmacology.

3.4 Lead Candidate Selection

If the target does not present significant potential liability, and single-dose pharmacology studies do not indicate concerns, manufacturing of the therapeutic proceeds, and more formal in vitro and animal studies are conducted as appropriate. A lead compound is selected once a cross-functional group comprised of discovery, manufacturing, and translational sciences understand risks and agree on bringing the compound forward. Once this lead compound is selected, a given company will fund the project according to given governance and resourcing decisions. Most companies have various gating points where the project is reviewed and agreement by senior management is needed to continue development. For example, single-dose pharmacology studies are conducted during the discovery phase, but more formal multiple-dose toxicology studies are conducted later in development to support potential human dosing.

3.5 Regulatory Guidance

Various International Commission on Harmonisation (ICH) guidelines are helpful with respect to pharmacology and toxicology studies (https://www.ich.org). The most general or overarching guideline for translation of drugs and biologics into and through clinical development is ICH M3(R2), which is titled "Guidance on nonclinical safety studies for the conduct of human clinical trials and marketing authorization for pharmaceuticals." This was first adopted in 1997, and the most recent revision was in 2009. For the purposes of this chapter, the part dealing with requirements for administering drugs to humans for the first time will be discussed rather than all studies needed at the time of marketing authorization. The guidance was designed to facilitate the timely conduct of trials as well as being consistent with 3R (reduce/refine/replace) to minimize the use of animals. The timing of studies applies for biologics. Pharmaceuticals under development for life-threatening diseases (e.g., advanced cancer) also warrant more of a case-by-case approach, and ICH S9 addresses nonclinical studies for these situations.

3.6 General Approach to Studies

The goals of the nonclinical safety assessment include identification and characterization of toxicity and of particular target organs, dose response, relationship of toxicity to exposure, and reversibility as appropriate. It is not always necessary to identify a maximum tolerated dose (MTD), and demonstration of a sufficient margin over and above what is considered an appropriate concentration in humans may be sufficient, for example, a multiple of ten times as per ICH S6 (R1). Similarly, a maximal feasible dose assessment may also suffice depending on given circumstances such as restrictions in concentration or volume to the target site.

When initial clinical trials involve multiple dosing, the duration of toxicity studies is dependent on the planned clinical trial, and whether the drug is likely to be administered short term (e.g., a growth factor to prevent febrile neutropenia) or long term (e.g., a disease-modifying agent for rheumatoid arthritis). Technically speaking, a single-dose clinical study could be conducted, for example, in the USA based on single-dose toxicology/pharmacology. However, this rarely happens and is best utilized when a go/no-go decision is to be made based on these data, such as a micro-dose study with an exploratory IND (see FDA 2006). On the other hand, for a biologic with a long duration of action, a single dose could have pharmacologic effects for several months. While theoretically this could suffice, in practice regulators like to see multiple doses.

Typically, FIH studies for both small molecules and biologics commence with a single-ascending-dose (so-called SAD) study followed by a multiple-ascending-dose (MAD) study which generally last for a week or two up to a month depending on the duration of activity. Most sponsors will conduct a 1-month nonclinical study since 30 days of exposure is required for marketing authorization even for a drug that is only planned to be administered for 14 days ("planning for success").

Pharmacokinetics (PK)/toxicokinetics is typically required to evaluate serum or plasma levels of the biologic in the toxicology studies. Exceptions occur, for example, with small interfering or silencing RNA (siRNA) molecules where pharmacodynamic (PD) responses only are available. For single- or multiple-dose studies, the assay may or may not be developed, but plasma can be stored for later evaluation and sometimes to help choose a dose and schedule for later studies. AUC_{0-t}, C_{max}, and Ct (a given time after dosing often trough levels) are measured (ICH S3A 1994). Plasma levels can be related to pharmacologic and toxicologic findings and safety margins calculated or estimated prospectively from animals to humans. Once human PK data are available, a more accurate estimate of the presumptive safety margin can be confirmed or re-calculated.

3.7 Safety Pharmacology

Pharmacology studies for safety and PD are defined in ICH S7A. The core studies evaluate the effects of single doses on the cardiovascular system, respiratory system, and central nervous system (CNS) and are typically conducted prior to human studies and before GLP toxicology studies. However, these studies can also be incorporated into the GLP toxicology studies for biologics and in the oncology therapeutic area. Similarly, ICH S7B outlines the testing strategy for "The non-clinical evaluation of the potential for delayed ventricular repolarization (QT interval prolongation) by human pharmaceuticals." This generally only applies to small molecules, and since biologics act extracellularly and do not directly affect ion channels, these studies are not typically needed.

3.8 Dose Extrapolation

When estimating the first dose in humans, "All of the relevant nonclinical data, including the pharmacological dose response, the pharmacological/toxicological profile, and pharmacokinetics, should be considered when determining the recommended starting dose in humans" (ICH M3(R2)).

For biotechnology-derived products or biotherapeutics, ICH S6 1997, R1 2011, and addendum 2012 outline differences from the small-molecule approach. The approach is defined as case-by-case justified by the science. One of the main differences relates to expression of the target in the species chosen for toxicology studies (Chapter 2). Rodents, for example, often do not express the target so there is no point in selecting rodent as a relevant toxicology species. Species such as the cynomolgus monkey is commonly selected, and it may be possible to proceed with only one species for toxicology studies or even no formal toxicologic studies if no relevant species have been identified. It is also not uncommon to not see target organ toxicity, and the NOAEL (see Dorato and Engelhardt 2005) will turn out to be the highest dose tested. For example, adalimumab and infliximab, monoclonal antibodies to TNF, have no observable nonclinical toxicology findings (van Mierlo et al. 2014). Toxicologic findings where present tend to relate to exaggerated pharmacology since there are less off-target effects with biologics (Sullivan and Hamadeh 2015). Many biologics or novel compounds have a prolonged duration of action, and a long washout period may be needed in toxicology studies to demonstrate reversibility of findings. For example, etelcalcetide (Parsabiv) is a peptide with a long duration of action that modulates the calcium receptor and is an effective

treatment for secondary hyperparathyroidism (Parsabiv FDA package insert 2017). Animal and human studies demonstrate that hypocalcemia is the main toxicity, and studies indicate that reversal of hypocalcemia occurs within a month in humans. Many studies with biologics may be difficult to conduct since most are immunogenic when given to animals and antibodies to human proteins may increase clearance of the therapeutic of interest making it difficult to maintain appropriate serum concentrations. Similarly, antibody immune complexes may produce pathologic findings such as vasculitis which would not be translatable to humans. Accordingly, appropriate interpretation of findings is of paramount importance.

3.9 First in Human (FIH) Studies

When selecting a biologic to be administered to humans, the general approach is to administer to healthy subjects if this is feasible. The reasons relate mainly to operational efficiencies. They are relatively easy to recruit, are willing to be housed under constant observation, and do not have background disease or medications which can confound assessment of adverse effects. The studies can be completed more quickly and at lesser cost than using a patient population. That being said, at times it is necessary to recruit patients when the risk to subjects is considered high and exceeds "risks of daily living." Overall, biologics (antibodies in particular) tend to have a longer duration of effect than small molecules. An example of where it typically would not be acceptable to administer a drug to healthy volunteers would include a situation where toxicologic findings were considered to be serious, unmonitorable, or irreversible. In these circumstances, it would only be considered acceptable to administer to patients if the potential benefits were considered to outweigh the risks (e.g., a life-threatening disease without other reasonable treatment options).

ICH S9 addresses toxicology studies for life-threatening diseases (typically advanced cancer patients) who have exhausted known effective treatment options and applies to both small molecules and biologics. Accordingly, the type, timing, and flexibility needed in the design of nonclinical studies can differ from those for non-life-threatening diseases (Chapter 29). For small molecules, a common approach is to set a starting dose at one-tenth the severely toxic dose in 10% of the animals (STD10) in rodents. If non-rodents are the most appropriate species, as is more usual for biologics, then one-sixth of the HNSTD is typically chosen. FIH studies in this population begin with multiple doses. If a patient responds to treatment (or at least does not have disease progression), he or she will stay on treatment until it is apparent that he or she is no longer receiving benefit. Accordingly, the duration of exposure in humans may well exceed that in animals.

3.10 Dose Selection

When selecting a dose to be administered to healthy volunteer humans for the first time, a variety of approaches have been taken and have generally been safe. The FDA guidance (2005) takes the approach of outlining a process for deriving the maximum recommended starting dose (MRSD). Alternative approaches place emphasis on animal PK data and modeling (Mahmood et al. 2003; Reigner and Blesch 2002; FDA Exposure Response Guidance 2003). However, this presupposes that there are adequate PK data from animal studies which may or may not be the case. There should be at least trough concentrations at the NOAEL. This is defined as the highest dose level that does not produce a significant increase in adverse effects in comparison with the control group. In other words, it is the dose level that is tested below that which produces effects considered to be "adverse" (Dorato and Engelhardt 2005). After the NOAEL has been determined in the toxicology studies, a human equivalent dose (HED) is calculated. Both EMA (2007) and FDA (2005) emphasize that the selected starting dose for humans be based on the NOAEL from the toxicology study in the most appropriate species. This typically defaults to the most sensitive species unless otherwise scientifically justified. This conversion to a HED relies on multiplication of the mg/kg dose at the NOAEL in the appropriate species to a mg/kg dose in humans based on body surface area (BSA) conversion factor between the species of interest and humans. For example, if a NOAEL of 10 mg/kg is determined in cynomolgus monkeys, the HED based on a BSA normalization would be 10 divided by 3.1, the BSA conversion factor for monkeys to humans, producing an HED of 3.2 mg/kg. For a more detailed discussion of the various assumptions underlying these calculations, see FDA (2005). For large-molecule biologics such as monoclonal antibodies (>100 KD), direct scaling by body weight is appropriate. In the example above, for instance, the HED would be 10 mg/kg. BSA calculations tend to arrive at a more conservative dosing strategy. Other approaches rely on PK modeling to arrive at a comparable area under the curve (AUC) for the NOAEL between a given species and human.

When the actual dose to be administered to humans is calculated, the dose should almost always be a fixed or flat dose unless the therapeutic window is narrow and actual mg/kg or BSA adjusted dosing is needed. For evaluation of how to do this for monoclonal antibodies, see Wang et al. (2013). In practice, it is rare that either mg/kg or BSA adjustments can typically be justified in adult humans even with cytotoxic drugs, and it is not usually necessary to adjust for body weight in adult studies. Retrospective studies for marketed drugs have generally demonstrated that fixed doses are just as safe as either mg/kg or BSA calculated doses (Sawyer and Ratain 2001; Grochow et al. 1990). Subjects that are obese tend to be "overdosed" when the amount of antibody to be administered is calculated on a mg/kg basis since biotherapeutics are not typically distributed into fat and do not have a high volume of distribution. On the other hand, smaller and lighter individuals will tend to be exposed to higher concentrations when using a fixed or flat dose (Yang et al. 2019). It is not typically a problem for small molecules administered orally, since usually only a few tablet or capsule sizes are manufactured, and the base case is for a fixed dose. It is more of an issue for biologics or non-orally administered small molecules since it is practically easier to administer mg/kg dosing for parenteral therapeutics, and animals tend to be dosed on a mg/kg basis. Many cancer drugs given parenterally are still administered on a mg/kg or BSA

basis, but this is mostly for historical reasons and usually was the regimen utilized for original marketing approval. When rigorously evaluated, a fixed dose would generally be more appropriate (Sawyer and Ratain 2001; Grochow et al. 1990). The reason that a fixed or flat dose is more appropriate (assuming scientific justification) relates to medication error and efficiency of manufacturing shelf-keeping units (SKUs). It is well established that human errors occur even with relatively simple calculations. Fewer steps and calculations minimize dosing errors (Nolan 2000). Furthermore, it is wasteful to develop unnecessary SKUs to cover weight-based dosing.

3.11 Pharmacologic Endpoints

The use of pharmacologic endpoints for HED has been proposed based on the observations that on occasion, a benign toxicology profile in animals is associated with profound toxicity profile in humans (EMA 2007). Events related to the FIH study of TGN1412 (TeGenero AG, Würzburg, Germany) provided a dramatic example of the shortcomings of extrapolating animal to human data (Expert Scientific Group 2006; Suntharalingam et al. 2006). A cohort of healthy volunteers at Parexel (a contract research organization with a phase 1 unit in the UK) were all dosed on the same day within an hour or so and received a super-agonist antibody against the T-cell target, CD28, and experienced an unexpected "cytokine storm" which resulted in intensive care hospitalization and prolonged morbidity in some volunteers (Suntharalingam et al. 2006). Considering the mechanism of action, a case could well have been made that the events were not unexpected. Consequently, the EMA, via its Committee for Medicinal Products for Human Use (CHMP), issued a "Guideline on Strategies to Identify and Mitigate Risks for First-In-Human Clinical Trials with Investigational Medicinal Products" (EMA 2007), a document targeted toward identifying and mitigating the risks associated with FIH trials in healthy volunteers. The TeGenero experience resulted in proposals regarding other endpoints for consideration, namely the PAD and the MABEL. Descriptions of these endpoints are comparable (EMA 2007; FDA 2005) and have been described as interchangeable (Visich and Ponce 2008). There is, however, a lack of clear difference between the two. They both describe a concentration associated with a pharmacologic response. Pharmacologic endpoints differ from a NOAEL, the latter being a dose and the former a concentration. MABEL, on the other hand, is a dose gleaned from more than one source and estimated projection of human PK data "anticipated to have minimal biologic effects." There is no clear algorithm for arriving at a MABEL (Tibbitts et al. 2010). In the TeGenero experience, the initial dose given to humans was based on NOAEL. In retrospect, had it been based on a MABEL, a lower dose would have been given since the initial dose given to humans was projected to have had greater than 50% receptor occupancy. The relationship between receptor occupancy and clinical effect is of course highly variable, but selection of an initial dose would have been one with low receptor occupancy. A further example would be romiplostim, which is a peptibody that acts on the c-mpl receptor to increase platelets. Dosing in humans was based more on a presumptive pharmacologic effect (increase in platelets) or MABEL and interspecies scaling rather than a NOAEL (Wang et al. 2004).

3.12 Determination of Safety Factors

The next step in the process is to provide a safety factor on top of the HED assessment. This is typically a factor of 10 (FDA 2005), but may vary depending on issues such as the novelty of the target, estimated toxicity margin, nature of identified toxicities, demonstrated reversibility of toxicity, population being studied, steepness of dose–response relationships, and linearity of PK. The intent is to select a dose that is either homeopathic or at the low end of the dose–response curve in normal volunteers. Consideration should clearly also be given to safety margins in selecting these doses for FIH studies. The safety margin is the ratio between the planned PK exposure measure (typically AUC) at the NOAEL and the projected exposure measure/AUC at the various doses planned in humans. The higher the margin, the greater the presumptive safety.

3.13 Clinical Study Protocol

After selecting the first dose to take into humans, writing a protocol, an informed consent form (ICF), an investigator brochure (IB), and obtaining approval from an ethics committee (EC)/institutional review board (IRB) and regulatory authority, as appropriate, are necessary. The protocol details the instructions to the investigator on how to carry out the trial including selection of subjects, procedures that include blood tests or other special investigations, and how and where to report adverse events (AEs). The protocol should also outline doses, including maximum planned dose and stopping rules for both the individual and the cohort. As previously outlined, the first dose will usually be administered to a healthy volunteer and will be a dose that is homeopathic without expected effects or at the low end of the therapeutic range with minimally anticipated effects. Initially, a SAD protocol is written, and this is followed by a MAD phase that may or may not be a separate protocol. The SAD and MAD are conducted sequentially. Historically, many FIH trials in healthy subjects were conducted dosing a full cohort (typically 6–8 subjects) on the same day with doses staggered by 10- to 30-minute intervals by subject. However, following the TeGenero experience (see above) where subjects sequentially developed severe cytokine release according to the dosing order (the first subject did not develop symptoms until after the last subject had been dosed), most sponsors now dose only one or two subjects on the first day. Often one subject is on active treatment, while the other is on matched placebo. This so-called sentinel dosing pair may be operative for the first subjects of the first cohort or can be completed for each new cohort. This approach provides insurance against an unsafe dose being administered to more subjects than is necessary. Similarly, it may also be applied to the multiple-dose phase cohorts depending on emergent findings and perceived level of risk. Most phase 1 healthy volunteer studies are conducted under double-blind conditions to ensure that the adverse effect profile is captured as accurately as possible. Many mild AEs are not drug related. Some sponsors conduct partially blinded studies where the subjects and investigator are blinded but the sponsor is not. Nevertheless, all protocols have instructions that allow the principal investigator (PI) to exercise medical judgment and break the blind should there be a need to urgently know whether the subject has received active treatment. Similarly, the protocol may be written in a manner that allows the sponsor to unblind for safety reasons prior to completion of the study. This scenario makes it easier for sponsors to comply with the FDA IND rule (2012) where aggregate data for emergent safety signals need to be reported on an ongoing basis. Ideally, PK data by cohort should be available also. For practical reasons, this may or may not be implemented, and a decision on this is usually a judgment call based on anticipated risk. For small molecules, it is important to establish that the kinetics are linear especially in the presumptive therapeutic range, and to understand the concentration–response relationships (which are often more instructive than dose response). There tends to be a close relationship between PK and PD. It is rare these days to develop a small molecule that does not have linear kinetics. For biologics, this is less of a concern since there tends to be much more of a lag between PK and PD. For example, darbepoetin (Aranesp) will have an increase in hemoglobin 2–6 weeks after either a single intravenous or subcutaneous dose (FDA package insert). Most monoclonal antibodies have nonlinear kinetics at low dosages (with greater-than-dose-proportional increases) and then develop linearity as receptor occupancy becomes saturated. At high doses, nonlinearity may again be observed (in the direction of less-than-dose-proportional increases) as subcutaneous absorption mechanisms become more important determinants of PK. If possible, it is also important to measure PD and understand the relationship with PK. This can often help in selecting doses and schedules for later-stage trials where outcome measures are needed. PD and other biomarkers often have a strong relationship to efficacy and safety.

The protocol should outline how dose escalation decisions are made. At a minimum, the PI will need to agree and typically personnel from the sponsor as well as the PI make this decision. The protocol is usually written in a manner such that a study may be stopped, a cohort repeated, or a dose other than that originally planned may be substituted (such as an intermediate rather than full dose escalation). Company personnel involved in dose escalation decisions typically include the medical monitor and may include appropriate team members such as a biostatistician or a PK scientist as well as a representative from outside the team such as a safety physician (to help provide more objectivity). Occasionally, an external data monitoring committee can be set up to make dose escalation decisions (usually at the request of a regulator) for FIH trials. In selecting doses for testing in FIH trials, usually half-log dose increments are selected since most dose–response relationships in biology follow a geometric rather than arithmetic progression. However, as higher doses are tested, it is customary to decrease the increment at higher doses to ensure greater safety for subjects. As far as highest planned dose is concerned, typically the NOAEL will not be exceeded. However, depending on what is seen at lower doses and what is anticipated to be a therapeutic dose in patients, the NOAEL may be exceeded if this can be scientifically and medically justified and can be safely implemented. The overall objective is to explore the dose–response and concentration–response relationships as best one is able to, in phase 1. It is important to have studied high doses in phase 1 under controlled conditions (such as in an inpatient facility where subjects are closely observed) before subjecting higher numbers of patients under outpatient conditions in later-stage trials. Ideally, one should have studied at least one higher dose in phase 1 than that planned in a phase 2 trial. This is because small numbers are studied in phase 1, and if important AEs that are frequent and drug related are to occur, you will tend to see them at high doses.

3.14 Safety Assessment in FIH Trials

With respect to safety in phase 1 trials, there is a high bar and risks should generally be no greater than the risks a normal person takes in daily life. While thousands of healthy volunteers have taken part in phase 1 trials, there are few publications on safety of these studies. While many early-stage trials are not published, the most recent comprehensive assessments indicate that phase 1 trials are indeed relatively safe. Johnson et al. (2016) conducted a systematic review of published phase 1 healthy volunteer trials from January 1, 2008, to October 1, 2012. In 475 trials enrolling 27,185 subjects, there was a median of zero serious or severe AEs (interquartile range=0–0)/1,000 treatment group participants/day of monitoring. Most subjects reported mild or moderate AEs. The authors concluded that phase 1 trials caused mild and moderate harms but posed low risk of severe harm. Emmanuel et al. (2015) summarized data from 11,028 participants in 394 phase 1 studies conducted at three phase 1 study sites run by Pfizer (Belgium, Singapore, USA). The majority of these studies included an investigational compound and were conducted mostly in males and with small molecules (12% female and 3% biologics). Thirty-four serious AEs (0.31%) occurred, and none were life-threatening or fatal. Eleven events were considered by the investigator to be related to drug, seven to study procedures, and 16 (including 4 on placebo) to be unrelated events. Four thousand (36.3%) of the study drug participants experienced no AEs. Seven thousand and twenty-eight (7,028 or 63.7%) experienced 24,643 AEs. Overall, 85% (n=20,840) of AEs were mild and 1.0% (n=255) were considered severe. The overall conclusion was that "Concerns about the high risks of serious harms in non-oncology phase 1 trials do not seem to be borne out." While there is a lack of publications on healthy subjects and biologics, the experience of the writer indicates that novel biologics are not importantly different to novel small molecules with respect to safety in this population.

In order to conduct a phase 1 trial, an IB and ICF are required, and these documents along with the protocol need to be approved by an IRB or EC, as well as usually a national regulatory authority. The IB is a document that communicates the known safety profile to the investigator conducting the trial. It summarizes nonclinical safety data and provides guidance to the investigator about risks to subjects. The ICF provides a summary of possible risks for subjects that is ideally written in lay language at a grade level that most of the population can understand. These documents are updated at regular intervals according to emergent safety data.

It is necessary to select a PI and site to conduct phase 1 studies. Some larger pharmaceutical companies have their own in-house phase 1 units in which experienced staff that work for the company conduct the healthy volunteer studies according to good clinical practice (GCP). However, most sponsors do not have their own sites and need to contract out their studies. It is important to select an investigator with experience and good judgment and who also has the appropriate support staff with experience in conducting these studies. It is important to adhere closely to the protocol and make appropriate judgments about subjects including assessments of AEs. Similarly, patient studies are contracted out to usually several investigators that have experience in dealing with the patient population of interest. They must have access to the population and particular expertise in the disease area (especially in oncology). Those that have a track record of being able to recruit appropriate patients are usually selected. It is important to avoid selecting investigators that do not have the appropriate expertise or support staff since clinical research is expensive and patient studies are often difficult to recruit to. You want to avoid having to close sites (and waste scarce research funds) that cannot recruit appropriate patients.

3.15 Specific Considerations for FIH Trials in Cancer and Life-Threatening Diseases

For FIH trials involving patients using the ICH S9 approach, the initial dose selected will be a potentially therapeutic dose and will be based on either the STD10 or HNSTD (see above). These trials are typically conducted in patients with advanced cancer who have exhausted the standard of care for that particular tumor type. Accordingly, multiple doses are given initially to small cohorts (often three patients) based on a 28-day cycle. Treatment is continued until the patient develops disease progression (as determined by investigator using various criteria including tumor size with RECIST or other measures as outlined in the protocol) or unacceptable adverse effects or elects to discontinue treatment. Often the study design uses a modified Fibonacci design where an estimate of MTD will be determined (Eisenhauer et al. 2000). If one dose-limiting toxicity (DLT) event occurs in the first three subjects, another three will be enrolled, and if no further DLTs occur, dose escalation will go ahead for the next cohort. If, however, two out of the first three patients develop a DLT, then that dose will be declared a non-tolerated dose and the MTD will be the lower dose previously tested. With such small numbers, the confidence in the designation of a DLT is not high, and accordingly, there are many iterations on this general approach. The most recent full assessment of the safety and efficacy of phase 1 trials in advanced cancer patients showed response rates (complete and partial) of around 10% and toxicity-related deaths of 0.49% (Horstmann et al. 2005), which are higher than those reported previously with cytotoxic agents of response rates of 4%–6% and toxicity-related deaths of 2.5% (Sekine et al. 2002). More recent studies especially with immunomodulators or studies with background known effective therapies give higher response rates (stable disease or better in up to 44.7%) and lesser toxicities (Kurzrock and Benjamin 2005).

3.16 Regulatory Considerations

It is important to recognize the role of the regulator in dosing for FIH trials. Most countries require regulatory assent for phase 1 trials. Regulations evolve and changes are often based on tragedies. For example, the 1937 sulfanilamide experience in which the excipient ethylene glycol was responsible for more than 100 deaths resulted in the "Food Drug and Cosmetic Act" (1938) that in the USA required demonstration of safety for the first time. Similarly, the thalidomide disaster resulted in the 1962 Kefauver Harris law that required demonstration of efficacy for the first time in the USA. More recently, the TeGenero incident resulted in new EMA guidelines for phase 1 trials in 2007. "It identifies factors influencing risk for new investigational medicinal products and considers quality aspects, non-clinical and clinical testing strategies and designs for first-in-human clinical trials. Strategies for mitigating and managing risk are given, including the calculation of the initial dose to be used in humans, the subsequent dose escalation, and the conduct of the clinical trial." More recently, following the unfortunate experience from the French Bial phase 1 trial in which there was a fatality from CNS toxicity due to a small molecule targeting fatty acid amide hydrolase (Report by the Temporary Specialist Scientific Committee 2016, Kerbrat et al. 2016), the EMA guideline above has been revised (EMA 2017). It now addresses both FIH and integrated early-phase trials to further assist in identifying risk factors for new investigational medicinal products. "Strategies for mitigating and managing risks are given, including principles on the calculation of the starting dose to be used in humans, the subsequent dose escalations, the criteria for maximum dose and the conduct of the trial inclusive of multiple parts."

In summary, careful evaluation of nonclinical data, writing a protocol based on appropriate judgment in dose selection and escalation, will ensure relative safety for both healthy subjects and patients participating in phase 1 trials.

REFERENCES

Aranesp (darbepoetin) package insert FDA 2001. https://www. accessdata.fda.gov/drugsatfda_docs/label/2001/darbamg091701LB.htm.

Communicating Toxicogenomics Information to Nonexperts: A Workshop Summary. The National Academies Press US, 2005. https://www.nap.edu/read/11179/chapter/2#3

Dorato, MA, Engelhardt, JA, 2005. The no-observed-adverse-effect-level in drug safety evaluations: use, issues, and definition(s). *Regulatory Toxicology and Pharmacology* 42(3): 265–274.

Eisenhauer EA, et al., 2000. Phase 1 clinical trial design in cancer drug development. *Journal of Clinical Oncology* 18: 684–692.

EMA, 2007. Guideline on strategies to identify and mitigate risks for first-in-human clinical trials with investigational medicinal products. Vol. EMEA/CHMP/SWP/28367/07.

EMA, 2017. Guideline on strategies to identify and mitigate risks for first-in-human and early clinical trials with investigational medicinal products. EMEA/CHMP/SWP/28367/07 Rev. 1.

Emmanuel JE, et al., 2015. Quantifying the risks of non-oncology phase I research in healthy volunteers: meta-analysis of phase I studies. *BMJ* 350: h3271. doi:10.1136/bmj.h3271

Expert Scientific Group, 2006. *Expert Scientific Group on Phase One Clinical Trials.* Norwich, UK.

FDA Guidance for Industry, 2003. Exposure-response relationships — Study design, data analysis, and regulatory applications(CDER,CBER).https://www.fda.gov/regulatory-information/search-fda-guidance-documents/exposure-response-relationships-study-design-data-analysis-and-regulatory-applications

FDA Guidance for Industry, 2005. Estimating the maximum safe starting dose in initial clinical trials for therapeutics in adult healthy volunteers. https://www.fda.gov/regulatory-information/search-fda-guidance-documents/estimating-maximum-safe-starting-dose-initial-clinical-trials-therapeutics-adult-healthy-volunteers.

FDA Guidance for Industry, Investigators and Reviewers. Exploratory IND Studies 2006. https://www.fda.gov/regulatory-information/search-fda-guidance-documents/exploratory-ind-studies.

FDA Guidance for Industry and Investigators, 2012. Safety reporting requirements for INDs and BA/BE studies. http://www.fda.gov/Drugs/GuidanceComplianceRegulatoryInformation/Guidances/default.htm

Grochow LB, Baraldi C, Noe D, 21 February 1990. Is dose normalization to weight or body surface area useful in adults? *JNCI: Journal of the National Cancer Institute* 82(4): 323–325. doi:10.1093/jnci/82.4.323

Hamadeh HK, Bushel PR, Jayadev S, et al., 2002. Gene expression analysis reveals chemical-specific profiles. *Toxicological Sciences* 67(2): 219–231.

Horstmann E, McCabe MS, Grochow L, et al., 2005. Risks and benefits of phase 1 oncology trials, 1991 through 2002. *The New England Journal of Medicine* 352: 895–904.

ICH M3(R2), 2009. Guidance on nonclinical safety studies for the conduct of human clinical trials and marketing authorization for pharmaceuticals. ICH M3 (R2) Non-clinical safety studies for the conduct of human clinical trials for pharmaceuticals | European Medicines Agency. https://www.ema.europa.eu/en/ich-m3-r2-non-clinical-safety-studies-conduct-human-clinical-trials-pharmaceuticals

ICH S3A, 1994. Note for guidance on toxicokinetics: the assessment of systemic exposure in toxicity studies. https://database.ich.org/sites/default/files/S3A_Guideline.pdf.

ICH S4, 1998. Duration of chronic toxicity testing in animals (rodent and non-rodent toxicity testing). https://database.ich.org/sites/default/files/S4_Guideline.pdf.

ICH S6, 1997. Preclinical safety evaluation of biotechnology-derived pharmaceuticals. In CPMP/ICH/384/95 (ed.). Available from: http://www.ich.org/LOB/media/MEDIA503.pdf.

ICH S6 (R1), 2011. Preclinical safety evaluation of biotechnology-derived pharmaceuticals. European Medicines Agency. Available from: http://www.ema.europa.eu/docs/en_GB/document_library/Scientific_guideline/2009/09/WC500002828.pdf.

ICH, 2012. Addendum to ICH S6: nonclinical safety evaluation of biotechnology-derived pharmaceuticals S6(R1) current step 2 version. http://www.fda.gov/downloads/Drugs/GuidanceComplianceRegulatoryInformation/Guidances/UCM194490.pdf.

ICH S7A, 2000. Safety pharmacology studies for human pharmaceuticals. http://www.ema.europa.eu/docs/en_GB/document_library/Scientific_guideline/2009/09/WC500002831.pdf

ICH S7B. The non-clinical evaluation of the potential for delayed ventricular repolarisation (QT Interval Prolongation) by Human Pharmaceuticals CPMP/ICH/423/02. https://www.ema.europa.eu/en/ich-s7b-non-clinical-evaluation-potential-delayed-ventricular-repolarization-qt-interval.

Johnson RA, et al., 2016. Risks of phase I research with healthy participants: a systematic review. *BMJ* 13: 149–160.

Kerbrat A, et al., 2016. Acute neurologic disorder from an inhibitor of fatty acide amide hydrolase. *The New England Journal of Medicine* 375: 1717–1725. doi:10.1177/1740774515602868

Kurzrock R, Benjamin RS, 2005. Risks and benefits of phase 1 oncology trials, revisited. *The New England Journal of Medicine* 352: 930–931.

Mahmood I, Green MD, Fisher JE, 2003. Selection of the first-time dose in humans: comparison of different approaches based on interspecies scaling of clearance. *Journal of Clinical Pharmacology* 43(7): 692–697.

Nolan TW, 2000. System changes to improve patient safety. *BMJ* 320(7237): 771–773.

Parsabiv (etelcalcitide) FDA package insert 2017. https://www.accessdata.fda.gov/drugsatfda_docs/label/2017/208325Orig1s000Lbledt.pdf

Reigner BG, Blesch KS, 2002. Estimating the starting dose for entry into humans: principles and practice. *European Journal of Clinical Pharmacology* 57: 835–845.

Report by the Temporary Specialist Scientific Committee (TSSC), 2016. "FAAH (Fatty Acid Amide Hydrolase)", on the causes of the accident during a Phase 1 clinical trial in Rennes in January 2016. http://ansm.sante.fr/var/ansm_site/storage/original/application/744c7c6daf96b141bc9509e2f85c227e.pdf

Sawyer M, Ratain MJ, 2001. Body surface area as a determinant of pharmacokinetics and drug dosing. *Invest New Drugs* 19: 171.

Sekine I, Yamamoto N, Kunitoh H, et al., 2002. Relationship between objective responses in phase I trials and potential efficacy of non-specific cytotoxic investigational new drugs. *Annals of Oncology* 13: 1300–1306. doi:10.1023/A:1010639201787

Sullivan J, Hamadeh H, 2015. Overview of safety evaluation and quantitative approaches during preclinical and early phases of drug development. In Jiang Q, Xia HA (Eds.), *Quantitative Evaluation of Safety in Drug Development. Design Analysis and Reporting.* CRC Press, Taylor & Francis Group, Boca Raton, FL, pp. 321–337.

Suntharalingam G, et al., 2006. Cytokine storm in a phase 1 trial of the anti-CD28 monoclonal antibody TGN1412. *The New England Journal of Medicine* 355: 1018–1028.

Tibbitts J, Cavagnaro JA, Haller CA, Marafino B, Andrews PA, Sullivan JT, 2010. Practical approaches to dose selection for first-in-human clinical trials with novel biopharmaceuticals. *Regulatory Toxicology and Pharmacology* 58: 243–251.

van Mierlo GJD, Cnubben NHP, Wouters D, et al., 2014. The minipig as an alternative non-rodent model for immunogenicity testing using the TNFα blockers adalimumab and infliximab, *Journal of Immunotoxicology* 11(1): 62–71. doi:10.3109/1547691X.2013.796023

Visich J, Ponce R, 2008. Science and judgement in establishing a safe starting dose for first-in-human trials of pharmaceuticals. In Cavagnaro J (Ed.), *Preclinical Safety Evaluation of Biopharmaceuticals: A Science-Based Approach to Facilitating Clinical Trials.* Wiley, New Jersey, pp. 971–984.

Wang B, Nichol J, Sullivan JT, 2004. Pharmacodynamics and pharmacokinetics of AMG 531, a novel thrombopoietin receptor ligand. *Clinical Pharmacology Therapeutics* 76: 628–638.

Wang DD, Zhang S, Zhao H, Men AY, Parivar K, 2013. Fixed dosing versus body size—Based dosing of monoclonal antibodies in adult clinical trials. *Journal of Clinical Pharmacology* 49: 1012–1024. doi:10.1177/0091270009337512

Yang B, Gozzi P, Sullivan JT, 2019. Pharmacokinetics of anakinra in subjects of heavier vs lighter body weights. *Clinical and Translational Science* 12: 371–378. doi:10.11/cts.12622

4

Ready, Aim, Fire! The Importance of Strategic Drug Development Plans

Patricia D. Williams
IND Directions. LLC

CONTENTS

4.1 The Planning Principle

Would you develop a drug without a plan? Yes, No, Maybe? Before you answer that question, would you build a house without a blueprint? The consequences of that could be quite dangerous! Or would you take a trip across country without a roadmap? That could be a very long trip! Or would you attempt to prepare a gourmet dessert without a recipe? If so, you may be eating it alone! This chapter will discuss the strategic planning process and ask you the question again later.

Before we do, we first need to acknowledge that the drug development process is complex, with multiple moving parts as shown in Figure 4.1. What steps can be conducted in parallel, and what steps are dependent on each other?

DOI: 10.1201/9781003124542-5

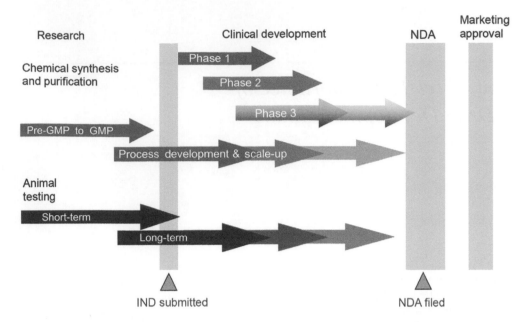

FIGURE 4.1   The drug development process.

4.2 The Strategic Drug Development Plan...*Ready, Aim!*

The strategic plan is the foundation (roadmap, blueprint, recipe) upon which your drug candidate's future depends (Figure 4.2; Tables 4.1 and 4.2).

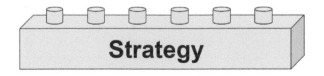

The strategic plan answers the following questions:

- What needs to be done?
- When will it be done?
- How much will it cost?
- Who will get it done?

4.2.1 What Needs To Be Done?

TABLE 4.1

Strategic Drug Development Plan – Table of Contents

Table of Contents	Page
1 Disease Background	
2 Biologic Therapies in Disease Indication	
3 Scope of Work	
4 Preclinical Studies	
4.1 Completed Pharmacology Studies	
4.2 IND-Enabling Preclinical Toxicology Studies	
5 Chemistry Manufacturing and Controls	
5.1 Biologic Substance	
5.2 Biologic Product	
6 Clinical Development	
6.1 Phase 1 Program	
6.2 Phase 2 Program	
6.3 Phase 3 Program	
7 Regulatory Support	
8 Program Management	
9 Proposed Timelines	
10 Budget 45	

4.2.2 When Does It Need To Be Done?

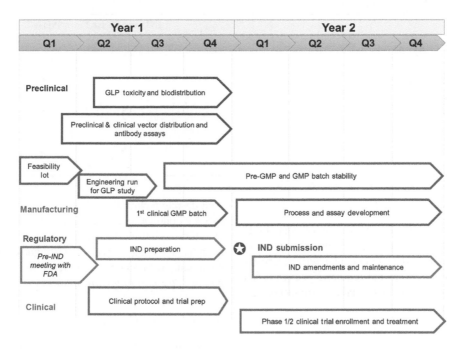

FIGURE 4.2   Biologic product: Phase 1 development timeline.

4.2.3 How Much Will It Cost?

TABLE 4.2

Budget Estimate for Drug Development Pla**n**

Program Task	IND and Phase 1	Phase 2	Phase 3 and NDA
1.0 Preclinical Studies			
Efficacy, Safety, and Biodistribution in Mouse Model of Disease	$		
GLP Toxicology/Biodistribution in Non-human Primate (NHP)	$		
qPCR Assay Validation (mouse, NHP, human)	$		
Antibody Assay Validation (mouse, NHP, human)	$		
Total for Preclinical Phase	$		
2.0 Manufacturing Biologic Substance and Product			
Manufacturing Process Development and Analytical Assays	$		
Non-GMP Engineering Run for Pivotal Toxicology	$		
Phase 1 Clinical Trial Supplies	$		
Phase 2 Clinical Trial Supplies		$	
Phase 3 and BLA Manufacturing			$
GMP Stability	$	$	$
Total for Manufacturing	$	$	$
3.0 Regulatory Sponsorship			
Orphan Product Designation Application	$		
Pre-IND Meeting	$		
IND Submission	$		
End-of-Phase 2 Meeting		$	
Pre-BLA Meeting			$
BLA Filing			$
Total for Regulatory	$	$	$

(Continued)

TABLE 4.2 (*Continued*)

Budget Estimate for Drug Development Plan

Program Task	IND and Phase 1	Phase 2	Phase 3 and NDA
4.0 Clinical Development Program			
Phase 1 Trial (CRO and site costs)	$		
Phase 2 Trial (CRO and site costs)		$	
Phase 3 Trial(s) (CRO and site costs)			$
Total for Clinical Development	**$**	**$**	**$**
5.0 Program Totals			
5.1 Subtotals	$	$	$
6.0 Grand Total		**$**	

4.2.4 Who Will Get It Done?

A good strategic plan also provides options and recommendations regarding the resources needed to implement drug development plans. The author of the strategic plan will be familiar with the company's organization and general capacity to manage a development program and can make recommendations for project management.

4.2.4.1 Company Resources

The expertise of employees in the company is a good place to start, but experience may be focused on one particular aspect of development (e.g., strength in cell biology or clinical trial management). And for very small ("virtual") companies, there is not the "luxury" of having one person for every discipline. So, it is not unusual that companies must look outwardly for resources to manage and conduct drug development activities.

Above all, it is important to *know what you don't know!* That admission is hard for some, but not being honest with your capabilities has consequences. When you don't know what you don't know, the tendency is to:

• Do more than is necessary
• Conduct activities in series rather than in parallel
• Worry more than necessary
• Become confused by varying opinions

4.2.4.2 Contract Organizations

Contract research organizations (CROs) and contract manufacturing organizations (CMOs) can provide as-needed services that would never be affordable for virtual to small organizations, such as preclinical studies, manufacturing, and conduct of clinical trials. However, while the technical expertise of contract organizations is assumed, there are vast differences in expertise in planning or strategy, and such "added services" should be scrutinized carefully for their foundation. Also, do not assume because of technical expertise that CROs or CMOs have the knowledge or experience to provide strategic advice. And unfortunately, because service industries have a vested interest in "recommending" programs that may be overly conservative, if not excessive, one should be wary of proposals that benefit their bottom line while harming yours.

And despite technical expertise being a given, it is also wise to ask a contract organization if they have performed the specific tasks you want done, and if so, how many times and how recently. They may express a willingness to do whatever you need done, with no prior experience in doing so! *Past performance is the best predictor of future success!*

4.2.4.3 Consultants

Consultants can bridge a variety of gaps in expertise for companies or offer a sounding board for ideas generated internally. However, more consultants do not necessarily lead to a better outcome, and the paralysis of analysis is a real danger. As with any service provider, past experience is the best predictor of future success, and so with consultants. Her expertise is limited to what she's actually done. Consultants who have worked in the discovery and early development of new drugs may be more appropriate for development through initial clinical trials, but those with later-stage experience through drug approvals may be more suited for Phase 3 and commercialization. It can be very harmful to the drug's future to apply late-stage commercial standards to early-stage development programs. This is because advancing to clinical proof of concept and product decision as soon as possible is the key objective of early drug development. And lastly, not all consultants have experience in implementing drug development plans. Some may be excellent at strategizing, while others are skilled at overseeing and managing development activities.

4.3 Implementation…*Fire!*

Implementation is all about *Making It Happen* and converting strategic plans into action.

4.3.1 Select a Compound!

The quality of your drug development pipeline depends on the criteria applied to selecting a compound, through in-licensing or internal discovery efforts. These criteria may include assessments of the feasibility of manufacture ("drugability"), marketing analysis, and intellectual property status. But in the end, whether a drug succeeds or fails resides in its ability to treat a disease without causing unacceptable harm. The therapeutic index (TI) provides a measure of the safety margin that exists between doses producing efficacy and those causing adverse effects or toxicity. Thus, obtaining information on the TI with a candidate *before selecting it* for development is paramount; this information can be obtained in in vitro systems or in animals. Having data on efficacy and safety in a relevant animal model of disease is ideal, since safety in normal, healthy animals can underestimate the toxic potential in diseased animals (and humans).

4.3.2 Getting into the Clinic

Entering the clinic in the United States requires a regulatory vehicle called an Investigational New Drug (IND) that is regulated by the US Food and Drug Administration (FDA). INDs are not approved as many misstate, but rather they are *allowed to proceed*. IND allowance marks the beginning of a drug's clinical development and is in place for the duration of the drug's (development) lifetime.

Prior to the IND submission, it is desirable to obtain input on the adequacy of the drug development plan, including manufacturing, preclinical studies, and the design of the first-in-human (FIH) trial. This is accomplished through the Pre-IND process. The Pre-IND will enhance the probability of success of the IND by providing feedback on all aspects of the IND plan. In addition, it is good to become familiar with the individuals at FDA reviewing your drug candidate.

The Pre-IND process is outlined in Figure 4.3. The entire process from request to receiving FDA final meeting minutes is ~90 days; however, one should add at least 30 days to draft the Pre-IND Information Package prior to making the meeting request. Since the Pre-IND Information Package must be submitted 30 days in advance of the Pre-IND meeting, making sure the package is ~75% complete when making the request

will ensure that the package can be completed and submitted within 30 days. The Pre-IND meeting may take the form of a face-to-face meeting, teleconferences, or written responses, and FDA will make the decision regarding the forum when granting the meeting. The central feature of the Pre-IND request and meeting is Sponsor questions to FDA which can be general or specific, but must be based on the information provided in the Pre-IND Information Package. Refer to "Formal Meetings Between the FDA and Sponsors or Applicants of PDUFA Products – Guidance for Industry (December 2017)."

For the actual IND, FDA Guidance on the Content and Format of Investigational New Drug Applications (INDs) for Phase 1 Studies of Drugs, Including Well-Characterized, Therapeutic, Biotechnology-Derived Products, is available.

Regulatory guidances on requirements for INDs and subsequent development that can be consulted include the following:

- M3(R2) Nonclinical Safety Studies for the Conduct of Human Clinical Trials and Marketing Authorization for Pharmaceuticals (2010)
- Gene and cell therapy
    - Preclinical Assessment of Investigational Cellular and Gene Therapy Products (2013)
    - Chemistry, Manufacturing, and Control (CMC) Information for Human Gene Therapy Investigational New Drug Applications (INDs). Guidance for Industry (2020)
    - Content and Review of Chemistry, Manufacturing, and Control (CMC) Information for Human Somatic Cell Therapy Investigational New Drug Applications (INDs) (2008)
- Human Gene Therapy for Rare Diseases (2020)

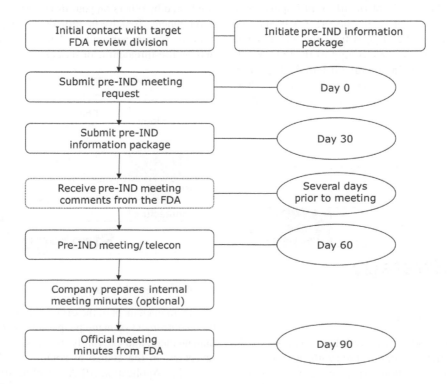

FIGURE 4.3 Pre-IND process.

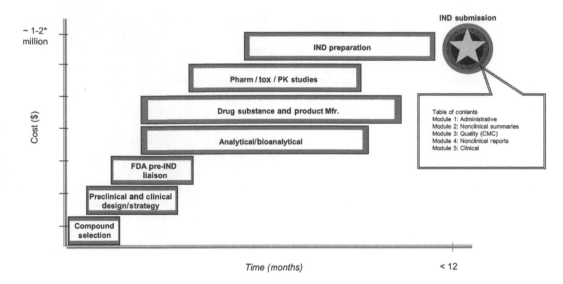

FIGURE 4.4   From compound selection to the IND.

From compound selection to the IND submission, the time-frame is usually within 1 year with a cost of ~$1–2 million (Figure 4.4).

With the strategic plan as the foundation, the formal development of the drug is initiated to the IND milestone.

With respect to chemistry, manufacturing, and controls (CMC), these activities are often critical path for the IND. A common misconception is the need for GMP (Good Manufacturing Practices) material for nonclinical safety studies; typically, a pre-GMP engineering run is used for the pivotal GLP (Good Laboratory Practices) toxicology studies. It is more important that the process and impurity profiles of preclinical vs. clinical material are properly aligned. Having higher levels of or different impurities in clinical GMP material relative to the pre-GMP material utilized in toxicology studies jeopardizes the integrity and validity of the toxicology studies to support the IND. While the formulation of the drug in pivotal, GLP toxicology studies should parallel clinical formulation, there may be flexibility if the clinical formulation contains only compendial excipients.

toxicology studies supporting the duration of the clinical trials. This will require conducting toxicology studies in parallel with clinical trials to support the next phase of clinical testing. In addition, reproductive and carcinogenicity studies may be required for marketing approval and therefore need to be initiated before or during pivotal Phase 3 clinical trials. For biotechnology products, additional toxicology studies beyond IND-enabling studies may not be necessary depending on the duration of use and patient population. For protein therapeutics that may be used on a chronic basis, longer term studies are typically required where with single-dose products such as gene or cell therapy, no repeat-dose studies are warranted.

It is important to remain vigilant regarding animal studies conducted by others on your drug during the clinical phase of development. Toxicity in animals can impact on the ongoing clinical program particularly if unexpected findings occur that may be life-threatening or serious.

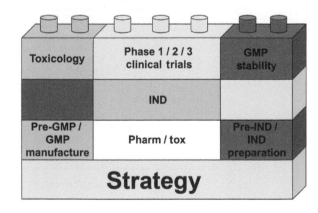

4.3.3 Staying in the Clinic

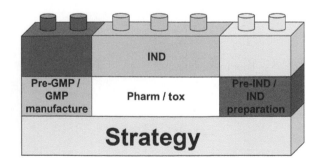

After the IND is active and clinical trials have commenced, the focus is how to keep the drug in the clinic without delays in the overall timeline. For conventional small molecules, this typically involves paying attention to the duration of the preclinical

4.3.4 Project Management

Project management of the drug development process involves the management of many people [internally: scientists, senior management; and externally: vendors, consultants, regulators, inventors) in the course of completing IND- and Biologics Licensing Application (BLA)-enabling studies and activities. It is also important to manage expectations and obstacles that appear along the way. It takes real skill to make projects run smoothly, and the best project managers make it look easy. The project manager is "point of contact" for all issues and information and generates project operations plan. The project manager helps to define roles and responsibilities of project team members and all critical processes and communicates project timelines, metrics, and milestones to the project team. Project managers typically manage and track the project budget and schedule project team meetings and teleconferences.

4.4 Special Considerations for Biologics Strategic Planning

4.4.1 Overview

Biologics commonly mimic human proteins or cells or provide the technology to deliver human genes or proteins; thus, their activity is often species-specific for human receptors. Thus, strategic planning is all about relevance: relevance in terms of pharmacological activity in the species to be tested for safety prior to human clinical trials. And because technologies are focused on very specific receptors or processes, toxicities are often limited to exaggerated pharmacological activity rather than target organ toxicity. The need for two species for preclinical safety is also dependent on the specificity of the biologic and availability of animal models of disease (AMD). In contrast, the development of conventional, small-molecule therapeutics follows a more prescribed course of preclinical requirements, with two species typically employed for safety testing, along with extensive pharmacokinetics and metabolism (PK/ADME), genetic toxicology, and reproductive toxicology testing. Biologics development also focuses on PK but less on metabolism, and with certain classes of agents (e.g., cells, gene therapy), biodistribution of cells and vectors is a key safety issue. Because biologics by nature frequently lack target organ toxicities, the demonstration of pharmacological activity in either AMD or normal animals validates the relevance of the species and studies to support human testing.

4.4.2 Safety Pharmacology

Safety pharmacology (i.e., effects on CNS and cardiovascular and respiratory systems) is still incorporated into pivotal toxicology studies for biologics (S7A Safety Pharmacology Guidance 2001), but issues such as QT interval prolongation and arrhythmogenic potential observed with small molecules are not generally raised.

And unlike small-molecule development, FIH trials with biologics are typically in patients with the disease targeted in the therapeutic indication. Thus, the importance of efficacy and safety data in AMD, if available, is paramount.

4.4.3 GLP Compliance

When conducting IND-enabling toxicology studies with biologics in AMD, it is not always feasible to conduct these studies according to GLP regulations. In those cases, studies can still be acceptable as pivotal safety studies with third-party oversight and auditing. Having a prospective study protocol and good documentation of study conduct from animal receipt to postmortem assessments is key for acceptance of non-GLP studies. In addition, often postmortem assessments such as histopathology and tissue biodistribution can be conducted by contract laboratories in full GLP compliance.

4.4.4 Examples

Examples of IND-enabling preclinical studies for a variety of biologics are provided in Tables 4.3–4.5. The diversity of packages illustrates the need to approach biologics in a case-by-case manner, tailoring the program to address specific issues unique to each class or compound. Each program is tailored to the duration of intended use, species specificity, and unique class-related issues. This diversity underscores the importance of having a pre-IND dialogue with FDA prior to initiating IND-enabling studies.

TABLE 4.3

Protein Therapeutics

Protein Product	Antibody	Enzyme	Protein Conjugate
Delivery	Systemic	Systemic	Systemic
Duration of Therapy	Chronic	Once	Subchronic

Example of Preclinical Package for the IND	• Species receptor binding affinity
	 • Twenty-eight-day toxicology in NHP with TK
	 • Tissue cross-reactivity – humans, animals
		• Fourteen-day toxicology with TK and recovery
		  • Rat
		  • NHP
			• Twenty-eight-day toxicology with TK:
			  • Rats
			  • NHP
			 • Tissue cross-reactivity – humans, animals

BLA-Enabling Preclinical Studies?	• Six-month toxicology with TK	• None	• Three-month toxicology with TK
Drug Development Plan Focus and Issues	• Off-target binding • Infusion reactions	• Species homology and activity	• Stability • Immunogenicity

TABLE 4.4

Cellular Therapeutics

Cell Product	Bacteria	Human Cell (Autologous)	Human Cells (Heterologous)
Delivery	Topical	Local	Local
Duration of Therapy	Subchronic	Once	Once

Example of Preclinical Package for the IND	• Single-dose IV toxicity in rabbits
	• Twenty-eight-day dermal toxicity in rabbits
	• Cytokine release in human peripheral blood mononuclear cells (PBMCs)
		• Single-dose efficacy, safety and biodistribution in porcine AMD
		  • Human cells
		  • Porcine cells
			• Single-dose toxicity in rats
			• Single-dose efficacy, safety, and biodistribution in porcine AMD
			  • Human cells
			  • Porcine cells

BLA-Enabling Preclinical Studies?	• None	• None	• Tumorigenicity in rodents

Drug Development Plan Focus and Issues	• Pro-inflammatory cytokine release	• Delivery devices
		  • Correlation to human
		  • Compatibility with therapeutic
			• Tumorigenicity
			• Delivery devices
			  • Correlation to human
			  • Compatibility with therapeutic

TABLE 4.5

Gene Therapies

Gene Therapy	AAV	AAV	AAV/Gene Editing
Delivery	Systemic	Local	Systemic
Duration of Therapy	Once	Once	Once

Example of Preclinical Package for the IND	• Single-dose small AMD pharm/tox
	• Single-dose small normal animal tox, biodistribution
		• Single-dose small AMD pharm/tox
		• Single-dose large normal animal tox, biodistribution
			• Single-dose small animal AMD pharm, tox
			• Single-dose large animal AMD pharm, tox, biodistribution
			• Off-target assessments
			  • In silico
			  • In vitro
			  • In vivo

BLA-Enabling Preclinical Studies?	• None	• None	• None

Drug Development Plan Focus and Issues	• Immunogenicity
	• Distribution, persistence
	• Gene expression
		• Delivery devices:
		  • Correlation to human
		  • Compatibility with therapeutic
		• Gene expression
			• On-target gene editing
			• Off-target genetic damage
			• Immunogenicity

4.5 Other Strategic Regulatory Considerations

The regulatory pathway for biologics can be enhanced by taking advantage of programs for expedited development. The FDA has designated four programs, listed in the subsections below, which are intended to facilitate and expedite the development and review of new drugs to address unmet medical needs in the treatment of serious or life-threatening conditions. These programs are intended to help ensure that therapies for serious conditions are approved and available to patients as soon as it can be concluded that the benefits justify the risks.

While all four of the programs share this overall goal, each program has different qualifications and may be applicable only to a specific facet of the development or review of a new drug. Three of these programs have existed for many years, but the Breakthrough Therapy Designation (BTD) is relatively new, dating from 2012. Because there is some overlap in the programs, FDA recently updated a Guidance for Industry entitled "Expedited Programs for Serious Conditions – Drugs and Biologics" in which each of the programs is discussed in detail (FDA 2020).

4.5.1 Fast Track Designation

The key feature of fast track designation is that it may be requested by the sponsor early in development based on preclinical or clinical data that demonstrate the potential to address an unmet medical need in the treatment of a serious condition. Fast track designation can be requested at the time of the IND or any time after the IND is active but no later than the pre-NDA meeting, as its features (more frequent meetings with FDA as needed) are intended to expedite the development and review of the product while studies are ongoing under the IND.

4.5.2 Breakthrough Therapy Designation (BTD)

The key feature of BTD is that it must be based on preliminary clinical evidence that indicates that the drug may demonstrate substantial improvement on a clinically significant endpoint over available therapies. The sponsor requests this designation with the IND (if prior clinical data exist that qualify the drug) or during development, ordinarily no later than the end-of-Phase 2 meeting. It is more valuable than the fast track designation because it must be based on clinical data and because the drug must demonstrate the potential to be superior to other therapies on a clinically significant endpoint. As a result, the FDA commits more of its resources to assist the sponsor in the development of a drug that has been designated as a Breakthrough Therapy.

For biologics, there is a designation similar to Breakthrough for regenerative medicines (Expedited Programs for Regenerative Medicine Therapies for Serious Conditions – February 2019). As described in Section 3033 of the 21st Century Cures Act, a drug is eligible for regenerative medicine advanced therapy (RMAT) designation if:

- The drug is a regenerative medicine therapy, which is defined as a cell therapy, therapeutic tissue engineering product, human cell and tissue product, or any combination product using such therapies or products, except for those regulated solely under Section 361 of the Public Health Service Act and part 1271 of Title 21, Code of Federal Regulations;
- The drug is intended to treat, modify, reverse, or cure a serious or life-threatening disease or condition; and
- Preliminary clinical evidence indicates that the drug has the potential to address unmet medical needs for such disease or condition

4.5.3 Accelerated Approval

Accelerated approval is not a "designation" but a path to approval for a drug that generally provides a meaningful advantage over available therapies and demonstrates an effect on a surrogate endpoint that is reasonably likely to predict clinical benefit or on a clinical endpoint that can be measured earlier than irreversible morbidity or mortality (IMM) (i.e., an intermediate clinical endpoint). There are several conditions attached to accelerated approval, including the requirement that the sponsor conduct confirmatory clinical trial(s) to verify and describe the anticipated effect on IMM or other clinical benefit. It is expected that these confirmatory trials will be ongoing if not fully enrolled at the time of accelerated approval.

4.5.4 Priority Review Designation

The sponsor may request priority review designation at the time of submission of the marketing application for a product that, if approved, would provide a clinically significant improvement in safety or effectiveness. The advantage of this designation is that FDA commits to reviewing the marketing application in 6 months instead of the standard 10–12 months.

4.6 Conclusions

The key to successful drug development is strategic planning (***Ready, Aim…***), knowing what you don't know, and implementing plans with dedicated project management (***Fire!***)

Acknowledge that obstacles and issues will occur, and have courage!

- Would you develop a drug without a strategic drug development plan? ***Never!***

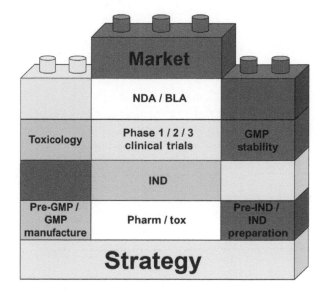

REFERENCES

Center for Drug Evaluation and Research Guidance Document: Expedited Programs for Serious Conditions— Drugs and Biologics. May 2014 (Updated 6/25/2020). https://www.fda.gov/regulatory-information/ search-fda-guidance-documents/expedited programs-serious-conditions-drugs-and-biologics

Chemistry, Manufacturing, and Control (CMC) Information for Human Gene Therapy Investigational New Drug Applications (INDs). Guidance for Industry. January 2020. https://www.fda.gov/regulatory-information/search-fda-guidance-documents/chemistry-manufacturing-and-control-cmc-information-human-gene-therapy-investigational-new-drug

Content and Review of Chemistry, Manufacturing, and Control (CMC) Information for Human Somatic Cell Therapy Investigational New Drug Applications (INDs). Guidance for Reviewers and Sponsors. April 2008. https://www.fda.gov/regulatory-information/search-fda-guidance-documents/content-and-review-chemistry-manufacturing-and-control-cmc-information-human-somatic-cell-therapy

Expedited Programs for Regenerative Medicine Therapies for Serious Conditions – Guidance for Industry. February 2019. https://www.fda.gov/regulatory-information/search-fda-guidance-documents/expedited-programs-regenerative-medicine-therapies-serious-conditions

Formal Meetings between the FDA and Sponsors or Applicants of PDUFA Products Guidance for Industry. December 2017. https://www.fda.gov/regulatory-information/search-fda-guidance-documents/formal-meetings-between-fda-and-sponsors-or-applicants-pdufa-products-guidance-industry

Human Gene Therapy for Rare Diseases. Guidance for Industry. January 2020.
https://www.fda.gov/regulatory-information/search-fda-guidance-documents/human-gene-therapy-rare-diseases

M3(R2) Nonclinical Safety Studies for the Conduct of Human Clinical Trials and Marketing Authorization for Pharmaceuticals. January 2010. https://www.fda.gov/regulatory-information/search-fda-guidance-documents/m3r2-nonclinical-safety-studies-conduct-human-clinical-trials-and-marketing-authorization

Preclinical Assessment of Investigational Cellular and Gene Therapy Products. Guidance for Industry. November 2013. https://www.fda.gov/regulatory-information/search-fda-guidance-documents/preclinical-assessment-investigational-cellular-and-gene-therapy-products

S7A Safety Pharmacology Studies for Human Pharmaceuticals. July 2001.
https://www.fda.gov/regulatory-information/search-fda-guidance-documents/s7a-safety-pharmacology-studies-human-pharmaceuticals

5

Global Regulatory Expectations and Interactions

Mary Ellen Cosenza
MEC Regulatory & Toxicology Consulting, LLC

CONTENTS

5.1 What Is a Biologic?

The Food and Drug Administration (FDA) and other regulatory agencies (Boards of Health) regulate products based on their intended use and modality. The FDA has one of the broadest mandates in that it regulates food, drugs, cosmetics, medical devices, and tobacco. For pharmaceuticals, there are differences based on indications/therapeutic area and on the type of product (traditional small molecules vs therapeutic proteins and monoclonal antibodies vs advanced therapies such as cell and gene therapies). How do you know if it is a "biologic"? This chapter will focus on those products that are classified as "biologics." In the USA, biologics are largely governed by the **Public Health Service Act (PHSA)**, not just the **Food, Drug, and Cosmetic Act (FDCA)**, with some exceptions. This difference is derived from their legislative and regulatory history (Korwek & Druckman, 2015). Biologics were first regulated via the Biologics Control Act of 1902, which focused on the "safety, purity, and potency of vaccines, serums, toxins, antitoxins, and similar products." This Act set the regulatory pathway for biologics and their manufacturing facilities and became recodified in 1944 as the PHSA. Biologics were regulated by different government services and agencies over the years and didn't move to the FDA from the National Institutes of Health (NIH) until 1972. The goal then was to apply both the PHSA and the FDCA (safe, effective, and not misbranded or adulterated) to the approval of biologics.

What medical products are now considered "biologics"? This category of products has grown tremendously in recent years. There are currently more than 250 biotechnology health care products and vaccines available commercially across the globe (www.bio.org). The PHSA states that "the term 'biologic product' means a virus, therapeutic serum, toxin, antitoxin, vaccine, blood, blood component or derivative, allergenic product, protein (except any chemically synthesized polypeptide), or analogous product, or arsphenamine or derivative of arsphenamine (or any other trivalent organic arsenic compound), applicable to the prevention, treatment or cure of a disease or condition of human beings" (42 United States Code 262(i)). They are medical products that can be made of sugars, proteins, or nucleic acids or complex combinations of these substances, or may be living entities such as cells and tissues. These would include cell and gene therapies, therapeutic viruses, and CAR T-cell and other cell therapies. Other common terms are biopharmaceuticals, biologics, and therapeutic proteins. It is clearly no longer just blood products and vaccines.

The primary difference between biopharmaceuticals and traditional pharmaceuticals is the method of manufacture and processing. Biologics are manufactured in living organisms such as bacteria, yeast, and mammalian cells, whereas traditional "small-molecule" drugs are manufactured through a series of chemical synthesis. [There is a gray area with chemically synthesized peptides.] Many biotechnology products are produced using recombinant DNA technology.

There are several subsets of biologics and this chapter will focus on the FDA designations, but it is worth mentioning some other jurisdictional definitions. The **International Council for Harmonisation (ICH)** first defined the term biologics in the ICH S6 guidance: Preclinical Safety Evaluation of Biotechnology-Derived Pharmaceuticals. In that guidance, biopharmaceuticals are defined as products derived from characterized cells including bacteria, yeast, insect, plant, and mammalian cells. Biopharmaceuticals include proteins, peptides, their derivatives, or products of which they are components. Examples include cytokines, proteins, growth factors, fusion proteins, enzymes, receptors, hormones, and monoclonal antibodies (International Council for Harmonisation, 1997).

The European Medicines Agency (**EMA**) generally follows the ICH definition of biologics, but it is worth noting that they have a **Committee for Advanced Therapies (CAT)**. This Committee is responsible for assessing the safety and efficacy of **advanced therapy medicinal products (ATMPs)**. These are defined as medicines for human use that are based on genes, cells, or tissue engineering (The European Parliament and The Council of the European Union, 2007).

Like drugs, some biologics are intended to treat diseases and medical conditions. Other biologics are used to prevent or diagnose diseases. Today, examples of biological products include the following: vaccines; blood and blood products for transfusion and/or manufacturing into other products; allergenic extracts, which are used for both diagnosis and treatment (e.g., allergy shots); human cells and tissues used for transplantation (e.g., tendons, ligaments, and bone); gene therapies; cellular therapies; and tests to screen potential blood donors for infectious agents such as HIV (U.S. Food and Drug Administration, 2017).

Evaluation and Research (**CBER**), and the **Center for Devices and Radiological Health (CDRH)**. "Biologics" may be regulated by CDER (e.g., therapeutic proteins and monoclonal antibodies), CBER (e.g., vaccines, blood products, and cell and gene therapies), or even CDRH (e.g., combination products).

Before 2003, most "biologics" were regulated by CBER and traditional pharmaceutical small molecules were regulated by CDER. The exceptions were hormones, oligonucleotides, and chemically synthesized peptides. In the early 2000s, there was a reorganization that led to the transfer of therapeutic proteins (**well-characterized proteins**), including monoclonal antibodies, to CDER. This move was designed to take advantage of the clinical disease-specific expertise in CDER as biopharmaceuticals became more prevalent and mainstream. CDER now regulates several categories of biological products including replacement proteins; monoclonal antibodies, including those modified by conjugation to small-molecule drugs (**antibody–drug conjugates or ADCs**) or parts of antibodies (Fc fusions); and cytokines, growth factors, enzymes such as thrombolytics, and immunomodulators (see Table 5.1). CBER is divided into offices based on modalities, for example, the Office of Blood Research and Review, the Office of Vaccines Research and Review, and the Office of Tissue and Advanced Therapies, which review cell and gene therapies. CDER is further divided into offices largely based on therapeutic areas (e.g., Office of Hematology and Oncology and the Office of Antimicrobial Products).

The licensing process for biologics still follows PHSA, even for products no longer regulated by CBER. Table 5.1 outlines the responsibilities of CBER and CDER with regard to biologics.

5.2 Which Center at the FDA Regulates Biologics? CBER or CDER?

In the USA, the FDA is divided into several offices (**Office of the Commissioner, Office of Foods and Veterinary Medicine, Office of Medical Products and Tobacco**), and then within each of these offices, there are centers. These centers focus on specific categories of products, for example, the **Center for Food Safety and Applied Nutrition (CFSAN)** or the **Center for Tobacco Products**. Medical products are divided into three main centers: the **Center for Drug Evaluation and Research (CDER)**, the **Center for Biologics**

5.3 What Is FDA's Role Regarding Biological Products?

FDA's regulatory authority for the approval of biologics resides in the PHSA and the Federal FDCA. CBER, under the FDCA's Medical Device Amendments of 1976, regulates some medical devices used to produce biologics. A combination of centers may be involved in the regulation of combination products, including CDRH. There is more discussion about combination products in Chapter 14 of this book.

Some of the direct responsibilities of FDA in regulating biologics include the review and approval of products for marketing;

TABLE 5.1

Regulation of Biotechnology Products

Products Regulated by CDER	Previously Regulated by CBER, Now by CDER	Products Regulated by CBER
Hormones	Proteins and modified proteins	Gene therapies
Chemically synthesized peptides	Cytokines	Cellular therapies
Oligonucleotides	Growth factors	Engineered tissue products
	Ligands and receptors	Vaccines
		Live biotherapeutics
	Antibodies	Blood and blood products
		Antitoxins
		Allergenics

inspections of manufacturing plants before product approval and on a regular basis thereafter; review and approval of new indications for already approved products; and monitoring the safety of biological products after they are marketed. As with drugs, the FDA also provides the public with information to promote the safe and appropriate use of biological products.

Specifics of the PHSA also give the FDA authority to approve biological products and immediately suspend licenses where there exists a danger to public health. It grants the FDA the power to procure products in the event of shortages and critical public health needs and to enforce regulations to prevent the introduction or spread of communicable diseases (U.S. Food and Drug Administration, 2009) (42 United States Code 262(i)).

Prior to 1997, biologics manufacturers had to file both a Product License Application (PLA) and an Establishment License Application (ELA) for approval to market their biologic product. In 1997, the Food and Drug Administration Modernization Act (FDAMA) attempted to harmonize the biologics and drug regulations. One change was consolidating the ELA and PLA into a single **Biologics License Application (BLA)**.

A BLA includes manufacturing information to demonstrate the company can properly and consistently manufacture the product and includes data and information regarding the biological product (animal and human studies). Data must demonstrate the product is safe and effective for its proposed use and can be manufactured consistently, meeting quality standards. The BLA also includes proposed labeling for uses for which it has been shown to be effective, possible risks, and how to use it. A BLA is very similar in approach to an NDA but generally includes more information on the manufacturing facility. As noted above, the PHSA authorized the issuance of a facilities license (dual licensing). This allows for rapid withdrawal of product from the market if a hazard arises.

5.4 How Do Biologics Differ from Conventional Drugs?

Most drugs consist of pure chemical substances, and their structures are known. Most biologics, however, are complex mixtures that are not easily identified or characterized (see Table 5.2). Biological products differ from conventional drugs in that they tend to be heat-sensitive and susceptible to

microbial contamination. This requires sterile processes to be applied from initial manufacturing steps. There are several preclinical parameters that differ as well. They can be immunogenic and are not metabolized, and their toxicity is often derived from their pharmacology.

5.4.1 Manufacturing, Quality, and Controls

Biologics are a category of medicinal products that includes a large variety of modalities. Some are clearly defined, such as blood product and vaccines, but others can be complex mixtures (cell therapies). Because biologics are derived from living matter, they can be variable in nature, and are often comprised of complex mixtures. They are not always easy to define or characterize and can be susceptible to contamination. Even replacement proteins such as erythropoietin and filgrastim (G-CSF) have been modified. Protein science groups have found ways to modify proteins through posttranslational modifications such as glycosylation and PEGylation or create new constructs such as Fc fusions and bispecifics. Because the products are derived from living organisms, their "manufacturing" is often extremely complex and requires additional controls. Many of the impurities are host proteins, nucleic acids, and viruses. The manufacturing must be conducted aseptically. An overarching theme often heard is that the "product is the process," which speaks to how small process changes can change the final product as well.

The unique characteristics of biologics contribute to the complication and challenges of manufacturing. In addition to the building blocks, amino acids and proteins have complex higher-order structures that are pivotal to the ensuring the correct activity of these molecules. There are a series of ICH guidelines (see Table 5.3) that address many of the specific **chemistry, manufacturing, and controls (CMC)** issues for biologics (International Council for Harmonisation, 1997). See Chapter 6 for more details.

These guidelines help address some of the unique biologic product challenges such as screening of starting materials; purification steps; virus removal steps; viral inactivation steps; and validation-viral clearance studies.

The PHSA emphasizes manufacturing control and adherence to processes. Novel biological products are on the cutting edge of medical science and research. New biologic constructs

TABLE 5.2

Differences between Biologics and Pharmaceuticals (Cosenza, 2010)

Parameter	Small-Molecule Pharmaceuticals	Biotechnology-Derived Pharmaceuticals
Size	<500 daltons	>1 kD (macromolecules)
Immunogenicity	Nonimmunogenic	Potential for immunogenicity
Metabolism	Metabolized	Degraded
Frequency of dosing	Daily	Variable
Toxicity	Often structure based	Exaggerated pharmacology
Half-life	Short	Long
Route of administration	Usually oral, some IV	Parenteral
Species specificity	Active in most species	Species specific
Synthesis	Organic chemistry (synthesized)	Genetic engineering (derived from living material)
Structure	Well defined	Often not fully characterized

TABLE 5.3

ICH Quality Documents for Biologics

Q5 A	Viral safety evaluation
Q5 B	Genetic stability (analysis of expression construct)
Q5 C	Product stability testing
Q5 D	Derivation and characterization of cell substrates
Q5 E	Comparability due to changes in manufacturing

often require new and novel manufacturing methods and quality control processes. Manufacturing processes for cell and tissue therapies, including autologous, allogeneic, or xenogeneic, often require close collaboration with regulatory agencies. Newer therapies, of genetically modified cells including CAR T cells and TCR T cells, need to develop their processes, specifications, and controls as these therapies are being developed.

Manufacturers of biologics must comply with the appropriate laws and regulations relevant to their biologics license and identifying any changes needed to help ensure product quality. All GMP regulations must be adhered to. Certain types of manufacturing and production problems must be reported to FDA's **Biological Product Deviation Reporting System (BPDR)**. There are established timeframes for reporting and corrective actions. There may be the need to recall or stop the manufacture of a product if a significant problem is detected.

5.4.2 Preclinical Development

The safety evaluation of biotechnology products has been an evolving process over the past three decades. **ICH S6 guideline (Preclinical Safety Evaluation of Biotechnology-Derived Pharmaceuticals)** is the principal ICH guideline to give guidance to preclinical scientists (in both industry and government) on how to approach preclinical development plans. In the future, the basic questions for these products will remain the same, but the challenges on how best to answer these questions may be greater as the molecules become more complicated. Global strategies for development of biopharmaceuticals are science driven and problem focused. If industry scientists want the reviewers at regulatory agencies to adhere to the scientific principles addressed in ICH S6, then the safety assessment industry scientist must be able to use science (e.g., target liability) to justify development plans as well. Not providing scientific justification is as imprudent as conducting traditional small-molecule pharmaceutical studies on biopharmaceuticals.

The overarching goal of any preclinical program is to evaluate the potential effects of these molecules and to provide guidance to inform the design of the clinical studies. Safety assessment approaches should have a strong scientific rationale and use the appropriate animal species judiciously. As with all pharmaceutical products, preclinical safety studies are expected to be conducted in compliance with **Good Laboratory Practices (GLPs),** and if there are deviations, they should be explained and justified. The product tested should be as comparable to the clinical product as possible (40 CFR 160 and 792, 1983).

There are specific preclinical challenges for developing biologics that differ from traditional small-molecule drugs. Some worthy of note here include **species selection, study design, route, and dose selection, and immunogenicity**. Many

of these topics were discussed in the original ICH S6 document of 1997 (International Council for Harmonisation, 1997) or later in the 2011S6 Addendum (International Council for Harmonisation, 2011).

5.4.3 Clinical Development

Over the past three decades, many biotechnology-derived products have been approved in the USA, Europe, Japan, and now globally. Innovations in molecular sciences have advanced research into a variety of therapeutics that target previously untapped ligands and receptors. These molecules and products hold the promise of treating unmet medical needs of patient with chronic and/or life-threatening diseases. The clinical development of these products is very similar to traditional small-molecule drugs and follows the same three study phases. Phase 1 focuses on safety and Phase 2 on efficacy and dose selection in patients, and then, Phase 3 trials are generally well-controlled trials in larger populations. ICH Efficacy guidelines (E1-E16) are generally all applicable, including those focused on compliance and **Good Clinical Practices (GCPs)** (International Council for Harmonisation, 2016).

There are a couple of unique aspects of biologics that can impact clinical development worth mentioning here. One is the difference in pharmacokinetics of these molecules. Many of these protein products, particularly monoclonal antibodies, have very long half-lives, sometimes days, weeks, or even months. This can change the study design and monitoring plans for early studies. It can also impact the populations selected (normal healthy volunteers vs. patients) for Phase 1 trials. Some molecules can cause rapid adverse reactions such as **infusion reaction** and **cytokine release phenomena**, yet others can lead to adverse effects that take time to manifest, due to the longer pharmacological actions (Haller, Cosenza, & Sullivan, 2008). Due to the highly targeted nature of the molecules, most adverse findings are due to exaggerated pharmacology. The most common off-target toxicity is **injection-site reactions** (Haller, Cosenza, & Sullivan, 2008).

Another unique concern with biologics is the formation of immunogenicity to the product itself. The more fully human a protein is, the less likely it is to be immunogenic, but there have been modifications in manufacturing and processing that have led to serious immunological consequences. Not all antibodies are clinically concerning. Some just bind without leading to serious effects. Others may lead to a more rapid clearing of the molecule, impacting the pharmacokinetics. The more serious antibodies are those that neutralize the effect of the product decreasing the intended efficacy of the biologic product. The most concerning are those antibodies that might cross-react with an endogenous protein as seen in clinical trials with megakaryocyte growth and development factor (MGDF) leading patients unable to generate platelets (Basser et al., 2002).

After the TeGenero incident (Horvath & Milton, 2009), the conduct of clinical trials with novel biologics has been modified to include slower dose escalation, sentinel dosing, and other safeguards to ensure such a disaster does not happen again. Safety reporting for biologics is also very important and is discussed more in the post-marketing section of this chapter.

5.5 The Regulatory Pathways

A sponsor who wishes to begin clinical trials with a biologic must submit an **Investigational New Drug application (IND)** to the appropriate division of the FDA. The IND describes the biologic, its method of manufacture, and quality control tests for release. Also included is information about the product's safety in animal testing, as well as the proposed clinical protocol for studies in humans. For vaccines, the ability to elicit a protective immune response in animals is also included.

Pre-marketing (pre-licensure) biologic or vaccine clinical trials are typically done in three phases, as is the case for any drug. Initial human studies, referred to as Phase 1, are safety and immunogenicity studies performed in a small number of closely monitored subjects. Phase 2 studies are dose-ranging studies and may enroll hundreds of subjects. Finally, Phase 3 trials typically enroll thousands of individuals and provide the critical documentation of effectiveness and important additional safety data required for licensing. At any stage of the clinical or animal studies, if data raise significant concerns about either safety or effectiveness, FDA may request additional information or studies, or may halt ongoing clinical studies.

5.5.1 Regulatory Agency Meetings

Robust and transparent meetings between sponsors and regulatory agencies are key to successful product development. In the USA, there are three categories of meetings (Types A, B, and C). Type A meetings are those that are meant to resolve urgent issues that are delaying FDA's product review. Type B meetings include most milestone meetings (e.g., pre-IND, EOP2, pre-BLA) and have Prescription Drug User Fee Act (PDUFA)-driven timelines associated with them. Type C meetings are any other product development meeting not covered by the other two categories. Both the CBER and CDER adhere to these categories, meeting processes and timelines. An important additional type of meeting that is available in CBER is the **IN**itial **T**argeted **E**ngagement for **R**egulatory **A**dvice on **CBER** Produc**T**s (INTERACT) meeting (U.S. FDA 2020).

The INTERACT meeting (formerly called a pre-pre-IND meeting) is available for novel cellular and gene therapy approaches, which are reviewed in CBER's **Office of Tissues and Advance Therapies (OTAT)**. This INTERACT discussion, focused primarily on manufacturing and preclinical issues, is not part of the IND meeting process, e.g., not a PDUFA (User Fee tracked). Because these products are so different than traditional drugs and biologics, OTAT strongly encourages early interaction with the Pharmacology/Toxicology staff. These programs are highly individualized, and OTAT is one of the groups that hold INTERACT. This advice is non-binding but can be extremely useful in planning the preclinical studies to support an IND. An INTERACT meeting does not replace the ability of a sponsor to request a pre-IND meeting with the FDA.

In Europe, Scientific Advice meetings can be held with individual national authorities. In addition, meetings can be held with the EMA to gain scientific advice and/or regulatory guidance. There are three EMA scientific committees that oversee the evaluation of products undergoing the centralized marketing authorization process: the Committee for Medicinal Products for Human Use (CHMP), the CAT, and the Pharmacovigilance Risk Assessment Committee (PRAC). The CAT oversees medicines based on genes, tissues, or cells. These meetings now take place at the EMA offices in Amsterdam.

5.5.2 Innovative and Expedited Pathways

All of the **expedited pathways** that apply to drugs are also applicable to biologics. These include **Fast Track**, **Accelerated Approval**, and **Breakthrough Therapy Designation**. Breakthrough Therapy Designation is one of the more recent of the expedited pathways that provides drug development sponsors more frequent interactions with FDA. This designation require sufficient clinical data to support. In addition, the FDA has recently developed a new designation: the **Regenerative Medicine Advanced Therapy (RMAT)** designation in 2017. Table 5.4 compares these designations. The RMAT designation was created as part of the 21st Century Cures Act. A drug is eligible for RMAT designation if:

- The drug is a regenerative medicine therapy, which is defined as a cell therapy, therapeutic tissue engineering product, human cell and tissue product, or any combination product using such therapies or products, except for those regulated solely under

TABLE 5.4

Comparison of RMAT and BT

	Breakthrough Therapy (BT) Designation	Regenerative Medicine Advanced Therapy (RMAT) Designation
Statute	Section 506(a) of the FDCA, as added by Section 902 of the Food and Drug Administration Safety and Innovation Act of 2012 (FDASIA)	Section 506(g) of the FDCA, as added by Section 3033 of the 21st Century Cures Act
Qualifying criteria	A drug that is intended to treat a serious condition, AND preliminary clinical evidence indicates that the drug may demonstrate substantial improvement on a clinically significant endpoint(s) over available therapies	A drug is a regenerative medicine therapy, AND the drug is intended to treat, modify, reverse, or cure a serious condition, AND preliminary clinical evidence indicates that the drug has the potential to address unmet medical needs for such disease or condition
Features	All fast track designation features, including actions to expedite development and review and rolling review Intensive guidance on efficient drug development, beginning as early as Phase 1 Organizational commitment involving senior FDA management	All Breakthrough Therapy Designation features including early interactions to discuss any potential surrogate or intermediate endpoints Statute addresses potential ways to support accelerated approval and satisfy post-approval requirements

Section 361 of PHSA and part 1271 of Title 21, Code of Federal Regulations;

- The drug is intended to treat, modify, reverse, or cure a serious or life-threatening disease or condition; and
- Preliminary clinical evidence indicates that the drug has the potential to address unmet medical needs for such disease or condition

Most of the products fall into the OTAT. The area of Regenerative Medicine is a rapidly expanding field that has the potential to treat serious conditions. CBER recognized the importance of these therapies and committed to helping ensure they are licensed by developing the RMAT designation. A draft guidance was issued in late 2017. This guidance is intended to facilitate development and review of regenerative medicine therapies intended to address unmet medical needs in those with serious conditions. It includes cell therapies, therapeutic tissue engineering products, human cell and tissue products, and combination products using any such therapies or products, with a few exceptions. It may also include genetically modified cells, that lead to a durable modification of cells or tissues that may meet the definition of a regenerative medicine therapy. **Combination products** may be eligible for RMAT designation if the regenerative medicine component provides the greatest contribution to the overall intended therapeutic effect.

Requests for both BT and RMAT can be submitted with the IND or after and ideally, no later than the end-of-Phase 2 meeting. The FDA is required to respond within 60 days after receipt of request. Both of these designations may be rescinded later in product development if the product no longer meets the designation-specific qualifying criteria (U.S. Food and Drug Administration, 2017).

With the outbreak of COVID-19 in early 2020 in the USA, the FDA created a new special emergency program for possible coronavirus therapies, the Coronavirus Treatment Acceleration Program (CTAP). The program uses every available method to move new treatments to patients as quickly as possible, while at the same time finding out whether they are helpful or harmful (https://www.fda.gov/drugs/coronavirus-covid-19-drugs/coronavirus-treatment-acceleration-program-ctap).

Other regulatory agencies have established expedited pathways as well. In Europe, the EMA established the **PRIority MEdicines (PRIME) regulatory scheme**, equivalent of the Breakthrough Therapy Designation in the USA. This scheme is designed to expedite and optimize the development of priority medicines (i.e., addressing unmet medical needs) in the **European Union (EU)**. The EMA PRIME appoints a CHMP's rapporteur who provides continuous support during the whole development. The PRIME takes advantage of the EMA-Scientific Advice (for early and enhanced dialogue) and Accelerated Assessment (for expedited MAA review). Similar to Breakthrough Therapy, PRIME is meant to help expedite the development of medicines of major public health interest, support therapeutic innovation, and target unmet medical needs (https://www.ema.europa.eu/en/human-regulatory/research-development/prime-priority-medicines).

In 2014, the MHLW of Japan established the SAKIGAKE (Ministry Project Team to Lead the World in the Practical Application of Innovative Medical Products). This designation program was developed to expedite the development of innovative medicines and medical devices that are developed first in Japan and offer "radical improvement" over existing therapies to treat critical diseases (https://www.mhlw.go.jp/english/policy/health-medical/pharmaceuticals/140729-01.html).

5.6 Submission and Review Process

To place a medicinal product, new drug, or biologic on the market in most countries, a company needs regulatory approval or marketing license. In the USA, this is done through the **NDA** or **BLA** process. In Europe, **Marketing Authorization (MA)** is either issued by the competent authority of country for its own territory (i.e., a national authorization) or can be granted for the entire Community (i.e., a community authorization).

5.6.1 United States

As discussed in previous sections of this chapter, the US FDA regulates biologics. The regulating center (**CBER or CDER**) will depend on the current classification of your biologic. The IND requirements (**21 CFR Part 312**) are all relevant, including format and content, financial disclosure, and clinical holds. The BLA process is similar to the NDA process discussed in Chapter 3 with the Establishment Licensing differences noted in previous sections of this chapter. In addition to the ICH guidelines already outlined, there are several FDA guidances and Points to Consider documents relevant to biologics that should be reviewed before embarking on the development of a new biologic. As many biologics are first-in-class, they may go to an **FDA Advisory Committee** for review and discussion during the BLA review process. The FDA publishes their review summaries for CDER here: https://www.accessdata.fda.gov/scripts/cder/daf/index.cfm

Similar information for cell and gene therapies can be found here: https://www.fda.gov/vaccines-blood-biologics/cellular-gene-therapy-products/approved-cellular-and-gene-therapy-products

5.6.2 Europe

The overarching regulatory agency in the EU is the EMA. In the EU, the **Centralized Procedure** is *mandatory* for biotechnological medicinal products derived from recombinant DNA technology, controlled gene expression, or monoclonal antibodies. It is also mandatory for orphan drug products and advanced therapies (e.g., gene and cell therapies) making this the route by which most "biologics" will be regulated. ATMPs have their own legislation found in Article 17 of Regulation (EC) No. 1394/2007. In addition to the mandated use of the Centralized Procedure for these products, they must also go through CAT for assessment.

A successful application under the Centralized Procedure delivers a single decision from the **European Commission (EC)** for marketing authorization valid throughout the EU. The current framework of legislation for this procedure is Regulation No. 726/2004. This regulation lays out the procedure for the authorization of medicinal products. The objective of the Centralized Procedure is to provide major innovative drug products with direct access to a community-wide market. Products approved through the Centralized Procedure have a common **Summary of Product Characteristics (SmPC, or SPC**; the EU equivalent of the US drug label) that must then be translated in all EU languages. Marketing authorizations are valid for 5 years and then must be renewed. European public assessment reports (EPARs) are searchable at the EMA website: https://www.ema.europa.eu/en/medicines/what-we-publish-when/european-public-assessment-reports-background-context

One area of particular concern in Europe for biotechnology products was the association of animal-derived products with **transmissible spongiform encephalopathy (TSE)**. Because of the seriousness of this disease as seen in bovine spongiform encephalopathy (BSE) and Creutzfeldt–Jakob disease (CJD), EU legislation required applicants to demonstrate that a medicinal product is manufactured in accordance with strict guidance (EMA/410/01 Rev3). The eventual goal is to replace ingredients of animal origin with vegetable-derived or synthetic materials.

The four principal parties involved in the Centralized Procedure review process include the company applying for the marketing authorization (MA), the EMA secretariat, the **CHMP**, and the **EC**. The EMA appoints a project team leader for each application, who is responsible for all communication and correspondence with the applicant. The CHMP appoints a rapporteur, and a co-rapporteur chosen from the CHMP members. The choice is based on the expertise required for the review of a certain therapeutic product area.

Release testing for products manufactured outside of the EU or **European Economic Area (EEA)** may also be required for every batch imported. It is therefore important to carefully consider the specifications selected for this testing. These tests can be more costly for biologics than for other products. For some biologics (e.g., vaccines), batch testing may be required even when produced within the EU or EEA.

5.6.3 Rest of the World (ROW)

Most countries now follow ICH guidelines for the development of biologics. Because many biologics, unlike traditional small-molecule pharmaceuticals, are single sourced, developing countries generally rely on the review and approval of these products in the major jurisdictions (the USA, EU, and Japan). They often require a **Certificate of Pharmaceutical Product (CPP)** from the exporting country's regulatory agency (e.g., FDA) before importing the product into their country. They may also require lot release or batch testing locally on imported biologics. Some countries require that local clinical trials be conducted as well. It is important to investigate the local regulations specific for biologics in all countries where a company plans on marketing their product.

5.7 Post-marketing Activities

There are several biologic-specific post-marketing activities worth mentioning. Many of these are related to the unique attributes of biologic manufacturing. They include lot releases; license revocation and suspension (related to Establishment licensure); recall orders (a provision of the PHSA for the recall of a specific batch lot or other quantity of a product; generally voluntary); and civil money penalties (rarely, if ever used). During the AIDS crisis, there were several court-ordered injunctions and consent decrees used against major US blood establishments.

In addition, the following activities are also worth noting:

- Post-approval **Manufacturing Change Supplements**: For some changes in biologics manufacturing, clinical data may be necessary due to the complexity of the process.
- **Establishment Inspections**: These are not specific to biologics, but because the manufacture is different, the FDA uses an approach called "Team Biologics" acknowledging the complexity of the manufacturing processes.
- **New indications**: New indications are filed as a supplemental BLA (sBLA). The regulations and processes for new indications and extensions are basically the same as for drugs.
- **New delivery devices**: Often as part of life-cycle management for therapeutic proteins or monoclonal antibodies, injection devices may be developed. For example, an injection pen to ease the self-injection process or reduce pain would be a combination product. The development of these types of products often involves multiple centers at the FDA.
- **Safety reporting**: For most biologics, this is similar to that for drugs, where adverse experience information must be reported on a timely basis depending on the seriousness and expectedness of the events. In addition, there are **Biological Product Deviation Reports (BPDRs)**. This reporting also applies to contract manufacturers, distributors, and other vendors in the production and distribution chain. This differs from drug manufacturing (field alert reporting). Of particular note is the **Vaccine Adverse Event Reporting System (VAERS)**, which the FDA and the Centers for Disease Control and Prevention (CDC) co-manage. This system covers those vaccines that are part of the **National Vaccine Injury Compensation Program (PHSA, tit. XXI, Subtitle 2)**. This system ensures that health care provides records and pertinent information for each vaccine administration.

5.8 Conclusions

Biologics and the biotechnology (now the biopharmaceutical) industry have grown tremendously. In the 1980s, there were very few INDs for these products per year. By 1990, there were over 200 open INDs, and now there are over 350 biologics in late-stage development. There are over 250 biotechnology health care products and vaccines available worldwide (Biotechnology Innovation Organization, 2017). Sales of biologics were estimated to be about $93 billion globally in 2009 (McCamish & Woollett, 2011). Biotechnology is now mainstream.

BIBLIOGRAPHY

42 United States Code 262(i). (n.d.). Regulation of Biological Products. *United States Code.*

Basser, R. L., O'Flaherty, E., Green, M., Edmonds, M., Nichols, J., Menchaca, D., . . . Begley, C. G. (2002). Development of pancytopenia with neutralizing antibodies to thrombopoietin after multicycle chemotherapy supported by megakaryocyte growth and development factor. *Blood, 99*(7), 2599–2602.

Biotechnology Innovation Organization. (2017). *What is Biotechnology.* Retrieved January 2, 2018, from Bio: https://www.bio.org/what-biotechnology

Cosenza, M. E. (2010). Safety assessment of biotechnology-derived therapeutics. In S. C. Gad (Ed.), *Pharaceutical Sciences Encyclopedia: Drug Discovery Development, and Manufacturing* (pp. 1–17). Hoboken, NJ: John Wiley & Sons, Inc.

Haller, C. A., Cosenza, M. E., & Sullivan, J. T. (2008, 08 13). Safety issues specific to clinical development of protein therapeutics. *Clinical Pharmacology & Therapeutics, 84*(5), 624–627.

Horvath, C., & Milton, M. (2009). The TeGenero incident and the duff report conclusions: A series of unfortunate events or an avoidable event? *Toxicologic Pathology, 37*, 372–383.

International Council for Harmonisation. (1995). *Q5B Analysis of the Expression Construct in Cells Used for Production of r-DNA Derived Protein Products.* International Council for Harmonisation.

International Council for Harmonisation. (1997). *Q5A: Viral Safety Evaluation of Biotechnology Products Derived from Cell Lines of Human or Animal Origins.* International Council for Harmonisation.

International Council for Harmonisation. (1997). *Q5D: Derivation and Characterization of Cell Substrates Used for Production of Biotechnological/Biological Products.* International Council for Harmonisation.

International Council for Harmonisation. (1997). *S6: Preclinical Safety Evaluation of Biotechnology-Derived Pharmaceuticals.* International Council for Harmonisation.

International Council for Harmonisation. (2004). *Q5E: Comparability of Biotechnological/Biological Products Subject to Changes in their Manufacturing Process.* International Council for Harmonisation.

International Council for Harmonisation. (2016). *Integrated Addendum to ICH E6(R1): Guideline for Good Clinical Practice E6(R2).* International Council on Harmonisation.

International Council for Harmonisation. (n.d.). *Q5C: Stability Testing of Biotechnological/Biological Products.* 1995: International Council for Harmonisation.

International Council for Harmonisation. (2011). *Preclinical Safety Evaluation of Biotechnology-derived Pharmaceuticals S6(R1).* International Council on Harmonisation.

Korwek, E. L., & Druckman, M. N. (2015). Human biologics. In D. G. Adams, R. M. Cooper, M. J. Hahn, and J. S. Kahan (Eds), *Food and Drug Law and Regulaton* (pp. 513–551). Washington, DC: FDLI.

McCamish, M., & Woollett, G. (2011, 03 01). Worldwide experience with biosimilar development. *mAbs, 3*(2), 209–217.

The European Parliament and The Council of the European Union. (2007, 11 13). Eur-Lex. *Regulation (EC) No. 1394/2007 of the European Parliament and of the Council of 13 November 2007 on Advanced Therapy Medicinal Products and Amending Directive 2001/83/EC and Regulation (EC) No. 726/2004.* Retrieved January 2, 2018, from Europa: http://eur-lex.europa.eu/legal-content/EN/ALL/?uri=CELEX%3A32007R1394

U.S. Food and Drug Administration. (2009, 09 15). *Public Health Service Act.* Retrieved January 2, 2018, from Regulatory Information: https://www.fda.gov/regulatoryinformation/lawsenforcedbyfda/ucm148717.htm

U.S. Food and Drug Administration. (2013, 06 14). *The Road to the Biologic Revolution – Highlights of 100 Years of Biologics Regulation.* Retrieved January 2, 2018, from About FDA: https://www.fda.gov/AboutFDA/WhatWeDo/History/CentennialofFDA/CentennialEditionofFDAConsumer/ucm096141.htm

U.S. Food and Drug Administration. (2017, 08 14). *CFR-Code of Federal Regulatons Title 21.* Retrieved January 2, 2018, from https://www.accessdata.fda.gov/scripts/cdrh/cfdocs/cfcfr/cfrsearch.cfm

U.S. Food and Drug Administration. (2017, 04 28). *Healthcare Providers (Biologics).* Retrieved January 2, 2018, from Vaccines, Blood & Biologics: https://www.fda.gov/BiologicsBloodVaccines/ResourcesforYou/HealthcareProviders/default.htm

U.S. Food and Drug Administration. (2017, 08 17). *Part 58: Good Laboratory Practice for Nonclinical Laboratory Studies.* Retrieved from CFR-Code of Federal Regulations Title 21: https://www.accessdata.fda.gov/scripts/cdrh/cfdocs/cfcfr/CFRSearch.cfm?CFRPart=58

U.S. Food and Drug Administration. (2017, 11 16). *Regenerative Medicine Advanced Therapy Designation.* Retrieved January 2, 2018, from Vaccines, Bood & Biologics: https://www.fda.gov/biologicsbloodvaccines/cellulargenetherapy-products/ucm537670.htm

U.S. Food and Drug Administration. (2020). *Interact Meetings.* https://www.fda.gov/vaccines-blood-biologics/industry-biologics/interact-meetings

Yang, L. (2013). Biologics submission. In *Fundamentals of US Regulatory Affairs* (pp. 273–298). Rockville, MD: Regulatory Affairs Professionals Society.

Part II

Practices

6

Key Considerations in the Chemistry, Manufacturing, and Controls of Biopharmaceuticals

Sara McKenzie and Ed Branson
PharmaDirections, Inc.

CONTENTS

6.1 Introduction

Regulatory approvals throughout the world are based on a risk-benefit assessment of the new therapeutic agent under review, and the basis for this assessment is very different for small molecule drugs and biopharmaceuticals. In the realm of chemistry, manufacturing and controls (CMC), methods of production differ greatly between small molecules and biopharmaceuticals and between various families of biopharmaceuticals. Multiple criteria for quality (and hence safety) are applied and highly dependent on the nature of the manufacturing process as well as the nature of the therapeutic agent.

This chapter describes the key considerations for different classes of biopharmaceutical products, with a focus on those that are manufactured using biotechnology processes, as opposed to those derived from tissues, blood, or blood products. The classes that are covered include proteins and large peptides; therapeutic live cells; and oligonucleotides. The manufacturing platforms include chemical synthesis (e.g., proteins or oligonucleotides chemically prepared from individual amino acids or nucleic acids); bacterial production systems (e.g., genetically engineered *E. coli*); whole cell (mammalian) production systems (e.g., genetically engineered Chinese hamster ovary [CHO] cells); and preparation of live cells for use in gene therapy or vaccines. Several other existing manufacturing platforms, such

DOI: 10.1201/9781003124542-8

as transgenic plants and animals, plant cell culture, insect cell culture, and avian eggs, are not discussed in this chapter but fall under the requirements for biopharmaceutical manufacturing discussed in the following sections. This chapter begins with a high-level description of the types of manufacturing platforms used for biopharmaceuticals. We then compare and contrast manufacturing and analytical methods applicable to all manufacturing platforms and include the key considerations to be taken into account when selecting a manufacturing process for a new biopharmaceutical. The chapter closes with a summary of useful regulatory guidance documents.

6.2 Manufacturing Systems Used for Biopharmaceuticals

6.2.1 Chemical Synthesis

Biopharmaceuticals such as peptide hormones or oligonucleotide-based drugs are made by chemical synthesis using well-defined chemical reactions such as solid-state peptide synthesis[1] or solid-state oligonucleotide synthesis.[2] These methods are used for smaller molecular weight compounds such as small interfering ribonucleic acids (siRNAs) and small peptides (Table 6.1). The time to manufacture these

compounds using automated equipment is relatively short compared with that using biological manufacturing systems. The purification processes are less complex, and there are no issues with viruses, host cell proteins, residual deoxyribonucleic acid (DNA), or removal of complex media components.

6.2.2 Mammalian Production Systems

Mammalian production platforms typically use a well-characterized cell line that has a copy or multiple copies of the DNA coding for the protein of interest. One of the most widely used cell lines is the CHO line. Mammalian-based systems are used for complex proteins that require post-translational modification such as the addition of specific carbohydrates to the protein chain(s). An example is the monoclonal antibody drug, HUMIRA®[3]. Challenges with mammalian systems include the cost of production, viral removal and inactivation and downstream processing due to the complexity of the media components, host cell protein removal, and endotoxin control. Mammalian systems are scalable with 15,000-liter bioreactors available for large volume biopharmaceuticals.[4]

In general, a biopharmaceutical is made in a complex series of steps, and the primary intermediate is contained in a mixture of related substances, reagents, and media components. This is

TABLE 6.1

Example: Manufacturing Process Flow for Chemical Synthesis

Step	Method	Purpose
Couple linker[a] to insoluble substrate (typically a resin)	This method depends on linker and resin	Provide a solid substrate on which the peptide will be synthesized
Remove protecting N^0 group	Chemical cleavage	To prepare resin and linker for coupling of amino acids
Wash	Solvent washing	Remove cleaved blocking group and other chemicals prior to next round of coupling
Couple protected amino acid to substrate(resin)	Chemical reaction	Addition of next amino acid in the protein/peptide sequence
Wash	Solvent washing	Remove unreacted blocked amino acids and coupling reagents
Remove protecting N^{0b} group	Chemical cleavage	To prepare for additional of next amino acid in protein/peptide sequence
Wash	Solvent washing	Remove cleaved blocking group and other chemicals prior to next round of coupling
Couple protected amino acid to substrate(resin)	Chemical reaction	Addition of next amino acid in the protein/peptide sequence
Repeat coupling, washing, and cleavage steps		To complete synthesis of protein/peptide
Final cleavage	Chemical reaction	To cleave protein/peptide from linker and resin and remove all amino acid protecting groups
Drying	Vacuum evaporation	To remove cleaving reagents
Washing	Solvent washing	To remove residual reagents
Solubilization and filtration	Aqueous acid solubilization of protein/peptide	To separate protein/peptide from resin
Drying	Lyophilization	To remove water from the purification process
Purification	Preparative high performance liquid chromatography (HPLC)	To remove residual reagents and chemicals from synthesized protein/peptide
Bulk API/drug substance	Packaging	Storage of the API until processed for further use

[a] Linkers are bifunctional molecules anchoring the growing peptide to the insoluble carrier.

[b] There are two classes of protecting groups—the N^0 group that protects the terminal amino group to which additional amino acids will be added and the side chain protecting groups that protect the various amino acid side chains from being modified during the synthesis process and are removed during the final cleavage step.

the upstream manufacturing process, and a complex mixture results whether it is chemically synthesized or produced by a live cell culture. Once sufficient material has been generated, downstream processing will purify the desired compound. Not surprisingly, the manufacturing processes and the in-process controls are quite different between the upstream and downstream stages of the manufacturing process.

An example process flow for a mammalian cell–based system in which the biopharmaceutical of interest is secreted is shown below in Table 6.2. Be aware that in some manufacturing companies, the harvest and recovery are considered part of the upstream process, whereas in other companies, harvest and recovery are considered downstream steps. Either approach is acceptable; it is simply a matter of how the contract manufacturing organization (CMO) has chosen to organize.

6.2.3 Microbial Production Systems

Microbial production systems commonly use *Escherichia coli* (*E. coli*)–based production platforms; however, other bacterial strains can also be used.

Common yeast strains used in the production of recombinant proteins are *Pichia pastoris* and *Saccharomyces cerevisiae*, but other strains are available.[5]

Microbial systems are scalable to 10,000 liters and have inexpensive media costs. They are easy to modify genetically, and their growth characteristics are straightforward and easy to optimize. They are used for less complex proteins such as alpha interferon and insulin that do not require extensive post-translational modifications for their bioactivity.

Microbial manufacturing platforms do not introduce concerns of viral contamination, which can be a significant benefit.

An example process flow for a microbial-based system is shown in Table 6.3. This process is based on *E. coli* that produces the protein of interest in inclusion bodies. In this system, the synthesized proteins go through a solubilization and refolding process whereas the mammalian CHO system noted above secretes the protein into the production medium. There are microbial systems that secrete proteins as well and do not require a refold step; *Pichia pastoris* (yeast) is one type of platform that secretes the engineered protein.

6.2.4 Live Cell Production

Cellular therapies involve the culture of cells, usually from humans, for therapeutic administration. Gene therapies involve the use of genetic vectors to genetically transform cells -either *ex vivo* gene therapy where cells are transformed, cultured, and administered to patients (the current predominant approach) or *in vivo* gene therapy, where the genetic vectors are administered directly into the patients. Cell/gene therapies may be classed based on their source/methods of manufacturing, with autologous therapies involving the administration of the patients' own cultured cells and allogenic therapies involving the administration of the same cells to multiple patients with their manufacture involving batches/lots larger than one patient unit.[6]

The Food and Drug Administration (FDA) provides the definition of cellular therapies as follows:

TABLE 6.2

Example: Manufacturing Process Flow for Cell Culture–Based Process

Step	Method	Purpose
Upstream Processing		
Process initiation	Cell bank thaw and flask/spinner inoculation	Inoculum prep for scale-up
Inoculum expansion	Cell passage into large flasks/spinners	Inoculum expansion
Bioreactor inoculation	Sterile transfer to the bioreactor	Start of scale-up
Biomass expansion	Nutrient feed	Generate suitable biomass for secretion of the product
Harvest	Centrifugation/filtration/tangential flow filtration (TFF)	Removal of cells from culture media
Downstream Processing[a]		
Product capture	Column chromatography[b]	Remove the API from culture media, the initial step in purification and product concentration
Purification step 1	Column chromatography[b]	Removal of impurities generated during the cell culture process
Purification step 2	Column chromatography[b]	Removal of impurities—endotoxins, fragmented product
Purification step 3	Column chromatography[b]	Removal of impurities—host cell proteins, DNA
Viral inactivation, removal[c]	• Inactivation by heat, chemicals, solvent detergents • Removal by nanofiltration	Removal/inactivation of viruses found in cell lines used for production or from external sources
Product concentration	Ultrafiltration/diafiltration	Concentrate purified API to desired range and add excipients and buffers
Bulk API filtration	Sterile filtration	Reduce potential bioburden of bulk for long-term storage
Bulk API storage	Low temperature storage $-20°C$ to $-80°C$.	Store bulk API under stable conditions until processed into a drug product

[a] Not all steps will be required for every manufacturing process.

[b] Not all chromatography steps require columns, as there are filter membranes with active ion exchange groups that perform the same function as traditional chromatography resins.

[c] Viral inactivation and removal are typically performed as two separate steps in downstream processing.

TABLE 6.3

Example: Manufacturing Process Flow for a Microbial-Based Process

Step	Method	Purpose
Upstream Processing		
Process initiation	Seed bank thaw and shake flask inoculation	Inoculum prep for scale-up
Inoculum expansion	Strain passage into large shake flasks or small fermenters	Inoculum expansion
Fermenter inoculation	Sterile transfer into the production fermenter	Start of biomass expansion
Biomass expansion	Nutrient feed	Generate initial biomass
Strain induction	Temperature drop and addition of induction agent	Production of inclusion bodies
Harvest	Centrifugation	Biomass collection
Downstream Processing		
Homogenization	High pressure shear	To rupture cells to release the inclusion bodies
Inclusion body isolation	Centrifugation	To separate inclusion bodies from rest of the biomass
Refold	Solubilization and diafiltration	To allow protein to refold into its bioactive conformation
Clarification	Depth filtration	To remove particulate matter in preparation for chromatography
Capture step	Column Chromatography	To capture the product of interest from refold process, removes bulk of impurities
Purification step 1	Column Chromatography	To remove additional impurities, endotoxins, residual DNA
Purification step 2[a]	Column Chromatography	To remove additional impurities, sometimes referred to as polishing
Drug substance concentration and buffer exchange	Ultrafiltration and diafiltration	Concentrate purified APIs to a desired range and add excipients and buffers
Bulk drug substance filtration	Sterile filtration	To reduce bioburden
Bulk drug substance storage	Filling into bulk containers and low temperature storage	Store bulk APIs under stable conditions until processed into a drug product

[a] Additional purification steps may be necessary for some proteins.

Somatic cell therapy is the administration to humans of autologous, allogeneic, or xenogeneic living cells which have been manipulated or processed *ex vivo*. Manufacture of products for somatic cell therapy involves the *ex vivo* propagation, expansion, selection … or pharmacologic treatment of cells, or other alteration of their biological characteristics. Such cellular products might also be used for diagnostic or preventive purposes.[7]

Process flows for live cell therapies will vary depending on the type of therapy, but in general, they may include various steps depending on the type of cells being manufactured and the source of the starting material. The process flow for cells isolated from a tissue sample taken from a donor is shown in Table 6.4. A list of approved cellular products and brief description of the manufacturing process are shown in Table 6.5.

6.3 General Manufacturing Considerations

Not infrequently, the CMC activities required for an original Investigational New Drug (IND) submission for a biopharmaceutical are on the critical path. But with careful planning and allotment of sufficient time for manufacturing process

development of unique therapeutics, clinical trial materials can be generated in parallel with other IND-enabling activities.

There are key considerations for any type of biopharmaceuticals made with any type of manufacturing platforms. They are described in broad terms below. Topics that are specific to each type of manufacturing systems are individually summarized following the discussion of the general manufacturing considerations.

6.3.1 "Fit for Purpose" Active Pharmaceutical Ingredient and Drug Product

In early stages of development, it is desirable to minimize investment of time and money prior to understanding whether the drug candidate has a reasonable safety profile in humans. Thus, quantities of active pharmaceutical ingredients (APIs) are often produced for testing in animals and for formulation development, without making a large investment in manufacturing process development. The API should be "clean enough" to be a representative of the drug that will eventually be used in the clinic, but it does not have to be made under current good manufacturing practice (cGMP) conditions or meet tight specifications. In fact, there is a school of thought that it is desirable to use an API in nonclinical toxicology studies that is somewhat "dirtier" than the clinical batches. This approach

TABLE 6.4

Example: Manufacturing Process Flow for Live Cells[a]

Step	Method	Purpose
Tissue or cell collection	Depending on the tissue/cell type: leukapheresis, surgery, biopsy	Provide starting material for manufacturing process
Tissue sample is cleaned of extraneous material	Extraneous material can be removed using physical manipulation, scalpel, scissors, etc.	Prep tissue sample for isolation of desired cells
The clean tissue sample is reduced to smaller pieces	Mechanical grinding	To increase the surface area for enzymatic digestion
Enzymatic digestion of the tissue	Use proteases, collagenases, and lipases to digest the tissue	Release cells from the tissue matrix
Termination of enzymatic digestion	Addition of protease inhibitors or other quenching agents	To stop further digestion of cells
Removal of cell debris	Filtration, centrifugation	Isolate desired cells from the digested tissue
Expansion of isolated cells[b]	Cell culture	Increase the mass of available cells for therapy
Harvest cells	Standard cell culture methods	Collect cells for storage or use
Cell preservation[b]	Cryopreservation	Storage until use

[a] This describes a generic process for manufacturing/collecting cells from a single donor and returning them to the original donor.
[b] This step may not be needed if cells are used immediately after the harvest step of cell culture.

TABLE 6.5

FDA-Approved CGT Products

Brand Name (Product)	Manufacturer	Manufacturing Platform	Description
ALLOCORD® (Hematopoietic progenitor cell (HPC) Cord Blood[a])	SSM Cardinal Glennon Children's Medical Center	Blood fractionation	Blood recovered from the umbilical cord and placenta is volume reduced and partially depleted of red blood cells and plasma using a closed system involving gravity settling and centrifugation. After collection, the cells are cryopreserved and stored until needed
GINTUIT® (allogeneic cultured keratinocytes and fibroblasts in bovine collagen)	Organogenesis Inc.	Live cell production	Autologous human fibroblasts and keratinocytes are cultured on a bovine collagen matrix
IMLYGIC® (talimogene laherparepvec)	BioVex, Inc., a subsidiary of Amgen Inc.	Mammalian cell culture	A herpes simplex virus (cold sore virus) grown in a mammalian cell line (HeLa, Vero) using standard cell culture methods.[8] The virus is very contagious, and Biosafety Level -2 (BSL-2) containment is required
KYMRIAH® (tisagenlecleucel)	Novartis Pharmaceuticals Corp	Live cell production	A patient's T-cells are isolated and genetically modified with a virus to express a cluster of differentiation protein (CD-19) (a transmembrane protein) immunoreceptor. The T-cells are expanded using mammalian cell culture processes. Classified as a gene therapy, chimeric antigen receptor – T cell (CAR-T)
LAVIV® (Azficel-T)	Fibrocell Technologies	Live cell production	Patient-specific fibroblasts are grown from a patient's skin biopsy using mammalian cell culture processes and are harvested and injected into the patient
LUXTURNA® (voretigene neparvovec-rzyl)	Spark Therapeutics, Inc.	Mammalian cell culture	Adeno viruses are modified with the gene of interest and infused into a patient where the virus vector delivers the missing gene to the target cell. A variation of gene therapy
MACI® (autologous cultured chondrocytes on porcine collagen membrane)	Vericel Corp.	Live cell production	Chondrocytes harvested from a patient's own cartilage are cultured on a porcine collagen membrane using mammalian cell culture process. The collagen membrane covered with the patient's chondrocytes is used to repair damaged knee cartilage
PROVENGE® (sipuleucel-T)	Dendreon Corp.	Live cell production	Patient's immune cells (antigen presenting cells) are collected by leukapheresis (centrifugation), modified with a prostate cancer antigen and infused back into the patient as a vaccine targeting cancer cells. A variation of gene therapy

(Continued)

TABLE 6.5 (*Continued*)

FDA-Approved CGT Products

Brand Name (Product)	Manufacturer	Manufacturing Platform	Description
YESCARTA® (axicabtagene ciloleucel)	Kite Pharma, Inc.	Live cell production	Patients' T-cells are collected by leukapheresis and activated. The chimeric antigen receptor (CAR) gene is inserted into the activated T-cells and the T-cells are expanded by mammalian cell culture processes and infused back into the patient. A variation of gene therapy
ZOLGENSMA® (onasemnogene abeparvovec-xioi)	AveXis, Inc.	Viral vector production in live cells	A normal copy of the SMN1 gene is transfected in vitro into a genetically engineered virus capsid, adeno-associated viral vector (AAV9). Upon intravenous administration to patients, the viral vector delivers the SMN1 transgene to affected motor neurons, leading to an increase in the survival motor neuron (SMN) protein

[a] Additional approved products for HPC Cord Blood include Clevecord, Ducord, Hemacord, and HPC Cord Blood from Clinimmune Labs, MD Anderson Cord Blood Bank, Lifesouth Community Blood Centers, and Bloodworks.

For the most current listing of FDA-approved cellular therapies, see this listing:

https://www.fda.gov/vaccines-blood-biologics/cellular-gene-therapy-products/approved-cellular-and-gene-therapy-products.

automatically qualifies the safety of the impurities at higher levels than are intended for use in the clinical batches and can be a useful approach to take while additional information is gathered regarding long-term stability of the API.

A common practice for supply of a test article for pivotal toxicology and safety pharmacology studies is to utilize the demonstration (or engineering) batch of drug substance which is generally produced as the last step prior to actual good manufacturing practice (GMP) manufacturing. Hence, this test article is "fit for purpose" and meets the immediate needs of the stage of development, without imposing unnecessary cost and requirements for purity or manufacturing process and scale.

6.3.2 Manufacturing API and Drug Product in a Continuous Process

In the manufacture of small molecule drugs, an API is often made in a facility or CMO that specializes in organic chemistry and related purification and analytical methods. It is made and stored in bulk until such time as it is shipped for the manufacture of the final drug product. A drug product is made in facilities that specialize in the production of tablets, capsules, or parenteral drugs. Thus, the skill sets required for successful API and drug product manufacture are quite different.

In the case of biologics, the final drug product often consists of APIs in a single-use vial, manufactured in a continuous process. It may not be practical to hold bulk APIs for any period of time (e.g., large volumes of dilute solutions of proteins or peptides; live cells used for vaccines), and the API is immediately converted into a drug product. An additional requirement if the API is held for further processing is the implementation of a stability program to demonstrate that the API meets all of its release criteria for the duration of the storage time. This can add cost and time to a development program but may be necessary if the CMO chosen to manufacture the API does not have the capability to manufacture the drug product. There are no real downsides to this approach; it is simply something to be aware of.

When writing the CMC section of the original IND, all data can be included in the API section, with the drug product section making reference to the pertinent sections for the API. This might be true, for example, for the release tests and specifications.

6.3.3 In-Process Controls

For the upstream part of a cell culture–based manufacturing process, the critical in-process control parameters will include temperature, pH, agitation rate, dissolved oxygen, sterility, cell density, cell viability, and product titer. At the end of the cell culture part of the manufacturing process, microbial purity and genetic stability may also be critical parameters to monitor.

The downstream part of the manufacturing process typically has numerous steps that will have some common parameters, such as product titer and product purity, that will be measured but may have different requirements for pH, ionic strength, flow rates, and temperature. One common requirement for all cGMP processes is the requirement for step yield and overall process yield.

6.3.4 Cell Banking for Live Cell–Based Manufacturing

Regardless of the type of the parent cell that might be used for manufacturing, long-term production can only be guaranteed by the creation of cell banks. A research cell bank should initially be created during the development phase of a program. Once a particular cell line or strain is selected for further development, the master cell bank (MCB) and working cell bank (WCB) should each be generated.

The MCB is created first to establish a long-term source of identical, original cells that are highly characterized. A quantity of original cells is cultured and fully characterized as regards stability of the transfected construct, genotypic and phenotypic characteristics, and purity as well as freedom from undesirable adventitious agents. These cells are cryopreserved and serve as the source of all future batches of the desired biopharmaceutical.

From the MCB, the WCB is created to provide the seed stock for each manufacturing run. One or more frozen vials of the MCB are cultured and again analyzed for production of the desired therapeutic agent and genetic characteristics as previously done for the MCB. The resulting WCB is also cryopreserved. Each time a manufacturing run is conducted, one or more vials of the WCB are thawed and cultured as the initial step of the manufacturing process. Once the WCB is depleted, vials of cells from the MCB are thawed and cultured to establish a new WCB.

6.3.5 Adventitious Agents

"Adventitious agents are a class of living contaminants of the exogenous origin that may get introduced during production of biotherapeutic products. These include viruses, bacteria, fungi, mycoplasma, transmissible spongiform encephalopathies (TSEs), and other such entities, many of which can propagate to high titers."[9]

Even prior to transfer of the cells to a CMO, the cell line used for production of the therapeutic agent must be demonstrated to be free of contaminating viruses, bacteria, and fungi and phage for bacterial-based systems. Monitoring and testing are required throughout manufacturing process development and cGMP manufacturing to assure that no such agents are introduced into the cell culture system.

New adventitious agents are being continually discovered and add to the complexity of biologics manufacturing. TSE and BSE are examples of such agents; they are the agents which were discovered to lead to "mad cow" disease. It is important to have certification that any bovine-derived products (such as fetal bovine serum [FBS] used in the tissue culture) are free of TSE and bovine spongiform encephalopathies (BSE).

6.3.6 Genetic Stability of Cell-Based Manufacturing Systems

Whether production is conducted using mammalian, bacterial, yeast, or insect cell systems, the genetic material for the therapeutic agent must be stably transfected into the parent cell line. The stability of this transfection must be supported by data from both the MCBs and WCBs, as noted above, and throughout the production cycle. Genetic stability is typically monitored throughout the upstream process with a final determination on the end-of-production cells to demonstrate that there is a consistent level of stability during manufacturing. These stability indicators are an intact gene of interest, a consistent copy number from beginning to end, and comparable expression levels throughout the production. A diploid cell strain should remain diploid throughout. If such characteristics are not stable, then it must be demonstrated that the instability does not adversely impact manufacturing, product consistency, or quality of the final biotherapeutic.

For mammalian-based production systems, the genetic stability at the end of the upstream culture stage can vary so long as it is consistent from run to run. Some microbial systems have a two-stage upstream process which in the first stage is the accumulation of biomass. In the second stage of the upstream process, the biomass is "turned on" or induced to make the molecule of interest. This induction process can involve a change in media composition, pH, and temperature and the addition of an inducting agent. During this second stage, the induction process can create a loss of genetic stability due to the rapid synthesis of the biological molecule of interest. An example is the use of *E. coli* during which the biomass is rapidly expanded using a medium rich in carbon (such as glucose or glycerol). After the desired level of biomass is reached, the temperature is reduced (generally from 37°C to 26°C), the glucose feed is increased, and the inducting agent, for example, isopropyl-β-D thiogalactopyranoside, is added. At the end of the induction period, the genetic purity of the *E. coli* can be less than 30%.

For methods to assess a cell substrate's genetic stability, a reference is made to the International Conference on Harmonization (ICH) Q5B and Q5D documents.[10]

6.3.7 Product Characterization

6.3.7.1 Analytical Methods

All manufacturing processes require testing and analysis of the manufacturing process, final product (both the API and drug product), and ongoing stability. There are numerous standard methods available from the *United States Pharmacopeia* (USP), such as pH, protein content, water content, and sterility, but in many cases, product-specific assays must be developed. The primary assays required for biologics include identity, purity, safety, potency (biological activity), and quality. Of all the assays required to characterize and release the API (drug substance), the potency assays typically are the most challenging to develop and qualify. Some potency assays are product specific and require the creation of product-specific cell lines that must go through the same process of generating MCBs and WCBs (see below, Section 6.3.7.4.). Furthermore, there may be multiple assays in each category. Table 6.6 lists some common methods currently used, but other methods may be suitable depending on the biopharmaceutical.

The development of analytical methods will be stage-appropriate with qualified methods used during development, preclinical lots, and engineering runs, transitioning to fully validated methods by the time the commercial manufacturing process is in place.

6.3.7.2 Related Impurities

During the manufacturing and/or storage of certain biopharmaceuticals, a number of related impurities may be generated and include some of the following types: degraded forms (fragments), aggregated forms, subunits, misfolded proteins, and incompletely synthesized forms (truncates) of the drug substance.[11] Additional impurities may include deamidated, oxidized, phosphorylated, sulfated, or N-terminally cyclized forms of a protein drug product.[12] During the downstream purification process, these related impurities may be reduced in concentration or removed entirely. These remaining product related impurities that are not removed during processing must be identified and characterized to ensure they do not impact the safety, efficacy, or potency of the desired drug substance.[13]

TABLE 6.6

Analytical Methods for Cell and Microbial Based Manufacturing Systems

Attribute	Common Methods	Purpose
Identity	ELISA, HPLC, SDS-PAGE, amino acid/oligo sequence, amino acid/oligo analysis, peptide map	Prove the product is what it claims to be
Purity	ELISA, HPLC, SDS-PAGE, amino acid/oligo sequence, amino acid /oligo analysis, peptide map, GC-MS	Demonstrate that the product has a predetermined chemical purity free from reagents and processing aids and is free of solvents and antibiotics
Potency	Ligand binding, enzymatic assays, cell-based assays, animal-based assays	Demonstrate the product has the desired biological activity
Safety	• Sterility (e.g., USP <71>) • Endotoxin (e.g., USP<85> LAL) • Viral safety (virus-specific assays required)	• Demonstrate the product is sterile and free of microbiological contaminants • Demonstrate the product has an acceptable level of endotoxins per patient dose • Demonstrate the product is free from potential contaminating viruses
Quality	• DNA (by PCR or qPCR) • Host cell protein (by ELISA or western blot)	• Demonstrate an acceptable level of DNA • Demonstrate an acceptable level of host cell protein

ELISA, enzyme linked immunosorbent assay; SDS-PAGE, sodium dodecyl sulphate polyacrylamide gel electrophoresis; GC-MS, gas chromatography-mass spectrometry; PCR, polymerase chain reaction; LAL, limulus amebocyte lysate.

6.3.7.3 Endotoxin

Bacterial endotoxins are lipopolysaccharide complexes associated with the outer cell wall of gram-negative bacteria. They elicit a variety of inflammatory responses in animals, including humans, and thus, quantities must be controlled in drugs that are intended for injection.

Validation of the bacterial endotoxins test must be conducted for each drug formulation to assure that the formulation does not interfere with the assay by providing either a false positive or false negative result. It is not uncommon for a formulation to require dilution in order to avoid any such assay interference.

The appropriate method for establishing the endotoxin limit for a specific biologic is to use the calculation methods described in the USP monograph <85>. The acceptable level of endotoxin is determined by the formula K/M, where K is the threshold pyrogen dose for humans, and M is the maximum human dose per kilogram body weight. If the product is injected at frequent intervals or infused continuously, M is the maximum dose administered in a single hour period. The value of K is set at 5.0 EU/kg for parenteral injection and 0.2 EU/kg for intrathecal injection. The value of M depends on the individual product.

6.3.7.4 Potency Assays

One of the more critical and often challenging aspects of the analytical process supporting the development of biopharmaceuticals is the identification and development of potency assays. These assays demonstrate that the drug product elicits the intended biological effect. The methods used for the measurement of biological activity during manufacturing and product release are typically biological in nature and range from *in vitro* enzymatic assays to *in vivo* animal assays. By way of example, a list of such assays for already approved biopharmaceuticals is shown in Table 6.7.

Additional guidance on the development of biological assays can be found in the USP with general principals in Chapter <111>, "Design and Analysis of Biological Assays." The FDA guidance "Potency Tests for Cellular and Gene Therapy Products" (January 2011) also contains important information.

6.3.7.5 Characterization Requirements

The regulatory requirements for the type of characterization of a biopharmaceutical depend primarily on the manufacturing platform used. A comparison of these requirements for different classes of biopharmaceutical products is provided below in Table 6.8.

TABLE 6.7

Examples of Potency Assays in Use for Approved Biopharmaceuticals

Biopharmaceutical	Drug Product	Analytical Method
RECOMBINATE™	Recombinant factor VIII	• One-stage clotting assay • Chromogenic substrate
HUMULIN®	Recombinant insulin	• Rabbit glucose test • Embryonic fibroblasts 3T3 L1 cells
ALTEPLASE®	Tissue plasminogen activator (tPA)	• Clot lysis • Chromogenic substrate
HUMIRA®	Anti-TNF monoclonal antibody	• Cell viability of L929 cells via neutralization of TNF by HUMIRA®
EPOGEN®	Erythropoietin	• Reticulocyte production in normocythemic mice

TABLE 6.8

Comparison of Characterization Requirements for Classes of Biopharmaceuticals

Attribute	Characterization Method	Chemical Peptide Synthesis	Chemical Oligo Synthesis	Microbial (*E. coli*)	Yeast (*Pichia pastoris*)	Mammalian (CHO Cells)
Identity	ELISA	X		X	X	X
	HPLC	X	X	X	X	X
	SDS-PAGE	X		X	X	X
	Amino acid/oligo sequence	X	X			
	Amino acid/oligo content analysis	X	X	X	X	X
	Peptide map			X	X	X
Purity	ELISA	X		X	X	X
	HPLC	X	X	X	X	X
	SDS-PAGE	X	X	X	X	X
	Amino acid/oligo sequence	X	X			
	Amino acid/oligo analysis	X	X	X	X	X
	Peptide map			X	X	X
	GC-MS (residual solvents)	X	X	X	X	X
Potency	Any method			X	X	X
Safety	Sterility (e.g., USP <71>)	X	X	X	X	X
	Endotoxin (e.g., USP <85> LAL)	X	X	X	X	X
	Viral safety (virus-specific assays)					X
Quality	Host cell DNA (by PCR or qPCR)			X	X	X
	Host cell protein (by ELISA or western blot)			X	X	X

"X" indicates that a method is highly recommended/required for this particular product class.

6.3.8 Reference Standards

Product reference standards are required to support the development of analytical methods and to run routine analytical checks during processing or final release testing. They are needed to ensure that the test methods are performing as expected each time the assay is performed. Reference standards are made with the same manufacturing process to be used for the preparation of clinical materials and can be sourced from the final GMP lots.[14] Development of analytical procedures may proceed with reference material from engineering or development batches, but the final reference material should come from the final GMP process.

Additional information can be found in the following ICH guidance documents:

- **ICH Q6B specifications**: Test Procedures and Acceptance Criteria for Biotechnological/Biological Products, March 1999
- **ICH Q7A**: Good Manufacturing Practice Guide for Active Pharmaceutical Ingredients, November 2000
- **ISO guide 30:1992/Amd 1:2008**: Revision of Definitions for Reference Material and Certified Reference Material.

6.3.9 Process Validation

The development of a robust manufacturing process is critical to the successful creation of any biological therapeutic. The validation of the manufacturing process starts with the Installation Qualification, Operational Qualification, and Performance Qualification of the processing equipment, utilities, and environmental controls, grouped together as the "facility." After the utilities and manufacturing equipment have been validated, the manufacturing process can undergo process validation (PV). PV will take place at the end of process development and prior to the initiation of the Phase III manufacturing.

The GMP manufacturing process can be modified concurrently with the conduct of Phase I and II of the clinical trials but must be finalized (or "locked") prior to the start of Phase III pivotal trials. The drug product manufactured in support of Phase III studies should represent, as close as possible, the drug product that will be commercialized. Hence, the manufacturing process used for drug supply of Phase III is considered the commercial process and will be submitted to the regulatory agencies for approval.

Additional parts of the validation of a manufacturing process include cleaning and environmental monitoring (EM). There must be established cleaning procedures for the common spaces in the facility (warehouse, laboratories, and building utilities that support the manufacturing process). There will be specialized, product-specific cleaning procedures that will be developed as part of the manufacturing process and will be part of the overall validation process. The use of single use/disposable equipment (bioreactor, media and buffer bags, columns and filters) eliminates the need for much of the cleaning validation and can simplify the overall manufacturing process and CMC documentation. The use of disposable equipment and consumables has continued to grow over recent years and offers an alternative to traditional hard-piped stainless steel manufacturing plants.

A well-established program for the routine EM of the particulates, both viable and nonviable, is also required for ensuring the quality of the biopharmaceuticals produced. Monitoring is ongoing during passive/static phases of facilities operation

TABLE 6.9

Example of Drug Product Stability Program at 5°C

Assay	Months of Stability								
	0	0.25	1	3	6	9	12	18	24
Appearance	X	X	X	X	X	X	X	X	X
Identity	X						X		X
Purity	X	X	X	X	X	X	X	X	X
Potency	X	X	X	X	X	X	X	X	X
Product content	X	X	X	X	X	X	X	X	X
Endotoxin	X								X
Sterility	X								X

when there is no active manufacturing taking place as well as during the active/dynamic phases during which manufacturing operations are occurring.

6.3.10 Stability Programs

A stability program is required for all drug products to ensure that the product is safe and efficacious during the drug's proposed shelf life. The program chosen will depend on the storage conditions of the finished dosage form and will include temperature, humidity, and time. All programs should be conducted on the container closure system to be used for commercial purposes and at the doses to be contained in the final container system, single use or multiple use vials or syringes.

A typical stability program is shown in Table 6.9 for a 24-month long study at one storage condition, 5°C (typical for a refrigerated biopharmaceutical), with an example of some of the assays that might be performed. All assays do not need to be performed at every time point; for example, sterility would only need to be done at time zero (the manufacturing and/or product release date) and at the last time point in the study. Stability studies can consume large quantities of product and the length of the study, and the number of assays to be run needs to be factored into the initial demonstration lot or clinical lots to ensure sufficient material is available to complete the study. This should include an overage of 30% or more to cover failed tests or repeat testing. Additionally, if the API is to be held before manufacturing the drug product, a stability program would need to be implemented to provide documentation that the API is stable until the drug product is produced. Additional details indicating other storage conditions are listed in the ICH guidelines on stability.[14]

6.4 Selecting a Manufacturing System

6.4.1 API Manufacturing

As noted above, there are several manufacturing platforms for producing biopharmaceuticals, from chemical synthesis to microbial and mammalian cell–based processes. All of these systems have common elements in the manufacturing process with the manufacturing being divided between the upstream processing and the downstream processing. The upstream process consists of the steps needed to generate the starting material containing the API or drug substance whereas the downstream process consists of the steps for purification of the desired API. A third phase that converts the API into the final drug product consists of the formulation and fill-finish processes that may involve addition of excipients and buffers to stabilize the drug and the filling of the formulated product into the final dosage containers. Additional steps including lyophilization, spray drying or freezing, and storage at low temperatures may be part of the drug product manufacturing process.

The choice of the manufacturing system depends on several variables:

- The cost of production, including media, processing aids (such as filters and chromatographic resins), reagents, the number of processing steps, and the processing equipment availability.
- Media cost for microbial systems are inexpensive salt solutions and yeast extracts whereas mammalian systems require media that may contain specific growth factors and FBS which is limited in supply.
- The scalability of the manufacturing process is driven by the quantities of material needed to treat the proposed patient population, the manufacturing platform chosen (microbial, mammalian, fungal, plant), the complexity of the manufacturing process, and equipment limitations (such as column sizes and resin availability)
- Molecular complexity of the biopharmaceutical being produced: Is post-translational modification required? These modifications can take the form of glycosylation, refolding, enzymatic modification, and assembly of multiple components (such as monoclonal antibodies and heme-containing globulins).
- In-process safety controls including viral clearance and inactivation, TSE contamination, and also reliable product assays, particularly, cell-based potency assays.
- Production steps such as cycle time, complexity of the downstream processing, and equipment availability.
- Availability of existing genetically engineered platforms, e.g., microbial, yeast, and mammalian systems that have previously been used to manufacture approved biological drugs.

See Table 6.10, below, for a summary of these factors.

TABLE 6.10

Factors to Consider when Selecting a Manufacturing Platform

Consideration	Chemical Synthesis	Microbial (*E. coli*)	Yeast (*Pichia pastoris*)	Mammalian (CHO Cells)
Type of product	Short peptide or Oligo	Large peptide or protein	Large protein	Protein requiring post-synthetic modifications
Cost	Expensive components (nucleic acids and amino acids)	Inexpensive media: salts	Inexpensive media: salts, yeast extract	Custom media: expensive components, inclusion of FBS[a]
Scalability	Easily scalable	Bioreactors available in 10,000 liters	Bioreactors available in 10,000 liters	Bioreactors available in 10,000 to 15,000 liters
Post-translational modifications	Not included; can be a concern for certain proteins	Enzymatic cleavage of preproteins, glycosylated proteins	Enzymatic cleavage of preproteins, some glycosylation	Enzymatic cleavage of preproteins, complex glycosylation, folding and assembly of proteins
Adventitious agents	No viral issues	No viral issues	No viral issues	Viral clearance and inactivation
Cycle time	Short upstream cycling (days)	Short upstream cycling (days)	Short upstream cycling (days to week)	Long upstream cycling (weeks to months)
Downstream processing	Less extensive processing (no cellular components)	Extensive processing	Extensive processing	Extensive processing
Genetic engineering	Not required	Easily manipulated	Easily manipulated	Easily manipulated
Timeline for manufacturing process development	Peptide: 3–6 months Oligo: 6–9 months[b]	12–18 months	12–18 months	18–24 months

[a] Use of FBS or any other mammalian source of reagents can lead to potential issues with regulatory agents due to ongoing concerns of transmission of spongiform encephalitis. Custom serum free and/or chemically defined media are replacing serum-based media.

[b] Oligo products can require longer lead times because of small numbers of qualified manufacturers. Each project competes with many others for scheduling in the manufacturing facility.

6.4.2 Drug Product Manufacturing

Manufacturing the final drug product can be a simple sterile filtration and fill into individual dosage containers (vials, syringes), or it may require additional formulation before the final filling process. In addition to liquid fill, some biopharmaceuticals are lyophilized as the final step before labeling and packaging.

The complexity of the manufacturing process is dependent on the type of biopharmaceutical being produced. A chemical synthesis–based production system using solid phase peptide synthesis is a relatively simple process with the primary step(s) being the coupling of the individual amino acids into the desired peptide followed by the removal of solvents and excess reagents. There will be numerous cycles of amino acid addition, but there are fewer impurities to remove (e.g., host cell protein or residual DNA; antibiotics). The chemical

synthesis of oligonucleotides is similar to peptide synthesis. Cell culture–based production of monoclonal antibodies is considered very complex with numerous purification steps and requires a large number of supporting analytical methods.

6.5 CMC Regulatory Requirements

The US FDA and the ICH have published numerous guidance documents to assist the industry in meeting regulatory requirements for all manner of new drug development and manufacturing. These documents include requirements for everything from development and validation of analytical methods to testing for pyrogens, setting drug specifications, and manufacturing (see Table 6.11).

TABLE 6.11

Manufacturing Systems for Select Biopharmaceuticals

Biologic	Molecular Type	Manufacturing Platform	System Description
Recombinant factor VIII	Blood clotting factor	CHO	Mammalian cell—based system
Insulin[16]	Peptide hormone	*E. coli* *Saccharomyces cerevisiae*	Microbial and yeast
Tissue plasminogen activator (tPA)	Enzyme	CHO	Mammalian cell-based system
Anti-tumor necrosis factor (TNF)	Monoclonal antibody	CHO	Mammalian cell-based system
Erythropoietin	Hormone, growth factor	CHO	Mammalian cell—based system
Shingles vaccine	Vaccine	MCR-5	Stem cell, human fibroblast
Fibrin sealant	Biological glue for wound closure	Human plasma fractionation	Isolation of components from human plasma
Peptide hormones[17]	Hormones	*Pichia pastoris*	Methanolic yeast
Hepatitis vaccines	Vaccine	*Saccharomyces cerevisiae*	Yeast-based system
Calcitonin	Peptide hormone	Peptide synthesis	Chemical synthesis
Fomivirsen	Nucleic acid	siRNA synthesis	Chemical synthesis

Biopharmaceutical manufacturing facilities, whether built and managed by CMOs or company owned, also must operate under strict standards defined in the FDA regulations as GMPs (or cGMPS). The US-focused guidance documents from FDA governing the cGMPs are designed to be stage appropriate for the life cycle of the drug product, providing more flexibility at the beginning of drug development and manufacturing and stricter compliance for manufacturing as the process moves through the various stages (Phase I–III) of the approval process.

A short list of the US FDA guidance documents with the broadest applicability is noted below in Table 6.12. A much longer, complete list of CMC and cGMP guidance documents can be obtained from the FDA website.

European regulations include more stringent requirements for cGMP at early stages of development and are codified in guidance documents produced by the ICH. These regulations must be taken into account if any of the proposed clinical trials will include investigative sites in the European Union (EU). (Note: at the time of this writing, Great Britain's exit from the EU had not yet occurred. However, the regulators of medicinal products in the UK have assured the public that there will be no major deviations from EU regulations at least for a few years following the UK's transition out of the EU.)

A partial list of important ICH guidance documents for CMC and cGMPs is included below in Table 6.13.

Finally, there are also guidance documents that are focused on the newest types of biotherapeutics, such as cellular and gene therapies (CGTs). One in particular focuses on the concept of somatic cell therapy using cells that are minimally manipulated for homologous use (e.g., human cells or tissues intended for implantation, transplantation, infusion, or transfer into human patients).

A short list of FDA guidance documents for these types of drugs is provided below in Table 6.14.

6.6 Summary

Biologics fall into a number of different chemical biological classes. Hence, not unexpectedly, the manufacturing specifics related to each type of the investigational agent will differ. This chapter attempts to provide some insight into the various factors to be considered when manufacturing the various types of biologic therapeutics. We summarized the general aspects of manufacturing that are broadly applicable to any production platform that might be utilized and then provided some specific information related to the various platforms.

TABLE 6.12

Partial List of FDA Guidance Documents for CMC and cGMP

Guidance	Type	Date
Preparation of investigational new drug products (human and animal)	Final guidance	Nov 1992
Sterile drug products produced by aseptic processing	Final guidance	Sept 2004
Quality systems approach to pharmaceutical cGMP regulations	Final guidance	Sept 2006
cGMP for phase 1 investigational drugs	Final guidance	July 2008
Process validation: general principles and practices	Final guidance	Oct 2011
Questions and answer on cGMPs for drugs	Final guidance	Dec 2011
Guidance for industry: pyrogen and endotoxins testing	Final guidance	June 2012
cGMP requirements for combination products	Final guidance	Jan 2017
Container closure systems for packaging human drugs and biologics	Final guidance	May 1999
Container closure systems for packaging human drugs and biologics—questions and answers	Final guidance	May 2002
INDs for phase 2 and phase 3 studies CMC information	Final guidance	May 2003
Analytical procedures and methods validation for drugs and biologics	Final guidance	July 2015

TABLE 6.13

Partial List of ICH Guidance Documents for CMC and cGMP

Guidance	Type	Date
Q1A-Q1F stability	Final guidance	Feb 2003
Q2(R2)/Q14 analytical procedure development and validation	Concept paper	Nov 2018
	Final guidance	Nov 1996
Q3A-Q3D impurities	Final guidance	2006–2018
Q5A-Q5E quality of biotechnology products	Final guidance	1995–2004
Q6B specifications for biotechnological/biological products	Final guidance	Mar 1999
Q7 good manufacturing practice guide for active pharmaceutical ingredients	Final guidance	Nov 2000
Q9 quality risk management	Final guidance	Nov 2005
Q10 pharmaceutical quality system	Final guidance	June 2008
Q11 development and manufacturing of drug substances	Final guidance	May 2012
Q13 continuous manufacturing of drug substances and drug products	Concept paper	Nov 2018

TABLE 6.14

Guidance Documents for Tissue, Cell, and Gene Therapies

Guidance	Type	Date
Regulatory considerations for human cells, tissues, and cellular and tissue-based products: minimal manipulation and homologous use[18]	Final guidance	Dec 2017
Early clinical trials with live biotherapeutic products: CMC information	Final guidance	June 2016
Guidance for human somatic cell therapy and gene therapy	Final guidance	Mar 1998
CMCs information for human gene therapy IND applications	Draft guidance	Jul 2018
Potency tests for cellular and gene therapy products	Final guidance	Jan 2011
Current good tissue practices and additional requirements for manufacturers of human cells, tissues, and cellular and tissue-based products	Final guidance	Dec 2011

New technological advances and new scientific discoveries are made continuously. As a consequence, it will be important for any developer to understand not only the basic considerations listed here but also to be aware of investigational agents that are currently in development as well as recent regulatory approvals. The development approaches and the bases for regulatory approvals provide important insight into the current thinking on the part of regulatory agencies. Such insights will only contribute to a more efficient and effective approach to the manufacturing and testing of new biologic therapies.

REFERENCES

1. Solid-Phase Peptide Synthesis, Bachem Group February 2016, https://www.bachem.com/knowledge-center/white-papers/
2. Oligonucleotide Synthesis Application Note.pdf - Fisher Scientific, www.thermofishersci.in/lit/Oligonucleotide%20Synthesis%20Application%20Note.pdf
3. Hyunah Kim, Su Jin Yoo, Hyun Ah Kang, Yeast synthetic biology for the production of recombinant therapeutic proteins, FEMS Yeast Research, 2015, 15:1–16.
4. https://www.bioprocessonline.com/doc/overcoming-the-manufacturing-hurdles-of-cell-gene-therapy-0001
5. Guidance for Human Somatic Cell Therapy and Gene Therapy, U.S. Department of Health and Human Services Food and Drug Administration Center for Biologics Evaluation and Research March 1998.
6. Anthony Mire- Sluis, Nadine Ritter, Barry Cherney, Dieter Schmalzing and Markus Blumel. Reference standards for therapeutic proteins current regulatory and scientific best practices and remaining needs, part 1, *BioProcess International*, March 2014, 12(3):26–36.
7. Anurag S. Rathore. The scare of adventitious agents in therapeutic products, *PDA Journal of Pharmaceutical Science and Technology*, 2014, 68:192.
8. Nabih A. Baeshen, Mohammed N. Baeshen, Abdullah Sheikh, Roop S. Bora, Mohamed Morsi M. Ahmed, Hassan A. I. Ramadan, Kulvinder Singh Saini, and Elrashdy M. Redwan. Cell factories for insulin production, *Microbial Cell Factories*, 2014, 13:141 (recombinant insulin).
9. Paul W. Tebbey, Amy Varga, Michael Naill, Jerry Clewell, and Jaap Venema. Consistency of quality attributes for the glycosylated monoclonal antibody, *Humira (adalimumab) mAbs*, September/October 2015, 7(5):805–811.
10. John A. Blaho, Elise R. Morton, and Jamie C. Yedowitz. Herpes simplex virus: propagation, quantification, and storage, *Current Protocols in Microbiology*, 2005: 14E.1.1–14E.1.23. https://doi.org/10.1002/9780471729259.mc14e01s00
11. Hyunah Kim, Su Jin Yoo, and Hyun Ah Kang. Yeast synthetic biology for the production of recombinant therapeutic proteins, Hyunah Kim, Su Jin Yoo and Hyun Ah Kang. *FEMS Yeast Research*, 2015, 15(1):1–16.
12. ICH Harmonised Tripartite Guideline Stability Testing of New Drug Substances and Products Q1A(R2), Current Step 4 Version, 6 February 2003.
13. Guidance for Industry Characterization and Qualification of Cell Substrates and Other Biological Materials Used in the Production of Viral Vaccines for Infectious Disease Indications, U.S. Department of Health and Human Services Food and Drug Administration Center for Biologics Evaluation and Research, February 2010.
14. Samsung BioLogics: The Story of the World's Largest Biologics Manufacturing Facility, https://www.bio-pharma-reporter.com/Headlines/Promotional-Features/Samsung-BioLogics-The-story-of-the-world-s-largest-biologics-manufacturing-facility, 01 April 2018.
15. ICH Harmonised Tripartite Guideline; Impurities in New Drug Products Q3B(R2) [Current Step 4 version dated 2 June 2006].
16. Guidance 18: Impurities in drug substances and drug products, Office of Medicines Authorisation, 09/08/2013 Australian Register of Therapeutic Goods (ARTG). Therapeutic Goods Administration, http://www.tga.gov.au
17. ICH Harmonised Tripartite Guideline; Specifications: Test Procedures and Acceptance Criteria for Biotechnological/Biological Products Q6B, 10 March 1999.
18. Regulatory Considerations for Human Cells, Tissues, and Cellular and Tissue-Based Products: Minimal Manipulation and Homologous Use, Guidance for Industry and Food and Drug Administration Staff, FDA, December 2017.

7

Preclinical Toxicology Testing Paradigms

Joy A. Cavagnaro
Access BIO, LC

CONTENTS

7.1 Standardized Approach

Experience in preclinical safety evaluation of small molecules (new chemical entities [NCEs]) over the last half century or more has shown that relatively standardized or conventional approaches (Table 7.1) have generally been sufficient to support the design of clinical trials and to safeguard the safety of subjects, both healthy volunteers and patients, participating in these trials. Standardized approaches are those defined by regulatory guidance as well as approaches considered to be company practice, historically and/or deliberately, and in some cases exceed regulatory guidance. The rationale for exceeding regulatory guidance is often presented as a way to mitigate regulatory risk and potential delays in development timelines. Thus, the standardized approach may be viewed as "conducting studies" to ensure regulatory acceptance, i.e., prioritizing predictions of acceptability, rather than designing studies to improve predictions for clinical relevance.

The relevance of preclinical data has often been the subject of debate among innovators, developers, clinicians, and regulators. Opinions range from those who consider preclinical data to have high predictive value and relevance to humans to those who believe they have low predictive value or even no relevance. Ironically, the judgement is often correlated with the endpoint being evaluated. For example, results of animal efficacy studies are often believed and interpreted as having a high predictive value, whereas the opposite is true for toxicity data, even when using the same test species that was used for efficacy studies. When toxicology studies are positive—that is, toxicity is observed in animals, the first question often asked is whether the finding could be species specific and therefore not of relevance to humans (Cavagnaro, 2002). Animals allow evaluation of endpoints that are not easy or possible in humans (e.g., histology, pregnancy outcome), but will never be more predictive than humans for informing clinical safety in the intended clinical population especially since most safety testing is conducted in normal animals.

The animal–human concordance for toxicity has been studied by various groups over the years. In the 1990s, Newell et al. studied 25 cancer drugs and concluded that the routine use of nonrodent species in preclinical toxicology studies for cancer therapeutics prior to initial clinical trials was not necessary because rodent-only toxicology studies provided a safe and rapid means of identifying the phase 1 trial starting dose and predicting commonly encountered dose-limiting toxicities (Newell et al., 1999). The seminal report by Olson et al. in 2000 reported a 70% concordance rate for observations in any species (Olson et al., 2000) when toxicities seen clinically were looked for retrospectively in animals. A more recent study examined the ability of animal adverse observations to predict human clinical adverse events observed in drug development programs demonstrating a strong association with some but far less strong association with others. The study also examined the relationship between animals and clinical observations and proposed a model to predict drug withdrawal based on these observations (Clark, 2013). The focus of concordance studies has been the comparison of similar toxicities observed in animals and humans, the positive-predictive value. Ironically, a successful preclinical program, observing toxicity in animals and not in humans, would by definition be nonconcordant. Toxicity would be characterized in animals, or a safety margin determined to support dose and dosing regimens, and safety parameters identified to guide clinical monitoring of safety in humans to avoid or manage toxicity/adverse events.

Retrospective reviews of the various types of preclinical studies have been useful in identifying best practices by providing an understanding of the relevance of the information to enhance predictivity and reduce animal use through efficiency improvements or streamlined processes (Monticello, 2015). Real-time assessments, i.e., providing an integrated safety assessment to include both clinical and preclinical safety data

DOI: 10.1201/9781003124542-9

TABLE 7.1

Standardized Approach vs. Case-by-Case Approach

Testing	Drug (NCE)	Biological Drug (NBE)
Off-target screening	• Required[a]	• Required for mAbs and mAb derivatives except for cancer indications
• Metabolic profiling	• Required	• Generally not required
• Genetic toxicity	• Required	• Generally not required
• Safety pharmacology	• Stand-alone studies (rodent or nonrodent) generally required; in some cases, can incorporate in general toxicity	• Endpoints generally incorporated as technically feasible in general toxicity
• General toxicity	• Required (2 species; rodent and nonrodent); up to 6 months rodent required; 9 or 12 months for nonrodent required	• Required (2 relevant species; rodent and nonrodent if both are relevant); up to 6 months in a single species • Surrogate molecule if no relevant species • Animal models of disease may be considered in some cases
• Reproductive and developmental toxicity	• Required (2 species)	• If needed, may be conducted in a single species • Surrogate molecule may be used • Written/literature assessment of reproductive risk may be conducted (WOE)
• Carcinogenicity	• Required (2 species) • ICH discussions ongoing	• Written/literature assessment of carcinogenic risk generally conducted (WOE)
• Local tolerance	• Required	• Generally incorporated into general toxicity studies
• Phototoxicity	• Required for drugs that absorb in the 290–700 nM range	• Not conducted

[a] In the United States, regulatory guidance is considered as suggestions or recommendations unless specific regulatory or statutory requirements are cited. For the purpose of this document, the term required is used to mean expected.
NCE-new chemical entity; NBE-new biological entity; WOE-weight of evidence.

at the time of approval, could serve to not only better communicate risks in the product label but also to make recommendations for the set of questions that should be asked and the relevance of studies to be conducted for the next product in the class.

7.2 Considerations Based on Product Attributes

It was recognized that conventional approaches to toxicity testing of pharmaceuticals may not be appropriate for biopharmaceuticals because of the unique and diverse structural and biological properties of the latter that may include species specificity, immunogenicity, and unpredicted pleiotropic activities (ICH S6). Over the years, however, there has been a blurring of product attributes—"product continuum" based on size and complexity of molecular structure, i.e., increasing for small molecules and decreasing for large molecules.

The "case-by-case" approach means that each new product or product class would have a science-based testing program customized for that product based on its chemistry, pharmacology, pharmacokinetics/distribution, and biological properties and effects, in addition to its clinical indication (Table 7.2). This approach is expected to be iterative; preclinical scientists should learn from and adapt testing to what has been learned from all previous testing with the product and from general advances in biological, physiological, immunological, and pathological understanding. "Science-based" means that the testing program for each new product is defendable in terms of the scientific understanding of the biological effects of the

product, and the testing is performed with an appropriate scientific rationale. References to case-by-case considerations, alternative approaches, are now explicitly stated in guidance documents including those for cancer (Guidance for Industry 2010), rare disease (Guidance for Industry 2017, 2019c), and enzyme replacement therapies (Guidance for Industry 2019b). In all cases, approaches should be justified for the specific indication. Understanding that there is not a one-size fits all testing paradigm, significant progress has been made in implementation of a case-by-case approach when there is early collaboration with regulatory authorities to optimize the scope and timing of the supportive studies (Allamneni et al., 2016).

The case-by-case approach is also being explored in the design of clinical trials. To satisfy a mandate under section 3021 of the 21st Century Cures Act (Cures Act), guidance was developed for interacting with FDA on complex innovative trial design (CID) for drugs and biological products. CID includes trial designs that have rarely or never been used to date to provide substantial evidence of effectiveness in new drug applications or biologics license applications. The guidance does not indicate whether specific novel designs are or are not appropriate for regulatory use, as such determinations are made on a case-by-case basis depending on the reasons for which the design is being proposed, its validity in the specific setting, and factors unique to a given development program. As such, a CID proposal that may be appropriate for one product class in one indication may not be appropriate for another product class or in another indication. Similar to alternative preclinical testing strategies discussed above, because certain cases may involve novel scientific review considerations, early

TABLE 7.2

Case-by-Case Approach is Based on Product Attributes

Product Attribute	Drug	ODN[a]	Biological Drug	Gene Therapy (Vector-Based)	Cell Therapy
Manufacture	Chemical synthesis	Chemical synthesis	Cell culture; rDNA technology	Cell culture; rDNA technology	Cell culture; sometimes rDNA technology
• Test article	Clinical candidate	Clinical candidate—sometimes animal analog	Clinical candidate—sometimes animal analog	Clinical candidate—sometimes animal analog (transgene)	Clinical candidate—sometimes animal analog (e.g., MSCs)
• Purity	Single to few	Few to several	"homogeneous"	"heterogeneous"	"heterogeneous"
• Impurities	Easy to qualify	Generally easy to qualify	Generally easy to qualify	May be difficult to qualify	May be difficult to qualify
• Potency	Not needed	Not needed	Needed	Needed; may be difficult	Needed; may be difficult
• Formulation	Often complex	May be complex	Simple	Simple; sometimes device	Simple or complex; sometimes device
• Half-life/PD effect	Minutes to hours	Minutes to hours (days to weeks in tissues)	Days to weeks	Months to years, potentially, lifetime	Days to years
• Dose interval	Often daily	Intermittently	Weekly to monthly	Generally, once	Once or intermittent
• Species Specificity	Relatively species independent (similar metabolism)	Sometimes	Generally, often NHP only relevant species	Sometimes; sensitive to infection and pathological consequences of wild type vector; sensitivity to biology of transgene	Access of anatomic site with intended delivery device, chemically modified or genetically modified or surgical model
• Toxicity	Often unpredictable; metabolites may have unique toxicities	Hybridization dependent and independent effects; sometimes predictable based on chemistry	Related to exaggerated pharmacology or nontoxic	Usually related to MOA and/or host response, immunogenicity	Usually related to MOA and/or host response, immunogenicity
• Immunogenicity	Rare	Rare	Often	Often	Sometimes

[a] Oligonucleotides (ODNs) are regulated as drugs as they are chemically synthesized; they are not functional genetic material that can insert, replicate, be transcribed or otherwise effect change in the genome and thus are not considered gene therapy.

rDNA, Recombinant DNA; MSCs, mesenchymal stem cells; PD, pharmacodynamics; MOA, mechanism of action; NHP, non-human primate

interaction with the agency is encouraged. It is also helpful to explain how the novel design provides advantages over conventional trial designs for the particular product and indication (FDA, 2019a).

7.3 Principles vs. Practices

As previously discussed in Chapter 1, the principles of safety evaluation remain as for conventional pharmaceuticals; however, in practice, differences exist based on product attributes. Table 7.3 provides highlights of general comparisons for illustrative purposes. Specific details are discussed in the various product-specific chapters of this book.

The design of safety evaluation programs should be question- and science-based, data-driven, and practical. Most questions are relevant across all modalities: Is the mechanism of action known and is it novel? Are animal models available? Can proof-of-concept be demonstrated? What is the optimal procedure/route/anatomical site/timing for product delivery? Is there relevant safety information about the proposed clinical delivery device or delivery procedure for the product? What is the proposed optimum regimen, duration? Where does the

product go? What are the target organs of toxicity? Is toxicity monitorable, delayed, or reversible? Is there precedence i.e., product class effects and are the adverse effects relevant to the clinical population? What is the risk/benefit for the planned clinical population? Is there potential to see any activity in early trials? Is the proposed first-in-human (FIH) trial in a vulnerable population? If the initial trial is a pediatric trial, are there pharmacodynamic data, including changes in known disease-specific biomarkers in addition to safety data that suggest the prospect of direct benefit? Should drugs used to mitigate toxicity in clinical trials also be used preclinically?

7.4 Right-Sizing Preclinical Safety Evaluation Programs

As previously mentioned, the case-by-case approach is not a minimalist approach but rather a scientifically justified, rational, and targeted approach. Explicit in ICH S6 is the recommendation that toxicity studies in nonrelevant species may be misleading and thus discouraged (Guidance for Industry, 1191, 2100). Optimizing the design and scope of animal studies is even more critical with the increasing pressures to reduce

TABLE 7.3

Principles vs. Practices Based on Product Attributes

Principle	Practice Drug	Practice ODN	Practice Biologic Drug	Practice Gene Therapy (Vector-Based)	Practice Cell Therapy
Dose administration (ROA and regimen)	Multiple ROAs including oral; multiple doses; (sometimes more than 1× per day)	Several ROAs; rate of delivery; multiple intermittent doses	Often IV, SC or IM; rate of delivery; multiple doses; various regimens	Many novel ROAs; volume and location considered, generally single dose	Multiple ROAs; concentration, volume, rate of delivery considered; single cell suspension, patch or sheet; encapsulated; often single dose
• Tissue distribution	Wide	Wide	Often limited	Generally limited	Generally limited
• PK/ADME	Metabolism; often short half-life	Catabolism; can be long acting	Catabolism; often long half-life	Biodistribution—peak level and persistence of gene expression; transduction efficiency, transgene expression, integration; vector shedding; long half-life	Paracrine activity or cell engraftment (site for intended activity) and migration outside target ("fate"), persistence; short or long-half life
• Dose levels	MTD, sometimes MFD, HNSTD, NOAEL	MTD, sometimes MFD, HNSTD, NOAEL	MTD, MFD, HNSTD, PAD, MABEL, NOAEL	Often MFD, NOAEL	Often MFD, NOAEL
Dose extrapolation (HED)	Based on BSA	Generally based on BSA; ideally based on BW	Based on BSA < 100 kDa; based on BW >100 kDa	BW, BSA, target organ (area or volume); previous human experience similar vectors	BW, BSA, target organ (area or volume); previous human experience similar cells

ROA, route of administration; HED, human equivalent dose; MTD, maximum tolerated dose; MFD, maximum feasible dose; HNSTD, highest non severely toxic dose; PAD, pharmacologically active dose; MABEL, minimal anticipated biological effect level; NOAEL, no observable effect level; BSA, body surface area; BW, body weight; IV, intravenous; SC, subcutaneous; IM, intramuscular

animal testing in favor of in vitro testing and computational predictive methods.

The topic of species selection has been reviewed (Prior et al., 2020b), specifically, the scientific justification and other considerations that are taken into account that ensure the most appropriate animal species are used for toxicity studies to meet regulatory requirements and provide the most value for informing project decisions. The assessment of predictive value was outside the scope of the paper. The authors recommended that species selection should take into account opportunities to apply the 3Rs (replace, reduce, refine) within toxicology studies including refinements within study designs to benefit animal welfare and study data and reduction in animals by optimizing group sizes and study designs (Prior et al., 2020b). The regulatory, scientific, and ethical aspects underlying the selection of appropriate nonrodent species in various preclinical toxicity studies have also been described (Son et al., 2020). It has also been acknowledged that industry and government agencies are working to provide alternative methodologies to decrease reliance on animal studies while trying to improve the predictivity of safety assessments (Prior et al., 2020b; Wange et al., 2021).

ICHS6 allows for the use of a single species for longer duration studies in cases where two relevant species are used to initiate clinical trials. It is important to consider how to determine which species will be the most appropriate to take into longer term toxicity studies. However, in practice, nonhuman primates (NHPs) are generally used largely based on the higher potential for immunogenicity in rodents. While a more robust data set is currently needed to provide clear, evidence-based

recommendations for extension of the practice to small molecules or other modalities where two species are currently recommended for longer duration studies, emergence of non-animal technologies (such as in silico modeling and in vitro 3D tumor models) might be able to provide more relevant and predictive data and thus replace the need for data in a second species in the future (Prior et al., 2020a).

7.5 Current Opportunities for Implementation of the 3Rs

Implementing novel preclinical testing paradigms is not only science-based but also experiential-based. It is important to consider not only what has been done or can be done but also a continued focus on improving the predictive value and relevance to humans. It was reasoned that biopharmaceuticals that are structurally and pharmacologically comparable to a product for which there is wide experience in clinical practice may need less extensive toxicity testing (ICH S6). It was also acknowledged that although all regions have adopted a flexible, case-by-case, and science-based approach to preclinical safety evaluation, there is a need for common understanding and continuing dialogue among the regions to ensure global acceptance, given this is a rapidly evolving scientific area.

As we continue to implement the 3Rs while improving the predictive value of our preclinical studies, there are several opportunities we can immediately consider. A central tenet of ICH S6 is the use of only relevant species; in practice, NHPs have generally been the principal species. Over recent years, there have been requests by some regulatory authorities, or self-imposed by developers/sponsors, to increase the group size of 3/sex to 4/sex for the main study endpoint. Since neither group size (3/sex or 4/sex) is statistically relevant, adding an additional animal across all dose groups does not appear to be scientifically justified. It is also unclear whether there has been clinical relevance, in arbitrarily increasing group sizes and the number of dose levels in an effort to increase the percent of animals exposed to a drug if clearing antidrug antibodies or "dosing-through" to overwhelm the amount of antidrug antibody so that there is still exposure to the drug. Furthermore, we also need to recognize that deimmunizing strategies to derisk clinical immunogenicity, confirmed by in silico and in vitro assays, can lead to more immunogenic products in animals including NHPs. Additional considerations include the following:

- Determine how best to interpret and translate toxicities secondary to immunogenicity, importantly, how best to communicate risk and inform clinical trials.
- Extend the acceptability of using patient cells as well as animal models of disease for assessing both efficacy and safety when scientifically justified, especially in cases where toxicity is more severe in normal animals (Cavagnaro and Silva-Lima, 2015; Do et al., 2021).
- More broadly consider the acceptability of an animal model of disease as a second species, even when two species are relevant (Allamneni et al., 2016).
- Recognize that when NHPs are deemed a relevant species, it may not be possible to assess pharmacological activity. This may also be the case with normal human volunteers where the pharmacological activity is only observed in the disease state.
- Revaluate translational value of 3 month toxicology study for biologics used in cancer when NHP is the only relevant species.
- Refrain from designing worse-case scenarios (e.g., studies performed not using the intended route of administration) where toxicities when observed are ultimately rationalized as not relevant because they are worse case.
- Consider platform approaches, including leveraging data within a product class. The principles and practices outlined in a guidance intended for developing antisense oligos may ultimately be applicable to developing other types of individualized drug products (FDA, 2021a, 2021b).
- Reevaluate the need for even a short-term study in rodents for monoclonal antibodies (mAbs) to exogenous targets when there is no binding to human tissues as toxicities observed have only been secondary to immune responses to the human product.
- Gain consensus on the acceptability of 10× safety margins to support initial clinical studies and that

maintenance of a 10× safety margin for longer duration studies is not needed as long as a no observable effect level is defined and is not exceeded in the clinic.

- Once in the clinic, we need to monitor for comparable toxicity and/or be informed by data with similar products to determine whether the most sensitive species is also the most relevant species.
- Assessments of reproductive risk and carcinogenicity risk focusing on the weight of evidence rather than conducting dedicated studies have been acceptable in some cases and are consistent with implementation of the principles of the 3Rs. We now need to determine how best to communicate these assessments in informed consent documents and product labels.
- Continually learn from retrospective analyses, informed by exceptional cases but not default to standardization because of them. Real-time integrated safety assessments of preclinical and clinical safety of individual products at the time of approval should help us learn more quickly.

Finally, we need to acknowledge that no drug is or will be 100% safe. Managing human risk includes determining better ways to maximize benefit, collaborating on improving quality of care, finding new tools to manage risk, developing effective risk communication, increasing healthcare provider and patient/consumer understanding and management of risk, and improving the predictive value of preclinical toxicology studies. Maintaining an open dialogue among scientists in academia, industry, and regulatory authorities will continue to be critical in ensuring that new products that are safe and effective are made available without unnecessary delay. Informed patients and patient advocacy groups also have important roles as neutral facilitators. How translational scientists respond to the challenges ahead will influence whether we will continue to seize the opportunity to advance toxicology and take full advantage of scientific and medical progress.

REFERENCES

Allamneni KP, Parker S, O'Neill CA, et al. (2016). Workshop proceedings: streamlined development of safety assessment programs supporting orphan/rare diseases - are we there yet? Int J Tox 35: 393–409.

Cavagnaro J. (2002). Preclinical safety evaluation of biotechnology-derived pharmaceuticals. Nat Rev Drug Disc 1: 469–475.

Cavagnaro J and Silva-Lima B. (2015). Regulatory acceptance of animal models of disease to support slinical trials of medicines and advanced therapy medicinal products. Eur J Pharm 752: 51–62.

Clark M. (2013). Prediction of clinical risks by analysis of preclinical and clinical adverse events. J Biomed Inform 54: 167–173.

Do M-H T, Cavagnaro J, Butt M, Terse PS, and McKew JC (2021). Use of an animal model of disease for toxicology enables identification of a juvenile no observed adverse effect level for cyclocreatine in creatine transporter deficiency Regul Toxicol Pharmacol. 123:104939 https://doi.org/10.1016/j.yrtph.2021.104939

Guidance for Industry: Pediatric Rare Diseases-A Collaborative Approach for Drug Development Using Gaucher Disease as a Model. (2017). https://www.fda.gov/regulatory-information/search-fda-guidance-documents/pediatric-rare-diseases-collaborative-approach-drug-development-using-gaucher-disease-model-draft

Guidance for Industry: Interacting with the FDA on Complex Innovative Clinical Trial Designs for Drugs and Biological Products. (2019a). https://www.fda.gov/regulatory-information/search-fda-guidance-documents/interacting-fda-complex-innovative-trial-designs-drugs-and-biological-products

Guidance for Industry: Investigational Enzyme Replacement Therapy Products: Nonclinical Assessment. (2019b). https://www.fda.gov/regulatory-information/search-fda-guidance-documents/investigational-enzyme-replacement-therapy-products-nonclinical-assessment

Guidance for Industry: Rare Diseases: Common Issues in Drug Development. (2019c). https://www.fda.gov/regulatory-information/search-fda-guidance-documents/rare-diseases-common-issues-drug-development-guidance-industry

Guidance for Sponsor-Investigators: IND Submissions for Individualized Antisense Oligonucleotide Drug Products: Administrative and Procedural Recommendations. (2021a). https://www.fda.gov/regulatory-information/search-fda-guidance-documents/ind-submissions-individualized-antisense-oligonucleotide-drug-products-administrative-and-procedural

Guidance for Sponsor-Investigators: Nonclinical Testing of Individual Antisense Oligonucleotide Drug Products for Severely Debilitating or Life-Threatening Diseases. (2021b). https://www.fda.gov/regulatory-information/search-fda-guidance-documents/nonclinical-testing-individualized-antisense-oligonucleotide-drug-products-severely-debilitating-or

ICH S6 Preclinical Safety Evaluation of Biotechnology-derived Pharmaceuticals. (1997, 2011). https://www.fda.gov/regulatory-information/search-fda-guidance-documents/s6r1-preclinical-safety-evaluation-biotechnology-derived-pharmaceuticals

ICH S9 Nonclinical Evaluation for Anticancer Pharmaceuticals. (2010). https://www.fda.gov/regulatory-information/search-fda-guidance-documents/s9-nonclinical-evaluation-anticancer-pharmaceuticals

Monticello T. (2015). Drug development and nonclinical to clinical translation databases: past and current efforts. Toxicol Pathol 43: 57–61.

Newell DR, Burtles SS, Fox BW, Jodrell D, and Connors TA. (1999). Evaluation of rodent-only toxicology for early clinical trials with novel cancer therapeutics. Br J Cancer 81: 760–768.

Olson H, Betton G, Robinson D, et al. (2000). Concordance of the toxicity of pharmaceuticals in humans and in animals. Regul Toxicol Pharmacol 32: 56–67.

Prior H, Baldrick P, Been S, et al. (2020a). Opportunities for use of one species for longer-term toxicology testing during drug development: a cross-industry evaluation. Reg Tox Pharm 113: 104624.

Prior H, Haworth R, Labra B, Roberts R, Wolfreys A, and Sewell F. (2020b). Justification for species selection for pharmaceutical toxicity studies. Tox Res 9: 758–770.

Son YW, Choi H-N, Che J-H, Kang B-C, and Yun J-W (2020). Advances in selecting appropriate non-rodent species for regulatory toxicology research: policy, ethical and experimental considerations. Reg Tox Pharm 116: 104757.

Wange RL, Brown PC, and Davis-Bruon KL. (2021). Implementation of the principles of the 3Rs testing at CDER: past, present and future Regul Toxicol Pharmacol. 123:104953. https://doi.org 10.1016/j.yrtph.2021.104953.

8

Inhalation Delivery of Biologics

Stephanie F. Greene
Consulting Toxicologist

Gregory L. Finch
Independent Toxicologist

CONTENTS

8.1 Introduction and Background

Given the current importance of biologics in the pharmaceutical industry, research and development is focused on developing noninvasive routes of systemic delivery, which includes the inhalation route. Preclinical inhalation studies in laboratory animals support pharmacology, pharmacokinetics, and toxicity evaluations of biologics intended for pulmonary delivery in humans. Biologic therapeutics encompass peptides, proteins, fusion molecules, monoclonal antibodies, cell and gene therapies, and vaccines. As an important and growing class of available and effective drugs, most commercially available biologics are small peptides, proteins, monoclonal antibodies, new biologic modalities, such as nucleotide-based therapeutics, and viral gene therapies, which are rapidly maturing toward widespread clinical use (Anselmo, 2018). There are several examples of successful inhaled biologics in development and as approved, marketed products. Although there are several approved biologics and vaccines that are delivered via the intranasal or upper respiratory tract route (e.g., calcitonin, oxytocin, nafarelin, desmopressin, and FluMist), this review will examine biologics intended for delivery to the deep lung (lower airways) as deep lung absorption provides opportunities for local and systemic treatment.

Therapeutic small molecule aerosol delivery has been a primary means of treating lung conditions, particularly asthma, for more than 3500 years. Over this entire period, atropine and related compounds have played an important role in therapeutic aerosol delivery and remain crucial in the treatment of lung diseases today. In ancient times, therapeutic aerosols were often delivered by smoking or placing herbal mixtures in a heated container and inhaling the resulting vapor. Advances in manufacturing capabilities during the industrial revolution led to more sophisticated techniques for generating therapeutic

DOI: 10.1201/9781003124542-10

vapors or nebulizing medicated solutions and a subsequent shift from therapeutic aerosols to devices produced by large-scale manufacturers.

The first metered dose inhaler (MDI) was introduced in 1956 and dramatically advanced the landscape of therapeutic aerosol delivery. The first dry powder inhaler (DPI) was developed in the mid-19th century, but DPIs did not gain market prominence until the 1990s. The signing of the Montreal Protocol in 1987 led to a surge in innovation in inhaler development that has shaped the current inhaler market (Stein, 2017). In the future, technologically advanced solutions to improve drug delivery and patient compliance will likely lead to market acceptance of smart inhalers. The demand for such inhalers will supplement the MDI and DPI market as these existing therapies will likely remain important components of therapeutic aerosol delivery.

Pulmonary administration provides direct drug delivery for respiratory tract diseases such as asthma, chronic obstructive pulmonary disease (COPD), and cystic fibrosis. Inhalation therapy has also been applied to treating nonpulmonary-related diseases, including diabetes (Table 8.1). There are clear advantages of pulmonary delivery over other routes of administration as the highly vascular lungs provide a large surface area for rapid drug absorption. Pulmonary delivery also avoids the first-pass hepatic metabolism that orally delivered drugs undergo. Furthermore, inhalation is less invasive than injection, which is the conventional delivery method for many proteins. Thus, interest in developing inhaled biologics for systemic treatments has increased in recent times.

To maximize the therapeutic effect and/or evaluation of potential toxicities of biologic therapies administered via inhalation, it is key to assess the physical characteristics of the therapeutic which may be unique to pulmonary delivery. Particle size and distribution of the biologic, along with temperature and humidity, are important components of the delivery system. Thus, the use of pulmonary delivery devices and excipients that are fit for purpose for the unique properties of each biotherapeutic (e.g., Technosphere particles) are key to the success of pulmonary delivery. The following sections will discuss the advantages and limitations of macromolecule inhalation delivery, advances in inhalation therapies, safety, and clinical/regulatory applications of biologics via pulmonary delivery.

TABLE 8.1

Selected Clinical Trials and Approved Products for the Inhalation Delivery of Biologics to the Lower Airways

Name (Company)	Delivery Approach	Biologic	Application/Indication/ Comment	Reference
FDA-Approved Products				
Pulmozyme™ (Genentech)	Oral inhalation (nebulizer)	Dornase alfa	Cystic fibrosis	FDA SBA (1994)
Exubera™ (Pfizer)	Oral inhalation (dry powder)	Human insulin	Diabetes mellitus (withdrawn 2007)	FDA SBA (2006)
Afrezza™ (MannKind)	Oral inhalation (dry powder)	Human insulin	Diabetes mellitus	FDA SBA (2014)
Investigational Programs				
AER-501 (Aerami [formerly Dance Biopharm])	Oral inhalation (aqueous solution)	Human insulin	PhII. PK/PD properties	NCT04100473 and others
AIR insulin (Lilly)	Oral inhalation (dry powder)	Human insulin	PhIII. Terminated 2008	NCT00355849 and others
AERx (Novo Nordisk)	Oral inhalation (aqueous solution)	Human insulin	PhIII. Terminated 2008	NCT00411892 and others
Growth hormone (Lilly)	Oral inhalation (dry powder)	Human growth hormone	Ph1 completed 2009; apparently terminated	McElroy et al (2013)
MVA85A (Oxford University)	Aerosol	Recombinant modified vaccinia	PhI. Tuberculosis vaccine	NCT02532036 and others
PUR003 (Pulmatrix)	Nebulizer	Not listed	Ph1. Flu vaccine	NCT00947687
Ad5Ag85A (McMaster Univ.)	Aerosol	Recombinant human adenovirus	Ph1. Tuberculosis vaccine	NCT02337270
Molgradex (Savara)	Oral inhalation (nebulized solution)	Recombinant human GM-CSF	PhIII. Autoimmune pulmonary alveolar proteinosis	NCT02702180
MRT5005 (Translate Bio)	Oral inhalation (nebulized solution)	mRNA	PhI/II.	NCT03375047
ALX-0171 (Ablynx)	Oral inhalation (nebulized solution)	Nanobody	PhI/IIa. Respiratory syncytial virus	NCT02309320
SB010 (Sterna Biologicals)	Oral inhalation (nebulized solution)	DNAzyme (enzymatic antisense oligonucleotide)	PhII. Allergic asthma	NCT01743768

Source: Adapted/expanded from Anselmo et al. (2018), Table 5.

PhI, Phase 1; PhII, Phase 2; PhIII, Phase 3; FDA, US Food and Drug Administration; SBA, FDA Summary Basis of Approval; NCT, US Clinicaltrials.gov identifier number; GM-CSF, granulocyte macrophage colony-stimulating factor; mRNA, messenger RNA; PK, pharmacokinetics; PD, pharmacodynamics.

8.2 Mechanisms of Absorption and Barriers with Inhalation Delivery

As noted above, inhaled macromolecules may be indicated for treating either pulmonary or systemic diseases. Following a brief review of the respiratory tract structure, this section focuses on the absorption of biopharmaceutical drugs from the lungs into systemic distribution.

8.2.1 Lung Structure and Morphology

The gross and microscopic anatomy of the respiratory tract has been extensively studied; the interested reader is referred to various texts and review papers on this topic (for example, see Phalen et al., 1996). The nasal and oral cavities are the first sites encountered by inspired air. Nasal airways are complex but are not considered in this review because the deep lung is the primary target for macromolecule deposition for ultimate absorption.

Airstreams encounter an approximate 90-degree redirection in the nasopharyngeal and oropharyngeal compartments, then pass through the larynx and trachea before being split for delivery to right or left lungs at the carina. Upon entering the lobar bronchi, the airstream enters the lung where in humans, some 16 branching generations of successively smaller bronchi and bronchioles deliver the airstream deeper into the lung. Upon passing terminal bronchioles, the airstream reaches the respiratory bronchioles and alveolar ducts, constituting airway generations 17–23, then distally to the alveolar sacs.

The entire respiratory tract is covered by an epithelial surface, the nature of which changes markedly as a function of airway generation. In head airways, the trachea, and bronchi and bronchiolar airways, the relatively thick epithelium consists of pseudostratified columnar cells interspersed with mucus-secreting goblet cells, ciliated cells, and underlying basal cells (Figure 8.1). Cilia work in tandem to continuously propel mucus, and particles deposited on the mucosal surfaces, from distal airways up to the throat (via the so-called mucociliary escalator) where the mucus can be swallowed. More distally, both the epithelial layer and the mucus blanket are thinner, until the bronchiolar airways where mucus clearance becomes progressively slower. Even more distally, the mucus is no longer present, and the alveolar spaces are lined by a thin (0.1–0.2 μm) layer of surfactant fluid containing a complex mixture of phospholipids and proteins, the purpose of which is to retain airspace patency. In the alveolar spaces, the epithelium consists of Type 1 and Type 2 cells and has an approximate surface area in man of 100 m². The thickness of the barrier for gas exchange between the airspaces and the blood (alveolar epithelium, interstitium, and capillary endothelium) is only on the order of 0.2 μm (Figure 8.2). The alveolar surfaces are patrolled by alveolar macrophages; cells that are mobile, and are capable of internalizing, destroying, and/or removing foreign material.

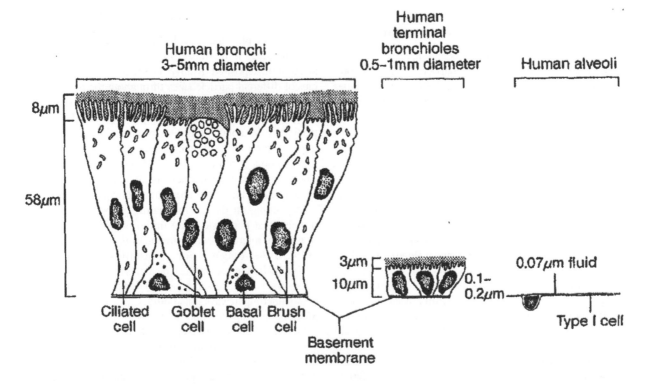

FIGURE 8.1   Schematic depictions of the pulmonary epithelium (from Patton, 1996; Figs 3 and 7). The relative epithelial cell size and fluid thickness in different regions of the human lung.

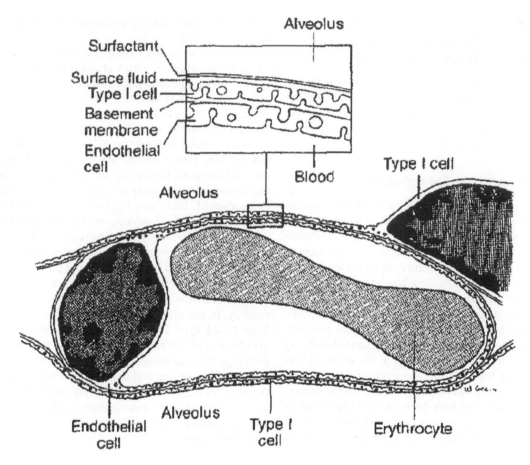

FIGURE 8.2   Schematic depictions of the pulmonary epithelium (from Patton, 1996; Figs 3 and 7). The cross-section of an alveolar septum showing a capillary, with blow-up showing type 1 endothelial cell interface and numerous caveoli in both cells.

8.2.2 Mechanisms of Macromolecule Absorption from the Respiratory Tract

The alveolar epithelium, basement membrane, and capillary endothelium, collectively the alveolar barrier, is likely the predominant site for absorption of a variety of macromolecules (Patton, 1996; Wolff, 1998, 2020). The relatively high alveolar surface area and the thin barrier between the airspaces and blood makes this seem logical. However, this has not been definitively proven. There are scant data defining the relative contribution of absorption across the thicker epithelial barriers found in the conducting airways although Mathias et al. (1996) found comparable transepithelial absorption rates across airway epithelium for hydrophilic solutes. Patton (1996) stated that the predominant mechanism is thought to be paracellular transport, consisting of passive diffusion of insulin across the alveolar epithelium through extracellular tight junctions (Figure 8.3). This would likely result from passive diffusion down a concentration gradient. Although transcytosis has also been demonstrated for the absorption of proteins from the lung, this mechanism may involve transport within alveoli and is probably more important for proteins of 40kDa or larger (Patton, 1996; Crandall and Matthay, 2001). Indeed, absorption of proteins from the lung is complex and dependent on a variety of factors, including molecular size, charge, enzymatic activity, site of deposition, and whether diffusion is active or passive (Byron and Patton, 1994; Patton, 1996). Other host factors, such as cigarette smoking status discussed below, also plays a role.

8.2.3 Role of Appropriate Particle Size

In order for pharmaceutical macromolecules to be absorbed from the deep lung, the aerosol particles must be sufficiently sized to be deposited distally. The relative deposition efficiencies of different particle sizes throughout the respiratory tract have been well described and are outside the scope of this chapter; see, for example, Schlesinger (1995). Briefly, larger particles (over about 10 μm) are preferentially deposited in the upper respiratory tract, whereas particles under that size (and ideally about 3–5 μm) are most likely to reach the deep lung. There are species differences in the particle deposition efficiencies in various respiratory tract subcompartments.

Depending on their aerodynamic properties, particles and droplets that penetrate these initial obstacles will deposit by impaction, interception, sedimentation, and diffusion (Gonda, 2019). If the residence time is insufficient for diffusion and sedimentation of the smallest particles to the walls of the respiratory tract, then they may be exhaled. Once particles deposit on conducting airways, mucociliary clearance will start translocating them upward and they may ultimately get swallowed.

Several studies have suggested that absorption from the deep lung is important in insulin absorption. Pillai et al. (1996) measured the bioavailability of two different inhaled insulin particle sizes using gamma camera imaging. At comparable inhaled doses, the smaller-sized aerosol, having relatively increased deep-lung deposition, produced a greater bioavailability and a greater bioefficacy as determined by blood

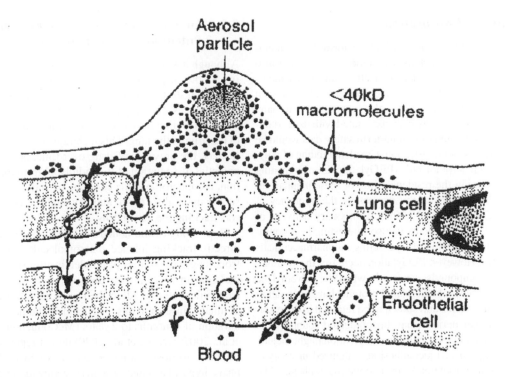

FIGURE 8.3 Schematic depiction of the absorption of relatively small macromolecules (<40 kDa) across the barrier between the alveolar lumen and capillaries (from Patton 1996, Fig 15.B). Passive diffusion by paracellular transport is believed to account for most of the absorbed insulin; transcytosis is thought to play only a minor role.

glucose lowering. Using gamma scintigraphy and pharmaco-kinetic monitoring in rabbits, Colthorpe et al. (1992) showed a greater peripheral deposition and a 10-fold greater bioavailability for inhaled versus intratracheally instilled insulin. These results translate clinically; Laube et al. (1998) used gamma camera imaging to show that relatively greater basal deposition, compared with apical deposition, was associated with greater percentage decreases in blood glucose levels.

8.2.4 Absorption Barriers

After bolus inhalation, the initial absorption of a macromolecule into the systemic circulation and its disappearance from the circulation over time should mirror removal of the drug from the lung. Derendorf et al. (2001) reached this conclusion for inhaled insulin. Although substantial deposition onto conducting airways would result in mucociliary clearance and swallowing, macromolecule absorption in the gastrointestinal tract would be negligible. Wolff (1998) noted that for soluble proteins, clearance of protein from the lung closely parallels absorption into blood.

However, macromolecule degradation in the lung tissue can occur owing to either a nonspecific or drug-specific enzymatic activity. As examples of nonspecific degradation, several ecto-peptidases were described in rat alveolar epithelial cells, A549 cells, and pulmonary macrophages, and the aminopeptidase activity, in particular, was seen as constituting a significant metabolic barrier to systemic delivery of peptides via the lung (Forbes et al., 1999). Evidence for the importance of enzymatic activity in intrapulmonary insulin bioavailability was

provided by Shen et al. (1999) who showed degradation could be inhibited by the enzyme inhibitors bacitracin and sodium cholate, and Komada et al. (1994) who showed glycocholate, a surfactant-like agent reported to suppress aminopeptidase activity, increased relative bioavailability by approximately 5-fold in rats receiving intratracheal instillations of aqueous insulin.

Macromolecule-specific enzymatic activity has been described for intrapulmonary insulin; Duckworth et al. (1998) concluded that insulin degrading enzyme, a 110 kDa metallo-proteinase, is the primary degradative mechanism for removal of insulin. In contrast, despite containing a wide range of lytic enzymes, alveolar macrophages do not appear to constitute an important clearance mechanism compared with absorption (Wolff, 1998), presumably since phagocytosis is more important in clearing relatively insoluble materials from the lung. Conversely, the presence of molecule-specific receptors could enhance absorption. However, despite the characterization of insulin receptors in lung cells *in vitro*, it appears that *in vivo* insulin receptors (if present) may not appreciably facilitate insulin absorption (Iozzo et al., 2002).

Absorption across the alveolar barrier is apparently not exclusively a one-way process. In a clinical study, Mendivil et al. (2015) found biologically relevant concentrations of some 19 proteins, including enteric and metabolic hormones, apolipoproteins, adipokines, and cytokines, in the alveolar lining fluid of healthy individuals. The authors concluded that protein charge may influence trafficking and compartmentalization to the alveolar airspace more than molecular weight or hydrophobicity.

8.2.5 Modifiers of Absorption

Physicochemical modifications can include formulation alterations to include molecules such as penetration enhancers or also modifications to the macromolecule itself. Many experiments have investigated the role of absorption enhancers. Although such agents can increase absorption, it has also been noted that many of these agents have historically been associated with tissue damage (Patton et al., 1999), and thus, long-term safety data would be needed to support product registration. Covalent binding of polyethylene glycol to a macromolecule (PEGylation) is an interesting approach for sustaining the residence time of these biopharmaceuticals in the lungs and thereby decreasing the frequency of administration (Guichard et al., 2017). Pulmonary delivery of PEGylated peptides and proteins is also interesting as a noninvasive route of administration of long-acting biopharmaceuticals to the bloodstream. However, PEGylation decreases the systemic absorption of the compounds, especially when the polyethylene glycol size is large. Several PEGylated proteins have been delivered to the lungs in rodents and shown to be retained in the respiratory tract for longer periods than unconjugated counterparts. Mechanisms involved in their pulmonary retention might include increased molecular size, mucoadhesion, enhanced proteolytic resistance, and escape from uptake by alveolar macrophages. The authors noted that potential safety concerns could include alveolar macrophage vacuolization and pulmonary inflammation.

Particle-based approaches can afford molecular level control over interactions between the particles and the lung (Anselmo, 2018). Strategies to improve lung delivery barriers include mucopenetrative and mucoadhesive methods to include retention time or diffusion. Chemical or permeation enhancers such as surfactants, polymers, and sugars are being investigated to aid in the transport of biologics across the lung epithelium. Cell-penetration peptides may also improve biologic transport, pulmonary deposition, and absorption. Long-term safety data will be key to the successful development of these approaches.

Cigarette smoking has been shown by numerous investigators to increase the permeability of the human lung to tracer compounds including macromolecules such as albumin. Although data in nonclinical species exposed to both smoke and intrapulmonary macromolecules are scant, clinical data clearly show an effect of smoking status on resulting pharmacokinetic and pharmacodynamic endpoints. In the case of inhaled insulin, Becker et al. (2006) showed that in comparison with nonsmokers, active smokers had significantly greater postinhalation C_{max} and AUC. Following a 1-week smoking cessation period, these parameters were reduced, but still not returned to levels seen in nonsmokers. The safety and efficacy of Afrezza in patients who smoke has not been established (Afrezza package insert). The use of Afrezza is not recommended in patients who smoke or who have recently stopped smoking.

Interestingly, acute passive cigarette smoke exposure modestly decreased the bioavailability of inhaled insulin (Fountaine et al., 2008); the reasons for this apparent discrepancy are uncertain. In addition, McElroy et al. (2013) noted that asthma and COPD can decrease insulin absorption. Clearly, any inhaled macromolecule development program needs to evaluate the effect of lung disease and smoking on the inhaled drug.

8.2.6 Lung Concentrations Achieved and Potential for Accumulation

Although it would be of interest to have a complete understanding of the disposition of inhaled macromolecules from the lung, such studies are difficult and further complicated by the need to access the deep lung. Most commonly, techniques such as ^{99m}Tc labeling have been used to image the initial deposition of the drug in the lung. This technique is of questionable utility to track the presence of drug over time, however, because of potential dissociation of the radiolabel from the drug. In addition, the macromolecule could be partially degraded either in situ or upon absorption, and it would not be certain that one was tracking the active drug.

Even though little nonclinical data appear in the literature directly tracking inhaled macromolecules, indirect evidence from long-term studies of inhaled insulin suggests drug accumulation in lung, if any, does not lead to adverse findings. Nonclinical studies (described in more detail in Section 8.6) of inhaled insulin in rats, dogs, and nonhuman primates with a duration of 6 months to 2 years (McConnell et al., 2006; Vick et al., 2007; Greene et al., 2020) do not report any suggestion of "lung overload," a phenomenon in which alveolar macrophage hyperplasia and/or hypervacuolization occur in chronic studies of relatively insoluble particles, especially in rodents (Schlesinger, 1995).

There are, however, clinical data regarding levels of insulin in the lung. Mendivil et al. (2012) evaluated the disposition of insulin by measuring trough levels in bronchoalveolar lavage (BAL) fluid following 12 weeks of inhaled insulin treatment. Compared with subjects receiving subcutaneous insulin, subjects receiving inhaled insulin had increased trough insulin levels (approximately 12 hours after the last dose) in BAL. The increase did not correlate with any clinical or laboratory parameters, and the investigators concluded the residual insulin had no significant biological action. Similarly, in a clinical study involving sequential BAL fluid analysis, Cassidy et al. (2011) estimated a clearance halftime of approximately 1 hour for a Technosphere inhaled insulin and its excipient and concluded that the potential for accumulation upon chronic administration was minimal.

8.3 Advantages and Challenges of Inhalation Delivery

There are many advantages of pulmonary delivery of biologics. The highly vascular and large surface area of the lung and thin alveolar epithelium provide an advantageous route for systemic exposure as discussed above. The human lung is an excellent platform to deliver drugs both locally and systemically, and the lungs provide a promising, noninvasive way to deliver biologics.

Inhaled biologics are administered to humans using either MDIs or DPIs or nebulizers. To successfully deliver the biologic into the deep lung, each device type requires a different formulation. DPIs have some advantages over other inhalers in that they utilize formulations that provide superior stability and are easy to use although there are development challenges for macromolecular as compared with small molecule powders. Also, generally, DPIs consistently deliver the theoretical or desired dose. Appropriate use of the device requires training for the patient and follow-up with healthcare experts to ensure that the proper technique is utilized.

Some challenges of using the respiratory route for delivery of biologics is overcoming pulmonary clearance mechanisms and metabolic pathways that protect against foreign particles or proteins. These endogenous defense pathways may reduce the effectiveness or overall systemic exposure of the therapeutic. Preclinical animal studies can use different dry powder delivery devices which may include nose-only, whole-body, insufflation, and intratracheal administration. Unfortunately, these delivery platforms usually lead to variable powder deposition in the respiratory tract of animals (Price, 2019).

Another significant challenge involves incorporating the biologic drug into an appropriate form that allows for generation of an appropriately sized aerosol. This is in marked contrast to, for example, the incorporation of a stable small molecule drug into a lactose-based formulation for a DPI. It is important that the macromolecule retain the physicochemical characteristics that are important to its biological activity; for example, the retention of the 2- and 3-dimensional structure of proteins/peptides. Accordingly, for dry powder biologic drugs, relatively "advanced" techniques may be needed; spray drying is one such example (Deshmukh et al., 2019). Also, it may be necessary to include the use of novel excipients in a biologic drug formulation for inhalation in order to provide improved stability, bioavailability, or therapeutic benefits, and this would likely entail the need of a toxicological qualification of the novel excipient(s) as well.

8.4 Considerations for Dose Administration

To determine the dose administration parameters for each delivery system, aerosol particle properties related to their potential biological effect or absorption are evaluated prior to dosing. These properties include chemical composition, mass concentration, aerodynamic size, size distribution, and geometric size. There are advantages and disadvantages associated with various modes of inhalation exposure in animals (Table 8.2).

Basic aerosol generation and exposure atmosphere validation requirements for animal studies are conceptually identical for inhaled biologics and for small molecules. Robust validation is particularly important for pivotal toxicity studies under Good Laboratory Practices regulations. However, it cannot be assumed that techniques suitable for small molecules are necessarily appropriate for the inhaled biotherapeutic. This is because the large molecule formulation may be unique or might be sufficiently delicate such that the strong forces used in some aerosol generation methods may be too energetic. For example, McElroy et al. (2013) noted that recirculation in conventional jet nebulizers and heat from ultrasonic nebulizers might adversely affect the biological activity of the macromolecule. Furthermore, although it is optimal to use the intended clinical device for animal studies, the relatively large material requirements for a study might be cost or logistically prohibitive. Thus, as for all aspects of a biotherapeutic development program, selection of appropriate generation methods for the aerosol should be on a case-by-case basis.

Direct pulmonary delivery requires endotracheal delivery into the lung, whereas passive delivery uses a nose-only or

TABLE 8.2

The Major Advantages and Disadvantages Associated with Various Modes of Inhalation Exposure in Animal Toxicity/Pharmacokinetic Studies

Mode	Advantages	Disadvantages
Whole body (rodents)	A large number of animals can be tested	Dermal, eye, and oral exposure, in addition to inhalation
	Suitable for chronic studies	High test article demand
	Minimal restraint	Expensive
	Labor efficient	Excreta can interact with the test article and alter PK if coprophagy occurs
Head only (rodents)	Repeated exposure	Animal stress
	Minimal skin contamination	Large test article loss
	Efficient dose delivery	Neck seal imperfect
	Better control of dose	Labor intensive
Nose/mouth only (large animal)	No skin contamination	Can be stressful to the animal
	Repeated exposure	Face seal required
	Uses less test article	Technically difficult
	Exposures can be pulsed	Labor intensive
	Minimal contamination	
Lung only (pulmonary instillation or insufflation) (rodents)	Precision of dose	Anesthesia or tracheostomy required; stressful to animals
	Uses least amount of test article (efficient)	Bypasses nose
		Artifacts in deposition and response
		Technically difficult

Source: Adapted/expanded from Phalen (1996), Table 5.1.
PK, pharmacokinetics.

a whole-body chamber. Endotracheal delivery of therapeutics and vaccines allows investigators to deliver the payload directly into the lung without the limitations associated with passive pulmonary administration methods (Price, 2018). Additionally, endotracheal delivery can achieve deep lung delivery without the involvement of other exposure routes and is more reproducible and quantitative than passive pulmonary delivery in terms of accurate dosing (Price, 2018).

For direct administration into the lungs, intratracheal administration, pulmonary instillation (liquid), or insufflation (dry powder) methods can be used as an alternative to inhalation (Driscoll et al., 2000). These methods require placement of the device into the trachea or bronchi once the animal is lightly anesthetized, followed by administration of aerosolized liquid or dry powder. Once dispensed, the test article is delivered directly to the upper airways with subsequent deposition in the lower airways for absorption. These methods mimic the single inhalation from a clinical device, whereas nose-only inhalation methods generally require longer dosing durations to achieve similar exposure levels achieved clinically.

Whole body exposure (or immersion) systems employ chambers in which the animals can move about, either unrestrained or in cages (Phalen, 1996). These systems allow for larger sample size, are relatively nonstressful for the animal, allow for longer dosing durations, and are less difficult to manage. The disadvantages of these whole-body systems are that they expose all surfaces of the body and require much larger amounts of the test article. Head-only exposure systems permit insertion of the head into the inhalation chamber. The advantages of head-only exposure systems are they can be used in repeat dose studies and expose less of the body to the test article and require less test article than whole-body systems. The disadvantage of head-only systems is that they require more technical labor and can be less accurate. Nose-only or mouth-only exposure systems include tapered cones (rodents), masks (dogs, rabbits, nonhuman primates), or oropharyngeal cannula that position an exposure system tube inside the mouth (requires anesthesia) (Phalen, 1996). These systems are labor intensive; however, they are very efficient in delivering accurate amounts of test article.

In animals, oral inhalation can be mimicked by intratracheal instillation, intratracheal inhalation, pulmonary instillation, or pulmonary insufflation. The most common method used in laboratory is the intratracheal instillation. In animal studies, intratracheal instillation has frequently been used to assess the pulmonary absorption and systemic bioavailability, especially regarding the precise dosing and effectiveness associated with this method (Patil, 2012). However, intratracheal instillation is not a physiological route for application, and results obtained from these studies may not be transferable to aerosol inhalation in animals, let alone humans. Inhalation methods using aerosol techniques such as nose-only in rodents provide a more uniform distribution of the aerosol, assuming the appropriate particle size. However, this method is more costly and technically challenging, and it is difficult to measure the exact dose delivered to the lungs.

Several techniques have been used to circumvent the rapid elimination of biopharmaceuticals from the lungs (Guichard et al., 2017). Nanoparticles and liposomes do not permit the delivery of high doses or proteins via the pulmonary route and their preparation can be stressful for the biopharmaceutical.

8.5 Advances in Pulmonary Delivery Systems

Biologics formulated for DPIs have included powder drugs, vaccines, and immunotherapeutics delivered by the pulmonary route (Ruge et al., 2013). Pulmonary delivery to the deep lung in animal models can be performed using either direct administration methods or by passive inhalation.

There are several preclinical methods to evaluate pulmonary delivery of biologics. Evaluation of inhaled drug delivery can be predicted using in silico and in vitro methods. Ex vivo and in vivo models can be implemented using in silico models or aerosol deposition and cascade impactor data to estimate drug dose, delivery, and deposition. Newer models include advanced cell culture using multiple cell layers, lung-on-chip technology, lung imaging, and pharmacokinetic modeling. Preclinical testing is not to be separated from clinical evaluation, as small proof-of-concept clinical studies or conversely large-scale clinical data may inform which preclinical models are most appropriate or relevant for longer versus shorter term studies. The extend of expertise required for such translational research is unlikely to be found in one single laboratory (Cazzola et al., 2020).

More and more therapeutic proteins are developed for an administration by inhalation to treat respiratory diseases. Local pulmonary delivery of biotherapeutics may offer advantages for the treatment of lung diseases. Delivery of the therapeutic entity directly to the lung has the potential for a rapid onset of action, reduced systemic exposure and the need for a lower dose, as well as needleless administration. However, formulation of a protein for inhaled delivery is challenging and requires proteins with favorable biophysical properties suitable to withstand the forces associated with formulation, delivery, and inhalation devices.

Nanobodies are the smallest functional fragments derived from a naturally occurring heavy chain–only immunoglobulin. They are highly soluble and stable and show biophysical characteristics that are particularly well suited for pulmonary delivery. There are advantages of using nanobodies for inhaled delivery to the lung as illustrated by ALX-0171, a nanobody in clinical development for the treatment of respiratory syncytial virus (RSV) infections (Van Heeke et al., 2017).

8.6 Toxicity Considerations with Lung Delivery

Numerous studies of single- or repeat-dose administration of macromolecules to the respiratory tract have been reported. Many use nonphysiologic routes of exposure, such as intratracheal instillation. A review of this work is beyond the scope of this chapter; the interested reader is referred to Wolff (1998), Finch (2005), McElroy et al. (2013), and Wolff (2020). Below, we discuss chronic inhalation toxicity studies with clinical drug formulations and the relevance to humans.

8.6.1 Chronic Toxicity Studies

Several investigators have reported results of chronic inhalation of clinical formulations of inhaled insulin powder. McConnell et al. (2006) exposed rats and cynomolgus monkeys to the Exubera®

inhaled insulin powder or excipients alone for 6 months up to hypoglycemia-limited maximum tolerated doses (up to 40× for rats and 4× for monkeys compared with a clinical starting dose). There were no toxicologically relevant findings, no effects on respiratory or pulmonary function parameters, no histopathologic responses in lung or lung-associated lymph nodes, nor in bronchiolar or alveolar cell proliferation markers. Vick et al. (2007) dosed Beagle dogs daily for 26 weeks with either human insulin (Eli Lilly discontinued program) or placebo powder and observed the expected pharmacodynamic effects of insulin. There were neither any toxic effects on a variety of standard toxicologic parameters nor any effects on pulmonary endpoints including respiratory function, BAL lavage assessments, or histologic findings including cell proliferation indices. Chronic inhalation toxicology studies were conducted with Afrezza inhaled insulin and with the novel excipient, Technosphere particles, 26 weeks in rats and 39 weeks in dogs and an inhalation carcinogenicity study in rats. Microscopic findings in rats exposed to Afrezza were attributed to the Technosphere particle component, were confined to nasal epithelia, and consisted of eosinophilic globules and nasal epithelial degeneration. There were no Afrezza-related changes in pulmonary proliferating cell nuclear antigen (PCNA) labeling indices in alveoli, large bronchioles, or terminal bronchioles. Afrezza did not exhibit carcinogenic potential in the 2-year study in rats (Greene et al., 2020).

The animal studies in which no pulmonary BAL findings were shown are consistent with a lack of findings clinically (Liu et al., 2008). In contrast to the chronic animal studies, however, clinical studies have shown some treatment-related effects on forced expiratory volume in 1 second (FEV1); see for example (Teeter and Riese, 2006). The clinical effects were small, evident within 2 weeks of inhaled insulin therapy, nonprogressive, and reversible. However, animal pulmonary function studies are difficult, involve forced ventilatory maneuvers, and are thus not equivalent to human subjects providing FEV1 measurements. In addition, the clinical effects were small, with approximately 1% differences between inhaled insulin versus non-inhalation subject groups. Thus, the apparent discrepancy should not be viewed as a deficiency of animal models, but rather that such small differences cannot be detected with the relatively low number of toxicity study animals using differing procedures from those in the clinical setting.

Green (1994) included inhalation toxicity studies for up to 6 months in rats and monkeys in a larger series of studies supporting the registration of Pulmozyme (recombinant human deoxyribonuclease I [rhDNase] for cystic fibrosis). No respiratory rate findings were reported, and respiratory tract findings included perivascular lymphocytic cuffing, lymphoid hyperplasia, and terminal airway bronchiolitis/alveolitis, the severity of which appeared to be associated with the titer of antibody response to rhDNase. The findings were not considered adverse in recognition that the treatment-related pulmonary findings were primarily consistent with an expected host response to the foreign human protein. Similarly, Bussiere et al. (1997) showed minimal eosinophilic cell infiltration in bronchial mucosa of cynomolgus monkeys inhaling an anti–immunoglobulin E (IgE) antibody in a 60-day inhalation toxicity study; an anti-IgE antibody response was also observed in the serum. McElroy et al. (2013) noted that no adverse effects to the lung were observed in 1- and 6-month inhalation toxicity studies of inhaled human growth hormone although specific details were not described.

8.6.2 Immunogenicity

Regarding immunogenicity of macromolecules delivered via the respiratory tract, long-term toxicity studies of inhaled insulin in animals demonstrated either weak or equivocal anti-insulin antibody responses (McConnell et al., 2006; Vick et al., 2007). There were no exposure-related changes in any histologic or functional endpoints in these studies which might be indicative of immune-mediated adverse effects. These data do not suggest any marked difference in response based on the inhalation route of delivery although there are scant data comparing antidrug antibody responses in animals when biotherapeutics were delivered to the respiratory tract versus more conventional routes. Thus, the anti-insulin antibody responses, where observed, were likely due to a response to a human peptide and not a response to the inhalation delivery itself. Interestingly, clinical data have demonstrated increased immunogenicity, as measured by positive antibody responses, for inhaled insulin versus subcutaneous insulin comparator therapy (Fineberg et al., 2007). However, the observed antibody increases were not associated with any adverse effects on tolerability, safety, or efficacy through 2 years of exposure (Cefalu et al., 2008; Yu et al., 2010; Bode et al., 2015). Thus, neither the preclinical data nor clinical data suggest any deleterious effect of potential immunogenicity that might be unique to the inhalation delivery route. Wolff (1998) reached the same conclusion based on a review of a variety of macromolecules delivered to the respiratory tract.

8.7 Extrapolation for FIH Dose

It is challenging to extrapolate the inhaled doses administered in animal toxicity studies to humans (Wolff, 2020). A variety of assumptions are required, and in addition, it can be challenging to measure the actual doses of drug administered to the respiratory tract of animals. Prestudy aerosol/exposure system validation work is essential to accurately quantify the amount of drug delivered to the breathing zone of the animals. Smaller species tend to have higher specific metabolic rates than larger species, so they have a higher ventilation rate per kilogram. Some of the important parameters, such as respiratory rate and/or minute volume, can be measured at one or a few points during the animal toxicity study. Others such as the fraction of inhaled drug delivered to various subcompartments of the respiratory tract involve assumptions based on the particle size and size distribution. A further complicating factor includes the recognition that the deep lung appears to be the predominant site of absorption into systemic distribution, and the deposition fractions of an inhaled aerosol are different among the various toxicology species and humans (for example, see Schlesinger, 1995; Wolff, 2020).

Green (1994) presented a detailed approach to dose extrapolation to humans for their inhalation toxicity studies of rhDNase described above. The assumptions used were clearly delineated, and the author concluded that while determination of exact doses delivered in inhalation studies is difficult, reasonable estimations of comparative doses on a mg/kg basis can be made. In another study conducted in cynomolgus monkeys in conjunction with an inhaled measles virus vaccine program, MacLoughlin et al. (2016) demonstrated that variation in respiratory tidal volume was the most important determinant in inhaled dose variability. These examples show it is important that the sponsor of any inhaled macromolecule program clearly presents the assumptions made, in order to build confidence in the extrapolation of inhaled doses in animals to those anticipated in humans. Once scientifically justified estimates of toxicity study doses delivered in comparison to humans, some comfort can be taken in the recognition that with a few exceptions (e.g., the number of lung lobes, or the presence/absence of terminal bronchioles), the respiratory tract structure and the types of cells present are reasonably similar between typical toxicity study species and humans.

8.8 Regulatory Considerations for Inhaled Biologics

Safety evaluations of biologics administered by the pulmonary route is covered by existing guidelines for biotechnology products, such as ICH S6 (Preclinical Safety Evaluation of Biotechnology-Derived Pharmaceuticals). Preclinical studies in support of clinical trials and registration should utilize the same route of administration as is intended for human use. In animals, dose administration and exposure evaluations should be similar to methods intended to be used clinically. In some cases, substantial safety margins may not be feasible via the pulmonary route (i.e., animal Institutional Animal Care and Use Committee [IACUC] limitations or exaggerated pharmacology); therefore, a scientific rationale should be provided to justify other routes of administration that may be used (i.e., subcutaneous injection). Furthermore, as described above, it may be necessary to incorporate novel excipients into the formulation of an inhaled biologic drug, and this would entail inclusion of additional toxicity studies as described in "Nonclinical Studies for the Safety Evaluation of Pharmaceutical Excipients" (FDA, 2005a).

8.8.1 Guidelines

In addition to regulatory guidance for the specific biotherapeutic, a sponsor needs to follow a variety of guidelines (established by authorities such as the European Medicines Agency and the US Food and Drug Administration [FDA]) on the development of pulmonary drug delivery products. These considerations include matters such as device performance, aerosol characteristics, dose reproducibility and reliability, and others (Deshmukh et al., 2019). Such performance characteristics are particularly important when therapeutic indices between efficacious versus toxic doses may be small. Further safety evaluation of device components such as plastics and rubberized gaskets may be needed (for example, under US Pharmacopoeia or International Organization for Standardization [ISO] testing protocols) for issues such as biocompatibility, irritation potential, and leachable/extractable chemicals.

The goal of the preclinical safety evaluations is to extrapolate from the dose-response data to identify a no-observable-adverse-effect level (NOAEL) (ICH M3(R2)). In addition to toxicity studies, respiratory safety pharmacology studies should be conducted for all compounds administered by the pulmonary route whether or not the target organ is the lung (Gad, 2016). At a minimum, respiratory function (rate and tidal volume in conscious animals) and pulmonary function (rate, tidal volume, minute volume, compliance, and resistance in anesthetized, ventilated animals) should be included in the preclinical safety program. By applying a safety factor to the NOAEL obtained from multiple dose toxicology studies, a safe clinical starting and maximum dose can be proposed and evaluated (FDA Guidance, 2005b).

8.8.2 Device Guidelines

In the United States, FDA's Center for Devices and Radiological Health is responsible for regulating medical devices used for pulmonary delivery. Inhalation devices are classified and based on the classification; regulatory requirements are delineated. Most Class II devices require Premarket Notification 510(k); and most Class III devices require premarket approval. For combination products which are biologic-device products, they are assigned to an agency center that will have primary jurisdiction for that combination product's premarket review and regulation (Draft ICH, 2019). Assignment of a combination product to a lead center is based on a determination of which constituent part provides the primary mode of action (PMOA) of the combination product. If the PMOA of a device-biologic product, a combination product, is attributable to the biological product, the center responsible for premarket review of such a biological product would have primary jurisdiction for the regulation of the combination product. The agency center with primary jurisdiction works with other agency centers to ensure adequate premarket review.

8.9 Future of Inhalation Delivery of Biologics

8.9.1 Biologics

Delivery of pharmacologically active compounds to the lung for systemic effects is well known and recently has entered a new era with several products achieving regulatory approval. Delivery of drugs to the lung for the treatment of pulmonary diseases such as asthma, COPD, pulmonary arterial hypertension, cystic fibrosis, rhinitis, and allergies are dominated by small molecules. Local delivery of biologics to the lung may be advantages to diseases of the pulmonary system. Delivery of drugs to the lung for the treatment of nonpulmonary diseases has shown promise in recent years as well with the registration of inhaled insulins.

The respiratory tract has many protective mechanisms that act as barriers to entry of foreign materials as well as other mechanisms that act to remove materials that penetrate beyond these barriers (Gonda, 2019). Combinations of drugs, such as decongestants, bronchodilators, mucolytics, and nondrug therapies, such as physiotherapy, prior to biologic delivery, are examples of how some of these reversible obstacles can be overcome. Minimizing deposition of the biologic in the oropharynx is important for drugs where efficiency and precision of delivery are important. Macrophages, and possibly other phagocytotic cells, can also ingest these particles which can be advantageous if they are the therapeutic target.

From a safety perspective, inhalation delivery of biologics directly to the sites of therapeutic action in the respiratory tract reduces the potential for systemic distribution and thus systemic side effects. An example is recombinant human DNase for the treatment of cystic fibrosis.

The growing importance of protein and peptide-based drugs as therapeutics is reflected by new drug approval statistics (FDA new drug approvals, 2019) and analysis of the current pharmaceutical pipeline (Clarke, 2017). Biologic-based drugs, targeting neutralization or inhibition of immune/inflammatory mediators, have provided new treatments for severe, persistent allergic asthma (anti-IgE, omalizumab) and severe eosinophilic asthma (IL-5 antagonists, mepolizumab, and reslizumab), and other cytokine antagonists are in late-stage clinical development (McGregor et al., 2019). The search for alternate noninvasive delivery routes to improve patient compliance has been a major objective of technology innovation within the field of pharmaceutical sciences. To date, three inhaled biologics have been approved, Pulmozyme® (dornase alfa for cystic fibrosis), Exubera® (insulin - withdrawn 2007), and Afrezza® (insulin). Concerns remain over long-term safety for the approved inhaled insulin product, reflected in a boxed warning regarding use in patients with extant respiratory disease (asthma and COPD) and smokers due to risk of acute bronchospasm as well as a postmarketing commitment to evaluate, through a randomized clinical trial, the potential risk of pulmonary malignancy, cardiovascular risk, and long-term effect on pulmonary function (Afrezza, prescribing information). Although carcinogenicity has been a potential concern with inhaled insulins (Gatto et al., 2019), clinical data do not support a greater risk with inhalation insulin versus subcutaneous injection.

The indications that are being targeted by inhaled therapies indicate a major focus on local lung disease (Borghardt et al., 2018). Other respiratory diseases targeted by biologics include cystic fibrosis, idiopathic pulmonary fibrosis, bronchiectasis, and treatment/prophylaxis of infection with respiratory pathogens (RSV, tuberculosis, pseudomonas spp., influenza) (Brenner, 2017; Chow, 2020). The inhaled route may also prove to be an appropriate portal for delivery of small interfering ribonucleic acid (siRNA) therapies (Liang, 2015a, b; Aguilo et al., 2015). Inhaled vaccines have been demonstrated to invoke effective mucosal immunoglobin A (IgA) and systemic immunoglobin G (IgG) immune responses and offer a number of advantages for large-scale administration (Omri, 2015; Tonnis et al., 2012). Another example includes the class of inhaled oligonucleotides (ONs). Several of these have reached clinical investigation over the last decade (for example, SB010, an antisense ON being investigated for allergic asthma). Preclinical data describing the respiratory tract effect of ON constructs have been summarized by Alton et al. (2012). Following relatively high doses, findings include accumulation of alveolar macrophages, interstitial macrophage/mononuclear cell infiltration and accumulation in the lung, occasional hemorrhage possibly secondary to inflammation, and fibroplasia and metaplasia in the lung or lung-associated tissues, usually with pronounced inflammation. Translation of these effects to the clinical setting is largely unknown; clinical trials to date have been of relatively short duration and lower doses. The ability to monitor research subjects receiving these inhaled ONs is also a challenge because of the relative inaccessibility of the lungs.

Genome-editing technologies such as clustered regularly interspaced short palindromic repeats (CRISPRs)/CRISPR-associated protein 9 systems provide potential precise genome-editing technology as a novel therapeutic strategy in many diseases, including pulmonary disorders such as cystic fibrosis and α-1 antitrypsin deficiency. Pulmonary delivery of therapeutic genes by inhalation requires the specific biopharmaceutical to be delivered in the form of an aerosol (Chow et al., 2020). Progress has been made in the development and identification of genome targets, optimization of delivery vectors and transfection efficiency, reduction of off-target effects, and improvement in safety profile. Inhalation delivery of suitable CRISPR formulations is an ongoing challenge. Selective lung-targeted delivery by lipid nanoparticles has shown potential for the safe and efficient delivery of genome-editing elements. Aerosolizable genome-editing delivery systems with either viral or nonviral vectors also contribute to the development of optimal formulation for lung genetic disorders (Wan and Ping, 2020).

8.9.2 Devices

The demand for cost effective inhalers competes with new inhalers with improved capabilities. For example, devices for MDI, DPI, and nebulizer products have been commercialized for MDI products (MD Turbo developed by Respirics, propellers developed by Propeller Health, smart inhalers developed by Adherium Ltd.) (Stein and Thiel, 2017). Some new features of these devices include providing reminders to take a dose or order a new inhaler, providing breath actuation, training the patient on the appropriate inhalation maneuver, and recording the time and location of each dose to evaluate adherence to the prescribed dosing regimen. Some device systems provide Bluetooth functionality to sync with apps on mobile devices and allow the patient to share treatment data with others so that family members or physicians can monitor adherence or even control the disease state. Future improvements and added features of inhalation devices are intended to improve therapeutic outcomes and ease of use.

8.10 Conclusion

There are several examples of successful inhaled biologics in development and as approved, marketed products. The ability of a drug to bypass hepatic metabolism provides an advantage over other routes of administration and in some cases, greatly increases bioavailability. The inhalation route provides a noninvasive route to administer a therapeutic which is attractive to certain populations who may have difficulty swallowing pills/tablets or have an aversion to injections. The lungs provide an extensive surface area for rapid drug delivery;

however, there are multiple challenges with pulmonary delivery which include intrinsic barriers such as mucus, enzymes, and immune cells. To successfully deliver a biologic therapeutic through the inhalation route, it is important to consider the particle formulation, size and delivery method. In general, pulmonary formulations are more stable than injectables and thus, may be better suited for widespread distribution. Devices that deliver inhaled biologics are pressurized MDIs, DPIs, or nebulizers. Over the years, these devices have become more sophisticated and compact to facilitate ease of use and increase successful delivery. The future of inhaled biologics will see technologically advanced delivery devices, improved formulations, and successful use of the pulmonary route for multiple therapeutics. Despite considerable investigation over the last few decades, many specific aspects of absorption of biologics from the respiratory tract are incompletely understood.

REFERENCES

Aguilo, N., Alvarez-Arguedas, S., Uranga, S., Marinova, D., Monzón, M., Badiola, J., Martin, C. 2015. Pulmonary but not subcutaneous delivery of BCG vaccine confers protection to tuberculosis-susceptible mice by an interleukin 17-dependent mechanism. *Journal of Infectious Diseases.* 212 (11):831–839. doi: 10.1093/infdis/jiv503.

Alfagih, I., Kunda, N., Alanazi, F., Dennison, S.R., Somavarapu, S., Hutcheon, G.A., Saleem, I.Y. 2015. Pulmonary delivery of proteins using nanocomposite microcarriers. *Journal of Pharmaceutical Sciences.* 104 (12):4386–4398. doi: 10.1002/jps.24681.

Alton, E.W., Boushey, H.A., Garn, H., Green, F.H., Hodges, M., Martin, R.J., Murdoch, R.D., Renz, H., Shrewsbury, S.B., Seguin, R., Johnson, G., Parry, J.D., Tepper, J., Renzi, P., Cavagnaro, J., Ferrari, N. 2012. Clinical expert panel on monitoring potential lung toxicity of inhaled oligonucleotides: consensus points and recommendations. *Nucleic Acid Therapeutics.* 22(4):246–254.

Anselmo, A.C., Gokarn, Y., Mitragotri, S. 2018. Non-invasive delivery strategies for biologics. *Nature Reviews Drug Discovery.* 18 (1):19–40. doi: 10.1038/nrd.2018.183.

Aragao-Santiago, L., Hillaireau, H., Grabowski, N., Mura, S., Nascimento, T.L., Dufort, S., Coll, J.-L., Tsapis, N., Fattal, E. 2016. Compared in vivo toxicity in mice of lung delivered biodegradable and non-biodegradable nanoparticles. *Nanotoxicology.* 10 (3):292–302. doi: 10.3109/17435390.2015.1054908.

Afrezza Package Insert: https://www.accessdata.fda.gov/drug-satfda_docs/label/2014/022472lbl.pdf.

Becker, R.H.A., Sha, S., Frick, A.D., Fountaine, R.J. 2006. The effect of smoking cessation and subsequent resumption on absorption of inhaled insulin. *Diabetes Care.* 29: 277–282.

Brenner, J.S. 2017. Nanomedicine for the treatment of acute respiratory distress syndrome: The 2016 ATS Bear cage award-winning proposal. *Annals of the American Thoracic Society.* 14 (4):561–564. doi: 10.1513/AnnalsATS.201701-090PS.

Borghardt, J.M., Kloft, C., Sharma, A., 2018. Inhaled therapy in respiratory disease: The complex interplay of pulmonary kinetic processes. *Canadian Respiratory Journal.* 2018, Article ID 2732017.

Bussiere, J. 2008. Species selection considerations for preclinical toxicology studies for biotherapeutics *Expert Opin Drug metab Toxicol.* 4(7): 871–877. doi: 10.1517/17425255.4.7.871.

Bussiere, J.L., Gross, M.C., Ruppel, J.M., Marian, M.L., Placke, M.E., Turner, N.A. 1997. 60-day repeated dose inhalation toxicity study of an anti-IGE antibody in Cynomolgus monkeys. Abstract Presented at the Society of Toxicology 36th Annual Meeting, March, 1997, Cincinnati, Ohio. *The Toxicologist.* 36;271. Abstract 1376.

Byron, P.R., Patton, J.S. 1994. Drug delivery via the respiratory tract. *Journal of Aerosol Medicine and Pulmonary Drug Delivery.* 7:49–75.

Bode, B.W., McGill, J.B., Lorber, D., Gross, J.L., Chang, P.C., Bregman, D.B. 2015. Inhaled Technosphere Insulin compared with injected prandial insulin in Type 1 Diabetes: A randomized 24-week trial. *Diabetes Care.* 38: 2266–2273.

Cassidy, J.P., Amin, N., Marino, M., Gotfried, M., Meyer, T., Sommerer, K., Baughman, R.A. 2011. Insulin lung deposition and clearance following Technosphere® insulin inhalation powder administration. *Pharmaceutical Research.* 28(9):2157–2164.

Cazzola, M., Cavalli, F., Usmani, O.S., Rogliani, P. 2020. Advances in pulmonary drug delivery devices for the treatment of chronic obstructive pulmonary disease. *Expert Opinion on Drug Delivery.* 17 (5): 635–646. doi: 10.1080/17425247.2020.1739021.

Cefalu, W.T., Bohannon, N.J., Fineberg, S.E., Teeter, J.G., Schwartz, P.F., Reis, J.M., Krasner, A.S. 2008 Assessment of long-term immunological and pulmonary safety of inhaled human insulin with up to 24 months of continuous therapy. *Current Medical Research and Opinion.* 24(11):3073–3083.

Chow, M.Y.T., Chang, R.Y.K., Chan, H.-K. 2020. Inhalation delivery technology for genome-editing of respiratory diseases. *Advanced Drug Delivery Reviews.* doi: 10.1016/j.addr.2020.06.001.

Chung, S.W., Hil-Lal, T.A., Byun, Y. 2012. Strategies for non-invasive delivery of biologics. *Journal of Drug Targeting.* 20 (6):481–501. doi: 10.3109/1061186X.2012.693499.

Clarke, J.G. 2017. Where have all the inhaled biologics gone? Drug Delivery to the Lungs (DDL2017). Accessed August 1, 2021 at https://ddl-conference.com/ddl2017/conference-papers/inhaled-biologics-gone/

Colthorpe, P., Farr, S.J., Taylor, G. et al. 1992. The pharmacokinetics of pulmonary delivered insulin: A comparison of intratracheal and aerosol administration to the rabbit. *Pharmaceutical Research.* 9:764–768.

Crandall, E.D., Matthay, M.A. 2001. Alveolar epithelial transport. Basic science to clinical medicine. *American Journal of Respiratory and Critical Care Medicine.* 162:1021–1029.

D'Angelo, I., Costabile, G., Durantie, E., Brocca, P., Rondelli, V., Russo, A., Russo, G., Miro, A., Quaglia, F., Petri-Fink, A., Rothen-Rutishauser, B., Ungaro, F. 2018. Hybrid lipid/polymer nanoparticles for pulmonary delivery of siRNA: Development and fate upon in vitro deposition on the human epithelial airway barrier. *Journal of Aerosol Medicine and Pulmonary Drug Delivery.* 31 (3):170–181. doi: 10.1089/jamp.2017.1364.

Derendorf, H., Hochhaus, G., Mollmann, H. 2001. Evaluation of pulmonary absorption using pharmacokinetic methods. *Journal of Aerosol Medicine and Pulmonary Drug Delivery.* 14(Suppl 1):S9–S17.

Deshmukh, R., Bandyopadhyay, N., Abed, S.N., Bandopadhyay, S., Pal, Y., Deb, P.K. 2019. Strategies for pulmonary delivery of drugs. *Drug Delivery Systems*. 85–129. doi: 10.1016/B978-0-12-814487-9.00003-X.

Driscoll, K., Costa, D., Hatch, G., Henderson, R., Oberdorster, G., Salem, H., Schlesinger, R. 2000. Intratracheal instillation as an exposure technique for the evaluation of respiratory tract toxicity: uses and limitations. *Toxicological Sciences*. 55:24–35.

Duckworth, W.C., Bennett, R.G., Hamel, F.G. 1998. Insulin degradation: progress and potential. *Endocrine Reviews*. 19(5):608–624.

FDA. 1994. FDA Summary Basis for Approval (SBA) for Pulmozyme. Accessed July 31, 2021 at https://www.accessdata.fda.gov/scripts/cder/daf/index.cfm?event=overview.process&ApplNo=103532

FDA. 2005a. Guidance for Industry Nonclinical Studies for the Safety Evaluation of Pharmaceutical Excipients.

FDA. 2005b. Guidance for Estimating the Maximum Safe Starting Dose in Initial Clinical Trials for Therapeutics in Adult Healthy Volunteers.

FDA. 2006. FDA Summary Basis for Approval (SBA) for Exubera. Accessed July 31, 2021 at https://www.accessdata.fda.gov/drugsatfda_docs/nda/2006/021868_exubera_toc.cfm

FDA. 2014. FDA Summary Basis for Approval (SBA) for Afrezza. Accessed July 31, 2021 at https://www.accessdata.fda.gov/drugsatfda_docs/nda/2014/022472Orig1s000SumR.pdf

FDA. 2019. New Drug Approvals. https://www.fda.gov/drugs/new-drugs-fda-cders-new-molecular-entities-and-new-therapeutic-biological-products/new-drug-therapy-approvals.

Finch, G.L. 2005. "Nonclinical Pharmacology and Safety Studies of Insulin Administered to the Respiratory Tract", Chapter 25 in *Inhalation Toxicology*, 2nd ed., H.E. Salem, ed., Boca Raton, FL: Taylor & Francis, pp. 603–614. doi: 10.1201/9781420037302.

Fineberg, S.E., Kawabata, T.T., Krasner, A.S., Fineberg, N.S. 2007. Insulin antibodies with pulmonary delivery of insulin. *Diabetes Technology & Therapeutics*. 9 (Suppl 1):S102–S110.

Forbes, B., Wilson, C.G., Gumbleton, M. 1999. Temporal dependence of ectopeptidase expression in alveolar epithelial cell culture: Implications for study of peptide absorption. *International Journal of Pharmaceutics*. 180:225–234.

Fountaine, R., Milton, A., Checchio, T., Wei, G., Stolar, M., Teeter, J., Jaeger, R., Fryburg, D. 2008. Acute passive cigarette smoke exposure and inhaled human insulin (Exubera) pharmacokinetics. *British Journal of Clinical Pharmacology*. 65(6):864–870.

Gad, S. 2016. "Safety Assessment of Therapeutic Agents Administered by the Respiratory Routes". Chapter 22 in *Inhalation Toxicology* 3rd ed., Salen H. and Katz S., Boca Raton, FL: Taylor & Francis, pp. 537–581. doi: 10.1201/b16781.

Gatto, N.M., Koralek, D.O., Bracken, M.B., Duggan, W.T., Lem, J., Klioze, S., Koch, G.G., Wise, R.A., Cohen, R.B., Jackson, N.C. 2019. Lung cancer-related mortality with inhaled insulin or a comparator: Follow-up study of patients previously enrolled in Exubera controlled clinical trials (FUSE) final results. *Diabetes Care*. 42(9):1708–1715.

Gaul, R., Ramsey, J.M., Heise, A., Cryan, S.-A., Greene, C.M. 2018. Nanotechnology approaches to pulmonary drug delivery: Targeted delivery of small molecule and gene-based therapeutics to the lung. *Design of Nanostructures for Versatile Therapeutic Applications*. 221–253. doi: 10.1016/B978-0-12-813667-6.00006-1.

Gonda, I. 2019. Is there a future for the respiratory delivery of biologics? *On Drug Delivery Magazine*. 96: 6–10.

Green, J.D. 1994. Pharmaco-toxicological expert report Pulmozyme rhDNase Genentech, Inc. *Human & Experimental Toxicology*. 13 (Suppl 1):S1–S42.

Greene, S., Nikula, K., Poulin, D., McInally, K., Reynolds, J. 2020. Long-term nonclinical pulmonary safety assessment of Afrezza, a novel insulin inhalation powder. *Toxicologic Pathology*. Supplemental Article: 1–15. doi: 10.1177/0192623320960420.

Guichard, M.-J., Leal, T., Vanbever, R. 2017. PEGylation, an approach for improving the pulmonary delivery of biopharmaceuticals. *Current Opinion in Colloid and Interface Science*. 31:43–50. doi: 10.1016/j.cocis.2017.08.001.

Heinemann, L., Baughman R., Boss A., Hompesch M. 2017. Pharmacokinetic and pharmacodynamic properties of novel inhaled insulin. *Journal of Diabetes Science and Technology*. 11(1):148–156.

Hidalgo, A., Cruz, A., Pérez-Gil, J. 2015. Barrier or carrier? Pulmonary surfactant and drug delivery. *European Journal of Pharmaceutics and Biopharmaceutics*. 95:117–127. doi: 10.1016/j.ejpb.2015.02.014.

ICH Draft Guidance Combination Products 2019. Bridging for Drug-Device and Biologic-Device Combination Products Guidance for Industry.

ICH Draft Guidance 2019. Principles of Premarket Pathways for Combination Products Guidance for Industry and FDA Staff.

ICH M3(R2) 2010. Nonclinical Safety Studies for the Conduct of Human Clinical Trials and Marketing Authorization for Pharmaceuticals.

ICH S6(R1) Preclinical Safety Evaluation of Biotechnology-Derived Pharmaceuticals 5/17/2012.

Iozzo, P., Osman, S., Glaser, M., et al. 2002. In vivo imaging of insulin receptors by PET: preclinical evaluation of iodine-125 and iodine-124 labelled human insulin. *Nuclear Medicine and Biology*. 29:73–82.

Kolte, A., Patil, S., Lesimple, P., Hanrahan, J.W., Misra, A. 2017. PEGylated composite nanoparticles of PLGA and polyethylenimine for safe and efficient delivery of pDNA to lungs. *International Journal of Pharmaceutics*. 524 (1–2):382–396. doi: 10.1016/j.ijpharm.2017.03.094.

Komada, F., Iwakawa, S., Yamamoto, N., et al. 1994. Intratracheal delivery of peptide and protein agents: Absorption from solution and dry powder by rat lung. *Journal of Pharmacological Sciences* 83:863–867.

Kourmatzis, A., Cheng, S., Chan, H.-K. 2018. Airway geometry, airway flow, and particle measurement methods: implications on pulmonary drug delivery. *Expert Opinion on Drug Delivery*. 15 (3):271–282. doi: 10.1080/17425247.2018.1406917.

Kumar, A., Mansour, H.M., Friedman, A., Blough, E.R. 2013. Nanomedicine in drug delivery. *Nanomedicine in Drug Delivery*. 1–431. doi: 10.1201/b14802.

Laube, B.L., Benedict, G., Dobs, A. 1998. Time to peak insulin level, relative bioavailability, and effect of site of deposition of nebulized insulin in patients with non-insulin dependent diabetes mellitus. *Journal of Aerosol Medicine and Pulmonary Drug Delivery.* 11:153–173.

Liang, W., Chow, M.Y.T., Lau, P.N., Zhou, Q.T., Kwok, P.C.L., Leung, G.P.H., Mason, A.J., Chan, H.-K., Poon, L.L.M., Lam, J.K.W. 2015a. Inhalable dry powder formulations of siRNA and pH-responsive peptides with antiviral activity against H1N1 influenza virus. *Molecular Pharmaceutics.* 12 (3):910–921. doi: 10.1021/mp500745v.

Liang, Z., Ni, R., Zhou, J., Mao, S. 2015b. Recent advances in controlled pulmonary drug delivery. *Drug Discovery Today.* 20 (3):380–389. doi: 10.1016/j.drudis.2014.09.020.

Liu, Q., Guan, J., Qin, L., Zhang, X., Mao, S. 2020. Physicochemical properties affecting the fate of nanoparticles in pulmonary drug delivery. *Drug Discovery Today.* 25 (1):150–159. doi: 10.1016/j.drudis.2019.09.023.

Liu, M.C., Riese, R.J., Van Gundy, K., Norwood, P., Sullivan, B.E., Schwartz, P.F., Teeter, J.G. 2008. Effects of inhaled human insulin on airway lining fluid composition in adults with diabetes. *European Respiratory Journal.* 32(1):180–188.

MacLoughlin, R.J., van Amerongen, G., Fink, J.B., Janssens, H.M., Duprex, W.P., de Swart, R.L. 2016. Optimization and dose estimation of aerosol delivery to non-human primates. *Journal of Aerosol Medicine and Pulmonary Drug Delivery.* 29(3):281–287. doi: 10.1089/jamp.2015.1250.

Mathias, N.R., Yamashita, F., Lee, V.H.L. 1996. Respiratory epithelial cell culture models for evaluation of ion and drug transport. *Advanced Drug Delivery Reviews.* 22:215–249.

McConnell, W.R., Finch, G., Elwell, M., Kawabata, T., Moutvic, R., Shaw, M., Stammberger, I. 2006. Toxicological Investigations on Inhaled Insulin. Abstract #619, The Toxicologist, 45th Annual Meeting of the Society of Toxicology, San Diego, CA; March 2006.

McElroy, M.C., Kirton, C., Gliddon, D., Wolff, R.K. 2013. Inhaled biopharmaceutical drug development: nonclinical considerations and case studies. *Inhalation Toxicology.* 25(4):219–232.

McGregor, M.C., Krings, J.G., Nair, P., Castro, M., 2019. Role of biologics in asthma. *American Journal of Respiratory and Critical Care Medicine.* 199(4): 433–445.

Mejías, J.C., Roy, K. 2019. In-vitro and in-vivo characterization of a multi-stage enzyme-responsive nanoparticle-in-microgel pulmonary drug delivery system. *Journal of Controlled Release.* 316:393–403. doi: 10.1016/j.jconrel.2019.09.012.

Mendivil, C.O., Teeter, J.G., Finch, G.L., Schwartz, P.F., Riese, R.J., Brain, J.D. 2012. Trough insulin levels in bronchoalveolar lavage following inhaled human insulin (Exubera) in patients with diabetes mellitus. *Diabetes Technology & Therapeutics.* 14(1):50–58.

Mendivil, C.O., Koziel, H., Brain, J.D. 2015. Metabolic hormones, apolipoproteins, adipokines, and cytokines in the alveolar lining fluid of healthy adults: compartmentalization and physiological correlates. *PLoS One.* 10(4): e0123344.

Omri, A. 2015. Pulmonary drug and vaccine delivery: Therapeutic significance and major challenges. *Expert Opinion on Drug Delivery.* 12 (6):853–855. doi: 10.1517/17425247.2015.1044277.

Paranjpe, M., Müller-Goymann, C.C. 2014. Nanoparticle-mediated pulmonary drug delivery: A review. *International Journal of Molecular Sciences.* 15 (4):5852–5873. doi: 10.3390/ijms15045852.

Patil, J.S., Sarasija, S. 2012. Pulmonary drug delivery strategies: A concise, systematic review. *Lung India.* 29(1): 44–49.doi: 10.4103/0970-2113.92361.

Patton, J.S. 1996. Mechanisms of macromolecule absorption by the lungs. *Advanced Drug Delivery Reviews.* 19:3–36.

Patton, J.S., Bukar, J., and Nagarajan, S. 1999. Inhaled insulin. *Advanced Drug Delivery Reviews.* 35:235–247.

Phalen, R.F., Yeh, H.-C., Prasad, S.B. 1996. Morphology of the Respiratory Tract. In *Concepts in Inhalation Toxicology,* McClellan RO and Henderson RF, editors. Washington, DC: Taylor and Francis.

Pillai, R.S., Hughes, B.L., Wolff, R.K., et al. 1996. The effect of pulmonary-delivered insulin on blood glucose levels using two nebulizer systems. *Journal of Aerosol Medicine and Pulmonary Drug Delivery.* 9:227–240.

Price, D.N., Kunda, N.K., Muttil, P. 2019. Challenges associated with the pulmonary delivery of therapeutic dry powders for preclinical testing. *KONA Powder and Particle Journal.* 36:129–144. doi: 10.14356/kona.2019008.

Price, D.N., Muttil, P. 2018. Delivery of therapeutics to the lung. *Methods in Molecular Biology.* 1809:415–429. doi: 10.1007/978-1-4939-8570-8_27.

Qiu, Y., Man, R.C.H., Liao, Q., Kung, K.L.K., Chow, M.Y.T., Lam, J.K.W. 2019. Effective mRNA pulmonary delivery by dry powder formulation of PEGylated synthetic KL4 peptide. *Journal of Controlled Release.* 314:102–115. doi: 10.1016/j.jconrel.2019.10.026.

Röhm, M., Carle, S., Maigler, F., Flamm, J., Kramer, V., Mavoungou, C., Schmid, O., Schindowski, K. 2017. A comprehensive screening platform for aerosolizable protein formulations for intranasal and pulmonary drug delivery. *International Journal of Pharmaceutics.* 532 (1):537–546. doi: 10.1016/j.ijpharm.2017.09.027.

Ruge, A.C., Kirch, J., Lehr, C.-M. 2013. Pulmonary drug delivery: From generating aerosols to overcoming biological barriers-therapeutic possibilities and technological challenges. *The Lancet Respiratory Medicine.* 1 (5):402–413. doi: 10.1016/S2213-2600(13)70072-9.

Schlesinger, R.B. Deposition and clearance of inhaled particles. 1995. In *Concepts in Inhalation Toxicology.* McClellan RO and Henderson RF, editors. Washington, DC: Taylor and Francis.

Shen, A., Zhang, Q., Wei, S., et al. 1999. Proteolytic enzymes as a limitation for pulmonary absorption of insulin: in vitro and in vivo investigations. *International Journal of Pharmaceutics.* 192:115–121.

Stein, S.W., Thiel, C.G. 2017. The history of therapeutic aerosols: A chronological review. *Journal of Aerosol Medicine and Pulmonary Drug Delivery.* 30 (1):20–41. doi: 10.1089/jamp.2016.1297.

Teeter, J.G., Riese, R.J. 2006. Dissociation of lung function changes with humoral immunity during inhaled human insulin therapy. *American Journal of Respiratory and Critical Care Medicine.* 173(11): 1194–1200.

Tonnis, W.F., Kersten, G.F., Frijlink, H.W., Hinrichs, W.L.J., De Boer, A.H., Amorij, J.-P. 2012. Pulmonary vaccine delivery: A realistic approach? *Journal of Aerosol Medicine and Pulmonary Drug Delivery.* 25 (5):249–260. doi: 10.1089/jamp.2011.0931.

Van Heeke, G., Allosery, K., De Brabandere, V., De Smedt, T., Detalle, L., de Fougerolles, A. 2017. Nanobodies® as inhaled biotherapeutics for lung diseases. *Pharmacology and Therapeutics.* 169:47–56. doi: 10.1016/j.pharmthera.2016.06.012.

Vick, A., Wolff, R., Koester, A., Reams, R., Deaver, D.R., Heidel, S. 2007. A 6-month inhalation study to characterize the toxicity, pharmacokinetics, and pharmacodynamics of human insulin inhalation powder (HIIP) in beagle dogs. *Journal of Aerosol Medicine and Pulmonary Drug Delivery.* 20(2):112–126.

Wan, T. and Ping, Y. 2020. Delivery of genome-editing biomacromolecules for treatment of lung genetic disorders *Advanced Drug Delivery Reviews.* Article in Press.

Wolff, R.K. 1998. Safety of inhaled proteins for therapeutic use. *Journal of Aerosol Medicine and Pulmonary Drug Delivery.* 11(4):197–219.

Wolff, R.K. 2020. Perspectives on lung dose and inhaled biomolecules. *Toxicologic Pathology.* 192623320946297. doi: 10.1177/0192623320946297.

Woods, A., Patel, A., Spina, D., Riffo-Vasquez, Y., Babin-Morgan, A., De Rosales, R.T.M., Sunassee, K., Clark, S., Collins, H., Bruce, K., Dailey, L.A., Forbes, B. 2015. In vivo biocompatibility, clearance, and biodistribution of albumin vehicles for pulmonary drug delivery. *Journal of Controlled Release.* 210:1–9. doi: 10.1016/j.jconrel.2015.05.269.

Yu, W., Marino, M., Cassidy, J.P., Boss, A.H., Fineberg, S. 2010. Insulin antibodies associated with Technosphere Insulin, *Diabetes.* 59 (Suppl 1) #216-OR.

9

Nonclinical Considerations for Biopharmaceutical Comparability Assessment[*]

C. E. Ellis
DPT-ID, CDER, US-FDA

M. T. Hartsough
Hartsough Nonclinical Consulting LLC

CONTENTS

9.1 Introduction

In this chapter, nonclinical considerations for product comparability assessments, following manufacturing changes, to support clinical trials and marketing applications for biopharmaceuticals are presented and discussed. This chapter focuses on general strategies and considerations for nonclinical comparability assessment and not on providing specific, prescriptive recommendations; applies only to nonclinical considerations for manufacturing changes for biopharmaceuticals occurring during the course of clinical development (*i.e.*, before biologics license application submission) or postapproval (*i.e.*, licensed under section 351(a) of the Public Health Service [PHS] Act) and not specifically to section 351(k) of the PHS Act (*i.e.*, biosimilar) applications (see Chapter 13); and is generally applicable only to proteins intended for therapeutic indications and not to vaccines, blood products, cell, tissue, or gene therapies. Various aspects and perspectives regarding biopharmaceutical comparability have been discussed elsewhere and may be consulted (Lewis, 2008; Lewis and Cosenza, 2010; Putnam et al., 2010; Wright et al., 2018; and Grampp et al., 2018).

The term "biopharmaceutical" applies to protein therapeutic, diagnostic, and prophylactic products derived from expression systems such as bacteria, yeast, insect, plant, and mammalian cells and produced by cells in culture or by recombinant DNA technology, including transgenic plants and animals (refer to ICH S6(R1) Preclinical Safety Evaluation of Biotechnology-Derived Pharmaceuticals [2012]). Biopharmaceuticals (*e.g.*, monoclonal antibodies, cytokines, growth factors, recombinant plasma factors, enzymes, and hormones) are heterogeneous mixtures of high molecular weight molecules (often 10 to >160 kD) defined by process-specific attributes, and so are not single-defined molecular entities. Because these products are essentially defined by the manufacturing methods used, it stands to reason that the product characteristics could change (*i.e.*, not be "highly similar") based on changes in manufacturing occurring during the course of clinical development. Heterogeneity of protein products is due to not only the presence of host cell impurities, etc. but also varying amounts of specific post-translational modifications (*e.g.*, glycosylation, acetylation, acylation, deamidation, oxidation, phosphorylation), amino acid substitutions, truncations, degree of multimerization, etc. Thus, biopharmaceutical products will likely consist of complex mixtures containing many types of protein modifications that determine tertiary structure, function, and, therefore, the overall product characteristics. These product-specific attributes can have safety and functional implications by influencing a variety of properties, including absorption, distribution, metabolism and/or excretion (ADME) characteristics, immunogenicity, pharmacology, and/or toxicity of the product.

The initial comparability assessment is typically related to the product quality (*i.e.*, Chemistry, Manufacturing and Controls). Documents that discuss various aspects of biopharmaceutical comparability have been published and should be consulted, including ICH Q5E "Comparability of Biotechnological/Biological Products Subject to Changes

---

[*] The opinions expressed in this chapter are those of the authors and should be viewed accordingly, unless specific regulatory or statutory requirements are cited.

in their Manufacturing Process" (2005), the European Medicines Agency (EMA) draft "Guideline on comparability of biotechnology-derived medicinal products after a change in the manufacturing process, —nonclinical and clinical issues" (2007), and the Food and Drug Administration (FDA) Guidance "Demonstration of comparability of human biological products, including therapeutic biotechnology-derived products" (1996). These documents focus primarily on product quality aspects of comparability assessment and, so only, address some limited nonclinical considerations for product comparability assessments. Although there is no comprehensive FDA guidance addressing nonclinical comparability assessments, the expected timing and framework for conducting nonclinical studies for biopharmaceuticals have been described in ICH M3(R2) Guidance on Nonclinical Safety Studies for the Conduct of Human Clinical Trials and Marketing Authorization for Pharmaceuticals (2010), ICH S6(R1), and ICH S9 Nonclinical Evaluation of Anticancer Pharmaceuticals (2010) (see Chapter 28). Nonclinical studies for product comparability assessments are often not needed. Considerations for the need, extent of testing, and types of studies conducted when needed are discussed throughout this chapter. As stated explicitly in ICH S6(R1), biopharmaceutical safety assessments must be made using a case-by-case approach, and it is expected that nonclinical studies intended for product comparability assessment would likewise follow this flexible approach. For this reason, it is strongly recommended for those developing biopharmaceuticals (and thus making manufacturing changes during clinical development or after approval) to work closely with the appropriate regulatory authorities when developing a nonclinical program.

9.2 Comparability Principles and Practices

9.2.1 General Product Quality– Related Considerations

There are a wide variety of manufacturing changes that may occur over the course of product development. Many of these changes such as process-related changes due to "scale up" can be anticipated, whereas others may be a bit more unpredictable. Some general categories for manufacturing changes include introducing a new cell line or master cell bank, changing cell culture conditions (*e.g.*, media, fermentation, method), formulation changes (lyophilization, liquid form, excipient changes), introducing new raw materials or reagents, new purification processes, changes in manufacturing site, facilities, equipment, or storage conditions, or some combination of the above. Each of these changes can be associated with different levels of risk regarding their potential to alter product attributes. Thus, a thorough understanding of the new manufacturing process(es) could help one to anticipate how specific changes may affect critical product quality characteristics (*i.e.*, identity, strength, overall quality, purity, potency, stability, consistency). Overall, it is important to have confidence that the manufacturing change is expected to produce a product where the existing nonclinical and clinical data can be relied upon.

Owing to the heterogeneous nature of biopharmaceuticals and the common occurrence of changes in manufacturing, the biopharmaceutical used in nonclinical studies does not have to be identical to what is used in clinical trials but does have to be "highly similar" to be considered comparable (refer to ICH Q5E). In order for prechange and postchange products to be comparable, the physicochemical properties, biological activity, and immunochemical properties must be "highly similar," and when physicochemical or biological differences are detected, these changes should have no adverse impact on the safety or efficacy of the biopharmaceutical. An initial comparability assessment considers whether manufacturing changes are expected to significantly impact critical product quality attributes to warrant additional testing; however, the extent of data collection to inform comparability assessments can vary considerably. Depending on the specific circumstances of the manufacturing change, additional data collection to inform comparability assessments are not always needed. For example, additional testing may not be needed when manufacturing changes are considered minor or occur prior to collection of pivotal in vivo data, as a key reason for conducting a formal assessment is to establish the basis to rely upon previous nonclinical and clinical efficacy and/or safety data. Although minor manufacturing changes are less likely to have a significant impact on product quality characteristics (and so likely to be "highly similar" and comparable), a series of minor changes could have a significant impact, so the decision to conduct product quality–related comparability studies (*i.e.*, side-by-side evaluation of the prechange and postchange material) is made on a case-by-case basis. When additional testing is needed, this is always initiated by product quality–related comparability studies. Note that detailed discussion of product manufacturing and quality assessment methods and/or procedures related to comparability is beyond the scope of this chapter. The goal of this section is simply to provide a broad overview of this type of assessment, including introducing some key issues and considerations regarding product quality data when determining the potential need for nonclinical assessment following a manufacturing change.

Product quality–related comparability assessments typically consist of a series of side-by-side comparisons of the prechange and postchange material using various methods designed to evaluate the physiochemical and biological attributes of the product. Physiochemical and biological characterization consist of rigorous in vitro functional comparisons designed to determine the similarity of structural folding, post-translational processing, carbohydrate content, impurity profile, potency, and other endpoints as appropriate (refer to ICH Q5E). These assays are conducted to determine whether manufacturing changes may affect the safety, identity, purity, or efficacy of the biopharmaceutical.

Critical quality attributes are "a physical, chemical, biological, or microbiological property or characteristic that should be within an appropriate limit, range, or distribution to ensure the desired product quality" [refer to ICH Q8(R2) Pharmaceutical Development (2009)]. Determination of critical product quality attributes of biopharmaceuticals can be both process and product dependent. Thus, utilizing a science-based risk approach is often an iterative process and may change over the course of product development as more information becomes available. Therefore, defining how critical certain product characteristics are by leveraging knowledge about the manufacturing process and how product attributes affect product function help in the selection of assays considered essential for comparability assessment. The types of quality attributes typically evaluated as part of rigorous physiochemical characterization include product-related variants (*e.g.*, size, charge, oxidation, glycosylation, structural), process-related impurities (*e.g.*, host cell proteins), raw materials, leachable compounds, drug product–specific attributes (*e.g.*, subvisible and visible particles, sterility), adventitious agents (*e.g.*, viruses, bacterial endotoxins, and other microbiological impurities) and other general attributes (*e.g.*, appearance, excipients, buffer and protein content, osmolality, pH).

Unlike physiochemical characterization, quality attributes evaluated as part of a typical biological characterization are entirely dependent on information available regarding the biological function of the product (refer to ICH Q6B Specifications: Test Procedures and Acceptance Criteria for Biotechnological/Biological Products [1999]). Assessment is intended to focus on clinically relevant product attributes by evaluating certain critical aspects of biological function(s) using various bioassays. Potency assays are a subset of biological assays that reflect the biological activity of the product (*i.e.*, based on primary mechanism of action(s) [MOA]) and are used to set lot release specifications. However, the most appropriate potency assay is often not selected, identified, and/ or developed until later in clinical development and so may not be available for comparability assessments conducted early in product development. Thus, it may be advisable to develop potency assays early in product development to help facilitate comparability assessments. Biological characterization assays can include binding assays, assays designed to evaluate a specific activity (*e.g.*, complement-dependent cytotoxicity, antibody-dependent cell cytotoxicity), and/or more direct functional assays (*e.g.*, cell culture assays, neutralization assays). Binding assays are typically target-directed binding assays (*i.e.*, evaluate binding characteristics to the intended biological target), including receptor binding assays, but can also assess binding to other proteins that may affect biological activity of the product, including proteins that affect pharmacokinetic (PK) characteristics and effector function for monoclonal antibody (mAb) products. It should also be noted that assay performance characteristics (*e.g.*, selectivity, sensitivity, variability) differ among assays so the most appropriate assays regarding functional assessment may not be the most robust or sensitive assay to measure subtle differences between prechange and postchange material.

Comparison of product quality attributes between the prechange and postchange product, based on predefined criteria, should allow an objective assessment of whether the product is comparable or not. Often analytical testing (physiochemical and biological characterization) is sufficient to demonstrate comparability of the product following a manufacturing change (see outcome #1 below). As stated in ICH Q5E, "If a manufacturer can provide assurance of comparability through analytical studies alone, nonclinical and clinical studies with the postchange product are not warranted." The ICH Q5E

guidance then proceeds to describe various outcomes that the product sponsor/manufacturer may be faced with following analytical study assessments (as briefly summarized below):

1. Postchange product considered "highly similar" and, therefore, comparable
2. Postchange product appears "highly similar" but analytical testing insufficient
3. Postchange product appears "highly similar" and considered comparable (following appropriate justification provided that no adverse impact expected for the observed product differences)
4. Postchange product appears "highly similar" (but possible adverse impact of observed product differences cannot be excluded).
5. Postchange product not "highly similar" and therefore not comparable

Of the potential five outcomes described in ICH Q5E, typically, nonclinical and/or clinical studies may be considered as part of additional testing to support comparability assessment for only outcome #2 and 4. In fact, the only outcome where nonclinical studies should always be considered is when a possible adverse impact of product quality–related differences on the safety or efficacy profiles of the postchange product cannot be excluded (*i.e.*, outcome #4). If the postchange product is not considered comparable based on product quality characteristics (*i.e.*, outcome #5), nonclinical studies to support the comparability assessment are not expected (*i.e.*, nonclinical data would not change the overall assessment). Although it is conceivable that existing nonclinical data with the prechange product could still be used to help support the safety of the postchange product, this decision would be made on a case-by-case basis. Further discussion of this scenario (*i.e.*, outcome #5) is beyond the scope of ICH Q5E and this chapter.

9.2.2 Considerations for Determining the Need for Nonclinical Assessment

The need for nonclinical studies to support a comparability assessment depends primarily on the perceived risk of the product, based on the type(s) and extent of manufacturing change(s), the sensitivity of analytical testing to detect changes that may be of potential significance, general product characteristics, clinical development considerations, as well as the actual results of product quality–related assessment (*i.e.*, physiochemical and biological characterization). It is, therefore, important to leverage not only all available product quality–related data and knowledge regarding the new manufacturing process but also information on general product characteristics and clinical development considerations. It is anticipated that detailed product characteristic information would be available from existing nonclinical and clinical data using the prechange product and from the literature (*e.g.*, biological pathway data). Considering all available information, one may conclude that the product risk level is low, but sometimes, the product may be considered high risk due to specific causes for concern, based on identified safety risk(s) from available information.

Potential causes for concern that may support the conclusion that the product has increased risk, include products with severe, nonmonitorable, and/or irreversible toxicity; variable bioavailability or in other PK-related measurements (e.g., nonlinear PK); steep, inadequate, or poorly defined dose-response relationship; novel target(s) or target(s) with known concerns based on the MOA or product class; and when the product is evaluated in animal models with limited utility (*i.e.*, no pharmacologically relevant species or a species thought to be insensitive/incapable to predict human response). These general product safety concerns are described in ICH Q5E, the FDA Guidance "Demonstration of comparability of human biological products, including therapeutic biotechnology-derived products" (1996), and/or in the FDA Guidance for Industry "Estimating the maximum safe starting dose in initial clinical trials for therapeutics in adult healthy volunteers" (2005). For example, a product may be considered high risk if it belongs to a product class with known concerns due to a narrow therapeutic window for a severe, nonmonitorable, and/or irreversible toxicity. In addition, products that function through novel targets or pathways can be of increased concern given the smaller knowledge base available (*i.e.*, less data and/or experience with target/pathway) and so may pose a higher risk for unexpected findings and/or outcomes. Similarly, a higher risk for unexpected safety outcomes may exist when nonclinical data are obtained from an animal model with limited utility, given the uncertainty about the value of data obtained from these models. Of course, the lack of these specific safety concerns may also support the opposite conclusion that the product may be of lower risk. For example, a product expected to exhibit a benign safety profile for a well-established biological pathway/mechanism of action, shallow dose response (*i.e.*, small changes in product exposure do not clearly alter activity) may be considered low risk. Overall, this benign profile makes it less likely that any small differences in product characteristics following a manufacturing change will have a clinically significant effect on the safety or efficacy of the product. Thus, this safety-related information may influence the decision regarding the need, extent, design, and type of nonclinical (or clinical) studies considered for comparability assessment.

Several additional considerations may also influence decisions regarding nonclinical (or clinical) comparability assessment following a manufacturing change, as well as downstream clinical decisions, including the timing of manufacturing changes as they relate to the clinical phase of product development (during Phase I, II, III, IV), characteristics of the disease or indication to be treated (*e.g.*, life threatening, severely debilitating disease, rare disease with orphan drug designation), medical need of the biotherapeutic, availability and/or features of existing therapies, the intended patient population (population size, age, etc.), and the feasibility of conducting trials in the intended clinical population. In general, making major manufacturing changes late in clinical development is associated with more risk than those made early in development because there is more nonclinical and clinical data available with the prechange product to rely upon. Thus, manufacturing changes made early in development are less likely to require as extensive of a comparability assessment as those made during Phase III. In addition, the more severe

the indication to be treated and the greater the medical need for novel therapies for the indication or patient population, the more flexibility that may be anticipated regarding the extent of comparability assessment. Of course, regulatory decisions based on these general clinical considerations for any given product depend on the specific circumstances (*i.e.*, decisions made on a case-by-case basis).

The need for nonclinical studies to support a comparability assessment often depends on the product quality–related assessment. In most cases, comparison of the in vitro quality attributes of prechange and postchange products is sufficient to establish comparability (*i.e.*, outcome #1 and 3 from ICH Q5E), and nonclinical studies are not necessary. However, sometimes, product quality data may be insufficient, and nonclinical studies in an appropriate animal model may be considered. In this latter scenario, nonclinical data could be collected to help establish comparability (*i.e.*, contribute to the overall comparability assessment) and/or to support clinical evaluation of the postchange material, if there are specific safety concerns based on available data. As discussed previously, situations where nonclinical (or clinical) studies to establish comparability may be considered include the following: when analytical testing is insufficient for comparison of safety and/or efficacy with the reference (prechange) biopharmaceutical (*i.e.*, outcome #2) and where a possible adverse impact on the safety or efficacy profile of the postchange product cannot be excluded when product quality–related alterations are identified (*i.e.*, outcome #4). Regarding outcome #2, it should be noted that although in some cases, analytical testing may be insensitive to detect more subtle changes that could affect product PK/ADME, animal studies may also be insensitive, particularly when a relevant species is not available or when nonhuman primates (NHPs) are the only relevant species (given the low numbers of animals used in these studies). For this and other reasons, we recommend that one should consider collecting additional product quality–related data (physiochemical and/or biological characterization data) to support the comparability assessment for outcome #2, prior to considering conducting animal studies to help resolve any remaining product uncertainties. However, it should be noted that a nonclinical study may be needed if the final biopharmaceutical formulation is changed (*e.g.*, to include a new excipient) or a different route of administration (ROA) is planned (refer to FDA Guidance for Industry "Nonclinical studies for the safety evaluation of pharmaceutical excipients" (2005) and "Nonclinical safety evaluation of reformulated drug products intended for administration by an alternate route" [2015]). In these circumstances, the endpoints may not be related to product comparability, but rather local tolerance, PK differences, etc. that are associated with a ROA change.

In situations where product quality–related alterations have been identified (outcome #4), sometimes, adverse impacts of the alterations cannot be excluded because of the nature or type of changes identified, with some known to have potential effects on product safety or efficacy. For example, some specific biochemical alterations identified in the active moiety may be known to potentially affect biopharmaceutical exposure in vivo (*e.g.*, glycosylation, charge) or may influence other in vivo characteristics. In these situations, particularly when manufacturing changes have occurred later in clinical development, clinical data to support the comparability assessment may be needed, regardless of the outcome of any nonclinical studies conducted. Thus, in many of these situations, nonclinical data may not contribute significantly to the overall comparability assessment (given the availability of clinical data), so collecting it may not be worthwhile. However, one may decide to conduct a nonclinical study to support the safety of the proposed clinical trial for higher risk products, if needed. Over the last several years, product sponsors have been utilizing ever more creative clinical approaches to take advantage of any available clinical data, however limited, including clinical PK modeling approaches and nonpowered clinical PK and/or pharmacodynamic (PD) trials, in lieu of more traditional clinical PK comparability assessment studies. Thus, there are ways to collect and assess clinical data that provide more relevant information for comparability assessment than data obtained in animals.

Depending on the nature of the product quality alterations of the postchange material (in outcome #4), there could be some limited situations where collecting nonclinical data could be used to help limit the scope of clinical assessment (*e.g.*, if manufacturing change occurring early in clinical development) and so could be useful for comparability assessment purposes. For example, for high-risk products with significant product quality–related changes, nonclinical assessment can be considered to answer specific questions. Ultimately, the decision regarding the need for nonclinical evaluation of a postchange product should be made on a case-by-case basis using a risk-based approach. Regrettably, in many cases, it seems that this decision is made by some product sponsors prior to the availability of sufficient product quality–related comparability data, and so based more on product timeline considerations and perhaps regulatory uncertainty regarding the need for such studies. When nonclinical studies are conducted, they should be designed to answer a specific question or safety concern, so conducting animal studies for comparability assessment should not be the default position (*i.e.*, collected just in case the data are needed or requested). In this regard, we recommend contacting the appropriate regulatory authority (*e.g.*, US FDA, EMA, MHRA, PMDA) prior to study conduct to discuss the need for specific nonclinical evaluation of the postchange product.

A series of questions to ask oneself when deciding whether nonclinical studies may be needed for comparability assessment are included in Table 9.1. These questions should be considered carefully prior to conducting any nonclinical study to ensure that the data obtained from a PK, PD, and/or toxicology comparability study is expected to be both useful (*i.e.*, used to answer an important question) and necessary (*i.e.*, information considered critical to make product development decisions). For example, if a nonclinical comparability study is expected to address an important knowledge gap and/or improve the overall risk assessment of the postchange product, then the study may be considered useful. However, if the outcome of the nonclinical study will not be used to make product development decisions, then it would seem to be unnecessary. It is also important to recognize that nonclinical comparability studies are not always needed. For example, when the prechange and postchange products are not considered comparable based on product quality characteristics, nonclinical data would not be sufficient to change the overall comparability determination.

9.2.3 Nonclinical Comparability Assessment

The types of nonclinical studies that may be considered to help establish comparability (*i.e.*, contribute to the overall comparability assessment) and/or support clinical administration (when needed) of a postchange product include PK, PD, toxicology, and/or immunogenicity. Historically, the strategies and practices for nonclinical comparability assessment have been quite varied among different product sponsors, indications, and product types. Please refer to the following publications for discussion and specific examples regarding these strategies and how nonclinical studies have or have not contributed to the overall comparability assessment (Lewis and Cosenza, 2010; Putnam et al., 2010; Wright et al., 2018; Grampp et al., 2018).

There are many unique aspects of biopharmaceuticals that necessitate special considerations when designing nonclinical studies intended for comparability assessment. Biopharmaceuticals are typically foreign proteins to the species selected for nonclinical evaluation that when administered to animals can elicit an immune response (see Chapter 10).

TABLE 9.1

Questions to Consider Before Conducting Nonclinical Comparability Studies

- Are the prechange and postchange products considered comparable based on product quality assessment?

If the prechange and postchange products appear "highly similar" but a possible adverse impact of product quality–related differences on the safety or efficacy profiles of the postchange product cannot be excluded, then additional questions to consider include the following:

- Is the product considered a high safety risk based on available data?
- What are the characteristics of the disease or indication to be treated? Is it a life-threatening or severely debilitating disease? Is there an unmet medical need for the biotherapeutic?
- Are there other important clinical development issues to consider?
- What are the knowledge gaps based on available data and could nonclinical PK, PD, and/or toxicology studies help address the gaps and/or improve the risk assessment of the postchange product?
- Is the risk associated with the information gaps significant enough to warrant conducting animal studies?
- What is the purpose of conducting the nonclinical study? Is it to help establish comparability and, therefore, contribute to the overall comparability assessment or to support the safety of clinical administration? Is it to reduce the level of uncertainty regarding potential safety, PK or PD effects of specific product quality–related differences between the prechange and postchange products?
- What are the intended next steps regarding clinical evaluation? For example, will clinical PK studies be conducted regardless of the outcome of any nonclinical PK study? If so, is the nonclinical PK study needed?
- What are the specific objectives of the nonclinical study and how will the outcome be used to make downstream product development decisions?

The resulting immune response can alter the PD, PK, and/or toxicity profiles of biopharmaceuticals. Thus, immunogenicity is an important general consideration for nonclinical study design and interpretation. Another unique aspect of biopharmaceuticals is that they are often species specific (see Chapter 2). Thus, pharmacological and toxicological consequences of biopharmaceutical exposure may only be observed in animals sharing a close phylogenetic relationship with humans. This aspect is important because adverse effects of biopharmaceuticals are typically due to an exaggerated pharmacology-associated response. These unique aspects of biopharmaceuticals must be considered when selecting a species for pharmacology, PK, and toxicology studies intended for comparability assessment. Species selected should typically be a pharmacologically relevant species. Although this is imperative for nonclinical safety assessments, occasionally, a nonpharmacologically relevant species may be considered for some limited PK studies, when target-independent mechanisms are thought to be an important component of product exposure (*e.g.*, mAb recycling through FcRn).

PK bridging studies are the most commonly conducted nonclinical study to assess comparability, as manufacturing changes can result in alterations of the active moiety that may affect biopharmaceutical exposure *in vivo*. For example, glycosylation changes can influence the PK of a protein due to changes in clearance rates through the asialoglycoprotein or mannose/GlcNAc receptor–mediated pathways (Park et al., 2005). The goal of PK analysis for biopharmaceuticals is to define the ADME characteristics of the product and the relationship of systemic and/or local exposure to the PD and toxicity observations. However, the size, composition, and structural characteristics of biopharmaceuticals typically limit their diffusion into tissues and so are confined primarily to the circulating vasculature but can also distribute to the extravascular space. Therefore, biopharmaceuticals usually have limited absorption and distribution characteristics and are administered either by intravenous (IV), subcutaneous (SC), or intramuscular (IM) routes or directly to the site of action. Additionally, biotransformation and elimination mechanisms of most biopharmaceuticals are limited, ultimately being catabolized to amino acids. Biopharmaceutical clearance, although often limited by the molecular size, typically can occur by renal filtration mechanisms. Given these unique characteristics, the primary endpoints in PK bridging studies are typically the maximum serum concentration (C_{max}), area under the curve (AUC), half-life ($T_{1/2}$), and clearance and so rarely measure potential changes in distribution. Although other PK/ADME evaluations including absorption and bioavailability can be considered for products administered by IM, SC, or other more unique routes of administration or sites of action, these are not typically evaluated in nonclinical PK comparability studies. Although a bit atypical, evaluating PK in nonpharmacologically relevant models (*e.g.*, humanized FcRn mice) has occurred, particularly when nontarget-mediated PK effects are suspected based on available product quality–related data. Adding PD (if pharmacologically relevant model with established endpoints available) and immunogenicity endpoints to these studies should also be considered. PK comparisons made between two independent studies, one with the postchange product and one with the prechange product, are difficult to interpret and are not typically considered appropriate. Thus, a direct comparison of PK parameters of the prechange and postchange products in a pharmacologically relevant animal species is preferable. Although a reasonable number of animals for a PK study could demonstrate, statistically, a 20% difference with 80% power (refer to the FDA Guidance for Industry "Statistical approaches to establishing bioequivalence" [2001]), there is no specific regulatory guidance or expectation regarding the appropriate number of animals to use for these studies. Comparability assessments are not intended to be the same as PK bioequivalence studies for small molecule drugs. Moreover, when the only relevant animal model is an NHP and/or the animal species chosen is known to develop antidrug antibodies (ADAs) that may limit the usefulness of the study, flexibility in the study design may be appropriate. We recommend leveraging all available information regarding the PK characteristics of the prechange product to help design the PK study with the postchange product. In the majority of cases, these PK (or PK/PD) comparisons provide sufficient information to either contribute to the totality of evidence supporting the comparability assessment or to allow for clinical dose adjustments (when a specific safety concern was identified) and additional nonclinical studies are typically not necessary.

In some instances, additional nonclinical studies may be considered to establish comparability or support clinical administration (when needed) of a postchange product. As discussed previously, the need for these studies is dependent upon the safety profile of the reference (prechange) biopharmaceutical, the magnitude of the manufacturing change(s), and any identified differences in product purity, structure, or in vitro activity. PD comparisons may include additional in vitro assays such as receptor binding (if not already evaluated as part of the product quality–related biological characterization assessment) or in vivo studies in an animal model of disease. For example, it may be useful to conduct PD comparison with the prechange and postchange products when a major alteration in the active moiety occurs and in vitro potency appears to be altered. However, applying the 20% difference/80% power rule for PD comparability studies is not expected or necessary.

Nonclinical safety/toxicology studies are usually not needed for a typical comparability assessment. With few exceptions, toxicology studies when conducted are intended to support safe administration of the postchange material in a clinical trial. Alterations of the biopharmaceutical that could potentially result in a significant shift in the risk/benefit ratio that cannot be solved by modifications to the clinical trial (*e.g.*, altering the clinical dose to account for potential potency or PK differences) may warrant conducting a toxicology study. This may be particularly important if there is a steep dose-response curve for a severe or unmonitorable clinical toxicity or if a small safety margin was established with the prechange product in initial toxicology studies. If a toxicology study is needed, selection of the dose level, regimen, duration, and species should provide a meaningful safety comparison between the prechange and postchange product. Typically, these studies consist of a single, short duration (*e.g.*, 1 month) study with the postchange product in a pharmacologically relevant species, if considered a sensitive model for evaluating the specific safety risk. However, the duration of this study may be shorter or longer depending on product characteristics. Ideally, these studies are designed to include the prechange product in a comparator arm, which is why it is important to retain sufficient samples from production lots.

Immunogenicity comparability assessment, including animal studies and/or ex vivo/in vitro studies typically consisting of various adaptive and/or innate immune response assays, can also be considered if comparing the prechange and postchange material directly. Prior to conducting an immunogenicity comparability study in animals, the likelihood of the study informing clinical decision-making, the utility of the study compared with clinical assessment, the type of data to be collected and evaluated, the animal model, and predictive potential of the results should all be carefully considered. These studies are often insensitive because of the low number of animals used and interanimal variability (*e.g.*, differences in time of onset, persistence, type of antibody produced, incidence, titer). Considerations for including comparative immunogenicity endpoints in a comparability study can include changes in the postchange product that are thought to increase immunogenicity, such as presence of certain leachables and increase in bacterial protein contaminants (*i.e.*, endotoxin) or high-order biopharmaceutical aggregates. Of note, greater clinical concern exists for induction of ADAs that have the potential to neutralize nonredundant endogenous protein function (for detailed discussion, refer to Shankar et al., 2007). Although these assessments can sometimes be of limited utility, if immunogenicity comparative endpoints are included in a nonclinical comparability study, then antibody titer along with the number of animals affected for prechange and postchange products should be compared side by side. Typically, these assessments would be conducted as part of a PK comparability study. When a detailed assessment is not conducted, we would recommend collecting samples for possible ADA analysis to help interpret the results of the PK, PD, and/or toxicology study with the postchange product.

9.3 Conclusion

Manufacturing changes occurring over the course of product development are inevitable. These changes could potentially affect critical product quality characteristics because biopharmaceuticals are heterogeneous mixtures defined by process-specific attributes (*i.e.*, the manufacturing methods employed), but they should have no adverse impact on the safety or efficacy of the biopharmaceutical. Comparability assessment considers whether manufacturing changes are expected to impact critical quality attributes and, if so, the types of additional testing that may be needed. This iterative process initially utilizes analytical testing (and occasionally nonclinical and/or clinical evaluation) to help ensure that the physicochemical properties, biological activities and immunochemical properties of the postchange product are "highly similar" (*i.e.*, comparable) to the prechange product. The decision regarding the need for nonclinical comparability assessment should be made on a case-by-case basis using a risk-based approach, after considering all product

quality–related comparability data (*i.e.*, analytical testing) as well as general product characteristics and clinical development considerations. When nonclinical studies are conducted, they should be designed to answer a specific question or safety concern. Contacting the appropriate regulatory authorities is highly recommended, prior to conducting a nonclinical study with the postchange product, to discuss the need for nonclinical comparability assessment and the most appropriate study design to address any safety concerns.

REFERENCES

EMEA: 2007. Guideline on Comparability of Biotechnology-Derived Medicinal Products after a Change in the Manufacturing Process, Non-Clinical and Clinical Issues.

Grampp, G., McElroy, P.L., Camblin, G. and Pollock, A. 2018. Structure-function relationships for recombinant erythropoietins: A case study from proposed manufacturing change with implications for erythropoietin biosimilar study designs. *Journal of Pharmaceutical Sciences* 107: 1512–1520.

ICH M3(R2): 2010. Guidance on Nonclinical Safety Studies for the Conduct of Human Clinical Trials and Marketing Authorization for Pharmaceuticals.

ICH Q5E: 2005. Comparability of Biotechnological/Biological Products Subject to Changes in their Manufacturing Process.

ICH Q6B: 1999. Specifications: Test Procedures and Acceptance Criteria for Biotechnological/Biological Products.

ICH Q8(R2): 2009. Pharmaceutical Development.

ICH S6(R1): 2012. Preclinical Safety Evaluation of Biotechnology-Derived Pharmaceuticals.

ICH S9: 2010. Nonclinical Evaluation of Anticancer Pharmaceuticals.

Lewis R.M. 2008. Chapter 8: Demonstration of comparability of a licensed product after a manufacturing change, In Cavagnaro, J.A. (Ed) *Preclinical Safety Evaluation of Biopharmaceuticals: A Science-Based Approach to Facilitating Clinical Trials*, John Wiley & Sons, Inc.

Lewis R.M. and Cosenza, M.E. 2010. Summary of DIA workshop: Comparability challenges: Regulatory and scientific issues in the assessment of biopharmaceuticals, *Drug Information Journal* 44:485–504.

Park, E.I., Yiling M., Unverzagt C., Gabius H-J and Baenziger, JU. 2005. The asialoglycoprotein receptor clears glycoconjugates terminating with Sialic Acidα2, 6GalNAc. *Proceedings of the National Academy of Sciences* 102: 17125–17129.

Putnam, W.S., Prabhu, S., Zheng, Y., Subramanyam, M., and Wang, Y.M.C. 2010. Pharmacokinetic, pharmacodynamic and immunogenicity comparability assessment strategies for monoclonal antibodies. *Trends in Biotechnology* 28: 509–516.

Shankar, G., Pendley, C. and Stein, K.E. 2007. A risk-based bioanalytical strategy for the assessment of antibody immune responses against biological drugs. *Nature Biotechnology* 25(5): 555–561.

US FDA Guidance for Industry: 1996. Demonstration of Comparability of Human Biological Products, Including Therapeutic Biotechnology-Derived Products.

US FDA Guidance for Industry: 2001. Statistical approaches to establishing bioequivalence.

US FDA Guidance for Industry: 2005. Estimating the Maximum Safe Starting Dose in Initial Clinical Trials for Therapeutics in Adult Healthy Volunteers.

US FDA Guidance for Industry: 2005. Nonclinical Studies for the Safety Evaluation of Pharmaceutical Excipients.

US FDA Guidance for Industry: 2015. Nonclinical Safety Evaluation of Reformulated Drug Products and Products Intended for Administration by an Alternate Route.

US FDA Guidance for Industry: 2016. Comparability Protocols for Human Drugs and Biologics: Chemistry, Manufacturing and Controls Information.

Wright, T., Li, A., Lotterhand, J., Graham, A.R., Huang, Y., Avila, N., and Pan, J., 2018. Nonclinical comparability studies of recombinant human arylsulfatase A addressing manufacturing process changes. *PLoS ONE* 13(4): e0195186 https://doi.org/10.1371/journal.pone.0195186.

10

Immunogenicity of Therapeutic Proteins

Steven J. Swanson
Steven J Swanson Consulting, LLC

CONTENTS

10.1 Introduction

Protein therapeutics have become an important option for physicians to help their patients. However, there are many unique challenges that must be considered when using a protein therapeutic. In order to understand clinical immunogenicity, it is vital to first understand the immunogenicity profile of a new therapeutic as defined by nonclinical studies. While traditional small-molecule drugs are invisible to the immune system, there is a strong potential that protein therapeutics could be recognized as foreign agents and trigger an immune response based upon their large size. It is important to understand that modifications to a native protein, including pegylation, fusion with another moiety, and conjugation with another moiety, can impact the inherent immunogenicity of the target protein. That impact could either enhance or suppress the protein's inherent immunogenicity.

When considering modified proteins, it is often very useful to understand if the product's immunogenicity is targeting the modification or the target protein. The consequences of initiating an immune response can vary from (1) having no effect, to having clinical relevance by (2) sustaining the drug in circulation, (3) clearing the drug more quickly from the circulation, (4) neutralizing the biological activity of the therapeutic, and (5) neutralizing an endogenous protein. It is not possible to predict with absolute certainty whether a given patient will mount an immune response against a protein therapeutic. Therefore, it is important that when these drugs are developed, that attention be paid to both understanding how likely the drug is to trigger an immune response and what the consequences of an immune response could be. When immunogenicity of a therapeutic protein is described, it is in the context of the reported clinical outcome observed in the clinical trials leading to the approval of the drug. It is generally reported as the percentage of patients that mount

DOI: 10.1201/9781003124542-12

an immune response, and often is further described by relating the percentage of patients that mount a neutralizing response to the drug. As methodologies for detecting antidrug antibodies continue to improve, it is apparent that many protein-based therapeutics induce a relatively high rate of patients that develop antibodies, yet the therapeutics still provide value for the patient and their usage is continued. The importance and significance of an immune response is unique to each protein therapeutic and must be evaluated as such. The difference between an immune response and a neutralizing immune response is important and defined by the analytical procedures that were used to detect the antibodies. An immune response indicates that an immunoassay (capable of detecting any antibody that binds to the therapeutic protein) was positive in the patient, whereas a neutralizing response indicates that the assay measured an antibody response capable of neutralizing the biological activity of the drug. Most neutralizing assays are forms of biological assays or bioassays, although exceptions are made when the only biological action of the drug involves binding to a target (such as with some antibody therapeutics) or if the function of the drug can be tested in a non-cell-based system. Of note, even if an immune response is not indicated as neutralizing, the overall effect of having the drug rapidly cleared because of antidrug antibodies in the patient, is in fact a response that may render the drug ineffective for the patient due to the rapid and thorough clearance. It can often be important to differentiate between a "clearing" antibody defined as an antibody that enhances the clearance of the drug as determined by pharmacokinetic studies, and a "neutralizing" antibody defined as an antibody capable of neutralizing or abrogating the biological effect of the drug.

Physicians that are caring for patients being treated with protein therapeutics should understand that an immune response could develop in the patient at any time they are being treated, and be aware that an immune response could be responsible if a patient fails to respond to the therapeutic. The physician may also have options to co-administer therapeutics that could block or suppress the immune response in order to prevent the antidrug antibody response from interfering with the biological effect of the protein therapeutic. An immune response could also occur when patients are treated with drugs whose reported immunogenicity is very low. While most immune responses to therapeutic proteins develop within a couple months of treatment initiation, it is possible that the response may not be triggered until much later. In order to keep immunogenicity information in proper context, it is important to remember that most patients being treated with protein therapeutics never display signs of immunogenicity toward that therapeutic even in the presence of antidrug antibodies.

It is also important to understand the potential for immunogenicity in nonclinical animal studies. The ICHS6 guidance describes the regulatory expectation that in repeat-dose toxicity studies, the immunogenicity should be monitored to help explain any observed toxicities. This is especially relevant if a toxicity is observed that is possibly linked to an immune response. The immunogenicity evaluation can help in designing the clinical trial strategy, especially if the therapeutic is strongly immunogenic or the presence of antibodies results in significant consequences. It is well understood that nonclinical immunogenicity is not an absolute predictor of what happens when the drug is exposed to humans, and often overpredicts a clinical immune response. However, there is a significant value in understanding the immune response in each animal tested, as this will allow a proper interpretation of any toxicological findings as well as the correct interpretation of pharmacokinetic parameters.

10.2 Regulatory Recommendations to Consider

When designing a strategy for assessing the immunogenicity of a therapeutic protein, care should be taken to meet or exceed the expectations of the regulatory agencies where the drug is targeted for approval. Requirements for immunogenicity testing are available at FDA and EMA websites, and the most current guidance documents should be strictly followed unless there are strong scientific justifications for deviations. The guidance documents have been prepared after thorough consideration of industry white papers published on immunogenicity assessment (Mire-Sluis, et al. 2004; Koren, et al. 2008; Shankar, Arkin and Devanarayan, et al. 2015; Shankar, Arkin and Cocea, et al. 2014; Gupta, et al. 2007). These are titles of some of the relevant documents from FDA and EMA websites:

Guidance for Industry, Investigators, and Reviewers Exploratory IND Studies (FDA.gov)

Guidance for Industry Immunogenicity Assessment for Therapeutic Protein Products (FDA.gov)

FDA Guidance for Industry: Assay Development and Validation for Immunogenicity Testing of Therapeutic Protein Products (FDA.gov)

Guideline on Immunogenicity assessment of therapeutic proteins (ema.europa.eu)

Guideline on immunogenicity assessment of monoclonal antibodies intended for in vivo clinical use (ema.europa.eu)

While guidance documents by definition provide guidance only and are not strictly mandated, regulatory agencies expect that their guidance will be followed and any deviations will likely cause comment, require a careful explanation, and the approach may not be approved. Guidance documents are prepared by the regulatory agencies after careful consultation with experts in the field and are generally applicable to new protein therapeutics. However, it is important to note that there may be strong scientific reasons why the guidance documents cannot be strictly followed for any given new drug. In addition, many companies have adopted a risk-based approach for immunogenicity testing. The basis for this strategy is that those proteins that are either at a high risk for developing antibodies (likely to be viewed as very foreign by the immune system) and those drugs where the consequences of developing an immune response are high (drugs that mimic a nonredundant endogenous counterpart) would have a more rigorous testing strategy. Examples of drugs that would be very likely to induce an immune response are those drugs whose genetic sequence is markedly different than an endogenous counterpart or in cases where a genetic abnormality prevents the subject from producing the endogenous equivalent (such as with many enzyme replacement therapies). Those therapeutic proteins that are considered very low risk would have more abbreviated testing. It is always helpful when following this risk-based approach to have careful conversations with the relevant regulatory agencies prior to the implementation of this strategy to ensure agreement. It is strongly recommended that when deviating from regulatory guidance that detailed conversations be held with the relevant regulatory agencies prior to submission for approvals to avoid unwanted surprises.

Regulatory agencies need to understand from the company prior to granting marketing approval for a new protein therapeutic the immunogenicity profile for the drug. The testing during clinical development must be robust and use appropriate analytical procedures that have been properly validated for their intended use. There are likely many justified approaches for determining the immunogenicity for any therapeutic protein rather than a single pathway that must be followed. The critical components of a successful assessment include the use of validated assays (immunoassays as well as biological assays, when warranted), testing patients at appropriate times during the clinical trials, testing a sufficient number of patients (must be statistically justified), and properly interpreting the immunogenicity data. When testing in nonclinical studies, the immunogenicity testing must also be robust and thorough. It is expected that testing follow Good Laboratory Procedure guidelines and that validated assays be used for immunogenicity assessment in both nonclinical studies and clinical trials.

Validated assays are important since a failure to understand assay performance, which is established during the validation process that is carefully outlined in FDA guidance, can result in improper interpretation of the results from that assay. For example, if an assay lacks a sufficient sensitivity, a negative result in the assay would suggest the subject did not mount an immune response, when in fact, the subject may have mounted a significant immune response that the poorly designed assay failed to detect. Each portion of the assay validation helps to interpret how the assay will respond under certain circumstances and allows a correct interpretation of the result from that assay. Without the confidence gained during validation, regulatory agencies will not be able to assess the merits of the analytical procedures used for the testing. The regulator's expectations regarding assay validation have been clearly described in guidance documents.

The timing for when samples are taken is very important in both nonclinical studies and clinical trials. An immune response takes time to develop and is easily masked by the presence of high levels of circulating drug. It is also possible that a subject may mount a transient immune response that could wane and be undetected if testing is performed too long after the cessation of treatment. It is always valuable to perform immunogenicity testing throughout the course of a trial to understand if an immune response might have been responsible for either a pharmacokinetic anomaly or an adverse event. If testing is only performed prior to initial dose (predose) and after conclusion of all dosing, it will not be possible to determine if the presence of an immune response had an impact on the subject as there will be no knowledge when the immune response occurred during the course of treatment.

When testing during early nonclinical studies, it is not uncommon for the assay to have less than ideal characteristics and the performance of the assay may still benefit from modifications and improvements. This is especially true when considering assay sensitivity. When IND-enabling studies are performed, it is expected that analytical procedures have been well examined and validations have been successfully performed. Fit-for-purpose assay validation is a concept where partial validations are used for early studies, and then full validation is performed prior to the IND-enabling studies. It is important to realize that early validation does not preclude further assay development, although any modifications in the procedure would warrant additional validation. While additional validations can be time-consuming and result in additional expense, it is very important to have the best assay available whenever possible. Assay validation is a value-added exercise because the nonclinical immunogenicity procedures can lay the groundwork for the clinical assays to follow. The experience gained in performing these procedures and analyzing their results is invaluable for the development of the required clinical assays.

During early clinical trials for a protein therapeutic, it will be possible to determine a likely range for the drug's immunogenicity incidence. Using this information and in consultation with statisticians, it can be determined how many patients need to be tested in the Phase 3 trial to provide sufficient data to report an immunogenicity rate and describe consequences of a patient's immune response. In most cases, it will be required that immunogenicity assessment be performed on all patients during clinical trials in order to understand immunogenicity and the effects on efficacy and safety. In rare cases, the real-time immunogenicity assessment may be required to provide the physician with necessary information for the patient being treated in case a clinically relevant immune response is generated.

The type of information that should be compiled in an immunogenicity report for drug approval includes how many animals or subjects developed an immune response at any time during treatment; how many developed a transient response (only present for a short time and no longer evident at the end of dosing); how many developed a persistent response (present at the end of dosing or persisting throughout multiple time points); how many developed a neutralizing antibody response (if the immunogenicity assessment plan includes testing for neutralizing antibodies); the association between pharmacokinetics and immune response; and any correlation between adverse events and those animals or subjects that developed an immune response. The collection of these data requires that all relevant data be compared, immunogenicity, pharmacokinetic, and safety.

10.3 The Immune System

The immune system has developed to protect from foreign invaders and threats that begin within the body. The cells comprising the immune system are derived from bone marrow and are replenished throughout the lifetime of an animal. At the core of the immune system is the ability to recognize "self vs non-self." Meaning, it is the job of the immune system to identify anything entering the body that does not belong there and to attempt to remove it. We are protected from foreign invaders such as bacteria, viruses, and other parasites. We are also protected from problems arising from internal challenges such as gene mutations that can lead to cancer. The immune system is also very tightly controlled. When control of the immune system breaks down such that it is too tightly controlled or suppressed, threats can escape resulting in infections and disease. Autoimmune disorders occur when the immune system's control fails and healthy tissue is attacked rather than ignored.

The immune system also plays a role when therapeutic proteins are administered to a patient and especially when administered to a test animal. Unfortunately, despite the fact that we want to administer these to benefit the patient, the patient's immune system may still identify the administered protein as a foreign threat and try to destroy it. The most common way for the immune system to interact with protein therapeutics is to produce antibodies to bind and eliminate them. Because the molecular weight threshold for the recognition of a foreign invader is between 1,000 and 2,000 daltons, traditional small-molecule therapeutics do not engage the human immune system. However, the larger size of protein therapeutics makes them susceptible to immune system intervention. All of the components of the immune system are derived from hematopoietic stem cells in the bone marrow. In addition to the bone marrow, the cells comprising the immune system can be found throughout the body, including in circulation and in lymphoid tissue, including the thymus, spleen, and lymph nodes. Because the majority of therapeutic proteins are based on human biology, they are almost always recognized as foreign in test animals during nonclinical studies. The immune response in these test animals can have a profound effect on the fate of the therapeutic and can make the interpretation of study findings quite complicated. It has often been observed that toxicities associated with an immune response in test animals do not always translate in clinical trials. This is primarily due to a combination of higher doses in test animals and a much more robust immune response in animals than is observed clinically.

10.3.1 Innate Immunity

The innate immune response consists of preformed cells that do not increase after exposure to a foreign agent. These preformed cells do not require a period for induction and are always available. The innate immune response consists of the first defense for the body against pathogens and includes cells comprising an epithelial barrier and cells that can phagocytize and destroy foreign agents. These cells have the ability to recognize and ignore self-proteins while responding to foreign agents. The cells comprising the innate response can also trigger the activation of the adaptive immune response. Triggering innate immunity can be a potential mechanism that can explain some early injection-site reactions.

10.3.2 Adaptive Immunity

The adaptive immune response is triggered after the recognition of a foreign invader by the innate response. The adaptive response requires an induction period of several days, but then provides a very robust and specific response to battle the

foreign invader. The adaptive immune response involves the interaction of lymphocytes in response to a foreign antigen and results in an immunological memory of the foreign agent. The memory response allows a much more rapid and robust response if the foreign antigen is encountered again. The adaptive immune response against therapeutic proteins can lead to the production of antibodies that can bind and potentially neutralize any effect of the therapeutic protein.

10.3.3 Phagocytic Cells

The first protective layer of the body that acts to prevent infection is the epithelial system. With therapeutic proteins, this layer of defense is avoided by the administration of the therapeutic across this epithelial layer. The first cellular component of the immune system that encounters an administered therapeutic protein is the group of cells classified as phagocytic cells. Phagocytic cells, including macrophages, polymorphonuclear leukocytes, and dendritic cells, are able to ingest foreign proteins, break them down, and present pieces of the foreign protein onto their surface to initiate further activation of the immune system. It is the dendritic cells that are present in the subcutaneous space that most often encounter and initiate an immune response against therapeutic proteins.

10.3.4 Lymphocytes

The immune system produces two types of lymphocytes: B lymphocytes (B cells) and T lymphocytes (T cells). Each of these cell types works together to trigger an immune response against a therapeutic protein. B cells are responsible for producing antibodies. B cells have a receptor on their surface (B-cell antigen receptor) that is antigen-specific and when activated causes the B cell to differentiate into an antibody-producing cell. The antibodies produced have the same specificity as the antigen receptor on the cell surface. T cells are defined by their development in the thymus and their heterodimeric receptors. T cells can be classified as cytotoxic (CD8+), helper, or regulatory (CD4+). Cytotoxic T cells can directly kill target cells expressing the antigen recognized by their T-cell receptor. Helper T cells are important in the activation of B cells to produce antibodies, and regulatory T cells are responsible for controlling adaptive immune responses.

10.3.5 Production of Antibodies

Antibodies are produced when circulating B cells encounter a foreign protein that matches their B-cell receptor. The interaction with the antigen causes the B cell to begin producing antibodies. The first class of antibody produced is IgM. If the B cell then interacts with a helper T cell, the immune response is magnified and amplified with more identical B cells being produced. Class switching can also occur, causing the B cells to start producing IgG instead of IgM. It can take up to 2 weeks for the first circulating antibodies to be detected, which is due to the lag phase required for the B cells to multiply and produce sufficient antibody to exceed the detection limit of the assay. In addition to producing more B cells to increase the amount of circulating antibody, some of the B cells and T cells become memory cells. It is the memory cells that allow a much more rapid secondary response characterized by a very short lag phase that allows detectable antibody by the second day after reintroduction of the antigen. The antibodies that comprise this secondary response are typically IgG, have higher binding affinity, are produced at a higher concentration, and often recognize additional regions of the foreign agent. While the initial antibody response to a therapeutic protein is often muted and may not be detectable, the secondary response is what is more likely to have an impact on the efficacy of the treatment. This is why it is important to test for the presence of antidrug antibodies at multiple time points after treatment with the agent when assessing the immunogenicity of a therapeutic protein.

10.4 Description of Immunoglobulins

There are five classes of immunoglobulins produced by humans and most mammals. These classes are IgM, IgG, IgA, IgD, and IgE. Each immunoglobulin is comprised of two heavy chains and two light chains that are linked by disulfide bonds. It is the heavy chain constant region from each class of antibody that distinguishes those antibodies as belonging in that class. These heavy and light chains contain both constant regions (identical across the class of antibody) and variable regions (unique for each antibody and provides the unique specificity of binding for the antibody). The basic immunoglobulin unit is Y-shaped and is comprised of a base (Fc or constant region) and two Fab (antibody-binding) regions. The molecular weight for each of these antibody units ranges from 146 to 188 kDa. It is the two Fab regions that are responsible for binding to the antigen. Antibodies are bivalent, and each antibody is generally capable of binding to two identical antigens. This allows antibodies to cross-link and form a large mesh-like complex of antibodies and antigens. These large complexes can then trigger further interaction by effector cells in the immune system to clear out the complexes.

IgM forms polymers of five antibody units forming a circular pentameric structure with a molecular weight of 970 kDa. IgA can form a dimeric structure where two of the antibody units are attached. The other three antibody classes are only found as monomeric units. IgG is the most common class of antibody found in circulation and can be further subdivided in humans into four subclasses: IgG1, IgG2, IgG3, and IgG4.

IgM is often the first antibody produced in response to a therapeutic protein. IgM is characterized by its large molecular weight (due to its pentameric configuration), having relatively low binding affinity, and having a half-life in circulation of approximately 10 days.

If the immune response continues to mature, class switching occurs and IgG antibodies are produced. These IgG antibodies would tend to have greater affinity for the target. Through a phenomenon known as epitope spreading, additional epitopes on the target would be recognized and antibodies would be produced that could bind to those epitopes. IgG1 through IgG4 would be produced depending on the maturity of the immune response. These IgG antibodies in addition to being produced in larger quantities, and with higher affinity, also have a longer half-life (3 weeks) in circulation. All of this adds up to a much more robust immune response that could have a significant impact on the efficacy of a therapeutic protein that was the target of the immune response.

It is IgE class antibodies that are associated with allergic or hypersensitivity responses. IgE antibodies are the class of antibody that has the lowest circulating level. When an IgE antibody binds to its target antigen, it rapidly binds to mast cells causing a robust release of histamine, which then induces a strong allergic response in the patient. While it is not common for a therapeutic protein to induce an IgE response, it is important to recognize that this is a possibility. Due to the very low level of circulating IgE antibodies, it is necessary to utilize special testing methods that are sensitive enough to detect this class of antibody, and due to the very short half-life of IgE antibodies, samples must be taken very soon after a suspected allergic reaction has occurred.

IgA antibodies are most often found in secretions and would not normally be expected to be relevant in assessing immunogenicity of therapeutic proteins. IgD antibodies have not been associated with immune responses to therapeutic proteins.

10.5 Reasons for Immunogenicity against Therapeutic Proteins

There are multiple reasons why a protein therapeutic can elicit an immune response from the patient (Schellekens 2003; Swanson 2007) and those reasons can be generally categorized as falling into one of these criteria: sequence differences with an endogenous counterpart, structural, impurities, stability, route of administration, and modifications to a native protein. While the net result of immunogenicity that is observed appears binary (**yes**, the subject mounts an immune response or **no**, the subject does not), the factors leading to that outcome are very much incremental and related. Each of these categories is described below; however, a given therapeutic may exhibit characteristics that fall into multiple categories. The subject's immune system is charged with recognizing the difference between "self vs non-self." Proteins recognized as being produced by the subject are essentially ignored by the immune system. When the immune system recognition breaks down, antibodies are formed against self-proteins and the subject experiences an autoimmune phenomenon that may progress into one of several autoimmune diseases.

Sequence differences Many protein therapeutics are designed to mimic an endogenous protein that the subject either fails to produce, produces at an insufficient quantity, or produces a version of the protein that is ineffective and fails to function properly. If there is an amino acid sequence difference between the endogenous protein and the therapeutic protein, it is possible that the amino acid difference could be significantly enough to be recognized as foreign by the subject's immune system and elicit an immune response. Unfortunately, there is currently not an algorithm that can reliably and accurately predict when an amino acid change is significant enough to trigger such an immune response. Factors to consider when developing a therapeutic protein with amino acid changes include the following:

(1) the amino acid changes on the surface of the molecule (more likely to induce an immune response), (2) the amino acid change affects the hydrophilicity of the region of the molecule, (3) the amino acid change alters the structure of the protein, and (4) the amino acid change creates a new "T-cell epitope" (described later in this chapter). The reasons for making amino acid sequence changes may be quite compelling and include the following: (1) increase half-life of the drug, (2) improve a binding interaction, or (3) possibly remove a known antigenic region to reduce immunogenicity. However, it is valuable to always consider the overall effect of these sequence changes on the immunogenicity of the therapeutic protein.

Structural Just as an amino acid change from an endogenous counterpart can allow the immune system to recognize the drug as foreign, structural differences in the drug can also elicit an immune response. Structural changes can expose regions of the drug to the immune system that were previously hidden and can also create novel regions or discontinuous epitopes that could be viewed as foreign to the immune system.

Impurities The goal for the manufacture of therapeutic proteins is to have a product that does not contain any impurities. Unfortunately, due to the complex nature of manufacturing therapeutic proteins, impurities are often present. Impurities are defined as any item remaining from the manufacture of the therapeutic other than the therapeutic itself. Impurities can consist of items, including bacterial fragments, media components, or breakdown products. Most of these impurities have no effect on stimulating an immune response; however, there are some very important exceptions. Both the amount and the nature of these impurities can influence the immunogenicity of the drug (e.g., host cell proteins, endotoxin). One method of action that can lead to impurities increasing an immune response is that they act as adjuvants. An adjuvant is a compound that augments an immune response. This augmentation could be the result of creating a stimulus to activate the immune system by recruiting cellular components of the immune system to the site of injection, it could directly stimulate the action of antigen-presenting cells, or it could elicit cytokine production that further augments the action of the immune system. Another mechanism of action is that the impurities could form an adduct with the protein therapeutic, which would create an unwanted variant of the protein therapeutic that may have different biological properties from the therapeutic. Impurities are often reduced during process development such that the version of the protein therapeutic that is released for commercial use is often much more pure than versions used during preclinical and often, early clinical trials. An important point is that manufacturing anomalies may occur even during commercial manufacturing that can result in a different impurity profile for any given batch of drug. This different impurity profile might result in a change in the overall immunogenicity of the drug for that batch. For this reason, it is very important for manufacturers to maintain strict quality control, including the monitoring of impurities throughout the life cycle of the therapeutic protein. This point also comes into play with biosimilar protein therapeutics. Another potential source of impurities is the container the drug is stored in, especially if that container is a prefilled syringe. There have been reports of tungsten fragments from needle placement in the syringe that have mediated important immune responses.

Stability When protein therapeutics break down or lose stability, their immunogenicity profile often changes. The changes that occur when the protein begins degradation often make it appear as foreign to the immune system and an immune response is generated. While not always occurring, the antibodies raised against the degrading protein may also bind and interact with the intact therapeutic protein. These antibodies could then render the protein therapeutic ineffective, and due to the long-term memory of the immune system, future administrations of the therapeutic protein may also be ineffective for the patient.

Route of administration The route of administration can have a profound effect on whether a therapeutic protein induces an immune response. The two most common routes of administration used for therapeutic proteins are intravenous and subcutaneous. It is acknowledged that in general, the subcutaneous route is more likely to induce an immune response than is the intravenous route (Matucci, Vultaggio and Danesi 2018). The reason for the difference in immunogenicity rate is due to the presence of dendritic cells in the subcutaneous space. It is the dendritic cells that are the most likely scavenging cells that would act as antigen-presenting cells to initiate an immune response, and placing the drug where these potent immune cells exist increases the opportunity to induce an immune response. In addition, the drug tends to reside longer in the subcutaneous space before being systemically distributed than when administered intravenously. The opportunity to encounter an antigen-presenting cell in the intravenous space prior to system delivery is much smaller than for drug administered into the subcutaneous space. While it is generally true that subcutaneous administration is more immunogenic than intravenous, this can vary by drug and should be established during trials for each protein therapeutic. It also should not be assumed that intravenous administration is incapable of initiating an immune response.

Modification from a native protein When a protein is modified such as when being conjugated to another moiety, pegylated, glycosylation pattern altered and other modifications, there is chance that the modification alters the inherent immunogenicity of the product when compared to the native protein. While it is sometimes the case that these modifications act to decrease immunogenicity (can often be seen when adding glycosylation sites), it is more likely that the modification will enhance immunogenicity by making the protein more likely to be viewed as "foreign" by the immune system.

10.6 Analytical Methodology

10.6.1 Immunoassays

Immunoassays are a large group of analytical procedures that are capable of identifying the presence of antidrug antibodies that bind to the therapeutic protein. They capitalize on the antibody's ability to specifically bind to the therapeutic protein. As long as the antibody can remain bound to the therapeutic protein throughout the course of the assay, this analytical procedure will detect its presence. In general, an immunoassay starts with an immobilized form of the therapeutic protein, either directly immobilized or captured. A high level of purity of the therapeutic protein is necessary to provide a specific assay. Any impurity in the immobilized protein could result in antibodies against that impurity being falsely identified as antibodies against the therapeutic protein. A serum sample (or sometimes plasma) is then added to the immobilized protein. This sample is often diluted since undiluted samples can result in a higher level of nonspecific cooperative binding and be interpreted as positive even if specific antibodies were not present in the sample. The sample is allowed to interact with the immobilized protein for a period of time (optimum timing is determined during assay development but is typically 1 hour or longer). Depending on the nature of the immobilized therapeutic protein, incubation can occur at ambient temperature (most common), a higher temperature that supports more binding events, or a reduced temperature that tends to suppress binding but can have the benefit of lower nonspecific binding. During the incubation period, if antidrug antibodies are contained in the sample, they can then bind to the immobilized protein therapeutic. One variation of this theme is a fluid-phase assay where both the therapeutic protein and the sample are allowed to interact without first immobilizing the therapeutic protein. Once the binding of the antibodies has occurred, the unreacted parts of the patient's sample are washed away, leaving the immobilized therapeutic protein with any antidrug antibodies now bound to the surface. The next step is to add a labeled reagent that will bind to the captured antibody (but will not bind to the immobilized protein). This labeled reagent varies depending on the type of immunoassay utilized. The label is a reagent that will elicit a signal that can be detected during the last step of the analytical procedure. An example of a label is an enzyme that induces a colorimetric change upon the addition of specific media and the intensity of the induced color is proportional to the amount of antidrug antibody that is bound to the therapeutic protein.

One of the challenges facing developers of analytical procedures to detect antidrug antibodies is that the presence of circulating drug frequently interferes with the ability of the assay to detect antibodies. This challenge is magnified in nonclinical studies where higher doses of the therapeutic protein are often used. In many cases, this is because the antibodies produced by the animals bind to the drug in circulation forming small immune complexes. These immune complexes are not detectable in most antidrug antibody assays. One solution is to perform an acid pretreatment step, which breaks the immune complexes and frees the antibodies to be detected in the assay (Patton, et al. 2005). Drug tolerance is the measure of how much circulating drug can be present with the assay still being able to detect a positive antibody sample and is an important assay characteristic that is tested during assay validation.

Other assay characteristics that are defined during assay validation include sensitivity, specificity, reproducibility, stability, and sample interference. Assay sensitivity determines the least amount of positive control that can reliably be detected in the samples tested. Specificity determines if any other entities could result in a positive assay result that are not consistent with antidrug antibodies. Reproducibility measures the variation resulting when identical samples are repeatedly tested. Both intra-assay variability and interassay variability are typically determined. Stability evaluates if there is a change in signal when the sample is reanalyzed after various lengths of storage time. This provides confidence that samples analyzed after lengthy periods of time after collection will still produce reliable and correct results. Sample interference evaluates if sample conditions such as lipemia or hemolysis have an effect on assay results. The purpose of assay validation is to allow an appropriate interpretation of an analytical result by fully understanding the characteristics and limitations of the analytical procedure.

There are multiple types of analytical procedures available to test for antidrug antibodies as shown in Figure 10.1. None of these methods are perfect, and each has its own set of

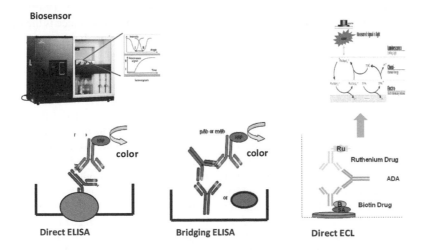

FIGURE 10.1 Common technologies utilized for immunoassays include biosensor, enzyme-linked immunosorbent assay (ELISA), and electrochemiluminescent Assay (ECL). The biosensor instruments depicted here utilizes surface plasmon resonance which produces an increase in signal as antidrug antibodies bind to immobilized drug on the surface of a sensorchip. This increase is reflected in real-time as the sample is binding and is proportional to the amount of antibody contained in the sample. Both the direct ELISA and the bridging ELISA utilize plate technology, and a signal is produced that is proportional to the amount of enzyme that is captured during the process of the assay. The resulting change in color is proportional to the amount of antibody in the sample that was bound to the drug. The ECL assay utilizes a modified ELISA where the resulting electrochemiluminescent signal is proportional to the amount of antibody contained in the sample.

advantages and disadvantages. It is important when devising a testing strategy that the optimal combinations for evaluating the immunogenicity of the therapeutic protein be determined.

ELISA The enzyme-linked immunosorbent assay (ELISA) has been a mainstay for the detection of antibodies since its development over 30 years ago (Voller, Bidwell and Bartlett 1980). This platform is based upon first immobilizing the therapeutic protein onto a microtiter plate through passive adsorption, covalent coupling, biotinylation, or other methods. After the drug is attached, a blocking step is performed where an irrelevant protein such as bovine serum albumin is added to the wells of the plate for a period of time to occupy or block any region of the well not coated with the drug. This blocking step is critical to prevent nonspecific sticking of subsequent reagents that could be perceived as antidrug antibodies. After the wells are blocked, a dilution of sample serum (or sometimes plasma) is added to the well and antibodies specific for the therapeutic protein are allowed to bind to the immobilized drug. After the unbound serum components are washed away, a labeled secondary reagent capable of binding to antibodies that have bound to the immobilized drug is added. This secondary reagent could be an anti-(test species) immunoglobulin reagent that has been conjugated to the enzyme phosphatase or peroxidase. After incubation and the removal of unbound reagents through a washing step, the substrate for the conjugated enzyme is added and the colorimetric result of the enzymatic reaction is monitored. The color observed is proportional to the amount of antidrug antibody that has been bound to the immobilized therapeutic protein on the plate. Another version of the ELISA uses labeled therapeutic protein as the detector. This bridging format takes advantage of the bispecific nature of antibodies and is a very specific way of detecting antibodies as it is less likely to demonstrate nonspecific binding. A disadvantage of the bridging platform is that it tends to be less sensitive than the direct ELISA and has limitations detecting antidrug antibodies if those antibodies have low affinity and a rapid dissociation rate. This is because antibodies with a rapid dissociation rate often leave the immobilized therapeutic protein prior to the final detection step.

The ELISA platform is preferred by many investigators because it is an easy technique to learn and requires minimal equipment. ELISAs can be very sensitive and robust analytical procedures. Care must be taken when developing an ELISA that the assay is specific, only detects antibodies that can bind to the therapeutic protein, and does not demonstrate a high degree of false-positive results. If the ELISA plate is improperly blocked or if reagents are chosen that demonstrate cross-reactivity, it is possible for the assay to falsely identify samples as positive when that sample does not contain antidrug antibodies. An additional concern with the ELISA is that antibodies that have low affinity and tend to rapidly dissociate from the target after binding may not be identified as positive. The inability of ELISAs to detect low-affinity antibodies is likely related to the multiple washing and incubation steps inherent with this method. These low-affinity antibodies could dissociate from the target and then be rinsed away during a subsequent wash cycle.

ECL Electrochemilluminescent (ECL) assays have many features in common with an ELISA (Wu, et al. 2013). The method for the detection of antibodies is different since ECL assays utilize the detection of light that is emitted proportional to the amount of antibody contained in the subject's sample. One version of this assay relies on immobilization of the therapeutic protein onto special microtiter plates. The plates can be blocked with bovine serum albumin or other nonreactive reagents and are then ready for analysis. The subject's serum sample is added to the plates, and any antibodies in the sample specific for the protein therapeutic have the opportunity to bind. Because antibodies are bivalent, there is still one binding site available after the antibody has bound to the immobilized target. This free site can then bind to soluble drug that has been coupled to ruthenium. This complex is then placed in the presence of the luminescence reagent, and light is emitted when an electrical pulse is made. The amount of light emitted is directly proportional to the amount of antidrug antibody present in the original sample.

This assay is very sensitive and typically very specific and can be automated to provide a high throughput. The ECL assay in this format is able to detect all classes of antibodies because the antibody in the serum sample creates a bridge between the therapeutic protein immobilized on the microtiter plate and the drug that is soluble and conjugated to ruthenium. A challenge with this assay lies in the detection of low-affinity antibodies; however, a thorough careful examination of washing parameters, this assay platform is capable of detecting low-affinity antibodies and is often superior at detecting these antibodies than an ELISA. Another challenge with this assay is that a hook effect can occur. A hook effect occurs when the signal produced in the assay peaks at a given concentration of antibody but instead of plateauing, the signal decreases in the presence of more antibody. The net result is that a very high concentration of antibody is erroneously recorded as having little or no antibody because very high levels of antibody produce lower signals in the assay than some samples containing far less antibodies. This hook effect is more common in nonclinical studies because animals tend to produce more antidrug antibodies when exposed to human therapeutics than humans do.

Biosensor One example of a biosensor instrument that relies on surface plasmon resonance is the BIAcore™. This platform relies on first coupling the therapeutic protein to a sensorchip. The sensorchip is a glass slide covered with a gold film that has carboxymethyl dextran attached to it. This provides an advantage to coupling the therapeutic protein nonspecifically to a polysorbate plate, given that the attachment to carboxymethyl dextran is less likely to distort the conformation of the molecule. Having less distortion presents the drug to any antibodies in a way that is more like the way the antibody sees the drug *in vivo*. As the drug immobilizes onto the surface, the instrument provides a read-out in the form of a sensorgram that is proportional to the mass accumulation on the surface of the sensorchip. This provides data confirming the drug has in fact immobilized to the surface of the sensorchip.

Once the drug has been immobilized onto the sensorchip, the serum sample can be added, and if antibodies in the sample bind to the drug, the instrument generates an increase in the sensorgram signal that is proportional to the amount of antibody that binds. The instrument thereby provides a real-time assessment of binding events as they occur. Unlike more traditional immunoassay platforms such as ELISA and ECL, this instrument does not wait until the conclusion of an assay to provide data. This feature makes the BIAcore better suited for the detection of low-affinity antibodies or antibodies that dissociate quickly from the immobilized drug. There have been instances where low-affinity or rapidly dissociating antibodies have been clinically important, and therefore, it is important for any immunoassay platform to be designed in a way to promote the detection of these antibodies.

After the antibody has bound to the immobilized drug on the sensorchip, it is possible through the addition of specific isotyping reagents to determine what class of antibody has been captured. It is important to verify by experimental testing that these isotyping reagents are indeed antibodies that specifically bind to the immunoglobulin class specified and there is no evidence of nonspecific binding to other classes. There have been reports where some commercial isotyping reagents have not been truly specific leading to false results. The first or primary antibody that is typically produced in response to a foreign protein is IgM. After subsequent exposure to the therapeutic protein, in cases where a robust immune response is generated, IgG is produced. The ability to monitor the class of antibody that is circulating in response to the drug can help in the understanding of the progression of the immune response.

This technology offers the advantages of automated sample analysis, real-time detection to better enable the detection of low-affinity antibodies, sample immobilization that better preserves the native conformation of the drug, and the ability to further characterize the immune response (Lofgren, et al. 2007). When the second-generation products are investigated, the BIAcore allows the detection of antibodies to four different entities from the same serum sample in the same analytical run. This feature allows an analysis of both the original therapeutic and the second-generation therapeutic simultaneously. The BIAcore is considerably more expensive than the equipment required for other assay platforms and is somewhat limited by throughput in that a typical assay of 100 samples could take over 8 hours. A further limitation of this instrument is in assay sensitivity. It is generally possible to achieve greater sensitivity for antibody assays using other platforms, but the advantages offered by this platform in many instances outweigh the deficiencies. The BIAcore has been documented to have identified a population of antibodies in patients undetected by other technologies.

10.6.2 Biological assays

Biological Assays Assays that can detect antibodies that impact the biological activity of a therapeutic protein are classified as biological assays. As their name implies, the output of these assays measures more than just a binding event. Every therapeutic protein is administered to patients because it can exert some biological effect on the patient. The best biological assay is able to measure that effect and determine if an antibody is able to interfere or block that effect. Likewise, in nonclinical studies, a bioassay can determine if the animal produced antibodies capable of interfering with the observed biological effect of that drug. Most biological assays are distinguished from immunoassays because of their ability to monitor biological activity rather than just a binding event. However, that capability comes at a cost. Biological assays are typically less

sensitive, more labor intensive, have lower throughput, more difficult to automate, and have inherent higher variability than corresponding immunoassays. For these reasons, it is most common to perform an immunoassay to detect samples that contain antibodies and then test only those immunoassay-positive samples with the biological assay. This approach is standard and recognized by regulatory agencies as being acceptable.

The bioassay is important because it is the only way to understand if a serum sample contains an antibody that can neutralize the effects of the drug. Neutralizing antibodies are typically of greater concern to the physician because it strongly suggests that the patient has lost or will soon lose the biological effect of the drug. In nonclinical studies, neutralizing antibodies are more likely to have impacted effective exposure of the animal to the test agent.

There are many biological effects that can be used as the basis for a bioassay. One of the most common endpoints used is cell proliferation (Wei, Swanson and Gupta 2004). In this case, when the cells are exposed to the drug, they respond to that exposure by proliferating. The presence of neutralizing antibodies are able to block the drug-induced proliferation as depicted in Figure 10.2. One disadvantage of the cell proliferation bioassay is that it may take multiple days for the cells to respond sufficiently to increase the number of cells sufficiently to provide a reliable quantitation. Cell proliferation is certainly not the only parameter that can be evaluated in a bioassay. Other examples that have been used include receptor phosphorylation, apoptosis, ADCC (antibody-dependent cellular cytotoxicity), mRNA expression, gene expression (Yu, et al. 2006), and protein expression. The common theme for all of these bioassays is that a cell responds to the administration of drug in a way that can be reliably measured and when the response is blocked by a neutralizing antibody, the blocked response is statistically different than the control case where no antibody is present.

Cell-based Biological assays that are cell-based differ from immunoassays in that they rely on the interaction of the cell-based system. In this form of bioassay, a cell line is identified that is capable of responding to the therapeutic protein in a way that can be measured. The types of cellular response that have been used as measurements include cell proliferation, production of a cytokine, apoptosis, and production of specific mRNA. To perform a bioassay for neutralizing antibodies, cells, the drug and the patient's serum sample are added together and incubated. If there is an antibody present in the serum sample that is capable of neutralizing the biological effect of the drug, the measured response of the cells is reduced compared with the negative control. The negative control contains the cells, drug, and a serum sample known to be negative for the presence of neutralizing antibodies. The positive control for this assay would substitute a known positive sample for the sample serum.

Since most cells require time to exert the biological response from the drug, these assays take on average 2–3 days to complete. Because this type of bioassay is a cell-based system, there is more variability associated with this type of assay than is observed with most immunoassay platforms. Understanding the variability of a bioassay is very important

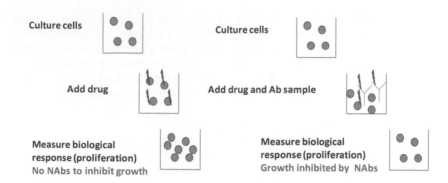

FIGURE 10.2 A typical cell-based bioassay for neutralizing antibodies is depicted. In this example, cells are used which respond to the therapeutic protein by increasing in number. The cell growth is proportional to the amount of drug which is added. When a sample containing neutralizing antibodies is added along with the drug to the cells in culture, the drug induces cell growth. If neutralizing antibodies are present in the sample, those antibodies bind and neutralize the added drug preventing it from stimulating the growth of the cells. If no antibodies are present in the sample, or if the antibodies present are not neutralizing, then the cells are able to respond to the added drug by proliferating. While this example uses cell proliferation, any response the cells make to the drug which can be reliably measured can be utilized in a cell-based bioassay.

to the interpretation of results obtained from that assay. When designing a bioassay, it is often difficult to identify a cell line that has a robust measurable response to the therapeutic protein. In some of these cases, it is necessary either to engineer a cell line that can respond or occasionally to use primary cells. The use of primary cells is a powerful technique because it better accounts for population variability and is many times a more accurate model; however, primary cell assays tend to be less reproducible than assays relying on the well-characterized cell lines. When conducting an entire development program for a therapeutic protein, it is important to have consistent assays. When a large degree of assay variability occurs, it is possible to misinterpret assay results that lead to incorrect assumptions on a drug's immunogenicity. When validating a cell-based assay, some additional parameters that must be evaluated are related to cell culture conditions. How many passages the cells can be subjected to and still produce consistent results is an important characteristic during validation. In addition, it is important to determine if cells need to be used when they are in a specific stage of their growth cycle. The viability and number of cells used are also characteristics evaluated during validation.

Non-cell-based In some instances, it is possible to measure the intended biological effect of a protein therapeutic without needing a cell-based system. An example of this would be a monoclonal antibody therapeutic whose only function is to bind and block an epitope or specific region of a target. In this case, the only biological effect is to bind to the specific region of the target. This type of biological activity can easily be monitored with a simpler immunoassay. A non-cell-based assay would still be different than a screening immunoassay – the screening assay would detect the presence of any and all antidrug antibodies that bind to the therapeutic, and the biological assay would only detect those antibodies specific for the active portion of the monoclonal antibody therapeutic. The expectations for sensitivity, specificity, and precision would be similar to the expectations for a traditional antidrug antibody immunoassay. Another example would be an enzyme functional assay. In this case, the drug is an enzyme that catalyzes a specific reaction. The assay for neutralizing antibodies would add the sample to the enzyme and substrate and determine if

the ability of the enzyme to catalyze the reaction had been inhibited. It is important to note that given a choice, regulators tend to prefer a traditional cell-based system for neutralizing antibody determination. This is because a cell-based system is usually a better approximation and model for what is happening in a test subject. When it is not possible to develop a cell-based bioassay, a non-cell-based system can provide a reasonable alternative.

10.7 Testing Strategy

The most traditional and cost-effective approach for testing for the immunogenicity of a protein therapeutic is shown in Figure 10.3 and includes testing all samples in the screening immunoassay (Swanson and Bussiere 2012). Those samples that are positive in the screening assay may either be further tested with a confirmatory assay if the screening assay suffers from a high rate of false-positive samples, or moving directly to testing using the biological assay for neutralizing antibodies. The ideal confirmatory assay uses a different scheme than the screening assay and is more than just a repeat of the screen. Samples positive in the immunoassay would be classified as binding antibodies and those that test positive in the biological assay would be classified as neutralizing antibodies. Using this paradigm, all neutralizing antibodies would also be considered binding antibodies, but binding antibodies may or may not be neutralizing. In some cases, it will be important to further characterize the antibodies. For example, it is often very valuable to understand how much antidrug antibody is present and determine the titer (inverse of the dilution of the sample that still scores positive in the assay, i.e., a sample that is positive at a 1:100 dilution but negative in a 1:150 dilution would have a titer of 100). While not absolutely quantitative, the titer provides a standard expression for the relative amount of antidrug antibody that is present in a sample. In most cases, the more antibody that is present, the more likely those antibodies will demonstrate an effect in the animal. Other examples of characterization that are often performed include antibody isotype determination. This can be done most conveniently using a biosensor instrument and will let investigators know the isotypes

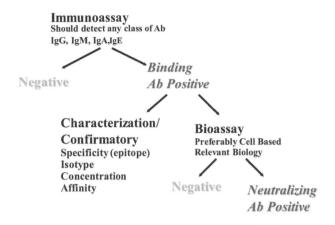

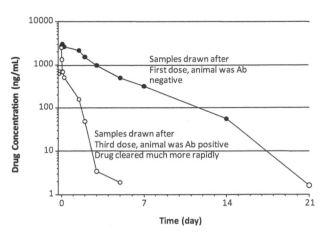

FIGURE 10.3 A testing paradigm for immunogenicity assessment of a therapeutic protein is shown. All samples are first tested in an immunoassay screening assay. It is very important that the assays have sufficient sensitivity (typically in low ng/ml range) and be able to detect all classes of antibodies that may be produced by the test animal. Samples that are positive in the immunoassay can be further confirmed and characterized if warranted. Characterization can include relative quantitation (typically the titer of the sample is determined for this purpose), isotype analysis, and in rare instances the relative binding affinity can be assessed (typically only performed using a biosensor). Any antibody confirmed positive is then further tested in a bioassay to determine if any antibodies are capable of neutralizing the biological effect of the drug. Samples are defined as antibody negative if the initial screening assay is negative and if samples positive in the screening assay are not confirmed as positive during the confirmation step (if utilized). Samples are binding antibody positive if they are positive in the screening assay and are confirmed positive in the confirmatory assay (if utilized). Samples are classified as neutralizing if they are positive in the bioassay for neutralizing antibodies. Note: samples that are negative in the bioassay are still considered to be binding antibody positive using this testing paradigm.

FIGURE 10.4 This figure demonstrates the pharmacokinetics observed in the presence of a clearing antibody. The line representing drug levels after the first administration of a therapeutic protein shows the expected slow clearance of the drug when there are no (or very few) circulating antibodies. The drug is present at a concentration greater than 10 ng/ml 14 days after drug administration. In contrast, the line representing drug levels in an animal administered the drug after the animal had produced circulating antibodies as a result of prior exposure to the drug shows the drug is cleared much more rapidly. In the animal with antibodies, the level of circulating drug drops below 10 ng/ml as early as day 3 post-administration.

of antibody are present. This can have relevance because if only IgM antibodies are present, it suggests an early and immature immune response. These antibodies tend to have lower binding affinity and are produced in lower numbers than a more mature IgG response. Another example where isotyping can be important is when determining if a hypersensitivity-like reaction is mediated by IgE antibodies. In rare instances, it may be important to know the relative binding affinity of the antidrug antibodies. A biosensor is ideal for this determination. When an antidrug antibody binds to the drug in a biosensor assay, there is a real-time record of the binding event as well as the subsequent dissociation phase. In the case of mature IgG antibody responses, the dissociation rate is very low with most of the antibody remaining tightly bound to the drug. However, in some cases, the binding affinity is quite low and the dissociation phase is marked by a rapid decrease in antibody bound. This occurs when the relative binding affinity of the antidrug antibodies is low.

10.8 Consequences of Immunogenicity

10.8.1 Effects of an Immune Response on Pharmacokinetics

The most common effect of antidrug antibodies on the pharmacokinetics of a protein therapeutic is to reduce the circulating level of the drug as demonstrated in Figure 10.4.

This is observed as a lower half-life of the drug and a reduced maximum drug concentration available after administration. This type of an immune response is classified as a clearing response because it facilitates a more rapid clearance of the drug. Antidrug antibodies with high affinity and avidity for the protein therapeutic remain bound to the drug long enough to facilitate an additional clearance mechanism for the drug via the Fc region of the antibody.

In some instances, the antidrug antibodies can increase the concentration of the circulating protein therapeutic, resulting in an increased half-life and an increased maximum concentration of circulating drug shown in Figure 10.5. The mechanism for this action is likely due to the antidrug antibodies preventing the drug from being cleared but not binding tightly enough, or long enough to facilitate clearance via the Fc portion of the antibody. Antidrug antibodies with lower affinity and avidity toward the protein therapeutic do not remain bound to the drug long enough to facilitate such clearing. These antibodies can be referred to as sustaining antibodies as they sustain the drug in circulation (Chirmule, Jawa and Meibohm 2012).

The magnitude of the effect on pharmacokinetics depends upon the following factors that are associated with the maturation of the immune response: what class of antidrug antibody is present; how much antidrug antibody is present in circulation; the affinity that the antidrug antibody has for the therapeutic protein; and where the antidrug antibodies are binding to the therapeutic protein. As the immune response matures, the type and amount of antibodies produced against the protein therapeutic changes and tends to be more effective at blocking the effects of the drug. When an antidrug antibody response is produced in an animal, that response is diverse. There are typically more than one class of antibody generated, multiple regions

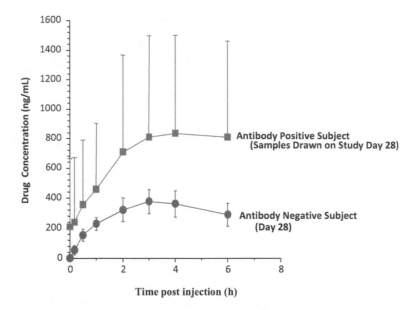

FIGURE 10.5 The pharmacokinetics of a sustaining antibody are shown. The drug concentration of circulating drug in an animal that does not have antidrug antibodies is shown in blue. The green line represents circulating drug levels in an animal that tested antibody positive. Unlike the profile shown in Figure 4 where the antidrug antibodies resulted in a more rapid clearance of the drug, in this case, the antibodies delayed clearance and supported a higher level of circulating drug. While not the most common response, this sustaining phenomenon has been observed in many animal studies. A likely explanation is that the antidrug antibodies bind with low affinity and remain bound long enough to protect the drug from normal clearance but are not bound long enough to support Fc-mediated clearance.

or epitopes on the therapeutic protein are recognized, and the affinity of the antidrug antibody binding is also variable. As the immune response matures, a phenomenon referred to as epitope spreading occurs and more regions of the protein therapeutic are recognized by the antidrug antibodies produced.

The first class of antibody produced in response to therapeutic protein is typically IgM. These IgM antibodies are characterized by their large molecular weight and low binding affinity. IgM antibodies are rarely associated with neutralizing ability or the ability to have a negative impact on pharmacokinetics. As the immune response matures, isotypes of the IgG form are produced and in humans may include subtypes IgG1, IgG2, IgG3, and IgG4. IgG antibodies tend to have higher affinity and are produced in higher concentrations. It is generally the IgG antibodies that have the most impact on the pharmacokinetics of the drug.

The amount of antidrug antibodies often increases upon subsequent exposure to the protein therapeutic. When more antibodies are produced, there is a greater chance that there will be an impact on the pharmacokinetics of the therapeutic protein. In addition to producing more antibodies as the immune response matures, the antibodies tend to have an increasing binding affinity and these higher-affinity antibodies are more likely to affect pharmacokinetics by promoting more rapid clearance of the drug.

10.8.2 Effects of an Immune Response on Efficacy and Safety

Antidrug antibodies can impact the efficacy of the protein therapeutic by either neutralizing the drug, binding to the biologically active region of the drug and blocking its function, by promoting a rapid clearance of the drug, or by preventing

clearance and sustaining high levels of the drug in circulation. The net result for the animal of neutralizing or clearing antibodies is that the drug is not able to perform its biological activity and loses efficacy. The efficacy of the drug can return when the immune response wanes. If the antibodies sustain the drug in circulation, increased toxicity can be observed because the drug is not being cleared as efficiently. The timing of the immune response is also an important consideration. In some cases, there is an immune response during treatment; however, the animal subsequently stops producing antidrug antibodies and the immune response is only transient. Cases of transient antibody production are common and often missed during trials because insufficient samples are taken to test for antibodies throughout dosing. Transient immune responses are often not significant for the animal since the effect of the antibodies is short-lived. When a response is not transient, the antibody response often progresses throughout dosing of the protein therapeutic with more antibodies and antibodies with higher affinity produced. These persistent immune responses are likely to have an impact on the animal's ability to derive an effect and/or assess the true safety of the therapeutic.

A more important consequence of antidrug antibodies occurs when antibodies produced by the animal against the protein therapeutic can bind and subsequently either clear or neutralize an endogenous protein. This can happen when the protein therapeutic is designed to mimic and replace the function of an endogenous protein. There are many examples of endogenous proteins that are mimicked by protein therapeutics, and these include erythropoietin and interferon. Any time that an endogenous protein is blocked by antidrug antibodies, there can be significant consequences for the animal. Fortunately, these occurrences are not common, but they are possible any time a protein therapeutic mimics an endogenous protein. When the endogenous protein performs a critical function and there are no redundant pathways the body can use to circumvent the loss of this endogenous protein, very careful attention must be made to monitor and minimize any immune response to the therapeutic protein that mimics the endogenous protein. Important considerations when considering immunogenicity include both the severity and consequences of the immune response in those animals that produce antidrug antibodies and also what percentage of animals treated with the drug generate an immune response. When the consequences of an immune response are significant, the threshold for how many animals mount an immune response is quite low. There is more tolerance for those drugs that induce an immune response if the consequences of that immune response are minor and transient.

10.9 Clinical Case Studies on Clinically Relevant Immunogenicity

Thrombopoietin is required for the body to produce platelets. In some disease conditions including immune thrombocytopenia, thrombopoietin levels are ineffective to maintain sufficient platelets in circulation. A drug was designed, megakaryocyte growth and development factor (MGDF), to mimic

thrombopoietin and stimulate platelet production. In nonclinical studies, it was observed that some animals developed antibodies that appeared to neutralize not only the drug (MGDF), but also some of the animal's endogenous thrombopoietin. The antibodies were anticipated because MGDF is a human analogue and would be expected to be viewed as foreign in the animals. It was not anticipated that MGDF would have a similar effect in clinical trials. Unfortunately, during an early clinical study in healthy volunteers, it was observed that antibodies were generated in several of the subjects (Wang, et al. 2008; Li, et al. 2001). These antibodies were able to neutralize not only the administered MGDF drug, but also circulating endogenous thrombopoietin. The clinical result was that since the subjects did not have any circulating thrombopoietin (it was neutralized by antibodies as soon as it entered the circulation), their platelet levels plummeted, an example is shown in Figure 10.6, and many subjects in the trial required platelet transfusions. In some of these subjects, the platelet transfusions were required for many years. The important message from this example is that sometimes, nonclinical immunogenicity provides a window into what the presence of antidrug antibodies could mean for patients. This is not a common occurrence in drug development, but an important cautionary anecdote to help drive drug development decisions when it comes to immunogenicity. After years of study by multiple drug companies and academic

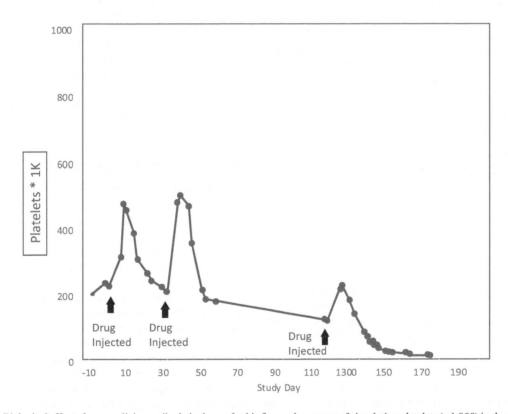

FIGURE 10.6 Biological effect of a neutralizing antibody is shown. In this figure, the amount of circulating platelets (x 1,000) is shown over 170 days. The drug used stimulates platelet production and the days when the drug was administered are shown. The first two doses of the drug resulted in a rapid rise in circulating platelets. However, the level of circulating platelets began to drop a few days after the second dose, and the response to the third dose was significantly suppressed with the level of circulating platelets barely reaching the level seen prior to first dosing. In addition, the level of circulating platelets dropped dramatically after the third dose and never returned to pre-study normal levels. What caused this phenomenon was a developing antidrug neutralizing antibody response. As can be seen, the antibodies were able to not only suppress the effect of the drug by the third administration, but they also neutralized endogenous thrombopoietin which prevented any new platelet formation.

researchers, it has been determined that thrombopoietin is an inherent immunogenicity risk and contains multiple regions on the molecule that are likely to induce a robust immune response.

Erythropoietin is also an endogenous protein and is produced in the kidney. Erythropoietin is absolutely required for the production of red blood cells. In certain diseases, including kidney disease and some cancers, insufficient erythropoietin is produced by the patient to support red blood cell production, which results in anemia. Erythropoietin has been produced by multiple manufacturers and was first approved by the FDA in 1989. Its safety profile related to immunogenicity had been exemplary until the early 2000s. It was discovered that a version of erythropoietin manufactured for distribution in Europe and Australia was responsible for several patients developing antibody-mediated pure red cell aplasia (Casadevall, et al. 2002). In these patients, the erythropoietin drug was immunogenic and patients began producing antibodies. Upon careful examination, it was determined that these antibodies were in fact able to neutralize endogenous erythropoietin produced by the patients as well as the erythropoietin drug that they were administered (Swanson, Ferbas, et al. 2004). It was not obvious what caused the drug to suddenly become immunogenic, and multiple changes were made by the manufacturer in response to the findings which has returned the drug to its previous status of being immunogenic in only very rare instances. The important message from this case is that manufacturers must remain vigilant to maintain their processes to prevent this type of unexpected immunogenicity. It also points out the need for these drug manufacturers to maintain laboratories capable of performing antibody tests on patients that suddenly and unexpectedly lose response to their drug as this may be the result of new neutralizing antibodies. The tests for antibodies against protein therapeutics are sophisticated and not available routinely in clinical laboratories, which places the burden for these tests with the manufacturer of the drug in order to protect patient safety.

10.10 Hypersensitivity Reactions

Hypersensitivity reactions can occur when a pharmaceutical product is administered and the immune system responds in an abnormal and enhanced manner (Murphy, Travers and Walport 2008). Four distinct types of hypersensitivity have been described, and each type has been reported on multiple occasions as an adverse event after a drug administration (Mayorga, et al. 2019). In addition, a phenomenon named CARPA or complement activation-related pseudoallergy, has been described during nonclinical studies whose symptoms closely mimic some symptoms observed during hypersensitivity reactions.

10.10.1 Type I: Immediate

This is the classic form of hypersensitivity that many people think of when they hear the term "allergic reaction." It can occur within minutes of exposure to an antigen (the actual entity that you are allergic to, such as pollen). It is characterized by the presence of large amounts of IgE antibodies directed against the antigen (or allergen, in this case), which are coating mast cells and basophils that are cross-linked by contact with free antigen. This cross-linking results in cell degranulation and release of histamine as well as other inflammatory mediators. The magnitude of the response is mediated by both the amount of IgE present and the amount of antigen encountered by the subject. Each subsequent encounter with the allergen further sensitizes the subject and results in more specific IgE being produced. Examples include food allergies, pollen allergies, bee stings, and some drug reactions. An important diagnostic feature for this type of hypersensitivity is the presence of a large amount of IgE antibodies and a large histamine release. It is important to remember that these IgE antibodies are short-lived and will likely only be detectable for a short time (hours) after symptoms are evident. In order to conclusively determine the subject has had a Type I hypersensitivity reaction, it is critical to obtain a serum sample within hours of the event to be able to detect the high level of IgE antibodies present. Symptoms from this type of hypersensitivity can have a very rapid onset and can be quite severe including airway obstruction that requires immediate medical intervention. It is also important to realize that each subsequent exposure to the antigen can result in increasingly severe reactions.

10.10.2 Type II: Cytotoxic

Type II hypersensitivity is characterized by the presence of IgG or IgM antibodies binding to antigens on cells. This can result in the activation of the complement system, which in turn results in the lysis and phagocytosis of cells. An example is antibody-dependent cell-mediated cytotoxicity by natural killer (NK) cells. Some examples include autoimmune hemolytic anemia, hemolytic disease of the fetus and newborn, Grave's disease, myasthenia gravis, and immune thrombocytopenia. The key finding is that IgG or IgM antibodies mistakenly bind to cells that should be ignored and the result is a cytotoxic (meaning death of cells) autoimmune reaction.

10.10.3 Type III: Immune Complex

Type III immune complex hypersensitivity occurs after the deposition of immune complexes in tissues or blood vessels. Normally, when an antibody binds to its soluble target antigen, a small immune complex is formed that is quickly removed from the circulation by phagocytic cells in circulation. However, in this type of hypersensitivity, these immune complexes are not cleared, but instead are allowed to increase in size. This increase in size occurs as the initial antibody-antigen complex continues to have more antibodies bind to it and have more antigen captured by the increasing amount of bound antibodies. This results in large and inconsistent sizes of immune complexes. Due to the bivalent nature of each antibody molecule (10 binding sites for an IgM antibody), each antibody molecule can bind either one or two antigens and each antigen could be bound by one or multiple antibody molecules, resulting in a matrix that can become large enough to fall out of circulation and deposit in tissues or on the surface of blood vessels (Krishna and Nadler 2016; Theofilopoulos and Dixon 1980). Examples of this include serum sickness and Arthus reaction (local inflammatory skin reaction at the site of a vaccination such as with tetanus toxoid).

10.10.4 Type IV: Delayed and Cell-Mediated

Type IV, delayed and cell-mediated hypersensitivity, is the result of T cells. Once an antigen has entered the body, it is processed and taken to lymph nodes where it "educates" T cells. Subsequent exposure to the antigen results in these sensitized T cells inducing the release of cytokines and lymphokines that cause an inflammatory reaction. Examples include contact dermatitis (when an agent such as poison oak, nickel, latex, some soaps, some cosmetics comes in contact with the skin and results in a rash which can be severe), organ transplant rejection, and drug reactions such as Stevens-Johnson syndrome. Type IV hypersensitivity can be systemic and quite severe, potentially life-threatening.

What distinguishes CARPA from the four types of hypersensitivity is that CARPA does not leverage the immune system to cause the symptoms, it is the result of direct complement activation (Zhang, et al. 2018). Whereas hypersensitivity reactions require prior exposure to the antigen for priming purposes, CARPA can occur during the first contact with the pharmaceutical product. Hallmarks of CARPA include normal levels of IgE but elevated levels of complement activation markers.

When injection reactions occur during the course of nonclinical studies, it is very important to correctly determine the mechanism for the reaction and determine if it is due to CARPA or one of the hypersensitivity reactions. In some instances, these injection reactions may also occur during clinical dosing, while others will be unique to the nonclinical setting.

10.11 Importance of Immunogenicity Assessment in Nonclinical Studies

Looking at immunogenicity of human therapeutics in nonclinical studies serves three functions. First, it can provide data to help predict how immunogenic a therapeutic protein may be in a clinical setting. Interestingly, while this was initially a very important driver to perform immunogenicity assessment in animal studies, it is actually the least compelling argument and these studies typically do not predict clinical immunogenicity. Second, it can be very useful in providing insight as to the consequences of an immune response, especially if that immune response is robust and results in adverse events. Finally, and most importantly, understanding of an immune response can help and may be required to interpret toxicity findings.

Predicting a response in a clinical setting: While there is some value in using nonclinical data to predict what an immune response would look like in a clinical study, that value is actually quite limited. The biggest reason for the limitation is that all animals will view a human therapeutic as a foreign protein, and in the vast majority of cases, the animals do mount an immune response as expected, and that response is likely more robust because of the species differences. It is very simple and straightforward for the immune system of the animals to recognize the amino acid sequence of the therapeutic as originating in a different species and therefore identify the protein as being foreign, resulting in the production of antibodies against it. However, in humans, because the amino acid sequence of the protein therapeutic originates from humans, it is more difficult for the patient's immune system to recognize the protein as foreign and to produce antibodies against it. The ability to predict how immunogenic a therapeutic protein might be was a major driver in performing immunogenicity assessments in early studies of protein therapeutics. The data accumulated throughout years of nonclinical studies using a wide range of protein therapeutics suggest that nonclinical studies do not accurately predict the immunogenicity of a protein therapeutic in a clinical setting. The rate of animals producing an immune response is almost always higher in nonclinical studies than is seen in clinical studies. This finding underscores the fact that a sequence difference between the therapeutic protein and endogenous protein produced in the patient is an important risk factor for inducing an immune response.

Predicting the consequences of an immune response: Animals in nonclinical studies not only demonstrate a higher rate of immunogenicity than seen in clinical studies with the same therapeutic protein, but the magnitude and robustness of that immune response is also typically greater than observed in clinical studies. This is predominately due to the therapeutic being more foreign in nonclinical studies than in clinical studies. The more foreign a protein is, the more likely it is to have multiple epitopes recognized by the immune system. This variety of epitopes results in a more aggressive immune response both in the number of antibodies produced and also by the diversity of epitopes recognized on the therapeutic protein. However, there is still value in understanding what the consequences of an immune response during a nonclinical trial are. Even though the response is most likely greater in nonclinical studies, the same consequences could be observed clinically. Those consequences can include a loss in efficacy because of enhanced clearance of the drug, enhanced toxicological findings due to sustained circulation of the drug, complications resulting from immune complex deposition, and perhaps most worrisome, the loss of an endogenous function. The loss of efficacy is the classic expectation of an immune response and occurs when antibodies produced in the test animals react to bind and/or neutralize the drug before it can exert its biological function. Rapid drug clearance is by far the most common consequence of an immune response that is observed in nonclinical studies, and when considering that many protein therapeutics do not exhibit any efficacy in healthy animals, this rapid clearance is often the only effect observed. A less commonly observed occurrence is when the toxicology of the drug is enhanced because antibodies are binding to the drug but rather than enhancing clearance, these antibodies protect the drug from being cleared. This protection results in enhanced pharmacokinetic profiles and elevated drug levels. While rarely seen in clinical studies, this phenomenon has often been observed in nonclinical settings. When there are very high levels of antibodies produced in the animals and the studies include high levels of drug being administered, especially when the drug is administered intravenously, there is a strong opportunity for immune complexes to be formed. This occurs when there is an equivalence of circulating drug and circulating antibodies against the drug. The antibodies will recognize and bind to the drug and because of the large number of drug and antibody molecules, and their equivalence in the circulation, rather large immune complexes can form which then deposit into vasculature walls or in target tissues. These immune complexes, once deposited, can result in severe pathology due to complement activation or further immune system intervention. This phenomenon can occur clinically; however, it is much less common. The clinical setting rarely induces as robust an immune response as seen nonclinically, and the levels of drug administered are typically lower. Thus, in the clinical setting, there are far fewer circulating antibodies and far fewer drug molecules circulating. When immune complexes form in this setting, they are most always smaller and more easily cleared without consequence. The most worrisome case of consequences from an immune response against a therapeutic protein is when that protein mimics an endogenous protein that performs a critical and nonredundant function. If an immune response is generated against this therapeutic protein, it is possible that these antibodies would bind and possibly neutralize not only the therapeutic protein but also the endogenous protein the therapeutic was modeled after. This could result in a loss of efficacy not only to the therapeutic protein, but also to the endogenous counterpart. An example of this occurred with MGDF, a protein that mimicked thrombopoietin. Antibodies formed against MGDF were able to bind and neutralize not only MGDF, but also endogenous thrombopoietin. This neutralization translated into the animals being unable to produce platelets. Even though the consequences of an immune response in clinical trials are most often much less severe than those observed in nonclinical studies, it is very important that investigators identify and understand what the consequences of an immune response are in their nonclinical studies. This understanding will help them de-risk their therapeutic in clinical trials by being prepared for early indications of critical consequences and having an appropriate risk management plan in place to respond to early clinical signals. Failure to understand consequences of an immune response in nonclinical studies can be a fatal flaw for a program.

Proper interpretation of nonclinical studies requires an immunogenicity assessment: There has been a very troubling trend to de-emphasize preclinical immunogenicity testing in nonclinical studies. This trend is the result of flawed thinking that it is expected all animals administered a human therapeutic will robustly raise antibodies and the data are of no value. This trend to de-emphasize the need for nonclinical immunogenicity assessment has been further strengthened by many nonclinical studies employing analytical methodology that was not ideal and failed to answer the important question of exactly which animals produced antibodies, and when they were produced. The argument put forward for de-emphasizing testing was that antibody testing was expensive and burdensome and did not add value to the trial. In fact, not every animal does raise an immune response, and although very many do, it is not reasonable to assume that an animal produced antibodies if the animal was not tested. Further, methodology has significantly improved and continues to improve to rapidly and accurately identify those animals that produced antibodies. The main value in knowing the immune status of each animal is to determine if the administered drug had an effect on the animal. Simply put, if it is not clear whether or not antibodies were generated in an animal, it is impossible to assess toxicological effects in that animal. The presence of antibodies, and just as important, an indication of the magnitude of that immune response, is vital to determine if the animals were exposed to the drug for sufficient time to evaluate safety. Further, it is completely unreasonable to assume certain findings in a nonclinical trial are the consequence of an immune response if that immune response was never assessed/measured. Therefore, despite the fact that nonclinical immunogenicity is a poor predictor of a clinical response, it remains very important to thoroughly test and evaluate immunogenicity in nonclinical studies that employ therapeutic proteins. In rare cases, the consequences of a robust immune response in nonclinical studies warrants that the real-time immunogenicity assessment be utilized for clinical trials. This could be the case if neutralizing antibodies are detected that could neutralize an endogenous counterpart with a critical and nonredundant function.

One final benefit of assessing the immune response during nonclinical studies is that the data obtained can be very beneficial in preparing an Immunogenicity Risk Mitigation Plan. This is a component that regulatory agencies are frequently requesting as soon as during an IND submission. This plan evolves over time as more data are available and typically contains sections describing (1) what is the probability of the therapeutic inducing an immune response in humans; (2) what are the possible and likely consequences of an immune response should it occur in humans; and (3) what are the sponsor's plans to minimize the risk and to respond in the event of a severe clinically relevant immune response that occurs. The probability of an immune response section includes degree of similarity to a human endogenous protein; identification of potential T-cell epitopes that might increase the risk of immunogenicity; manufacturing risks including aggregation and stability; route, frequency, and amount of drug administered; posttranslational modifications; nonclinical data on immunogenicity; and clinical data on immunogenicity as it becomes available. The potential consequences of an immune response include the following: If there is an endogenous counterpart to the therapeutic, what would the consequences be if this endogenous protein was neutralized; what would the consequences be if the therapeutic were rapidly neutralized and/or removed from circulation; are there any similar entities that antibodies generated against the therapeutic might also bind and influence; and what would happen if the therapeutic induced hypersensitivity. The risk mitigation portion contains topics including: are assays robust, sufficiently sensitive, reproducible, able to detect all clinically relevant antidrug antibodies and identify those antibodies capable of neutralizing the biological effects of the drug; plans to intervene in the event of a severe immune response; timing and logistics of testing (both when will samples be taken and when will results from analysis be available, since in very rare circumstances it may be necessary to provide antidrug antibody data prior to patient receiving their next dose of drug); plans for any concomitant medication to reduce potential and/or consequences of an immune response; plans for cessation of dosing in a study due to clinically significant immune response; and plans to deimmunize the therapeutic. This document is typically submitted with the IND and is modified as data are collected with a final submission going in with the BLA.

10.12 Predicting an Immune Response

It is evident that nonclinical studies will not be effective in predicting clinical immunogenicity. There are times during drug development when it is very important to understand the likelihood and potential consequences of clinical immunogenicity prior to the conduct of any clinical trials (Rosenberg and Sauna 2017). In these instances, it can be helpful to evaluate the amino acid sequence of the therapeutic candidate with any of several databases that have been established to help predict immunogenicity (Vita, et al. 2010). The way these databases work is they have compiled a listing of known amino acid sequences that have been identified as T-cell epitopes. When a foreign body is phagocytized by the immune system effector cells, small pieces of the genetic sequence are transported to the receptor of these cells. If any of these sequences are recognized by T cells, an immune response can be initiated that can eventually result in antibodies being formed against that sequence and ultimately, against the foreign material that was phagocytized. *In silico* immunogenicity prediction is based on the ability to identify the presence of known T-cell epitopes (typically ~7 amino acids in length) throughout the genetic sequence of the therapeutic protein (Koren, et al. 2007). The *in silico* prediction tools then identify how many of these potential matches occur and how close the sequence matches these known T-cell epitopes. Higher numbers of T-cell epitopes being present along with very close matches of known epitopes correlate with a higher risk of immunogenicity. It is important to understand some of the limitations of this exercise. In nature, conformational epitopes exist when certain amino acids are not linear in sequence, but due to the three-dimensional structure of the protein are brought together and a new epitope is formed that is different than the linear sequence would suggest. These epitopes are not likely seen in prediction models. Further, these T-cell epitope models work best for regions of the protein that are on the surface. While antibodies may well be produced against a strong epitope, if that epitope is not present on the surface of the molecule, any antibodies against it will not be able to bind and the presence of the epitope will be irrelevant. In addition, cellular assays can be performed that further test the interaction of cells in the immune system with potential epitopes. Despite current limitations of these models, there is potential value when immunogenicity is a big concern, such as with therapeutics mimicking a critical endogenous protein, of utilizing a prediction algorithm. If this algorithm is used early in development, it may be possible to engineer out any T-cell epitope(s) without severely impacting the efficacy of the therapeutic (Baker and Jones 2007). These models have been known to underpredict immunogenicity in some cases and overpredict in others, which can be frustrating.

10.13 Summary

Immunogenicity assessment is an important component of nonclinical studies. Because most therapeutic proteins are human-based, it is common for these drugs to produce significant levels of antidrug antibodies in nonclinical test species.

While not necessarily predictive of the level and magnitude of the immunogenicity that will occur in clinical settings, it remains important to fully understand the immune response that occurs in these test animals. The ability to interpret toxicological findings in any animal absolutely requires that the immune status of that animal be fully understood.

It is important to carefully develop and validate the analytical procedures to identify and characterize binding and neutralizing antibodies against the therapeutic being tested. Only through the validation process are the parameters and characteristics of an analytical procedure defined sufficiently to correctly interpret assay results.

While the consequences of a robust immune response in a nonclinical species may not reflect what occurs clinically, understanding the animal response will prepare the investigator for clinical consequences that may occur so they can be prepared and patients monitored closely to facilitate a rapid response if necessary. Because overall safety determination is a primary objective of nonclinical studies, immunogenicity assessment is one of the critical attributes of safety that should be carefully evaluated.

BIBLIOGRAPHY

Baker, M, and T Jones. 2007. "Identification and removal of immunogenicity in therapeutic proteins." *Current Opinion in Drug Discovery and Development* 10 219–227.

Casadevall, N, J Nataf, B Viron, A Kolta, J-J Kiladjian, P Martin-Dupont, P Michaud, et al. 2002. "Pure red cell aplasia and anti-erythropoietin antibodies in patients treated with recombinant erythropoietin." *New England Journal of Medicine* 346 469–475.

Chirmule, N, V Jawa, and B Meibohm. 2012. "Immunogenicity to therapeutic proteins: impact on PK/PD and efficacy." *The AAPS Journal* 14 no. 2 296–302.

Gupta, S, S R Indelicato, V Jethwa, T Kawabata, M Kelley, A R Mire-Sluis, S M Richards, et al. 2007. "Recommendations for the design, optimization, and qualification of cell-based assays used for the detection of neutralizing antibody responses elicited to biological therapeutics." *Journal of Immunological Methods* 321 1–18.

Koren, E, A DeGroot, V Jawa, K Beck, T Boone, D Rivera, L Li, et al. 2007. "Clinical validation of the "in silico" prediction of immunogenicity of a human recombinant therapeutic protein." *Clinical Immunology* 124 26–32.

Koren, E, H W Smith, E Shores, G Shankar, D Finco-Kent, B Rup, Y-C Barrett, et al. 2008. "Recommendations on risk-based strategies for detection and characterization of antibodies against biotechnology products." *Journal of Immunological Methods* 333 1–9.

Krishna, M, and S G Nadler. 2016. "Immunogenicity to biotherapeutics - the role of anti-drug immune complexes." *Frontiers in Immunology* 7 1–13.

Li, J, C Yang, Y Xia, A Bertino, J Glaspy, M Roberts, and D J Kuter. 2001. "Thrombocytopenia caused by the development of antibodies to thrombopoietin." *Blood* 98 3241–3248.

Lofgren, J A, S Dhandapani, J Pennucci, C M Abbott, D T Mytych, A Kaliyaperumal, S J Swanson, and M C Mullenix. 2007. "Comparing ELISA and surface plasmon resonance for assessing clinical immunogenicity of panitumumab." *The Journal of Immunology* 178 no. 11 7467–7472.

Matucci, A, A Vultaggio, and R Danesi. 2018. "The use of intravenous versus subcutaneous monoclonal antibodies in the treatment of severe asthma: a review." *Respiratory Research 19* 154–164.

Mayorga, C, T D Fernandez, M I Montanez, E Moreno, and M J Torres. 2019. "Recent developments and highlights in drug hypersensitivity." *Allergy 74* no. 12 2368–2381.

Mire-Sluis, A R, Y C Barrett, V Devanarayan, E Koren, H Liu, M Maia, T Parish, et al. 2004. "Recommendations for teh design and optimization of immunoassays used in the detection of host antibodies against biotehnology products." *Journal of Immunological Methods 289* 1–16.

Murphy, K, P Travers, and M Walport. 2008. *Janeway's Immunobiology*. New York: Garland Science.

Patton, A, M C Mullenix, S J Swanson, and E Koren. 2005. "An acid-dissociation bridging ELISA for detection of antibodies directed against therapeutic proteins in the presence of antigen." *Journal of Immunological Methods 304* 189–195.

Rosenberg, A, and Z Sauna. 2018. "Immunogenicity assessment during the development of protein therapeutics." *Journal of Pharmacy and Pharmacology 70* no. 5 584–594.

Schellekens, Huub. 2003. "Immunogenicity of therapeutic proteins." *Nephrology Dialysis Transplantation 18* 1257–1259.

Shankar, G, S Arkin, L Cocea, V Devanarayan, S Kirshner, A Kromminga, V Quarmby, et al. 2014. "Assessment and reporting of the clinical immunogenicity of therapeutic proteins and peptides-harmonized terminology and tactical recommendations." *The AAPS Journal 16* no 4 658–673.

Shankar, G, S Arkin, V Devanarayan, A Quarmby, V Kromminga, S Richards, M Subramanyam, and S Swanson. 2015. "The quintessence of immunogenicity reporting for biotherapeutics." *Nature Biotechnology 33* no. 4 334–336.

Swanson, S J. 2007. "Immunogenicity in the development of therapeutic proteins." *International Journal of Pharmaceutical and Medicinal Research 21* 207–216.

Swanson, S J, and J Bussiere. 2012. "Immunogenicity assessment in non-clinical studies." *Current Opinions in Microbiology 15* 337–347.

Swanson, S J, J Ferbas, P Mayeux, and N Casadevall. 2004. "Evaluation of methods to detect and characterize antibodies against recombinant human erythropoietin." *Nephron Clinical Practice 96* 88–95.

Theofilopoulos, A N, and F J Dixon. 1980. "Immune complexes in human diseases: a review." *The American Journal of Pathology 100* no. 2 529–594.

Vita, R, L Zarebski, J Greenbaum, H Emami, I Hoof, N Salimi, R Damle, A Sette, and B Peters. 2010. "The immune epitope database 2.0." *Nucleic Acids Research 38* 854–862.

Voller, A, D Bidwell, and A Bartlett. 1980. Enzyme-linked immunosorbent assay. In: Rose N R, Friedman H, eds. *Manual of Clinical Immunology*. Washington, DC: American Society of Microbiology.

Wang, J, J Lozier, G Johnson, S Kirshner, D Verthelyi, A Pariser, E Shores, and A Rosenberg. 2008. "Neutralizing antibodies to therapeutic enzymes: considerations for testing, prevention and treatment." *Nature Biotechnology 26* 901–908.

Wei, X, S J Swanson, and S Gupta. 2004. "Development and validation of a cell-based bioassay for the detection of neutralizing antibodies against recombinant human erythropoietin in clinical studies." *Journal of Immunological Methods 293* 115–126.

Wu, Y, X Liu, Y Chen, R Woods, N Lee, H Yang, P Chowdury, L Roskos, and W I White. 2013. "An electrochemiluminescence (ECL)-based assay for the specific detection of anti-drug antibodies of the IgE isotype." *Journal of Pharmaceutical and Biomedical Analysis 86* 73–81.

Yu, Y, C Piddington, D Fitzpatrick, B Twomey, R Xu, S J Swanson, and S Jing. 2006. "A novel method for detecting neutralizing antibodies against therapeutic proteins by measuring gene expression." *Journal of Immunological Methods 316* 8–17.

Zhang, B, Q Li, C Shi, and X Zhang. 2018. "Drug-induced pseudoallergy: a review of the causes and mechanisms." *Pharmacology 101* 104–110.

11

Testing for Off-target Binding

Diana M. Norden and Benjamin J. Doranz

Integral Molecular

CONTENTS

11.1 Introduction

Off-target binding occurs when a drug binds to an unexpected and/or unwanted target. Specificity, which is the avoidance of off-target binding, is an important part of toxicity assessments and is critical for the safety of biopharmaceuticals, including monoclonal antibodies (MAbs), antigen-binding fragments (Fabs), single-chain variable fragments (scFvs), fusion proteins containing an immunoglobulin G (IgG)–based variable chain, and nanobodies.[1] Peptides, biologics, and biologic fusions (proteins designed with an IgG-based crystallizable fragment (Fc)) also need proper specificity testing. Moreover, absolute specificity is vital for chimeric antigen receptor (CAR) T cell therapies, antibody-drug conjugates (ADCs),

and bispecifics, where the therapeutic is usually designed to kill the target cell, and off-target interactions can have severe detrimental effects. MAbs are generally valued for their exquisite specificity compared with small molecules. However, emerging data from profiling panels of MAbs for lead selection suggest that 20%–25% of MAbs bind proteins in addition to their intended targets (Sullivan et al., 2020), potentially causing adverse reactions and failed clinical trials. Proper assessment of specificity early in development will contribute to more efficient clinical programs, safer trials, and more successful therapeutics.

11.2 Polyspecific vs. Polyreactive Compounds

Off-target binding can occur as a result of specific ("polyspecific") or nonspecific ("polyreactive") target interactions. Polyspecific binding occurs using two or more clearly defined epitopes, whereas polyreactive binding occurs through nonantigen-specific interactions (Figure 11.1). Polyreactive

---

[1] We refer primarily to MAbs throughout this chapter but most of the guidelines for MAbs apply to all of these modalities. Similarly, we primarily refer to the US Food and Drug Administration (FDA) throughout this chapter, but most of the guidelines for the FDA also apply to other regulatory agencies and ICH guidelines.

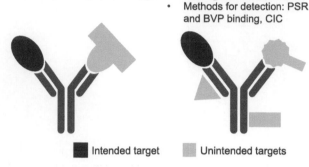

Polyspecific

- Antigen specific epitope
- Shared epitopes
- CDR-mediated binding
- Methods for detection: TCR studies, cell expression arrays

Polyreactive

- Non-specific binding (proteins, carbohydrates, surfaces)
- Interactions due to hydrophobic, charged residues
- Binding not limited to CDR
- Methods for detection: PSR and BVP binding, CIC

■ Intended target   ■ Unintended targets

FIGURE 11.1 Polyspecific and polyreactive monoclonal antibodies. Both polyspecific and polyreactive compounds will have off-target binding, but through different mechanisms. While polyspecific cross-reactivity is antigen specific, polyreactive compounds can display nonspecific binding to several different off-targets. Complementarity-determining regions (CDR), tissue cross-reactivity (TCR), polyspecific reagent (PSR), baculovirus particle (BVP), cross-interaction chromatography (CIC).

specificity (polyspecificity), as methods to assess polyreactivity are common and easier to interpret (Gunti and Notkins, 2015; Notkins, 2004; Starr and Tessier, 2019).

11.3 Importance of Specificity

11.3.1 Significance of Antigen Specificity

Off-target binding can cause unintended cellular toxicity, adverse events, and clinical trial failures. Even if not harmful directly, off-target binding may affect drug efficacy and pharmacokinetics with unfavorable results. For diagnostic MAbs, nonspecific interactions can give rise to false-positive diagnostic results.

While the exact impact of off-target binding by biotherapeutics has not yet been quantified, off-target binding is the single largest cause of failed small molecule preclinical trials and early clinical trials. A retrospective analysis of the AstraZeneca small molecule pipeline determined that 62% of all of their preclinical failures were caused by off-target binding (Cook et al., 2014) (Figure 11.2). Off-target safety problems were also the primary cause of their early-stage clinical trial failures. A recent analysis indicates that 10% of FDA-approved cancer drugs do not act through their intended target, but instead cause nonspecific toxicity that inadvertently benefits cancer patients (Lin et al., 2019). In another case, two purported KRAS inhibitors (peptides) were not specific for KRAS and instead induced unfolding of another protein to inhibit cell proliferation (Ng et al., 2020). These studies highlight the importance of accurately identifying the targets of a drug for its safety and for understanding its mechanism of action.

compounds are often characterized as "sticky" and bind to undefined proteins, carbohydrates, or surfaces. Polyreactivity is a significant factor in the developability of a MAb, as it can influence bioavailability, pharmacokinetics, manufacturing, formulation, and concentration. One study indicated that polyreactivity is the single most critical factor in determining success through clinical trials (Jain et al., 2017; Starr and Tessier, 2019). Testing for polyreactive binding typically occurs at the lead candidate selection phase and is done via traditional biochemical and biophysical methodologies, such as binding assays with the polyspecific reagent (PSR) and baculovirus particle (BVP), cross-interaction chromatography (CIC), and enzyme-linked immunosorbent assay (ELISA) with commonly used antigens. For the purpose of this review, we will discuss methods (i.e., traditional tissue cross-reactivity [TCR] studies and cell expression arrays) to determine antigen

11.3.2 Polyspecificity of Clinical MAbs

Despite the presumed specificity of monoclonal antibodies, emerging data indicate that MAbs frequently display polyspecificity (Bumbaca et al., 2011; Finton et al., 2013; Ma et al., 2012). For example, human clinical trials with the anti-programmed cell death protein 1 (PD1) antibody camrelizumab resulted in severe capillary hemangioma in

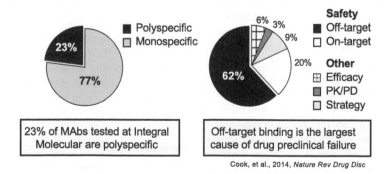

23% of MAbs tested at Integral Molecular are polyspecific

Off-target binding is the largest cause of drug preclinical failure

Cook, et al., 2014, *Nature Rev Drug Disc*

FIGURE 11.2 Off-target reactivity is the single leading cause of preclinical and early clinical failure. Analysis of specificity testing of lead panels of MAbs using a cell-based membrane proteome array found that approximately 20%–25% of MAbs tested demonstrate off-target binding, almost always to unpredicted membrane proteins with no significant sequence homology to the intended target (Integral Molecular's membrane proteome array internal database). A retrospective analysis by AstraZeneca found that 62% of their preclinical failures were due to off-target binding that caused safety problems (Cook et al., 2014). This study focused on their small molecules; a comparable study of antibody therapeutics is not yet published.

Phase 1 due to off-target binding to the vascular endothelial growth factor receptor (VEGFR) (Finlay et al., 2019; Mo et al., 2018). Importantly, the study directors specified that the capillary hemangioma was an unexpected adverse event that was not observed in preclinical nonhuman primate (NHP) studies, indicating that even NHPs do not fully represent the human condition. Our own specificity profiling of lead candidate MAbs suggests that approximately 20%–25% display polyspecific off-target binding (Figure 11.2). To determine whether polyspecificity is also prevalent among clinical MAbs and, most importantly, whether off-target reactivity can explain adverse events in patients, we conducted comprehensive specificity characterization of nearly all late-stage clinical and FDA-approved MAbs. This analysis found potentially harmful off-target reactivity present in MAbs at all stages of clinical development that, in many cases, may explain their adverse events. For example, one MAb currently in clinical trials demonstrated off-target binding to a widely expressed protein that would be predicted to result in adverse events due to MAb-mediated toxicity (Figure 11.3a). Another MAb was withdrawn from clinical trials because of the death of several patients and demonstrated off-target binding to a checkpoint protein that may explain its severe toxicity (Figure 11.3b). Finally, an FDA-approved MAb that has FDA black box warnings demonstrated off-target binding that may explain its severe side effects (Figure 11.3c). In each case, the original MAb developers were presumably unaware of these particular off-target binding events, and the specificity testing methods used (primarily TCR studies) did not identify the off-target interactions that could have averted clinical failures and drug safety issues.

11.3.3 CAR T and Other T Cell Therapies Require Absolute Specificity

Specificity profiling is especially important for biotherapeutics designed to be highly toxic to target cells (e.g., cancer cells), such as CAR T cell therapies, antibody-drug conjugates, and bispecifics that recruit T cells. In particular, CAR T cells are designed to kill cancerous cells through receptor engagement but cannot differentiate between on- and off-target engagement. Off-target interactions will therefore induce CAR T cell activation just as an on-target interaction would, and cells expressing the off-target will be destroyed. Moreover, the main adverse effect of CAR T cells is immune cell activation and cytokine storm (cytokine release syndrome). Any off-target interaction would increase cytokine release and contribute to enhanced immune activation. The difficulties associated with safety testing of CAR T cells lie in the fact that CAR T cell therapies must be evaluated in animal models of cancer (i.e., to achieve CAR T cell proliferation), so cannot be assessed in healthy animals including nonhuman primates. Rodent studies can determine some aspects of safety but may not adequately assess toxicity due to off-target binding, as human CAR T cells will not necessarily recognize off-target binding sites in animals.

Despite the potential for severe side effects, CAR T cell therapy is a major emerging biotherapeutic class for cancer treatments. In 2017, the first CAR T cell therapy (Kymriah) was approved by the FDA. Since then, the number of CAR T cell therapies entering development and clinical trials has increased dramatically, with nearly 200 CAR T clinical trials in progress and even more planned including for noncancer indications. Unfortunately, not all trials have had successful outcomes. For example, Juno Therapeutics' JCAR015 CD19 CAR T molecule was withdrawn after five patients died during Phase 1 safety trials. Moreover, a clinical trial to test engineered T cells in myeloma and melanoma patients was quickly halted as the first two treated patients developed cardiogenic shock and died within a few days of T-cell infusion. It was later found that the toxicity was due to recognition of an epitope on an unrelated protein expressed in normal cardiac tissue (Linette et al., 2013). These case studies highlight the potentially severe outcome of off-target interactions for CAR T and related cell therapy modalities. Rigorous specificity analysis prior to initiating CAR T cell clinical development programs can help avoid safety pitfalls.

11.3.4 Mechanisms of Polyspecificity: Off-target Interactions Are Unexpected and Cannot Be Predicted

Two factors that contribute to the high specificity of biotherapeutics are the propensity of most biotherapeutics, such as MAbs, to recognize a specific conformational epitope and the relatively large surface area required for target binding. The surface area of antibody contact residues typically ranges from 500 to 750 Å^2 (Finlay and Almagro, 2012),

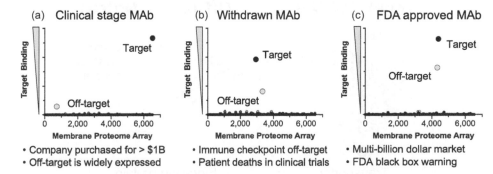

FIGURE 11.3 Off-targets identified in late-stage therapeutic MAbs. Integral Molecular's membrane proteome array (MPA) was probed with (a) a clinical-stage MAb intended to kill cancer cells, (b) a MAb withdrawn after clinical trials, and (c) an FDA-approved MAb currently on the market. The correct target was identified for all MAbs, but all three MAbs also showed off-target binding (greater than three standard deviations above average reactivity levels) that may explain their adverse events and reasons for withdrawal. The off-target proteins identified for each are completely unrelated human membrane proteins that could not have been predicted by sequence homology (i.e., not immediate protein family members).

compared with small molecule contact surface areas of 50–100 Å² (Pardridge, 2005). Moreover, MAbs are usually derived from immunizations with the target antigen, so in principle should only recognize that target.

So how can a MAb become polyspecific? One way is through molecular mimicry of a MAb's epitope. For example, in a previous study of a panel of antibodies against SLC2A4 (GLUT4), a 12-transmembrane (TM) insulin sensitive glucose transporter (Tucker et al., 2018), we found one MAb that demonstrated low-level reactivity to the unrelated signaling protein, Notch1. This was unexpected as SLC2A4 and Notch1 are structurally unrelated (12-TM vs. 1-TM) and share less than 7% sequence identity. High-resolution shotgun mutagenesis epitope mapping revealed the MAb's amino acid level epitope on a loop-constrained LGXXGP sequence motif on SLC2A4. Despite being completely unrelated in sequence and structure, the exact same LGXXGP motif was shared on a disulphide-constrained loop of Notch1 (Figure 11.4). After uncovering this cross-reactivity, the SLC2A4 candidate was deprioritized. In a similar case, T cells engineered to recognize the tumor antigen, MAGE-A3, were retrospectively found to cross-react with the off-target protein, titin, using the same EXDPIXXXY motif (Cameron et al., 2013; Raman et al., 2016). The off-target protein, titin, is expressed in cardiac muscle cells and the clinical trial resulted in fatal cardiac toxicity (Linette et al., 2013). These unpredicted cross-reactivities show the limitations of specificity testing against family members alone, as these cross-reactivities did not involve closely related family member proteins. These case studies also highlight that such cross-reactivity is based on structural conservation of small conformational regions, rather than simply sequence homology across a linear span of amino acids, so it is very difficult to predict.

A second mechanism of polyspecificity is through complementarity-determining region (CDR) flexibility. For example, a broadly neutralizing anti-HIV antibody, 4E10, cross-reacts with several autoantigens, primarily types 1, 2, and 3 inositol trisphosphate receptors (Finton et al., 2013). Crystal structures of 4E10 showed significant restructuring of the CDR binding site that enabled the antibody CDRs to adapt to more than one antigen. Moreover, other studies have demonstrated polyspecificity through the use of different CDR residues contributing to distinct, but overlapping, paratopes (Bostrom et al., 2009). These studies show that high flexibility in the CDR can increase the potential for off-target binding.

In addition to off-target toxicity, polyspecificity can also impair the generation of neutralizing antibodies following immunizations against exogenous antigens (viruses, bacteria, or tumor neoantigens). For example, cross-reactivity with autoantigens is thought to hinder generation of antibodies like the neutralizing anti-HIV MAb 4E10 during B cell development following immunization. This is likely due to a tolerance mechanism, where B cells with self-antigens undergo negative selection. A similar study suggested that autoreactivity due to structural mimicry limits the generation of neutralizing antibodies against influenza hemagglutinin (HA) (Bajic et al., 2019). These examples suggest that cross-reactivity can hinder antibody generation and result in poor vaccine responses.

11.4 Tissue Cross-reactivity Studies

Because of the potential adverse consequences of off-target interactions, specificity profiling is a requirement for advancing MAbs and other biotherapeutic categories into the clinic. The specific guidance documents are the International Council for Harmonisation of Technical Requirements for Pharmaceuticals for Human Use (ICH) S6 (ICHS6) and the FDA's Points to Consider in the Manufacture and Testing of Monoclonal Antibody Products for Human Use (US FDA [Center for Biologics Evaluation and Research (CBER)], first published in 1983 and last updated on February 28, 1997). These guidelines describe the use of *in vitro* TCR studies for specificity testing, which was the most relevant assay available at the time of guidance. As such, TCR studies have become a standard inclusion in filings to the FDA and other international regulatory agencies to support clinical development. TCR studies involve screening human tissues to identify unexpected off-target binding and unknown sites of on-target binding, and binding is determined by immunohistochemical (IHC) staining. If positive results are found in unexpected human tissues, then additional studies are performed with tissues from one or more animal species to determine the relevance of the species

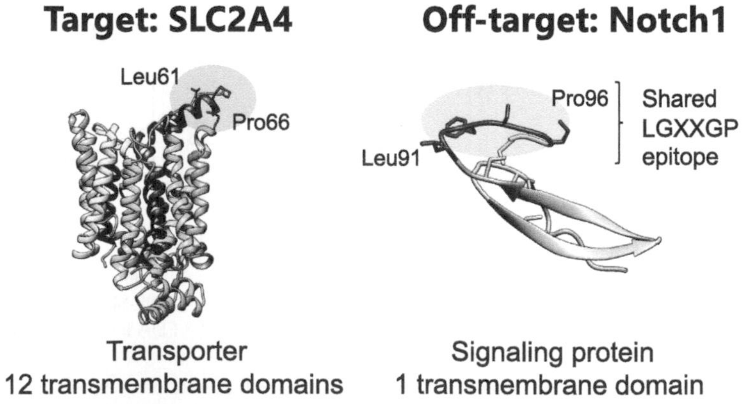

Target: SLC2A4 | **Off-target: Notch1**

Leu61 · Pro66 · Transporter 12 transmembrane domains

Pro96 · Leu91 · Shared LGXXGP epitope · Signaling protein 1 transmembrane domain

FIGURE 11.4 Unexpected cross-reactivity between SLC2A4 (GLUT4) and Notch1 is due to epitope mimicry. The MPA identified cross-reactivity of an SLC2A4 MAb with the unrelated signaling protein, Notch1. Shotgun mutagenesis epitope mapping studies identified the binding site on SLC2A4. The epitope structure is visualized on SLC2A4 (left) and the exact same sequence motif is found on the EGF-like domain of Notch1 (right).

for assessing the potential *in vivo* consequences of this unexpected binding (Leach et al., 2010). Additionally, both the FDA guidance document and ICHS6 guidance suggest that other technologies could be employed in place of IHC-based TCR studies as they became available and validated.

11.4.1 Tissue Cross-reactivity Study Technical Requirements

Technical requirements and suggestions for TCR studies have been well described in the literature (Leach et al., 2010) and are summarized here (Table 11.1). Human tissue samples are obtained from autopsy or surgical specimens. The tissue section needs to be large enough and of adequate quality to sufficiently represent the organ (which generally excludes tissue microarrays [TMAs]). Standard TCR studies use tissues from adults, as pediatric tissues are difficult to obtain and are only used if relevant for the therapeutic application. For animal tissue comparisons, at least three donors are recommended, with the exception of inbred rodent strains where two donors are sufficient. Sections should be prepared fresh and fixed in a manner that preserves antigen integrity. Similarly, blood smears should be prepared fresh and allowed to dry prior to fixation.

Standard ICH methods often need to be optimized for each MAb to decrease background staining while maintaining a robust positive signal. The method used to preserve the tissue (fixed or frozen) can have a major impact on MAb reactivity and often must be optimized in advance. Moreover, samples must be blocked to decrease nonspecific background binding to endogenous Fc receptors and IgG found within the tissue, as well as endogenous detectors (e.g., endogenous biotin, alkaline phosphatase, or peroxidase). Ideally, TCR studies should be performed with the therapeutic to be used in the clinic, without any modifications to the antibody, for instance, to improve detection by IHC methods. However, using the unmodified antibody requires some consideration because it is not labeled but needs to be detected by IHC. If the MAb is humanized, detection using an antihuman IgG secondary will yield excessive background staining due to the presence of endogenous human IgG. Therefore, the therapeutic is often directly labeled, and it is important to confirm that the labeling did not interfere with CDR-mediated binding to the target. Staining of the test compound should be evaluated under two different concentrations. One concentration should be the lowest concentration that produces maximum binding to the target antigen (the ideal concentration), and the other should be the highest feasible concentration to detect any low-level off-target binding.

Isotype and negative controls are important for defining specificity. Ideally, the isotype control is identical to the test antibody but with a different CDR to identify positive staining due to non-CDR–mediated binding. At the least, the negative control antibody needs to be the same isotype as the therapeutic MAb. An assay control includes screening a control slide *without* the primary antibody to detect any background staining resulting from the secondary antibody. To ensure proper sensitivity of the assay, positive and negative tissue controls should also be used. Positive tissue controls should express the target antigen, whereas negative tissue controls should have no or minimal target expression. If the target antigen is not normally expressed on a healthy, nondiseased tissue, then other approaches should be used to ensure that the test article can be detected when encountering its target. These options include diseased tissue, cell lines expressing the target antigen, or purified protein. Purified protein should only be used if the target is an exogenous target that cannot be expressed in cells, such as viral and bacterial components.

TABLE 11.1

Study Design for TCR Studies

Criteria	Approach or Technique
Tissue samples	38 human tissues/organs from three unrelated, nondiseased donors 2–3 animal donors Large enough physical section to represent the full organ Equally represent male and female
Tissue preparation	Optimized fixation methods (acetone, methanol, neutral-buffered formalin, or paraformaldehyde) to preserve tissue morphology and target antigen detection Optimized antigen retrieval processes to ensure target detection by the test article
Limit background	Block with serum to reduce binding to endogenous Fc receptors or endogenous IgG Block endogenous reaction enzymes (peroxidases, alkaline phosphatases, etc.) and detectors (biotin)
Test compound	Good manufacturing practice (GMP)-level material Non-GMP material can be used to preview target distribution and inform subsequent studies
Controls	Isotype control matched closely to the test MAb Assay control (no primary antibody added) Tissue positive and negative controls
Concentrations	0.5–50 μg/mL, with typical concentrations 2–10 μg/mL Two concentrations are to be tested Lowest concentration that produces maximum binding to the target (ideal concentration) Highest acceptable concentration used to best detect low affinity off-target reactivity Concentration may be decreased if high background staining prevents meaningful interpretation of the results
Detection	Immunohistochemistry (IHC) Direct label, secondary, or tertiary antibodies Biotin or fluorescence labels

11.4.2 Outcomes of Tissue Cross-reactivity Studies

TCR staining patterns must be carefully evaluated by a trained pathologist. Positive staining should confirm binding to the expected tissues expressing the intended target. Staining in unexpected tissues can be the result of two different scenarios. Unexpected staining can result from cross-reactive binding to an unrelated protein; this scenario is considered a polyspecific "off-target interaction." Alternatively, the intended target may be expressed in tissues that were previously unknown; this scenario is termed "off-target organ reactivity." Unfortunately, experimentally differentiating these scenarios can be difficult using TCR studies alone. Based on the staining pattern, the pathologist can conjecture on the potential identity of the off-target. In some cases, competition assays can be conducted by adding purified target antigen or another competing antibody to the assay.

The intensity of staining can also provide insight into potential toxicity, but this will depend on the MAb's affinity and the target's expression level in each tissue. Low-intensity staining can be caused either by low affinity or low expression levels. In these cases, RNA expression levels (available from online RNAseq databases) can provide an indication of the expression of a target protein in any given tissue. However, RNAseq and protein expression levels are not always directly correlated, and RNAseq across an entire tissue may not reflect protein expression levels in individual cell types within that tissue.

When staining of human tissue indicates potential off-target binding, results can be compared with tissues from other species (e.g., mouse, rat, or nonhuman primates) to determine which animals are most relevant for assessing off-target binding *in vivo*. In these cases, TCR results are considered in conjunction with other binding assays (*in vitro* and *in vivo* binding and activity) to support species selection. In some cases, such as when the MAb is directed to an exogenous target such as a tumor neoantigen or virus, TCR results have been used as the sole criterion for species selection of toxicology. Notably, TCR studies can also rule out species that are *not* appropriate or relevant for safety studies (e.g., nonhuman primates).

11.4.3 Limitations of Tissue Cross-reactivity Studies for Evaluating Target Specificity

Although there are important benefits to TCR studies, they also have well recognized limitations. The primary limitation of TCR analysis is that the molecular identity of positive binding is not known. For unexpected off-target tissue reactivity, the identity of the stained target protein is not determined. Moreover, on-target tissue reactivity may provide false reassurance if a cross-reactive target protein is expressed within the same tissue. The use of tissue for specificity analysis is also not ideal, with high variability in endogenously expressed, secreted, and disease-relevant proteins. Most tissue samples are fixed or frozen (desiccated) onto glass slides, potentially altering the conformation and misrepresenting the native structure of proteins (especially membrane proteins that are highly sensitive to folding conditions). High background binding is also frequently a problem due to native Fc receptors and endogenous IgG found throughout human tissues. Owing to these limitations, abundant examples can be found throughout the literature where TCR assays and *in vivo* toxicity studies do not correlate (Leach et al., 2010; MacLachlan et al., 2021).

Results used in Investigational New Drug (IND) filings are scored by trained pathologists, so they are based on their observations and interpretations. Ideally, more quantitative approaches should be implemented to increase consistency and feasibility of statistical analysis between studies to ensure reproducibility (Geoly, 2014). Optimizing the staining protocol and completing TCR studies typically require at least 12 weeks. Tissue microarrays (TMAs) of up to 1,000 tissue samples on a slide can make tissue staining easier and faster and provide a preliminary specificity assessment (Hewitt, 2004; Warford et al., 2004). However, TMAs are not recommended by the FDA for IND filings because they represent very limited tissue cross sections (<2 mm) that do not faithfully represent all elements of the originating tissues (Leach et al., 2010). To accelerate product development timelines, animal TCR studies are frequently conducted in parallel with human TCR studies to ensure that the species selected for toxicity assessment also have the potential to assess any toxicity that might be related to off-target binding. In most cases, nonhuman primates will be the relevant species (and in some cases, the only relevant species), and in such cases, TCR can be limited to nonhuman primates. In practice, nonhuman primates are almost always used for safety testing of biotherapeutics regardless of TCR results, a practice that both the FDA and NIH discourage because of ethical considerations (Chapman et al., 2009; Sewell et al., 2017).

11.5 *In Vitro* Specificity Screening Using Cell Expression Arrays

11.5.1 Cell-based Membrane Proteome Arrays

Both the ICHS6 and FDA's Points to Consider guidelines allow that alternative technologies can be used to demonstrate target binding as they become available, and in recent years, there has been progress in the development of new *in vitro* technologies. "Cell expression arrays" can provide comprehensive specificity analysis against native human membrane proteins. These types of arrays use cDNA plasmid expression systems to test MAb interactions with each individual protein target within living cells. Cell arrays are created by reverse-transfecting arrayed expression plasmids into eukaryotic cell lines (Doranz, 2001; Ziauddin and Sabatini, 2001). Target binding is determined by high-throughput flow cytometry on unfixed cells (Tucker et al., 2018) or immunofluorescence on fixed cells (Freeth and Soden, 2020). Screening against the cellular membrane proteins of the proteome is especially important as these targets will impact any off-target cellular toxicity.

A specific membrane proteome array (MPA) has been developed that expresses the entire human membrane proteome in a cell expression array format and has emerged as a novel approach to test the specificity of biotherapeutics (Integral Molecular). Cell expression arrays have been used to determine the specificity of nearly all major biotherapeutic modalities to date, including IgG, IgM, scFv, single variable domains on heavy chain (VHH) nanobodies, bispecifics, peptides, RNA aptamers, and whole CAR T cells (Figure 11.5). These types

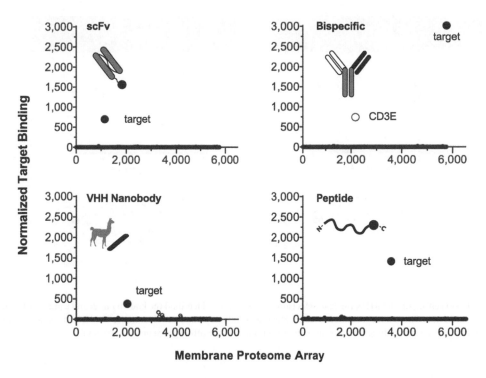

FIGURE 11.5 Biotherapeutic modalities screened on the MPA. The MPA has been used to determine the specificity of diverse biotherapeutic modalities, including scFvs, bispecifics, V_{HH} nanobodies, and peptides.

of arrays are especially useful during the lead selection phase of development. For example, two lead candidate MAbs that bound to the same target were tested on the MPA. One of these demonstrated polyspecificity with strong binding to a completely unrelated off-target protein (Figure 11.6). When biodistribution studies in mice were conducted on the same MAbs, both localized to the thyroid (the location of the primary target), but the polyspecific MAb also localized to the adrenal medulla (where the off-target protein is expressed), thereby prioritizing the highly specific MAb as the lead candidate for preclinical development and IND filing.

11.5.2 Recommendations for the Use of Cell Expression Arrays

Cell arrays use standardized and reproducible methods for reliable and unbiased specificity testing (summarized in Table 11.2). Individual plasmids are overexpressed in live cells to allow each protein target to be individually tested. Expression in live cells allows each protein to fold in its native conformation, including proper post-translational modifications, glycosylation, partner proteins, and multimerization (if applicable), which is essential for testing conformationally sensitive MAbs. Importantly, MAbs are tested on unfixed cells as fixation usually alters the conformation of multispanning membrane proteins. Indeed, fixation of cells can significantly mask epitopes and cause important off-target binding to be missed, such as observed for a CD19 antibody (Figure 11.7). Binding is measured by high-throughput flow cytometry, allowing for high-sensitivity readouts and statistically quantified results. To be considered specific, MAbs should bind only one target, with all other target proteins binding below preset

statistical thresholds (e.g., three standard deviations of mean binding across the library).

Both on-target and off-target binding interactions identified using cell expression array screens should be validated for cellular binding using antibody titration. For off-targets, follow-up studies can suggest the impact of the off-target protein on safety. For example, is the target or binding epitope intracellular and, therefore, inaccessible? Is binding to the target of low affinity, which may impact the therapeutic window less than a high affinity interaction? Would binding of the biotherapeutic to cells expressing the off-target result in cell killing? In addition, some cell expression array data points may reveal low reactivity with an off-target that needs to be investigated further, for instance, to differentiate real low affinity interactions from artifactual false-positive results. Such low off-target reactivity can be genuine, based on the affinity of the interaction and expression levels of the off-target, and can be confirmed using biosensor measurements to demonstrate a real but low affinity interaction. Alternatively, low off-target reactivity could also be a false-positive artifact, the result of normal statistical variability among the thousands of proteins measured. In this case, such variability can be distinguished from a true off-target in a follow-up validation assay with additional statistical power and controls.

To be considered reliable, cell expression arrays must be validated and controlled to ensure consistent and reliable results. For example, in the MPA, all target proteins are cloned with a C-terminal V5 epitope tag to measure full-length protein expression, and many clones are optimized for expression, trafficking, and reduced toxicity. Especially for data that will be included in IND submissions, a closely related isotype control should be tested in parallel. An isotype control with the

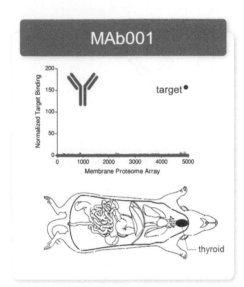

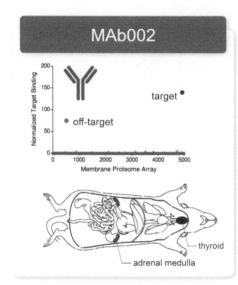

FIGURE 11.6 **Specificity screening on the MPA for lead selection**. Binding results identified the known target and a previously unknown off-target binder for two potential lead MAbs. These data predicted MAb localization results in animal studies, where MAb002 accumulated in the target organ (thyroid) as well as in an off-target organ (adrenal glands, the site of expression of the off-target membrane protein).

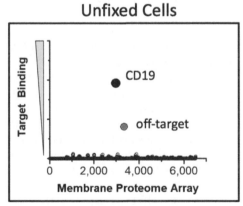

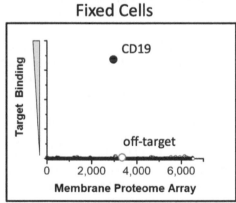

FIGURE 11.7 **Cell fixation can mask epitopes**. An anti-CD19 MAb was screened on the MPA using both unfixed and fixed cells in parallel. Both conditions identified the target, but the fixed cells failed to identify an important off-target interaction. Binding to the off-target protein was validated in follow-up studies, suggesting that the altered epitopes under fixed conditions can result in missed interactions.

TABLE 11.2

Study Design of Cell Expression Arrays

Criteria	Approach or Technique
Binding conditions	Unfixed cells to preserve native protein conformation and post-translational modifications
Controls	Binding controls: Fc-receptors and membrane-tethered protein A included in the array
	Assay controls: Transfection controls for each cell, plate-to-plate measurement controls to verify experimental consistency, and sensitivity controls to ensure maximum detectability
	Negative control: Isotype-matched molecule containing identical Fc and constant domains, produced using same methodology and from same cell type as test molecule
Expression validation	Epitope tags to confirm full-length expression of each protein in the array
Quantitative analysis	Results statistically analyzed for hits (three standard deviations above average reactivity across the array)
Cell type	Human embryonic kidney (HEK)-293 cells for human expression, avian or other cell types to reduce background if the target is endogenously expressed on HEK-293 cells
Concentration	20 μg/mL, or highest possible based on each MAb's background (2–20 μg/mL typical)
Detection	Flow cytometry for highest sensitivity, single-cell detection and quantitative, statistically controlled data

same Fc and constant domains is especially important because endogenous Fc receptors and lectins are also included in cell expression arrays, and these will inevitably be identified as "hits." Binding to such membrane proteins does not indicate nonspecific binding, but rather actual binding of the antibody by naturally occurring proteins in the human membrane proteome. Isotype controls that are precisely matched to the same format and production process as the molecule of interest can differentiate between protein interactions with the constant and variable domains of an antibody.

11.5.3 Advantages of Cell Expression Arrays

Cell expression arrays provide significant advantages for specificity analysis compared with TCR studies (summarized in Table 11.3). The key feature of cell expression arrays is that human proteins can be individually expressed and tested in their native state directly within human cells. This allows proteins to retain their structural integrity and native post-translational modifications. Moreover, cell expression arrays allow for high expression of proteins with variable or disease-dependent expression patterns that may not be found in normal tissue samples. Most importantly, cell expression arrays determine the identity of any cross-reactive, off-target protein. Knowing the identity of the off-target is critical for assessing its associated biological relevance and safety concerns and can also guide potential re-engineering of the lead molecule. The FDA has recognized the advances of cell expression arrays and has accepted IND filings that include cell expression array data alone (MacLachlan et al., 2021).

If used correctly, cell expression arrays can significantly shorten biotherapeutic development timelines. Screening several lead candidates early in discovery allows for selection of leads with no off-target liabilities. In our experience, many companies choose to screen their top 3–5 final lead candidates. Screening later when a single lead candidate has already been chosen could

reveal unexpected off-target binding that requires additional antibody engineering, new candidate selection, or, at the least, a detailed understanding (and explanation) of the potential safety concerns associated with the off-target interaction. A second screen on cell expression arrays is often conducted later to provide data, figures, experimental conditions, and auditability of data records that is compliant with IND filing requirements. Cell expression array screens themselves are typically completed in 4–6 weeks, with several candidates evaluated simultaneously.

Cell expression arrays can also considerably reduce the use of nonhuman primates for toxicity studies, especially in cases where the target is an exogenous antigen, as noted above. Decreasing the number of nonhuman primates used for safety testing is a major goal of the FDA and NIH (Chapman et al., 2009; Sewell et al., 2017). MAbs that do not bind unintended human targets would not be expected to have any off-target safety liabilities. On-target safety liabilities could still exist and must be tested for, but potentially in animal studies focused primarily on on-target liabilities. For MAbs with exogenous targets (e.g., against viral proteins), on-target safety concerns are not expected, and therefore, compelling cell expression array data showing no off-targets could completely eliminate the need for *in vivo* toxicity screening in nonhuman primates.

11.5.4 Use of Cell Expression Array Results to Guide Toxicity Studies

Human cell expression arrays identify the exact proteins (on-target and off-target) to which the molecule binds. The array itself, however, does not identify the tissue of positive binding, nor does it determine what species are most relevant for toxicity studies. Therefore, results from cell expression array studies guide subsequent toxicity studies using a different process compared with those from TCR studies. For selecting a relevant species for toxicity studies using cell expression array data, species orthologs of both the on-target

TABLE 11.3

Comparison of TCR and Cell Expression Array Studies

Purpose	TCR Studies	Cell Arrays
Regulatory		
IND filing	Recommended by FDA since 1983 for biotherapeutics safety testing	Newer technology that is being accepted to demonstrate off-target/binding site distribution
Guide toxicity studies	Identifies tissues to watch during toxicity testing	Identifies off-targets to be aware of during toxicity testing
Guide species selection	Used to confirm species with similar off-target binding	Identifies target and off-targets to be tested against species orthologs
CAR T testing	Limited to measuring scFv binding, not final product	Three methods: scFv binding, CAR T cell binding, CAR T cell activation
Timing of use	Used to support IND filing	Used to guide lead selection (3–5 candidates) and/or to support IND filing
Technical		
Target specificity	Off-target tissues identified for both human and animal species	Off-target proteins identified at molecular level
Sensitivity	Low sensitivity (IHC, secreted proteins washed away, high background due to native Fc receptors and IgG)	High sensitivity over-expression system with flow cytometry (low background, highly quantitative, low rate of false positives)
Native target reactivity	Fixed and frozen tissue can alter conformational epitopes	Native conformation of targets if used with unfixed cells
Analysis	Results interpreted by pathologist	Quantitative statistical analysis

and any off-targets should be tested for binding. This can be completed by cloning the genes for the relevant mouse, rat, or nonhuman primate targets, transfecting them into cells and testing for binding. TCR studies could also be performed to identify relevant species for toxicity testing. To determine which tissues express the on-target and any off-targets, the expression can be predicted using RNAseq and protein expression databases, or the expression can be tested by tissue staining with specific antibodies (the test molecule or other specific antibodies).

11.5.5 Screening of Soluble Proteins

Cell expression arrays traditionally focus on membrane proteins, due to these proteins' importance in targeting MAbs to the correct cell type, but secreted proteins can also be included in cell expression arrays. The inclusion of secreted proteins enables specificity profiling against the complete extracellular compartment, encompassing nearly every protein that a biotherapeutic will encounter. While secreted protein off-target interactions are usually not an issue for toxicity, they can impact the pharmacokinetics and dosing of therapeutics. For example, MAbs that bind highly prevalent off-target circulating proteins can display rapid clearance, poor target tissue biodistribution, and limited efficacy (Bumbaca et al., 2011).

11.6 Screening CAR T Cells for Specificity *In Vitro*

While FDA's 2013 guidance on Preclinical Assessment of Investigational Cellular and Gene Therapy Guidance provides general guidance, there is currently no product class–specific guidance for specificity testing of CAR T and other T cell therapies. The final therapeutic (a living cell) is simply not amenable to the same types of assays as chemically defined proteins and other drugs. TCR assays can be used with scFv (the typical targeting moiety for CAR T), and this approach is accepted by the FDA for IND filings. However, monomeric scFv binding to tissues can have low sensitivity, especially if the antibody has low affinity. CAR T cells can be activated by even very low affinity interactions that IHC-based binding assays may not detect, potentially resulting in unidentified off-targets. Cell expression arrays are also accepted by the FDA and other regulatory agencies owing to their value in predicting off-targets. Three different methods for determining CAR T specificity are used on cell expression arrays: (1) scFv binding, (2) CAR T cell binding, and (3) CAR T cell functional activation (Figure 11.8a). scFv binding is conducted similarly to other antibody binding protocols. For cell binding assays, fluorescently labeled CAR T cells are added and allowed to bind, followed by washing; remaining bound CAR T cells

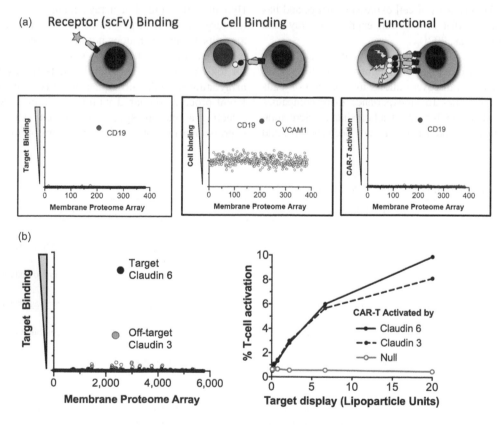

FIGURE 11.8 The specificity of CAR T cells can be detected three different ways on cell expression arrays. (a) Specificity of CAR T cells can be examined by receptor binding, cell binding, or functional activation. Here, a CD19 scFv was tested for binding on Integral Molecular's membrane proteome array (MPA). CAR T cells targeted with this scFv were also tested for binding and activation on the MPA. (b) Low levels of off-target binding can cause full CAR T cell activation. Screening of a CLDN6 MAb on the MPA identified low level cross-reactivity with CLDN3. CAR T cells targeted with this scFv had identical activation (CD69 expression) curves following CLDN6 and CLDN3 stimulation.

are detected by flow cytometry. For functional assays, live CAR T cells are incubated on the array, and activation markers on the CAR T cell are detected using flow cytometry. When using whole cells, a CAR T cell expressing an unrelated scFv should be used as a negative control.

The most directly relevant approach for CAR T cell specificity analysis is determining cell activation. For example, a CD19 scFv was tested for binding on the MPA and showed no off-targets (Figure 11.8a, left panel). CAR T cells targeted with this same scFv were also tested for binding and activation on the MPA. Positive cell binding was detected for CD19, but sensitivity in this assay was poor by comparison (Figure 11.8a, middle panel). In addition, CAR T cell binding to a nonactivating adhesion molecule, VCAM-1, was also detected, which complicates the interpretation of cell binding assays. Testing of specificity by CAR T cell activation resulted in very high sensitivity and detection of only the relevant CD19 interaction, so is the most relevant mechanism for detecting the final CAR T cell drug product (Figure 11.8a, right panel). In another example, a recently isolated (now deprioritized) claudin 6 (CLDN6) MAb was tested on the MPA and exhibited low-level cross-reactivity with the highly homologous claudin 3 (CLDN3) protein (Figure 11.8b). CAR T cells targeted using this antibody were fully activated by both its on- and off-target binding proteins. Thus, even minimal antibody cross-reactivity in a CAR T format can result in misdirected cell killing. These examples suggest that functional screens are the most sensitive and relevant for detecting CAR T cell specificity.

11.7 Other Methods for Detecting Biotherapeutic Specificity

A number of other methods are used to determine the specificity of biotherapeutics, especially in the early stages of drug discovery research. Initial profiling almost always includes screening against a small number of homologous family members with high sequence identity. Tissue-based lysates screened by western blotting can also provide some early information on target reactivity. For more comprehensive screening, spotted protein arrays are sometimes used, in which recombinant or purified proteins are spotted on a solid surface, and the test molecule is screened for binding (Diehnelt et al., 2010; Michaud et al., 2003; Poetz et al., 2005). Protein arrays provide a fast and low-cost screen for target binding but have inherent limitations, including denaturation, altered protein conformation, and unnatural surface interactions. Traditional protein arrays are particularly problematic for screening against multipass membrane proteins, as most such proteins require a lipid bilayer to maintain their native structure. Therefore, spotted protein array results should be interpreted with caution. In addition to protein-based methods for antibody characterization, a number of gene-based techniques, such as CRISPR-Cas9 or short-interfering RNA (siRNA) knockdowns have been applied for validating target specificity.

11.8 Interpreting Specificity Testing Results

11.8.1 Risk Assessment of Off-target Proteins Identified Using Cell Expression Arrays

If off-target binding is revealed during specificity testing, a thorough risk analysis should be undertaken to determine whether a molecule warrants reconsideration or if further progression through development is still appropriate. Decision factors fall into four categories: polyreactivity, polyspecificity lead selection, accessibility, and toxicity analysis (Figure 11.9).

1. **Polyreactivity evaluation**: First, compounds that are polyreactive with high background binding (e.g., "sticky" MAbs) should be reconsidered, as high polyreactivity is inversely correlated with clinical success.

2. **Polyspecificity lead selection**: If a small panel (3–5) of lead candidates is screened early enough in discovery, a lead candidate without any off-target liability should be relatively easy to identify and progress into preclinical trials. Our profiling of MAbs indicates that ~75% of lead MAbs are truly specific for their intended target, so monospecific leads are common.

If a preferred lead does reveal an off-target interaction, then there are additional considerations. Should an off-target always deprioritize the candidate? Or is there such a thing as an acceptable off-target? Some off-target proteins may indeed be perfectly acceptable with very low risk for safety issues in humans based on accessibility, target biology, and modality (discussed below).

3. **Accessibility**: To begin, the accessibility of the off-target needs to be evaluated. For example, many membrane proteins are expressed solely intracellularly, in the nucleus, Golgi, endoplasmic reticulum, and other intracellular membranous structures. Membrane proteins in the central nervous system are also generally inaccessible to MAbs in most patients. The binding epitope of the off-target interaction could also be located on the intracellular side of the membrane protein. In other cases, off-target proteins may be naturally expressed at very low levels.

4. **Toxicity analysis**: For lead candidates with accessible off-targets, focused investigation into the functional relevance of the off-target binding can be completed and risk potentially alleviated (Lee et al., 2020). Any off-target binding must be analyzed in the context of the target biology, dosing, and therapeutic modality. Would binding of the antibody have a biological effect based on the natural function of the off-target protein? Is the dosing (amount, chronic vs. acute administration) and modality of the intended therapeutic a safety risk? For example, CAR T, ADCs, and bispecifics are usually designed to kill cancer cells that they bind (so would also kill any off-target cell type). Moreover, antagonist or agonist

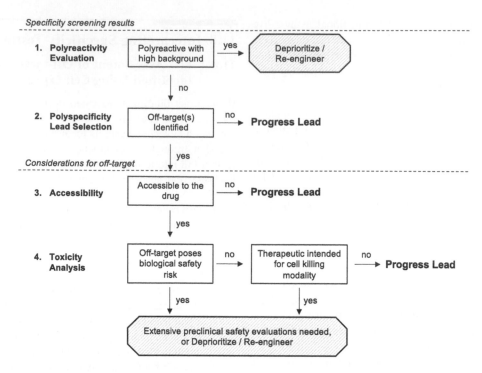

FIGURE 11.9   Decision tree for off-targets identified from cell expression arrays. Four major decision points guide the use of information from cell expression arrays.

MAbs that are designed to modulate the function of a target protein may or may not alter the function of an off-target protein. If the off-target does pose a potential safety risk, developers may choose to ameliorate these risks with extensive safety preclinical evaluations, by re-engineering the molecule or by selecting a back-up candidate with a clean specificity profile if polyspecificity screening is performed early enough in lead selection.

11.8.2   Risk Assessment of Off-target Tissues Identified Using TCR Assays

TCR studies are capable of identifying the tissue(s) of drug binding and target reactivity, but the target identity of the positive staining may not be known. If an off-target protein is identified, then the decision tree above can be used (Figure 11.9). If the off-target protein is not known, preclinical safety evaluations are conducted to identify the impact of off-target tissue staining. Several published case studies illustrate the shortcomings of using TCR studies for predicting *in vivo* safety (Brennan et al., 2018; Leach et al., 2010). For example, some antibodies with clear off-target TCR tissue staining patterns have not demonstrated any *in vivo* toxicity. In contrast, other antibodies demonstrated *in vivo* toxicity even though the TCR study showed only expected staining patterns. Surveys of pharmaceutical and biotechnology companies regarding the use and value of TCR studies highlight the limitations of TCR data in practice (Bussiere et al., 2011; MacLachlan et al., 2021). The surveys found that TCR results did not influence the development strategy of 92-95% of biologics. Only 2% of biotherapeutics used TCR studies as the only determinant for predicting toxicity in humans, whereas only 27% used TCR studies as the only determinant for selecting relevant species for toxicity studies (Bussiere et al., 2011).

With the development of cell expression arrays, it is possible to replace TCR studies in IND filings if ample *in vitro* specificity screening is provided. This is especially the case for CAR T and other cell therapies. Informal and published surveys of cell expression array usage by ourselves and others have found that about one-third of IND filings that include cell expression array data did not include TCR data (MacLachlan et al., 2011). We expect this percentage to rise over time as cell expression assays are increasingly validated and data are beginning to demonstrate their predictive value for identifying potential safety risks, both preclinically and clinically.

11.9   Summary and Future Considerations

TCR studies have been used since the 1980s to identify whether there is unintended target expression or off-target binding to tissues. However, in many cases, even if unexpected binding is observed, there is no correlation with toxicity. Cell expression arrays are now sufficiently accepted, based on existing FDA and ICH guidance, to be used to assess potential off-target toxicity. These arrays can determine individual protein targets, but do not identify the specific tissue(s) of target expression. Small panels (3–5) of potential clinical candidates can be screened using cell expression arrays prior to selecting a lead candidate to ensure a monospecific final lead. If off-targets are identified and cannot be avoided, then a decision matrix for determining the impact of the off-target should be employed, which considers the off-target biology, distribution, and therapeutic modality.

Cell expression arrays are currently the only option for testing final CAR T cell products and other gene-modified targeted cell therapies. Importantly, functional testing of live CAR T cells is the most relevant method of detecting off-target interactions that cause CAR T activation. Decreasing biotherapeutic cross-reactivity should improve likelihoods of succeeding in preclinical and clinical trials.

REFERENCES

Bajic, G., van der Poel, C.E., Kuraoka, M., Schmidt, A.G., Carroll, M.C., Kelsoe, G., and Harrison, S.C. (2019). Autoreactivity profiles of influenza hemagglutinin broadly neutralizing antibodies. *Sci Rep 9*, 3492.

Bostrom, J., Yu, S.F., Kan, D., Appleton, B.A., Lee, C.V., Billeci, K., Man, W., Peale, F., Ross, S., Wiesmann, C., *et al.* (2009). Variants of the antibody herceptin that interact with HER2 and VEGF at the antigen binding site. *Science 323*, 1610–1614.

Brennan, F.R., Cavagnaro, J., McKeever, K., Ryan, P.C., Schutten, M.M., Vahle, J., Weinbauer, G.F., Marrer-Berger, E., and Black, L.E. (2018). Safety testing of monoclonal antibodies in non-human primates: case studies highlighting their impact on human risk assessment. *MAbs 10*, 1–17.

Bumbaca, D., Wong, A., Drake, E., Reyes, A.E., 2nd, Lin, B.C., Stephan, J.P., Desnoyers, L., Shen, B.Q., and Dennis, M.S. (2011). Highly specific off-target binding identified and eliminated during the humanization of an antibody against FGF receptor 4. *MAbs 3*, 376–386.

Bussiere, J.L., Leach, M.W., Price, K.D., Mounho, B.J., and Lightfoot-Dunn, R. (2011). Survey results on the use of the tissue cross-reactivity immunohistochemistry assay. *Regul Toxicol Pharmacol 59*, 493–502.

Cameron, B.J., Gerry, A.B., Dukes, J., Harper, J.V., Kannan, V., Bianchi, F.C., Grand, F., Brewer, J.E., Gupta, M., Plesa, G., *et al.* (2013). Identification of a Titin-derived HLA-A1-presented peptide as a cross-reactive target for engineered MAGE A3-directed T cells. *Sci Transl Med 5*, 197ra103.

Chapman, K., Pullen, N., Coney, L., Dempster, M., Andrews, L., Bajramovic, J., Baldrick, P., Buckley, L., Jacobs, A., Hale, G., *et al.* (2009). Preclinical development of monoclonal antibodies: considerations for the use of non-human primates. *MAbs 1*, 505–516.

Cook, D., Brown, D., Alexander, R., March, R., Morgan, P., Satterthwaite, G., and Pangalos, M.N. (2014). Lessons learned from the fate of AstraZeneca's drug pipeline: a five-dimensional framework. *Nat Rev Drug Discov 13*, 419–431.

Diehnelt, C.W., Shah, M., Gupta, N., Belcher, P.E., Greving, M.P., Stafford, P., and Johnston, S.A. (2010). Discovery of high-affinity protein binding ligands – backwards. *PLoS One 5*, e10728.

Doranz, B.J. (2001). Elucidation of Gene Function (US patent 10/476,297).

Finlay, W.J., and Almagro, J.C. (2012). Natural and man-made V-gene repertoires for antibody discovery. *Front Immunol 3*, 342.

Finlay, W.J.J., Coleman, J.E., Edwards, J.S., and Johnson, K.S. (2019). Anti-PD1 'SHR-1210' aberrantly targets pro-angiogenic receptors and this polyspecificity can be ablated by paratope refinement. *MAbs 11*, 26–44.

Finton, K.A., Larimore, K., Larman, H.B., Friend, D., Correnti, C., Rupert, P.B., Elledge, S.J., Greenberg, P.D., and Strong, R.K. (2013). Autoreactivity and exceptional CDR plasticity (but not unusual polyspecificity) hinder elicitation of the anti-HIV antibody 4E10. *PLoS Pathog 9*, e1003639.

Freeth, J., and Soden, J. (2020). New advances in cell microarray technology to expand applications in target deconvolution and off-target screening. *SLAS Discov 25*, 223–230.

Geoly, F.J. (2014). Regulatory forum opinion piece: tissue cross-reactivity studies: what constitutes an adequate positive control and how do we report positive staining? *Toxicol Pathol 42*, 954–956.

Gunti, S., and Notkins, A.L. (2015). Polyreactive antibodies: function and quantification. *J Infect Dis 212 Suppl 1*, S42–S46.

Hewitt, S.M. (2004). Design, construction, and use of tissue microarrays. *Methods Mol Biol 264*, 61–72.

Jain, T., Sun, T., Durand, S., Hall, A., Houston, N.R., Nett, J.H., Sharkey, B., Bobrowicz, B., Caffry, I., Yu, Y., *et al.* (2017). Biophysical properties of the clinical-stage antibody landscape. *Proc Natl Acad Sci U S A 114*, 944–949.

Leach, M.W., Halpern, W.G., Johnson, C.W., Rojko, J.L., MacLachlan, T.K., Chan, C.M., Galbreath, E.J., Ndifor, A.M., Blanset, D.L., Polack, F., *et al.* (2010). Use of tissue cross-reactivity studies in the development of antibody-based biopharmaceuticals: history, experience, methodology, and future directions. *Toxicol Pathol 38*, 1138–1166.

Lee, J., Lundgren, D.K., Mao, X., Manfredo-Vieira, S., Nunez-Cruz, S., Williams, E.F., Assenmacher, C.A., Radaelli, E., Oh, S., Wang, B., *et al.* (2020). Antigen-specific B-cell depletion for precision therapy of mucosal pemphigus vulgaris. *J Clin Invest. 130*, 6191–6753.

Lin, A., Giuliano, C.J., Palladino, A., John, K.M., Abramowicz, C., Yuan, M.L., Sausville, E.L., Lukow, D.A., Liu, L., Chait, A.R., *et al.* (2019). Off-target toxicity is a common mechanism of action of cancer drugs undergoing clinical trials. *Sci Transl Med 11*, eaaw8412.

Linette, G.P., Stadtmauer, E.A., Maus, M.V., Rapoport, A.P., Levine, B.L., Emery, L., Litzky, L., Bagg, A., Carreno, B.M., Cimino, P.J., *et al.* (2013). Cardiovascular toxicity and titin cross-reactivity of affinity-enhanced T cells in myeloma and melanoma. *Blood 122*, 863–871.

Ma, D., Baruch, D., Shu, Y., Yuan, K., Sun, Z., Ma, K., Hoang, T., Fu, W., Min, L., Lan, Z.S., *et al.* (2012). Using protein microarray technology to screen anti-ERCC1 monoclonal antibodies for specificity and applications in pathology. *BMC Biotechnol 12*, 88.

MacLachlan, T.K., Price, S., Cavagnaro, J., Andrews, L., Blanset, D., Cosenza, M.E., Dempster, M., Galbreath, E., Giusti, A.M., Heinz-Taheny, K.M., *et al.* (2021). Classic and evolving approaches to evaluating cross reactivity of mAb and mAb-like molecules - A survey of industry 2008-20019. *Regul Toxicol Pharmacol 121*, 104872.

Michaud, G.A., Salcius, M., Zhou, F., Bangham, R., Bonin, J., Guo, H., Snyder, M., Predki, P.F., and Schweitzer, B.I. (2003). Analyzing antibody specificity with whole proteome microarrays. *Nat Biotechnol 21*, 1509–1512.

Mo, H., Huang, J., Xu, J., Chen, X., Wu, D., Qu, D., Wang, X., Lan, B., Wang, X., Xu, J., *et al.* (2018). Safety, anti-tumour activity, and pharmacokinetics of fixed-dose SHR-1210, an anti-PD-1 antibody in advanced solid tumours: a dose-escalation, phase 1 study. *Br J Cancer 119*, 538–545.

Ng, S., Juang, Y.-C., Chandramohan, A., Kaan, H.Y.K., Sadruddin, A., Yuen, T.Y., Ferrer-Gago, F.J., Lee, X.E.C., Liew, X., Johannes, C.W., *et al.* (2020). De-risking drug discovery of intracellular targeting peptides: screening strategies to eliminate false-positive hits. *ACS Med Chem Lett 11*, 1993–2001.

Notkins, A.L. (2004). Polyreactivity of antibody molecules. *Trends Immunol 25*, 174–179.

Pardridge, W.M. (2005). The blood-brain barrier: bottleneck in brain drug development. *NeuroRx 2*, 3–14.

Poetz, O., Ostendorp, R., Brocks, B., Schwenk, J.M., Stoll, D., Joos, T.O., and Templin, M.F. (2005). Protein microarrays for antibody profiling: specificity and affinity determination on a chip. *Proteomics 5*, 2402–2411.

Raman, M.C., Rizkallah, P.J., Simmons, R., Donnellan, Z., Dukes, J., Bossi, G., Le Provost, G.S., Todorov, P., Baston, E., Hickman, E., *et al.* (2016). Direct molecular mimicry enables off-target cardiovascular toxicity by an enhanced affinity TCR designed for cancer immunotherapy. *Sci Rep 6*, 18851.

Sewell, F., Chapman, K., Couch, J., Dempster, M., Heidel, S., Loberg, L., Maier, C., Maclachlan, T.K., Todd, M., and van der Laan, J.W. (2017). Challenges and opportunities for the future of monoclonal antibody development: improving safety assessment and reducing animal use. *MAbs 9*, 742–755.

Starr, C.G., and Tessier, P.M. (2019). Selecting and engineering monoclonal antibodies with drug-like specificity. *Curr Opin Biotechnol 60*, 119–127.

Sullivan, J.T., Harmon, D., Navia, C., Screnci, B., Fong, R., Willis, S., Rucker, J., Doranz, B. J. (2020). Screening the membrane proteome to determine antibody specificity and de-risk CAR-T cell development. Paper presented at: 2020 PEGS Boston Virtual Summit.

Tucker, D.F., Sullivan, J.T., Mattia, K.A., Fisher, C.R., Barnes, T., Mabila, M.N., Wilf, R., Sulli, C., Pitts, M., Payne, R.J., *et al.* (2018). Isolation of state-dependent monoclonal antibodies against the 12-transmembrane domain glucose transporter 4 using virus-like particles. *Proc Natl Acad Sci U S A 115*, E4990–E4999.

Warford, A., Howat, W., and McCafferty, J. (2004). Expression profiling by high-throughput immunohistochemistry. *J Immunol Methods 290*, 81–92.

Ziauddin, J., and Sabatini, D.M. (2001). Microarrays of cells expressing defined cDNAs. *Nature 411*, 107–110.

12

Reproductive, Developmental, and Juvenile Toxicity Assessments

Christopher J. Bowman
Pfizer, Inc.

Gerhard F. Weinbauer
Labcorp Early Development Services GmbH

CONTENTS

12.1 Background

The purpose of specific safety assessments of reproductive, developmental, and juvenile toxicity is to identify and inform potential risk of male and female infertility, adverse pregnancy outcomes including fetal harm, and supporting safe use in pediatric populations. The risk should be assessed through one complete life cycle (from conception in one generation through conception in the following generation) where possible and where relevant to the intended population. For example, not all stages need to be assessed for an exclusively postmenopausal female patient population or in exclusively hospitalized settings where pregnancy can be excluded. In addition to patient population, unique attributes of biopharmaceuticals (such as limited off-target toxicity of monoclonal antibodies (mAbs) and extensive availability of on-target toxicity information based on literature or existing data), a case-by-case safety assessment of reproductive, developmental, and juvenile toxicity may be appropriate without one or more additional animal studies (Bowman and Chapin, 2016; Morford et al., 2011). This weight of evidence evaluation should be considered for all assessments to determine which, if any, animal studies are needed to identify and inform potential risk of male and female infertility, adverse pregnancy outcome including

fetal harm, and supporting safe use in pediatric populations. If experimental animal studies will not impact the human risk assessment due to either known risks based on target modulation or existing data, then the sponsor should negotiate risk communication (labeling) language with health authorities to confirm some or all animal studies are not needed. If animal studies are conducted, timing of specific developmental and reproductive toxicity (DART) study and juvenile animal study (JAS) is dependent on the clinical study population, phase of pharmaceutical development, and risk management during clinical trials (e.g., contraception). The past several years there has been increased regulatory acceptance of weight of evidence and case-by-case approaches for these types of assessments, particularly for biopharmaceuticals as described in ICH S5(R3), ICH S6, and recent publications (Barrow, 2018; Barrow and Clemann, 2021; Rocca et al., 2018).

When experimental data are needed to complement the assessment of DART, testing is commonly done in rodents (mice and rats) and rabbits. When needed and pharmacologically relevant, rodents are also preferred for JAS with biopharmaceuticals. According to ICH S5(R3), rats, mice, and rabbits are considered the routine species for DART testing, nonhuman primates (NHPs) and minipigs are nonroutine species, whereas hamsters and dogs are limited-use species.

While this is true for drug development of small molecules, the demand for DART studies and JAS in NHPs is higher since NHPs are frequently the only pharmacologically relevant species for highly human-specific biopharmaceuticals. This holds particularly true for the development of mAbs for which it is reported that over 70% of compounds have NHPs as the relevant animal model (Brennan et al., 2018; Iwasaki et al., 2019; SCHEER, 2017; van Meer et al., 2013). In such cases, ICH S6(R1) allows restriction to a single animal species for safety assessment including DART testing (single-species testing strategy).

12.2 Species Selection

The concept of species selection for biopharmaceuticals (and oligonucleotides) in general and in the specific context of DART evaluation has been the subject of comprehensive reviews (Cavagnaro et al., 2014; Martin et al., 2009; Rocca et al., 2018) and species selection is specifically addressed in Chapter 2 in this book. Target protein sequence alignment across species, tissue cross-reactivity studies, and/or binding assays can be helpful tools but alone can be misleading regarding pharmacologic activity. In general, evaluation of pharmacologic activity in vitro or in vivo should be confirmed in species selected for toxicity studies if possible. For antibody-related products directed at foreign targets (such as bacterial or viral), there typically is not a pharmacologically relevant toxicology animal model and as such ICH S6(R1) states that DART studies may not be warranted. Interestingly, for prophylactic vaccines targeting infectious diseases, there is still a regulatory requirement for a DART study despite no endogenous target of the immune response. Relevant species for vaccines are those that elicit an adequate immune response to the clinical vaccine product. In addition to pharmacological relevance, consideration of physiological relevance in pharmacologically relevant species compared with humans should be considered. For DART and juvenile animal testing, it is generally assumed that developmental and reproductive biological pathways are reasonably well conserved across species, but it is advisable to research any known species reproduction differences, particularly in the pathway targeted by the biopharmaceutical. There are few known examples where DART effects were observed in rodents but not in NHPs and in NHPs but not in rats. Administration of a soluble IL-4 receptor to pregnant NHPs resulted in increased abortion and embryofetal death while subsequent evaluation of the effects on reproduction in a murine surrogate model did not confirm the observations in the NHP (Carlock et al., 2009). For an IgG4 mAb against a cytokine (BIO-5), an enhanced pre- and postnatal development (ePPND) study in NHP revealed prolongation of gestation, mortality at delivery, dystocia caused by placental retention, and infant mortality likely associated with dystocia while studies in knockout mice and homolog mAb mice did not yield adverse reproductive findings (Brennan et al., 2018). For an IgG4 mAb antagonist of a receptor present on a subpopulation of macrophages (BIO-4), administration to knockout mouse caused an osteopetrotic phenotype and impaired fertility and reproduction but dosing of NHP did not impair female

and male reproductive endpoints and – albeit bone metabolism was altered – bone density and architecture remained unaltered (Brennan et al., 2018).

While the tenants of species selection are not different for DART and JAS compared to general toxicology, how sponsors determine relevant species and when it is done during drug development can introduce some challenges. It is not uncommon to screen rodents and NHPs for pharmacologic activity early in drug development; but if either or both are relevant, then rabbits, guinea pigs, minipigs, or other animal models are often not considered at that stage. Since DART study and JAS data are not typically needed until after first-in-human (FIH) trials, the impact of species selection decision made earlier in drug development often comes up again when the sponsor realizes the limitations, time, and cost of conducting a developmental toxicity study in NHPs compared with other species. Because both ICH S5(R3) and S6(R1) indicate developmental toxicity should only be conducted in NHP when it is the only relevant species, a re-evaluation of species relevance prior to conducting DART studies may identify additional relevant species. If mice or rats are not pharmacologically relevant, species such as the rabbits, guinea pigs, and minipigs could be considered for evaluation before committing to a NHP developmental toxicity study. If mouse or rat was a pharmacologically relevant species, it may have been deemed not feasible due to immunogenicity that reduces exposure. If that is the case, there are still options for conducting some or all DART studies in rodents. These options may include dosing higher (dosing through immunogenicity), adding animals to account for those with reduced exposure (depending on the percentage of animals with reduced exposure), and window dosing where multiple cohorts of animals are used to cover different developmental windows needed for a complete evaluation. When no relevant species can be identified, the use of surrogate molecules or transgenic models can be considered as described in ICH S5(R3) and S6(R1). DART studies with human antisense oligonucleotide therapeutics have used a hybrid approach since many are specific for human sequences. For these studies, both the clinical candidate and species-specific surrogate antisense molecules are evaluated for chemistry/off-target-based toxicity and on-target pharmacological-based toxicity, respectively (Cavagnaro et al., 2014) (Chapter 24 of this book). If an animal model of a pediatric disease exists (e.g., for enzyme replacement therapy) and is being used to support pharmaceutical development, appropriate safety endpoints (e.g., histopathology, clinical pathology) can be incorporated in these studies as part of a weight of evidence, potentially providing sufficient information without conducting a dedicated JAS.

If NHPs constitute the only pharmacologically relevant animal model, it is possible to use the NHP for all DART and JAS testing, but there are a limited number of laboratories that have the expertise to conduct these specialized studies. Because of the specialized nature of NHP DART and JAS testing, it is advisable to consider the pros and cons as part of species selection. The pros and cons for various species including NHPs are provided in ICH S5(R3) for DART and in ICH S11 for JAS. For DART, advantages of the NHP model are physiological similarity to humans and a higher likelihood of having similar pharmacology to humans, similarity to human placentation, data available from repeat-dose toxicity studies, and similarity of antibody transfer across the placenta to humans. Disadvantages for DART include business (time and cost) and scientific considerations of comparatively smaller group sizes associated with low statistical power and variability across groups; single offspring; spontaneous pregnancy and infant loss; limited availability of breeding animals (no commercial supply of time-mated animals); long menstrual cycle (30 days) and gestation (165 days); low fecundity and late implantation, hence impractical for fertility (mating) studies; limited evaluation of F1 reproduction function due to late sexual maturity (around 3–6 years of age); and sourcing/confirming sexually mature animals for DART studies.

For JAS in NHPs, advantages include similarity of many developmental milestones to humans, similarity of neonates/infants for human organ systems (e.g., gastrointestinal, immune system, cardiovascular, renal and special sense (eye and ear) development), comparatively large birth weight for macaques, availability of extensive reference and historical background data from birth onward, the similarity of maternal transfer of immunoglobulin to humans (infants are born with passive immunity derived from serum IgG), often the most pharmacologically relevant animal model for highly targeted therapies, and the feasibility of using rhesus monkey and marmoset (in addition to long-tailed macaques) (Morford et al., 2011). Disadvantages for JAS in NHPs are protracted development (~3–6 years for sexual maturity, ~5–8 years for skeletal maturity in macaques) rendering JAS impractical to cover all developmental phases; single offspring for macaques with high inter-individual variability in growth and development; small offspring in marmosets (although typically 2 offspring) that require both maternal and paternal care in preweaning phase; maturity of neonatal NHPs that are precocious relative to human neonates in terms of musculoskeletal, central nervous system (CNS), endocrine, and respiratory system; lack of synchronized breeding; and ethical reservations requiring strong rationale for using juvenile NHP for toxicity testing.

12.3 Guidelines and General Considerations

As a key regulatory reference on the safety assessment of biopharmaceuticals, ICH S6(R1) provides guidance on the appropriate application of case-by-case strategies on many topics including DART assessments. ICH S6(R1) indicates the use of rodents and rabbits where relevant and as described in ICH S5, but importantly provides details on how to optimize DART evaluations when NHP is the only relevant nonclinical species, including the ePPND study. For those biotherapeutics only relevant in the NHP, dedicated embryofetal development (EFD) studies are not required anymore per ICH M3(R2), ICH S6(R1) and now ICH S5(R3); as the ePPND study design is a pre- and postnatal development (PPND) study in which key elements of an EFD study (external, skeletal and visceral examination) are being investigated in newborns and offspring rather than in the fetus (Stewart, 2008, 2009; Weinbauer et al., 2011, 2013). Another critical component with NHP only assessments relates to the conduct of dedicated female and male fertility studies. ICH S6(R1) specifically states that *When the NHP is*

the only relevant species, the potential for effects on male and female fertility can be assessed by evaluation of the reproductive tract (organ weights and histopathological evaluation) in repeat-dose toxicity studies of at least a 3-month duration using sexually mature NHPs. If there is a specific cause for concern based on pharmacological activity or previous findings, specialized assessments such as menstrual cyclicity, sperm count, sperm morphology/motility, and male or female reproductive hormone levels can be evaluated in a repeat-dose toxicity study. Although this guidance recommendation is subject to interpretation (e.g., when an assessment was needed, and how such an assessment should be conducted), it is important to note that dedicated fertility studies are typically *not* conducted but are replaced by a repeat-dose toxicity study of 3–6-month duration in sexually mature NHPs. In this case, histopathological examination of the reproductive organs from both male and female animals should be comprehensive as detailed on Note 1 of ICH S5(R3). It is also important that sexual maturity should be confirmed *prior to* study initiation rather than expecting animals to mature during study conduct (ICH S5(R3)).

While the primary ICH guideline for DART assessment is S5, it was not until the 3rd revision (R3) was released in 2020 that it was appropriately updated and aligned with ICH S6 for biopharmaceuticals. Together now, ICH S5(R3) and S6(R1) provide both strategies and study designs appropriate to inform human safety at all stages of reproduction and development for biopharmaceuticals. The strategies described in both ICH S5 and S6 include using a scientific basis for assessing the potential effects on reproduction and development that includes mechanistic studies indicating similar effects to a particular class of compounds (e.g., interferons) and this evaluation may obviate the need for formal DART studies. Figure 12.1 illustrates the DART study design dosing and nondosing periods and how they map to the stages of reproduction and development as described in ICH S5. Once the appropriate selection of pharmacologically and physiologically relevant species is complete and a weight of evidence assessment for DART and JAS determines which study or study types are needed for human risk assessment as described earlier, there may still be different experimental options for completing the appropriate DART assessment. Figure 12.2 shows some example DART study packages based on species relevance assuming studies are needed to address all stages of reproduction.

What has been conspicuously absent until recently, was harmonized guidance on nonclinical safety support of pediatrics, such as when to conduct JAS and appropriate JAS design considerations. In 2020, ICH S11 was adopted and provided the detailed weight of evidence considerations for whether a JAS is needed when it is a follow-on to an adult indication, JAS design elements consisting of core and triggered endpoints, and lastly the considerations for JAS to support pediatric first or only drug development (no prior adult indication/data). Not only does S11 provide the latest scientific understanding of species- and organ-specific postnatal development to help inform a weight of evidence and appropriate study design, but it also provides detailed considerations unique to JAS and specifies which core endpoints should be included in all JASs and which endpoints should be added only to address identified concerns.

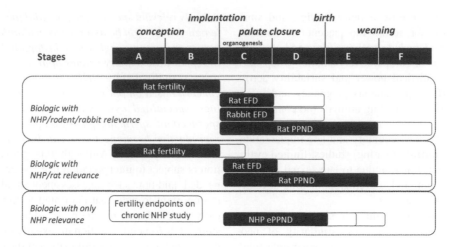

FIGURE 12.1   Example DART packages based on species relevance and stages of reproduction and development outlined in ICH S5(R3).

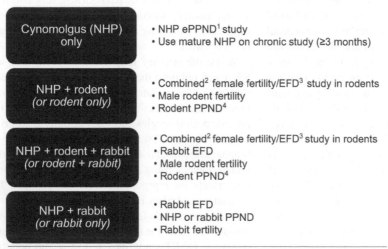

¹ ePPND = enhanced prenatal/postnatal development
² If female reproductive toxicity anticipated then would separate into separate female fertility and EFD studies
³ EFD = embryo-fetal development
⁴ PPND= prenatal/postnatal development

FIGURE 12.2   Example DART study packages based on species relevance.

Timing of DART and JAS dependents on the patient population in clinical trials over the course of drug development. Developmental toxicity data help to inform risk of adverse pregnancy outcomes and may inform/reduce pregnancy testing/contraception requirements where appropriate. Where possible, EFD data are desirable before enrolling women of childbearing potential (WOCBP), but specific criteria regarding the number of women, duration of the trial, and applicable geographical regions are described in more detail in ICH M3(R2). ICH S5(R3) includes additional options for the timing of EFD data relative to specific clinical trials. As described in ICH S6(R1), for NHP-only programs, no NHP EFD study is required, but instead, an ePPND study is recommended and is only needed to support registration. Typically, if a JAS is needed to support pediatric trials, then those nonclinical studies would be conducted prior to dosing humans and this is described further in ICH S11.

As described in Chapter 28 of this book, there are unique considerations for drug developmental programs supporting advanced cancer indications. The strategy for both DART and JAS is impacted when the patient population has advanced cancer because the benefit–risk considerations are so different. ICH S9 specifically states that fertility and PPND studies are not needed and that effects on reproductive organs from repeat-dose toxicity studies are the basis of the fertility assessment. Interestingly, the 2018 US Food and Drug Administration (US FDA) Guidance on reproductive toxicity testing of oncology pharmaceuticals states that a general toxicity study in sexually mature NHPs is not warranted to assess fertility. ICH S9 also states that assessment of EFD risk is only needed to the point of identifying a clinically relevant risk of malformations and/or embryofetal lethality and is only needed to support registration, not clinical trials. For biopharmaceuticals, assessment in one relevant species is usually sufficient. In practice, this means that if there is sufficient supporting information and data for a robust weight of evidence assessment, it may be possible to inform human risk without any DART studies (Rocca et al., 2018). If there is not sufficient data, then the DART strategy may appropriately focus on confirming expected risk using smaller numbers of animals (e.g., a small dose range-finding (DRF) study in pregnant animals may be sufficient) and/or alternative design strategies (e.g., surrogate molecules and or transgenic animal models).

Although ICH S5(R3) describes multiple options for dose selection including evidence of slight maternal toxicity, for most biopharmaceuticals the doses for DART studies are based on human exposure multiples and/or maximum exposure/pharmacology. As specified in both ICH S6(R1) and ICH S5(R3), a 10× human exposure multiple is sufficient justification for high-dose selection in a pharmacologically relevant species. When doing DART and JAS in species that were used in repeat-dose toxicity studies, the exposure and toxicity profile is typically already characterized so there is often little reason to conduct DRF studies for biopharmaceuticals unless off-target toxicity is expected and/or if the pharmacological target has a key role in pregnancy maintenance or placental development/function. In which case, pilot work in pregnant animals may be useful and ICH S5(R3) describes some different options if rats and/or rabbits are relevant species.

An important consideration when dosing animals with biopharmaceuticals specific to human targets is the potential for immunogenicity to those targets. This immunogenicity, or antidrug antibody (ADA) responses, may have no impact on the toxicity study but if present may result in neutralizing activity that reduces exposure and/or target pharmacology. Immunogenicity may also lead to immune complex-related effects that have the potential to confound data interpretation as both immunogenicity and immune complex disease may or may not be relevant to human safety because the translation of immunogenicity is notoriously difficult to predict (see Chapter 10 for more details on immunogenicity and immunotoxicity assessments). Because DART studies are typically conducted in species used for repeat-dose toxicity studies, there should be data available indicating the incidence of ADA and whether systemic exposure is affected. Based on this, DART study designs can be adapted accordingly to ensure appropriate data interpretation. In general, if the biopharmaceutical has been shown to induce ADA, it is considered good practice to collect blood samples for potential ADA analysis from all-dose groups, including the control group, and these should be collected concurrently with samples for toxicokinetic analysis. A sample taken prior to the initiation of dosing and a sample taken at the end of dosing are generally adequate. Based on previous data on incidence or other considerations, it may make sense to collect samples from all animals or simply a representative number of animals per dose group. If exposure data are unexpectedly low and/or there are toxicities potentially associated with immune complex disease, then those samples can be analyzed for ADA to aid the interpretation of the study data.

Biodistribution during pregnancy is also an important consideration. Based on ICH S5(R3), maternal systemic exposure should be evaluated during gestation, particularly if dose selection is based on human exposure multiples. There is no regulatory requirement to measure embryofetal exposure in EFD studies as human embryofetal exposure is not typically available, and for small molecules, these exposures are usually expected to be similar to maternal exposures based on simple diffusion. Biopharmaceuticals are large molecules (>5 kDa) and generally do not cross the placenta; however, Fc-containing modalities do cross the placenta with a species-specific profile over the course of gestation (Bowman et al., 2013; DeSesso et al., 2012). Monoclonal IgG antibodies are a common type of Fc-containing modality and available experimental data demonstrate low placental transfer in the first trimester and increases in the second and third trimester in NHPs (Catlin et al., 2020; Moffat et al., 2014; Wang et al., 2016). Similar experiments have been conducted in rats that also demonstrate low placental transfer during organogenesis and increasing in the fetal growth phase (Bowman et al., 2012; Coder et al., 2013). These data suggest that while the placental transfer of mAbs is low during organogenesis but with highly potent molecules and high doses, it is plausible that embryos could be exposed to biologically active concentrations during organogenesis. On the contrary, reports are also available of effects of mAbs observed during an (e)PPND study but not in the EFD study. Denosumab is a mAb that targets RANKL for inhibition of bone resorption; no effects were observed on pregnancy and embryofetal development in an EFD study with dosing during GD20 to 50, while in a PPND study with dosing from GD20 to parturition, increased stillbirths and postnatal mortality, decreased body weight gain, and decreased growth/development were encountered (Bussiere et al., 2013b). The observed effects were consistent with the pharmacological action of denosumab. For other biopharmaceutical modalities, if insufficient data exist on placental transfer or where fetal exposure cannot reasonably be understood, it can be helpful to measure fetal exposure if results are unexpected and/or to confirm fetal exposure when no effects are observed.

Much like fetal exposure, there is no regulatory requirement to measure biopharmaceutical exposure in maternal milk or offspring during lactation. While milk concentration in animals is not considered predictive of milk concentration in humans, the presence of milk in animals does suggest that it may be present in human milk. Potentially more useful than exposure in milk is confirmation of biopharmaceutical exposure in offspring following maternal administration because this can have a direct impact both on data interpretation of the specific study, but also to potentially provide safety data to support pediatrics depending on the concentration and duration of exposure in offspring. Some examples of NHP ePPND studies that measured mAbs in milk and offspring include denosumab (Bussiere et al., 2013b), tabalumab (Breslin et al., 2015b), and tanezumab (Bowman et al., 2015).

12.4 When Rodent and/or Rabbit are Pharmacologically Relevant

12.4.1 Considerations

If pharmacologically relevant, the rat is the most common and preferred rodent species for evaluation of all stages of reproductive development including fertility, pregnancy, lactation, and PPND. Sprague Dawley and Wistar strains are the most common based on the use in general toxicity studies and therefore can be the most valuable due to the large amount of historical background data available for all DART study types. The mouse, typically the CD-1, can also be used as a rodent species for DART studies if the rat is not appropriate, as historical background data are also available in this species and strain. For the purposes of EFD evaluation, if a second mammalian nonrodent, nonprimate species is pharmacologically relevant, then both should be evaluated. The rabbit has historically served this purpose since its value has been previously proven in identifying human teratogens not detected in rodents. Common rabbit strains include the New Zealand White, Dutch-belted, and Japanese white. According to ICH S6(R1), if both rodents and rabbits are pharmacologically relevant, then both should be subject to EFD evaluation; but if only rat and NHP are relevant, then a rat-only DART package can be sufficient and NHP should only be used if they are the only relevant species.

Even by controlling the age, weight, and parity in DART studies, many endpoints have a wide degree of variability in the population and a specific group of animals on a study (including control groups) may not always represent the normal data range for a particular endpoint. For this reason, the number of animals per group in definitive DART studies is a balance of scientific judgment from many decades of experience and ethical considerations on the appropriate use of animals. For DART studies in rodents and rabbits, 16–20 litters per group provide consistency across studies as experience indicates that below 16 per group, the results are less reproducible, and that above 20–24 litters per group, consistency is not much improved. In addition, contemporary historical control data collected at the test facility using consistent criteria and standard operating procedures can be important for differentiating test item-related effects from normal background variability. This is particularly true for fetal morphological evaluations in the EFD study where malformations are rare but do occur in the background population. The study should be conducted at a test facility experienced in DART studies because it is critical not only for high-quality evaluations but also for the application of their historical control database in the species and strain evaluated to enable robust data interpretation that routinely is communicated directly in labeling as a risk for humans.

12.4.2 Male and Female Fertility

The objective of the fertility study is to evaluate effects related to exposure during reproductive stages A (premating to conception) and B (conception to implantation) as described in ICH S5(R3). Stage A encompasses adult male and female reproductive functions, development, and maturation of gametes, mating behavior, and fertilization. For males, this includes detection of functional effects (such as epididymal sperm maturation) that are not evaluated in general toxicity (nonmating) studies. Stage B encompasses adult female reproductive functions, preimplantation development, and implantation. For females, this includes effects on cyclicity and tubal transport. The vast majority of fertility studies are conducted in rats and sometimes mice, as such the information provided here is specific to rodents. However, if rats or mice are not

relevant but rabbits are, there is limited experience conducting male and female fertility studies in rabbits including with biopharmaceuticals such as tabalumab (Breslin et al., 2015a). The primary difference with rabbits is that females do not spontaneously cycle or ovulate, rather ovulation is induced by mating with the male.

For the integrated male reproductive toxicity assessment, the appropriate qualitative "stage-aware" microscopic evaluation of the testis is an important component (Creasy, 2001; Lanning et al., 2002; Vidal and Whitney, 2014), and this is typically done in repeat-dose toxicity testing. The male fertility study is needed to detect other functional effects unrelated to testicular sperm production such as post-testicular sperm maturation, behavior, libido, and fecundity (Ulbrich and Palmer, 1995). The male fertility study involves dosing males prior to and during mating with treatment-naïve females until evidence of mating in females, with females evaluated mid-gestation for confirmation of pregnancy and viability of embryos. In the male fertility study, male reproductive organs are weighed and preserved for potential future evaluation. If there is no effect on male reproductive organs in the repeat-dose rodent toxicity study, a 2-week premating dosing period is sufficient in the male rodent fertility study. Importantly, this 2-week dosing prior to mating can detect post-testicular effects on sperm, accessory male organ function, male libido, and male copulatory function. This is supported by the approximate 2-week post-testicular transit time in rats as it is these post-testicular sperm that are ejaculated during the subsequent mating period. Key examples of this include alpha-chlorohydrin and ornidazole, which have no overt effects on testicular weights or histopathology but do cause male infertility via effects on sperm maturation (motility and capacitation) in the epididymis (Jones and Cooper, 1999; Takayama et al., 1995). If there is a potential for male reproductive toxicity, then 10-week premating dosing and assessment of sperm at necropsy are appropriate to better characterize the functional consequence of toxicity. Sperm assessment can be a useful complementary endpoint to potential effects on male fertility (functional mating) and morphologic changes in male reproductive tissues. Sperm assessment can be a more sensitive measure of effects on spermatogenesis than fertility in rodents because there is a large sperm reserve in these species such that as much as a 90% decrease in sperm count may still result in normal fertility (Blazak et al., 1993; Meistrich, 1982; Takayama et al., 1995). As such, without sperm evaluation, a post-testicular effect on sperm maturation may be missed in rodents (Marien et al., 2016). However, for effects on spermatogenesis in the testis, microscopic evaluation is still considered the most sensitive endpoint (Cappon et al., 2013; Creasy, 2001; Vidal and Whitney, 2014).

The female fertility study involves dosing females prior to mating, during mating with treatment-naïve males, and into gestation until implantation. Female rodents should be monitored prior to and during mating for the stage of estrous until mated. Estrous evaluation in the mouse or rat is relatively noninvasive as both have short, regular estrous cycles that can easily be monitored by examining cytologically from a daily vaginal smear (Goldman et al., 2007; Vidal and Filgo, 2017). Some considerations unique to mouse are that vaginal smears can be more difficult to obtain and that the presence of males in adjacent cages can facilitate normal cycling. In a rodent fertility study, the mating trial pairs the one treated female with one male for a set period of time, typically 2 weeks, until evidence of mating is confirmed by copulatory plug in the vagina or sperm present in a vaginal smear. The animals are unpaired, and the mated female is allowed to progress through gestation until Cesarean section typically in mid-gestation. The primary fertility endpoints include pregnancy confirmation, calculation of reproductive indices (mating and fertility), enumeration of corpora lutea (ovulation), implantation confirming successful development of preimplantation stage of the embryo, and the number of viable and nonviable conceptuses relative to the number of implantation sites. The limited apical endpoints calculated in rodent mating trials include time to mating and several different types of reproductive indices such as mating index ([number of females with evidence of mating (or females confirmed pregnant)/ total number of females used for mating] × 100) and fertility index ([number of pregnant females/ total number of females used for mating]×100).

Depending on when data are needed and anticipated effects, the male and/or female fertility study can be combined with other study types. A common combination is dosing both sexes at the same time and mating them to each other. This combined fertility study may be useful if no effects on male or female reproduction are anticipated based on literature or previous studies. If an effect on fertility is detected, it can be difficult to attribute to which or both sexes. It is also possible to start with a female fertility study mated with treatment-naïve males and then dose those same males for a male fertility study mated with treatment-naïve females. Another possible combination is a female fertility study with EFD; in this study design, females keep dosing to the end of organogenesis and fetuses are evaluated at the end of gestation. This can be an attractive approach if no effects on female fertility are anticipated but if fertility is affected it can compromise the EFD evaluation. Combining the male fertility study with the 3- or 6-month repeat-dose study can also be done, as this only requires mating study males with treatment-naïve females and conducting a mid-gestation Cesarean section.

A critical component of experimental test systems to appropriately evaluate potential effects on male and female fertility is that the test system should be sexually mature. An immature or developing testis can in many ways resemble types of testicular toxicity and at best confound an otherwise adequate assessment of test item-related toxicity (Lanning et al., 2002). Based on microscopic evaluation of the male reproductive tract including sperm evaluation, the Wistar and Sprague Dawley rats are considered sexually mature by 10 weeks of age (Campion et al., 2013), but it is common for functional fertility evaluations to mate rats between 12 and 24 weeks of age, as that seems to represent peak male reproductive capacity in most rat strains; younger and older than that there is more variability as males first mature, and then, as they age, their reproductive capacity appears to slowly decline (Auroux et al., 1985; Blazak et al., 1985; Jarak et al., 2018; Saksena et al., 1979; Takakura et al., 2014). Based on microscopy of the testis, it is recommended that mice be older than 7 weeks of age at termination (Lanning et al., 2002). For female rodents

that are not yet sexually mature (still in puberty) or too old (reproductively senescent), cyclicity and fertility can be inconsistent and is likely to confound the interpretation of test item-related effects. In rats there is some variability in maturation of estrous cyclicity even out to 8 weeks old, and, although they are likely to mature by 10 weeks old, it is common to conduct the mating trial in a functional fertility study using female rats at least 12 weeks of age. Importantly, female rats should cycle normally (4–5 days per cycle) between 3 and 6 months of age. Although during this span abnormal estrous cycles can occur occasionally, the number and duration of abnormal cycles start increasing further around 6 months of age, and soon thereafter fertility indices start decreasing, including embryo loss (Ishii et al., 2012; Mitchard and Klein, 2016).

12.4.3 Pregnancy, Lactation, and Developmental Toxicity

To address reproductive stages C (pregnancy-organogenesis) through stage F (weaning to sexual maturity of offspring) as described in ICH S5(R3), multiple study types are typically conducted in the rodent and/or rabbit. Specifically, the EFD study addresses stage C by dosing pregnant animals during organogenesis and evaluating prenatal developmental toxicity in fetuses just prior to delivery. The EFD study data inform the safety risk of enrolling women of child-bearing potential in clinical studies. The PPND study addresses stages C through F by dosing pregnant and lactating animals during organogenesis through parturition to weaning and evaluating postnatal developmental toxicity in offspring through sexual maturity. This latter study is typically completed to support product registration concurrent to Phase 3 clinical testing. This PPND study evaluates adult female reproductive functions including parturition and lactation, as well as pre- and postweaning development of offspring including survival, growth, the onset of puberty, and sexual maturity and function. Route of administration can be an important consideration as the intended clinical route may not always be most appropriate, depending on the species. Because the risk assessment in pregnancy generally relies on animal studies, comparing systemic exposure between the animal species and human usually provides the most meaningful translation of risks to the fetus. Therefore, systemic routes of exposure are typically used for DART studies, even if the clinical route may not be (e.g., intravitreal, intrathecal).

The dose paradigm for EFD studies is consistent across species; however, the specific gestation dosing days are different due to species-specific differences in the days of implantation and closure of the hard palate (Wise et al., 2009). For biotherapeutics with potential off-target toxicity or target-based concern specific for maternal, placental, or developmental toxicity; it can be useful to conduct DRF studies to ensure an appropriate dose selection for the definitive EFD study. This can be particularly helpful if rabbit is a relevant species since often this is the first study in the rabbit and preliminary toxicity and exposure data can be helpful. However, since most biotherapeutics do not have anticipated developmental toxicity or off-target effects, it is possible to forego the DRF study if there is available exposure data from the repeat-dose toxicity studies.

Typically, there is no need for DRF studies for PPND dose selection as the EFD study usually is appropriate for that purpose. If there is a potential for toxicity in parturition or early postnatal development based on available information, then a modified PPND DRF using fewer animals and taking the study to weaning can usually provide confidence in dose section prior to the definitive PPND study.

The objective of the definitive EFD study is to assess maternal toxicity and to evaluate potential effects on embryofetal lethality, intrauterine growth, and fetal morphological development (Wise et al., 2009). Clinical observations; body weight; body weight gain; food consumption; and blood collection for immunogenicity, bioanalytical, and toxicokinetic analyses are the typical in-life observations. In addition, clinical pathology or other pharmacodynamic markers could be evaluated in maternal or fetal samples for cause, to confirm expected pharmacology, and/or to evaluate potential effects in pregnancy. There are relatively few published examples of EFD studies in rodents or rabbits with clinical pathology or other markers contributing to the interpretation of an EFD study with biotherapeutics (Breslin et al., 2015a; Campion et al., 2015; Crawford and Friedman, 2019; Katavolos et al., 2018). It is important to be aware of potential differences in any endpoints between early and late gestation and whether pregnant or not (Honda et al., 2008; Liberati et al., 2004; Mizoguchi et al., 2010; Wells et al., 1999); as such control data and/or historical control data can be critical for the interpretation of such endpoints. Required postmortem evaluations include maternal macroscopic evaluation (including placenta and any gross lesions) and Cesarean section for the collection of gravid uterine weights, enumeration of corpora lutea, implantation sites, and live and dead conceptuses, and early and late resorptions. Body weight, sex, and external, visceral, and skeletal evaluation are completed for all fetuses if possible. Although maternal gross lesions and/or target tissues may be collected and preserved, they are not typically evaluated microscopically unless there is a specific rationale that informs the interpretation of the study for risk assessment purposes. If collecting maternal tissues for a possible pathology, it is important to collect corresponding tissues from control animals.

The most technical aspect of these studies is the fetal evaluations. These fetal evaluations are specialized evaluations that require very specific training, sometimes considered fetal pathology but microscopic evaluations are rarely completed. These are specialized morphological evaluations of external, visceral, and bone structures. There are several techniques used to examine visceral structures, including fresh (Stuckhardt and Poppe, 1984), frozen (brain) (Astroff et al., 2002), or free-hand sections (Wilson, 1973)/gross examinations following fixation. A recent comparison between fresh and fixed evaluation of brain and eye illustrated the value of fresh examination (Ziejewski et al., 2015). Evaluations of the skeletal bones are typically performed following an alizarin red staining procedure (Redfern and Wise, 2007). Terminology is variable among laboratories although there are published lexicons based on international scientific discussions (Makris et al., 2009) and future electronic data submissions to FDA indicate standardization of fetal terminology. All laboratories independently classify all fetal anomalies as malformations,

variations, and in some cases additional categories such as gray zone anomalies or incomplete ossification. There is no strict standardization of how specific anomalies are classified as the adversity of many specific malformations and variations are not well understood but have been the subject of scientific debate for many years and continues to this day (Solecki et al., 2013, 2015). Generally, permanent structural changes likely to adversely affect survival or health are considered malformations and developmental variations are expected to occur within the normal population under investigation and are unlikely to adversely affect survival or health (including those findings that may be transient). Each endpoint/fetal observation is tabulated and statistically analyzed on a litter basis since fetuses are not directly dosed. Litter-based calculations (e.g., litter percent postimplantation loss, live litter size, and fetal percent per litter of specific anomalies) help normalize uneven litter sizes across animals and provide a more appropriate comparison across animals, groups, and studies. Hopefully apparent by the complicated procedures described above, having EFD studies conducted by personnel and laboratories with years of experience can be critical for appropriate and defined criteria for data collection, and to reduce the potential for technical error that could compromise data interpretation.

The objective of the definitive PPND study is to assess maternal toxicity following exposure during gestation, parturition, and lactation as well as impact to the offspring including viability, altered growth and development, and functional deficits such as sexual maturation, reproductive capacity, sensory functions, motor activity, and learning and memory (Bailey et al., 2009). The study design itself is conducted primarily in rodents, specifically the rat although mice can be a suitable alternative if rats are not appropriate. There is also limited experience in the rabbit if neither rodent model is relevant (Breslin et al., 2017). Interestingly, DART studies with vaccines include a delivery phase and many of those are rabbit studies (Paoletti et al., 2008); although those studies do not typically extend past weaning. The in-life portion of the standard PPND study typically takes longer than 4 months. The endpoints are typically broken into maternal (F0) data, litter data, and offspring (F1) data. Maternal evaluations include clinical observations, body weight, body weight gain, food consumption, and macroscopic findings at necropsy including the number of former implantation scars in the uterus. Litter data include gestation length, evidence of dystocia (parturition difficulties), maternal care of pups, live litter size, pup survival, pup clinical signs including the presence of milk bands (evidence of normal nursing), pup body weights and body weight change, and preweaning landmarks of development and reflex ontogeny such as eye-opening, pinna unfolding, surface righting, and response to light. Postweaning offspring endpoints evaluated include landmarks of sexual maturation (vaginal opening and preputial separation), functional tests that assess sensory functions, motor activity, learning and memory, and lastly reproductive performance that includes F1 female cycling data, mating, and fertility indices usually ending with F1 male gross necropsy and female C-section at mid- or end of gestation for confirmation of F2 viability. There is little guidance regarding which specific functional tests, but pragmatically those tests with some confidence and capability to detect changes (Crofton et al., 2008) are available at select laboratories and experience and historical control in the test system are preferred. In addition, clinical pathology, toxico-kinetic, or pharmacodynamic markers could be evaluated in maternal or pup samples for cause, to confirm expected phar-macology, and/or to evaluate potential effects in pregnancy, lactation, or in offspring. In rodent and rabbit PPND studies, there are typically no scheduled tissue collections in F0 or F1 unless for cause. However, at the gross necropsy for both F0 and F1 animals, routinely any gross lesions will be collected along with corresponding control tissue for possible micro-scopic examination.

12.4.4 Juvenile Animal Studies

With the recent adoption of the new ICH S11 guidance, it was made clear that JASs are conducted for one of two reasons. Either JAS are done in young animals to support dosing the pediatric population as the primary patient population or they are done to fulfill a data gap necessary to support dos-ing pediatrics in addition to existing nonclinical and likely clinical data in adults. In the primary instance, JASs should be conducted in one rodent and one nonrodent, assuming both are pharmacologically relevant. These are also completed as full-repeat-dose toxicity studies as would be done for a normal development program. The latter example can be more com-plicated since in that scenario there is already existing data in young adult animals and humans. In this case, a deliberate weight of evidence is conducted to determine whether a juve-nile animal study is warranted. If such a study is warranted, ICH S11 describes study design considerations, core end-points, and additional endpoints to address specific concerns in pediatrics as described below.

When possible and pharmacologically relevant, rodents are the preferred species for JAS since it is possible to evaluate all aspects of postnatal development up to sexual maturity due to the compressed developmental schedule compared with primates (2 months in rodents compared with many years in primates). DRF studies are recommended due to uncertainties with age-specific exposure and target organ sensitivity. The age of animals at dosing initiation should developmentally correspond to the youngest intended patient age based on the organ system(s) of toxicological concern. At very young ages, the route of administration in animals may need to be modi-fied for technical reasons to optimize exposure that would be relevant for human safety assessment. Special considerations of how animals are allocated to study groups and endpoint subsets need to be made, particularly when dosing preweaning animals that are still part of litter. There are many potential approaches, but the aim is to reduce potential confounding fac-tors such as maternal care, genetics, and litter size. ICH S11 describes different approaches for this purpose. The number of animals per group should be similar to repeat-dose toxicity testing (e.g., ten animals/sex/group at the end of dosing). The dosing regimen should include exposures during the develop-mental periods of concern for the pediatric patient population, not necessarily directly corresponding to clinical treatment duration. In general, a recovery period is recommended not only to understand persistence, reversibility, or progression of

effects observed during dosing but also to evaluate the poten-tial for delayed-onset effects.

As defined in ICH S11, each JAS should generally include core endpoints and additional endpoints as appropriate to address safety concerns. The core endpoints include mortal-ity, clinical observations, growth (including long bone length at necropsy), food consumption, sexual development (vaginal opening and balanopreputial separation), clinical pathology, microscopic evaluation of major organs and previously identi-fied target organs, and toxicokinetics. Additional endpoints to address identified safety concerns include other growth end-points (e.g., crown rump length, body length, and X-ray), bone assessments (e.g., biomarkers, bone mass, and histomorphom-etry), clinical pathology (e.g., urinalysis and coagulation), additional tissues for microscopic evaluation, ophthalmologic examination, various assessments of CNS structure and/or function, reproductive evaluations (e.g., cycling, sperm assess-ment but not typically mating assessments), and immunologi-cal assessments as described in ICH S8.

12.5 Only NHP Pharmacologically Relevant

12.5.1 Considerations

The cynomolgus monkey (*Macaca fascicularis*) is by far the most frequently used NHP species for the safety assessment of biopharmaceuticals. This macaque species derives from Southeast Asia and is known under additional names – e.g., Macaca irus, crab-eating macaque, and long-tailed macaque. The current scientific common name for *M. fascicularis* is long-tailed macaque (Rowe, 2016), since the tail in this spe-cies is particularly long relative to body length. Long-tailed macaques originate from equatorial latitudes without a dis-tinct summer and winter and, therefore, are fertile and sexu-ally active throughout the entire year. Another advantage of the long-tailed macaque is that male and female animals are socially highly compatible even after having reached sexual maturity. Larger-scale breeding institutions for NHPs are located in the Asia mainland (e.g., Cambodia, China, and Vietnam) and on Mauritian island. It is generally assumed that animals with island origin are likely more different than those with mainland origin due to genetic isolation. For example, Mauritian-origin NHPs attain sexual maturity faster than ani-mals from the Asia mainland (Luetjens and Weinbauer, 2012). On the contrary, experience with developmental toxicity eval-uation of NHPs with Asia mainland and Mauritian origin does not suggest relevant differences for study outcomes such as pregnancy success and infant survival (Luetjens et al., 2015).

Marmoset monkeys (*Callithrix jacchus*), whose natural hab-itat is Brazil, are occasionally used as an alternative NHP spe-cies. New World monkeys such as the marmoset are now well studied in terms of reproductive physiology and endocrinol-ogy (Abbott et al., 2003; Li et al., 2005; Luetjens et al., 2005; Wistuba et al., 2013). However, the reproductive physiology and endocrinology of the marmoset are substantially different from those of human and Old World monkeys; among these differences are lack of menstrual bleeding, multiple ovula-tion (two to four ova per cycle), twin pregnancies as default, common chorion/anastomoses leading to hematopoietic XX/XY chimerism, and absence of luteinizing hormone (LH). The latter seems to be a common feature of New World monkeys (Muller et al., 2004). In essence, the pituitary produces and releases chorionic gonadotropin (CG) instead of LH, and CG stimulates gonadal steroid hormone production. Marmosets and tamarins seem to be the only anthropoid primate species that regularly exhibit multiple ovulations per cycle (Tardif et al., 2003). Because of these substantial differences, the clinical relevance of the marmoset for DART assessment has been questioned, and unless there is no other choice, using this species for DART evaluation is not recommended.

However, there is precedence and limited historical data available for DART assessment in the marmoset with canakinumab (FDA, 2009). Canakinumab targets IL-1β and is prescribed for the therapy of a variety of periodic fever syndromes. For that particular mAb, long-tailed macaques and rhesus monkeys were not acceptable due to lack of target binding while IL-1β from marmosets shares 96% identity with human IL-1β, the mAb has full cross-reactivity to marmoset IL-1β, and bioactivity of marmoset IL-1β is effectively neutralized by canakinumab. Canakinumab has been shown to produce delays in fetal skeletal development in a marmoset EFD study. Similar delays in fetal skeletal development were observed in mice administered a murine analog of canakinumab. These delays in skeletal ossification are changes from the expected ossification state in an otherwise normal structure/bone and, hence, these findings are generally reversible or transitory and not considered detrimental to postnatal survival.

Rhesus monkeys (*Macaca mulatta*) are meanwhile rarely used in regulatory safety studies for a variety of reasons, one being that the reproductive physiology is distinctly seasonal in this species, and reproductive function may be diminished or suppressed for approximately half of the year (Bansode et al., 2003; VandeVoort et al., 2015). It is crucial to consider that the annual rhythmicity of reproductive cycles can persist for years in captivity, despite conditions of controlled, indoor, and artificial light patterns.

12.5.2 Male and Female Fertility

In rodents, fertility is typically investigated by test article administration to male and female animals during a premating period and throughout mating, and dosed male animals are mated with untreated females and vice versa. In contrast, mating studies for assessing fertility are not recommended in long-tailed macaques because fertility rates are comparatively low. Pregnancy rates are in the range of 25% to 45% per ovarian cycle and 60% per animal. Preimplantation losses are around 25% and overall pregnancy loss can achieve 45% (Chellman et al., 2009b; Jarvis et al., 2010; Luetjens et al., 2020). Twin pregnancies/births are common in marmosets but extremely rare in macaques, with an overall incidence of twin live births around 0.1% (Hendrie et al., 1996; Jarvis et al., 2010). Hence, it is recognized that physical mating studies are not practical in NHPs. Therefore, assessments of potential test item effects on female and male fertility are assessed in toxicity studies using reproductive parameters as surrogates for fertility examination. As described in ICH S6(R1), a general toxicity study

of at least 3-month duration in sexually mature NHP can be used for fertility assessment using the evaluation of reproductive organ weight and histopathology as fertility endpoints. If there is a specific cause for concern based on pharmacological activity or previous findings, specialized assessments such as menstrual cyclicity, semen parameters, and male or female reproductive hormone levels can be evaluated. It should be mentioned, however, that physical mating studies are feasible and have rarely been conducted in the NHP if the test article is already suspected to interfere directly with mating behavior, fertilization, or implantation.

Male sexual maturity should be proven using functional maturity endpoints, i.e., the presence of sperm in a semen sample and at least two consecutive menstrual bleedings (Luetjens and Weinbauer, 2012; Mecklenburg et al., 2019). The onset of sexual maturity in the male long-tailed macaque is highly variable such that even in comparatively large animals of more than 5 years of age and more than 5 kg body weight, the likelihood of testicular maturity is only 90% (Lawrence, 2009; Smedley et al., 2002). An investigation in more than 900 animals revealed that the youngest animal with mature spermatogenesis histology was 3.4 years and the oldest animal with immature spermatogenesis diagnosis was 5.1 years; based on the presence of sperm in a semen sample, the age range was 2.8–7.1 years (Luetjens and Weinbauer, 2012). Hence, the use of functional endpoints such a presence of sperm in a semen sample will reveal the maturity of younger animals and reduce the burden on the supply of NHP colony.

Default reproductive parameters are organ weight and histology. Beyond that, daily vaginal swabs are recommended for females since information on the ovarian cycle phase at necropsy can provide very helpful information of the interpretation of ovarian histology findings. For male animals, it is recommended to record testis volume by sonography (e.g., at baseline and necropsy). Ultrasound-based testicular volume determination compares well with testis weight (Ramaswamy and Weinbauer, 2014) and allows a direct comparison of effects on testis size within the same animal. This can be particularly helpful if testicular histopathology is present and the question arises as to whether there has been a decline of testicular function during the study. Stage-aware analysis of spermatogenesis can be applied, and currently, a 12-stage system is being used (Dreef et al., 2007; Mecklenburg et al., 2019). Testis tissue can also be frozen at necropsy for later testicular cell quantification by flow cytometry (Mecklenburg et al., 2019). Blood collection in male animals, for potential analysis of reproductive hormones at a later stage, can easily be incorporated albeit in the authors' experience, there has been rarely a need for the analysis of these samples. For females, only if there is a cause for concern, blood collection for potential reproductive hormone analysis should be conducted owing to the need for frequent blood sampling.

For biopharmaceuticals, a minimum of two-dose groups are being used in order to collect safety information at exposures comparable to and at some higher multiple of anticipated clinical exposures (Chapman et al., 2012). A group size of at least five animals (typically separated into three animals that will be euthanized directly after test article exposure and an additional two animals that are used to investigate recovery) should be employed in long-tailed macaque studies indirectly investigating female and male fertility. This means a group size of three for terminal parameters and a group size of five for in-life parameters during the drug exposure phase. The group size of three to five animals yields low statistical power for some male reproductive endpoints, but it is acceptable for a number of parameters (see Table 12.1). Statistical power is 10% to 35% for reproductive organ weights, below 10% for ejaculate volume and sperm number, but over 70% for sperm morphology and motility. It is below 20% for LH and testosterone concentrations in serum, but over 50% for concentrations of FSH and inhibin B. For female hormones, statistical power is generally low. Therefore, in most cases, interpretation needs to be based on a weight-of-evidence approach rather than statistical significance. Power for testicular/epididymal histopathology has not been determined but is considered to be acceptably high (ICH S5(R3)).

With a statistical power below 10% for sperm number in a semen sample, a group size of five animals can only reveal major changes in sperm numbers, that is, changes that would also likely be evident in testicular and epididymal histology. This is in concordance with sperm analysis in humans, where a group size of 200 subjects in order to detect a 50% change is recommended by the FDA draft guidance on testicular toxicity (FDA, 2018). Therefore, semen evaluations are not routinely needed in toxicity studies indirectly addressing male fertility, unless a strong scientific rationale is evident. On the contrary, statistical power is remarkably high (> 80%) for ovarian cycle duration (Bussiere et al., 2013a; Mecklenburg et al., 2019). Since the power of female reproductive organ weight and hormones is generally low, the addition of ovarian cycle monitoring – albeit not requested by the respective guidelines – can aid in data interpretation. Another argument for the examination of the ovarian cycle in these studies is the

TABLE 12.1

Statistical Power Estimates for Various in-life and Terminal Parameters to Detect a 50% Change in Male and Female Long-Tailed Macaques

In-Life Parameters (n=5)	Statistical Power (%)
Semen Parameters	
Ejaculate weight[a]	<10
Sperm count[a]	<10
Sperm motility[a]	>90
Sperm morphology[a]	>70
Male Reproductive Hormones	
Testosterone[a]	<20
Luteinizing hormone[a]	10
Follicle-stimulating hormone[a]	>90
Inhibin B[a]	>50
Female Reproductive Hormones	
Estradiol	35
Progesterone	19
Luteinizing hormone	22
Follicle-stimulating hormone	37
Female Ovarian Cycle	
Cycle duration	99–100
Terminal Parameters (n=3)	
Testes weight[a]	30
Epididymides weight[a]	35
Seminal vesicles weight[a]	13
Prostate weight[a]	18
Epididymal sperm motility	96
Testis flow cytometry[b]	20/99/97/94/74
Ovaries weight	17
Uterus (incl. cervix) weight	20

Based upon a group size of three animals for terminal parameters and a group size of five animals for in-life parameters. Analysis with a two-sided two-sample t-test at p <.05

[a] Parameters derived from Cappon et al. (2013)

[b] Flow cytometry yields five testicular cell populations (HC/1C/2C/S-ph/4C) with close to or acceptable statistical power of 80% except for HC cell population (power is 20%) which contributes <10% of cells. Modified from Mecklenburg et al. (2019)

fact that mature female animals will have substantial cycle disturbances resulting from transport, altered housing environment, when switched between single/pair/group housing or when groups of females are being altered these altering social hierarchies (e.g., if a sick animal needs to be isolated) (Bussiere et al., 2013a; Weinbauer et al., 2008).

12.5.3 Pregnancy, Lactation, Developmental Toxicity

As outlined above, for the assessment of developmental toxicity of biopharmaceuticals in the NHP model, it is sufficient to conduct an ePPND study rather than an EFD study followed by a PPND study or a combined EFD/PPND approach. Typically, the ePPND study is conducted during Phase 3 for registration and ICH S6(R1) also offers to submit an interim study report comprising the data until postnatal day (PND) 7 of the study to inform Phase 3 as appropriate. Since pregnancy duration in the long-tailed macaque is around 160 days (Grossmann et al., 2020) and since it can take several weeks or months for accrual of the required number of pregnant animals, the in-life part of an ePPND study can last 12–18 months – also depending on the chosen animal number and the duration of the postnatal infant observation period. Unlike for studies in pregnant rodents and rabbits, DRF studies or preliminary PPND studies are not needed for pregnant NHPs.

Reviews on ePPND study design options are available (Chellman et al., 2009b; Weinbauer et al., 2015, 2011, 2013). Beyond that, ICH S6(R1) and ICH S5(R3) provide very specific and detailed recommendations for developing an appropriate and acceptable ePPND study design. Typically, two-dose groups are being used following ICH S6(R1). For biotherapeutics with preexisting scientific knowledge, a single-dose group may be sufficient, e.g., for mAbs targeting B cells. The minimal postnatal observation period is one month with growth, behavior, and external examination being covered. For analysis of the immune system, the minimum postnatal observation period is three months, and the maximal duration is 6 months with immunophenotyping being done at about one month. For learning and memory assessment, clinical behavioral observations are considered sufficient and instrumental learning is not recommended since this would extend the postnatal period to at least nine months. However, in the authors' experience (GFW), instrumental learning is still being demanded if there is concern about adverse effects on brain function. Within the first 2 weeks, neurobehavioral functions are being tested on at least one occasion and grip strength within the four weeks. Also, an infant image for skeletal evaluation (e.g., by X-ray) is compulsory and is being collected at one month of age or later. For mAbs, there is no need for milk collection since IgG transfer/uptake in the infant via breast milk is negligible in primates. In case of specific concerns and/or driven by the mode of action of the test item, more targeted parameters can be added, e.g., for the examination of the cardiovascular system, bone metabolism, and the ocular system. At infant necropsy, a visceral examination should be performed. It is also important, to collect and evaluate placentas – if available – since test item-related placental dysfunction has been observed. For example, treatment with onartuzumab, a mAb that targets the MET receptor and prevents hepatocyte growth factor signaling, was associated with decreased gestation length, decreased birth weight, and increased fetal and perinatal mortality (Prell et al., 2018). Placental infarcts with hemorrhage in the chorionic plate, chorionic villus, and/or decidual plate limited to placentas from onartuzumab-treated animals were identified as a potential cause for the observed effects. Administration of a mAb against insulin-like growth factor 1 (IGF-1, figitumumab) during the period of organogenesis was associated with pregnancy loss and fetal growth deficits (Bowman et al., 2010). Fetal malformations were also observed and were considered secondary to altered placental function and/or reduced fetal growth due to impaired IGF-1 signaling although a direct inhibition of IGF signaling in the conceptus could not be ruled out. Another example is a set of two studies with an antinerve growth factor mAb (tanezumab) in pregnant monkeys that resulted in a higher incidence of stillborn, infant death, and developmental neurotoxicity in the absence of maternal toxicity (Bowman et al., 2015).

As detailed above, preimplantation losses are around 25% and overall pregnancy loss can achieve 45% in the NHP model (Chellman et al., 2009b; Jarvis et al., 2010; Luetjens et al., 2020). Therefore, group size for NHP developmental toxicity studies is an important consideration as well as the distinction of spontaneous/background pregnancy/infant losses versus effects related to administration of a test item. Typically, test item-related effects on pregnancy success are assessed by using historical data ranges, i.e., average/median, minimal, and maximal losses. The limit of this approach comes when very low/high pregnancy losses have been encountered in some historical control/vehicle groups. In the case of a very low loss control group, a median loss in a test item group might be relevant. Conversely, a high loss in a test item group may be neglected since there is a historical control group with a comparable loss. To relive that dilemma, it has been tried to use the entirety of historical data and to determine the likelihood of pregnancy losses and use these probabilities for NHP developmental toxicity study interpretation. The so-called normograms were developed that provided – relative to the chosen group size – data and figures for likelihoods and the chosen criteria were "likely", "can occur", "unusual", "unlikely", and "not observed" (Jarvis et al., 2010). These normograms facilitated data interpretation and also permitted monitoring of the developmental toxicity study – e.g., whether abortion rate is within background likelihood. The normograms provided by Jarvis et al., comprised EFD and PPND studies, were based on singly housed animals and only covered the postnatal period until day 7 (Jarvis et al., 2010). Normograms for group-housed animals became available recently (Grossmann et al., 2020). Since there has been a shift from EFD toward ePPND studies, enhanced normograms were developed that provide an extended postnatal period up to three months, a new concept of separate normograms for the prenatal and the postnatal period, specific information on the perinatal phase events, a prediction of expected number of live infants for group size management, and the option to evaluate effects on pregnancy duration through the distinction of live births and infant losses (Grossmann et al., 2020).

As per ICH S6(R1), pregnant animal numbers for ePPND studies should enable 6–8 live infants/group on PND 7, and

TABLE 12.2

Estimated Probability (%) for Achieving At Least 6, 7, or 8 Live Infants on Postnatal Days (PND) 2–7 and PND 51–90 Relative to the Number of Pregnant Animals at Study Start

Number of Pregnant Animals	Number of Live Infants (PND 2–7)			Number of Live Infants (PND 51–90)		
	6	7	8	6	7	8
10	87	69	43	86	67	40
12	97	91	77	96	89	74
14	99	97	93	99	97	91
16	99	99	98	99	99	97
18	99	99	99	99	99	99
20	100	100	100	100	100	100

The number of pregnant animals refers to study start. The number of 6, 7, or 8 infants is derived from recommendations in ICH S6(R1) (2011). Based upon Grossmann et al. (2020).

ICH S5(R3) recommends approximately 16 pregnant females and notes that *Group sizes in ePPND studies should yield a sufficient number of infants in order to assess potential adverse effects on pregnancy outcome, as well as dysmorphology and postnatal development, providing the opportunity for specialist evaluation if warranted (e.g., immune system)* … These authors are unaware of statistical power estimates for detecting dysmorphology in the NHP model. However, there are reports that a group size of eight animals for TDAR (Lebrec et al., 2011) and a group size of six to eight animals for lymphocyte immunophenotyping (Krejsa et al., 2013) provide acceptable statistical power for detecting alterations. It has also been demonstrated for learning and memory testing in juvenile animals that a group size of eight animals yields sufficient statistical power (Rose et al., 2015). A recent review on pregnancy success (Luetjens et al., 2020) and data derived from enhanced normograms (Grossmann et al., 2020) indicate that an initial group size of 14 pregnant animals per group for an ePPND study will yield six infants on PND 90 with 99% likelihood and eight infants on PND 90 with 91% likelihood (Table 12.2). Hence, an initial group size of 14 pregnant animals per group for an ePPND study should generally be sufficient to comply with the guideline's requirements.

12.5.4 Juvenile Animal Studies

The ICH S11 guideline contains important new perspectives on the use of NHPs for JAS. Since juvenile rather than neonatal animals are typically used in NHP JAS, it is important to consider whether organ system gaps will be relevant, and if so which ones, when trying to cover the period from birth until adolescence. ICH S11 states that there can be limited value in performing a JAS in postweaning NHPs (> ~6 months old) because organ system maturity is generally beyond that relevant for many pediatric ages. Most organ systems are well developed or mature at birth or shortly thereafter in NHPs, and with the advent of more ePPND studies being conducted for mAbs, the question arises as to whether a stand-alone JAS is needed to bridge the age gap between DART studies and general toxicity studies. Some specific approaches are still being considered to obtain younger NHPs for JAS, such as using some of the infants from an ePPND study to conduct a juvenile "spin-off" study or breeding/holding NHPs at the test site to generate infants specifically for a neonatal/juvenile toxicity study. Similar to humans, postnatal maturation and development of the cynomolgus monkey can be divided into distinct phases and show marked individual variation. In ICH S11, new demarcation points have been provided, and for the long-tailed macaque these are neonate, first solid food, weaning, puberty, and adulthood at ages of <1 month, ~3 months, ~6 months, ~3–4 years, and ~4 years, respectively.

During preclinical testing of mAbs, ePPND studies are being conducted in the NHP model. Because of specific IgG placental transport mechanisms in primates, the late fetus is massively exposed to mAbs such that at and after birth, the neonates and even infants may demonstrate relevant exposure for some months (Bowman et al., 2015; Breslin et al., 2015b; Bussiere et al., 2019; Clarke et al., 2015). Therefore, early postnatal exposure during the conduct of an ePPND study has been used to derive data and information for consideration of human pediatric trials and in order to obtain a waiver for a separate JAS. Also, infants from ePPND studies can be allocated toward specific juvenile toxicity assessments. In this particular case study (Weinbauer and Korte, 2015), at the age of six months, the mid-dose group of infants from an ePPND study was maintained with their cage mates but underwent dosing for about one month in order to address specific pediatric safety concerns. Quite a number of investigations were applied including clinical signs, body weight, clinical pathology, echocardiography, and advanced in vivo imaging. In all cases, the maternal animals tolerated repeated handling of infants, and the infants were already familiar with some procedures and handling from the previous ePPND study postnatal phase. Such investigations in a subset of infants/juveniles from an ePPND study may in some circumstances provide an opportunity to address specific pediatric concerns, although in general juvenile spin-off investigations from an ePPND are not a preferred approach since study design and execution are challenged by many practical limitations. Also, a spin-off study cannot duplicate the sample size or gender mix of a stand-alone JAS.

If NHPs <6–9-month-olds need to be tested in a JAS, "breed and hold" may provide an option to obtain the neonatal age NHPs required. In specific cases, e.g., concern about adverse effects on CNS and brain development, a JAS in very young animals may be needed, and in such cases, study animals need to be generated at the test site. The experimental approach is similar to that for an ePPND study except that timed mating is not needed (meaning that potentially more efficient mating approaches can be used – e.g., one or more male animals co-housed over time with several female animals instead of 1:1 timed mating), and maternal animals are not dosed and are handled minimally, thereby potentially reducing any handling-related pregnancy loss rate. Otherwise, group size planning will be similar to that for an ePPND study. Besides the added time frame (pregnancy duration in long-tailed macaque is around 160 days), another potential caveat of this approach is the lack of control of gender distribution. In a recent review, the male:female infant ratio on PND7 was on average 1.24 (median: 1.20) and ranged from 0.6 to 3.5 (Luetjens et al., 2020). However, precise gender distribution may only be critical for JAS with test items known to have gender-specific effects/indications.

There has been a gradual evolution in NHP juvenile study design from simply being a general toxicity study in immature animals, to case-by-case study designs (Chellman et al., 2009a; Morford et al., 2011). Supported by ICH S11, case-by-case design has evolved from this focus on *age* to a focus on matching the *stage* of organ system development between the animal model and the intended age range of pediatric patients. If a biopharmaceutical is known to target a particular organ system, it may be more appropriate to evaluate age-related, organ-specific functional endpoints rather than focus on matching a particular clinical age (Morford et al., 2011). In the event that target organ(s) is/are not known, a JAS may be warranted because there may be effects on one of the developing organ systems; since the study cannot be designed based on the stage of the development of a known target organ system nor on associated specialty endpoints, it should be based on an optimal age match of the NHPs with the intended age of pediatric patients and of a design similar to a general toxicity study. In addition, ICH S11 now specifies core and trigger endpoints as discussed earlier for rats and rabbits in this chapter. The ICH S11 guideline states that only in rare cases is the value of a JAS conducted in preweaning NHPs justifiable (e.g., pharmaceuticals with first and primarily neonatal clinical use, inadequate exposure from an ePPND study, and/or where alternative approaches to nonclinical safety assessment are not feasible). In one author's laboratory (GFW), 18 studies were initiated between 2004 and 2017. One study used marmoset and the remaining studies used long-tailed macaque. In 12/18 studies, the test item was a pharmaceutical and in 6 studies, biopharmaceuticals/oligonucleotides had been tested. Between 2018 and 2020, 29 JASs were initiated/planned in long-tailed macaques. One study used a pharmaceutical as test item and the remainder were mAbs, antisense-oligonucleotides, or gene therapy vectors. For two of the 29 JASs, animals were bred in house.

12.6 Summary

The assessments of potential adverse effects on pregnancy, development, and fertility are an important part of the safety evaluation of biopharmaceuticals because these specialized assessments are typically not directly evaluated in clinical trials and thus are included in product labels of approved products. The need for a juvenile animal study depends on the clinical plan and the availability of relevant data to inform safety. The assessment starts with a careful evaluation of the target pathway in reproduction and development using all available information to establish a weight of evidence regarding potential risks and to what extent additional experimental studies in pharmacologically and physiologically relevant species will inform the human risk assessment. This evaluation is completed on a case-by-case basis for each product and depends on many factors including species selection, patient population, type of biopharmaceutical, and availability of information on the mechanism of action. For biopharmaceuticals, it is preferable to use rodents for developmental, reproductive, and juvenile toxicity testing where possible. However, NHPs may be the only pharmacologically and physiologically relevant species and a complete safety assessment can be conducted despite limitations to the evaluation of fertility (no mating studies), pregnancy/development (limited testing options that are expensive, use mature NHPs, and can take a year or more to complete), and juvenile testing (cannot span infant to adulthood in one study). The weight of evidence approach and detailed experimental considerations to address any data gaps in pregnancy, development, fertility, and juvenile safety of biopharmaceuticals are described in detail in ICH guidance S5(R3) and S11, both recently approved in 2020. For both guidance documents, the basic principles and concepts for biotherapeutics safety assessment build on and align with ICH S6(R1).

REFERENCES

Abott, D.H., Barnett, D.K., Colman, R.J., Yamamoto, M.E. and Schultz-Darken, N.J., 2003. Aspects of common marmoset basic biology and life history important for biomedical research. *Comp Med*. 53, 339–50.

Astroff, A.B., Ray, S.E., Rowe, L.M., Hilbish, K.G., Linville, A.L., Stutz, J.P. and Breslin, W.J., 2002. Frozen-sectioning yields similar results as traditional methods for fetal cephalic examination in the rat. *Teratology*. 66, 77–84.

Auroux, M., Nawar, N.N. and Rizkalla, N., 1985. Testicular aging: vascularization and gametogenesis modifications in the Wistar rat. *Arch Androl*. 14, 115–21.

Bailey, G.P., Wise, L.D., Buschmann, J., Hurtt, M. and Fisher, J.E., 2009. Pre- and postnatal developmental toxicity study design for pharmaceuticals. *Birth Defects Res B Dev Reprod Toxicol*. 86, 437–45.

Bansode, F.W., Chowdhury, S.R. and Dhar, J.D., 2003. Seasonal changes in the seminiferous epithelium of rhesus and bonnet monkeys. *J Med Primatol*. 32, 170–7.

Barrow, P., 2018. Review of embryo-fetal developmental toxicity studies performed for pharmaceuticals approved by FDA in 2016 and 2017. *Reprod Toxicol*. 80, 117–125.

Barrow, P. and Clemann, N., 2021. Review of embryo-fetal developmental toxicity studies performed for pharmaceuticals approved by FDA in 2018 and 2019. *Reprod Toxicol*. 99, 144–151.

Blazak, W.F., Ernst, T.L. and Stewart, B.E., 1985. Potential indicators of reproductive toxicity: testicular sperm production and epididymal sperm number, transit time, and motility in Fischer 344 rats. *Fundam Appl Toxicol*. 5, 1097–103.

Blazak, W.F., Treinen, K.A. and Juniewicz, P.E., 1993. Application of testicular sperm head counts in the assessment of male reproductive toxicity, in: Chapin, R.E. and Heindel, J.J. Eds.), *Methods in Toxicology*. Academic Press, Inc., San Diego, CA, pp. 86–94.

Bowman, C.J., Breslin, W.J., Connor, A.V., Martin, P.L., Moffat, G.J., Sivaraman, L., Tornesi, M.B. and Chivers, S., 2013. Placental transfer of Fc-containing biopharmaceuticals across species, an industry survey analysis. *Birth Defects Res B Dev Reprod Toxicol*. 98, 459–85.

Bowman, C.J. and Chapin, R.E., 2016. Goldilocks' determination of what new in vivo data are "Just Right" for different common drug development scenarios, Part 1. *Birth Defects Res B Dev Reprod Toxicol*. 107, 185–194.

Bowman, C.J., Chmielewski, G., Oneda, S., Finco, D., Boucher, M.A. and Todd, M., 2010. Embryo-fetal developmental toxicity of figitumumab, an anti-insulin-like growth factor-1 receptor (IGF-1R) monoclonal antibody, in cynomolgus monkeys. *Birth Defects Res B Dev Reprod Toxicol*. 89, 326–38.

Bowman, C.J., Evans, M., Cummings, T., Oneda, S., Butt, M., Hurst, S., Gremminger, J.L., Shelton, D., Kamperschroer, C. and Zorbas, M., 2015. Developmental toxicity assessment of tanezumab, an anti-nerve growth factor monoclonal antibody, in cynomolgus monkeys (Macaca fascicularis). *Reprod Toxicol*. 53, 105–18.

Bowman, C.J., King, L.E. and Stedman, D.B., 2012. Embryo-fetal distribution of a biopharmaceutical IgG2 during rat organogenesis. *Reprod Toxicol*. 34, 66–72.

Brennan, F.R., Cavagnaro, J., McKeever, K., Ryan, P.C., Schutten, M.M., Vahle, J., Weinbauer, G.F., Marrer-Berger, E. and Black, L.E., 2018. Safety testing of monoclonal antibodies in non-human primates: case studies highlighting their impact on human risk assessment. *MAbs*. 10, 1–17.

Breslin, W.J., Hilbish, K.G., Cannady, E.A. and Edwards, T.L., 2017. Prenatal and postnatal assessment in rabbits with evacetrapib: a cholesteryl ester transfer protein inhibitor. *Birth Defects Res*. 109, 486–96.

Breslin, W.J., Hilbish, K.G., Martin, J.A., Halstead, C.A. and Edwards, T.L., 2015a. Developmental toxicity and fertility assessment in rabbits with tabalumab: a human IgG4 monoclonal antibody. *Birth Defects Res B Dev Reprod Toxicol*. 104, 117–28.

Breslin, W.J., Hilbish, K.G., Martin, J.A., Halstead, C.A., Newcomb, D.L. and Chellman, G.J., 2015b. An enhanced pre- and postnatal development study in cynomolgus monkeys with tabalumab: a human IgG4 monoclonal antibody. *Birth Defects Res B Dev Reprod Toxicol*. 104, 100–16.

Bussiere, J.L., Davies, R., Dean, C., Xu, C., Kim, K.H., Vargas, H.M., Chellman, G.J., Balasubramanian, G., Rubio-Beltran, E., MaassenVanDenBrink, A. and Monticello, T.M., 2019. Nonclinical safety evaluation of erenumab, a CGRP receptor inhibitor for the prevention of migraine. *Regul Toxicol Pharmacol*. 106, 224–238.

Bussiere, J.L., Moffat, G., Zhou, L. and Tarlo, K.S., 2013a. Assessment of menstrual cycle length in cynomolgus monkeys as a female fertility endpoint of a biopharmaceutical in a 6 month toxicity study. *Regul Toxicol Pharmacol*. 66, 269–78.

Bussiere, J.L., Pyrah, I., Boyce, R., Branstetter, D., Loomis, M., Andrews-Cleavenger, D., Farman, C., Elliott, G. and Chellman, G., 2013b. Reproductive toxicity of denosumab in cynomolgus monkeys. *Reprod Toxicol*. 42, 27–40.

Campion, S.N., Carvallo, F.R., Chapin, R.E., Nowland, W.S., Beauchamp, D., Jamon, R., Koitz, R., Winton, T.R., Cappon, G.D. and Hurtt, M.E., 2013. Comparative assessment of the timing of sexual maturation in male Wistar Han and Sprague-Dawley rats. *Reprod Toxicol*. 38, 16–24.

Campion, S.N., Han, B., Cappon, G.D., Lewis, E.M., Kraynov, E., Liang, H. and Bowman, C.J., 2015. Decreased maternal and fetal cholesterol following maternal bococizumab (anti-PCSK9 monoclonal antibody) administration does not affect rat embryo-fetal development. *Regul Toxicol Pharmacol*. 73, 562–70.

Cappon, G.D., Potter, D., Hurtt, M.E., Weinbauer, G.F., Luetjens, C.M. and Bowman, C.J., 2013. Sensitivity of male reproductive endpoints in nonhuman primate toxicity studies: a statistical power analysis. *Reprod Toxicol*. 41, 67–72.

Carlock, L.L., Cowan, L.A., Oneda, S., Hoberman, A., Wang, D.D., Hanna, R. and Bussiere, J.L., 2009. A comparison of effects on reproduction and neonatal development in cynomolgus monkeys given human soluble IL-4R and mice given murine soluble IL-4R. *Regul Toxicol Pharmacol*. 53, 226–34.

Catlin, N.R., Mitchell, A.Z., Potchoiba, M.J., O'Hara, D.M., Wang, M., Zhang, M., Weinbauer, G.F. and Bowman, C.J., 2020. Placental transfer of (125) iodinated humanized immunoglobulin G2Deltaa in the cynomolgus monkey. *Birth Defects Res*. 112, 105–117.

Cavagnaro, J., Berman, C., Kornbrust, D., White, T., Campion, S. and Henry, S., 2014. Considerations for assessment of reproductive and developmental toxicity of oligonucleotide-based therapeutics. *Nucleic Acid Ther*. 24, 313–25.

Chapman, K.L., Andrews, L., Bajramovic, J.J., Baldrick, P., Black, L.E., Bowman, C.J., Buckley, L.A., Coney, L.A., Couch, J., Maggie Dempster, A., de Haan, L., Jones, K., Pullen, N., de Boer, A.S., Sims, J. and Ian Ragan, C., 2012. The design of chronic toxicology studies of monoclonal antibodies: implications for the reduction in use of non-human primates. *Regul Toxicol Pharmacol*. 62, 347–54.

Chellman, G.J., Bussiere, J.L., Makori, N., Martin, P.L., Ooshima, Y. and Weinbauer, G.F., 2009a. Developmental and reproductive toxicology studies in nonhuman primates. *Birth Defects Res (Part B)*. 86, 446–62.

Chellman, G.J., Bussiere, J.L., Makori, N., Martin, P.L., Ooshima, Y. and Weinbauer, G.F., 2009b. Developmental and reproductive toxicology studies in nonhuman primates. *Birth Defects Res B Dev Reprod Toxicol*. 86, 446–62.

Clarke, D.O., Hilbish, K.G., Waters, D.G., Newcomb, D.L. and Chellman, G.J., 2015. Assessment of ixekizumab, an interleukin-17A monoclonal antibody, for potential effects on reproduction and development, including immune system function, in cynomolgus monkeys. *Reprod Toxicol*. 58, 160–73.

Coder, P.S., Thomas, J.A., Stedman, D.B. and Bowman, C.J., 2013. Placental transfer of (125)Iodinated humanized immunoglobulin G2Deltaa in the Sprague Dawley rat. *Reprod Toxicol*. 38, 37–46.

Crawford, D. and Friedman, M., 2019. Evaluation of the developmental toxicity of vedolizumab, an alpha4beta7 receptor antagonist, in rabbit and nonhuman primate. *Int J Toxicol.* 38, 395–404.

Creasy, D.M., 2001. Pathogenesis of male reproductive toxicity. *Toxicol Pathol.* 29, 64–76.

Crofton, K.M., Foss, J.A., Hass, U., Jensen, K.F., Levin, E.D. and Parker, S.P., 2008. Undertaking positive control studies as part of developmental neurotoxicity testing: a report from the ILSI Research Foundation/Risk Science Institute expert working group on neurodevelopmental endpoints. *Neurotoxicol Teratol.* 30, 266–87.

DeSesso, J.M., Williams, A.L., Ahuja, A., Bowman, C.J. and Hurtt, M.E., 2012. The placenta, transfer of immunoglobulins, and safety assessment of biopharmaceuticals in pregnancy. *Crit Rev Toxicol.* 42, 185–210.

Dreef, H.C., Van Esch, E. and De Rijk, E.P., 2007. Spermatogenesis in the cynomolgus monkey (Macaca fascicularis): a practical guide for routine morphological staging. *Toxicol Pathol.* 35, 395–404.

FDA, 2009. Ilaris (canakinumab) Drug Approval Package, Pharmacology Review Part 3.

FDA, 2018. Testicular Toxicity: Evaluation During Drug Development, Guidance for Industry.

Goldman, J.M., Murr, A.S. and Cooper, R.L., 2007. The rodent estrous cycle: characterization of vaginal cytology and its utility in toxicological studies. *Birth Defects Res B Dev Reprod Toxicol.* 80, 84–97.

Grossmann, H., Weinbauer, G.F., Baker, A., Fuchs, A. and Luetjens, C.M., 2020. Enhanced normograms and pregnancy outcome analysis in nonhuman primate developmental toxicity studies. *Reprod Toxicol.* 95, 29–36.

Hendrie, T.A., Peterson, P.E., Short, J.J., Tarantal, A.F., Rothgarn, E., Hendrie, M.I. and Hendrickx, A.G., 1996. Frequency of prenatal loss in a macaque breeding colony. *Am J Primatol.* 40, 41–53.

Honda, T., Honda, K., Kokubun, C., Nishimura, T., Hasegawa, M., Nishida, A., Inui, T. and Kitamura, K., 2008. Timecourse changes of hematology and clinical chemistry values in pregnant rats. *J Toxicol Sci.* 33, 375–80.

Ishii, M., Yamauchi, T., Matsumoto, K., Watanabe, G., Taya, K. and Chatani, F., 2012. Maternal age and reproductive function in female Sprague-Dawley rats. *J Toxicol Sci.* 37, 631–8.

Iwasaki, K., Uno, Y., Utoh, M. and Yamazaki, H., 2019. Importance of cynomolgus monkeys in development of monoclonal antibody drugs. *Drug Metab Pharmacokinet.* 34, 55–63.

Jarak, I., Almeida, S., Carvalho, R.A., Sousa, M., Barros, A., Alves, M.G. and Oliveira, P.F., 2018. Senescence and declining reproductive potential: Insight into molecular mechanisms through testicular metabolomics. *Biochim Biophys Acta Mol Basis Dis.* 1864, 3388–3396.

Jarvis, P., Srivastav, S., Vogelwedde, E., Stewart, J., Mitchard, T. and Weinbauer, G.F., 2010. The cynomolgus monkey as a model for developmental toxicity studies: variability of pregnancy losses, statistical power estimates, and group size considerations. *Birth Defects Res B Dev Reprod Toxicol.* 89, 175–87.

Jones, A.R. and Cooper, T.G., 1999. A re-appraisal of the posttesticular action and toxicity of chlorinated antifertility compounds. *Int J Androl.* 22, 130–8.

Katavolos, P., Prell, R., Zane, D., Deng, R. and Halpern, W., 2018. Resolution of unexpected pregnancy-related findings in a rat embryofetal development and toxicokinetic study of monoclonal antibodies specific for hCMV. *Birth Defects Res.* 110, 1347–1357.

Krejsa, C.M., Neradilek, M.B., Polissar, N.L., Cox, N., Clark, D., Cowan, L., Bussiere, J. and Lebrec, H., 2013. An interlaboratory retrospective analysis of immunotoxicological endpoints in non-human primates: flow cytometry immunophenotyping. *J Immunotoxicol.* 10, 361–72.

Lanning, L.L., Creasy, D.M., Chapin, R.E., Mann, P.C., Barlow, N.J., Regan, K.S. and Goodman, D.G., 2002. Recommended approaches for the evaluation of testicular and epididymal toxicity. *Toxicol Pathol.* 30, 507–20.

Lawrence, W.B., Saladino, B.H., 2009. Correlation of age and bodyweight, and testicular weight with degree of sexual maturity in male cynomolgus macaques with emphasis on peripubertal animals. *Vet Pathol.* 46, P235.

Lebrec, H., Cowan, L., Lagrou, M., Krejsa, C., Neradilek, M.B., Polissar, N.L., Black, L. and Bussiere, J., 2011. An interlaboratory retrospective analysis of immunotoxicological endpoints in non-human primates: T-cell-dependent antibody responses. *J Immunotoxicol.* 8, 238–50.

Li, L.H., Donald, J.M. and Golub, M.S., 2005. Review on testicular development, structure, function, and regulation in common marmoset. *Birth Defects Res B Dev Reprod Toxicol.* 74, 450–69.

Liberati, T.A., Sansone, S.R. and Feuston, M.H., 2004. Hematology and clinical chemistry values in pregnant Wistar Hannover rats compared with nonmated controls. *Vet Clin Pathol.* 33, 68–73.

Luetjens, C.M., Fuchs, A., Baker, A. and Weinbauer, G.F., 2020. Group size experiences with enhanced pre- and postnatal development studies in the long-tailed macaque (Macaca fascicularis). *Primate Biol.* 7, 1–4.

Luetjens, C.M., Fuchs, A. and Weinbauer, G.F., 2015. Developmental toxicity evaluation in the cynomolgus monkey (Macaca fascicularis): Does Mauritian origin matter? 54th Annual Meeting of the Society of Toxicology. San Diego, CA.

Luetjens, C.M. and Weinbauer, G.F., 2012. Functional assessment of sexual maturity in male macaques (Macaca fascicularis). *Regul Toxicol Pharmacol.* 63, 391–400.

Luetjens, C.M., Weinbauer, G.F. and Wistuba, J., 2005. Primate spermatogenesis: new insights into comparative testicular organisation, spermatogenic efficiency and endocrine control. *Biol Rev Camb Philos Soc.* 80, 475–88.

Makris, S.L., Solomon, H.M., Clark, R., Shiota, K., Barbellion, S., Buschmann, J., Ema, M., Fujiwara, M., Grote, K., Hazelden, K.P., Hew, K.W., Horimoto, M., Ooshima, Y., Parkinson, M. and Wise, L.D., 2009. Terminology of developmental abnormalities in common laboratory mammals (Version 2). *Birth Defects Res B Dev Reprod Toxicol.* 86, 227–327.

Marien, D., Bailey, G.P., Eichenbaum, G. and De Jonghe, S., 2016. Timing is everything for sperm assessment in fertility studies. *Reprod Toxicol.* 64, 141–50.

Martin, P.L., Breslin, W., Rocca, M., Wright, D. and Cavagnaro, J., 2009. Considerations in assessing the developmental and reproductive toxicity potential of biopharmaceuticals. *Birth Defects Res B Dev Reprod Toxicol.* 86, 176–203.

Mecklenburg, L., Luetjens, C.M. and Weinbauer, G.F., 2019. Toxicologic pathology forum*: opinion on sexual maturity and fertility assessment in long-tailed macaques (Macaca fascicularis) in nonclinical safety studies. *Toxicol Pathol.* 47, 444–60.

Meistrich, M.L., 1982. Quantitative correlation between testicular stem cell survival, sperm production, and fertility in the mouse after treatment with different cytotoxic agents. *J Androl.* 3, 58–68.

Mitchard, T.L. and Klein, S., 2016. Reproductive senescence, fertility and reproductive tumour profile in ageing female Han Wistar rats. *Exp Toxicol Pathol.* 68, 143–7.

Mizoguchi, Y., Matsuoka, T., Mizuguchi, H., Endoh, T., Kamata, R., Fukuda, K., Ishikawa, T. and Asano, Y., 2010. Changes in blood parameters in New Zealand White rabbits during pregnancy. *Lab Anim.* 44, 33–9.

Moffat, G.J., Retter, M.W., Kwon, G., Loomis, M., Hock, M.B., Hall, C., Bussiere, J., Lewis, E.M. and Chellman, G.J., 2014. Placental transfer of a fully human IgG2 monoclonal antibody in the cynomolgus monkey, rat, and rabbit: a comparative assessment from during organogenesis to late gestation. *Birth Defects Res B Dev Reprod Toxicol.* 101, 178–88.

Morford, L.L., Bowman, C.J., Blanset, D.L., Bogh, I.B., Chellman, G.J., Halpern, W.G., Weinbauer, G.F. and Coogan, T.P., 2011. Preclinical safety evaluations supporting pediatric drug development with biopharmaceuticals: strategy, challenges, current practices. *Birth Defects Res B Dev Reprod Toxicol.* 92, 359–80.

Muller, T., Gromoll, J., Simula, A.P., Norman, R., Sandhowe-Klaverkamp, R. and Simoni, M., 2004. The carboxyterminal peptide of chorionic gonadotropin facilitates activation of the marmoset LH receptor. *Exp Clin Endocrinol Diabetes.* 112, 574–9.

Paoletti, L.C., Guttormsen, H.K., Christian, M.S., Hoberman, A.M. and McInnes, P., 2008. Neither antibody to a group B streptococcal conjugate vaccine nor the vaccine itself is teratogenic in rabbits. *Hum Vaccin.* 4, 435–43.

Prell, R.A., Dybdal, N., Arima, A., Chihaya, Y., Nijem, I. and Halpern, W., 2018. Placental and Fetal Effects of Onartuzumab, a Met/HGF Signaling Antagonist, When Administered to Pregnant Cynomolgus Monkeys. *Toxicol Sci.* 165, 186–97.

Ramaswamy, S. and Weinbauer, G.F., 2014. Endocrine control of spermatogenesis: Role of FSH and LH/ testosterone. *Spermatogenesis.* 4, e996025.

Redfern, B.G. and Wise, L.D., 2007. High-throughput staining for the evaluation of fetal skeletal development in rats and rabbits. *Birth Defects Res B Dev Reprod Toxicol.* 80, 177–82.

Rocca, M., Morford, L.L., Blanset, D.L., Halpern, W.G., Cavagnaro, J. and Bowman, C.J., 2018. Applying a weight of evidence approach to the evaluation of developmental toxicity of biopharmaceuticals. *Regul Toxicol Pharmacol.* 98, 69–79.

Rose, C., Luetjens, C.M., Grote-Wessels, S. and Weinbauer, G.F., 2015. Feasibility of repeated testing for learning ability in juvenile primates for pediatric safety assessment. *Regul Toxicol Pharmacol.* 73, 571–7.

Rowe, N., Myers, M., 2016. *All the World's Primates*, Pogonia Press, Charlestown, RI.

Saksena, S.K., Lau, I.F. and Chang, M.C., 1979. Age dependent changes in the sperm population and fertility in the male rat. *Exp Aging Res.* 5, 373–81.

SCHEER, 2017. Final Opinion on 'The need for non-human primates in biomedical research, production and testing of products and devices (update 2017)'. Scientific Committee on Health, Environmental and Emerging Risks.

Smedley, J.V., Bailey, S.A., Perry, R.W. and CM, O.R., 2002. Methods for predicting sexual maturity in male cynomolgus macaques on the basis of age, body weight, and histologic evaluation of the testes. *Contemp Top Lab Anim Sci.* 41, 18–20.

Solecki, R., Barbellion, S., Bergmann, B., Burgin, H., Buschmann, J., Clark, R., Comotto, L., Fuchs, A., Faqi, A.S., Gerspach, R., Grote, K., Hakansson, H., Heinrich, V., Heinrich-Hirsch, B., Hofmann, T., Hubel, U., Inazaki, T.H., Khalil, S., Knudsen, T.B., Kudicke, S., Lingk, W., Makris, S., Muller, S., Paumgartten, F., Pfeil, R., Rama, E.M., Schneider, S., Shiota, K., Tamborini, E., Tegelenbosch, M., Ulbrich, B., van Duijnhoven, E.A., Wise, D. and Chahoud, I., 2013. Harmonization of description and classification of fetal observations: achievements and problems still unresolved: report of the 7th Workshop on the Terminology in Developmental Toxicology Berlin, 4–6 May 2011. *Reprod Toxicol.* 35, 48–55.

Solecki, R., Rauch, M., Gall, A., Buschmann, J., Clark, R., Fuchs, A., Kan, H., Heinrich, V., Kellner, R., Knudsen, T.B., Li, W., Makris, S.L., Ooshima, Y., Paumgartten, F., Piersma, A.H., Schonfelder, G., Oelgeschlager, M., Schaefer, C., Shiota, K., Ulbrich, B., Ding, X. and Chahoud, I., 2015. Continuing harmonization of terminology and innovations for methodologies in developmental toxicology: Report of the 8th Berlin Workshop on Developmental Toxicity, 14–16 May 2014. *Reprod Toxicol.* 57, 140–6.

Stewart, J., 2008. Developmental/reproductive toxicology study design options for monoclonal antibodies, in: Weinbauer, G., Vogel, F. (Ed.), *Critical Contributions of Primate Models for Biopharmaceutical Drug Development.* Waxmann Verlag GmbH, Munster, Germany, pp. 101–12.

Stewart, J., 2009. Developmental toxicity testing of monoclonal antibodies: an enhanced pre- and postnatal study design option. *Reprod Toxicol.* 28, 220–5.

Stuckhardt, J.L. and Poppe, S.M., 1984. Fresh visceral examination of rat and rabbit fetuses used in teratogenicity testing. *Teratog Carcinog Mutagen.* 4, 181–8.

Takakura, I., Creasy, D.M., Yokoi, R., Terashima, Y., Onozato, T., Maruyama, Y., Chino, T., Tahara, T., Tamura, T., Kuroda, J. and Kusama, H., 2014. Effects of male sexual maturity of reproductive endpoints relevant to DART studies in Wistar Hannover rats. *J Toxicol Sci.* 39, 269–79.

Takayama, S., Akaike, M., Kawashima, K., Takahashi, M. and Kurokawa, Y., 1995. Studies on the optimal treatment period and parameters for detection of male fertility disorder in rats–introductory summary. *J Toxicol Sci.* 20, 173–82.

Tardif, S.D., Smucny, D.A., Abbott, D.H., Mansfield, K., Schultz-Darken, N. and Yamamoto, M.E., 2003. Reproduction in captive common marmosets (Callithrix jacchus). *Comp Med.* 53, 364–8.

Ulbrich, B. and Palmer, A.K., 1995. Detection of effects on male reproduction- A literature survey. *J Am Coll Toxicol.* 14, 293–327.

van Meer, P.J., Kooijman, M., van der Laan, J.W., Moors, E.H. and Schellekens, H., 2013. The value of non-human primates in the development of monoclonal antibodies. *Nat Biotechnol.* 31, 882–3.

VandeVoort, C.A., Mtango, N.R., Midic, U. and Latham, K.E., 2015. Disruptions in follicle cell functions in the ovaries of rhesus monkeys during summer. *Physiol Genomics*. 47, 102–12.

Vidal, J.D. and Filgo, A.J., 2017. Evaluation of the estrous cycle, reproductive tract, and mammary gland in female mice. *Curr Protoc Mouse Biol*. 7, 306–25.

Vidal, J.D. and Whitney, K.M., 2014. Morphologic manifestations of testicular and epididymal toxicity. *Spermatogenesis*. 4, e979099.

Wang, H., Schuetz, C., Arima, A., Chihaya, Y., Weinbauer, G.F., Habermann, G., Xiao, J., Woods, C., Grogan, J., Gelzleichter, T. and Cain, G., 2016. Assessment of placental transfer and the effect on embryo-fetal development of a humanized monoclonal antibody targeting lymphotoxin-alpha in non-human primates. *Reprod Toxicol*. 63, 82–95.

Weinbauer, G.F., Bowman, C.J. and Halpern, W.G., 2015. Developmental and Reproductive Toxicity Testing, in: J., B. et al. (Eds.), *The Nonhuman Primate in Nonclinical Drug Development and Safety Assessment*. Academic Press, Amsterdam.

Weinbauer, G.F., Fuchs, A., Niehaus, M. and Luetjens, C.M., 2011. The enhanced pre- and postnatal study for nonhuman primates: update and perspectives. *Birth Defects Res C Embryo Today*. 93, 324–33.

Weinbauer, G.F. and Korte, S.H., 2015. Juvenile toxicity testing: Experience using nonhuman primate models, in: Weinbauer, G.F. and Vogel, F. (Eds.), *Primate Biologicals Research at a Crossroads*. Waxmann Verlag, Munster/New York, pp. 61–78.

Weinbauer, G.F., Luft, J. and Fuchs, A., 2013. The enhanced pre- and postnatal development study for monoclonal antibodies. *Methods Mol Biol*. 947, 185–200.

Weinbauer, G.F., Niehoff, M., Niehaus, M., Srivastav, S., Fuchs, A., Van Esch, E. and Cline, J.M., 2008. Physiology and Endocrinology of the Ovarian Cycle in Macaques. *Toxicol Pathol*. 36, 7S–23S.

Wells, M.Y., Decobecq, C.P., Decouvelaere, D.M., Justice, C. and Guittin, P., 1999. Changes in clinical pathology parameters during gestation in the New Zealand white rabbit. *Toxicol Pathol*. 27, 370–9.

Wilson, J.G., 1973. *Environment and Birth Defects*, Academic Press, New York.

Wise, L.D., Buschmann, J., Feuston, M.H., Fisher, J.E., Hew, K.W., Hoberman, A.M., Lerman, S.A., Ooshima, Y. and Stump, D.G., 2009. Embryo-fetal developmental toxicity study design for pharmaceuticals. *Birth Defects Res B Dev Reprod Toxicol*. 86, 418–28.

Wistuba, J., Luetjens, C.M., Ehmcke, J., Redmann, K., Damm, O.S., Steinhoff, A., Sandhowe-Klaverkamp, R., Nieschlag, E., Simoni, M. and Schlatt, S., 2013. Experimental endocrine manipulation by contraceptive regimen in the male marmoset (Callithrix jacchus). *Reproduction*. 145, 439–51.

Ziejewski, M.K., Solomon, H.M., Rendemonti, J. and Stanislaus, D., 2015. Comparison of a modified mid-coronal sectioning technique and Wilson's technique when conducting eye and brain examinations in rabbit teratology studies. *Birth Defects Res B Dev Reprod Toxicol*. 104, 23–34.

13

Biosimilar Products—A Review of Past and Current Regulatory Approval Standards for Preclinical Safety Studies

A. Kimzey, K. Mease, B. Mounho-Zamora, and M. Wood
ToxStrategies, Inc.

CONTENTS

13.1 Introduction

With the patents for biotechnology-derived medicines (also known as biological products or biotherapeutics) being near or past their expiration, pharmaceutical and biopharmaceutical companies have been ardently pursuing the development of biosimilar products. A biosimilar is a biotherapeutic product demonstrated to be "highly similar" to the innovator (reference) product (RP), and for marketing approval, there can be no clinically meaningful differences between the biosimilar and the RP, in terms of its safety, purity, and potency, although there may be minor differences in clinically inactive components (P. Declerck, Danesi, Petersel, & Jacobs, 2017; EMA, 2015a; FDA, 2015b, 2015c, 2016; Panesar, 2016). Demonstrating that a biosimilar candidate is highly similar to the RP in terms of physiochemical properties, quality, pharmacological function, efficacy, and safety involves a combination of complicated and rigorous testing (i.e., analytical, nonclinical, clinical) using advanced, cutting-edge technology to reduce manufacturing costs, which ultimately leads to a cost reduction for patients (P. Declerck et al., 2017; Khraishi, Stead, Lukas, Scotte, & Schmid, 2016; Sullivan & DiGrazia, 2017). Over the years, the regulatory standards for the approval of biosimilar products have been an area of discussion, debate, and controversy

among interested parties, including the pharmaceutical/biopharmaceutical industry, regulatory health authorities, academic institutions, and healthcare providers. The discussion and debate over the approval of biosimilars continue today, with the emergence of new data, advancing technology, and revised and/or new regulatory guidelines. Inherent differences exist between biotherapeutics and traditional, small molecule pharmaceutics, such as their respective molecular size (biotherapeutics are generally greater than 30 kD and are significantly larger than small molecule drugs, which are generally less than 1 kDa), manufacturing processes (biotherapeutics are derived from living organisms, whereas small molecule products are chemically synthesized), and structural and physicochemical properties (biotherapeutics are substantially more complex than small molecule drugs). Owing to the fundamental differences between biotherapeutics and small molecule medicines, legislators and regulatory health authorities around the world have acknowledged that the regulatory pathways for the approval of generic medicines (chemically derived pharmaceutics demonstrated to be an exact copy of the innovator drug) are not scientifically appropriate for biosimilars. Over time, distinguishing between generic medicines and biosimilars has resulted in established regulatory standards and guidelines specific to the approval of biosimilars in various regions around to the world, including Europe, Australia,

Canada, Japan, the United States, and regions of rapidly growing economies or "emerging markets," such as Brazil and India. Additionally, the World Health Organization (WHO) established guidelines in 2009 for national regulatory authorities considering the approval of biosimilars in their regions (WHO, 2013). European Union (EU) has been and continues to be recognized as the pioneer in establishing legal and regulatory standards for the approval of biosimilar products, and in 2005 and 2006, the European Medicines Agency (EMA) released the first regulatory guidelines for the approval of biosimilars. Subsequently, other regions followed EU and issued regulatory guidelines for biosimilar products; although many general principles and scientific standards are similar across the various regional guidelines, some differences in scientific data requirements do exist. With emerging analytical, preclinical, and clinical data provided by sponsors over the years, the regulatory authorities have gained tremendous experience in what data are critical in the demonstration of biosimilarity for the approval of biosimilar products. Additionally, the manufacturing processes and analytical technology for biotherapeutics (novel and biosimilars) continue to advance, with manufacturing processes generating higher product yields with lower cost of goods and more sensitive analytical techniques that enable further characterization of the complex structural properties of biotherapeutics. As a result, the regulatory authorities have issued new guidelines or revised either specific sections or the entire document of existing guidelines to reflect the "lessons learned" from the emerging data and the advancement in technology (EMA, 2012, 2014, 2015a, 2015b, 2017; FDA, 2012, 2014a, 2014b, 2014c, 2015a, 2015b, 2015c, 2016, 2018a, 2018b, 2019a, 2019b, 2019c, 2020a; WHO, 2016, 2018).

This chapter provides a general review of biosimilar products and how they differ from generic small molecule medicines and why a new regulatory pathway to receive marketing approval for biosimilars was necessary. In addition, this chapter will review the history of the regulatory pathways for the approval of biosimilar products in different regions of the world, how regulatory standards have evolved over the years, and how the current standards have changed compared with the initial guidelines, with specific emphasis on the preclinical studies needed for the demonstration of biosimilarity.

13.2 Biosimilars vs. Generic Medicines: The Scientific and Regulatory Differences between Generic Medicines and Biosimilar Products

Although different terms have been used in different regions for facsimiles of innovator biotherapeutic products, such as subsequent entry biologics (SEBs) or similar biological medicinal products, "biosimilar" is the most widely accepted. A biosimilar is a version of a marketed innovator biotherapeutic product (whose patent and data exclusivity period have expired) that claims to be highly similar based on demonstration of similarity in physiochemical characteristics, efficacy, and safety to a marketed biotherapeutic product or RP (McKinnon & Lu, 2009; Schellekens, 2009; Weise et al.,

2011). In the context of this book chapter, biotherapeutic products refer to biotechnology-derived (recombinant DNA technology) protein therapeutics such as recombinant proteins, monoclonal antibodies, fusion proteins, growth factors, and replacement enzymes. The patents and regulatory data protection (data exclusivity) period for many innovator biotherapeutic products have or soon will reach expiration, and consequently, many manufacturers are pursuing development and marketing of biosimilar versions of these innovative products (GaBI, 2019b).

Over the past 30 years, advances in recombinant DNA technology (biotechnology) and manufacturing processes have led to the development of numerous biotherapeutic products for the treatment of numerous diseases. In contrast to traditional small molecule pharmaceuticals, which are chemically derived, biotherapeutics are derived from complex processes that utilize the expression of a living (host) cell system to express the therapeutic protein of interest (Crommelin et al., 2005; Mounho-Zamora, 2013). Because biotherapeutics are derived from living organisms, several variables in the manufacturing process, such as the type of expression system (such as Chinese hamster ovary [CHO] cells or bacteria such as *E. coli*), growth conditions, purification processes, and post-translation modifications (e.g., glycosylation, methylation, phosphorylation) influence the biological activity (efficacy) and safety of the final product (FDA, 2015c). Additionally, the inherent variability of the living cells/organisms and manufacturing processes results in a structurally complex product that has an inherent degree of variability (microheterogeneity) that may be difficult to fully characterize (Paul Declerck, 2012; Sullivan & DiGrazia, 2017; Weise et al., 2012). Unlike biotherapeutics, the manufacturing processes for small molecule drugs consist of a series of well-characterized chemical reactions that produce a final product that is well-defined, stable, and highly reproducible and that can be fully characterized analytically.

The fundamental differences between biotherapeutics and small molecule pharmaceuticals in their manufacturing processes, size, and structural/physiochemical properties have been acknowledged by legislators and regulatory authorities around the world, and because of these differences, they have recognized that the regulatory pathways for attaining approval of copies of small molecule medicines (generics) are not scientifically appropriate for copies (biosimilars) of biotherapeutic products (Paul Declerck, 2012; Mounho-Zamora, 2013).

Generic medicines contain active substance(s) that are identical to the RP (P. Declerck et al., 2017; P. J. Declerck, 2007; Hennessy, Leonard, & Platt, 2010; Roger & Mikhail, 2007). Thus, because generic medicines have the identical active substance(s) as the RP, the regulatory pathways for the approval of generics are predicated on the demonstration of sameness between the generic copy and the RP (Gottlieb, 2008; Kingham & Lietzan, 2008). Generic medicines that are demonstrated to be pharmaceutically equivalent to the RP through comparative analytical tests are considered to be therapeutically equivalent to the RP. Thus, the data required for generic manufacturers to gain market approval for their generic medicine are generally limited to comparative (i.e., head-to-head) analytical tests demonstrating that the generic medicine is absorbed into the body at an extent and rate similar to those of the RP (i.e., clinical bioequivalence). In addition, bioequivalence can generally be demonstrated in healthy volunteers (rather than the patient population for which the RP is approved). Thus, clinical efficacy and safety studies are generally not necessary for the approval of generic medicines (Carver, Elikan, & Lietzan, 2010; Strober et al., 2012). Hence, the abbreviated approval process for generic medicines significantly reduces their development costs. For example, the abbreviated new drug application (ANDA) pathway for generic medicines falls under the Drug Price Competition and Patent Term Restoration Act enacted in 1984 (also known as the Hatch-Waxman Act). The act—following demonstration that the active ingredient of the generic is identical to the RP—allows the sponsor to rely on or reference the FDA's previous finding of efficacy and safety of the approved RP, and thus, demonstration of therapeutic equivalence in clinical trials is not required (P. Declerck et al., 2017; Mounho et al., 2010; Mounho-Zamora, 2013).

Although the active substance of the biosimilar may be similar to that of the RP, it is not identical because of the differences that inevitably exist in certain product attributes (e.g., post-translation modifications, three-dimensional structure) (Minghetti, Rocco, Del Vecchio, & Locatelli, 2011). Therefore, biosimilars are not generics, and a clinical bioequivalence study that is generally sufficient for the approval of generic medicines under the ANDA pathway is not appropriate for biosimilars because it would not be sufficient to determine the impact of any differences in product attributes on the quality, efficacy, and safety (immunogenicity) of a biosimilar candidate (P. Declerck et al., 2017; Mounho-Zamora, 2013; Olech, 2016; Schellekens, 2009; Sullivan & DiGrazia, 2017; Weise et al., 2011). Therefore, under abbreviated approval pathways such as the US Biologics Price Competition and Innovation Act (BPCIA) of 2009, demonstration of highly similar clinical efficacy and safety in the patient population of interest is required for the approval of biosimilar products (the extent of the clinical studies depends on the sponsor's demonstration of analytical similarity between the proposed biosimilar and the RP (FDA Guidance on Scientific Considerations, April 2015c) (Weise et al., 2011). Although seeking the approval of a biosimilar product allows sponsors to follow an abbreviated regulatory pathway, developing biosimilar products encompasses numerous challenges, and compared to generics, are more costly and require more data and studies by the regulators in the United States and other regions (which will be described further in this chapter).

13.3 Biosimilar Guidelines in the United States

Twenty-nine biosimilars have been approved in the United States as of the end of 2020, of which 20 were monoclonal antibodies (FDA, 2020b). The first biosimilar approved in the United States was Zarxio (filgrastim—Sandoz) in 2015, which along with other early products, served as test cases, allowing the FDA to develop a regulatory process for biosimilar approval.

There are now 15 biosimilar guidance documents listed on the FDA's website (FDA, 2021) to inform developers on current FDA recommendations. One of the first of these biosimilar guidances, "Reference Product Exclusivity for Biological Products Filed Under Section 351(a) of the PHS Act," was issued in 2014 and has not yet been finalized. It addresses RPs and provides guidance on the appropriate use of the RPs in light of the US law, as outlined in the Public Health Service Act (PHS Act) and BPCIA (FDA, 2014b). The appropriate use of RPs is clarified further in a series of final 2015–2016 guidances (FDA, 2015b, 2015c, 2016):

- Scientific Considerations in Demonstrating Biosimilarity to a Reference Product
- Quality Considerations in Demonstrating Biosimilarity of a Therapeutic Protein Product to a Reference Product
- Clinical Pharmacology Data to Support a Demonstration of Biosimilarity to a Reference Product.

Per the PHS Act, a biosimilar "product is highly similar to the RP notwithstanding minor differences in clinically inactive components," and "There are no clinically meaningful differences between the biological product and the RP in terms of the safety, purity, and potency of the product" (FDA, 2015c). This set of guidances as a group is designed to clarify the nontrivial challenge of demonstrating that a biosimilar is truly highly similar to the RP (FDA, 2015b, 2015c, 2016). This challenge was the major cause of the delay in the approval of biosimilars in the United States relative to the EU, where the initial biosimilar guidances were published in 2005–2006. Defining "similar" was the subject of considerable discussion between the FDA, industry, and the public when the drafts of these guidances were first released in 2012–2014, and discussions regarding best practices continue to this day.

To further address the concerns of the biosimilar industry and the public, the FDA issued a Q&A guidance. This guidance has been an evolving document that addresses frequently asked questions (FAQs) about biosimilars that have not been addressed adequately in other guidances. The initial Q&A document was issued in a draft form in 2012 (FDA, 2012). Some but not all of the FAQs in this original guidance were finalized in 2015 (FDA, 2015a). That same year, the draft version of Revision 1 was issued. In 2018, the final version of Revision 1 was issued, and, simultaneously, the draft version Revision 2 was released (FDA, 2018a, 2018b). Finally, in November 2020, the FDA released another Q&A guidance: "Biosimilarity and Interchangeability: Additional Draft Q&As on Biosimilar Development and the BPCI Act" (FDA, 2020a). Most of these new questions are designed to clarify the interchangeable guidance (described below). The need for this series of ever-evolving Q&As exemplifies the changing landscape surrounding the biosimilar regulatory pathway in the United States.

One of the major components included in regulatory submissions to define whether or not a proposed biosimilar is, in fact, highly similar to the RP is comparative analytical assessments. The FDA issued a 2019 draft guidance, "Development of Therapeutic Protein Biosimilars: Comparative Analytical Assessment and Other Quality-Related Considerations," on this topic as a companion to earlier guidances. Among the concerns that this guidance addresses are expression systems, manufacturing processes, physiochemical properties, functional activity, target binding, and impurities. The FDA evaluates the totality of the analytical data to determine similarity. In addition, it is important to reiterate that, owing to the inherent variability in biological systems, highly similar does not mean identical (FDA, 2019c).

Another important consideration for biosimilar safety evaluation is immunogenicity. All of the minor differences between the biosimilar and the RP, whether identified by the comparative analytical assessment or undetected, have the potential to lead to a different immunogenicity profile for the biosimilar product versus the reference molecule. The regulators are concerned about the possibility that immunogenicity may be worse in the biosimilar than in the RP; however, it is important to note that it is also possible that the biosimilar may have an improved immunogenicity profile relative to the RP. Immunogenicity has the potential to be a very serious adverse event, resulting in, for example, induction of autoimmune disorders, anaphylaxis, and death. Therefore, the FDA has historically recommended that a clinical immunogenicity evaluation be conducted as part of the biosimilar approval process. However, the FDA recently updated its recommendations on immunogenicity in a new 2019 guidance, "Clinical Immunogenicity Considerations for Biosimilar and Interchangeable Insulin Products." Specifically, the FDA now recommends that "if a comparative analytical assessment based on state-of-the-art technology supports a demonstration of "highly similar" for a proposed biosimilar or interchangeable insulin product, there would be little or no residual uncertainty regarding immunogenicity; in such instances, the proposed biosimilar or interchangeable insulin product, such as the RP, would be expected to have minimal or no risk of clinical impact from immunogenicity." However, the FDA reserves the right to request clinical immunogenicity studies on a case-by-case basis. This change was based on real-world data from biosimilar products. In practice, the risk of differential immunogenicity between highly similar products has turned out to be low (FDA, 2019a). Note that insulin products previously have occupied a regulatory grey area, sometimes considered drugs, other times considered biologics. However, insulin is now officially considered a biologic in the United States (ADA, 2020).

Interchangeability is the next major area that recent FDA guidances have addressed. The FDA issued a guidance in 2019 specifically addressing this subject: "Considerations in Demonstrating Interchangeability with a Reference Product (Final)." In addition, recommendations on interchangeability are found as a subsection in many other biosimilar guidances. The PHS Act states that interchangeability means that "the biological product may be substituted for the reference product without the intervention of the health care provider who prescribed the reference product" (FDA, 2019b). Legally, the product must be "biosimilar to the RP" and "can be expected to produce the same clinical result as the RP in any given patient," and also that, "for a biological product that is administered more than once to an individual, the risk in terms of safety or diminished efficacy of alternating or switching between use of the biological product and the RP is not greater than the risk of using the RP without such alternation or switch." This legal definition is rather broad, and the lack of clarity has contributed to the dearth of interchangeability applications. These guidances are designed to clarify what these statements mean in the real world and to help guide sponsors on what data they need to submit. One of the key data sets is a "switching study" (either as a stand-alone study or incorporated as an arm in another study) in which patients are switched from the RP to the interchangeable product, demonstrating no clinically meaningful differences from the patients in the switched cohort in comparison with patients who remained on the RP (FDA, 2019b).

13.4 Biosimilar Guidelines in Europe

The EU was the first major region to establish a formal regulatory pathway for the approval of biosimilars. The EU has approved 77 biosimilar products as of 2020 (GaBI, 2021b). The first EU biosimilar guideline was published in October 2005, titled, "Guideline on similar biological medicinal products" (EMA, 2015a). In January 2006, two additional guidelines from the EU became effective—the guideline that specifically addresses nonclinical and clinical issues and the guideline on quality issues, which have both since been updated (EMA, 2014, 2015b). These guidelines were proceeded by the first EU biosimilar approval in April 2006, Omnitrope by Sandoz GmbH, for the reference compound "somatropin," a growth hormone. Prior to the 2013 EU approval of two infliximab biosimilars (>100,000 Daltons), the prior EU-approved biosimilar molecules were lower molecular weight (<40,000 Daltons) growth hormones and growth factors (Schiestl, Zabransky, & Sorgel, 2017; Tabernero et al., 2016). The regulatory framework for biosimilar approval in the EU is based on the scientific principles guiding manufacturing changes of approved originator biotherapeutics, where it is a process to allow manufacturing changes without requiring additional clinical development. This process is based on the comparability of the prechange and postchange products, demonstrating by analytical methods that the two molecules are highly similar, which allows marketing to continue under the same product label. In cases where analytical methods determine that there are differences, the manufacturer must further demonstrate that there is no adverse impact on safety, efficacy, or immunogenicity, which may include additional analytical, nonclinical, and/or clinical studies with the prechange and postchange molecules. The EU regulatory framework evolved further with time as biosimilar product class-specific guidelines were developed, and it continues to be revised. Although earlier versions of biosimilar guidelines recommended *in vivo* pharmacokinetic (PK) and repeat-dose studies, the 2010 directive in the EU on the protection of animals used for scientific purposes, which took full effect in 2013, highlighted the use of nonhuman primates (NHPs), especially for the development monoclonal antibodies (van Aerts, De Smet, Reichmann, van der Laan, &

Schneider, 2014). This directive, in conjunction with the EU scientific review, found that most biosimilar quality and toxicities could be predicted by *in vitro* assays, rather than *in vivo* assays (van Aerts et al., 2014). The revised biosimilar guidelines reflect this change in scientific thinking on biosimilar approvals in the EU and on accepting regulatory packages without the additional head-to-head comparison of the RP and biosimilar product in *in vivo* toxicology studies; however, it is important to note that, for some member states within the EU, *in vivo* toxicology studies are still required for global approval (Chapman et al., 2016).

The EU does not have a regulatory pathway for the biosimilar designation of "interchangeability," which allows automatic substitution of biosimilar with a RP at the pharmacy level (Schiestl et al., 2017; Tabernero et al., 2016). The lack of a regulatory pathway to interchangeability by the EU includes not requiring a transition study (i.e., a clinical study in which patients on a reference material are switched to the biosimilar to demonstrate comparable safety), which is a requirement in the United States (Schiestl et al., 2017). EU member states are advised to consider the potential risks associated with interchangeability. Some EU member states support switching during the initial treatment or with the decision of the prescribing physician, but switching (also known as substitution) is not supported by all EU member states (O'Callaghan, Barry, Bermingham, Morris, & Griffin, 2019; Rugo, Rifkin, Declerck, Bair, & Morgan, 2019).

Extrapolation in clinical drug development is the process of using clinical study data for one indication to support another indication. This concept also applies to biosimilars and is important in reducing time and cost by limiting unnecessary clinical trials and generally expediting the regulatory pathway (Ogura, Coiffier, Kwon, & Yoon, 2017; Schiestl et al., 2017; Tabernero et al., 2016). When biosimilar comparability has been demonstrated in one indication for the RP, the biosimilar data package for this one indication can be extrapolated to other RP indications. The EMA has specifically stated, "If clinical similarity can be shown in a key indication, extrapolation of efficacy and safety data to other indication(s) of the reference product may be possible under certain conditions" (GABI, 2017; Weise, 2016). An example is Celltrion Healthcare's (Celltrion) rituximab biosimilar Truxima (CT-P10), an anti-CD20 (cluster of differentiate 20) monoclonal antibody approved for use in autoimmune and hematological cancer indications in the EU. Truxima was compared with the RP rituximab, based on the totality of the data, which included analytical, *in vitro*, and *in vivo* nonclinical data and clinical data in rheumatoid arthritis patients and advanced follicular lymphoma patients (Ogura et al., 2017). Extrapolation to chronic lymphocytic leukemia, granulomatosis with polyangiitis, microscopic polyangiitis, and diffuse large B-cell lymphoma was scientifically justified based on the known mode of action and the strength of clinical data in two patient populations with similar disease pathology in B-cell–related indications (Ogura et al., 2017). Another EU example of extrapolation is for the biosimilar Inflectra, for which the RP was infliximab. The phase III clinical trial for the biosimiliar registration was conducted in rheumatoid arthritis patients, but Inflectra is approved for all indications

of the RP, which also include ankylosing spondylitis, psoriatic arthritis, psoriasis, adult and pediatric Crohn's disease, and adult and pediatric ulcerative colitis (Mielke, Jilma, Koenig, & Jones, 2016; Reinisch, Louis, & Danese, 2015; Yoo et al., 2013). The scientific justification included a literature review of the indication and mechanism of action, and preliminary data in patients with either Crohn's disease or ulcerative colitis, and the application sponsor agreed to conduct additional postmarketing studies (Mielke et al., 2016; Reinisch et al., 2015).

13.5 Overview of Guidances: WHO, Canada, Australia, Japan, India, and "Rest of the World"

Biosimilar regulations have been a rapidly moving target with nearly constant regulatory changes around the globe. Generally, regulations in most rest of the world (ROW) countries (of those that have approved regulations) are based either on European guidances (either 2006 or 2012) or WHO guidances or a combination thereof. It is important to note, however, that "based on" does not mean "identical to" and in spite of the broad similarities, each country has its own regulatory idiosyncrasies.

The choice of the proper reference biotherapeutic is critical to the regulatory approval process. The WHO guidance recommends that only reference biotherapeutics based on a full regulatory package are acceptable (i.e., a biosimilar using another biosimilar as a reference biotherapeutic is not recommended). In general, most countries also require that the RP used must be approved in that country (Mounho et al., 2010). However, the guidances regarding acceptable RPs can vary by country, and there has been a recent trend toward slightly loosening and/or clarifying those requirements. For example, in India, an update to the biosimilar regulator guidance states that an acceptable RP, if not licensed in India, is one licensed in "an ICH country,[1]" whereas previously, if the reference biotherapeutic was not authorized in India, it was required to be both licensed and widely marketed for 4 years in a country with a "well-established regulatory framework" (Brennan, 2016; CDSCO, 2012, 2016).

13.5.1 WHO Guidance

The WHO guidances were adopted in 2009 (WHO, 2009) and were formally published as Annex 2 of Technical Report 977 (WHO, 2013). The 2009 guidance states that "a definitive version of this document, which will differ from this version in editorial but not scientific details, will be published in the WHO Technical Report Series," indicating that there is no significant difference between the two publications. Unlike more recent European and FDA guidances, the WHO

---

[1] An ICH country is one that is 1) a member of the International Council for Harmonisation of Technical Requirements for Pharmaceuticals for Human Use (ICH) or 2) an ICH observer. Refer to the following link for a current list of members and observers: https://www.ich.org/page/members-observers.

guidance "requires" an *in vivo* nonclinical toxicity study of some type, which was typical for the early guidances. Specifically, the 2009 WHO guidance recommends a minimum of one head-to-head *in vivo* repeat-dose toxicity study between the biosimilar and the reference biotherapeutic, including toxicokinetic (TK) and immunogenicity parameters in a relevant species.

With that said, however, although the 2009 WHO guidance was not withdrawn, the WHO issued an update to their guidance in 2016, which was formally published as Annex 2 of Technical Report 1004 in 2017. This guidance specifically addresses monoclonal antibody biosimilars, which are among the most common types of biosimilars, and the scope of this guidance specifically states that it is an expansion of the original 2009 guidance and not a replacement for it. The updated 2016 guidance notes that it is possible to change the expression system used for biosimilar manufacture relative to the RP (e.g., changing from a mouse cell line to a CHO or human cell line). This change poses risks, in that the biosimilar may not be "highly similar." However, there are benefits as well because some of the early monoclonal antibody therapeutics were manufactured in mouse cell lines that produce products that are more immunogenic than monoclonal antibodies manufactured in modern cell lines. In addition, as with the updated guidances in other regulatory regions, the 2016 monoclonal expansion guidance (WHO, 2016) relaxes the requirement for nonclinical *in vivo* evaluations, suggesting that the national regulatory authorities should consider waiving the *in vivo* requirement if the other parts of the data package provide sufficient evidence of similarity, based on the totality of the data presented, and specifically notes that repeat-dose NHP studies are rarely necessary. The updated guideline also reduces the emphasis on the nonclinical immunogenicity evaluation but continues to recommend a robust clinical immunogenicity evaluation (WHO, 2016).

The WHO also released a lengthy Q&A document in 2018 addressing FAQs in multiple areas, including RPs and nonclinical and clinical studies. The WHO notes that, in practice, "*in vitro* functional tests are more sensitive than clinical studies in detecting differences between the biosimilar and the RP," and that the clinical evaluation should be designed based on the *in vitro* data. These FAQs further emphasize WHO's updated 2016 recommendation that nonclinical studies are generally unnecessary, but they continue to recommend a robust clinical immunogenicity program (WHO, 2018).

13.5.2 Canada

The biosimilar (SEBs) guidance in Canada was updated in 2016 and 2017. The current Canadian guidance is similar to the current European guidances, in that it states that, if sufficient similarity between the RP and the biosimilar has been determined by *in vitro* assays, then head-to-head *in vivo* toxicity studies are not required. The guidances strongly recommend a presubmission consultation with regulatory authorities to determine whether the regulatory authorities agree with the sponsor that the *in vitro* data obtained to date are indeed sufficient. As of the end of 2020, 27 biosimilars have been approved in Canada (GaBI, 2021b).

13.5.3 Australia

The biosimilar guidances in Australia were updated in 2015 and 2018 (ARTG, 2018). These regulations state that EMA guidances are to be followed for the registration of biosimiliars. As of the end of 2020, 26 biosimilars have been approved in Australia (GaBI, 2021a).

13.5.4 Japan

The Japanese biosimilar (follow-on biological medicinal products) guidances were originally approved in 2009 and have been clarified/updated three times in Q&A documents issued in 2009, 2010, and 2015 (PDMA, 2009a, 2009b, 2010, 2015). The original 2009 guidance does not require a repeat-dose toxicity study with TKs for all products. However, it states that such studies are "useful" in understanding the toxicity profile of the biosimilar and that repeat-dose toxicity studies are required when the impurity profile of the biosimilar is "considerably" different from the impurity profile of the RP, or if there are new impurities. In the 2015 Q&A, the Japanese regulators further clarify that toxicology studies can be waived after a regulatory consultation if sufficient information regarding the characterization of the biotherapeutic is available.

If a toxicology study is conducted, the Japanese guidances recommend (but do not require) an evaluation of immunogenicity primarily for the purposes of TK interpretation. Similar to the WHO guidances, the Japanese guidances note that safety pharmacology, reproductive toxicity, genotoxicity, and carcinogenicity studies are "considered less needed" and are not recommended unless necessary because of the specific pharmacology of the therapeutic or the results of repeat-dose toxicity testing. At least 21 biosimilars have been approved in Japan (GaBI, 2019a).

13.5.5 India

India has approved the most biosimilars (similar biologics) of any country in the world, with more than 50 and possibly up to 98 approved biosimilars (depending on what is included) (GaBI, 2018; Jeremias, 2020). The majority of these biosimilars were approved on a case-by-case basis before the first formal guidances were enacted in 2012 (GaBI, 2018). These approvals did not necessarily meet international standards in all cases, as evidenced by noticeable difference in potency and efficacy between several similar biologics versus their RPs, for example, possibly due to the introduction of impurities through the manufacturing process, and the safety of some of these early biosimilars has been questioned (GaBI, 2016b, 2018). The current regulations in India are based on this prior experience, and both India's 2012 and 2016 biosimilar guidances are generally considered weaker than the European or WHO guidances, primarily because of less strict regulations regarding the clinical component (GaBI, 2016a). The 2016 guidance update "clarifies" the clinical guidances. Detailed summaries of this clarification are beyond the scope of this review but can be found at George 2016 (George, 2016). It is too soon to determine the practical impact of the clarifications in the 2016 guidance.

Both the 2012 and the 2016 guidances (CDSCO, 2012, 2016) recommend that comparative preclinical studies be conducted prior to the initiation of clinical trials. In general, the studies are recommended to be 28-day repeat-dose studies, with a 14-day recovery period in a relevant species, and to include TK endpoints with the high dose being set at least five times the human equivalent dose. The guidance contains a detailed set of protocol recommendations. Immunogenicity should be analyzed and compared with the RP. The guidances recommend that protocols be reviewed by regulators prior to the initiation of *in vivo* studies. With regard to preclinical studies, differences between the 2012 and 2016 guidances are minor. The differences primarily address species selection for preclinical studies in the absence of a pharmacologically relevant species.

13.5.6 Rest of the World

As noted above, the majority of the countries in the ROW generally follow European (either 2006 or 2012) guidances or WHO guidances or both. However, there are some exceptions. For example, in Columbia, in addition to the standard biosimilar approval pathway, there is a second abbreviated pathway (Cruz et al., 2017; Díaz Vera, 2014; GaBI, 2015, 2019c, 2020; Garcia & Araujo, 2016). The intent of this pathway appears to be to allow the rapid approval of biosimilars already known to be safe; however, the exact wording of the decree has been a cause for concern because it appears to have loopholes that may allow unsafe biosimilars to be approved (BIO, 2014; GaBI, 2015).

Biosimilars approved under regulations that do not meet international standards are generally referred to as "intended copies" rather than biosimilars. Intended copies may have incomplete similarity data, insufficient clinical trial data, or may lack sufficient direct comparisons with the RP. In many cases, they may not have safety and/or efficacy comparable to the originator product (Castañeda-Hernández et al., 2014; P. Declerck et al., 2017; Mysler et al., 2016). Significant clinical safety problems have been reported with some of these intended copies (Castañeda-Hernández et al., 2014; Mysler et al., 2016) (GaBI, 2016b; Halim et al., 2014; Jefferis, 2016). These products are often approved in countries with inadequate postmarketing surveillance; therefore, there is concern that problems with intended copies may be underreported (Al Ani et al., 2019; Mysler et al., 2016).

13.6 History of Regulatory Standards for Nonclinical Toxicology Studies

As described above, the EU was the first major region to establish a formal regulatory pathway for the approval of biosimilars. The EU guideline that specifically addresses nonclinical issues (titled "Guideline on similar biological medicinal products containing biotechnology-derived Proteins as active substance: non-clinical and clinical issues") was adopted in the EU in 2006 (EMEA/CHMP/BMWP/42832/2005) (EMA, 2006). This initial guideline described the general scientific principles and methods for the nonclinical (and also clinical,

but this section will focus on the nonclinical) safety assessment (toxicology) studies to be conducted for a biosimilar candidate. Specifically, the initial 2006 guideline states that the nonclinical toxicology studies should include *in vitro* and *in vivo* data and recommends that at least one repeat-dose toxicology study be conducted in a pharmacologically relevant animal species, with a sufficiently long duration to allow detection of relevant differences in toxicity and/or immune responses between the biosimilar candidate and the RP (EMA, 2006). Additionally, the study should be comparative (head-to-head with the RP) in nature, incorporating TKs and measurement of antidrug antibody (ADA) responses.

The first two biosimilars approved in the EU were versions of somatotropin—first Omnitrope® (2006), followed shortly by Valtropin® (2006; withdrawn by the manufacturer in October 2011). Following the initial 2006 EU guideline for nonclinical issues, the nonclinical toxicology studies performed for the marketing approval of both Omnitrope and Valtropin included animal studies. For Omnitrope, a 14-day toxicity study was performed in Sprague Dawley rats. In this study, Omnitrope was administered daily to rats by subcutaneous injection for 14 days, and the study included assessment of TK parameters (Sandoz, 2006). In addition, a 7-day local tolerance test evaluating two formulations of Omnitrope was conducted in male and female rabbits. The nonclinical toxicology studies conducted for Valtropin were more extensive and included two combined 28-day and 90-day repeat-dose toxicity studies, one performed in mice and the other in rats (the 28-day rat study was comparative with Humatrope® as the RP); these studies also incorporated TK assessments (Biopartners, 2006). Additional toxicology studies that were not required in the initial 2006 guidance were also conducted, including reproduction toxicity studies in rats and rabbits; safety pharmacology studies in mice, guinea pigs, and rabbits; and a battery of genotoxicity tests. Although it is unknown why the type and extent of toxicity studies conducted for the approval of Omnitrope vs. Valtropin were so vastly different and did not follow the recommendations in the initial 2006 EU guideline, it can be presumed that while the guidance was published in 2006, as these nonclinical studies were conducted prior to the initial guideline being adopted in 2006, the manufacturers of Omnitrope (Sandoz®) and Valtropin (Biopartners®) conducted more comprehensive battery of toxicity studies (than later required) to ensure that the nonclinical toxicology program was sufficient to receive marketing authorization. Several biosimilars that were approved a few years after the issuance of the initial 2006 EU guidance conducted nonclinical toxicology programs that were consistent with that recommended by the guideline. For example, Zarzio® (manufactured by Sandoz International Limited) is a biosimilar of Neupogen® and received marketing authorization in 2009 (Sandoz, 2009). As recommended by the initial 2006 EU guideline, the nonclinical toxicology program for Zarzio included a 4-week, comparative (RP was Neupogen®) toxicology study in male and female Wistar rats (a pharmacologically relevant animal species) with a 6-week recovery period, and incorporated TK and ADA analysis. A local tolerance study was also conducted in New Zealand white rabbits comparing different formulations of Zarzio with Neupogen administered by different routes (e.g., intravenous, subcutaneous, intramuscular, paravenous, intraarterial). Another Neupogen biosimilar is Nivestim® (manufactured by Hospira, Inc.), which received marketing authorization in 2010 (Hospira, 2010). The nonclinical toxicology program for Nivestim was similar to that for Zarzio, and included a 4-week, comparative (RP was Neupogen) toxicology study in male and female Sprague Dawley rats, followed by a 14-day recovery period and included both TK and ADA assessment.

A new directive was issued in the EU in 2010 and was in full effect by January 2013, which strengthened the legislation to improve and protect the welfare of animals used in nonclinical research and to firmly establish the principle of the "Three Rs"—to replace, reduce, and refine the use of animals in research (EU Directive 2010/63/EU) (EU, 2010). The key principle of this directive is that the use of animals for research purposes should be considered only when non-animal alternatives are not available; moreover, that the use of NHPs is exempted from animal studies whenever possible; and that scientific justification is required if the nonclinical study cannot be achieved with any animal species other than NHPs. Shortly following the issuance of the EU Directive 2010/63/EU, the EMA issued a guideline specific to biosimilar monoclonal antibodies, which became effective in December 2012 (EMA/CHMP/BMWP/403543/2010) (EMA, 2012). This EMA guideline recommends that a risk-based, step-wise approach be applied to the nonclinical studies for biosimilar monoclonal antibodies, emphasizing that *in vitro* studies should be conducted first, to determine whether animal studies, if any, are warranted. The general scientific principles of the EMA guideline for biosimilar monoclonal antibodies are consistent with the EU Directive 2010/63/EU, in that if nonclinical animal studies (e.g., toxicology) are warranted, a modified approach consistent with the principles of the 3Rs should be considered in the study design, and that it may not be necessary to terminate the animals at the end of the study, depending on the endpoints needed. Additionally, the EMA guideline for biosimilar monoclonal antibodies specifically states that repeat-dose toxicity studies in NHPs and toxicology studies in a nonpharmacologically relevant animal species (to evaluate nonspecific toxicity, such as impurity-related toxicity) are not recommended (EMA, 2012).

The EMA thinking on nonclinical studies for biosimilars has evolved considerably since 2006, when at least one repeat-dose toxicology study, even in NHPs, was expected. The new EMA paradigm for nonclinical development of biosimilars that emphasized comparative *in vitro* studies and did not require repeat-dose animal toxicology studies (especially NHPs), by default, is a result of various factors, particularly data and expertise gained since 2006 as well as the vast advances in biotechnology manufacturing and analytical instrumentation. Additionally, the experience-based knowledge gained by the EMA over the years on nonclinical data for biosimilars submitted by manufacturers has led to the regulators acknowledging that the predictable toxicity (i.e., adverse events associated with the pharmacology or "exaggerated pharmacology") of a biosimilar and the RP can be established *in vitro*, and thus, there is no need for a comparative animal

study that is likely less sensitive than the *in vitro* model (van Aerts et al., 2014). The EMA biosimilar guideline for nonclinical and clinical issues (EMEA/CHMP/BMWP/42832/2005) (EMA, 2006) was revised subsequently, came into effect in July 2015, and replaced the initial guideline (EMEA/CHMP/BMWP/42832/2005 Rev 1) (EMA, 2015b).

Similar to the EMA guideline for biosimilar monoclonal antibodies, the revised biosimilar guideline for nonclinical and clinical issues recommends that a stepwise approach be applied when evaluating what nonclinical studies are needed to support a biosimilarity determination, with an emphasis on conduct of comparative *in vitro* pharmacotoxicological studies first, prior to conducting any animal studies, if needed (EMA, 2015b). Additionally, the revised guideline notes that many of the of the *in vitro* assays may have been developed already as comparative quality-related assays, such as binding to the target and functional activity/cell viability assays. Furthermore, the guideline states that *in vitro* pharmacotoxicological assays (i.e., target binding and signal transduction and functional activity/viability in pharmacologically and toxicologically relevant cell populations) may be more specific and sensitive than animal studies to detect potential differences between the proposed biosimilar and RP, and therefore, the comparative pharmaco-toxicological *in vitro* assays can be considered the principal studies for the nonclinical comparability exercise. Clearly, the thinking of the EMA regulators on what nonclinical studies are necessary for biosimilar products has evolved from the initial biosimilar guideline, wherein a comparative animal toxicology study was generally expected (van Aerts et al., 2014).

As noted above, many biosimilar products have been approved in the EU since the issuance of the EMA guideline for monoclonal antibodies (EMA/CHMP/BMWP/403543/2010) (EMA, 2012) and the revised guideline for nonclinical and clinical issues (EMEA/CHMP/BMWP/42832/2005 Rev 1) (EMA, 2015b). Thus, one would expect that the nonclinical comparability exercise for many biosimilar products recently approved in the EU would have applied a stepwise approach consisting primarily of *in vitro* pharmacotoxicology studies and minimal to no animal toxicology studies.

This was not, however, the case for some earlier biosimilar products approved in the EU. For example, Riximyo®, a biosimilar to the monoclonal antibody, rituximab, was approved in June 2017; the nonclinical comparability exercise included both *in vitro* and animal studies, including studies in NHPs (Sandoz, 2017). *In vitro/ex vivo* studies included a human whole-blood B-cell depletion assay and an assessment of ADCC (antibody-dependent cellular cytotoxicity) potency in human peripheral blood NK (natural killer) cells as the effector cells against different immortalized B-cell lines, in addition to CD20 binding activity, CDC (complement-dependent cytotoxicity) activity, apoptosis, C1q binding, and interaction with FcRn (neonatal Fc receptor) and FcγR (Fc gamma receptor) family members. Studies in NHPs consisted of a comparative single-dose PK/PD (pharmacodynamic) study in which male cynomolgus monkeys were administered a single-dose intravenous (IV) dose (5 mg/kg) of either Riximyo or the RP

(MabThera) and a comparative GLP,[2] a 4-week toxicology study where cynomolgus monkeys were administered four IV doses of Riximyo or MabThera at 20 or 100 mg/kg once weekly, followed by a 6-month recovery phase; standard safety endpoints were included in the study, including histopathology, PK/PD, and ADA responses were also evaluated. The nonclinical comparability exercise for Truxima®, also a biosimilar to rituximab (approved in the EU February 2017 (Celltrion, 2017)), also consisted of *in vitro* and animal studies. *In vitro* studies consisted of an evaluation of CD20 binding affinity, apoptosis, interaction with FcRn and FcγR family members, C1q binding, ADCC and CDC activity, and a comparative tissue cross-reactivity assessment in human tissues. Animal studies included a GLP repeat-dose comparative toxicology study in which cynomolgus monkeys were administered a 20 mg/kg dose of Truxima or the RP (MabThera) by IV injection once weekly for 5 weeks (females) or 6 weeks (males), followed by a 2-week recovery period; standard safety endpoints, including histopathology, were assessed in this study, and PK/PD and ADA responses were evaluated. Despite the EMA guideline for biosimilar monoclonal antibodies recommending a stepwise approach to the nonclinical comparability exercise, starting with *in vitro* studies and minimizing animal studies, particularly NHP studies (when possible), it is unknown why the manufacturers of Riximyo and Truxima would perform comparative, repeat-dose toxicology studies in NHPs. One likely reason is that the nonclinical comparability exercise, including the toxicology studies, for Riximyo and Truxima had started, or even were completed, before the final EMA guideline for biosimilar monoclonal antibodies was issued; in this case, the manufactures may have conducted full comparative toxicology studies to ensure that their demonstration of similarity to the RP was accepted by the regulators. When the need for nonclinical studies is unclear, in some cases, risk-adverse companies may perform nonclinical studies rather than risk delays to or rejection of their biosimilar program by regulatory authorities.

As described above, the FDA published a scientific guidance for biosimilars in April 2015, which primarily reviews the nonclinical and clinical data necessary for establishing biosimilarity (FDA, 2015c). Similar to the principles of the EMA guideline for biosimilar monoclonal antibodies, the FDA scientific guidance recommends that a stepwise approach be applied to demonstrate biosimilarity, and notes that the FDA will consider the totality of the evidence provided by a sponsor when evaluating the sponsor's demonstration of biosimilarity. The FDA guidance states that rigorous comparative structural and functional studies that show minimal or no difference between the biosimilar candidate, and the RP will strengthen the sponsor's scientific justification for a selective and targeted approach to animal and/or clinical studies to support a demonstration of biosimilarity. Thus, if a sponsor has comparative analytical data demonstrating that the biosimilar candidate is highly similar to the RP, minimal or even no animal studies may be needed.

The FDA guidance does state, however, that data from animal toxicity studies may be useful when uncertainties about the safety of biosimilar candidate exist, based on the data of the comparative physiochemical and functional studies. If any animal studies are warranted (based on the analytical and/or *in vitro* pharmacology assays), the type and extent of the studies needed will depend on the similarities and differences identified between the proposed biosimilar and RP, as well as the information known about the biosimilar candidate and RP. In addition, the FDA guidance states that animal toxicity studies in a nonrelevant species are generally not useful; however, there may be some cases when PK studies using a nonrelevant animal species to show similar *in vivo* PK profiles may be supportive of clinical trials for biosimilar candidates that have not been tested previously in humans.

The FDA guidance (FDA, 2015c) recommends a stepwise approach to the nonclinical studies and emphasizes rigorous comparative *in vitro* assays (e.g., analytical and pharmacology) to demonstrate biosimilarity. Such assays may potentially minimize or remove the need for animal toxicology studies; however, animal toxicology studies, including studies in NHPs, have been conducted for biosimilar products approved in the United States. For example, similar to Rixiymo and Truxima, a comparative monkey toxicology study was conducted for Amejevita®, a biosimilar to adalimumab that was approved in the United States in September 2016 (Amgen, 2016). Specifically, this study was a GLP, comparative 4-week toxicology study where cynomolgus monkeys were administered Amejevita or the RP (Humira®) at 157 mg/kg by subcutaneous (SC) injection once weekly for 4 weeks; standard safety endpoints, including histopathology, were assessed in this study, and TK and ADA responses were evaluated. A GLP, comparative 4-week monkey toxicology study was also conducted for Erelzi®, which is a biosimilar of etanercept, which was approved in the United States in August 2016 (Sandoz, 2016). In this comparative toxicology study, cynomolgus monkeys were administered Erelzi or the RP (Enbrel®) at doses of 15 mg/kg by SC injection once every 3 days for 28 days; standard safety endpoints, including histopathology were assessed, and TK and ADA responses were evaluated. Again, it is unknown why the manufacturers would conduct full comparative toxicology studies in NHPs, where the animals are terminated, rather than at least modifying the study to a nonterminal study and assessing in-life and PK/PD parameters. It is likely, however, that these studies were also initiated or even completed before the final FDA guidance (FDA, 2015c) was issued. Therefore, to ensure the FDA's approval of the nonclinical comparability exercise by the FDA, some manufacturers may have decided to take a conservative approach and conducted a full comparative toxicology study.

FDA biosimilar guidance and the EMA's revised biosimilar guideline on nonclinical/clinical issues as well as the guideline on biosimilar monoclonal antibodies have been published for a number of years. As a result, more and more manufactures will rely on comparative *in vitro* pharmacotoxicological assays for the nonclinical comparability exercise, or in cases where animal studies are necessary, will apply a modified approach to assessing in-life parameters (e.g., clinical pathology, PK/PD parameters) without terminating the animals or performing studies in animal species other than NHPs.

---

[2] GLP = Good laboratory practice

13.7 Preclinical Data Translation to First In Human

Biosimilars are biologics and, therefore, technically have the same degree of translatability between nonclinical toxicology clinical adverse events as novel biologics (EMA, 2015b, 2017; FDA, 2015c). However, biosimilars differ from novel biologics, in that some of the answers to these translational questions can be extrapolated from the originator biologic if the biosimilar is similar enough. This leads to the important question, "How similar is similar?" As discussed above, at the dawn of the biosimilar field, no one knew the answer to that question, and thus, a conservative approach requiring significant *in vivo* preclinical toxicology testing was chosen. As data from more and more biosimilar packages were examined by the regulators, it became apparent that assuming that highly stringent criteria for similarity were in place (e.g., comparative analytical assessment data) and data from new comparative preclinical *in vivo* toxicology studies are not needed (Chapman et al., 2016; EMA, 2015a; WHO, 2016, 2018).

13.8 Conclusion

A great deal of the regulatory confusion associated with biosimilars has been due to the fact that biosimilars are a new therapeutic modality, and genuine safety concerns have been raised by experts in the field regarding their development. However, biosimilars are beginning to mature as a proven therapeutic modality, with steadily increasing numbers of biosimilars on the market in highly regulated countries, such as EU-member countries or the United States. The experience gained from the development of these biosimilars has been instrumental in the evolution of the current regulatory environment.

The future of biosimilars is promising. The regulatory environment is stabilizing, with critical global regulators such as the EMA, FDA, and WHO issuing consistent, harmonized regulations. The regulatory clarity, combined with the fact that biotherapeutics are at the end of their patent life, will most likely lead to the development of many more biosimilars which will ultimately lead to cost reduction for patients. Given the global nature of the pharmaceutical business and global patients' need, biosimilar manufacturers are lobbying the various governments to facilitate further harmonization of regulations.

REFERENCES

ADA. (2020). *Insulin Is Now a Biologic—What Does That Mean?* Retrieved from https://www.diabetes.org/blog/insulin-now-biologic-what-does-mean

Al Ani, N. A., Gorial, F. I., Al-Sulaitti, S., Humadi, J. A., Awadh, N. I., Mounir, M., . . . Sunna, N. (2019). Review of biologics, biosimilars, and intended copies in rheumatology, and current practice in Iraq. *Open Access Rheumatol, 11*, 1–9. doi:10.2147/oarrr.S176965

Amgen. (2016). *Amjevita, US Biologics License Application, Pharmacology Review.* Retrieved from https://www.accessdata.fda.gov/drugsatfda_docs/nda/2016/761024Orig1s000PharmR.pdf

ARTG. (2018). *Biosimilar Medicines Regulation.* Retrieved from https://www.tga.gov.au/publication/biosimilar-medicines-regulation

BIO. (2014). *Comments on Draft Ministry of Health and Social Welfare Decree: Regulating the Requirements and Procedure for Pharmaceutical and Pharmacological Evaluations of Biological Medicines for Sanitary Registration Purposes.* Retrieved from https://www.bio.org/sites/default/files/files/2014-07-25_BIO%20Comments%20to%20Colombian%20MoH%20on%205th%20Draft%20Biologics%20Decree_FINAL.pdf

Biopartners. (2006). *Valtropin European Public Assessment Report Scientific Discussion.* Retrieved from http://www.ema.europa.eu/docs/en_GB/document_library/EPAR_-_Scientific_Discussion/human/000602/WC500047158.pdf

Brennan, Z. (2016). India Releases New Biosimilars Guidance. *Regulatory Focus.* Retrieved from http://www.raps.org/Regulatory-Focus/News/2016/03/28/24638/India-Releases-New-Biosimilars-Guidance/

Carver, K. H., Elikan, J., & Lietzan, E. (2010). An unofficial legislative history of the Biologics Price Competition and Innovation Act 2009. *Food & Drug LJ, 65*, 671.

Castañeda-Hernández, G., Szekanecz, Z., Mysler, E., Azevedo, V. F., Guzman, R., Gutierrez, M., . . . Karateev, D. (2014). Biopharmaceuticals for rheumatic diseases in Latin America, Europe, Russia, and India: Innovators, biosimilars, and intended copies. *Joint Bone Spine, 81*(6), 471–477. doi:10.1016/j.jbspin.2014.03.019

CDSCO. (2012). *Guidelines on Similar Biologics: Regulatory Requirements for Marketing Authorization in India.*

CDSCO. (2016). *Guidelines on Similar Biologicals: Regulatory Requirements for Marketing Authorization in India.* Retrieved from https://cdsco.gov.in/opencms/opencms/system/modules/CDSCO.WEB/elements/download_file_division.jsp?num_id=NTU0NA==

Celltrion. (2017). *Truxima European Public Assessment Report.* Retrieved from http://www.ema.europa.eu/docs/en_GB/document_library/EPAR_-_Public_assessment_report/human/004112/WC500222695.pdf

Chapman, K., Adjei, A., Baldrick, P., da Silva, A., De Smet, K., DiCicco, R., . . . McBlane, J. (2016). Waiving in vivo studies for monoclonal antibody biosimilar development: National and global challenges. *MAbs, 8*(3), 427–435.

Crommelin, D., Bermejo, T., Bissig, M., Damiaans, J., Krämer, I., & Rambourg, P. (2005). Pharmaceutical evaluation of biosimilars: Important differences from generic low-molecularweight pharmaceuticals. *European Journal of Hospital Pharmacy Science, 11*(1), 11–17.

Cruz, C., Carvalho, A. V., Dorantes, G. L., Londoño Garcia, A. M., Gonzalez, C., Maskin, M., . . . Walt, J. (2017). Biosimilars in psoriasis: Clinical practice and regulatory perspectives in Latin America. *The Journal of Dermatology, 44*(1), 3–12.

Declerck, P. (2012). Biologicals and biosimilars: A review of the science and its implications. *GaBI-Generics and Biosimilars Initiative Journal, 1*(1), 13–16.

Declerck, P., Danesi, R., Petersel, D., & Jacobs, I. (2017). The language of biosimilars: Clarification, definitions, and regulatory aspects. *Drugs, 77*(6), 671–677. doi:10.1007/s40265-017-0717-1

Declerck, P. J. (2007). Biotherapeutics in the era of Biosimilars. *Drug Safety, 30*(12), 1087–1092.

Díaz Vera, L. (2014). *The Colombian Biological Medicines Decree*. Retrieved from http://propintel.uexternado.edu.co/the-colombian-biological-medicines-decree/.

EMA. (2006). *Guideline on Similar Biological Products Containing Biotechnology-Derived Proteins as an Active Substance: Nonclinical and Clinical Issues*. Retrieved from http://www.ema.europa.eu/docs/en_GB/document_library/Scientific_guideline/2009/09/WC500003920.pdf

EMA. (2012). *Guideline on Similar Biological Medicinal Products Containing Monoclonal Antibodies – Non-Clinical and Clinical Issues*. Retrieved from https://www.ema.europa.eu/en/documents/scientific-guideline/guideline-similar-biological-medicinal-products-containing-monoclonal-antibodies-non-clinical_en.pdf

EMA. (2014). *Guideline on Similar Biological Medicinal Products Containing Biotechnology-Derived Proteins as Active Substance: Quality Issues*. Retrieved from http://www.ema.europa.eu/ema/index.jsp?curl=pages/regulation/general/general_content_000886.jsp&mid=WC0b01ac058002956b

EMA. (2015a). *Guideline on Similar Biological Medicinal Products*. Retrieved from http://www.ema.europa.eu/ema/index.jsp?curl=pages/regulation/general/general_content_000887.jsp&mid=WC0b01ac058002956b

EMA. (2015b). *Guideline on Similar Biological Medicinal Products Containing Biotechnology-Derived Proteins as Active Substance: Non-Clinical and Clinical Issues*. Retrieved from http://www.ema.europa.eu/docs/en_GB/document_library/Scientific_guideline/2015/01/WC500180219.pdf

EMA. (2017). *Guideline on Immunogenicity Assessment of Biotechnology-Derived Therapeutic Proteins*. Retrieved from http://www.ema.europa.eu/docs/en_GB/document_library/Scientific_guideline/2017/06/WC500228861.pdf

EU. (2010). *Directive 2010/63/EU of the European Parliament and of the Council*. Retrieved from http://eur-lex.europa.eu/legal-content/EN/TXT/PDF/?uri=CELEX:32010L0063&from=EN

FDA. (2012). *Biosimilars: Questions and Answers Regarding Implementation of the Biologics Price Competition and Innovation Act of 2009*. Retrieved from https://www.pharmacy.umaryland.edu/media/SOP/wwwpharmacyumarylandedu/centers/cdpp/pdfs/Guidance_BioSimiliarsQA.pdf

FDA. (2014a). *Immunogenicity Assessment for Therapeutic Protein Products*. Retrieved from https://www.fda.gov/downloads/drugs/guidances/ucm338856.pdf

FDA. (2014b). *Reference Product Exclusivity for Biological Products Filed under Section 351(a) of the PHS Act*. Retrieved from https://www.fda.gov/media/89049/download

FDA. (2014c). *Scientific Considerations in Demonstrating Biosimilarity to a Reference Product*. Retrieved from https://www.fda.gov/downloads/drugs/guidances/ucm291128.pdf

FDA. (2015a). *Biosimilars: Questions and Answers Regarding Implementation of the Biologics Price Competition and Innovation Act of 2009*. Retrieved from https://patentdocs.typepad.com/files/ucm444661.pdf

FDA. (2015b). *Quality Considerations in Demonstrating Biosimilarity of a Therapeutic Protein Product to a Reference Product*. Retrieved from https://www.fda.gov/media/135612/download

FDA. (2015c). *Scientific Considerations in Demonstrating Biosimilarity to a Reference Product*. Retrieved from https://www.fda.gov/downloads/drugs/guidances/ucm291128.pdf

FDA. (2016). *Clinical Pharmacology Data to Support a Demonstration of Biosimilarity to a Reference Product*. Retrieved from https://www.fda.gov/media/88622/download

FDA. (2018a). *New and Revised Draft Q&As on Biosimilar Development and the BPCI Act (Revision 2)*. Retrieved from https://www.fda.gov/media/119278/download

FDA. (2018b). *Questions and Answers on Biosimilar Development and the BPCI Act Revision 1*. Retrieved from https://www.fda.gov/media/119258/download

FDA. (2019a). *Clinical Immunogenicity Considerations for Biosimilar and Interchangeable Insulin Products*. Retrieved from https://www.fda.gov/media/133014/download

FDA. (2019b). *Considerations in Demonstrating Interchangeability With a Reference Product*. Retrieved from https://www.fda.gov/media/124907/download

FDA. (2019c). *Development of Therapeutic Protein Biosimilars: Comparative Analytical Assessment and Other Quality-Related Considerations*. Retrieved from https://www.fda.gov/media/125484/download

FDA. (2020a). *Biosimilarity and Interchangeability: Additional Draft Q&As on Biosimilar Development and the BPCI Act*. Retrieved from https://www.fda.gov/media/143847/download

FDA. (2020b). *FDA-Approved Biosimilar Products*. Retrieved from https://www.fda.gov/drugs/biosimilars/biosimilar-product-information

FDA. (2021). *Search for FDA Guidance Documents Using the word "Biosimilar"*. Retrieved from https://www.fda.gov/regulatory-information/search-fda-guidance-documents#guidancesearch

GaBI. (2015). *Colombian Guidelines for Productos Bioterapéuticos Similares*. Retrieved from https://www.gabionline.net/layout/set/print/Guidelines/Colombian-guidelines-for-productos-bioterapeuticos-similares

GaBI. (2016a). *Low Costs and Less Stringent Regulatory Requirements in India*. Retrieved from http://www.gabionline.net/Biosimilars/Research/Low-costs-and-less-stringent-regulatory-requirements-in-India

GaBI. (2016b). *Safety Concerns Limit Similar Biologics Uptake in India*. Retrieved from http://www.gabionline.net/Biosimilars/Research/Safety-concerns-limit-similar-biologics-uptake-in-India

GaBI. (2017). *Scientific Rationale for Extrapolation of Cancer Indications*. Retrieved from http://www.gabionline.net/Biosimilars/Research/Scientific-rationale-for-extrapolation-of-cancer-indications?utm_source=GONL7&utm_campaign=4b6c5f55f7-GONL+V17H18-7&utm_medium=email&utm_term=0_b09051b624-4b6c5f55f7-64578753

GaBI. (2018). *'Similar Biologics' Approved and Marketed in India*. Retrieved from http://gabionline.net/Biosimilars/General/Similar-biologics-approved-and-marketed-in-India

GaBI. (2019a). *Biosimilars Approved in Japan*. Retrieved from http://www.gabionline.net/Biosimilars/General/Biosimilars-approved-in-Japan

GaBI. (2019b). *Patent Expiry Dates for Biologicals: 2018 Update*. Retrieved from http://gabi-journal.net/patent-expiry-dates-for-biologicals-2018-update.html

GaBI. (2019c). *Similar Biotherapeutic Products Approved and Marketed in Latin America*. Retrieved from https://www.gabionline.net/Biosimilars/General/Similar-biotherapeutic-products-approved-and-marketed-in-Latin-America

GaBI. (2020). *Amgevita Approved in Colombia*. Retrieved from https://www.gabionline.net/Biosimilars/News/Amgevita-approved-in-Colombia

GaBI. (2021a). *Biosimilars Approved in Australia*. Retrieved from http://www.gabionline.net/Biosimilars/General/Biosimilars-approved-in-Australia

GaBI. (2021b). *Subsequent Entry Biologics Approved in Canada*. Retrieved from http://www.gabionline.net/Biosimilars/General/Subsequent-entry-biologics-approved-in-Canada

Garcia, R., & Araujo, D. V. (2016). The regulation of biosimilars in Latin America. *Current Rheumatology Reports, 18*(3), 16.

George, B. (2016). Changes in regulatory requirements for biosimilar development in India. *Biosimilar Development*. Retrieved from https://www.biosimilardevelopment.com/doc/changes-in-regulatory-requirements-for-biosimilar-development-in-india-0001

Gottlieb, S. (2008). Biosimilars: Policy, clinical, and regulatory considerations. *American Journal of Health-System Pharmacy, 65*(14), S2–S8.

Halim, L. A., Brinks, V., Jiskoot, W., Romeijn, S., Praditpornsilpa, K., Assawamakin, A., & Schellekens, H. (2014). How bioquestionable are the different recombinant human erythropoietin copy products in Thailand? *Pharmaceutical Research, 31*(5), 1210–1218. doi:10.1007/s11095-013-1243-9

Hennessy, S., Leonard, C., & Platt, R. (2010). Assessing the safety and comparative effectiveness of follow-on biologics (biosimilars) in the United States. *Clinical Pharmacology & Therapeutics, 87*(2), 157–159.

Hospira. (2010). *Nivestim, European Public Assessment Report*. Retrieved from http://www.ema.europa.eu/ema/index.jsp?curl=pages/medicines/human/medicines/001142/human_med_001344.jsp&mid=WC0b01ac058001d124

Jefferis, R. (2016). Posttranslational modifications and the immunogenicity of biotherapeutics. *Journal of Immunology Research, 2016*, 5358272. doi:10.1155/2016/5358272

Jeremias, S. (2020). Part 1: India works on guidelines for biological products. *AJMC Peer Exchange*. Retrieved from https://www.centerforbiosimilars.com/view/india-works-on-its-guidelines-for-biological-products

Khraishi, M., Stead, D., Lukas, M., Scotte, F., & Schmid, H. (2016). Biosimilars: A multidisciplinary perspective. *Clinical Therapeutics, 38*(5), 1238–1249. doi:10.1016/j.clinthera.2016.02.023

Kingham, R., & Lietzan, E. (2008). Current regulatory and legal considerations for follow-on biologics. *Clinical Pharmacology & Therapeutics, 84*(5), 633–635.

McKinnon, R. A., & Lu, C. Y. (2009). Biosimilars are not (bio) generics. *Australian Prescriber, 32*(6), 146–147. Retrieved from https://www.nps.org.au/australian-prescriber/articles/biosimilars-are-not-biogenerics-editorial

Mielke, J., Jilma, B., Koenig, F., & Jones, B. (2016). Clinical trials for authorized biosimilars in the European Union: A systematic review. *British Journal of Clinical Pharmacology, 82*(6), 1444–1457. doi:10.1111/bcp.13076

Minghetti, P., Rocco, P., Del Vecchio, L., & Locatelli, F. (2011). Biosimilars and regulatory authorities. *Nephron Clinical Practice, 117*(1), c1–c7.

Mounho, B., Phillips, A., Holcombe, K., Grampp, G., Lubiniecki, T., Mollerup, I., & Jones, C. (2010). Global regulatory standards for the approval of biosimilars. *Food and Drug Law Journal, 65*(4), 819–837, ii–iii.

Mounho-Zamora, B. (2013). Regulatory standards for the approval of biosimilar products: A global review. In L. Plitnick & D. Herzyk (Ed.), *Nonclinical Development of Novel Biologics, Biosimilars, Vaccines and Specialty Biologics* (pp. 159–182). Cambridge, MA: Academic Press by Elsevier Inc.

Mysler, E., Pineda, C., Horiuchi, T., Singh, E., Mahgoub, E., Coindreau, J., & Jacobs, I. (2016). Clinical and regulatory perspectives on biosimilar therapies and intended copies of biologics in rheumatology. *Rheumatology International, 36*(5), 613–625. doi:10.1007/s00296-016-3444-0

O'Callaghan, J., Barry, S. P., Bermingham, M., Morris, J. M., & Griffin, B. T. (2019). Regulation of biosimilar medicines and current perspectives on interchangeability and policy. *European Journal of Clinical Pharmacology, 75*(1), 1–11. doi:10.1007/s00228-018-2542-1

Ogura, M., Coiffier, B., Kwon, H.-C., & Yoon, S. W. (2017). Scientific rationale for extrapolation of biosimilar data across cancer indications: Case study of CT-P10. *Future Oncology, 13*(15s), 45–53. doi:10.2217/fon-2017-0156

Olech, E. (2016). Biosimilars: Rationale and current regulatory landscape. *Seminars in Arthritis and Rheumatism, 45*(5 Suppl), S1–10. doi:10.1016/j.semarthrit.2016.01.001

Panesar, K. (2016). Biosimilars: Current approvals and pipeline agents. *U.S. Pharmacist, 41*(10), 26–29. Retrieved from https://www.uspharmacist.com/article/biosimilars-current-approvals-and-pipeline-agents

PDMA. (2009a). *Guidance for the Quality, Safety and Efficacy of Follow-on Biological Medicinal Products (English Translation)*. Retrieved from https://www.pmda.go.jp/files/000153851.pdf

PDMA. (2009b). *Questions and Answers (Q&A) Regarding the Guidance for the Quality, Safety, and Efficacy Assurance of Follow-on Biologics (Biosimilars) (English Translation)*. Retrieved from https://backup.jga.gr.jp/library/old/www.jga.gr.jp/common/img/eng/pdf/QA-Biosimilars01.pdf

PDMA. (2010). *Questions and Answers (Q&A) Regarding the Guidance for the Quality, Safety, and Efficacy Assurance of Follow-on Biologics (Biosimilars) (English Translation)*. Retrieved from https://backup.jga.gr.jp/library/old/www.jga.gr.jp/common/img/eng/pdf/QA-Biosimilars02.pdf

PDMA. (2015). *Questions and Answers (Q&A) Regarding the Guidance for the Quality, Safety, and Efficacy Assurance of Follow-on Biologics (Biosimilars) (English Translation)*. Retrieved from https://backup.jga.gr.jp/library/old/www.jga.gr.jp/common/img/eng/pdf/QA-Biosimilars03.pdf

Reinisch, W., Louis, E., & Danese, S. (2015). The scientific and regulatory rationale for indication extrapolation: A case study based on the infliximab biosimilar CT-P13. *Expert Review of Gastroenterology & Hepatology, 9 Suppl 1,* 17–26. doi:10.1586/17474124.2015.1091306

Roger, S. D., & Mikhail, A. (2007). Biosimilars: Opportunity or cause for concern. *Journal of Pharmacy and Pharmaceutical Sciences, 10*(3), 405–410.

Rugo, H. S., Rifkin, R. M., Declerck, P., Bair, A. H., & Morgan, G. (2019). Demystifying biosimilars: Development, regulation and clinical use. *Future Oncology, 15*(7), 777–790. doi:10.2217/fon-2018-0680

Sandoz. (2006). *Omnitrope European Public Assessment Report Scientific Discussion.* Retrieved from http://www.ema.europa.eu/docs/en_GB/document_library/EPAR_-_Scientific_Discussion/human/000607/WC500043692.pdf

Sandoz. (2009). *Zarzio, European Public Assessment Report.* Retrieved from http://www.ema.europa.eu/ema/index.jsp?curl=pages/medicines/human/medicines/000917/human_med_001170.jsp&mid=WC0b01ac058001d124

Sandoz. (2016). *Erelzi US Biologics License Application, Pharmacology Review.* Retrieved from https://www.accessdata.fda.gov/drugsatfda_docs/nda/2016/761042Orig1s000PharmR.pdf

Sandoz. (2017). *Riximyo European Public Assessment Report.* Retrieved from http://www.ema.europa.eu/docs/en_GB/document_library/EPAR_-_Public_assessment_report/human/004729/WC500232539.pdf

Schellekens, H. (2009). Assessing the bioequivalence of biosimilars The Retacrit case. *Drug Discovery Today, 14*(9–10), 495–499. doi:10.1016/j.drudis.2009.02.003

Schiestl, M., Zabransky, M., & Sorgel, F. (2017). Ten years of biosimilars in Europe: Development and evolution of the regulatory pathways. *Drug Design Development and Therapy, 11,* 1509–1515. doi:10.2147/dddt.s130318

Strober, B. E., Armour, K., Romiti, R., Smith, C., Tebbey, P. W., Menter, A., & Leonardi, C. (2012). Biopharmaceuticals and biosimilars in psoriasis: What the dermatologist needs to know. *Journal of the American Academy of Dermatology, 66*(2), 317–322. doi: 10.1016/j.jaad.2011.08.034

Sullivan, P. M., & DiGrazia, L. M. (2017). Analytic characterization of biosimilars. *American Journal of Health-System Pharmacy, 74*(8), 568–579. doi:10.2146/ajhp150971

Tabernero, J., Vyas, M., Giuliani, R., Arnold, D., Cardoso, F., Casali, P. G., . . . Ciardiello, F. (2016). Biosimilars: A position paper of the European Society for Medical Oncology, with particular reference to oncology prescribers. *ESMO Open, 1*(6), e000142. doi:10.1136/esmoopen-2016-000142

van Aerts, L. A., De Smet, K., Reichmann, G., van der Laan, J. W., & Schneider, C. K. (2014). Biosimilars entering the clinic without animal studies. A paradigm shift in the European Union. *MAbs, 6*(5), 1155–1162. doi:10.4161/mabs.29848

Weise, M. (2016). *Evolving Landscape on Data Requirements to Demonstrate Biosimilarity – the EU Perspective.* Paper presented at the 14th Annual Biosimilar Medicines Group Conference, London, UK.

Weise, M., Bielsky, M. C., De Smet, K., Ehmann, F., Ekman, N., Giezen, T. J., . . . Schneider, C. K. (2012). Biosimilars: What clinicians should know. *Blood, 120*(26), 5111–5117. doi:10.1182/blood-2012-04-425744

Weise, M., Bielsky, M. C., De Smet, K., Ehmann, F., Ekman, N., Narayanan, G., . . . Schneider, C. K. (2011). Biosimilars-why terminology matters. *Nature Biotechnology, 29*(8), 690–693. doi:10.1038/nbt.1936

WHO. (2009). *Guidances on Evaluation of Similar Biotherapeutic Products (SBPs).* Retrieved from http://www.who.int/biologicals/areas/biological_therapeutics/BIOTHERAPEUTICS_FOR_WEB_22APRIL2010.pdf

WHO. (2013). *Guidances on the Quality, Safety and Efficacy of Bio-therapeutic Protein Products Prepared by Recombinant DNA Technology.* Retrieved from http://who.int/biologicals/publications/trs/areas/biological_therapeutics/TRS_977_Annex_2.pdf

WHO. (2016). *Guidelines on Evaluation of Monoclonal Antibodies as Similar Biotherapeutic Products (SBPs).* Retrieved from https://www.who.int/biologicals/biotherapeutics/WHO_TRS_1004_web_Annex_2.pdf?ua=1

WHO. (2018). *WHO Questions and Answers: Similar Biotherapeutic Products.* Retrieved from https://www.who.int/biologicals/expert_committee/QA_for_SBPs_ECBS_2018.pdf?ua=1

Yoo, D. H., Hrycaj, P., Miranda, P., Ramiterre, E., Piotrowski, M., Shevchuk, S., . . . Muller-Ladner, U. (2013). A randomised, double-blind, parallel-group study to demonstrate equivalence in efficacy and safety of CT-P13 compared with innovator infliximab when coadministered with methotrexate in patients with active rheumatoid arthritis: The PLANETRA study. *Annals of the Rheumaatic Diseases, 72*(10), 1613–1620. doi:10.1136/annrheumdis-2012-203090

14

Nonclinical Safety Strategy for Combinations of Biopharmaceuticals or a Biopharmaceutical with a Small Molecular Weight Compound

Maggie Dempster
GlaxoSmithKline

Helen G. Haggerty
Janssen

CONTENTS

14.1 Introduction

Combination drug therapy continues to be an important tool in a pharmaceutical company's arsenal with which to treat complex diseases, such as cancer viral and autoimmune diseases, with the expectation that the pharmacodynamic interaction of the drug products will produce an improved efficacy and/or safety profile. Therefore, prior to any clinical investigation of the combination, an assessment of whether the interactions of the two drug products produce potential additive, synergistic, or antagonistic effects with respect to their pharmacodynamic, pharmacokinetic (PK), or toxicological properties is critical. For example, if both drug products exhibit similar target organ toxicity, they could result in increased toxicity and potentially lower safety margins. Potential for an interaction that could affect the PK, distribution, and/or metabolism of one or both drugs, thereby negatively affecting efficacy and/or safety, could also occur, or a new toxicity may be identified (FDA, 2006; 2020; EMEA, 2008).

The design of the safety strategy for the combination should be based on the extent of existing nonclinical and clinical data including comparator drugs in a similar pharmacological class (Birkebak et al., 2019). In addition, deficiencies in or absence of data for single components, changes in the intended indication (i.e., benefit risk ratio), and new impurities/degradants or novel excipients should be considered. As will be discussed below,

TABLE 14.1

Considerations for Combination Toxicity Testing

Scientific	Regulatory
Potential PD Interactions • Both agents affect same or closely related target/overlapping pathways leading to exaggerated pharmacologic response	**Comarketed products** • Fixed-dose combinations • Copackaged products • Labeling of products for couse • Exceptions, oncology, HIV, and HCV
Potential PK Interactions • One drug has the potential to affect absorption, distribution, or excretion of another drug based on animal or human data	**Minimal Animal or Clinical Data** • Lack of long-term nonclinical toxicity data for either compounds • Lack of adequate clinical safety data for either compound • Lack of adequate clinical experience of the combination
Potential Overlapping Target Organ Toxicity • Concerning overlapping toxicities for individual drugs based on animal toxicology studies and/or clinical data	**Safety Margins** • Narrow margin of safety or nonmonitorable toxicities for either compound • Concern that exposure with the combination cannot be reliably managed by dose adjustment without exceeding individual safety margins
Potential Chemical Interactions • One drug may chemically modify another drug that could result in new toxicities	**Inadequate exposure** • Systemic exposures expected in the clinical combination is not covered by existing data

depending on the indication and patient population, product types, and/or the amount of clinical experience with the combination, this strategy should begin with an assessment of the current nonclinical and clinical data together with a literature review and an understanding of current regulatory guidance, an assessment which may or may not result in the need for in vivo testing. When needed, combination toxicity studies should be designed to detect potential adverse interactions between the individual components of a combination product and to provide a risk benefit ratio (FDA, 2006; EMEA, 2008). Given the scientific and regulatory complexities of combination indications, it is prudent to consider proactive engagement with health authorities to gain alignment on your strategy.

The purpose of this chapter is to discuss the nonclinical safety strategy for the combination of drug products (either as a combination product or a combination regimen), focusing on the specific scientific and regulatory considerations for combinations that include at least one biopharmaceutical with a small molecular weight compound or two biopharmaceuticals together and how these considerations drive this strategy as detailed in Table 14.1. The scope of the chapter pertains primarily to those biopharmaceuticals governed by ICH S6(R1) (2011), ICH S9 (2009), and ICH S9 Q&A (2012) and, therefore, will not include gene therapy or vaccines. Small molecular weight compounds will be discussed but only in the context of a combination with a biopharmaceutical. Although a number of scenarios exist, the chapter will focus on combinations of two or more late-stage drug products (both from Phase 3 studies and/or postmarketing), one late-stage drug product with an early-stage entity (Phase 2 or less), and two early-stage entities; these scenarios will discuss two biopharmaceuticals as well as a biopharmaceutical with a small molecular weight compound (ICH M3(R2), 2009).

14.2 Regulatory Guidance

A combination treatment can include two or more drug products (either a biopharmaceutical or small molecular weight compound) that according to their labeling are to be used only with each other to achieve the intended efficacy and/or improved safety profile for a specific indication (ICH M3(R2), 2009). A combination product, as defined by the FDA, is a product that includes two or more drug entities such as drug/device, biologic/device, drug/biologic, or drug/device/biologic that can be either copackaged or the separate components (active pharmaceutical agents) can be combined in a single dosage form (fixed-dose combination product) (21 CFR 3.2, FDA, 2019; 2020). Adjunctive therapies are combination regimens for which patients who are being treated with one pharmaceutical agent are also treated with a second pharmaceutical agent that are used together but not necessarily dosed at the same time. Adjunctive therapy is not typically considered to be a combination product in the FDA regulatory guidance, unless if these combinations are already labeled for concomitant use, there is an intention to revise labeling to include concomitant use, or the combination poses a serious toxicity risk. It should be noted that adjunctive therapies can also be copackaged but may or may not be labeled for concomitant use (FDA, 2006).

Prior to inclusion in ICH guidelines, regional guidance documents from the FDA and EMEA (FDA, 2006; EMEA, 2008) provided recommendations for the nonclinical safety assessment strategy to support clinical development and subsequent registration of combination drug treatments. These regional guidance documents laid the foundation for the subsequent clarification and harmonization in several ICH guidelines regarding combination drug toxicity testing (ICH M3(R2), 2009; ICH M3(R2) Q&A, 2012; ICH S9, 2009; ICH S9 Q&A, 2012; ICH S11, 2019).

The scope of the nonclinical safety guidance documents covers most therapeutic areas except for oncology, tuberculosis, and antiviral products and includes small molecular weight drugs and protein-based biopharmaceuticals regulated by the Center for Drug Evaluation and Research (CDER) at the FDA. For biopharmaceuticals, ICH S6(R1) should be consulted for individual product evaluation; however, as combination safety strategy is not addressed in ICH S6(R1), the need for and design of combination toxicity studies should be based on the scientific principles of ICH S6(R1) and ICH M3(R2). While the regional guidance documents (FDA, 2006; EMEA, 2008) provide recommendations for when combination toxicity studies are warranted and at times, specific study designs, ICH M3(R2) focuses primarily on the timing and duration of nonclinical combination toxicity studies with respect to clinical development rather than recommending detailed study designs. The ICH M3(R2) guideline also serves to provide an agreed position among the ICH signatory countries, such as the United States, Europe, and Japan, and, therefore, should reflect each regulatory authority's current recommendations (ICH M3(R2), 2009).

Combination treatment scenarios can be grouped into the following three categories: (1) two or more late-stage or approved drug products, (2) at least one early-stage drug product and a late-stage or approved drug product and (3) two early-stage drug products. According to ICH M3(R2), a late-stage drug product is defined as having significant clinical experience (i.e., Phase 3 and postmarketing) whereas an early-stage drug product would be associated with limited clinical experience (i.e., Phase 2 or less). The concept is that the more clinical experience you have with each individual product, the better you will understand the potential risks that may be associated when the products are used in combination in the clinic and the less likely animal data will add to that understanding (ICH M3(R2), 2009).

14.2.1 Two Late-Stage or Approved Drugs

A combination drug toxicity study would not generally be required for two late-stage drug products with adequate nonclinical data for each product and sufficient clinical experience of the combination, given that each individual drug would have been fully tested in nonclinical toxicity studies (assuming no gaps in data) with both efficacy and safety having been assessed during clinical development. However, if there is a significant safety concern, such as that arising from a suspected toxicologic or pharmacodynamic interaction, a combination toxicity study, if needed, should generally be conducted prior to initiating a clinical trial with the combination.

When a combination toxicity study is recommended for two late-stage drug products because of inadequate clinical experience of the combination, the available data for the separate drug entities could support a small-scale or shorter duration clinical trial (Phase 2 study up to 3 months in duration), but a combination toxicity would be required prior to a large-scale or long-term clinical trial or registration (ICH M3(R2), 2009; ICH M3(R2) Q&A, 2012).

14.2.2 One Early-Stage Drug and Late-Stage or Approved Drug

In addition to the nonclinical toxicity studies required to support clinical development for an early-stage drug, a repeat-dose toxicity study of up to 90 days, depending on the duration of the proposed clinical indication, would be typically required to support a combination clinical trial and registration. However, if the combination includes an early-stage drug with clinical experience and a late-stage drug product for which there are no toxicological concerns, a combination toxicity study would not be required to support a clinical trial in which the duration does not exceed each individual product's clinical experience. A combination toxicity study would, however, be required to support a longer duration clinical trial. If results from the combination toxicity study indicate a toxicologic interaction such as overlapping toxicity and if the mechanism of toxicity is not well understood, investigative studies may need to be considered (ICH M3(R2), 2009).

14.2.3 Two Early-Stage Drugs

For two early-stage drug products, even though each drug product would be evaluated separately, a combination toxicity study would be expected prior to support the combination in clinical trials. However, if the two drug products will only be marketed as a combination treatment, studies on the combination should provide enough data to support clinical development and registration without conducting separate studies on each product (ICH M3(R2), 2009).

Combination genotoxicity, safety pharmacology, or carcinogenicity studies are not generally recommended assuming that both drug products, if required, would have been individually tested using current testing standards (ICH M3(R2), 2009). Although combination reproductive toxicity studies were required in the FDA guidance in 2006 when neither drug product posed a potential reproductive toxicity risk, they are not recommended in ICH M3(R2), unless based on the properties of the individual components, the combination of the two products could present a hazard for humans. In the situation, where a concern exists for the combination, a combination embryo-fetal toxicity study in one species should be available to support the marketing application with appropriate precautions ensuring an appropriately worded informed consent and barrier methods in place to protect women of childbearing potential (ICH M3(R2) Q&A, 2012). There may be other situations in which a reproductive hazard with one drug product is observed in a specific trimester of pregnancy, studies to assess the potential effect of the small molecular weight compound, or combination during the other trimesters may be required (FDA, 2006).

The potential need for combination juvenile toxicity studies is addressed in the ICH S11, which is the guideline for nonclinical safety testing for pharmaceuticals for use in pediatric populations (ICH S11, 2019). The nonclinical safety assessment strategy for combination products for pediatric indications should, in principle, follow the recommendations discussed in ICH M3(R2) and the weight of evidence approach as outlined in ICH S11 (2019), ICH M3(R2) (2009). This weight of evidence approach includes both nonclinical (i.e., pharmacology, pharmacodynamic, toxicity data) and clinical safety data (adult and/or pediatric) to provide an integrated overall hazard assessment. However, a combined juvenile toxicity study could be recommended if previous clinical and nonclinical data are not enough to proceed safely into pediatric development, or alternatively, a combined juvenile animal study is required to address a specific safety issue. There may, however, be situations in which a juvenile study with the combination could replace separate juvenile animal studies for each of the individual drug products, or the combination could be added as an extra group to a juvenile study with one of the drug products when the other drug product had already been assessed in a separate study (ICH S11, 2019).

14.2.4 Therapeutic Areas Outside the Scope of ICH M3(R2)

While the ICH M3(R2) guidance addresses the general need for nonclinical combination toxicity testing to support clinical trials of combination drugs, it is out of scope for pharmaceuticals under development for indications in life-threatening or serious diseases without current effective therapy such as advanced cancer and resistant human immunodeficiency virus (HIV) and hepatitis C virus (HCV). These indications are addressed by separate guidance documents as discussed below.

14.2.4.1 Oncology

The requirement for nonclinical studies for oncology agents to support advanced cancer indications differs from that of other indications because of the limited therapeutic options for these patients. Almost all cancer therapeutics are at some point delivered in combination regimens with other therapeutics to drive greater efficacy. Consequently, there are many industry- and investigator-sponsored investigational new drug (INDs) applications submitted for clinical trials with combinations, so many that it would not be practical to require combination toxicity studies to support each combination, and if they were required, it would likely impede the discovery and development of efficacious combinations. Before most anticancer agents are tested in combinations, they have some clinical safety data as a monotherapy from their first-in-human trial. These clinical data for each agent, when given as a monotherapy, can be limited (e.g., from a lead-in monotherapy phase or concurrent trial with monotherapy). However, clinical data with monotherapy have generally been found to provide more useful information to aid in the determination of the appropriate starting dose for the combination as compared with animal combination toxicity data. For these reasons, combination toxicity studies are generally not needed when toxicity data are available with each drug alone, and data are available to support the rationale of the combination to be investigated in humans (ICH S9, 2009).

ICH S9 is a globally harmonized guidance on the nonclinical evaluation for anticancer pharmaceuticals, (ICH S9, 2009; ICH S9 Q&A, 2018) for advanced cancer and sets the expectation for the nonclinical support for the development of combination oncology therapies. As described, if the human toxicity profile has been characterized for each drug in a completed Phase 1 or monotherapy arm within a Phase 1 trial, then nonclinical studies of the combination to assess toxicity are usually not needed. A scientific rationale should be provided that justifies the conduct of a combination clinical study based on data demonstrating that the combination increases antitumor activity with animal tumor models and/or in vitro or in vivo studies based on mechanistic understanding of the target biology. These data can be from sponsor-conducted studies or scientific literature. In those cases when at least one of the compounds is in early-stage development and its human toxicity profile has not yet been evaluated, a short-term toxicity study of the individual drugs (including small molecular weight compounds and biopharmaceuticals) and a nonclinical pharmacology study to support the rationale for the combination should be submitted. This study should provide evidence of increased antitumor activity with the combination in the absence of a substantial increase in toxicity, based on limited safety endpoints, such as mortality, clinical signs, and body weight. A determination can then be made as to whether a dedicated combination toxicity study of the combination is warranted.

If only the combination of the two drugs will be studied in the clinical Phase 1 trial, so no monotherapy clinical data will be available, then a combination toxicity study should be conducted along with the toxicologic evaluation of each individual agent. If the pharmacology data suggest a concern for synergistic toxicity of unpredictable magnitude which precludes clinical dose adjustments and suggest that clinical monitoring may be insufficient to mitigate the risk on its own, then a dedicated in vitro (e.g., cytokine release assay for some monoclonal antibodies [mAbs] that target immune cells) or an in vivo toxicology combination toxicity study should be considered. As can be the case with many therapeutic proteins (TPs), a relevant animal model may not exist to assess the efficacy and safety of the therapeutic. When the safety risk for the combination is a concern, an assessment of the combination toxicity can be based on relevant in vitro assays or in vivo studies based on mechanistic understanding of target biology. Therefore, the use of an alternative model such as a surrogate, animal model of disease and/or transgenic should be considered.

When an anticancer agent is being combined with another agent that has no anticancer activity itself, but the agent is designed to enhance the activity of the anticancer agent, data should be provided to show that the enhancer is nonactive as well as general toxicology, safety pharmacology, and reproductive toxicology assessments should be done for the combination. The enhancer alone may have a more limited safety assessment either as an arm in the general toxicology combination study or as a stand-alone general toxicology study of up to 1-month duration.

14.2.4.2 Human Immunodeficiency Virus and Hepatitis C Virus

Current treatments for both HIV and HCV often require a combination of antiviral agents to be most effective and reduce the potential for resistance to develop. FDA guidance has been developed to specifically address these indications when developing combination treatment regimens, which follow similar guiding principles with regards to their nonclinical safety testing strategy (FDA, 2015; 2017). When a new antiviral combination is not expected to offer benefits over currently effective therapies, the principles of ICH M3(R2) are expected to be followed to guide testing. However, similar to advanced cancer indications, combination toxicity studies are not generally warranted for HIV or HCV antiviral agents that are intended to treat patients who have limited or no treatment options or for which the combination is expected to improve response rates in patients at risk of serious morbidity or to provide a substantial improvement over other approved therapies. In these cases, the benefit of the combination is believed to outweigh the potential risks of foregoing the combination toxicity studies, provided there is no specific cause for concern based on in vitro, animal, or clinical data. These concerns for the combination can arise from the following: (1) mechanisms of action data or in vitro data of potential off-target effects (unless deemed not relevant) that suggest a potential for additive or synergistic toxicity of significant clinical concern; (2) animal or human absorption, distribution, metabolism, and excretion (ADME) studies that show the potential for an unmanageable drug–drug interaction (DDI) or serious toxicity; (3) toxicology studies of at least 3 months duration of the individual drug products that demonstrate concerning overlapping toxicities or a low safety margin for toxicities that are potentially serious and/or unable to be adequately monitored clinically; or (4) Phase 1 or 2 clinical data (if available) that reveal substantial or unmanageable safety concerns.

14.3 Considerations for Combination Toxicity Study Designs

14.3.1 Introduction

Biopharmaceuticals, given their size, complex biophysical characteristics, and mode of manufacturing, require a different approach with respect to their nonclinical safety assessment strategy than small molecular weight compounds (Todd and Dempster, 2013). The primary regulatory guidance document for biopharmaceuticals is ICH S6(R1), whereas the primary guideline for small molecular weight compounds is ICH M3(R2). As previously mentioned, recommendations for nonclinical combination toxicity are not addressed in ICH S6(R1), but both regional (FDA and EMEA) regulatory guidelines and ICH M3(R2) Q&A discuss when combination toxicity studies are needed including both biopharmaceuticals and small molecular weight compounds (FDA, 2006; EMEA, 2008; ICH M3(R2) Q&A, 2012). ICH S6(R1) should also be consulted when designing a combination toxicity strategy that includes a biopharmaceutical (ICH S6(R1), 2011).

14.3.1.1 Repeat-Dose Combination Toxicity Study Design

An in vivo combination toxicity assessment, when required, will typically include a repeat-dose combination toxicity study up to 90 days in a single species. The choice of species should be justified based on factors such as high concordance with human toxicity, similar target organ toxicities among species, and the species selected is relevant for human risk assessment. It should be noted, however, that health authorities may request a second species depending on the results of the study, particularly if a novel toxicity is observed in the combination toxicity study (ICH M3(R2), 2009). These studies can be thought of as "bridging" studies designed to detect potential adverse interactions between the individual drug products (FDA, 2006). In addition, the study should be designed to provide information to answer the following questions which include (1) are there

acceptable margins of safety for the proposed doses for the combination? (2) are there overlapping target organ toxicities? (3) are they any clinical data to suggest a potential negative interaction? and (4) is there a possibility of a pharmacodynamic interaction, e.g., affinity for the same receptor? (FDA, 2006).

14.3.1.1.1 Species Selection

Assessment of on- and off-target toxicity is important to be determined for small molecular weight compounds, and therefore, nonclinical toxicity studies are typically conducted in both rodent (rat) and nonrodent (dog) species to support clinical development (ICH M3(R2), 2009). Given that off-target toxicity is rare for biopharmaceuticals, selection of a pharmacologically relevant species is imperative and owing to their highly selective target affinity, often the sole relevant species is a nonhuman primate (NHP) (Todd and Dempster, 2013). Therefore, any combination toxicity study that includes a biopharmaceutical will need to be conducted in a pharmacologically relevant species. Given the selectivity of many biopharmaceuticals, species selection can be problematic, particularly, if the biopharmaceutical is combined with a small molecular weight compound that has been assessed in a rat and dog and the biopharmaceutical is not pharmacologically active in either species. Therefore, the combination toxicity strategy here may require that the small molecular weight compound be tested in a 2-week dose range-finding study in a NHP prior to assessment of the combination. Clearly, this can cause issues, for example, if the toxicity between the NHP and the dog differs, novel unique toxicity is observed in NHPs, and/or the results from the dog toxicity study exhibit better translation to humans. Another complication with a combination of small molecule with a biopharmaceutical that could arise is when although the biopharmaceutical is pharmacologically active in the rodent, the toxicity observed in the rodent for the small molecule did not translate to the clinic.

14.3.1.1.2 Dose Level Selection

The dose levels selected for a combination toxicity study should represent an exposure range that produces a sufficient level of toxicity that allows for the identification of additive or synergistic effects (FDA, 2006). A dose level that produces unacceptable toxicity could result in pharmacodynamic effects in animals not relevant for human safety (EMEA, 2008). However, dose levels will need to be high enough to produce exposure ratios that ensure an appropriate exposure margin at the intended clinical dose, but may not always be feasible because of differences in metabolism or greater sensitivity to the toxicity in animals versus human (FDA, 2006).

Although the principles for dose selection discussed above apply to both small and large molecular weight compounds, there are differences between them. For small molecular weight compounds, the high dose typically represents either the maximum tolerated dose (i.e., a dose that produces toxicity) or maximum feasible dose based on physiochemical properties of the drug product with the low dose level being near or at expected clinical efficacy exposure (ICH M3(R2), 2009), whereas for a biopharmaceutical, the high dose level should represent the maximum intended pharmacological effect that includes a 10-fold multiple over the intended maximal clinical exposure (ICH S6(R1), 2011; Todd and Dempster, 2013). Depending on the pharmacology of the biopharmaceutical, the high dose level may not result in overt target organ toxicity unlike what is expected for a small molecular weight compound. Therefore, for these types of mAbs, a combination toxicity with a small molecule and biopharmaceutical may combine the high dose of the biopharmaceutical with the three dose levels (low, mid, and high) of the small molecule, resulting in a total of four dose groups (including one group dosed with both vehicles). In general, the dose level and number of dose levels will need to be selected in order to identify potential new toxicity or to establish clinically relevant safety margins, particularly when assessing two early-stage therapeutics (ICH M3(R2) Q&A, 2012).

14.3.1.1.3 Study Duration

The guidance suggests that, in general, combination toxicity studies, if required, need to be of sufficient duration to produce the toxicity of concern but would not typically be longer than 90 days for a chronic clinical indication. For a clinical indication of shorter duration, a combination toxicity study less than 90 days could be used to support marketing registration. If the combination toxicity study addresses a specific safety toxicity concern of the combination, the duration of the study should be long enough to fully evaluate that toxicity (ICH M3(R2), 2009; ICH M3(R2) Q&A, 2012).

14.3.1.2 Animal Models of Efficacy/Pharmacology

Assessment of combined pharmacology using animal models of efficacy is not required to support combination therapy for nononcology indications. The advanced cancer indication in which combination pharmacology studies are recommended, is discussed in Section 14.2.4.1. However, results from these studies could identify potential areas of concern and inform on the general toxicity study design (ICH M3(R2), 2009). For example, if a combination is being developed in which one drug is thought to reduce the other drug's adverse side effects, the addition of toxicity endpoints should be considered for a combination pharmacology study, but regulatory guidance cautions that toxicity endpoints may not be adequately assessed in a pharmacology study and a combination toxicity study would still be warranted (ICH M3 (R2) Q&A, 2012). Because the toxicity of biopharmaceuticals is typically associated with exaggerated pharmacology, there may be situations in which endpoints in a combined pharmacology study may identify more subtle effects than what is typically measured in a general toxicity study. However, if this strategy is chosen, early interaction with a health authority is important.

14.3.1.3 Safety Pharmacology

Combined safety pharmacology studies, although not generally recommended, may be considered when both therapeutics target similar organ systems or when one or both therapeutics belong to a class of compounds or targets associated with a specific toxicity. Given that many biopharmaceuticals are highly specific for their target standalone safety pharmacology studies are rarely conducted for biopharmaceuticals but instead safety

pharmacology endpoints are added to the general toxicity study (ICH S7A, 2001). Therefore, combination safety pharmacology studies with two biopharmaceuticals would not typically be warranted. Although if both drug products affect the same functional process (e.g., QT prolongation), a combined safety pharmacology study could provide important data for clinical trial initiation (FDA, 2006; EMEA, 2008).

14.3.1.4 Genotoxicity and Carcinogenesis

Biopharmaceuticals (e.g., recombinant proteins and mAbs) composed of endogenous amino acids are unlikely to react with DNA or other chromosomal material, and therefore, combination genotoxicity studies are not required (ICH S6(R1), 2011). Although there are biopharmaceuticals such as antibody drug conjugates that contain organic linkers, where genotoxicity would be assessed, however, it is unlikely that a combination genotoxicity study would provide any additional information, and therefore, combined genotoxicity studies would not be recommended. (FDA, 2006; Todd and Dempster, 2013; ICH S6(R1), 2011). Although carcinogenicity studies are rarely conducted with biopharmaceuticals and combined bioassays would not be expected, the potential impact of the small molecular compound or other biopharmaceutical could be included in the carcinogenic assessment document completed for a biopharmaceutical intended for chronic use in the clinic (ICH S6(R1), 2011).

14.3.1.5 Reproductive Development Toxicity

When women of childbearing potential are included in the intended patient population, the current regulatory recommendation is that combined reproductive toxicity studies are not recommended if a potential human developmental hazard has already been identified for either agent alone or if nonclinical embryo-fetal development studies for each agent indicate that neither agent poses a potential developmental risk. However, there could be a situation for a combination in which neither drug product results in a reproductive risk alone but the interaction with the two targets could result in a potential risk. In this case, a combined reproductive development toxicity study could be considered. If a combined embryo-fetal development study is warranted, the study should be available for registration. In the meantime, appropriate precautions should be included in any clinical trial involving women of childbearing potential. (ICH M3 Q&A, 2012). Often with biopharmaceuticals, the NHP is the only relevant species for toxicity testing of the clinical candidate. As reproductive toxicity studies can be challenging in the NHP, one may want to consider the use of a surrogate in a rodent model as a viable alternative, especially if being combined with a small molecule that has not been evaluated in an NHP model. This approach should be scientifically justified and discussed with regulators.

14.3.1.6 Pharmacokinetics/ADME

Combination PK, and/or ADME studies for combination of two late-stage drug products would not typically be recommended because of available nonclinical and clinical data and, particularly, because most of these parameters can be monitored clinically (ICH M3(R2), 2009). However, given the lack of clinical experience with combinations consisting of at least one new drug product, combination PK/ADME studies could be considered to assess whether a PK interaction could result in one drug entity altering the absorption, distribution, and/or excretion of the other drug product or competition for serum protein binding affecting systemic exposure of unbound drug levels or competition for the same biologic target. Therefore, in addition, to further defining the safety profile, these data can provide valuable information to assist in the design of nonclinical toxicity studies and/or clinical combination trials. However, when the pharmacodynamic properties are known for the individual drug products, potential interactions can be anticipated and inform on the clinical trial design without the need for combination studies. See Section 14.3.2 below for more information on potential mechanisms of DDIs with biologics and examples of those interactions.

14.3.2 Drug–Drug Interactions

When a TP is to be used as a combination therapy with another drug, be it either a small molecule or a TP, the potential for a DDI and its impact on exposure needs to be considered. While this is especially important for the combination of two small molecular compounds, TP can also be impacted or have an impact on the disposition of other drugs, be they a TP or a small molecule, although it is less common. To assess for this potential, one needs to understand the clearance mechanisms of each agent. TPs can be cleared by specific receptor-mediated endocytosis either via binding to their target or, for Fc-bearing therapeutics such as mAbs or Fc-fusion proteins, binding to the FcRs; nonspecific pinocytosis; immunogenicity (antidrug antibodies [ADAs])-mediated clearance; and/or renal filtration. On the other hand, small molecules are often cleared by hepatic metabolism and biliary and renal clearance (Huang et al., 2010). Thus, when evaluating the potential for a DDI between TPs and small molecules or between TPs, it is necessary to take a science-driven approach based on the understanding of the mechanisms that may be in play for each agent. If a potential risk is identified and depending on the mechanism, its impact on exposure may be evaluated in combination animal studies or it may be best evaluated clinically. The FDA recently published a draft guidance for industry entitled "Drug-Drug Interaction Assessment for Therapeutic Proteins," which provides a systematic, risk-based approach to determining the need for DDI studies for TPs (FDA, 2020). Following are several examples of different sources of DDIs that involve TPs.

Hepatic drug-metabolizing cytochrome P-450 (CYP) enzymes and drug-transporter proteins play an important role in the disposition of many small molecular weight drugs, and their induction or inhibition can often lead to DDIs between small molecules (Huang et al, 2010). Owing to differences in mechanisms associated with the disposition of TPs and small molecule drugs, the risk for the DDI between them has been generally anticipated to be low. However, CYP enzymes and drug transporters are known to be down-regulated during inflammation largely due to the release of proinflammatory cytokines, such as interferons (IFN), TNFα, IL-2, and IL-6

(Lee et al., 2010; Evers et al., 2013; Fardel and Le Vée, 2009; Le Vee et al., 2009). Thus, TPs that are proinflammatory cytokines or cytokine modulators can alter the CYP expression or function and, thereby, potentially impact the exposure of small molecular weight drugs that are CYP substrates. Clinically relevant interactions have been reported with some therapeutic proinflammatory cytokines such as recombinant IFNs when administered with drugs that are CYP substrates (Christensen and Hermann, 2012). IFN-α administration in patients with hepatitis B has been shown to cause a 15% decrease of erythromycin metabolism (Craig et al., 1993), and patients monitored on warfarin required a dose reduction when IFN-α2b and IFN-β were given (Adachi et al., 1995). Conversely, TPs that treat inflammatory diseases may reverse cytokine-mediated suppression of CYP, indirectly leading to increased clearance of CYP substrates. This has been demonstrated by reduced exposure to simvastatin in patients with rheumatoid arthritis treated with tocilizumab, an antibody that blocks the IL-6 receptor, or adalimumab, an antibody that neutralizes TNF (Schmitt et al., 2011; Christensen and Hermann, 2012; Evers et al., 2013). Thus, regulatory guidance from both the FDA and EMA recommend that if an investigational TP is a proinflammatory cytokine or cytokine modulator that has known effects on CYP enzymes or transporter proteins, studies should be done to determine the magnitude of TP's effects on drugs that are substrates of the affected CYP enzyme or transporter (Evers et al., 2013). As in vitro and animal studies to date have shown limited translation value in the qualitative and quantitative projection of clinical interactions, clinical DDI studies are often recommended for these TPs.

Other known mechanisms for DDI interactions with TPs involve combination of TPs (mAb or Fc-fusion protein) that have an immunoglobulin G (IgG) Fc region with a molecule that compromises the function of neonatal Fc receptor (FcRn). FcRn is responsible for prolonging the half-life of IgG in the circulation by protecting it from lysosomal degradation and recycling it to the systemic circulation. For example, rozanolixizumab is an investigational humanized monoclonal IgG antibody that targets FcRn and is being developed for the treatment of myasthenia gravis, a neuromuscular condition thought to be triggered by an autoimmune response (Kiessling et al., 2017). Rozanolixizumab binds to FcRn, preventing the binding of endogenous IgG, but also other TPs containing an Fc region of human IgG, to FcRn. Treatment in humans and cynomolgus monkeys with rozanolixizumab demonstrated a significant reduction in serum IgG levels. One could hypothesize that if rozanolixizumab was administered in combination with another therapeutic IgG mAb or Fc-fusion protein, the exposure of the mAb or Fc-fusion protein would also be reduced. Similarly, high doses of intravenous immunoglobulin (IVIg), when administered in combination with the human anti-C5 mAb, tesidolumab, in end-stage renal disease patients, caused a 34% decrease in tesidolumab exposure, as well as a shortened period of full complement activity inhibition demonstrating reduced pharmacodynamic activity, as compared with when tesidolumab was given alone. These findings demonstrate that IVIg can have a clinically relevant impact on the clearance of other mAbs when given in combination likely due to competition for the FcRn salvage pathway (Jordan et al., 2020).

Another potential DDI is the combination of a TP whose PK is known to be affected by immunogenicity (ADA) with molecules that can impact immunogenicity by either suppressing or enhancing the immune response. For example, treatment with methotrexate has been shown to suppress the generation of antiadalimumab antibodies that can enhance the clearance of adalimumab (Farhangian and Feldman, 2015; Krieckaert et al., 2012). Conversely, treatment of TPs with immunostimulatory molecules might enhance humoral immune responses as seen with the combination of nivolumab and ipilimumab, two immunostimulatory mAbs (Statkevich et al., 2016). Immunogenicity has the potential to alter exposure or neutralize pharmacologic activity, resulting in the loss of efficacy, or increase the risk of safety via the induction of infusion-related adverse events. As the ADA response in animals to human TPs generally overpredict the risk of immunogenicity in humans, the concern for DDI associated with ADA is best evaluated in the clinic and/or addressed in the label.

14.4 Case Studies

14.4.1 Nononcology Case Studies with Combinations of a Biopharmaceutical and Small Molecule and Two Biopharmaceuticals

Autoimmune diseases are complex and heterogenous, and although there has been some progress made, approved therapies have only been partially efficacious with a considerable unmet medical need. Thus, combination treatments, which can impact multiple targets or pathways, will likely be needed to improve clinical responses either by increasing therapeutic activity directly or by allowing dose reduction to minimize adverse effects without loss of efficacy. Atacicept is a fully human recombinant Fc fusion protein that blocks the activity of B-lymphocyte stimulator (BLyS) and a proliferation-inducing ligand that was being evaluated in early clinical trials as a monotherapy for autoimmune diseases. Atacicept had a nonclinical safety package completed to support monotherapy indication, but to support its clinical use as adjunctive therapy with standard of care (marketed) immunomodulators, rituximab and mycophenolate mofetil (MMF), 13-week combination toxicity studies were conducted (Ponce, 2009). Atacicept is pharmacologically active in both mice and NHPs, and nonclinical studies in mice and cynomolgus monkeys demonstrated dose-dependent, reversible decreases in circulating Ig and reductions in mature B cells in the peripheral blood and lymphoid tissues. MMF is a small molecule, purine synthesis inhibitor, and rituximab is a chimeric mAb that binds CD20 expressed primarily on B cells and triggers cell death. In designing the combination toxicity studies, clinically relevant routes of administration for each agent and an allometrically scaled human equivalent dose and regimen for MMF and rituximab in combination with an exaggerated human-equivalent dose and regimen for atacicept were employed.

To support the combination of atacicept with MMF, a 13-week combination toxicity study with a 13-week recovery period was conducted in mice, a species for which its

pharmacologic activity and safety had been previously established with each agent. Four groups of mice (35–50 per sex per group) consisting of a control group (both vehicles), atacicept alone with MMF vehicle, MMF alone with atacicept vehicle, and MMF and atacicept combined were administered MMF (and its vehicle) orally once daily at 350 mg/kg and atacicept (and its vehicle) subcutaneously three times a week at 20 mg/kg. Four mice per sex were necropsied at the end of 5 or 13 weeks of treatment and 5 or 15 weeks of recovery.

The safety of atacicept and rituximab was evaluated in cynomolgus monkeys because the species-specific binding of rituximab for CD20 is restricted to primates and its pharmacologic activity, and safety had been previously established in the cynomolgus monkey. The combination toxicity study evaluated two different combination scenarios, atacicept in combination with rituximab for 13 weeks and the sequential administration of rituximab for 4 weeks followed by atacicept for 13 weeks, both with a 13-week recovery period. Five groups of monkeys (3-6 per sex per group) consisting of rituximab vehicle followed by atacicept vehicle; rituximab followed by atacicept vehicle; rituximab vehicle followed by atacicept; rituximab followed by atacicept; and rituximab and atacicept were administered once weekly rituximab (and its vehicle) via intravenous infusion at 20 mg/kg or atacicept (and its vehicle) subcutaneously at 20 mg/kg.

Overall, the combinations of atacicept with MMF or rituximab were well tolerated and did not appear to impact the exposure of atacicept. Combination therapy of atacicept with either MMF or rituximab demonstrated greater reductions in B cells in the periphery (MMF) or tissues (MMF and rituximab) compared with monotherapy. In addition, the combination treatment of atacicept with MMF resulted in enhanced reduction of serum Ig levels throughout the dosing period. Moreover, atacicept treatment did not augment MMF-induced reductions in red blood cells or platelets. These data suggest that combination treatment with atacicept may augment the effects of B-cell–targeted therapies without incurring novel or untoward toxicity. However, these nonclinical studies, which were conducted over short exposure periods in healthy animals, do not address the possible risk of infection associated with combination therapy, which would be best evaluated in the clinic.

Multiple sclerosis (MS) is an autoimmune disease characterized by inflammation leading to neurodegeneration. Avonex® is INF beta (IFNβ), a cytokine that by balancing the expression of pro- and anti-inflammatory cells in the brain results in an overall suppressed neuroinflammation (Kieseier, 2011). Natalizumab, is a humanized mAb that binds to α4β1 integrin and blocks its interaction with vascular cell adhesion molecule-1 (VCAM-1). Its primary mechanism of action is to inhibit leukocyte migration into the brain, thereby decreasing inflammation resulting in dampening formation of lesions (Rudick et al., 2006). Although Avonex® was effective as a monotherapy, patients still relapsed and the combination with natalizumab was found to be more effective in patients with relapsing MS (Rudick et al., 2006). As natalizumab and Avonex® would be expected to be used in combination, a 4-week combination toxicity with an 8-week recovery was conducted in rhesus monkeys. Six groups of rhesus monkeys

(5/sex/group) were administered vehicle control (both vehicles administered), Avonex® only (30 μg, intramuscularly), natalizumab only (30 or 60 m/kg intravenously), and Avonex® (30 μg) in combination with natalizumab at 30 or 60 mg/kg once weekly for 4 weeks. Natalizumab at 30 and 60 mg/kg, alone or in combination with Avonex®, had no effect on IFNβ1a serum levels nor did Avonex® administration have any effect on a4 integrin on peripheral blood cells. In addition, natalizumab serum levels were not impacted by Avonex®. Clinical pathology changes were limited to dose-independent natalizumab-related increases in lymphocytes and lymphocyte subsets (T-lymphocytes, T-helper, T-cytotoxic/suppressor, and B-lymphocytes), with lesser effects on monocytes, eosinophils, basophils, and secondary increases in white blood cell counts. Clear increases in nucleated red blood cells were associated with slightly increased reticulocyte numbers followed by lower increased incidence of anisocytosis and polychromasia. These effects were not noted in the Avonex® alone group and, therefore, felt to be indicative of natalizumab pharmacological activity; there was no evidence of an additive effect on the hematologic parameters. In general, all test-article changes were minimal to mild and reversible (Biogen, 2004). However, when natalizumab was studied in patients with relapsing MS given in combination with Avonex, two cases of progressive multifocal leukoencephalopathy (one of which was fatal) were diagnosed in patients, given the combination and with Avonex alone. This finding raised the concern for its long-term safety (Rudick et al., 2006), and highlighted the limitations of animal models to predict some clinical risks.

14.4.2 Oncology Case Studies with Two Biopharmaceuticals in Combination

Over the last decade a number of mAbs mAbs that target two immune checkpoints, cytotoxic T lymphocyte-associated antigen 4 (CTLA-4) and the programmed cell death protein 1 pathway (PD-1/PD-L1), have been approved for use as monotherapies in multiple tumor types given their significant clinical benefit for some patients. Nevertheless, there remains a need to expand the benefit to broader patient populations. Thus, many new targets continue to be explored, and it is becoming increasingly apparent based on nonclinical and clinical data that combination therapy with agents that intervene at different stages of the cancer-immunity cycle has the greatest potential to provide significant additional benefit (Chen et al., 2013). For example, combined blockade of PD-1/PD-L1 with other coinhibitors, such as CTLA-4, LAG-3, or TIM-3, has a synergistic effect in reversing T cell exhaustion and restoring the CD8+ effector function (Morrissey et al., 2016). However, with increased benefit comes increased risk for enhanced immune-mediated toxicities.

Given the strong efficacy and safety profile for the PD1/PDL1 mAbs, they have become the cornerstone for most combination anticancer regimens. The first approved combination of two checkpoint inhibitors is ipilimumab (anti-CTLA4 mAb) and nivolumab (anti-PD1 mAb) for the treatment of metastatic melanoma and, more recently, lung cancer. While both are checkpoint inhibitors, they have complimentary mechanisms of action. Ipilimumab helps to stimulate the activation of naive T cells and their proliferation, whereas nivolumab helps to reverse exhaustion in the periphery and continue the activity of these T cells in tumor tissues. This combined therapy in the clinic resulted in significantly longer progression-free and overall survival than ipilimumab alone (Wang et al., 2014). However, the increased benefit achieved with the combination in patients with advanced cancer was also associated with the increased risk for developing immune-related adverse events such as diarrhea/ colitis and hepatitis. Importantly, despite the higher incidence of grade 3 or 4 adverse events with combination therapy, no new types of adverse events were identified, and they were generally manageable.

To support the clinical development of ipilimumab in combination with nivolumab and prior to the issuance of ICH S9 guidance, a combination toxicity study was conducted in the NHP to evaluate the potential for enhanced toxicity (Selby et al., 2016). This was the first experience combining two mAbs that targeted checkpoint inhibitors whose complementary mechanisms could lead to enhanced immune stimulation. This combination was of particular concern given the TeGenero incident in 2006, in which an immunostimulatory mAb resulted in an acute cytokine storm, systemic inflammatory response, and multiorgan failure following the first dose to healthy volunteers in the FIH clinical trial, a response not predicted by preclinical toxicity studies (Suntharalingam et al., 2006). Given the highlighted risk associated with immune activation by mAb-targeting T cells, there was concern about the potential risk associated with the combination of two T-cell immunostimulatory mAbs in humans. Both ipilimumab and nivolumab as monotherapies had demonstrated immune-related adverse events in the clinic affecting multiple organ systems, whereas in toxicity studies conducted in the NHP (the only pharmacologically relevant toxicology species for each), each drug was well tolerated with no adverse findings when tested at a clinically relevant dose range.

In the combination toxicity study, three groups of cynomolgus monkeys (5/sex/group) consisting of a control group, a low-dose combination group (3 mg/kg ipilimumab and 10 mg/kg nivolumab), and a high-dose combination group (10 mg/kg ipilimumab and 50 mg/kg nivolumab) were treated intravenously once weekly for 4 weeks. Three per sex per group were necropsied on Day 30, whereas the remainder of the animals were necropsied following a 1-month recovery period. No significant alterations of lymphocyte subpopulations were observed in any group. Dose-dependent combination treatment-related effects were observed in the spleen (increased weight and lymphoid follicle hypertrophy and/or marginal zone expansion) and lymph nodes (decreased germinal centers and/or hypocellularity). A dose-dependent increase in diarrhea was also observed that correlated with a dose-dependent increase in the incidence and severity of inflammation in the large intestine (colitis) and associated decreases in albumin, increases in globulin, and/or increases in neutrophil and eosinophil counts. Given that similar inflammatory events were not observed in cynomolgus monkeys treated with ipilimumab (Keler et al., 2003) or nivolumab (Wang et al., 2014) alone, these findings suggested that combination therapy may further exacerbate self-reactive immune responses in patients. Still, a low incidence of other immune-related adverse events encountered in patients (in monotherapy or combination), such as hypophysitis, pneumonitis, rash, and increases in transaminases or lipases, was not seen in NHP combination toxicity studies. In addition, an in vitro cytokine release assay with human peripheral blood mononuclear cells (PBMCs) was conducted with the combination, and no impact was observed with the combination as compared with each agent alone.

Lymphocyte-activation gene 3 (LAG3) is another immune checkpoint pathway that negatively regulates effector T-cell function and is a marker of T-cell exhaustion. Relatlimab is an IgG4 mAb that blocks LAG3, and in nonclinical pharmacology studies, it demonstrated synergistic antitumor activity when given in combination with nivolumab. The Phase 1 clinical plan for relatlimab involved limited treatment of advanced cancer patients with LAG3 mAb alone prior to combination therapy with nivolumab, a marketed drug. As part of the nonclinical strategy to support the combined administration of nivolumab with relatlimab in the clinic, a combination NHP toxicity study was conducted. In the 1-month toxicity studies with anti-LAG3 mAb alone and in combination with nivolumab, immune-related toxicities, including moribundity with associated central nervous system (CNS) vasculitis and epididymitis in one animal, were observed for the high-dose combination whereas the low-dose combination and either mAb alone did not have findings (Herzyk and Haggerty, 2018).

It is important to note that, given the increased knowledge of the risks of combining two checkpoint inhibitors and in accordance with ICH S9, these combination toxicity studies would likely not be conducted today to support an advanced oncology indication. Indeed, many combination clinical trials have been safely executed without supporting combination toxicity studies for multiple checkpoint inhibitor programs that are in development.

14.5 Conclusion

Combination drug therapy, including combination products and combination regimens, will continue to grow as an important tool with which to combat complex diseases. However, concomitant with the promise of improved therapeutic efficacy, comes the challenge to ensure that sufficient nonclinical data are available to support safe progression into humans. A scientifically robust approach is needed to address safety potential concerns such as toxicologic or pharmacodynamic interactions. Recommendations from regional regulatory agencies drafted in the early 2000s provided initial guidance that was later updated in ICH M3(R2) provide a framework to assist with the nonclinical safety strategy.

A nonclinical combination safety strategy should begin with a critical review of the nonclinical and clinical data with the purpose of identifying areas of concern or significant safety gaps that prevent safe clinical progression. Although a combination toxicity study may be appropriate for some programs, other studies such as animal pharmacology, in vitro studies, or other special toxicity studies may be more informative (Birkebak et al., 2019). Therefore, the decision to conduct combination toxicity studies should be based on strong scientific rationale and understanding of regulatory guidance, together with a view to minimize animal use such that the data contribute to the understanding of patient safety. The data should provide a critical impact to the design of the clinical trial by adding appropriate safety biomarkers, modification to the starting clinical dose or clinical dose escalation, and/or change in dose regimen (Birkebak et al., 2019; Sacaan et al., 2020). Ideally, nonclinical combination toxicity strategy should be guided by scientific judgment coupled with proactive engagement with health authorities.

REFERENCES

Adachi, Y., Y. Yokoyama, T. Nanno, and T. Yamamoto. 1995. "Potentiation of warfarin by interferon." *BMJ (Clinical Research ed.)*, 311(7000):292. doi: 10.1136/bmj.311.7000.292a

Ascierto, Paolo Antonio, Ignacio Melero, Shailender Bhatia, Petri Bono, Rachel E. Sanborn, Evan J. Lipson, Margaret K. Callahan, Thomas Gajewski, Carlos A. Gomez-Roca, F. Stephen Hodi, et al. 2017. "Initial efficacy of anti-lymphocyte activation gene-3 (anti–LAG-3; BMS-986016) in combination with nivolumab (nivo) in pts with melanoma (MEL) previously treated with anti-PD-1/PD-L1 therapy." *J Clin Oncol* 35:15_suppl:9520–9520. doi: 10.1200/JCO.2017.35.15_suppl.9520

Biogen Inc. 2004. "Summary basis of approval of Tysabri (Natalizumab)." Application No: 125104. Freedom of Information Services, FDA. https://www.accessdata.fda.gov/drugsatfda_docs/nda/ 2004/125104s000_Natalizumab.cfm

Birkebak, Joanne, Lorrene A. Buckley, Donna Dambach, Eunice Musvasva, Karen Price, Sherry Ralston, and Aida Sacaan. 2019. "Pharmaceutical industry perspective on combination toxicity studies: Results from an intra-industry survey conducted by IQ DruSafe Leadership Group." *Regul Toxicol Pharmacol.* Mar;102:40–46. doi: 10.1016/j.yrtph.2018.12.012. Epub 2018 Dec 19. PMID: 30576687.

Chen, Daniel S. and Ira Mellman. 2013. "Oncology meets immunology: The cancer immunity cycle." *Immunity* 39(1):1–10. doi: 10.1016/j.immuni.2013.07.012

Christensen, Hege and Monica Hermann. 2012. "Immunological response as a source to variability in drug metabolism and transport." *Front Pharmacol.* 3:8. doi: 10.3389/fphar.2012.00008

Craig, Philip I., Michael Tapner M, and Geoffrey C. Farrell. 1993. "Interferon suppresses erythromycin metabolism in rats and human subjects." *Hepatology* 17:230–235. doi: 10.1002/hep.1840170212

European Medicines Agency, Committee for Medicinal Products for Human Use. 2008. "Guideline on the non-clinical development of fixed combinations of medicinal products." http://www.emea.europa.eu/pdfs/human/swp/25849805enfin.pdf.

Evers, Raymond, Shannon Dallas, Leslie J. Dickmann, Odette A. Fahmi, Jane R. Kenny, Eugenia Kraynov, Theresa Nguyen, Aarti H. Patel, J. Greg Slatter, and Lei Zhang. 2013. "Cytochrome P450-related therapeutic protein drug interaction white paper." *Drug Metab Dispos.* 41(9):1598–1609. doi: 10.1124/dmd.113.052225

Fardel Oliver and Marc Le Vée. 2009 "Regulation of human hepatic drug transporter expression by pro-inflammatory cytokines." *Expert Opin Drug Metab Toxicol.* Dec;5(12):1469–1481. doi: 10.1517/17425250903304056. PMID: 19785515.

Farhangian, Michael E. and Steven R. Feldman. 2015. "Immunogenicity of biologic treatments for psoriasis: Therapeutic consequences and the potential value of concomitant methotrexate." *Am J Clin Dermatol.* Aug;16(4):285–294. doi: 10.1007/s40257-015-0131-y. PMID: 25963062.

Food and Drug Administration, Center for Drug Evaluation and Research. 2006. "Guidance for industry: Nonclinical safety evaluation of drug or biologic combinations." http://www.fda.gov/cder/guidance/6714fnl.pdf.

Food and Drug Administration, Center for Drug Evaluation and Research. 2015. "Human immunodeficiency virus-1 infection: Developing antiretroviral drugs for treatment guidance for industry." https://www.fda.gov/media/86284/download

Food and Drug Administration, Center for Drug Evaluation and Research. 2017. "Chronic Hepatitis C virus infection: Developing direct-acting antiviral drugs for treatment guidance for industry." https://www.fda.gov/media/119657/download

Food and Drug Administration. 2019. "Code of federal regulations title 21, volume 1, subpart a section 3.2." https://www.accessdata.fda.gov/scripts/cdrh/cfdocs/cfcfr/cfrsearch.cfm?fr=3.2

Food and Drug Administration, Center for Drug Evaluation and Research. 2020. "Drug-drug interaction assessment of therapeutic proteins draft guidance for industry." https://www.fda.gov/media/140909/download

Food and Drug Administration, Office of Commissioner, Office of Clinical Policy and Programs, Office of Combination Products, Center for Drug Evaluation and Research, Center for Biologics Evaluation and Research, Center for Devices and Radiological Health. 2020. "Requesting FDA feedback on combination products, guidance for industry and FDA Staff." Docket Number FDA-2019-D-4739. https://www.fda.gov/regulatory-information/search-fda-guidance-documents/requesting-fda-feedback-combination-products

Herzyk, Danuta J. and Helen G. Haggerty. 2018. "Cancer Immunotherapy: Factors important for the evaluation of safety in nonclinical studies." *The AAPS Journal* Feb 7;20(2):28. doi: 10.1208/s12248-017-0184-3

Huang, S.-M., H. Zhao, J.-I. Lee, K. Reynolds, L. Zhang, R. Temple, and L. J. Lesko. 2010. "Therapeutic protein-drug interactions and implications for drug development." *Clin Pharmacol Ther.* Apr;87(4):497–503. doi: 10.1038/clpt.2009.308. Epub 2010 Mar 3. PMID: 20200513.

International Conference Harmonization. 2001. "S7 Guidance for industry safety pharmacology studies for human pharmaceuticals." https://www.fda.gov/media/72033/download

International Conference Harmonization. 2009. "M3(R2): Guidance on nonclinical safety studies for the conduct of human clinical trials and marketing authorization for pharmaceuticals." https://database.ich.org/sites/default/files/M3_R2_Guideline.pdf

International Conference Harmonization. 2009. "S9 Nonclinical evaluation for anticancer pharmaceuticals." https://www.ich.org/page/safety-guidelines

International Conference Harmonization. 2011. "Preclinical safety evaluation of biotechnology-derived pharmaceuticals S6 (R1)." https://database.ich.org/sites/default/files/S6_R1_Guideline_0.pdf

International Conference Harmonization. 2012. "M3(R2) Guideline: Guidance on nonclinical safety studies for the conduct of human clinical trials and marketing authorization for pharmaceuticals questions & answers (R2)." https://database.ich.org/sites/default/files/S9_Q%26As_Q%26As.pdf

International Conference Harmonization. 2018. 'S9 Guideline on nonclinical evaluation for anticancer pharmaceuticals - questions and answers. https://www.ich.org/page/safety-guidelines

International Conference Harmonization. 2019. "S11 Nonclinical safety testing in support of development of paediatric medicines core guideline." https://www.ich.org/page/safety-guidelines

Jordon, Stanley C., Klaus Kucher, Morten Bagger, Hans-Ulrich Hockey, Kristina Wagner, Noriko Ammerman, and Ashley Vo. 2020. "Intravenous immunoglobulin significantly reduces exposure of concomitantly administered anti-C5 monoclonal antibody tesidolumab." *Am J Transplant.* 2020;20:2581–2588. doi: 10.1111/ajt.15922

Keler, Tibor, Ed Halk, Laura Vitale, Tom O'Neill, Diann Blanset, Steven Lee, Mohan Srinivasan, Robert F. Graziano, Thomas Davis, Nils Lonberg, et al. 2003. "Activity and safety of CTLA-4 blockade combined with vaccines in cynomolgus macaques." *J Immunol.* 1;171(11):6251-9. doi: 10.4049/jimmunol.171.11.6251. PMID: 14634142.

Kieseier, Bernd C. 2011. "The mechanism of action of Interferon-β in relapsing multiple sclerosis." *CNS Drugs* 25:491–502. Jun 1;25(6):491–502. doi: 10.2165/11591110-000000000-00000. PMID: 21649449.

Kiessling, Peter, Rocio Lledo-Garcia, Shikiko Watanabe, Grant Langdon, Diep Tran, Muhammad Bari, Louis Christodoulou, Emma Jones, Graham Price, Bryan Smith, et al. 2017. "The FcRn inhibitor rozanolixizumab reduces human serum IgG concentration: A randomized phase 1 study." *Sci Transl Med.* 2017 Nov 1;9(414):eaan1208. doi: 10.1126/scitranslmed.aan1208. Erratum in: Sci Transl Med. 2017 Dec 6;9(419): PMID: 29093180.

Krieckaert, Charlotte L., Michael T. Nurmohamed, and Gerrit Jan Wolbink. 2012. "Methotrexate reduces immunogenicity in adalimumab treated rheumatoid arthritis patients in a dose dependent manner." *Ann Rheum Dis.* Nov;71(11):1914–1915. doi: 10.1136/annrheumdis-2012-201544. Epub 2012 May 14. PMID: 22586169.

Larkin, J., V. Chiarion-Sileni, R. Gonzalez, J. J. Grob, C. L. Cowey, C. D. Lao, D. Schadendorf, R. Dummer, M. Smylie, P. Rutkowski, et al. 2018. "Combined nivolumab and ipilimumab or monotherapy in untreated melanoma." *N Engl J Med.* Jul 2;373(1):23–34. doi: 10.1056/NEJMoa1504030. Epub 2015 May 31. Erratum in: N Engl J Med. 2018 Nov 29;379(22):2185. PMID: 26027431; PMCID: PMC5698905.

Le Vee, Marc, Valérie Lecureur, Bruno Stieger, and Olivier Fardel. 2009. "Regulation of drug transporter expression in human hepatocytes exposed to the proinflammatory cytokines tumor necrosis factor-alpha or interleukin-6." *Drug Metab Dispos.* 2009 Mar;37(3):685–693. doi: 10.1124/dmd.108.023630. Epub 2008 Dec 15. PMID: 19074973.

Lee, Jang-Ik, Lei Zhang, Angela Y. Men, Leslie A. Kenna, and Shiew-Mei Huang. 2010. "CYP-Mediated drug-therapeutic protein interactions: Clinical findings, proposed mechanisms and regulatory implications." *Clin Pharmacokinet.* 49:295–310. doi: 10.2165/11319980-000000000-00000. PMID: 20384392.

Morrissey, K. M., T. M. Yuraszeck, C.-C. Li, Y. Zhang, and S. Kasichayala. 2016. "Immunotherapy and novel combinations in oncology: Current landscape, challenges, and opportunities." *Clin Transl Sci.* 9(2):89–104. doi: 10.1111/cts.12391

Ponce, Rafael. "Preclinical support for combination therapy in the treatment of autoimmunity with atacicept." *Toxicol Pathol* 37(1) (January 2009):89–99. doi: 10.1177/0192623308329477

Rudick Richard A., William H. Stuart, Peter A. Calabresi, Christian Confavreux, Steven L. Galetta, Ernst-Wilhelm Radue, Fred D. Lublin, Bianca Weinstock-Guttman, Daniel R. Wynn, Frances Lynn, et al. 2006. "Natalizumab plus Interferon Beta-1a for Relapsing Multiple Sclerosis. *N Engl J Med* Mar 2;354(9):911–923. doi: 10.1056/NEJMoa044396. PMID: 16510745.

Sacaan, Aida S., Satoko Nonaka Hashida, and Nasir K. Khan. 2020. "Non-clinical combination toxicology studies: Strategy, examples and future perspective." *J Toxicol Sci.* 45(7):365–371. doi: 10.2131/jts.45.365. PMID: 32612005.

Schmitt, C., B. Kuhn, X. Zhang, A. Kivitz, and S. Grange. 2011. "Disease–drug–drug interaction involving tocilizumab and simvastatin in patients with rheumatoid arthritis." *Clin Pharmacol Ther* 89:735–740. doi: 10.1038/clpt.2011.35

Selby, Mark J., John J. Engelhardt, Robert J. Johnston, Li-Sheng Lu, Minhua Han, Kent Thudium, Dapeng Yao, Michael Quigley, Jose Valle, Changyu Wang, et al. 2016. "Preclinical development of ipilimumab and nivolumab combination immunotherapy: Mouse tumor models, in vitro functional studies, and cynomolgus macaque toxicology." *PLoS One.* Sep 9;11(9):e0161779. doi: 10.1371/journal.pone.0161779. Erratum in: PLoS One. 2016 Nov 18;11(11):e0167251. PMID: 27610613; PMCID: PMC5017747.

Suntharalingam, Ganesh, Meghan R. Perry, Stephen Ward, Stephen J. Brett, Andrew Castello-Cortes, Michael D. Brunner, and Nicki Panoskaltsis. 2006. "Cytokine storm in a phase 1 trial of the anti-CD28 monoclonal antibody TGN1412." *N Engl J Med.* 2006;355(10):1018–1028. doi: 10.1056/NEJMoa063842

Statkevich, P., C. Passey, J. Park, S. Saeger, A. Bello, A. Roy, S. G. Agrawal, M. Gupta. 2016. "Assessment of the immunogenicity of nivolumab (nivo) and ipilimumab (ipi) in combination and potential impact on safety and efficacy in patients with advanced melanoma." *Clin Pharmacol Ther.* 2016;99:S9.

Todd, Marque and Maggie Dempster. 2013. "Regulatory guidelines and their application in the nonclinical evaluation of biological medicines." In *Nonclinical Development of Novel Biologics, Biosimilars, Vaccines and Specialty Biologics.* doi: 10.1016/B978-0-12-394810-6.00002-2

Wang, Changyu, Kent B. Thudium, Minhua Han, Xi-Tao Wang, Haichun Huang, Diane Feingersh, Candy Garcia, Yi Wu, Michelle Kuhne, Mohan Srinivasan, et al. 2014. "In vitro characterization of the anti-PD-1 antibody nivolumab, BMS-936558, and in vivo toxicology in non-human primates." *Cancer Immunol Res.* 2(9):846–856. doi: 10.1158/2326-6066.CIR-14-0040

15

Due Diligence Regulatory and Preclinical Focus

Janet Nokleby

Janet Nokleby Consultant

CONTENTS

15.1 Introduction

Due diligence is a critical part of drug development. Before starting the review, both the company providing the data package and the review team need to understand the purpose of the review. The expectations for data and review may be different if the review is for acquisition of the sole asset or acquisition of the entire company or if the companies will share development of the asset. For the potential buyer, a thorough review of the data package can lead to the acquisition of important assets to add to the pipeline or elimination of molecules which may not be appropriate for acquisition. For the owner of the asset, a clear and thorough data package will provide a complete overview of the asset for the review team. Depending on the size and financial situation of the owner, a successful result from a due diligence review may impact the viability of the company. If the intended result of the review is to establish a collaborative development of the asset, the process of the review can help establish foundation for a working relationship for the companies.

This chapter will address the preclinical and regulatory aspects of the data and points to consider for a thorough due diligence review. In order to have a successful due diligence review, the companies should compile all the appropriate data and information together to understand the information that is available, strategy for development, and assessment of any gaps in the data. The goal of the owner of the asset should be to compile a data package that will fully inform the party considering the acquisition or deal of important issues and provide them with an in-depth understanding of the strategy for development and status of the program. This will allow the acquiring company to assess the thoroughness of the work

that has been done and assess what additional work is needed to support the program through the entire development life cycle. That assessment will help the acquiring company make informed decisions regarding the asset.

There are several factors which impact the type and content of a data package. Those factors include are the type of company that owns the asset, the type of asset under consideration, and the intended result of the review. Biotechnology products and emerging technology programs are very different from conventional pharmaceutical products. The team reviewing the data package needs to be familiar with the uniqueness of biotechnology products or the emerging technology. Also, the size of a company that owns the asset may impact the data that are available. A smaller company or university may have limited resources to support the asset and therefore may not have completed the same amount of work that a larger company would typically do. The owner of the data should also inform the reviewers if portions of the data have been redacted and the reasons for the redactions (e.g., confidentiality). If data that are redacted are critical for the assessment of the asset, the legal teams should get involved to work with the team to establish terms to allow mutually acceptable access to appropriate information. The reviewers must assess if the data that do exist are appropriate for the support of the asset at that stage of development.

15.2 Process Development/Manufacturing

When reviewing the manufacturing data, the reviewers should note important factors regarding the product which has been manufactured and understand the ability of that process to support manufacturing at a larger scale to supply large clinical trials and potentially support the commercial material. The reviewing team should be familiar with manufacturing for the specific modality under review. There are important differences in requirements and processes for differing modalities. For example, the process used to develop biotechnology products is unique for each product, and small changes to the process could lead to major differences in the final product.

It is important to note if the product is being manufactured at the company or if there is a contract manufacturing organization responsible for manufacturing. Also, it is important to understand the history of manufacturing (e.g., where the process was developed, transfer of the process, and if multiple sites were involved in manufacturing). When a contract manufacturing organization is involved, the agreement between the company and manufacturer should be available for review. It would be important for the reviewers to understand the conditions of that agreement to determine if it will be appropriate for the acquiring company to continue. When the company is manufacturing the product, the team must understand if the process is transferrable to another organization, especially if the intent of the review would lead to dissolving the company.

For early development assets, the review team should review the development of the formulation or cell line to determine if it is possible to use that process for large-scale production. If it is not possible to use that process for large-scale production, the review team should assess the impact of that on the potential development of the asset. In that case, the review team needs to understand the cost and potential timeline delay to develop a process that would be appropriate for large-scale production.

If the product has been manufactured at a larger scale to support larger trials, the data set should include appropriate data to support comparability of the various manufacturing runs. Should the comparability data not be available, it would be helpful to understand the comparability strategy in order to understand the needs to support future development of the product (reference comparability chapter 6). Additionally, the data should include what material was used for the toxicology studies and if that material appropriately represents what is used or is planned to be used in the clinical setting. The acquiring company must be able to assess if the formulation that exists is appropriate in the commercial setting. If the formulation for clinical trials is not intended for commercial use, the reviewers must understand if it is possible to produce a formulation that is commercially viable and to what degree a new formulation has been investigated.

15.3 Pharmacology

The preclinical setting provides unique challenges for biotechnology products as these are engineered to interact with a human biologic target, and nonclinical models may not be relevant to the target or disease in humans. The data package should include the relevant data to provide support for the preclinical species that were tested. A rationale should be provided for the types of studies that were done and provide explanation for studies that were not required to have been done. An overview of the strategy to support the choices of the preclinical studies, dose levels, and study designs should be provided. If there are several potential indications for the asset, the pharmacology studies should be done in appropriate models to support the potential indications. The reviewers should assess the completeness of the pharmacology data that have been included in the package. The data should clearly indicate the institution that has completed the work. It is important for the reviewers to know if the data are available electronically or in laboratory notebooks, if the data are available to transfer should the asset be acquired and if there are completed reports of the studies that were done. Also, a list of publications discussing the asset should be available. This information will support future filings for clinical trials or potential marketing applications.

15.4 Pharmacokinetics

Important information regarding the pharmacodynamics and pharmacokinetic behavior of the asset should be provided in addition to any pharmacokinetic and toxicokinetic data. The data necessary for supporting a program are highly dependent on the type of molecule that is under development. As with other types of nonclinical data, there may be limitations varying requirements for testing based on the modality or species specificity of the asset. Any of these limitations should be explained by the owner of the asset.

The pharmacokinetic data in the preclinical species are very helpful in understanding the results of the toxicology studies. The preclinical reviewer should look at the drug exposure data in relation to any findings in the toxicology studies. The safety margin should support clinical development, and differences in exposure in the toxicology species should be explained. In the absence of clinical data, the preclinical pharmacokinetic data can be useful to predict human exposure in the clinical studies and are important in establishing the initial clinical dose. The pharmacokinetic data should provide adequate information to justify the initial clinical dose and dose escalating strategy.

15.5 Toxicology

When reviewing the toxicology data, there are many important factors to understand. As noted above, it is important to understand rationales for the selection of the preclinical species for the toxicology studies. Some disease states require special toxicology studies or testing in model animals with disease. If this is the case for the asset in question, the data package should include rationales for special toxicology studies and the type of animal used in the toxicology package. Biologics are evaluated on a case-by-case basis, and the supporting toxicology package is customized based on the properties of the molecule. The reviewer must be aware of the requirements of the applicable guidance documents to aid in understanding the expectations of the health authorities. Before reviewing the data, the reviewers should be familiar with the appropriate International Council for Harmonisation (ICH) guidance such as ICHS6 safety guidance and ICH multidisciplinary guidance M3 (2010, 2012).

If the asset is either approaching the first clinical trials or in clinical trials, the toxicology data must appropriately assess the potential risks of the asset to support clinical development. The toxicity profile of the molecule should be characterized to the extent possible in the studies that have been done. The preclinical reviewer should work closely with the clinical reviewer to understand the safety-related events that have been noted clinically and closely review the toxicology data for relevant related observations in the toxicology studies. In the event that similar events were noted in the toxicology studies, the reviewers should pay special attention to the description of those events in the study reports. The preclinical reviewer should also work with the regulatory affairs reviewer to understand any issues or concerns noted in the correspondence with health authorities and the impact of those concerns on the development timeline or future clinical development of the asset.

15.6 Immunogenicity

The immunogenicity profile of a biotechnology product should be fully described. Data investigating the presence of antidrug antibodies and an assessment of the presence of antibodies on exposure should be available. Antidrug antibodies should be assessed for the impact on the drug levels, including the ability of the antibody to neutralize the drug. The data to represent the validation of the assays should be available for the reviewers. All assays should be validated to the extent necessary to support the preclinical and clinical programs. It is critical that the appropriate assays were done to adequately characterize the immunogenicity response in the preclinical studies. Although the presence of antibodies in a toxicology species does not predict the development of antibodies in the human, the immunogenicity data in the preclinical species are critical to assess the toxicology profile of biotechnology products.

15.7 Regulatory

All regulatory documents should be available for review. The initial Clinical Trial Application (CTA) or Investigational New Drug (IND) application provides useful information as to the documents that were included and the assessment of the preclinical package. These documents provide the initial rationale for the first indication to be investigated for the asset. The clinical sections provide insight as to the initial assessment of the potential clinical risks of the asset and proposed safety monitoring and mitigation.

Communications with health authorities provide insight into the issues or concerns of the reviewing agency. The reviewers from the acquiring company will need to review these documents to understand if the concerns raised by the health authorities were adequately addressed. Additionally, these documents will outline any commitments that that company has made to health authorities. The acquiring company should carefully review any commitments to ensure that these are reasonable and can be completed during the development of the asset.

If the company had any discussions with relevant health authorities regarding the preclinical data package (e.g., pre-IND or pre-CTA meetings), any minutes and communications of those discussions should be included in the data package. Those discussions aid the reviewers in understanding the rationale for the work that has been done and will help the reviewer understand concerns or the level of comfort the health authority has with the asset. As noted above, there may also be specific commitments that have been made to the health authority during meetings. Reviewers should pay special attention to those commitments as the health authority will expect that commitment to be fulfilled by the acquiring company.

Recognizing that factors outside of the asset in question may also play a role in the development of a program, general information regarding the company may be helpful for the reviewers. A list of relevant standard operating procedures, company policies, or training manuals that impact the program under review should be provided. To the extent that such documents exist, the company should make available any documents regarding regulatory inspections. The companies should be prepared to discuss general information regarding previous regulatory actions (i.e., review timeline and history, hold order discussions and documents, inspection documents, warning letters). The general relationship of the company with health authorities may be important for the program development.

15.8 Special Considerations

Novel therapies such as blood products, vaccines, and cell and gene therapies present many unique challenges. Often times, the preclinical package is limited due to the type of therapy, especially if the asset is an emerging technology as is the case with many cell or gene therapy assets. With assets in these areas, it is especially important to review any communications with health authorities as it is more likely that companies have reached out to discuss complicating aspects of development with health authorities (pre-IND communications). The developing company should be able to outline the development strategy and provide appropriate justification for the strategy.

Some types of therapies require companion diagnostic tests. The reviewers should be aware of the guidelines applicable in each region addressing these diagnostics. Specifically, the United States has requirements that other regions do not (https://www.fda.gov/medical-devices/vitro-diagnostics/companion-diagnostics). The strategy for development of the companion diagnostic needs to be outlined and any communications with the US Food and Drug Administration (USFDA) should be included in the data package. The development of the asset can be delayed if the diagnostic test is not considered and appropriate data are not acquired during the clinical trials.

The team should also understand if commercialization of the asset will require a device or combination with another molecule. If that is required, the data for that device or combination product should be available and reviewed. As with diagnostics, delays in development can occur if the development of the device or combination product have not been fully considered and implemented.

TABLE 15.1

Due Diligence Questionnaire

No.	Information Requested	Response

General Information

1   Describe the candidate's local reputation, as checked through the local regulatory authority and/or local consultants prior to the due diligence. Seek clarification of any findings with candidate during due diligence

2   Assess the candidate's knowledge of local regulations and its ability to develop and utilize local regulatory intelligence

3   Assess the candidate's familiarity with and understanding of the international regulatory environment

4   Describe the candidate's understanding of the potential challenges confronting regulatory approval of those products

5   Has the candidate's regulatory function been inspected or reviewed by a regulatory authority? If "yes," summarize the results of that inspection or review or provide a copy of the regulatory authority's report or findings. Assess the implications of the results on the candidate's qualifications

Regulatory Function

6   If the candidate has not provided written policies or procedures with respect to each of the following, describe in detail the candidate's procedures with respect to:
    1. Compilation, finalization, and submission of marketing authorization applications;
    2. Acquisition of local registration information;
    3. Completion of local registration application forms;
    4. Receipt and dissemination of regulatory authority questions during the marketing authorization application review period, including the submission of responses to such questions;
    5. Receipt of marketing authorizations; and
    6. Submission of Good Manufacturing Practice (GMP) certification documentation

7   Assess the candidate's working relationship with the local regulatory authority, including the candidate's access to and rapport with agency staff

8   Assess whether the candidate's past experience in seeking or obtaining marketing authorization for medicinal products indicates that the candidate will be able to meet expectations. State the facts upon which you rely and how those facts support your assessment

9   Describe the candidate's experience as the marketing authorization holder (MAH) for medicinal products, including:
    1. The products for which the candidate has been the MAH;
    2. The dates such marketing authorizations were granted and, if no longer held, the dates they were terminated or transferred;
    3. The nature of such products (e.g., small molecule, biological, device, etc.);
    4. The indications for which such products were approved;
    5. The geographical territories in which such authorizations were held; and
    6. Any significant regulatory actions taken with respect to such products (for example, the termination or restriction of the marketing authorization; a product recall; an instruction or recommendation with respect to an urgent safety matter; etc.), the reasons given therefor, and how the candidate responded to such regulatory action

10 Does the candidate typically prepare regulatory filings itself?

11 What assistance can the candidate provide in preparation of the regulatory filings?

12 Describe the candidate's capabilities and expertise to provide Regulatory Chemistry, Manufacturing and Controls (CMC) and/or Qualified Person (QP) support (local technical expertise, release testing requirements, GMP requirements) in developing a dossier. (As applicable, cite to any relevant documents provided by the candidate, such as organizational charts, staff Curriculum Vitae (CVs), and procedural documents)

(Continued)

TABLE 15.1 (*Continued*)

Due Diligence Questionnaire

No.	Information Requested	Response
13	Describe the candidate's average times for approval of large and small molecules and how this compares with industry expectations	
Wrap Up		
14	Has the candidate been subject to any regulatory enforcement action not already described in response to another question? If so, describe such enforcement action, the reasons therefor, and the candidate's response to such action	
15	Provide any additional information not otherwise contained in this due diligence report that you believe is relevant to the assessment of this candidate	

15.9 Organization

Many organizations have developed checklists to aid in the due diligence review. Table 15.1 is an example of a basic checklist. While these can be very useful in identifying general areas of the review, the reviewers should use appropriate discretion to expand the generic questions to fit the specific conditions of the asset under consideration.

The team should also be aware of competitors or approved molecules for the desired indication. The USFDA and European Medicines Agency publish summaries of the scientific review of approved therapies. The Summary Basis of Approval is published by the USFDA on the website (https://www.accessdata.fda.gov). For drugs approved in the European Union, the European Public Assessment Report is published on the website (https://www.ema.europa.eu/en/medicines/field_ema_web_categories%253Aname_field/Human/ema_group_types/ema_medicine). Team members should review those websites for health authority assessments of those molecules. Those documents are important to understand the strategy of the asset under review. If there are no competitors or approved molecules in the indication, the team can still use similar types of documents to help assess the proposed strategy for the asset, but the team should understand what is unique about the asset and how that will impact the development strategy.

15.10 Summary

While there is no one checklist or document that will cover the preclinical package required for all assets, there are many things that reviewers can look to in order to help with the due diligence review of an asset. Reviewers can look to precedent for approved molecules in a similar indication or similar modality as to guide them to assess the completeness of the data package. Documented discussions with health authorities are invaluable tools to assess the level of concern the agency has with the asset and if the developing company has developed strategies to address those concerns.

Ultimately, each molecule is unique. The owner of the asset facilitates a successful due diligence review by being transparent and providing as much of the documentation as is possible for review. The members of the acquiring team should educate themselves on the uniqueness of the asset under review, thoroughly review the information presented, and prepare questions to address the gaps that arise during the review. Successful due diligence reviews are collaborative and designed to help the acquiring company receive the information that is needed to make informed decisions.

REFERENCES

European Medicines Agency. Medicines. https://www.ema.europa.eu/en/medicines/field_ema_web_categories%253Aname_field/Human/ema_group_types/ema_medicine

International Council for Harmonisation. 2010. Guidance on Nonclinical Safety Studies for the Conduct of Human Clinical Trials and Marketing Authorization for Pharmaceuticals M3 (R2). https://database.ich.org/sites/default/files/M3_R2__Guideline.pdf

International Council for Harmonisation. 2012. Preclinical Safety Evaluation of Biotechnology-Derived Pharmaceuticals S6 (R1). https://database.ich.org/sites/default/files/S6_R1_Guideline_0.pdf

U.S. Food & Drug Administration. 2018. Companion Diagnostics. https://www.fda.gov/medical-devices/vitro-diagnostics/companion-diagnostics

U.S. Food & Drug Administration. Drugs@FDA: FDA-Approved Drugs. https://www.accessdata.fda.gov/scripts/cder/daf/

16

Cytokine Assessments

Florence G. Burleson, Stefanie C.M. Burleson, and Gary R. Burleson
Burleson Research Technologies, Inc.

CONTENTS

16.1 Cytokines: An Introduction

Cytokines are low molecular weight extracellular glycoproteins and polypeptides synthesized primarily by T cells, neutrophils, and macrophages although they can be produced by nearly all nucleated cells (Ferreira et al., 2018; Lin and Leonard, 2019). Cytokines serve as immunological mediators with critical roles in facilitating the cellular communication underlying signal-dependent immune responses and the regulation of immune cell homeostasis. They serve to orchestrate elaborate yet targeted and regulated responses, fundamental to multitudinous biological processes including both innate and adaptive responses to antigen, protective responses conferred by vaccines, stem cell differentiation, and embryonic development (Dinarello, 2007; Ferreira et al., 2018; Lin and Leonard, 2019).

Cytokine-mediated signaling may be autocrine (in which cytokines released by a particular cell bind to their own surface receptors), paracrine (in which cytokines released by a particular cell bind surface receptors of neighboring cells), or endocrine (in which cytokines are released into the circulation to affect a more systemic response upon binding surface receptors of distant targets) (Altan-Bonnet, 2019).

Cytokines interact with cells bearing appropriate receptors on the cell surface, and the receptor expression differs based on cell type, cell maturation status, and cell activation status (Burleson et al., 2015). Cytokine-receptor interactions elicit responses via initiation of intracellular signaling cascades and downstream gene activation, resulting in the growth, differentiation, recruitment, activation, deactivation, generation of cellular products, or death of specific cell subsets. The highly varied and numerous responses actuated by cytokine–receptor interactions are complex as the nature of these interactions are promiscuous, in that cytokine ligands are capable of interacting with multiple receptors and receptors may bind multiple ligands; functionally distinct, in that the genes that may be activated within a particular cell by a specific cytokine may differ from those activated within another cell type; and interactive, in that the presence of certain cytokines may amplify or suppress the effects of other cytokines (Toews, 2001; Burleson et al., 2015). Furthermore, certain cytokines not only function as classic ligands for specific receptors but also serve additional roles as transcription factors by binding DNA (as is the case with the N-terminal amino acids of the IL-1 α precursor) or repress transcription via chromatin binding (as observed with the N-terminal domains of IL-33) (Dinarello, 2007).

Cytokines include interleukins (ILs), interferons (IFNs), the tumor necrosis factor (TNF) family, colony stimulating factors (CSFs), growth factors, as well as chemokines; many with well-characterized specific functions and some with functions that have not yet been fully elucidated (Dinarello, 2007; Le et al., 2004; Ono et al., 2003; Turner et al., 2014). Some cytokine family members primarily function as modulators of proinflammatory or anti-inflammatory responses, some serve as lymphocyte growth factors, and others contribute to the adaptive immune response to an antigen; and although a multitude of individual responses are recognized, there is also notable redundancy in the function (Dinarello, 2007). The ILs comprise 33 members, with a third members of the IL-1 family. Functional overlap within the IL-1 family includes proinflammatory activity. The IL-6 family of cytokines induces the production of hepatic acute phase proteins. The IL-10 family includes interleukins that exhibit anti-inflammatory immune responses (Dinarello, 2007; Turner et al., 2014). The IFN Type I, Type II, and Type III family members exhibit redundancies with regard to proinflammatory and antiviral abilities (Ferreira et al., 2018; Abbas et al., 2014; Ank et al., 2006; Parham and Janeway, 2009; Platanias, 2005). The TNF family of cytokines includes over 20 constituents with individual functions yet a notable overlap in roles such as those involved in cell death. CSFs including IL-3, granulocyte-CSF, granulocyte-macrophage CSF (GM-CSF), and macrophage CSF also have closely related functions yet remain individual gene products with specific receptors. In addition, the many members of the chemokine family orchestrate the migration of cells from the blood compartment into the tissues (Dinarello, 2007; Turner et al., 2014).

This redundancy in the cytokine function within and across cytokine families is beneficial when viewed in the context of host survival. It is unlikely that a few or even a dozen cytokines would have had the capacity to mount a protective response when met with a lethal challenge. Upon facing an overwhelming invasion, the host will turn on most cytokine genes and, in doing so, mobilize multiple mechanisms to quickly and efficiently overcome the challenge.

16.1.1 Intended and Unintended Actions of Cytokines

Cytokine signaling networks are highly regulated, as aberrant or chronic activation of signaling pathways have the ability to disrupt homeostatic conditions and potentiate immunopathology and disease. Dysregulated cytokine signaling predicates a multitude of pathological and biological processes, including autoinflammatory disease, autoimmune disease, cytokine storms, and particular cancers (Rani et al., 2019; Chousterman et al., 2017; O'Shea and Lipsky, 2002; Burleson et al., 2015). Herein lies the conundrum, as cytokine responses are necessary for protection against antigenic challenge and host survival, yet they may also effectuate or worsen disease.

IFNγ, for instance, is essential in host defense and control of acute infections caused by influenza viruses, *Mycobacterium tuberculosis*, *Listeria monocytogenes*, lymphocytic choriomeningitis virus, vaccinia virus, and ectromelia virus, among others, *yet* is implicated in exacerbation of autoimmune and autoinflammatory responses (Burleson et al., 2015; Cytokines in the Balance, 2019; Toews, 2001; Buchmeier and Schreiber, 1985; Huang et al., 1993; Karupiah et al., 1993; Kolls, 2013; Sarawar et al., 1994; Spellberg and Edwards, 2001; Wille et al., 1989). Many patients diagnosed with autoimmune or autoinflammatory diseases have gene expression signatures related to IFN signaling (Barrat et al., 2019). Indeed, given the capacity for IFNγ to augment autoimmune disease, clinicians must exercise caution if selecting IFN as a treatment for hepatitis C virus (HCV)–infected patients with a history of autoimmune disease. Furthermore, occasional cases documenting the development of *de novo* autoimmune disease in patients with no prior history have been observed following treatment with IFN (Silva, 2012).

Cytokine storm is a potentially lethal phenomenon stemming from uncontrolled cellular activation and cytokine release. Severe cytokine storms are typically characterized by massive and sudden systemic inflammation resulting in tissue damage, edema, multiple organ dysfunction, and hypotension. Although the precise mechanisms underlying the generation of a cytokine storm are poorly understood, it is thought that highly virulent pathogens and superantigens, which can cause nonspecific mass T cell activation, are capable of initiating such activation (Canna and Behrens, 2012; Iwasaki and Medzhitov, 2011; Morens and Fauci, 2007; Tisoncik et al., 2012). Cytokine storms may also be initiated by superagonists such as TGN1412, a humanized anti-CD28 antibody manufactured by TeGenero that had undergone a Phase I clinical trial with the intent to treat B cell chronic lymphocytic leukemia and autoimmune disease, respectively, via expansion of T cell and regulatory T cell populations. During the clinical trial, however, it was found to circumvent T cell receptor (TCR)–mediated activation and activate T cells via coreceptor, CD28. Although TGN1412 was seemingly innocuous in nonhuman primate studies (NHPs), nonspecific T cell activation led to the hospitalization of six healthy male volunteers due to multiorgan failure resulting from a cytokine storm (Burleson et al., 2015; St. Clair, 2008; Horvath and Milton, 2009).

As with proinflammatory cytokines, cytokines involved in postchallenge healing, maintenance, and repair are no exception to the dual nature of cytokine function and the importance of balance in promoting homeostasis. Vascular endothelial growth factor (VEGF) is an example of a cytokine involved in angiogenic healing and repair processes, and yet, VEGF contributes to key aspects of cancer tumorigenesis (Goel, 2013). IL-7, best-known as a homeostatic cytokine that contributes to the development, maintenance, and survival of T and B lymphocytes in lymphoid tissues, may also precipitate leukemic transformation and survival in T or B cell acute lymphoblastic leukemia due to dysregulation of the IL-7Rα cytokine receptor in lymphoid progenitor cells. Divergent IL-7 and IL-7R signaling has also been observed in solid tumors including those arising in breast and prostate cancers, in which an elevated IL-7 expression is associated with poorer patient outcomes (Barata et al., 2019).

Owing to the beneficial as well as potentially pernicious effects of cytokine signaling, a thorough understanding of the pathways involved in health, disease, and dysfunction is of utmost importance.

16.2 Cytokines in Disease States

The fact that cytokines can contribute to pathology was acknowledged early in the characterization of their actions when IL-1 was described as an "endogenous pyrogen" (Duff and Durum, 1953). Since then, IL-1 and other cytokines have been shown to contribute to pathologies in a wide range of human diseases including autoinflammatory diseases, rheumatoid arthritis (RA), and neuroinflammation.

Cytokines have also been shown to be important in contributing to the pathogenesis of inflammatory bowel disease (IBD), including ulcerative colitis and Crohn's disease, through regulation of intestinal inflammation. The disease progression and tissue damage in IBD resulting from the imbalance between proinflammatory (TNF, IFN-γ, IL-6, IL-12, IL-21, IL-23, IL-17), and anti-inflammatory cytokines (IL-10, TGFβ, IL-35) limits the resolution of inflammation (Guan and Zhang, 2017).

Rheumatic diseases which include RA, juvenile idiopathic arthritis, and psoriatic arthritis as well as others are characterized by increased release of proinflammatory cytokines, including IL-6, IL-17, IL-21, IL-22, and IL-23, and down-regulation of anti-inflammatory cytokines, such as IL-10 (Woś and Tabarkiewicz, 2021). RA is a chronic and systemic autoimmune disease attacking multiple joints. Production of cytokines contributes to the pathogenesis of RA and systemic consequences that affect multiple other systems, including cardiovascular, pulmonary, psychological, and bone. IL-1α/β and TNF-α have been shown to initiate signaling pathways that result in activation of mesenchymal cells, recruitment of immune cells, and the activation of synoviocytes that play a crucial role in the pathogenesis of this disease and results in activation of cytokines (e.g., TNF-α, IL-1, IL-6, and IL-8), contributing to synovium inflammation and increased angiogenesis (Alam and Bukhari, 2017).

Multiple sclerosis (MS) is a demyelinating autoimmune neurological disease in which an abnormal expression of specific cytokines contributes to pathology. TNF is one of the cytokines that has been shown to play a pivotal role in MS, and there has been demonstrated involvement of TNF in the immune dysregulation, demyelination, and neuroinflammatory responses that contribute to this disease (Bullita et al., 2020; Fresegna et al., 2020).

Induction of proinflammatory cytokines and microglia inflammasome activation with IL-1 production in the brain have been shown to contribute to the pathology in brain tissue, resulting in neuroinflammation and neurodegeneration (Mantovani et al., 2019).

While there is a wealth of information on the contribution of various cytokines to disease states, it should be noted that it is challenging to determine diagnostic cutoff values for cytokines. Such a determination requires identification of abnormal levels and the establishment of a normal range. Normal ranges are typically calculated in a given study as a mean or median value with the application of two standard deviations to obtain lower and upper limits and generally only apply to the population of interest. This is not necessarily diagnostically reliable as individual variability in cytokine levels, cytokine release, and downstream effects are dependent on a number of parameters that include activating signals, cell targets, age, and physiological factors (Zhou et al., 2010; Kim et al., 2011). While cytokines have been evaluated in disease states and correlations of abnormal profiles have been established, cytokine cutoff values as biomarkers of disease have not been well studied. To determine clinically relevant diagnostic cutoff values that can differentiate "normal" from "abnormal," more studies are needed with healthy subjects from various populations, under conditions that control for factors contributing to the release and action of the cytokines of interest, while taking into account cytokine assay platform differences (Monastero and Pentyala, 2017).

16.3 Cytokines as Therapeutics, Therapeutic Targets, and Biomarkers

The cytokine network is important in the control of immune responses and regulation of the immune system. Cytokines and their receptors are variably released or expressed by multiple cell types and form a complex functional system that modulates the interaction of the effector and target cells as well as the magnitude and duration of activation. Cytokine research has introduced therapies for several diseases. These therapies are generally based on the administration of (1) the recombinant cytokine alone (e.g., CSFs and IFNs) or as a fusion protein, (2) molecules that stimulate certain cytokine pathways, or (3) therapeutics that decrease upregulated cytokines, such as the anti-TNF therapies in the treatment of RA or receptor blocking therapies (Berraondo et al., 2019; Silk and Margolin, 2019; Vilcek and Feldmann, 2004).

16.3.1 Therapeutic Use of Cytokines

As cytokines mediate proliferative signals and immune activation, they have long held promise as therapeutic agents. Some of the cytokine therapies examined have included IFNs, IL-2, IL-7, IL-10, IL-12, IL-15, IL-21, and GM-CSF (Conlon et al., 2019; Li et al., 2018; Silk and Margolin, 2019). IFNs are the first line of defense against viral infections and are key cytokines in establishing an antiviral response. The standard of care for chronic HCV infection between 2001 and 2011 was pegylated IFNs and ribavirin (Yau and Yoshida, 2014).

IFNβ therapies were the first approved, and still widely used, disease-modifying therapies for MS. When produced in high amounts, IFN-β has been shown to upregulate anti-inflammatory cytokines such as IL-4 and IL-10, while down-regulating proinflammatory cytokines including TNFα, IFNγ, and IL-2. In MS, where anti-inflammatory cytokines are reduced, the administration of IFNβ can upregulate anti-inflammatory cytokines and provide a beneficial effect (Dumitrescu et al., 2018, Kasper and Reder, 2014).

The use of IL-2 family cytokines, including IL-2, IL-7, IL-15, and IL-2, to activate immune responses in cancer patients is an important area of current cancer immunotherapy research. The infusion of IL-2 in patients with metastatic melanoma and renal cell carcinoma was the first successful immunotherapy and demonstrated that, under certain conditions, the immune system could eradicate the tumor cells (Sim and Radvanyi, 2014).

IL-11 interacts with a variety of hemopoietic and nonhemopoietic cells and stimulates proliferation and maturation of bone marrow stem cells and megakaryocytes. Recombinant human IL-11 (oprelvekin) was FDA approved in 1998 to treat severe thrombocytopenia caused by chemotherapy (Metcalfe et al., 2020).

Cytokines are potent and complex immune modulators. Owing to their pleiotropic effects on multiple cell types, there can be significant toxicities, and cytokine monotherapies are often blunt instruments. However, there is also promise in deploying cytokines as part of combination strategies with other monoclonal and gene cancer therapies, as additional efforts are expanded in confining the action of the cytokines to the site of action to avoid systemic inflammatory reactions. (Berraondo et al., 2019).

16.3.2 Cytokines and Their Receptors as Therapeutic Targets

As previously discussed, RA is a systemic autoimmune disease that culminates in joint destruction and disability. Proinflammatory cytokines (such as IL-1α/β, TNFα, IL-6) play a central role in the pathogenesis of RA. Many cytokines are involved in RA, including IL-1 α/β, TNF-α, IL-6, IL-17, and GM-CSF. TNF and IL-6 play a central role in the pathogenesis of RA and are both well-established targets in RA treatment (Alam et al., 2017; Noack and Miossec, 2017; Li et al., 2019). A healthy human IL-6 serum level is normally less than 4 pg/ml; however, in cases of RA and chronic inflammatory diseases, serum IL-6 can be elevated between 10 and 100 pg/ml or more (Narazaki et al., 2017). "*Table 16.1 shows*

approved disease-modifying RA drugs that target IL-1, TNF, and the IL-6 receptor."

Atopic dermatitis is a chronic, systemic, and inflammatory disease affecting the skin and is characterized by itching and redness. Atopic dermatitis is associated with an increase in IL-4 and IL-13, contributing to tissue inflammation and epidermal barrier dysfunction. Monoclonal antibodies targeting the cytokines and their receptors provide potential for therapeutic intervention. In March 2017, dupilumab, a human anti-IL4Ra antibody, was approved for the treatment of moderate to severe atopic dermatitis. Lebrikizumab and tralokinumab, anti-IL-13 monoclonal antibodies which bind different IL-13 epitopes, are in late-stage clinical trials (Moyle et al., 2019).

16.3.3 Modulation of Cytokine Pathways

Given the role of cytokine pathways signaling in cytokine effector functions and the numerous pathological conditions that can result from activation, there is general interest in the development of therapeutics that modulate cytokine pathways and inhibit the activation. Activity can be blocked at multiple points (1) by preventing the initial cell surface protein–protein interactions (binding of gp130) or (2) by targeting the components of the signal transduction pathway in the cell. The Janus kinase (JAK)/signal transducer and activator of transcription (STAT) pathway is the best studied cytokine activation pathway; however, alternate signaling pathways include nuclear factor-κB (NF-kB), mitogen-activated protein kinase (MAPK), and phosphatidylinositol 3-kinase (PI3K). JAK inhibitors, including tofacitinib and baricitinib, are used to treat RA. Nonspecific JAK inhibition can result in opportunistic viral infections. These pathways provide therapeutic opportunities for cytokine modulation with more selective targeting of the individual kinases and STAT activity (Metcalfe et al., 2020).

TABLE 16.1

Approved Disease-Modifying Drugs for Rheumatoid Arthritis Targeting Cytokines/Cytokine Receptors

Biologic Drug	Target	Mode of Action	Other Approved Indications
Anakinra (Kineret)	IL-1	And IL-1α and IL-1β and IL-1RA	Deficiency of the IL-1–receptor antagonist (DIRA; cryopyrin-associated periodic syndromes)
Etanercept (Enbrel)	TNF-α	Recombinant fusion protein of TNF-R moieties linked to human IgG1 Fc—binds TNF-α	Ankylosing spondylitis, plaque psoriasis, psoriatic arthritis, polyarticular juvenile idiopathic arthritis, active arthritis
Infliximab (Remicade)	TNF-α	Chimeric antibody to TNF-α—binds TNF-α	Crohn's disease, ulcerative colitis, ankylosing spondylitis, plaque psoriasis, psoriatic arthritis, idiopathic pulmonary fibrosis
Adalimumab (Humira)	TNF-α	Human monoclonal antibody to TNF-α—binds TNF-α	Crohn's disease, ulcerative colitis, ankylosing spondylitis, plaque psoriasis, psoriatic arthritis, juvenile idiopathic arthritis
Golimumab (Simponi)	TNF-α	Human monoclonal antibody to TNF-α—binds TNF-α	Ankylosing spondylitis, psoriatic arthritis, polyarticular juvenile idiopathic arthritis
Certolizumab (Cimzia)	TNF-α	Pegylated humanized antibody Fab' fragment of TNF-α monoclonal antibody—binds TNF-α	Ankylosing spondylitis, psoriatic arthritis, polyarticular juvenile idiopathic arthritis
Tocilizumab (Actemra)	IL-6R	Humanized monoclonal antibody to IL-6R—inhibits IL-6 signaling	Giant cell arteritis, polyarticular juvenile idiopathic arthritis, systemic juvenile idiopathic arthritis, cytokine release syndrome
Sarilumab (Kevzara)	IL-6R	Human recombinant monoclonal antibody to IL-6 receptor—inhibits IL-6 signaling	None

16.4 Cytokine Assessments

While additional work is required for diagnostic cutoff values for disease states, cytokines are measured in pharmacokinetic assessments or as pharmacodynamic markers in preclinical and clinical studies to confirm exposure, establish target doses and dosing regimens, and provide proof of mechanism/efficacy or safety. Cytokine assessments also provide valuable information on immune activation and mechanisms in the course of nonclinical and clinical studies. For example, if an increase in cytokines or infusion reaction is anticipated based on specific product attributes, serum or plasma cytokine measurements are included in the design of toxicology studies. For these evaluations, blood is generally collected before dosing to provide cytokine baseline measurements and at multiple timepoints after dosing up to at least 24 hours. IL-6 is a commonly elevated cytokine in infusion reactions although cytokines in general can be increased (Ramani et al., 2015; Mease et al., 2017).

Cytokines can also serve as biomarkers of potential drug toxicity (Tarrant, 2010; Lim et al., 2019). Although a number of biomarkers are capable of allowing correlations to the degree of tissue injury due to drug toxicity, cytokines do not always allow direct correlation. In the event that drug-related toxicity is targeted to a specific mechanism or organ system, it may be possible for early markers of inflammatory processes to correlate with toxicity and subsequent tissue injury. If multiple mechanisms or organ systems are involved, however, individual mechanisms or sites may affect cytokine values, resulting in difficulty attaining specificity for a particular inflammatory biomarker. Examples of circumstances that may preclude the identification of a particular biomarker following drug administration include a reduction in leukocyte numbers, resulting in alterations in cytokine production; renal or liver injury, resulting in changes in clearance; or liver damage, resulting in reduced production of binding proteins. In addition, subacute or chronic disease states coupled with multidose therapies may contribute to cyclical cytokine fluctuations that may not directly support the resulting related histology. Yet, under the correct circumstances, cytokine biomarkers to detect toxicity may be quite successful, as is the case for the measurement of serum IFN-γ to detect immunostimulation following administration of IV recombinant human IL-12. Human, cynomolgus macaque, and mouse data show correlations between recombinant IL-12–induced serum IFN-γ modulation and resulting tissue toxicity and death. Such biomarkers that precede pathology and predict patient outcomes are clearly valuable in the clinical setting and could contribute to risk assessment and dosing strategies (Tarrant, 2010).

16.4.1 Cytokine Release Assays

Cytokine assessments are important for therapies that modulate the immune system. Immunotherapies including monoclonal antibodies, chimeric antigen receptor modified T-cell(CAR-T), and bispecific T-cell receptor engaging (BiTE) have the potential to result in undesirable immune activation such as cytokine release syndrome (CRS) and its associated pathologies (Shimabukuro-Vornhagen et al., 2018). CRS is a rapid systemic response where proinflammatory cytokines, including IL-6, IL-8, TNF-α, and IFN-γ, are released from immune cells. CRS can occur at first exposure or upon subsequent administration of the therapeutic, and it is important to identify the potential risk of CRS prior to administration in humans.

Cytokine release assays (CRAs) have been developed and are routinely used in the preclinical safety assessment of new therapeutic monoclonal antibodies and therapies for hazard identification of CRS and its associated pathologies. Various formats are used for CRAs and include different cells (e.g., whole blood, human peripheral blood mononuclear cells (PBMCs), endothelial cells) and different cell densities. While the selection of CRA test concentrations can present difficulties as *in vitro* systems do not have the capacity to account for *in vivo* metabolism, tissue distribution, and the possibility of long-term exposure, concentrations should be selected in the range of those anticipated for use in clinical and preclinical studies. With regard to the investigation of postdose acute effects, the intended human dose level predicted maximum concentration (Cmax) may serve to inform assay concentrations (Brennan and Kiessling, 2017).

The presentation of the monoclonal antibody may be solution-based, captured to beads, or in plate-bound formats, and may include specific modifications to simulate the intended target populations. The selection of assay format and cytokines to be measured are dependent on the target and mechanism of action of the antibody tested although several antibodies that are associated with CRS increase IL-6, IL-8, and/or TNF-α in the CRA. There can be significant interdonor variability in CRA, but there is no current recommendation on the number of individual donors to be tested as this may also vary by assay read-out and performance (Finco et al., 2014; Grimaldi et al., 2016). Following the incubation of the test antibody and the cells, supernatants are collected, generally within 24–48 hours, and the concentration of cytokines determined. This is typically performed using a multiplex cytokine assay that allows the simultaneous determination of multiple cytokines in the same assay plate.

"Table 16.2 provides an overview of CRAs."

While there is no single recommended CRA method, the February 2020 US FDA Draft Guidance on Nonclinical Safety Evaluation of the Immunotoxic Potential of Drugs and Biologics Guidance for Industry recommends that the assessment of CRS potential be performed using unstimulated human cells in both plate-bound and soluble formats. CRA can also be performed using NHP cells; however, species differences and the mode of action need to be considered. (Grimaldi et al., 2016; Römer et al., 2011; Stebbings et al., 2007). An example of such *in vivo* species differences between human and cynomolgus monkeys resulted in the tragic TeGenero incident. It was demonstrated that TeGenero's TGN1412 was capable of TNF-α, IL-2, IL-6, IL-8, and IFN-γ release and superagonist activity when tested in a CRA on cell populations from humans, but not in a CRA using cells cynomolgus macaques, echoing the *in vivo* preclinical data in NHPs and the March 2006 Phase I clinical trial in humans (Stebbings et al., 2007). However, notwithstanding such exceptions and

TABLE 16.2

Cytokine Release Assays—An Overview

Criteria for Use and Selection of Cytokine Release Assay for Hazard Identification

- Drug can/does interact with the immune system
- Drug has strong ability to crosslink FcγR
- Drug targets membrane-bound receptors and antigens
- Mode of action of drug and mechanism of cytokine release
- Fc binding affinity and specificity of monoclonal antibody

Platforms	
Solution phase	Drug in solution phase
Immobilized	Drug immobilized on plate or beads
Wet coat	Non-tissue culture plates
Evaporation or warm air	Polypropylene or tissue culture polystyrene plates
Bead-based	Protein A immobilized on beads
Source of Cells	
Healthy patient/animal	Used in routine assays
Patient/disease specific	May be more appropriate if the expression of the relevant cellular antigen is patient- or disease-specific
Cell Types	
PBMC	Robust cytokine response, but some important factors (e.g., complement, platelets) may be missing. A variation uses PBMCs precultured at high density
Whole blood	More physiological (includes platelets and granulocytes)
Cocultures	When target is expressed in tissues or disease states, inclusion of relevant cell lines, primary fibroblasts, or endothelial cells may be warranted
Cytokines	
IL-2, IL-6, IL-8, TNF-α, IFN-γ	Usually included in panel
Additional cytokines	Selection is tailored to the mode of action of the drug

Considerations for Interpretation of Results

- Location of target
- Level of expression of target
- Degree of receptor occupancy
- Toxicopharmacological data
- Extrapolate with caution

allowing for varying degrees of translatability to the clinic, evaluation of cytokine release in nonclinical studies can be informative (Grimaldi et al., 2016).

To identify unanticipated CRS risk, calibrated and reproducible assay performance across CRA formats is required. While individual laboratories have used a variety of controls including lipopolysaccharide (LPS) and phytohemagglutinin (PHA) to stimulate cytokine release, the inclusion of a reference control antibody panel would increase confidence in assay performance and data interpretation. The National Institute for Biological Standards and Controls (NIBSC) positive and negative control monoclonal antibody reference panel consists of negative control antibodies as well as positive controls that cover different modalities with established clinical CRS risk. This panel was evaluated across different laboratories and assay formats. The negative (isotype) control antibodies were shown to cause little-to-no cytokine release whereas the anti-CD52, anti-CD3, and anti-CD28SA positive antibody control produced cytokine release. Notwithstanding interlaboratory variability and differences in absolute cytokine levels for different CRA methods, similar response patterns were observed (Vessilier et al., 2020). The selection of the positive controls for a particular assay should take into consideration the expected mode of action of the drug to allow a better comparison and extrapolation to the clinic (Brennan and Kiessling, 2017).

16.4.2 Sample Collection and Storage

Cytokine and cytokine receptor assessments can be performed in a variety of body fluids as well as tissues, cells, and cell culture supernatants. *In vivo* assessments are most readily obtained from blood collections and evaluation of the serum or plasma. Such collections provide the advantage of allowing multiple samplings over time and the comparison of posttreatment time points to baseline concentrations. However, cytokines measured in blood often are not reflective of the degree and type of local inflammation that exists in a specific organ; thus, the degree of inflammation in that organ could be misinterpreted. Obtaining a sample collection from an affected organ can therefore be important to characterize local inflammation (Kreiner et al., 2010; Valaperti et al., 2019).

For samples collected for cytokine analysis, the timing of the collection, method of sample collection, use of anticoagulant, type of anticoagulant, storage time and conditions between collection and processing, and storage conditions after processing can be important preanalytical aspects that can affect the data obtained. For example, when samples are collected in blood and processed to plasma or serum, variations in cytokine measurements can occur because of variability in blood processing procedures with increased cytokine production from blood activation, release from platelets, or degradation. The plasma concentrations of several cytokines, including ILs and growth factors, can increase during 2 hours of room temperature storage prior to centrifugation. Serum concentrations of selected cytokines, including IL-8, MIP-1α, and MIP-1β, can increase when centrifugation is delayed to 4 hours after collection (Skogstrand et al., 2008; Ayache et al., 2006; Lee et al., 2016, Aziz et al., 2016). While serum cytokines are generally increased when centrifugation is delayed, once processed to serum, cytokines (IL-4, -5, -6, -8, -12, -13, -17A, 23, IFN-γ, and TNF-α) are generally stable when stored for 24 hours at room temperature or at 4°C (Valaperti et al., 2019).

While some degradation can be seen for some cytokines stored for a year at −80°C, other cytokines remain stable within a 2-year period and then decrease 10%–20% per year thereafter. Multiple freeze–thawing cycles affect cytokines differently, with some having greater stability than others following freeze–thaws (Keustermans et al., 2013; de Jager et al., 2009). In a review of PubMed articles related to cytokine storage stability (Simpson et al., 2020), the authors determined that there is a wide range of reported stability, and although there is a clear consensus for some cytokines, more research needs to be done for many others. Caution should therefore be used when interpreting cytokine concentration results for samples that have been stored for a long period of time or following multiple freeze–thaw cycles.

Since not all cytokine responses can be evaluated systemically, appropriate cell and tissue processing from alternate sites or necropsies is also important. If cells need to be lysed, the choice of lysis buffer should be evaluated to confirm that tissue cytokine levels are not altered (Keustermans et al., 2013). For tissue immunohistochemistry, collection procedures should ensure that the structure and organization has been preserved properly.

Thus, even prior to sample analysis, it is important to have standardized procedures that ensure that cytokine variations are minimized during handling and preservation of samples.

16.4.3 Cytokine Assay Platforms

Many cytokine assay platforms are currently available to measure concentrations of cytokines or cytokine soluble receptor levels in blood, tissues, cells, or cell supernatants. They include bioassays, enzyme-linked immunosorbent assay (ELISA) immunoassays, multiparametric flow cytometry, bead-based flow cytometric assays, enzyme-linked immunospot (ELISPOT), immunostaining of cells and tissues, protein microarrays, and mRNA-based assays (Sachdeva and Asthana, 2007). While biological activity is measured in the bioassays, the remaining platforms measure the protein or the mRNA.

16.4.3.1 Bioassays

In bioassays, a biological system (cells, tissues, animals) serves as the indicator system, and the read-out is a measure of the function of the test material being evaluated. Cytokines are biologically active proteins and cannot be fully characterized solely by physicochemical procedures. Bioassays provide essential information on potency during the various stages of drug development of cytokines, including biological characterization, batch-to-batch lot release, appropriate formulations, and confirmation of stability. Bioassays can also be useful to confirm neutralization of activity in the presence of neutralizing antibodies. In the case of cytokines, whose biological effects can be observed in cell culture, bioassays have focused on quantification of activity/potency *in vitro*, using defined cell lines. Parameters measured may include increases in cell numbers or proliferation, inhibition of viral replication, inhibition of cell proliferation, induction of a specific cell function (e.g., stimulation of migration), increase in surface antigen expression or secretion of particular proteins, as well as induction of cytotoxicity or apoptosis. Although bioassays are useful to detect bioactive molecules and can be very sensitive, they have low specificity as the indicator cells are not specific to a particular cytokine, and other factors (e.g., rheumatoid factors or heterophilic antibodies) present in the sample can interfere with the assay. In addition, these assays are generally time-consuming. As bioassays are inherently variable, it is important that the biological measurement of a cytokine is made relative to a stable reference that allows assay validation and interlaboratory comparison. Such primary reference international standards and reference reagents have been developed over time and are available from the World Health Organization (WHO) (Meager, 2006; Corsini and House, 2018).

16.4.3.2 Immunoassays

Immunoassays measure the protein (cytokine or receptor) of interest in the context of antigen/antibody recognition and binding. The most common method used for the detection of cytokines in biological fluids is the ELISA. In these assays, the enzyme labels amplify the signal and result in high specificity, sensitivity, and reproducibility. Many companies commercially produce ELISA kits for the evaluation of cytokines and receptors in a number of species. The quality of the immunoassay is mostly dependent on the source, quality, and specificity of the capture and detection antibodies, which is why there can be significant differences in performance in immunoassays sold by different vendors. There is generally a lack of information provided by the manufacturer as to the exact components of the specific immunoassay that make comparisons across vendors difficult. Additional factors that affect the immunoassays are the specificity of the antibodies to different forms of the same cytokine (e.g., soluble vs. membrane-bound). Additional factors that can affect the assay include different forms of the cytokine, the degree of glycosylation, and the presence of autoantibodies or cytokine inhibitors in the sample (Galle et al., 2004; Sachdeva and Asthana, 2007). The sensitivity of the ELISA is also affected by the detection limit of the colorimetric, luminescent, or chemiluminescent substrate used by the manufacturer. While it does not provide information on potency and cannot provide information on the frequencies of individual cytokine-producing cells, the standard ELISA remains a useful tool to measure cytokine protein levels in biological fluids and culture supernatants.

Assays that measure individual cytokines are gradually being replaced by platforms that allow multiplex analyses. While these methods still cannot distinguish between bioactive and inactive molecules, their high sensitivity and low background while providing results for multiple analytes simultaneously and economizing on the sample volume have resulted in their increased use and popularity. The Meso Scale Discovery (MSD) is such a platform. The detection by electrochemiluminescence also results in a large dynamic range which further saves on the sample volume by avoiding retest of samples that would be out of the calibration curves of the standard sandwich ELISA (Keustermans et al., 2013; McKay et al., 2017).

16.4.3.3 Multiparameter Flow Cytometry

Multiparameter flow cytometry allows individual cells to be analyzed for several parameters simultaneously. The use of beads coated with the capture antibody provides the solid support to bind the cytokine of interest. This can be multiplexed to simultaneously detect multiple cytokines. Examples of these multiplex bead assays include the Luminex multianalyte profiling and the Becton Dickinson (BD) cytometric bead array. Multiparameter flow cytometry also has high specificity and sensitivity and a large dynamic range. It also only requires a small sample volume. Although multiplex bead assays result in significant advantages, these assays still suffer from the same limitations previously discussed for the ELISA (Khalifian et al., 2015).

16.4.3.4 Cytokine Production by Single Cells

Cytokine production by single cells can be measured by ELISPOT, and the intracellular cytokine staining (ICCS) of single cells for flow cytometric evaluation.

The ELISPOT is widely used for evaluating cytokine release from single cells and measures the frequency of cytokine-secreting cells. The cells are cultured in a 96-well plate format with surfaces coated with capture antibody. Cytokines produced in response to stimuli are captured by the antibody. Following incubation, the cells are removed, and the secreted antibody is measured using a detection antibody. Using a substrate with a precipitating product, each spot corresponds to a single cytokine-secreting cell. This assay is extremely sensitive (it can detect one cytokine producing cell per 10^5 cells) and is very useful to study small populations of cells in specific immune responses. Limited multiplexing is possible in this assay by using a precipitating product that results in different color spot, but there can be some difficulties in interpretation with multiple colors (Sachdeva and Asthana, 2007).

ICCS procedures use a protein transport inhibitor, fixation and permeabilization of the cells, and anticytokine antibodies that bind to the cytokines fixed in the cell. This method allows for evaluation of multiple cytokines from a single cell. Owing to fixation, there can be some artifacts and increased autofluorescence, and the permeabilization can result in nonspecific interactions unless the staining antibody is carefully titered. This method can detect complex phenotypes and also permits the concurrent evaluation of additional analytes and activation and viability markers (Yin et al., 2015).

16.4.3.5 Immunostaining of Cytokines in Tissues

Immunostaining of cytokines in tissues provides *in situ* information on the production of cytokines and associated pathologies. This allows local measurement when systemic levels in the blood or serum are not necessarily informative. Antibody selection is critical for immunostaining. The procedure requires fixation, a process that may alter the conformation of a cytokine, and the antibody selected must be able to recognize and bind to the cytokine after fixation. Isotype controls are used to control for nonspecific staining. Visualization is performed by light or fluorescent microscope, depending on the label on the conjugate. This method is low throughput but can provide valuable information as to the localization of the cells producing cytokines in the context of the pathologies observed in the tissues (Sachdeva and Asthana, 2007).

16.4.3.6 Protein Microarrays

Even though protein measurements are generally preferred to gene expression, protein microarrays are more challenging than DNA microarrays because there is no amplification step. Protein microarrays are similar to gene microarrays and provide expression profiling of cytokines and related proteins of interest. Protein microarrays allow protein profiling and is applicable to biomarker detection. Current challenges include short shelf life, maintaining sensitivity while reducing background noise, and difficulties in generating chips that hold the required tertiary structure that may be required for binding and activity (Utz, 2005; Keustermans et al., 2013).

16.4.3.7 mRNA Evaluations

In contrast to the various immunoassays previously described in this section, the mRNA assays are based on the detection of cytokine transcripts, not the protein itself, in the cells or tissues. Using real-time PCR, cytokine gene expression can be quantitatively compared between several targets. A variation utilizes *in situ* hybridization for cytokine transcripts and is useful for detecting protein expression in the cell that produces the transcripts (Sachdeva and Asthana, 2007).

16.5 Conclusions

Cytokine assessments, while critical to providing a wide range of information from mechanism of action in pathological states to drug development in the clinic, are not without challenges. Optimal assessment strategy, including selection of appropriate samples, sample timing, and handling and storage of sample collections, must be determined according to the nature of the particular cytokine(s) and the nature of the effects being measured. Preanalytical methodologies need to be understood and optimized, and proper platforms selected in order to obtain meaningful data. Available platforms and differing technologies capable of measuring cytokines of interest must be considered, as it can be difficult to evaluate resulting data across platforms because reproducibility and reliability are not consistent among different technologies, a point that becomes especially relevant when cytokines are measured in different laboratories and over time (Casaletto et al., 2018). With regard to relevance between nonclinical and clinical data, varying degrees of translatability have been shown between rats, NHPs, and humans, and species-specific differences and *in vitro* interdonor variability must be taken into account when extrapolating to humans (Grimaldi et al., 2016). In addition, interpretation of cytokine data may present challenges as it may not be possible to determine cutoff values that distinguish between mild and moderate responses in patients, or to define cytokine production parameters that will be predictive of serious pathophysiology in humans.

Despite these challenges, cytokine assessments provide valuable information on immune status, disease pathogenesis, therapeutic effects, dose and dose escalation, and potential toxicities during the course of nonclinical and clinical studies.

REFERENCES

Abbas AK, Lichtman AH, and S Pillai. 2014. *Cellular and Molecular Immunology*, 8th ed. Philadelphia: Elsevier Saunders; 535 p.

Alam J, Jantan I, and SNA Bukhari. 2017. Rheumatoid arthritis: recent advances on its etiology, role of cytokines and pharmacotherapy. *Biomed Pharmacother.* 92:615–633.

Altan-Bonnet G, and R Mukherjee. 2019. Cytokine-mediated communication: a quantitative appraisal of immune complexity. *Nat Rev Immunol.* 19:205–217.

Ank N, West H, Bartholdy C, Eriksson K, Thomsen AR, and SR Paludan. 2006. Lambda interferon (IFN-lambda), a type III IFN, is induced by viruses and IFNs and displays potent antiviral activity against select virus infections in vivo. *J Virol.* 80:4501–4509.

Ayache S, Panelli M, Marincola FM, and DF Stroncek. 2006. Effects of storage time and exogenous protease inhibitors on plasma protein levels. *Am J Clin Pathol.* 26(2):174–184.

Aziz N, Detels R, Quint JJ, Li Q, Gjertson D, and AW Butch. 2016. Stability of cytokines, chemokines and soluble activation markers in unprocessed blood stored under different conditions. *Cytokine.* 84:17–24.

Barata JT, Durum SK, and B Seddon. 2019. Flip the coin: IL-7 and IL-7R in health and disease. *Nat Immunol.* 20(12):1584–1593.

Barrat FJ, Crow MK, and LB Ivashkiv. 2019. Interferon target-gene expression and epigenomic signatures in health and disease. *Nat Immunol.* 20(12):1574–1583.

Berraondo P, Sanmamed MF, Ochoa MC, Etxeberria I, Aznar MA, Pérez-Gracia JL, Rodríguez-Ruiz ME, Ponz-Sarvise M, Castañón E, and I Melero. 2019. Cytokines in clinical cancer immunotherapy. *Br J Cancer.* 120(1):6–15.

Brennan FR, and A Kiessling. 2017. In vitro assays supporting the safety assessment of immunomodulatory monoclonal antibodies. *Toxicol In Vitro.* 45(Pt 3):296–308.

Buchmeier NA, and RD Schreiber. 1985. Requirement of endogenous interferon-gamma production for resolution of *Listeria monocytogenes* infection. *Proc Natl Acad Sci.* 82(21):7404–7408.

Bullitta S, Musella A, Rizzo FR, De Vito F, Guadalupi L, Caioli S, Balletta S, Sanna K, Dolcetti E, Vanni V, Bruno A, Buttari F, Stampanoni Bassi M, Mandolesi G, Centonze D, and A Gentile. 2020. Re-examining the role of TNF in MS pathogenesis and therapy. *Cells.* 9(10):2290.

Burleson, GR, Burleson, SCM, and FG Burleson. 2015. *Pulmonary Immunology of Infectious Disease. Comparative Biology of the Normal Lung*, 2nd ed. (ed. Parent, R.A.), Academic Press, pp. 581–600.

Canna SW and EM Behrens. 2012. Making sense of the cytokine storm: a conceptual framework for understanding, diagnosing, and treating hemophagocytic syndromes *Pediatr Clin North Am.* 59(2):329–344.

Casaletto KB, Elahi FM, Fitch R, Walters S, Fox E, Staffaroni AM, Bettcher BM, Zetterberg H, Karydas A, Rojas JC, Boxer AL, and JH Kramer. 2018. A comparison of biofluid cytokine markers across platform technologies: correspondence or divergence? *Cytokine.* 111:481–489.

Chousterman BG, Swirski FK, and GF Weber. 2017. Cytokine storm and sepsis disease pathogenesis. *Semin Immunopathol.* 39(5):517–528.

Conlon KC, Miljkovic MD, and TA Waldmann. 2019. Cytokines in the treatment of cancer. *J Interferon Cytokine Res.* 39(1):6–21.

Corsini E, and RV House. 2018. Evaluating cytokines in immunotoxicity testing. In: DeWitt J, Rockwell C, and C Bowman. (eds) *Immunotoxicity Testing. Methods in Molecular Biology*, vol. 1803. New York, NY: Humana Press.

Cytokines in the balance (editorial). 2019. Nat Immunol. 20: 1557.

de Jager W, Bourcier K, Rijkers GT, Prakken BJ, and V Seyfert-Margolis. 2009. Prerequisites for cytokine measurements in clinical trials with multiplex immunoassays. *BMC Immunol.* 10:52.

Dinarello CA. 2007. Historical insights into cytokines. *Eur J Immunol.* 37(Suppl 1):S34–S45.

Duff GW, and SK Durum. 1953. The pyrogenic and mitogenic actions of interleukin-1 are related. *Nature.* 304: 449–451.

Dumitrescu L, Constantinescu CS, and R Tanasescu. 2018. Recent developments in interferon-based therapies for multiple sclerosis. *Exp Opin Biol Therapy.* 18(6):665–680.

Ferreira VL, Borba HHL, Bonetti A, Leonart LP, and R Pontarolo. 2018. *Cytokines and Interferons: Types and Functions, Autoantibodies and Cytokines, Wahid Ali Khan*. IntechOpen. DOI: 10.5772/intechopen.74550

Finco D, Grimaldi C, Fort M, Walker M, Kiessling A, Wolf B, Salcedo T, Faggioni R, Schneider A, Ibraghimov A, Scesney S, Serna D, Prell R, Stebbings R, and PK Narayanan. 2014. Cytokine release assays: current practices and future directions. *Cytokine.* 66(2):143–155.

Fresegna D, Bullitta S, Musella A, Rizzo FR, De Vito F, Guadalupi L, Caioli S, Balletta S, Sanna K, Dolcetti E, Vanni V, Bruno A, Buttari F, Stampanoni Bassi M, Mandolesi G, Centonze D, and A Gentile. 2020. Re-Examining the Role of TNF in MS Pathogenesis and Therapy. Cells. 9(10): 2290.

Galle P, Svenson M, Bendtzen K, and MB Hansen. 2004. High levels of neutralizing IL-6 autoantibodies in 0.1% of apparently healthy blood donors. *Eur J Immunol.* 34(11): 3267–3275.

Goel HL, and AM Mercurio. 2013. VEGF targets the tumour cell. *Nat Rev Cancer.* 13(12):871–882.

Guan Q, and J Zhang. 2017. Recent advances: the imbalance of cytokines in the pathogenesis of inflammatory bowel disease. *Mediators Inflamm.* 2017:4810258.

Grimaldi C, Finco D, Fort MM, Gliddon D, Harper K, Helms WS, Mitchell JA, O'Lone R, Parish ST, Piche MS, Reed DM, Reichmann G, Ryan PC, Stebbings R, and M Walker. 2016. Cytokine release: a workshop proceedings on the state-of-the-science, current challenges and future directions. *Cytokine*. 85:101–108.

Horvath CJ, and MN Milton. 2009. The TeGenero incident and Duff Report conclusions: a series of unfortunate events or an avoidable event? *Toxicol Pathol*. 37:372–383.

Huang S, Hendriks W, Althage A, Hemmi S, Bluethmann H, Kamijo R, Vilcek J, Zinkernagel RM, and M Aguet. 1993. Immune response in mice that lack the interferon-gamma receptor. *Science*. 259(5102):1742–1745.

Iwasaki A, and R Medzhitov. 2011. A new shield for a cytokine storm. *Cell* 146(6):861–862.

Karupiah G, Fredrickson TN, Holmes KL, Khairallah LH, and RM Buller. 1993. Importance of interferons in recovery from mousepox. *J Virol*. 67(7):4214–4226.

Kasper LH, and AT Reder. 2014. Immunomodulatory activity of interferon-beta. *Ann Clin Transl Neurol*. 1(8):622–631.

Keustermans GC, Hoeks SB, Meerding JM, Prakken BJ, and W de Jager. 2013. Cytokine assays: an assessment of the preparation and treatment of blood and tissue samples. *Methods*. 61(1):10–17.

Khalifian S, Raimondi G, and G Brandacher. 2015. The use of luminex assays to measure cytokines. *J Invest Dermatol*. 135(4):1–5.

Kim HO, Kim H-S, Youn J-C, Shin E-C, and S Park. 2011. Serum cytokine profiles in healthy young and elderly population assessed using multiplexed bead-based immunoassays. *J Trans Med*. 9:113.

Kolls JK. 2013. CD4(+) T-cell subsets and host defense in the lung. *Immunol Rev*. 252(1):156–163.

Kreiner F, Langberg H, and H Galbo. 2010. Increased muscle interstitial levels of inflammatory cytokines in polymyalgia rheumatica. *Arthritis Rheum*. 62(12):3768–3775.

Le Y, Zhou Y, Iribarren P, and J Wang. 2004. Chemokines and chemokine receptors: their manifold roles in homeostasis and disease. *Cell Mol Immunol*. 1(2):95–104.

Lee JE, Kim JW, Han BG, and SY Shin. 2016. Impact of whole-blood processing conditions on plasma and serum concentrations of cytokines. *Biopreserv Biobank*. 14(1):51–55.

Li S-F, Gong M-j, Zhao F-r, Shao J-j, Xie Y-l, Zhang Y-g, and H-y Chang. 2018. Type I interferons: distinct biological activities and current applications for viral infection. *Cell Physiol Biochem*. 51:2377–2396.

Li X, Bechara R, Zhao J, McGeachy MJ, and SL Gaffen. 2019. IL-17 receptor-based signaling and implications for disease. *Nat Immunol*. 20:1594–1602.

Lim SY, Lee JH, Gide TN, Menzies AM, Guminski A, Carlino MS, Breen EJ, Yang JYH, Ghazanfar S, Kefford RF, Scolyer RA, Long GV, and RH Rizos. 2019. Circulating cytokines predict immune-related toxicity in melanoma patients receiving anti-PD-1-based immunotherapy. *Clin Cancer Res*. 25(5):1557–1563.

Lin J and WJ Leonard. 2019. Fine-tuning cytokine signals. *Annu Rev Immunol*. 37:295–324.

McKay HS, Margolick JB, Martínez-Maza O, Lopez J, Phair J, Rappocciolo G, Denny TN, Magpantay LI, Jacobson LP, and JH Bream. 2017. Multiplex assay reliability and long-term intra-individual variation of serologic inflammatory biomarkers. *Cytokine*. 90:185–192.

Mantovani A, Dinarello CA, Molgora M, and C Garlanda. 2019. Interleukin-1 and related cytokines in the regulation of inflammation and immunity. *Immunity*. 50(4):778–795.

Meager, A. 2006. Measurement of cytokines by bioassays: Theory and application. Methods 38:237–252.

Mease KM, Kimzey AL, and JA Lansita. 2017. Biomarkers for nonclinical infusion reactions in marketed biotherapeutics and considerations for study design. *Curr Opin Toxicol*. 4:1–15.

Metcalfe RD, Putoczki TL, and MDW Griffin. 2020. Structural understanding of interleukin 6 family cytokine signaling and targeted therapies: focus on interleukin 11. *Front Immunol*. 11:1424.

Monastero RN, and S Pentyala. 2017. Cytokines as biomarkers and their respective clinical cutoff levels. *Int J Inflam*. 2017:Article ID 4309485, 11 pages. https://doi.org/10.1155/2017/4309485

Morens DM, and AS Fauci. 2007. The 1918 influenza pandemic: insights for the 21st century. *J Infect Dis*. 195(7):1018–1028.

Moyle M, Cevikbas, F, Harden, JL, and E Guttman-Yassky. 2019. Understanding the immune landscape in atopic dermatitis: the era of biologics and emerging therapeutic approaches. *Exp Dermatol*. 28(7):756–768.

Narazaki M, Tanaka T, and T Kishimoto. 2017. The role and therapeutic targeting of IL-6 in rheumatoid arthritis. *Expert Rev Clin Immunol*. 13(6):535–551.

Noack M, and P Miossec. 2017. Selected cytokine pathways in rheumatoid arthritis. *Semin Immunopathol*. 39:365–383.

Ono SJ, Nakamura T, Miyazaki D, Ohbayashi M, Dawson M, and M Toda. 2003. Chemokines: roles in leukocyte development, trafficking, and effector function. *J Allergy Clin Immunol*. 111(6):1185–1199.

O'Shea JJ, Ma A, and P Lipsky. 2002. Cytokines and autoimmunity. *Nat Rev Immunol*. 2(1):37–45.

Parham P, and C Janeway. 2009. *The Immune System*, 3rd ed. London, New York: Garland Science; 506 p.

Platanias LC. 2005. Mechanisms of type-I- and type-II-interferon-mediated signalling. *Nat Rev Immunol*. 5:375–386.

Ramani T, Auletta CS, Weinstock D, Mounho-Zamora B, Ryan PC, and TW Salcedo. 2015. Cytokines: the good, the bad, and the deadly. *Int J Toxicol*. 34:355–365.

Rani A, Dasgupta P, and JJ Murphy. 2019. Prostate cancer: the role of inflammation and chemokines. *Am J Pathol*. 189(11):2119–2137.

Römer PS, Berr S, Avota E, Na SY, Battaglia M, ten Berge I, Einsele H, and T Hünig. 2011. Preculture of PBMCs at high cell density increases sensitivity of T-cell responses, revealing cytokine release by CD28 superagonist TGN1412. *Blood*. 118:6772–6782.

Sarawar SR, Sangster M, Coffman RL, and PC Doherty. 1994. Administration of anti-IFN-gamma antibody to beta 2-microglobulin-deficient mice delays influenza virus clearance but does not switch the response to a T helper cell 2 phenotype. *J Immunol*. 153(3):1246–1253.

Sachdeva N, and D Asthana. 2007. Cytokine quantitation: technologies and applications. *Front Biosci*. 12:4682–4695.

Shimabukuro-Vornhagen A, Gödel P, Subklewe M, Stemmler HJ, Schlößer HA, Schlaak M, Kochanek M, Böll B, and MS von Bergwelt-Baildon. 2018. Cytokine release syndrome. *J Immunother Cancer*. 6(1):56.

Silk AW, and K Margolin. 2019. Cytokine therapy. *Hematol Oncol Clin North Am*. 33(2):261–274.

Silva MO. 2012. Risk of autoimmune complications associated with interferon therapy. *Gastroenterol Hepatol (NY)*. 8(8):540–542.

Sim GC, and L Radvanyi. 2014. The IL-2 cytokine family in cancer immunotherapy. *Cytokine Growth Factor Rev*. 25(4):377–390.

Simpson S, Kaislasuo J, Guller S, and L Pal. 2020. Thermal stability of cytokines: a review. *Cytokine*. 125:154829. DOI: 10.1016/j.cyto.2019.154829

Skogstrand K, Ekelund CK, Thorsen P, Vogel I, Jacobsson B, Nørgaard-Pedersen B, and DM Hougaard. 2008. Effects of blood sample handling procedures on measurable inflammatory markers in plasma, serum and dried blood spot samples. *J Immunol Methods*. 336(1):78–84.

Spellberg B, and JE Jr. Edwards. 2001. Type 1/type 2 immunity in infectious diseases. *Clin Infect Dis*. 32(1):76–102.

St. Clair EW. 2008. The calm after the cytokine storm: lessons from the TGN1412 trial. *J Clin Invest*. 118(4):1344–1347.

Stebbings R, Findlay L, Edwards C, Eastwood D, Bird C, North D, Mistry Y, Dilger P, Liefooghe E, Cludts I, Fox B, Tarrant G, Robinson J, Meager T, Dolman C, Thorpe SJ, Bristow A, Wadhwa M, Thorpe R, and S Poole. 2007. "Cytokine storm" in the phase I trial of monoclonal antibody TGN1412: better understanding the causes to improve preclinical testing of immunotherapeutics. *J Immunol*. 179:3325–3331.

Tarrant JM. 2010. Blood cytokines as biomarkers of in vivo toxicity in preclinical safety assessment: considerations for their use. *Toxicol Sci*. 117(1):4–16.

Tisoncik JR, Korth MJ, Simmons CP, Farrar J, Martin TR, and MG Katze. 2012. Into the eye of the cytokine storm. *Microbiol Mol Biol Rev*. 76(1):16–32.

Toews GB. 2001. Cytokines and the lung. *Eur Respir J*. Suppl 34: 3s–17s.

Turner MD, Nedjai B, Hurst T, and DJ Pennington. 2014. Cytokines and chemokines: at the crossroads of cell signalling and inflammatory disease. *Biochim Biophys Acta*. 1843(11):2563–2582.

Utz PJ. 2005. Protein arrays for studying blood cells and their secreted products. *Immunol Rev*. 204:264–282.

Valaperti A, Bezel P, Vonow-Eisenring M, Franzen D, and UC Steiner. 2019. Variability of cytokine concentration in whole blood serum and bronchoalveolar lavage over time. *Cytokine* 123:154768.

Vessilier S, Fort M, O'Donnell L, Hinton H, Nadwodny K, Picotti J, Rigsby P, Staflin K, Stebbings R, Mekala D, Willingham A, Wolf B and participants in the study. 2020. Development of the first reference antibody panel for qualification and validation of cytokine release assay platforms. Cytokine:X 2:100042.

Vilcek J, and M Feldmann. 2004. Historical review: cytokines as therapeutics and targets of therapeutics. *Trends Pharmacol Sci*. 25(4):201–209.

Wille A, Gessner A, Lother H, and F Lehmann-Grube. 1989. Mechanism of recovery from acute virus infection. VIII. Treatment of lymphocytic choriomeningitis virus-infected mice with anti-interferon-y monoclonal antibody blocks generation of virus-specific cytotoxic T lymphocytes and virus elimination. *Eur J Immunol*. 19(7):1283–1288.

Woś I, and J Tabarkiewicz. 2021. Effect of interleukin-6, -17, -21, -22, and -23 and STAT3 on signal transduction pathways and their inhibition in autoimmune arthritis. *Immunol Res*. DOI: 10.1007/s12026-021-09173-9. Epub ahead of print. PMID: 33515210.

Yau AH, and EM Yoshida. 2014. Hepatitis C drugs: the end of the pegylated interferon era and the emergence of all-oral interferon-free antiviral regimens: a concise review. *Can J Gastroenterol Hepatol*. 28(8):445–451.

Yin Y, Mitson-Salazar A, and C Prussin. 2015. Detection of intracellular cytokines by flow cytometry. *Curr Protoc Immunol*. 110:6.24.1–6.24.18.

Zhou X, Fragala MS, McElhaney JE, and GA Kuchel. 2010. Conceptual and methodological issues relevant to cytokine and inflammatory marker measurements in clinical research. *Curr Opin Clin Nutr Metab Care*. 13(5):541–547.

17

"Regulatory Toxicology for Biopharmaceuticals: Preparing for Pre-IND Interactions and Avoiding IND Pitfalls for Oncology and Non-Oncology Products"

Janice Lansita
ToxAlliance LLC

Andrew McDougal and Jane Sohn
U.S. Food and Drug Administration (FDA)

Shawna L. Weis
Constellation Pharmaceuticals, Inc.

CONTENTS

DOI: 10.1201/9781003124542-19

17.1 Introduction

The original *Guidance for Industry ICH S6 Preclinical Evaluation of Biotechnology-Derived Pharmaceuticals*, which was first implemented in 1997, documented the principles of regulatory toxicology for the nonclinical safety assessment of biopharmaceuticals. At that time, biologic drug approvals included OKT3, a murine anti-CD3, the first monoclonal antibody (mAb) approved in 1986, and several growth factors (including insulin, erythropoietin, granulocyte colony-stimulating factor, etc.). Since that time, the range of biologic constructs has expanded dramatically and now encompasses an innovative array of proteins that range in complexity from mAbs to fusion proteins, bispecific antibodies (bispecifics), antibody-drug conjugates (ADCs), and bispecific T-cell engagers (BiTes, which are antibody-based receptor fusions; Spiess et al., 2015). The complexity of these molecules continues to evolve as developers aim to overcome intrinsic limitations of the various constructs to alleviate disease conditions. Key areas of emphasis include modifying constructs to improve pharmacokinetic (PK), pharmacodynamic (PD), tissue distribution, and immunogenicity properties of monoclonal antibodies (Spiess et al., 2015). To address safety concerns and streamline development of this ever-changing class of drugs, the ICH S6 guidance was revised in 2011. The resulting guidance, ICH S6(R1), and its addendum communicate current best practices for the nonclinical development of biotechnology products. Regulators and regulated industry have the same fundamental goal: to rapidly develop biologic drugs with good safety profiles and efficacy.

As a useful reference, the US Food and Drug Administration (FDA), Center for Drug Evaluation and Research (CDER) updates semi-annually an approved Therapeutic Biologic Products list.[1] In 2016, CDER[2] reported approving seven novel biologics, compared to 15 new molecular entity (NME) small-molecule drugs in the same year. In 2017, CDER approved 12 novel biologics, compared to 34 NME small-molecule drugs. In 2018, CDER approved 17 novel biologics, compared to 42 NME small-molecule drugs. In 2019, CDER approved 10 novel biologics, compared to 38 small-molecule products.[3] The FDA issued a final rule that defines a "protein" as "any alpha amino acid polymer with a specific, defined sequence that is greater than 40 amino acids in size."[4]

This chapter aims to describe common "pitfalls" in biologic drug development at the pre-Investigational New Drug submission (pre-IND) and Investigational New Drug submission (IND) stages to help current biologic drug developers avoid these potential issues. The terms "biologic" and "biologic drug" synonymously refer to "biologic product" (used in the Public Health and Safety/PHS Act) and "biotechnology-derived pharmaceutical" (used in ICH S6(R1)). While ICH S6(R1) applies to "products derived from characterized cells

[1] FDA: New Drugs and FDA: CDER's New Molecular Entities and New Therapeutic Biological Products. Accessed from https://www.fda.gov/drugs/developmentapprovalprocess/druginnovation/ucm20025676.htm

[2] CY 2016 CDER New Molecular Entity (NME) Drug & Original BLA Calendar Year Approvals as of December 31, 2016. Accessed from https://www.fda.gov/downloads/Drugs/DevelopmentApprovalProcess/HowDrugsareDevelopedandApproved/DrugandBiologicApprovalReports/NDAandBLAApprovalReports/UCM540569.pdf

[3] Compilation of CDER NME and New Biologic Approvals 1985–2020. Accessed from https://www.fda.gov/drugs/drug-approvals-and-databases/compilation-cder-new-molecular-entity-nme-drug-and-new-biologic-approvals

[4] Federal Register Volume 8, No. 35, 2/21/2020. Definition of the Term "Biological Product." Accessed from https://www.federalregister.gov/documents/2020/02/21/2020-03505/definition-of-the-term-biological-product

through the use of a variety of expression systems including bacteria, yeast, insect, plant, and mammalian cells," this chapter focuses on biologic drugs reviewed by FDA CDER (e.g., monoclonal antibodies, cytokines, enzymes, fusion proteins, bispecifics, ADCs). Biologics, including vaccines, cell therapies, and gene therapies, for example, regulated by the Center for Biologic Drug Evaluation and Research (CBER) at FDA are not covered in this chapter (See Chapters 23–27).

17.2 IND Submission for a Biologic Drug

17.2.1 General Principles of Development for Biologic Drugs

The basic principles outlined in ICH *S6(R1)* are discussed below. ICH S6(R1) covers scientific and technical challenges that are specific to biologics; for timing of studies needed to support the different phases of clinical development, ICH S6(R1) refers to ICH *M3(R2)*.

The main objective of the studies described in ICH S6(R1) is to characterize the pharmacology and toxicology of a biologic drug to support clinical development. The guidance includes sections on biologic activity/PD, species selection, study design aspects, immunogenicity, reproductive and developmental toxicity, and carcinogenicity. ICH S6(R1) advocates a "flexible, case-by-case, science-based approach" for the development of biologic drugs; thus, the nonclinical package to support clinical development of a biologic drug should be focused on defining the pharmacological, and toxicological aspects of the specific product. While some insights can be gleaned from regulatory reviews of previously approved products, published guidance or interactions with the appropriate Review Division are generally more informative about current regulatory expectations. FDA recommends that Sponsors seek concurrence from the relevant Review Division regarding the design of the nonclinical program.

The first stage of nonclinical development for a newly selected drug candidate is the selection of the most appropriate toxicology species. The selection of pharmacologically relevant species for nonclinical development should be scientifically justified, which for a biologic drug entails the demonstration of binding and PD activity in the intended nonclinical model (see Chapter 2). Because of differences in amino acid sequence homology that may have arisen across phyla, non-human primates (NHPs) are often the only pharmacologically relevant nonclinical species. While general toxicology studies are feasible in NHPs, other studies, such as carcinogenicity and reproductive toxicity studies, either are not practical (e.g., carcinogenicity) or are of sufficient technical difficulty (e.g., reproductive toxicity) that Sponsors should consider a modified approach to assess these endpoints (e.g., use of a surrogate molecule).

Regarding the assessment of carcinogenicity potential, ICH S6(R1) Section 17.6 (Carcinogenicity) encourages Sponsors to begin with a weight-of-evidence (WoE) approach considering all relevant information. In addition to the data sources explicitly stated in ICH S6(R1) that include published literature (animal model data), class effects, target biology, MOA, chronic toxicology and clinical data from subchronic toxicity studies and immunotoxicity studies may also be relevant. In many cases, sufficient data are available about the pathway and toxicity of the drug that additional studies are not requested, and the written carcinogenicity assessment can support product labeling. When the available data are not adequate, Sponsors should begin discussing testing strategies with FDA as early in product development as feasible (e.g., at or before the end of Phase 2 meeting) to ensure that acceptable data are available in time to support the marketing application. Early communication about the expectations for carcinogenicity assessment of a biotechnology product are particularly warranted when there is no relevant rodent species, as lifetime studies are not feasible in the primate.

Similarly, for programs in which the NHP is the only pharmacologically relevant species, ICH S6(R1) Section 17.5.3 recommends that Sponsors consider conducting a well-designed enhanced pre- and post-natal development (PPND) study in NHPs in lieu of stand-alone embryo-fetal development (EFD) and PPND studies.

Immunogenicity data from repeat-dose toxicology studies are used to assist in the characterization of toxicity. These data are especially helpful when dosing is associated with reduced PK exposure and/or PD responses, which may be caused by neutralizing antidrug antibodies (ADAs). FDA recognizes that ADA formation is not predictive of the potential for ADA formation in humans; however, these data are often important for the interpretation of study results, including the interpretation of a potential NOEL (no observed effect level) or NOAEL (no observed adverse effect level) in which the absence of a given finding may be complicated by ablation of exposure at that dose level. For some drugs, the highest non-severely toxic dose (HNSTD) may be another appropriate level to identify.

The principles mentioned above are repeated and are discussed in further depth below. This chapter does not discuss specification of the test article, which is outlined in ICH S6(R1).

17.2.2 Pharmacological Activity

The biological activity of the compound should be characterized through a series of *in vitro* and *in vivo* assays to demonstrate the intended mechanism of action. These studies aid in the selection of appropriate toxicology species for nonclinical safety evaluation and can provide useful biomarkers for the interpretation of toxicology and/or clinical studies that can inform decision-making throughout drug development.

Although the primary pharmacology of most biologic drugs is generally intended and targeted, "exaggerated pharmacology" often occurs and can be toxic. Exaggerated pharmacology occurs when a biologic causes an excessive modulation in a targeted pathway, which is beyond what is considered desirable for efficacy. Although not anticipated for most biologic drugs, secondary pharmacology (i.e., unintended, or "off-target" pharmacology) does occasionally occur and is a key theoretical concern particularly as it relates to cross-reactivity of the biologic to an unintended target.

Robust primary pharmacology and PD analyses early in the lead-optimization or lead-identification phases of development are important for characterizing clinically relevant biological activity. Selection of successful candidates can be aided by the well-designed nonclinical studies that elucidate the role of the target in normal physiology, characterize differences in the target in diseased tissues versus healthy tissues, define the role of the pathway for the disease being treated, identify compensatory pathways that may be modulated by the treatment, defining the steepness of the dose-response curve, and clarifying the PD range (e.g., PK targets for receptor saturation).

In vitro PD studies can be used to help predict the biological activity using cells from various species, including humans. For example, assays with recombinant proteins (e.g., surface plasmon resonance; assays using protein expressed in transfected cells) can address specific questions regarding binding affinity, which can be useful for identifying the relevant animal models. *In vitro* models can also characterize the functional activity (i.e., activation or inhibition), using cell types most relevant to the targeted disease.

In some cases, regulators may recommend disease model data to support the first-in-human (FIH) trial (e.g., a drug for which data in a healthy animal may grossly underestimate the toxicity of a product when administered to a person with the disease of interest). When adequate disease models are not already available in a pharmacologically relevant species, consideration should be given to developing a model.

Characterization of the mode of action is also important for the interpretation of toxicology studies and integration of multiple endpoints. For example, understanding the physiology and downstream pathways of a target can help to predict on-target toxicity, sometimes referred to as "exaggerated pharmacology." In addition, toxicokinetic (TK) data from toxicology studies allow for comparisons to *in vitro* concentration-response curves, helping to predict therapeutic doses in humans.

In general, the identification of a translatable nonclinical biomarker early in development will facilitate toxicology and clinical development by aiding in the selection of appropriate animal species, and identification of the optimal clinical dose range based on the totality of the pharmacology and toxicology data. A qualified biomarker[5] that directly relates to the disease indication (cause, severity, progression, or resolution) is optimal. In cases where no adequate PD marker is available prior to the FIH trial, Sponsors can measure exploratory endpoints (e.g., in serum or urine samples), to try to find PD markers for the longer-duration toxicology study and later-phase trials.

17.2.3 Troubleshooting Secondary (Off-Target) Pharmacology

The assessment of secondary pharmacology is generally evaluated in both *in vivo* toxicology studies and an *ex vivo* tissue cross-reactivity (TCR) study for biologics with complementarity-determining regions (CDR); to assess off-target binding and on-target binding in human tissues. Alternative technologies can also be considered for evaluating off-target binding such as tissue or protein arrays.[6] The assessment of off-target pharmacology can be challenging because the *in vivo* toxicology assessment may be limited to one (or fewer) species due to limited cross-reactivity. In addition, because the therapeutic under development is likely not optimized as an immunohistochemical reagent, the tissue cross-study can have problems both with specificity and with sensitivity (Leach et al., 2010).

Generally, the results in the TCR study for biologics confirm expectations for the target's distribution and expression. In a few rare cases, the tissue cross-reactivity study has identified tissues/cell types targeted by the biologic drug. In some cases, binding to highly sensitive tissues (e.g., the retina or the heart) could produce exaggerated pharmacology (e.g., antibody dependent cellular cytotoxicity (ADCC)) with outcomes of sufficient severity to affect patient safety.

The following case study illustrates the importance of understanding the pharmacology of the drug and the target cells across species. Unfortunately, a limited understanding of the target cell population in humans versus the animal species utilized in toxicological testing can lead to poor outcomes.

17.2.3.1 Case Study: Inadequate Understanding of Biological Activity in Nonclinical Species versus Humans

TGN1412 is an immunomodulatory drug that was originally developed for the treatment of B cell chronic lymphocytic leukemia. TGN112 was designed to bind to the CD28 receptor of T cells, but acted as a novel superagonist in clinical trials. In 2006, six male healthy volunteers were treated with the NME, resulting in multiple adverse events including systemic organ failures. The toxicities in humans were caused by cytokine storm, later determined to be due to cytokine release by effector memory T-cells.

Cytokine storm was not observed in studies in non-human primates (NHPs). It is now known that CD28 is not expressed on NHP memory T-cells, and the difference in CD28 expression between humans and NHPs may be one of the reasons that studies in NHPs did not predict cytokine storm in humans (Eastwood et al., 2010; Pallardy and Hunig, 2010). As a result of this experience and others like it, close attention is paid to the likelihood that the nonclinical species will predict the critical toxicities of the biologic drug in humans, and *in vitro* assays to detect cytokine storm are recommended on a case-by-case basis.

[5] US Food and Drug Administration. Biomarker Qualification Program. Accessed from https://www.fda.gov/Drugs/DevelopmentApprovalProcess/DrugDevelopmentToolsQualificationProgram/BiomarkerQualificationProgram/default.htm

[6] Lueking A, Beator J, Patz E, Müllner S, Mehes G, Amersdorfer P. Determination and validation of off-target activities of anti-CD44 variant 6 antibodies using protein biochips and tissue microarrays. *Biotechniques*. 2008;45(4). doi:10.2144/000112898.

Determining the specific amino acid sequence(s) targeted by a biologic is an important step in secondary pharmacology screening. Some antibodies are developed against a specific sequence, but techniques such as mutation analyses may be useful for highly polymorphic targets, as polymorphisms at the binding site may reduce the clinical activity in a subset of patients. While in general, the utility of this information is to mitigate risk by optimizing trial design (e.g., powering the trials sufficiently to include the patients most likely to derive benefit, and aiding in patient selection), in some cases, polymorphism data may be needed to assure safety (for example, in cases for which administration of the drug to a person with a different polymorphism – such occurs with certain tumor mutations – may lead to exacerbation of disease).

17.2.4 Species Selection: Demonstrating Pharmacological Relevance

As described in ICH S6(R1), biologic drugs should generally be tested in pharmacologically relevant species. mAbs have limited species cross-reactivity due to the specificity of the CDR. Historically, mAbs have had cross-reactivity to only NHPs. However, with more mAbs designed and screened to bind targets with higher binding affinity, more mAbs have broader cross-reactivity across species. For example, both rodents and nonrodents may be pharmacologically relevant species. Recombinant proteins such as hormones, growth factors, cytokines, and enzymes generally show broader cross-reactivity in more than one species based on pharmacological activity.

To evaluate species cross-reactivity, sponsors should evaluate relative binding affinity of the biologic drug to the target, target expression and degree of expression on cells and/or key tissues, as well as *in vitro* and/or *in vivo* functional activity in human and animal cells.

Although binding of a target on comparable cell types and the level of binding affinity are key requirements for justification of toxicology species, these data alone are insufficient to predict the drug's overall activity. For example, even if binding affinities are similar between two species, the downstream effects, or functional activity, of a molecule may be different between the two species. The following case study illustrates that similar binding affinities do not always translate to comparable outcomes in different species.

17.2.4.1 Case Study: Binding Affinities May Not Be Predictive of Functional Activity between Species

A mAb exhibited similar overall binding affinity in rats, but different on- and off-rates compared with humans and monkeys. In the pilot *in vivo* toxicology studies, the PD marker evaluated showed a very different profile in the rat with an increase in activity and not the anticipated decrease in activity as observed in the monkey. These data demonstrate that although the rat and monkey may both show similar binding affinity *in vitro* it is also important to evaluate the *in vivo* functional activity in both species if feasible.

In unique cases where the biologic drug has no relevant animal species, the toxicity package may be limited to *in vitro* studies using human cells, tissue cross-reactivity in human tissues, and a general toxicology study in a single species (e.g., rat) to rule out the potential toxicities unrelated to the intended target. This stratagem is described in ICHS6(R1) for mAbs to exogenous targets not expressed in human tissues (e.g., antiviral or antibacterial targets). For other indications, such as oncology, a study in an irrelevant animal model may not be required. The studies needed ultimately depend on the clinical indication and overall risk vs. benefit assessment (e.g., if the indication is serious and/or life-threatening). Other approaches to assess fundamental questions regarding the safety of a drug for which few (or no) toxicology models are available include use of a surrogate molecule in a rodent, or use of transgenic models (knock-in, knock-out and humanized mouse model). In some cases, a robust *in vitro* dataset may be all that is feasible for a particular biologic drug. In those cases, the clinical starting-dose and dose-escalation schema may be particularly conservative (e.g., the minimally active biological effect level, or MABEL, approach) and may require extensive clinical monitoring to assure patient safety in the absence of more predictive scientific data. The MABEL approach is discussed later in this section.

Once the number of relevant species has been determined, the overall nonclinical plan can be designed to support the clinical plan. The route, dose frequency, and toxicology study durations are driven by the clinical plan. The IND-enabling toxicology studies (typically 28-day studies) are conducted in a rodent and nonrodent species (assuming both are pharmacologically relevant). Following the initial IND-enabling toxicology studies, subsequent studies (e.g., subchronic or chronic studies) may be conducted in a single species, if the toxicity profiles were the same in both species. Under these circumstances, typically the most sensitive species is used to evaluate the longer-term effects. If there is no specific reason to choose the nonrodent (e.g., intractable immunogenicity in the rodent, etc.), the rodent is generally preferred.

For some chronic indications, following the standard Good Laboratory Practices (GLP) IND-enabling study(ies), some Sponsors have elected to conduct an intermediate duration toxicity study (e.g., a 13-week study) prior to the conduct of the 26-week study recommended by ICH S6(R1) for biologic drugs. The decision to conduct a 13-week study, or to include an interim sacrifice group in the chronic study, will depend on the timing of data needed to support the intended clinical plan, the toxicity profile of the drug, and the Sponsor's tolerance of risk for not defining an NOAEL in the subchronic toxicology study to support dose selection for the 26-week study.

For indications in which the inclusion of children is likely, it is important to determine whether juvenile toxicology studies are needed to support pediatric clinical trials. Considerations for needing to conduct a juvenile study include the pharmacological mechanism of action of the product (i.e., are pediatric patients more sensitive?), a novel route of administration or dose regimen (dose level or frequency), or inadequate clinical safety data. For example, if there is no existing clinical safety data and the FIH trial is in a pediatric population, a juvenile study may be needed.

For programs in which the NHP is the only relevant model, the cynomolgus monkey is usually the first choice, followed by the rhesus and the marmoset.[7,8,9,10] If no pharmacologically relevant model is found among these three monkey species, Sponsors might consider screening other species of NHPs and discussing alternatives with FDA.

The following case study illustrates how robust data are needed for proper species selection. Importantly, the case study is an example of a Sponsor being able to avoid unnecessary testing in primates.

17.2.4.2 Case Study: Biologic Testing in Relevant Species Based on Adequate Data for Functional Activity

Early research and development (R&D) work for a biologic drug produced potency data that appeared to show higher affinity for monkey target than for human target, with no activity against rodent, rabbit, or dog target. The Sponsor requested a pre-IND meeting to seek advice and concurrence on their plans for further nonclinical testing, including planned toxicology studies in a single species (cynomolgus monkey). The FDA Review Division noted that the Sponsor's summaries of the potency experiments stated that the studies were uncontrolled and conducted sequentially, and questioned the reproducibility of the results. The Sponsor decided to repeat the experiments, testing target protein from humans and each species head-to-head, to verify the data. The results of the second experiment found comparable activity across species. The Sponsor proposed to use two pharmacologically relevant species based on binding data for toxicology testing, and proposed not using the monkey. The Division concurred with the Sponsor's approach.

In some cases, no appropriate nonclinical species can be identified. When this occurs, the MABEL can be used to support the FIH clinical trial. The MABEL[11] approach is rarely used for small-molecule drugs and is occasionally used for

biologic drugs. MABEL is an alternative method for identifying a safe clinical dose in situations where the mechanism of action raises concern for severe toxicity, but the predictivity of the nonclinical models is limited. The MABEL is identified using the most relevant data (usually *in vitro* activity data) and is intended to provide a large safety margin from the exposure level expected to result in toxicity. When available, quantitative data about target expression should be considered. If a MABEL approach is being considered, a pre-IND meeting may be particularly helpful for concurrence on the adequacy of the data used to determine the MABEL dose, and the threshold of activity for the assay. For severe indications (e.g., oncology indications), a higher level of activity may be appropriate for selecting the MABEL (e.g., EC_{20} vs. EC_{10}). The following case study illustrates an example of when a MABEL approach is appropriate.

17.2.4.3 Case Study: Using the Minimally Active Biological Effect Level to Support First-in-Human Dosing

A Sponsor conducted toxicology studies in two non-primate species for a non-mAb biologic, but did not base species selection on adequate functional data. Intravenous bolus injection of a biologic drug caused cardiovascular toxicity and deaths in two species (rat and dog), with a NOAEL and clear-dose response curve identified across dose range-finding and GLP toxicology studies early in drug development. Because cardiovascular toxicity was consistent with exaggerated primary pharmacology, the Sponsor considered the toxicity as additional support for proof-of-concept for the efficacy of the candidate molecule.

The FDA Review Division noted the absence of data investigating the pharmacological relevance of the rat or dog models, and noted reports in the published literature that the target protein is only expressed in humans and chimpanzees; non-primates do not have an analogous pathway.

Because of the lack of adequate safety data in a pharmacologically relevant species, and the lack of characterization of an appropriate model, the IND was placed on clinical hold. In response to FDA's concerns, the Sponsor conducted binding affinity experiments, and verified the lack of a pharmacologically relevant model appropriate for toxicology testing using functional assays. Although the chimpanzee was found to be a pharmacologically relevant species, FDA does not recommend studies in chimpanzees because they are an endangered species.

Based on discussions with FDA, the Sponsor suspected that the observed cardiovascular toxicity was due to rapid administration (i.e., intravenous bolus) of the protein (i.e. non-specific toxicity, or possibly toxicity due to the protein's particular structure). Follow-up toxicology studies using slow intravenous infusion established a large dose margin for cardiovascular safety.

---

[7] The most frequently used primate models are the cynomolgus macaque (*Macaca fasciularis*) and rhesus macaque (*Macaca mulatta*). Both of these are Old World catarrhine monkeys (family *Ceropithecidae*).

[8] New World platyrrhine monkeys are nonstandard laboratory species. The Callitrichidae family has a small history of biomedical research use: Marmoset (*Callithrix jacchus*) and Tamarin (family *Callitrichidae*; genus *Saguinus*; many species). The *Cebidae* family includes squirrel monkey (genus *Saimiri*, 5 species) and capuchin monkey [genus *Cebus*, 9 species)]; owl monkey (family *Aotidae*, genus *Aotus*); howler monkey (family *Atelidae*, genus *Alouatta*, 10+ species).

[9] Other Old World monkeys with laboratory use are the vervet monkey (genus *Chlorocebus*, also known as the African green monkey), and baboon (genus *Papio*).

[10] As a disclaimer, Regulators strongly recommend against any use of non-human apes, or any endangered species.

[11] Muller PY, Brennan FR. Safety assessment and dose selection for first-in-human clinical trials with immunomodulatory monoclonal antibodies. Clinical Pharmacology & Therapeutics. 2009;85(3):247–258.

For this case, the Sponsor concluded that a transgenic model (i.e., knock-in mice) would not provide useful information, and the FDA Review Division concurred. In the absence of any pharmacologically relevant animal model, the Sponsor conducted additional pharmacodynamics studies to identify the minimally active biological effect level (MABEL) to support the first-in-human (FIH) clinical trial. The IND was allowed to proceed based on the MABEL approach using slow intravenous infusion.

The following case study illustrates a submission in which a Sponsor did not provide adequate support for their species selection. The Sponsor proposed to rely upon an approved biologic as a reference, without conducting a stand-alone nonclinical program, and proposed that the NHP was an appropriate species based on the reference product. The Sponsor based their decisions on data demonstrating that the amino acid sequence of the proposed molecule was identical to the reference product.

17.2.4.4 Case Study: Regulatory Consideration for Species Selection

A Sponsor submitted a pre-IND application proposing to develop Biologic Drug B to be licensed under 351(a) of the PHS Act. This pathway applies to biologic drugs seeking marketing approval without reference to previous FDA-licensed biologic products. The proposed drug was indicated for a severe, chronic, non-oncology indication. The Sponsor proposed the cynomolgus monkey as the only relevant species, based on similarity to approved innovator Drug A. Drug B had an identical amino acid sequence to Drug A, and the Sponsor provided binding and functional activity data using Drug A as a comparator. The proposed nonclinical program was limited to a 4-week toxicology study in NHPs. The proposed clinical protocol was a 12-week clinical bioequivalence study with Drug A as a reference product. Overall, the Sponsor proposed to bridge to the previously approved biologic to demonstrate safety and effectiveness.

It is clear from the submission that the Sponsor meant to rely upon comparability to an approved product for approval. The Sponsor could potentially develop their product under the 351(k) pathway, and license their product as a biosimilar. In contrast, under the 351(a) pathway, the goal is "stand-alone" development to demonstrate that the proposed product is safe and effective, without reliance on another drug for safety or efficacy. For example, drug development starts with nonclinical research, and progresses through clinical trials. Pivotal Phase 3 trials are conducted to show safety and efficacy. However, the 351(k) pathway is used to demonstrate biosimilarity between the proposed product and an approved reference product. The FDA guidance for industry *Scientific Considerations in Demonstrating*

Biosimilarity to a Reference Product provides an overview of FDA's approach to determining biosimilarity.

Further, when a Sponsor chooses the 351(a) pathway, the Sponsor should follow the recommendations in ICH S6(R1). For example, a Sponsor needs to provide adequate "stand-alone" data for species selection, without comparing to a reference product. Functional data prevails over sequence data alone when selecting pharmacologically relevant species, because functional data are more clinically relevant. If pharmacologically relevant rodent and nonrodent species are identified, the Sponsor should conduct studies in both species to support the dose levels and duration of the proposed clinical protocol, as recommended in ICH S6(R1).

17.3 Dose Selection: Pitfalls Arising from Target Specificity

The goals of general toxicology studies include identifying a maximum tolerated dose (MTD) and/or dose-limiting toxicity (DLT); however, overt toxicity may not be observed with biologics, as toxicity is usually the result of exaggerated pharmacology. Whereas small-molecule drugs can be tested for toxicity, the high dose for biologic drugs is often limited by other factors (maximum feasible dose [MFD], toxicity secondary to administration of protein). Per ICH *M3(R2)*, if no toxicity is observed, the high dose should be a saturating dose, the MFD, or provide a 50-fold exposure margin for small-molecule drugs. For biologic drugs, however, ICH S6(R1) is clear that the high dose should be based upon the maximum intended pharmacologic effect of the drug, or a 10-fold exposure margin over the clinical dose, whichever is higher, unless there are issues with feasibility:

> "A rationale should be provided for dose selection taking into account the characteristics of the dose-response relationship. Pharmacokinetic-pharmacodynamic (PK-PD) approaches (e.g., simple exposure-response relationships or more complex modeling and simulation approaches) can assist in high dose selection by identifying 1) a dose which provides the maximum intended pharmacological effect in the preclinical species; and 2) a dose which provides an approximately 10-fold exposure multiple over the maximum exposure to be achieved in the clinic. The higher of these two doses should be chosen for the high dose group in preclinical toxicity studies unless there is a justification for using a lower dose (e.g., maximum feasible dose)."

Ideally, a PD marker can be evaluated in general toxicology studies, to demonstrate and study in vivo pharmacologic activity. Frequently, however, a PD marker is not available.

For biologics that fail to demonstrate expected effects in general toxicology studies, the Sponsor should consider whether the dose range evaluated was sufficient, or whether the doses should have taken any differences in binding affinity into consideration when designing the study. Other concerns include whether the species selected is sufficiently relevant from a pharmacological perspective. This may occur either because of intrinsic differences in the physiology of the pathway between humans and animals, or between healthy and diseased animals. In the absence of a plausible biological mechanism, the Sponsor should evaluate whether ADA-mediated clearance may have affected the interpretation of the data.

In cases where the PD effect of a biologic drug cannot be shown in a GLP-compliant toxicology study with healthy animals, Sponsors may consider conducting GLP-compliant toxicology studies in a disease model; however, such approaches should be considered on a case-by-case basis and only after consultation with the appropriate Review Division. The decision should take into consideration the patient population, severity of the disease, and feasibility of obtaining useful information. The lack of the well-characterized models (e.g., models with limited historical control data) for most diseases contributes to the challenge of toxicity testing in a disease model. Further, understanding the predictivity of a particular animal disease model for human diseases may be challenging. Distinguishing treatment-related toxicity from disease-related effects in the animal study may also be difficult. In a few cases, Regulators have raised specific concerns and asked Sponsors to consider GLP-compliant toxicology testing in a disease model.

17.3.1 FIH Start Dose Calculation Examples

The FDA Guidance for Industry *Estimating the Maximum Safe Starting Dose in Initial Clinical Trials for Therapeutics in Adult Healthy Volunteers*[12] provides recommendations for calculating starting doses for clinical trials. The guidance includes a focus (in Section 17.5.1) on calculation of human equivalent doses (HEDs) based on drug distribution by body surface area (BSA), and provides (in Section 17.5.2) guidance for calculating HEDs based on body weight (mg/kg). Most biologic drugs distribute into the vascular space; thus, FDA recommends interspecies dose extrapolation based on body weight as more appropriate than extrapolation based on BSA for most biologic drugs. Extrapolation based on BSA may be appropriate for some biologic drugs (e.g., ADCs and particular mechanisms of action). The maximum recommended starting dose (MRSD) should be adjusted for species differences in potency (e.g., target binding affinity and PD activity), and should incorporate a safety margin, as described in ICH M3(R2), or the ICH guidance for industry S9 *Nonclinical Evaluation for Anticancer Pharmaceuticals* as appropriate.[13]

The following five examples illustrate how calculations for the start dose are performed for:

1. Calculating a MRSD using body weight extrapolation and the monkey as the only pharmacologically relevant species.
2. Calculating a MRSD using body weight extrapolation, with the monkey as the only pharmacologically relevant species, and adjusting the start dose based on potency differences observed in *in vitro* studies with monkey and human cells.
3. Calculating a MRSD using BSA extrapolation, which can be applicable for biologics conjugated to small molecules. Multiple species are pharmacologically relevant, and pivotal general toxicology studies are conducted in the dog and rat.
4. Calculating a MRSD using BSA extrapolation, from studies in two pharmacologically relevant species, and adjusting for potency.
5. Calculating the local MRSD for the ocular route of administration, using general toxicology data from single species, while considering local and systemic margins of exposure.

17.3.1.1 Calculation Example: MRSD Based on Dose (mg/kg) – Single Relevant Species

For an antibody-derived biologic (MW >100 kDa) with equal potency in human and cynomolgus monkey, the monkey was identified as a pharmacologically relevant species. No NHPs were pharmacologically relevant. In the four-week intravenous GLP-compliant toxicology study in the cynomolgus monkey, the high dose of 100 mg/kg/week was the NOAEL, supporting a clinical start dose of 10 mg/kg.

Species	NOAEL (mg/kg)	K_d Fold Difference from Human	HED (mg/kg)	Margin of Exposure (HED Divided by Clinical Dose) Clinical Start Dose = 10 mg/kg
Monkey	100	1×	100	10×

17.3.1.2 Calculation Example: MRSD Based on Dose (mg/kg) – Single Species, Adjusted for Potency

For an investigational monoclonal antibody (MW ~ 150 kDa) with the cynomolgus monkey identified as the only pharmacologically relevant species, the biologic was four-fold less potent in *in vitro* assays using the monkey receptor, compared to the human receptor. In the four-week intravenous GLP-compliant toxicology study in the cynomolgus monkey, the highest dose tested, 100 mg/kg/week, was the NOAEL. The Sponsor had initially planned for a clinical start dose of 10 mg/kg. Based on the patient population and the potential for toxicity based on exaggerated pharmacology, FDA provided recommendations on the start dose. The Sponsor recognized the importance of adjusting for potency and revised the clinical start dose to 2.5 mg/kg.

---

[12] Guidance for Industry. 2005. Estimating the Maximum Safe Starting Dose in Initial Clinical Trials for Therapeutics in Adult Healthy Volunteers. Accessed from https://www.fda.gov/downloads/drugs/guidancecomplianceregulatoryinformation/guidances/ucm078932.pdf

[13] Guidance for Industry. 2010. S9 Nonclinical Evaluation for Anticancer Pharmaceuticals. Accessed from https://www.fda.gov/downloads/Drugs/Guidances/ucm085389.pdf

Species	NOAEL (mg/kg)	K_d Fold Difference from Human	HED (mg/kg)	Margin of Exposure (HED Divided by Clinical Dose) Clinical Start Dose = 2.5 mg/kg
Monkey	100	4×	25	10×

17.3.1.3 Calculation Example: MRSD Based on Body Surface Area (mg/m²) – Multiple Species

For a drug-biologic conjugate, the mouse, rat, dog, minipig, and monkey were identified as pharmacologically relevant species. Toxicology testing was performed in the rat and dog. In both the rat and dog, the NOAEL was 1 mg/kg; toxicity at 10 mg/kg was attributed to the small-molecule conjugate. In both the rat and dog, toxicity consistent with the expected pharmacology of the biologic portion of the conjugate was observed at 100 mg/kg, but not at 10 mg/kg. Proposed clinical start dose of 0.016 mg/kg was supported by nonclinical data from two species.

Species	NOAEL (mg/kg)	Conversion Factor from Animal Dose in mg/kg to Dose in mg/m² (k_m)	HED (mg/m²) (mg/m²)	HED (mg/kg)[a]	Margins of Exposure (HED Divided by Clinical Dose) Clinical Start Dose=0.016 mg/kg
Rat	1.0	6	6.0	0.16	10×
Dog	1.0	20	20.0	0.54	33×

[a] To convert the human dose from mg/m² to mg/kg, divide by the reference k_m value of 37.

17.3.1.4 Calculation Example: MRSD Based on Dose (mg/kg) – Multiple Relevant Species

For an investigational monoclonal antibody, *in vitro* binding (K_d) and inhibition (IC_{50}) assays showed slight differences in affinity: 1× for the human and cynomolgus monkey, fivefold less potency against the dog target, and 1.5-fold less potency against the mouse and rat targets. The rat and dog were selected as pharmacologically relevant species for toxicology testing. Although the monkey exhibited the closest affinity, the dog was considered an acceptable non-primate second species. Dose selection took the differences in binding affinity into consideration. The NOAELs for the rat and dog extrapolate to a HED of 10 mg/kg. The nonclinical data supported a clinical start dose of 1 mg/kg. Subsequent higher dose levels were supported by the combination of nonclinical and early clinical data.

Species	NOAEL (mg/kg)	K_d Fold Difference from Human	HED (mg/kg)	Margins of Exposure (HED Divided by Clinical Dose) Clinical Start Dose=1 mg/kg
Rat	15	1.5×	10	10×
Dog	50	5×	10	10×

17.3.1.5 Calculation Example: Local MRSD for Intravitreal Dosing – Single Species

For drugs administered by the ocular route, local and systemic margins of exposure following ocular dosing should be considered. For intravitreal dosing, the ocular dose levels can be scaled based on vitreal volume, which is species-specific.

Species	Reference Vitreal Volume[14]
Adult human	4.0 mL
Human (infant ~ 6 months)	1.5 mL
Mouse	5 µL
Rat	50 µL
Rabbit	1.5 mL
Dog	3.0 mL
Minipig	3.0 mL
Monkey	2.0 mL

For a biologic drug (MW > 100 KDa), the monkey was identified as the only relevant species. A GLP-compliant intravitreal toxicology study identified 2.0 mg/eye as the NOAEL for ocular and systemic toxicity. Adjusting for vitreal volume, the equivalent human intravitreal dose would be 4.0 mg/eye. The ocular NOAEL provides a 1× exposure margin over the clinical high dose. The systemic NOAEL corresponded to a systemic dose margin of 20× (on a mg/kg body weight basis) from the clinical high dose. WoE for the biologic drug supported omitting a GLP systemic-route toxicology study (please see Section 17.8.2 of this chapter, below). The FIH clinical trial was allowed to proceed.

Species	NOAEL	Fold Difference in Vitreal Volume Compared to the Adult Human	HED (mg/eye)	Margins of Exposure[a] (HED Divided by Clinical Dose) Clinical Start Dose=0.4 mg/kg	Clinical Highest Feasible Dose=4 mg/eye
Monkey	2.0 mg/eye	2×	4	10×	1×

[a] Proposed clinical doses are 0.4, 0.8, 1.6, 3.2, and 4.0 mg/eye.

While high-dose selection is not the focus of this section, it is important to acknowledge that when previous clinical trial data are not available to guide dose selection, adequate justification should be provided from safety information in nonclinical studies. Higher exposure margins may be needed to support safety for biologic drugs shown to cause serious, unmonitorable adverse effects compared to drugs with no findings of concern in adequately conducted studies. The FDA Review Division may have specific advice regarding the exposure margins appropriate for the disease indication being investigated, taking into consideration the severity of the nonclinical findings.

---

[14] Personal communication, Authors/FDA's Division of Transplant and Ophthalmology Products (DTOP).

17.4 Immunogenicity: Mitigating Pitfalls with Nonclinical Data

Immunogenicity assessments in nonclinical studies are conducted to facilitate the interpretation of the nonclinical study results and to help design subsequent studies. Omitting ADA assessment may be a pitfall if the data are needed to interpret the nonclinical results. Blood samples can be collected for toxicology studies with biologic drugs and can be archived for possible ADA analysis if needed for future study interpretation. Human proteins (e.g., human antibodies, humanized antibodies, replacement proteins) can be recognized as foreign proteins for animals, resulting in ADA. For this reason, and because of intrinsic species differences in the adaptive immune response, the induction of ADA in animals is not predictive of the potential for ADA formation in humans (see ICH S6(R1)).

In some cases, ADA enhances clearance of the biologic drug. When the ADA response is strong enough to rapidly deplete blood levels of the biologic below the lower limit of quantitation (LLOQ), dosing is no longer useful, and the dosed animals are essentially in recovery. Often, this information is not known during the conduct of the study unless TK or biomarker assessments are conducted in real time. If the Sponsor is able to obtain samples to assess a biological effect (e.g., flow cytometry markers suggest that PD has been lost) sacrificing a limited number of animals before scheduled main-group necropsy may facilitate the observation of tissue effects before potential lesions have had time to recover. Assuming data can be evaluated in real time and depending on the number of animals affected and the study design, reassigning animals between the main and recovery groups may help to maximize the usefulness of the study (i.e., reassignment of animals to an earlier sacrifice may provide an adequate number of animals with recent drug exposure at the time of assessment). In other cases, ADA may prolong exposure. Although this may increase the inter-animal variability and can cause exaggerated effects in some animals, it would generally not impair the assessment of toxicity unless evidence suggested that ADA abrogated PD activity of the product (i.e., treatment-related diminution of PD effect that correlated with an onset of ADA and/or subsequent bioanalytical investigations demonstrated that the ADA were neutralizing).

For chronic studies, increasing the dose or dose frequency to "push through" ADA clearance should be considered. This approach has more flexibility if the top dose is not limited by toxicity, and the doses are below the MFD. Notably, since the goal of the toxicology study is to achieve clinically relevant exposures, adjusting the administered dose and dosing frequency can be challenging. Generally, maintaining exposure for hazard characterization outweighs the value of keeping the dose frequency and risking loss of exposure, which could invalidate the study.

The timing of observations may be helpful to distinguish species-specific responses from predictive responses. In general, toxicity observed immediately after dosing may be caused by hypersensitivity or cytokine release. In the absence of other explanations, an immune response coinciding with the T_{max} may generally be attributed to primary pharmacology. In contrast, ADA-mediated inflammation generally increases in incidence and severity, beginning after the second or third dose of a biologic drug. ADA-related toxicity can be dose-limiting. In cases where the attending veterinarian orders a humane dosing holiday, the animals may not tolerate subsequent re-dosing. In this case, collecting histopathology data (i.e., humane sacrifice and necropsy) as soon as possible after the last dose is generally advisable.

If treatment-related deaths or other serious toxicity occurs and immune complex deposition is suspected, then immunohistochemistry (to demonstrate the deposition of the biologic drug, ADA complexes, and/or complement at the site of injury) may be helpful. The human tissue cross-reactivity study may serve as an initial guide for distinguishing sites of primary activity or direct binding from potential sites of immune complex deposition. Importantly, routine fixation of tissues (for histopathology) can prevent efficient immunohistochemical detection. If an animal dies prematurely, Sponsors should consider immediate necropsy and flash freezing of tissues to preserve antigens for histological detection.

Importantly, toxicities associated with immune complex formation can be addressed by demonstrating a clear link between the toxicity and immunogenicity in the animal model. Because immunogenicity in animals is not always predictive of immunogenicity in humans (see ICH S6(R1)), toxicities associated with nonclinical immunogenicity can be addressed with adequate nonclinical data and careful clinical monitoring for immunogenicity. The following case study illustrates how nonclinical data partly addressed toxicities observed in mice and monkeys, associated with immune complex formation.

17.4.1 Case study: Verifying Cause of Death Associated with Immune Complex Formation

In this example, a Sponsor opened an IND application for the development of an NME humanized monoclonal antibody for the treatment of a common but serious disease. Previous human experience had been obtained outside of the United States and up to 1000 mg had been administered clinically for 4 weeks with no adverse clinical findings. In addition, GLP-compliant 1-month and 3-month studies in both cynomolgus monkey and mice were submitted. The proposed clinical protocol was a single-ascending dose (SAD) trial in healthy human volunteers. FDA review of the toxicology studies in mice and monkeys raised questions regarding safety.

In vitro binding studies and functional assays demonstrated that cynomolgus monkeys and mice were pharmacologically relevant species.

In the 1-month mouse study, animals developed tremors at all doses that were associated with decreased general activity. The development of tremors precluded the establishment of a NOAEL in this study. The Sponsor investigated if the tremors were associated with the formation of ADAs, but there was no clear correlation. Approximately half of the animals at the low-dose group developed ADAs, but only 4 of 20 animals at the mid-dose, and 2 of 20 animals at the high-dose developed ADAs.

In the 3-month mouse study, with a 3-month recovery, deaths were observed at the low-dose starting at day 15 of the study. There were no associated clinical signs. The Sponsor attributed these deaths to acute hypersensitivity, although no supportive data was provided. Due to the lack of supportive data, no NOAEL was established in the 3-month mouse study. ADA was noted in all dose groups, but was most prevalent in mice at the low-dose. The toxicokinetic data showed an association of ADA with lower drug exposure. The FDA concluded that immunomodulatory effects of the drug may have affected levels of antidrug antibody (ADA), resulting in inhibition of ADA response at the higher doses.

In monkeys, no concerning test-article related findings were observed in the 1-month study. In the 3-month monkey study with a 1 month recovery period, dose-dependent tissue swelling was observed in 4 out of 4 monkeys during the study, immediately after dosing. On Day 1, approximately 4 hours after intravenous (IV) infusion, one high-dose male and one high-dose female developed facial swelling, which was controlled with diphenhydramine treatment. Later during the study, two additional animals at the high-dose also developed swelling in other areas of the body. No dose-limiting findings were observed in control monkeys. The ADA assay in the monkey study was difficult to interpret, due to positive signals in control animals at pretest. Microscopic kidney lesions in IV-dosed monkeys were associated with immune complex formation in the glomeruli and tubular epithelia, based on immunohistochemistry assessments and histopathological evidence. Thus, the Sponsor determined the kidney lesions to be clinically irrelevant and FDA concurred.

Relying on the data from the 3-month mouse study, the nonclinical data were deemed inadequate to support clinical dosing by the IV route. However, clinical safety was demonstrated by the previous human experience at doses of up to 1000 mg for up to 4 weeks; thus, the proposed clinical protocol was allowed to proceed. The Division sent non-hold comments recommending that the Sponsor provide evidence to support the Sponsor's hypothesis attributing the deaths in the 3-month mouse study to hypersensitivity. Further, the Sponsor was asked to address the swelling in the 3-month monkey study. Additional information to address these concerns was requested to support repeat-dose clinical trials greater than 1 month in duration.

Later during development, the Sponsor submitted immunohistochemical data on tissues from the 3-month mouse study, providing compelling evidence that death in mice was associated with immune complex formation, and therefore, not clinically relevant. Tissues from multiple organs were assayed from control, low-dose and high-dose animals. Granular deposits were observed in the liver, kidney and spleen of animals that died at the low-dose in the 3-month mouse study. These deposits were not observed in animals that were euthanized for reasons unrelated to the test article, or in animals that survived to scheduled euthanasia.

Preliminary data were also submitted from an ongoing 6-month monkey study, suggesting that the swelling observed in the 3-month monkey study was due to perivascular swelling. The Sponsor notified FDA that immunohistochemical testing was ongoing to determine if immune complex formation was the root cause of vasculitis in the monkey.

In summary, immune complex formation led to different toxicities in mice and monkeys. FDA concurred that the deaths at the low-dose in the 3-month mouse study were not clinically relevant because they were associated with immune complex formation. However, the swelling in the 3-month monkey study correlated to findings of perivascular inflammation in the longer term 6-month monkey study. The Sponsor planned to provide data to support their hypothesis that the swelling was the result of immune complex-associated vasculitis. The swelling observed in monkeys remained a concern for patient safety.

17.5 Further Safety Considerations for General Biologic Drug Development

The following three case studies highlight strategies for overcoming safety issues during drug development that were not specifically addressed in the previous sections. FDA reviews situations on a case-by-case basis. Briefly, the first case study discusses how data from recovery animals can be used to enable dosing in clinical trials. The second case study illustrates how the proposed indication can be changed to align better with the benefit-risk assessment. Finally, the third case study discusses how historical control data can be used to address findings in a general toxicology study.

The first case study discusses how data from recovery animals can be used to enable single-dose clinical studies for a serious and life-threatening indication with no approved therapies. Such decisions are made on a case-by-case basis. ICH S6(R1) recommends that a recovery period should generally be included in studies to help determine if toxicities are reversible, or if there is delayed toxicity.

17.5.1 Case Study: Taking Reversibility into Account for Serious Indications for Single Dose Studies

A Sponsor submitted a new IND with a clinical protocol proposed to treat a population with a serious disease, and targeted patients who were refractory to the standard of care. Although the disease was

not life-threatening, it impacted the ability to perform routine daily tasks. The proposed biologic was
a new molecular entity (NME), Biologic Drug C, for
a first-in-human (FIH) single-ascending dose (SAD)
trial. The Division had several ongoing INDs for
NMEs targeting the same pathway.

For Drug C, the pivotal nonclinical studies were
1-month repeat-dose GLP-compliant toxicology
studies in monkeys and rats. In monkeys, treatment caused multiple toxicities, but the low-dose
was not associated with any toxicity, and was determined to be the NOAEL. In the 1-month rat study,
with a 2-week recovery period, animals developed
pancreatic inflammation at the mid-dose, with full
reversal at the end of recovery. At the high-dose,
pancreatic inflammation was associated with only
partial recovery. The rat was identified as the most
sensitive species. Relying on the dose-limiting pancreatic inflammation observed, the NOAEL was
determined to be the low-dose in rats.

For safety assessment of the SAD trial design,
reversibility of the pancreas finding was considered in FDA's benefit-risk assessment. In this case,
the disease being treated in the clinical trials was
serious, and there were no approved disease-
modifying drugs. Importantly, the pharmacology
studies were promising; therefore, the mid-dose in
the rat study was used to support administration
of a single clinical dose because the lesions at this
dose demonstrated full recovery after 1-month of
repeated dosing. The maximum supported clinical
dose, calculated based on mg/kg drug distribution
and an adequate safety margin, was lower than the
Sponsor's proposed high dose in the clinical protocol. As a result, the reviewing Division requested
that the Sponsor lower the highest dose in the proposed SAD study. The Sponsor's amended protocol
was determined to be safe to proceed.

Regarding future multiple ascending dose (MAD)
clinical studies, FDA communicated that the high
dose should be supported by NOAELs identified at
the end of the dosing period (i.e., in dose termination groups, not recovery groups) in animal studies. Reversibility of findings in nonclinical studies
would not be taken into account for MAD clinical
studies for the proposed indication.

The second case study below illustrates how the proposed
indication or clinical population can be changed to align
better with the toxicities observed, and the benefit-risk balance considered during drug development. FDA generally
does not list which indications are appropriate for a specific
benefit-risk assessment, but FDA Review Divisions will
inform Sponsors if a proposed indication may not be appropriate given available safety and efficacy data, and the current
standard of care for a disease or condition. The appropriateness of a Sponsor's clinical testing plan may also depend on
the specific toxicities observed; the potential impact on the
population proposed in clinical trials; and the population that
would be affected if the product were to be approved for the
proposed indication.

17.5.2 Case Study: No NOAEL Identified: Focusing on an Appropriate Serious, Life-Threatening Indication

A Sponsor proposed to develop a NME named
Biologic Drug D for two separate indications a the pre-
IND stage. The indications were different with regard
to the benefit-risk assessment, and certain toxicities
may be acceptable in one population that would not
acceptable in the other population. Specifically, the
first indication was serious, but had multiple approved
therapies, and was not life-threatening. The second
indication was serious and life-threatening, had no
approved therapies, and mainly affected women.

The meeting package summarized data that
NHPs were the only pharmacology relevant species.
Toxicities in GLP-compliant 1-month and 3-month
monkey toxicology studies were outlined in the
Meeting Package. The Sponsor identified testicular toxicity in the 3-monkey study, which included
germ cell injury leading to failure to produce viable
sperm. The Sponsor determined that no surrounding
cells in the testes were targeted.

FDA clinical and nonclinical teams met internally
and discussed the Sponsor's summary. No data had
been submitted because the application was at the pre-
IND stage of development. The Division determined
that the testicular toxicity may be acceptable in this
case for a serious and life-threatening disease with no
approved therapies; however, the Division considered
clinical trials with Drug D to be inappropriate for the
serious indication with multiple approved therapies;
approved therapies did not cause comparable toxicities.

The Division conveyed this decision to the
Sponsor and emphasized that the testicular findings
must be clearly described as adverse in the Clinical
Investigator's Brochure, and the Patient Informed
Consent. While the more serious indication predominantly affected women, it also occurred in men.
Therefore, the overall development program was
required to address both sexes.[15] If robust efficacy
was seen in female patients with a substantial benefit, a clinical trial in men may be appropriate. For
example, if the drug showed prevention or reversal of
organ damage and/or death in women, testicular toxicities may be an acceptable risk in informed male
patients. The Division noted that these comments
provided at pre-IND meeting were preliminary, and
based on the information provided by the Sponsor.
Further, no review of the data had been conducted,
and it was not clear if there was a safety margin
for the findings. The testicular toxicity would be a
review issue at the time of IND submission.

The third case study discusses how historical control data
can be used to address findings in a general toxicology study.
Sponsors may observe findings that appear to be test article

---

[15] FDA Guidances Relating to Testing and Characterization of Drugs in
Humans by Demographic Group Can Be Accessed from https://www.
fda.gov/ScienceResearch/SpecialTopics/WomensHealthResearch/
ucm131182.htm

related, based on a higher incidence in dose animals versus controls, with a clear dose response. In some situations, a clear dose response is not demonstrated (particularly if all dose levels produce saturating exposures), but the interpretation of the data can still be difficult. In such cases, historical control data from the same species, strain, sex, and the same laboratory and animal source may aid in the interpretation of findings. Data from other laboratories or animals from a different vendor are generally reviewed with caution.

17.5.3 Case Study: No NOAEL Identified: Use of Historical Control Data to Address Toxicities

A Sponsor opened an IND for an NME with a clinical protocol that did not have adequate nonclinical support, and lacked previous clinical experience to overcome the lack of nonclinical support. *In vitro* binding and functional data demonstrated that only NHP species were pharmacology relevant, but a NOAEL was not identified in the general toxicology study.

Briefly, the Sponsor submitted a 1-month monkey study in which FDA identified potential test article related toxicity at all doses. The submitted study report did not adequately address the finding, and an Information Request was sent to the Sponsor during the initial 30-day review period to address the finding. The Sponsor hypothesized that the finding was not test article related, but did not provide any historical control data or literature to support this hypothesis. Because the Sponsor did not adequately address the safety concerns during the 30-day IND safety review period, the IND was put on clinical hold.

To remove the clinical hold, the Sponsor was asked to address the toxicities in the monkey study, or to repeat the study with lower doses to identify a NOAEL. The Sponsor commissioned a third party to convene a Pathology Working Group (PWG) to review the finding in the monkey. The PWG clarified that the finding was a common background finding based on data from multiple labs and the literature, which were then submitted to the IND. Upon reviewing the PWG's data, FDA concurred with the PWG and the Sponsor. The original clinical protocol was determined to be safe to proceed.

Convening the PWG was important to gathering and sorting data sufficiently compellingly to address the safety concern. Expert opinions alone, however, generally do not address safety issues, in the absence of additional data.

17.6 Development of Biologic Drugs for Specific Indications

Special considerations for the nonclinical development of biologic drugs for specific disease indications: transplant, ophthalmology, and oncology, are provided below. In addition, Section 17.7.2 covers the transition of oncology drugs to a non-oncology indication.

17.6.1 Biologic Drugs for Transplant Indications

Transplant indications represent major unmet medical needs, and development of therapeutic biologics to treat transplant indications is encouraged.

Few biologic drugs are developed solely for transplant; most have a history of development for oncology, autoimmune disorders, or inflammation.

Muromonab-CD3 (Orthoclone OKT®) was the first monoclonal antibody approved by FDA (CBER) in 1985 (prior to the finalization of the first ICH S6 guidance). It is a murine antibody against CD3 and was approved to treat acute allograft in patients with renal, cardiac, and hepatic transplants.

The National Institute of Health's (NIH's) Clinicaltrials.gov provides public examples of approved therapies being tested for transplant indications, including biologics approved for hematological malignancies (e.g., rituximab, ofatumumab, alemtuzumab, eculizumab) and agents to treat multiple sclerosis, arthritis, colitis and Crohn's disease (e.g., natalizumab, infliximab, tocilizumab, and vedolizumab).

Therapies for transplant focus on three main areas: (1) preventing and reversing ischemic injury to the organ resulting from the transplant procedure, (2) modifying the patient immune system to maintain the graft and prevent rejection, and (3) addressing the underlying conditions that necessitated transplant. Biologics research for investigational transplant therapies has focused on ischemic injury and immunomodulation. For severe and life-threatening indications with unmet medical need, CDER's approach is analogous to the description in the Serious Conditions guidance[16] and in ICH S9.

17.6.2 Biologic Drugs for Ophthalmology Indications

Ophthalmologic product development is uniquely challenging. Although the surface of the eye can be easily dosed, the drug product is rapidly cleared away by the tear film and lasting efficacy is difficult to achieve. The tear film and cornea together prevent the penetration of biologic drugs into deeper ocular structures. For systemic (e.g., intravenous, subcutaneous) dosing of biologic products, the blood-ocular barriers greatly limit exposure of the eye (if not compromised by the underlying disease and inflammation, drug-induced inflammation, or vehicle). Additionally, concentrations in blood are relatively low compared to those that can be achieved by direct local administration of drug to the eye. Therefore, most ophthalmic biologic drugs are administered by intraocular injection (e.g., intravitreal, intracameral, subconjunctival, subretinal, sub-Tenon's space, peribulbar and retrobulbar injection) or intraocular implant.

Intraocular dosing faces major obstacles: (1) Since the eye is a closed space, the maximum volume of injection is limited by intraocular pressure, limiting the MFD, (2) the frequency of dosing is limited by the need for a clinical visit (due to the expertise needed to perform the procedure), the risks

---

[16] CDER/CBER. 2014a. Procedural Guidance for Industry. Expedited Programs for Serious Conditions – Drugs and Biologics. Accessed from https://www.fda.gov/downloads/Drugs/Guidances/UCM358301.pdf

TABLE 17.1

Flow Chart for Nonclinical Development of Biologic Drug Products for Ophthalmology

In vitro and *in vivo* PD studies, secondary pharmacology screen
↓
One systemic-route general toxicology study in a relevant species (to characterize systemic toxicity and TK)
↓
Ocular toxicology studies in two pharmacologically relevant species (if available)
- Using the clinical formulation
- Using the clinical route of exposure
- Standard endpoints for systemic toxicology studies (e.g., body weight, hematology, clinical chemistry, coagulation, urinalysis, blood TK, organ weights, full systemic histopathology)
- Ocular endpoints, including irritation, slit lamp biomicroscopy, fundoscopy, tonometry, ERG assessment, and full ocular histopathology.
↓
Ocular distribution study in one species using clinical formulation/clinical route
          ↓   ↓

If systemic exposure following ocular dosing is negligible	If systemic exposure following ocular dosing is **more than negligible**
↓	↓
Initiate clinical trials (with adequate contraception, as appropriate)	If adequate exposure margins (generally 10×, corrected[17]) over clinical dose were not achieved in the ocular toxicology studies, then conduct systemic-route general toxicity studies in second species to support clinical use.
↓	↓
	Safety pharmacology studies (usually incorporated into one or more of the toxicology study designs with time points covering the estimated systemic T_{max}; stand-alone testing can also be done)
	↓
	Initiate clinical trials (with adequate contraception, as appropriate)
	↓
Longer-term /chronic ocular toxicology studies in two relevant species to support long-term clinical use • ocular endpoints • systemic TK (confirm that systemic exposure following longer-term ocular dosing is still negligible).	Longer-term/chronic ocular toxicology studies in two relevant species to support long-term clinical use • ocular and systemic endpoints • systemic TK
↓	↓
	If adequate exposure margins (generally 10×, corrected[18]) over clinical dose were not achieved in the chronic ocular toxicology studies, then conduct chronic long-term systemic-route general toxicity studies in at least one species to support long-term clinical use.
	↓
Initiate Phase 3 clinical trials (with contraception, as appropriate)	
↓	↓
For the BLA: • Embryo-fetal development (EFD) studies in two relevant species, with TK • Formal request for waiver of carcinogenicity studies	For the BLA: • Full developmental and reproductive (DART) toxicology studies. • Carcinogenicity studies, if feasible

associated with the procedure, and procedure-related discomfort and inflammation. The potency, specificity, and long half-life of biologic drugs make them attractive, compared to small-molecule drugs, for intraocular dosing.

The nonclinical development path used by many Sponsors for ophthalmic biologic drugs can be summarized with this chart (Table 17.1):

Alternative approaches may be appropriate for some biologic drugs (e.g., a longer-term ocular toxicity study in one species rather than two species), depending on the mechanism of action and safety profile. Sponsors may find discussion of specific cases with regulators to be helpful, prior to study initiation.

17.6.2.1 Species Selection Considerations for Ophthalmic Biologic Drugs

The ICH S6(R1) guidance recommends testing biologic drugs in a rodent species "unless there is a scientific rationale for using nonrodents." Generally, the rodent is considered

---

[17] Corrected for differences between the patient population and test species for the biologic drug (e.g., differences in binding affinity or potency, differences in vitreal volume following intravitreal injection).
[18] ibid.

adequate if the target is expressed, the biologic drug binds the target with comparable affinity and is pharmacologically active in that species. However, physiological and anatomical differences between rodents and humans may limit the utility of the rodent model for ophthalmic products. The rabbit may be considered as a standard laboratory model that provides many of the advantages of rodent testing (e.g., relevant historical data, laboratory expertise, larger group sizes to detect pharmacology/toxicology). For example, the small intravitreal volume of the mouse eye (5 μL) discourages the use of the mouse for intravitreal dosing with a biologic drug candidate. The larger intravitreal volume of the rabbit (1.5 mL) makes intravitreal dosing feasible.

17.6.2.2 PK/TK Drives Nonclinical Program Design for Ophthalmology Biologic Drugs

Why conduct systemic route-toxicology studies to support ocular dosing? The purpose of the systemic-route toxicology studies is to identify toxicities, to characterize the dose response in systemic tissues, and to ensure an adequate exposure margin for systemic toxicity when selecting doses for the ocular-route studies.

In a few cases for biologic drug products empirically shown to have negligible systemic exposure in early PK studies, Sponsors have begun to omit the systemic-route GLP-compliant toxicology studies, instead relying on the systemic endpoints incorporated into the ocular-route GLP-compliant toxicology studies to support safety, when they can achieve adequate systemic exposure margins, corrected.[19] This approach necessitates adequate analytical methods.

For some biologic drug products, achieving an adequate dose margin by the ocular route may not be technically feasible (e.g., solubility or volume limitations; dose correction for species differences in potency). In some cases, Sponsors have learned, after conducting ocular-route studies, that their analytical methods were not yet sensitive enough to measure serum concentrations of their biologic drug. In these types of cases, the importance of GLP-compliant systemic-route toxicology studies in two species is clear. Generally, design of systemic-route toxicology studies to support ocular dosing should consider the guidance provided in ICH M3(R2) for dose selection and the *Guidance for Industry ICH S3A Toxicokinetics: The Assessment of Systemic Exposure in Toxicity Studies* for TK. When the biologic drug product is not detected systemically following ocular dosing, ideally the systemic route NOAEL will achieve systemic exposures at least 10× over the clinical LLOQ.

What is negligible systemic exposure for ocular dosing, and how is negligibility demonstrated without systemic data from toxicology studies? Usually, the *in vitro* and *in vivo* PD studies have identified an inactive concentration for the endpoint(s) measured (i.e., the intended pharmacology). These can be used to predict a systemic concentration below which activity would not be expected. This approach helps protect against toxicity caused by exaggerated primary pharmacology, but are inherently limited. Moreover, the early safety data for off-target

toxicity (e.g., secondary pharmacology screening, tissue cross-reactivity study in relevant human tissues) are even more limited. To protect patient safety, the default approach for ocular administration of biologic drugs is to assume that systemic exposure occurs (even if below the lower limit of detection) and reaches a high-enough concentration to cause toxicity. Therefore, systemic toxicology endpoints are recommended for the initial GLP toxicology studies.

The decision to omit systemic endpoints from clinical trial design and later nonclinical toxicology studies is necessarily case-by-case. The scientific justification for concluding that systemic exposure is negligible would be strengthened by sensitive analytical methods (i.e., low LLOD) and an understanding of the targeted pathway (e.g., previous experience from small molecule drugs or other biologics, knockout mouse data, natural disease models). Reliable *in vitro* assays (binding affinity, functional activity assays) are needed to bridge from the inactive concentration (under the *in vitro* conditions tested) to the systemic concentration (or LLOQ).

For topical ocular dosing, one pitfall is particularly notable for biologics: the drainage of drug product into the nasolacrimal duct, which may result in systemic absorption. For potent biologics, this exposure may be enough to cause systemic toxicity. Therefore, systemic PK or TK should be measured for topically administered biologic drugs, as well as for injected/implanted biologic drugs.

Maximum feasible intraocular dose is a key limitation for drugs (small-molecule and biologic drugs). Intraocular injection increases intraocular pressure. As a benchmark, a clinical intravitreal injection volume of 50 μL is commonly accepted, and ≤ 100 μL is the maximum dose volume for adult eyes. Divided dosing (e.g., two doses separated by a given time) can be considered, but increases the risk of procedure-related damage. Trying to inject too large a volume results in extrusion of the drug from the eye through the injection-site hole. Large volumes increase the likelihood of immediate procedure-related damage (e.g., retinal tear/detachment, cataract, IOP increase) as well as longer-term effects (e.g., damage to the optic nerve). Because many biologics have the potential to cause or worsen these types of damage, the protective default approach is to assume that toxicity in a treated eye is due to treatment.

Biologic drugs are frequently chosen as candidates over small-molecule drugs, because biologics' potency and relative longer elimination half-life increase their duration of pharmacological activity. In many cases, a clinical dose goal is identified, but the highest feasible dose is less than 10× of this goal. A conservative approach is to lower the FIH start dose to 1/10th the NOAEL, even if this is anticipated to be subtherapeutic. However, depending on the clinical indication and patient population, this may not be warranted and can be particularly challenging for biologic drugs where no toxicity has been observed. An additional pitfall arises when the biologic is less potent in the animal model than in humans (i.e., warranting dose adjustment based on potency differences). In all cases, the start dose and the MRSD for the FIH clinical trial should be scientifically justified.

Target saturation is a particularly important consideration for intraocular injections and implants of biologic drugs. The

---

[19] ibid.

eye is a relatively closed space, and the blood: ocular barriers slow distribution of the biologic into systemic circulation. Since target saturation causes a maximal pharmacological response, a higher dose will increase the duration of toxicity, but will not affect the magnitude of responses. Therefore, the dose margin is not increased beyond saturation, when calculating the maximum safe starting dose for clinical trials. Instead, the dose response is observed in the duration of effect.

For example, the labeling[20] for aflibercept (Eylea®) recommends a high-dose (2 mg administered by intravitreal injection every 4 weeks) for the first 12 weeks, followed by a low-dose (2 mg via intravitreal injection once every 8 weeks). Labeling notes that "additional efficacy was not demonstrated in most patients when EYLEA was dosed every 4 weeks compared to every 8 weeks. Some patients may need every 4 weeks (monthly) dosing after the first 12 weeks."

For biologic drugs whose mechanism and potency warrant a safety concern, a robust approach is to empirically assess target saturation, measuring free: bound target over multiple time points from the first dose until immediately prior to the second dose. Understanding target saturation is also important in the context of establishing exposure margins for labeling.

A pitfall for intraocular biologic drugs with very long elimination half-lives is the importance of accurately estimating the time to full clearance (e.g., 6 half-lives), to inform clinical trial design and follow-up. In one case, TK data from single-dose intravitreal toxicology studies predicted persistence of the biologic drug in the eye for ≥ 2 years. Because removing the drug product from the eye after administration is infeasible, the time commitment required to understand the kinetics is important for patients and investigators.

17.6.2.3 DART Considerations for Ophthalmic Biologic Drugs

For biologic drug products, the BLA should address potential toxicity to all aspects of development and reproduction, per ICH guidances S5A, S6(R1), and M3(R2). For ophthalmic biologic drugs intended to treat women of child-bearing potential (WOCBP), EFD studies are generally recommended even if systemic exposure appears negligible. Particularly, clinically relevant dosing is recommended. This recommendation is based on the potential for developing tissues and organs of the embryo and fetus to be much more sensitive than adult issues. Generally, target expression and function in developing embryos and fetuses is not well understood, and other methods to collect data are not available (e.g., age-appropriate cells for *in vitro* PD assays, age-appropriate tissues for cross-reactivity). Many proteins are only expressed during development, allowing the potential for off-target toxicity; compensatory/protective pathways may not yet be fully developed at embryonic or early fetal stages.

A relatively common pitfall for EFD studies to support ophthalmic indications is dose selection. The doses (and resulting systemic exposures) for systemic-route administration are generally orders-of-magnitude higher than the total dose and systemic exposure resulting from ocular dosing. A NOAEL value from a systemic-route EFD study may result in a large safety margin. However, if the systemic-route EFD studies fail to identify NOAEL values for each key endpoint, then the relevance of the high LOAEL concentrations to clinical safety may be unclear. In this case, repeating the EFD studies, to characterize developmental toxicity at lower doses relevant to clinical exposures, might be necessary. Three case examples of appropriate dose selection help illustrate this point.

17.6.2.3.1 Case Study: EFD Data for Ranibizumab

Ranibizumab[21] is administered to patients by intravitreal injection, 0.5 mg/eye. Labeling summarizes the embryofetal developmental toxicity study in cynomolgus monkeys. Pregnant animals were dosed by intravitreal injection every 14 days, from gestation day 20 to day 62, at doses of 0, 0.125, or 1 mg/eye. No skeletal anomalies were observed with the 0.125 mg/eye low dose, which resulted in "trough exposures equivalent to a single eye treatment in humans." The high dose, 1 mg/eye, was 13-times the predicted human exposure based on maximal serum trough levels (C_{max}), and caused skeletal abnormalities.

17.6.2.3.2 Case Study: EFD Data for Aflibercept

In contrast to the previous case study, aflibercept[22] was administered to pregnant rabbits systemically (intravenous or subcutaneous). Although no developmental NOAEL was identified, the developmental LOAEL (0.1 mg/kg subcutaneous) achieved systemic exposure relevant to the clinical dose (6 times higher by AUC). This approach was also adequate to characterize the risk for patients because the exposures achieved in rabbits were relevant to clinical exposures.

17.6.2.3.3 Case Study: EFD Data to Support a Change in Route of Administration

For a biologic drug, an EFD study in one non-primate species was conducted, with doses selected to support intravenous dosing to treat a life-threatening indication. Developmental toxicity was observed at all dose levels, with the lowest dose equivalent to 1x the clinical dose (on a mg/kg basis).

Subsequently, intravitreal dosing of this biologic drug was investigated to treat ophthalmic indications. Doses under consideration for the pivotal Phase 3 ophthalmic indication clinical trials were more than 120X lower than the previously evaluated clinical systemic doses. The Review Division was concerned that labeling based only on the previously

---

[20] Regeneron Pharmaceutical's BLA 125387 for Aflibercept. U.S. Package Insert was updated 5/26/2017. Accessed from https://www.accessdata.fda.gov/drugsatfda_docs/label/2017/125387s054lbl.pdf

[21] Lucentis' BLA 125156 for Lucentis® (ranibizumab) was approved in 2006. U.S. Package Insert was updated in 2017. Accessed from https://www.accessdata.fda.gov/drugsatfda_docs/label/2017/125156s114lbl.pdf

[22] Regeneron's BLA 125397 for Eylea® (aflibercept) was approved in 2011. U.S. Package Insert was updated in 2017. Accessed from https://www.accessdata.fda.gov/drugsatfda_docs/label/2017/125387s054lbl.pdf

completed EFD study at high exposures may not be relevant to the intravitreal route, may be misleading and does not address whether the drug is active or may not cause adverse effects on embryofetal development at lower exposures more relevant to the intravitreal indication. In order to generate relevant data to better inform the potential risks and benefits, the Review Division requested an additional study, with doses selected based on the clinical systemic exposure after intravitreal dosing. Results are not yet public.

17.6.2.3.4 Case Study: EFD Exposure Margin Based on Target Saturation

The issue of correcting for target saturation (discussed above) is particularly important when calculating the safety margins from DART studies of biologic drugs. *ICH S5(R3) Detection of Reproductive and Developmental Toxicity for Human Pharmaceuticals* (Section 6.1.2 Saturation of Systemic Exposure Endpoint) notes: "High dose selection based on saturation of systemic exposure measured by systemic availability of pharmaceutical-related substances can be appropriate. There is little value in increasing the administered dose if it does not result in increased plasma concentration". Calculations are straightforward when the biologic drug is not developmentally toxic, and/or the maximum recommended human ophthalmic dose (RHOD) results in negligible systemic exposure. For biologic drugs showing developmental toxicity, the true safety margin is generally not greater than the margin from the clinical C_{max} to the systemic concentration that results in target saturation. The importance of accurately conveying safety information is most important when the biologic drug is a potent developmental toxicant, and clinical dosing results in systemic exposure at or near target saturation (even if the C_{max} is transient).

For an antibody-derived antigen-binding fragment (Fab), intended to treat a serious chronic ocular condition, primary PD data included binding (K_D) and inhibition (IC_{50}, IC_{90}) values for human and animal models. The particular target afforded the opportunity to validate assays for plasma total Fab, total target, and Fab-target. For the two dose levels selected for Phase 3 clinical trials, systemic exposure was detected and predicted to have some transient pharmacological activity, but not achieve target saturation. Plasma AUC values could not be reliably calculated.

The rat was identified as the single relevant nonprimate species for assessment of developmental and reproductive toxicity. For the rat EFD and PPND studies, the low-dose was selected to achieve a C_{max} approximately equal to the C_{max} for the clinical high-dose. The mid-dose targeted a systemic exposure 10x the clinical C_{max}, and resulted in transient target saturation in the rat. The high-dose targeted a systemic exposure 25x the clinical C_{max}, and maintained near-complete target saturation.

The mid-dose was the developmental and maternal NOAEL. The high-dose was the developmental LOAEL (reduced fetal weight, visceral and skeletal malformations) and maternal LOAEL (reduced maternal weight gain and systemic target organ lesions). The Sponsor concluded that the observed toxicity reflected the duration of target saturation, and proposed that the study results were adequate to characterize safety; the Review Division agreed. The Sponsor proposed omitting summary of the high-dose results from labeling; a regulatory decision has not yet been reached.

17.6.2.4 Other Nonclinical Design Considerations for Ophthalmic Biologic Drugs

For ophthalmic biologic drugs, the maximum feasible duration of the ocular toxicology study may be limited. For human and humanized biologic drug products, the duration of nonclinical repeat-dose intraocular (e.g., intravitreal) studies is frequently limited by species-specific immune responses. This limitation does not preclude ocular clinical trials of longer duration than can be supported by nonclinical ocular toxicology data. If systemic exposure occurs following ocular dosing, then the longer-term/chronic systemic route toxicology may still be feasible, to characterize potential systemic toxicity. Conversely, if systemic exposure is negligible and chronic ocular dosing is not feasible, then a long-term toxicology study may not be needed.

In addition to species considerations for pharmacological relevance, the anatomy and physiology of the test species should be considered, as well as mechanism of action, route of administration, and predictivity for the clinical indication. The technical challenges of ocular dosing of rodents, and the anatomical differences of the rodent eye compared to the human eye, limit the practical use of rodent models for ophthalmic biologic drugs (e.g., to disease model PD studies, transgenic models). Frequently, the rabbit is used instead of rodent.

For both small-molecule drugs and biologic drugs administered by the ocular route, separate local (ocular) and systemic safety margins should be calculated to establish an appropriate MRSD. For intravitreal injection (and certain other intraocular exposures), calculating an ocular exposure margin corrected for species differences in vitreal volume is appropriate (please see the reference table and example below).

For biologic drugs, the tissue cross-reactivity study should be adequate to assess the eye and ocular adnexa. For products initially investigated for systemic administration, the previously completed tissue cross-reactivity study may not have assessed the eye in adequate detail to support the safety of ocular dosing.

ADA-related immunogenicity is common for ophthalmic dosing of animals with biologic drugs. As noted above, the species-specific response to human/humanized protein is not predictive of the patient response. Generally, treatment-related inflammation of the eye is monitorable, treatable, and resolves as the biologic drug clears. Frequently, the individual animal data show a correlation between ADA response and ocular inflammation.

When toxicity occurs that might be a species-specific immune response, a key question for understanding the toxicology study results is how to separate exaggerated pharmacology (primary and secondary) from species-specific immune responses. This challenge is especially difficult for biologics intended to target the immune system. Even when the goal is immunosuppression, the potential of partial activation (instead of inactivation) and compensatory inflammation should be considered. Likewise, for biologics intended to target the vasculature, toxicity due to immune-complex deposition seems consistent with potential toxicity.

For immunomodulators eliciting potent immunogenic responses in animal models, separating species-specific inflammation from unintended pharmacology may be difficult. When other approaches have been exhausted, two further approaches might be feasible toward demonstrating safety prior to the availability of clinical data. One possible approach to distinguish species-specific effects from direct pharmacology is the use of an isotype control arm. The goal would be to design a nonclinical study testing the candidate biologic drug compared to a sham-negative control (e.g., no treatment, saline treatment), and to a near-identical biologic that lacks the intended mechanism of action (e.g., an isotype control antibody, or a biologic with mutations to silence pharmacologic activity without intentionally affecting immunogenicity). For example, if a rabbit intravitreal toxicology study detects a higher severity of ocular inflammation for the candidate biologic drug compared to the isotype control, then the inflammation due to primary pharmacology can be distinguished from the rabbit response to the administration of humanized biologics. Some Sponsors have used the same antibody scaffold for multiple development programs, varying the antigen CDR, or making targeted amino acid changes (e.g., reduce immunogenicity, increase binding potency, reduce effector function). In several cases, the comparison of nonclinical and clinical data for previous products has helped interpret nonclinical data for the new products.

17.7 Oncology Drug Development for Biologic Drugs

The regulatory expectations regarding the development of anticancer pharmaceuticals are detailed in the ICH S9 guidance, entitled *Nonclinical Evaluation of Anticancer Pharmaceuticals* and its supplementary Q&A document (currently at Step 2 draft) (refer Oncology chapter). Because the safety of a biotechnology product is largely dependent upon its mechanism of action, careful justification is needed to support the pharmacological relevance of the selected toxicology species. A detailed description of the data needed to justify the selection of toxicologically species is provided in the ICH S6 Guidance entitled *Preclinical Safety Evaluation of Biotechnology-Derived Pharmaceuticals*, and its addendum.

Many of the regulatory expectations to support clinical development of biologic drugs intended for oncology indications are similar to those of non-oncology products; their key differences rest in timing and in the duration of studies needed to support longer-term clinical trials and marketing. For example, for an oncology indication, studies of up to 1-month duration are sufficient to support clinical administration until the initiation of registration-enabling trials. Longer-term studies (i.e., three-month toxicology studies) are not needed until the initiation of trials intended to support registration, and embryo-fetal toxicity studies are not needed until submission of a BLA.

Because most toxicities associated with the administration of a biologic are extensions of the intended pharmacology, a robust package of pharmacology data to demonstrate the drug's intended activity is needed to support clinical administration. As with small molecules, repeat-dose toxicology data in two species are expected to support a FIH study of a biotechnology product intended to treat patients with advanced cancer; however, the utility of these studies should also be supported by the potential for PD activity. For example, for many biopharmaceutical targets, the monkey is the only relevant toxicology species due to poor inter-species amino acid sequence homology that limits binding to rodent orthologues. In such cases, data demonstrating activity in the monkey, as well as data demonstrating a lack of activity in the rodent, are needed to support the FIH trial. For products that lack a relevant rodent species, a single-species general toxicology program in the monkey would be sufficient to support the development. If the product is active in both rodents and nonrodents and the toxicity profile is similar between the species, longer-term IND toxicology studies to support later clinical development and marketing may only be needed in a single species.

The toxicology data obtained should be augmented by a robust package of pharmacology studies to demonstrate the drug's intended mechanism of action. A typical pharmacology package for a monoclonal antibody that inhibits a growth-promoting receptor tyrosine kinase might include binding kinetic data against recombinant human and animal orthologues; effects of binding on downstream signaling in animal and human cells (e.g., pRTK inhibition by Western blot in transfected cells); demonstration of the drug's ability to block ligand binding and/or receptor activation; effects of the drug on cell proliferation and/or survival in cultured animal and human cells; effects of administration in a suitable disease model (e.g., a murine xenograft with cells that express the relevant target); and data from ADCC and complement dependent cytotoxicity (CDC) assays.

As stated in the ICH S9 guidance, assessment of a drug's potential embryo-fetal effects are needed to support marketing of drugs to patients with advanced cancer. For biologic drugs that lack a relevant toxicology species, Sponsors should seek FDA feedback about what data may be needed to support labeling for embryo-fetal risk. In some cases, literature data about the basic pharmacology of a given target may be sufficient to convey risk; however, Sponsors should consider the effects of partial pathway suppression as well as effects of complete pathway knockout, since in many cases, limited placental transport of biologic drugs may only be sufficient to reduce the activity of a given target in the developing fetus. In cases for which knockdown may lead to significant adverse reproductive effects (e.g., serious malformations or cognitive impairment), knockdown studies or studies with murine homologues (if available) may be most informative of risk to the developing fetus.

Because the toxicity of a biologic drug is often an extension of the drug's pharmacological mechanism of action, dose setting for FIH studies may involve the totality of pharmacology and toxicology data, particularly for drugs in which the toxicology species is likely to underpredict expected human toxicities. Immune-modulating products are an emerging class of drugs that highlight both the challenges intrinsic in biologic drug development and the need for a broad array of basic pharmacology data to support human safety. As such, the remainder of this section will emphasize examples from these types of products.

The recent success of CTLA4 and PD-1 inhibitors in the treatment of patients with highly refractory diseases has reinvigorated interest in immunostimulatory biologics, an area that was formerly hampered by concerns about significant clinical safety. These agents, collectively referred to as "cancer immunotherapies," aim to shift the patient's immunological tone from self-tolerance to tumor growth suppression, the side-effects of which can include auto-inflammatory diseases resulting from uncontrolled self-reactivity. These effects are idiosyncratic, frequently dose-limiting, potentially irreversible, and can be life-threatening or fatal; thus, while the growing understanding about interplay between cancer and the immune system has yielded a wealth of possible new drug targets, understanding the safe use of these drugs in a given patient is still in need of exploration. For approved anti-PD-1/PD-L1 inhibitors, the NHP toxicology studies conducted to support product approval have not predicted the observed toxicities in humans.[23]

The range of potential cancer immunotherapy targets varies widely from direct agonists of resting or activated T cells (e.g., anti-CD28 or anti-4-1BB and OX40) to inhibitors of immune-repressive pathways (e.g., anti-PD-1, -PD-L1/2 or -CTLA4 antibodies) and immunosuppressive cytokines like IL-10 and TGFβ or metabolic inhibitors and their downstream products like IDO-1. Still other targets include pathways to reduce the influx of myeloid-derived suppressor cells that can foster tumor cell immune evasion in the tumor microenvironment.

Because the monkey frequently underpredicts human safety with cancer immunotherapies, and because of the limited cross-reactivity with other species, much greater emphasis is placed upon the totality of pharmacology and toxicology data when making the overall safety determination for a FIH study with an immune-modulating target. Starting doses for FIH trials with cancer immunotherapy agents typically use a MABEL-based approach based on the totality of the pharmacology and toxicology data. The need to rely on this relatively conservative method to establish a safe starting dose has led to a concern from all parties that the early doses in these oncology dose escalation trials may be subtherapeutic. This concern has provoked interest in ways to streamline the early dose-escalation phase to minimize exposure of patients to subtherapeutic doses. Common approaches to address this issue in oncology trials include accelerated titration schemes and intra-patient dose-escalation plans, the details of which will depend

on the proposed schedule and PD mechanism of the drug and are best devised in consultation with the appropriate Review Division prior to submission of an IND application. For some drugs with the well-defined mechanisms of action, particularly when supplemented with directly comparative data with a similar agent, a higher degree of initial PD activity may be justified for a FIH trial.

Because the development schedule in oncology is often significantly truncated relative to many other therapeutic areas, timing of CMC and nonclinical activities may need to be accelerated to avoid delays in development and/or approval. As stated in the ICH S9 guidance, the reports of three-month studies are expected prior to the initiation of a Phase 3 trial; however, drugs that exhibit a high degree of clinical activity relative to currently available therapies may be granted accelerated approval before Phase 3. For drugs that exhibit a high degree of early clinical activity such as those granted breakthrough designation early in development, the Sponsor should consider the initiation of any studies needed to support registration-enabling trials as soon as possible.

As stated in the ICH S6 and S9 guidances, the purpose of toxicology studies is to identify a drug's target organs of toxicity. For some biologic drugs, such as inhibitory monoclonal antibodies targeting immune suppressive pathways, target organs may be difficult to extrapolate between animals and humans due to the relative insensitivity of the test system. In such cases, Sponsors should augment the toxicology studies with safety data from other sources (e.g., literature data; data with surrogate antibodies, if available; or data with knock outs, knockdowns, or knock-in models). For modulators of less well-characterized pathways, these data can be particularly useful in establishing the most appropriate starting dose and for formulating patient monitoring plans for a FIH trial.

For biologic drugs that stimulate the immune system (e.g., cytokine mixtures with the potential for synergistic toxicity; potent, pro-inflammatory cytokines fused to Fc fragments; bispecific agonist antibodies), the major concerns usually relate to the potency of the expected response. For this reason, it is important to evaluate the potential for a steep, even lethal, activity-response curve *in vivo*, and, particularly if the toxicology models are expected to underpredict toxicity, in *in vitro* models using human cells. Because most oncology trials escalate doses to the MTD in humans, doses may exceed those tested in animals; therefore, it is important for these types of products to characterize the toxicity dose response and to particularly evaluate the potential for a steep lethal dose response to occur at some point in the dose escalation.

In addition, during development, Sponsors should anticipate safety considerations of theoretical concern based on the pharmacological activity of the product. For example, one concern with some cancer immunotherapies is the potential for the drug to increase the magnitude of an immediate and/or memory responses to a foreign antigen (e.g., an influenza or tetanus vaccine), leading to severe inflammatory reactions following the initial or repeated vaccination. This evaluation is of particular concern if clinical trials have excluded routine vaccination. Another theoretical concern with some cancer immunotherapies is the potential to exacerbate chronic infections (e.g., tuberculosis). Given the accelerated nature of

[23] Ochoa de Olza M, et al. Early-drug development in the era of immuno-oncology: are we ready to face the challenges? *Annals of Oncology.* 2018;29(8):1727–1740.

many oncology development programs, only a few hundred patients may be treated prior to the drug receiving accelerated approval; thus, the trials may be incapable of detecting even serious safety effects if they occur at low frequencies in the intended patient population. In the absence of available data, Sponsor may expect requests to add language to the product label to address remaining safety uncertainties with the drug and/or post-marketing studies to assess outstanding safety concerns based on the drug's mechanisms that were not fully assessed in clinical trials.

With the recent approval of a PD-1/CTLA4 combination regimen, there is increased interest in developing novel combinations of immune-stimulating agents and/or chemotherapy regimens. In accordance with the ICH S9 guidance, combination *toxicology* studies are generally not warranted for use in patients with advanced cancer in part because combination clinical trials are typically not initiated until clinical data are available with each agent in the monotherapy setting. Monotherapy data can underpredict the activity of the drugs when used in combination, particularly if there is the potential for synergistic pharmacological effects; therefore, when Sponsors propose combination regimens for biologic products very early in development, providing *in vitro* or *in vivo* pharmacology data on the combination early in development can aid in dose selection and help support the safety of the proposed trial. Once limited clinical data are available with the individual agents, the totality of the clinical and nonclinical data can then justify dose setting for the combination.

As stated in the ICH S9 guidance, an assessment of embryofetal effects is needed to support a marketing application for drugs intended to treat patients with advanced cancer; however, in some cases, long-term administration sufficient to detect embryo-fetal effects in monkeys may be impractical (such as when an exposure-ablating ADA response precludes long-term administration and the high dose is tolerability-limited and cannot be increased to overcome immunogenicity). In these cases, an assessment based on data from alternative model systems may suffice, provided the model is sufficiently robust. For example, data from EFD studies using knockout or knockdown mice or in pregnant mice dosed with murine homologues might adequately inform human risk if the activity of the targeted pathway is sufficiently similar in humans and mice. FDA encourages Sponsors to seek feedback early in development about any alternative proposals for assessing the effects on EFD.

17.7.1 Oncology Case Studies

The following series of case studies illustrate some common difficulties encountered by Sponsors of cancer immunotherapy drug applications and are intended to serve as guides to current thinking about the development of cancer immunotherapies.

17.7.1.1 Case Study: Pharmacology Package Insufficient to Support Dose Selection

Biologic Drug H is an agonist monoclonal antibody that blocks the receptor of a novel pathway by which tumor cells downregulate the activity of tumor-infiltrating lymphocytes (TILs).

The Sponsor provided data from a four-week study in the monkey at weekly doses of 0, 10, 30, or 100 mg/kg. There were two preterm deaths at the low- and mid-dose levels during weeks 2 and 4 that were attributed to hypersensitivity. FDA considered the deaths treatment-related, as published data suggest that the pathway is associated with the development of hypersensitivity disorders.

On the basis of positive cytokine release data which produced levels comparable in magnitude to those of the positive control (anti-CD3 agonist antibody), the Sponsor was required to lower the starting dose to the expected EC_{20} for cytokine release. The Division also required revisions to the Investigator Brochure, Informed Consent Document, and clinical protocol to communicate the risk of hypersensitivity reactions and to provide appropriate provisions for safety.

17.7.1.2 Case Study: Lack of Pharmacologically-Relevant Toxicology Species

Biologic Drug I is a recombinant T-cell receptor-specific for a tumor-associated antigen fused to an agonist CD3 monoclonal antibody. By its mechanism of action, binding of the CD3 arm led to T-cell stimulation and redirected activity of the drug-bound T cells toward the epitope recognized by the recombinant TCR, which was not present in normal monkeys. Because the CD3 arm did not bind to endogenous monkey CD3, no pharmacologically relevant toxicology species was available.

The Sponsor provided tissue cross-reactivity, cytokine release, and data from a murine syngeneic mouse construct to support dose selection. The first clinical dose was based on a minimum-anticipated biological effect level (MABEL) of 1 pM, with an activity cutoff of 10% for target-cell cytotoxicity in co-cultures of T cells with target-expressing cells. The clinical starting dose was 0.2 μg, which was expected to produce exposures in the range of 1 pM.

17.7.1.3 Case Study: Insufficient Data to Support Toxicology Species Selection

Biologic Drug J is an inhibitory monoclonal antibody that was stated to bind and block signaling of a tumor-specific growth factor receptor. The Sponsor submitted the reports of four-week toxicology studies in the rat and the monkey conducted at twice-weekly IV doses of 0, 10, 30, or 50 mg/kg. There were no preterm deaths and no histopathological or clinicopathologic changes associated with treatment in either species, as was expected for a tumor-specific target. The Sponsor did not provide pharmacology data demonstrating the drug's target, binding affinity in humans or animals, or its PD activity.

Although the NOAELs for both toxicology studies were 50 mg/kg, the pharmacological relevance of the animal models had not been adequately established. In the absence of data to support the identity and safety of the intended target, there was insufficient information to support the safety of the proposed human trial. The IND was placed on clinical hold pending availability of adequate pharmacology data to characterize the drug's mechanism of action. The Sponsor was asked to provide data from *in vitro* pharmacology studies using transfected and non-transfected cells, to demonstrate target binding and downstream function, and to provide cross-species binding affinity data for Drug J against its intended target.

17.7.1.4 Case Study: Toxicokinetic Irregularities That Led to a Reduction in the Proposed Starting-Dose for an Antibody-Drug Conjugate (ADC)

Biologic Drug K is an antibody-drug conjugate (ADC). The Sponsor performed a four-week toxicology study in the monkey at doses of 0, 0.15, 0.3, 0.6, or 0.9 mg/kg every 3–4 weeks for 8 weeks (2 or 3 doses). At doses ≥0.6 mg/kg, all animals were euthanized in moribund condition after the second dose. The highest non-severely toxic dose (HNSTD) was 0.15 mg/kg due to severe target organ toxicity observed in animals treated at the 0.3 mg/kg dose level. The Sponsor-proposed starting dose was 8 μg/kg, which would have been supported by the data from animals treated at the 0.15 mg/kg dose level, but because of the steep lethal dose response and the apparent PK overlap between animals in the 0.15 and 0.3 mg/kg dose levels, the Sponsor was asked to lower the starting dose by 3× (1/18th of the BSA-adjusted HNSTD). The starting dose was reduced to 3 μg/kg.

17.7.1.5 Case Study: Insufficient Data to Characterize Toxicity

Biologic Drug L is a proinflammatory cytokine. The Sponsor provided data from a single-dose toxicology study in the mouse to support the FIH trial. The Sponsor provided a scientific justification for testing in only one species; however, the Division did not concur and recommended conducting a repeat-dose toxicology study in the monkey. Additionally, the doses selected for the mouse study were insufficient to characterize the potential toxicity of the drug over the anticipated clinical dose range. Repeat-dose toxicology data at doses up to the MTD or MFD in the monkey were needed to support the proposed clinical plan.

17.7.1.6 Case Study: Dose Setting for a Combination: Insufficient Monotherapy Data in Patients to Support Initiation of Clinical Development of Combinations

Biologic Drug M is an agonist-monoclonal antibody that blocks T-cell downregulation following the initial immune activation. The Sponsor provided *in vitro* binding and activity data, *in vitro* activity and cytokine release data, a tissue cross-reactivity study, and data from a four-week study in the monkey to support the initiation of a FIH study with Drug M. The proposed clinical plan included a short monotherapy run-in with Drug F with the initiation of a combination arm shortly thereafter. The combination arm proposed to administer Drug M with another monoclonal antibody that blocks a different T-cell inhibiting pathway. The IND was placed on a partial clinical hold for the combination arm, pending availability of both initial clinical monotherapy data as well as pharmacology data sufficient to support dose selection for the combination.

The *in vitro* pharmacology data provided demonstrated greater-than-additive PD activity for the two agents in combination (~5× increase in cytokine release vs. either agent alone). Data from the pharmacology and toxicology studies, in combination with clinical data from the two individual agents, were used to set the starting dose for the combination arm. For each agent, the starting dose based on clinical and pharmacology data and the dose escalation for the combination began at doses that were 3× lower than those evaluated and found to be clinically tolerable in the monotherapy setting.

17.7.1.7 Case Study: Reproductive Toxicology When More Than One Relevant Species Exists

Biologic Drug N is an inhibitory monoclonal antibody that targets a growth factor receptor. To support a potential marketing application, the Sponsor conducted 4- and 13-week toxicology studies in the rat and the monkey. At the end of Phase 2 meeting, the Sponsor provided a proposal to evaluate the reproductive toxicity of Drug N in the rat.

Data from the preliminary dose-ranging study in pregnant rats were negative for adverse reproductive effects; however, based on the pharmacological class, and a reduced binding affinity for the rat orthologue relative to humans or primates, the Sponsor was informed that a negative definitive study may not be sufficient to support labeling for Drug N and that additional studies (e.g., a study in the monkey) may be needed. The Agency recommended that the Sponsor request feedback on the proposed reproductive toxicology assessment in sufficient time to conduct another study if needed for inclusion in the BLA.

17.7.1.8 Case Study: Lack of Cytokine Release Data

Biologic Drug O is an inhibitor of the PD-1 pathway. The Sponsor provided data from a four-week toxicology study in the monkey at weekly doses of 50, 100, or 200 mg/kg, as well as data from an *in vitro* binding study; a murine xenograft study in mice reconstituted with human T cells; and a mixed lymphocyte reaction study. Although there were no treatment-related toxicities observed in the monkey study, the IND was placed on hold for the lack of cytokine release data. The Division requested that the Sponsor provide data from a cytokine release assay in cultured human PBMCs using both soluble and plate-bound formats.

In their Complete Response to Hold, the Sponsor provided data from an *in vitro* cytokine release assay using both the soluble and plate-bound formats, which employed both positive and negative controls. The data were considered acceptable to initiate the proposed study.

17.7.1.9 Case Study: Juvenile Toxicology Studies

Biologic Drug P is directed against a tumor-associated fusion protein expressed in a common childhood cancer, but which also exhibited a lower-degree of activity against the target's endogenous isoform. To support the proposed clinical study, the Sponsor submitted data from 28-day toxicology studies in the rodent and nonrodent. The nonrodent was considered the most-sensitive and pharmacologically relevant species. The doses evaluated in the nonrodent, were 0, 10, 30, and 50 mg/kg. Key toxicities were observed in the bone marrow, GI tract, and lymphoid organs, which were dose-limiting at 30 and 50 mg/kg. Because the intended patient population had already received the first-line standard-of-care treatment and there were no other therapies that were likely to offer substantial benefit to these patients, studies in juvenile animals were not considered necessary to support the initiation of the proposed trial in adolescent children ≥12 years of age.[24]

17.7.2 Development of Non-Oncology Indications, after Development in Patients with Advanced Cancer

Sponsors often develop drugs for an oncology indication first, and follow with a program for a non-oncology indication in a disease that may not be life-threatening. In the case of diseases that are not life-threatening and have existing therapies, sponsors should follow the ICH S6(R1) recommendations for the studies needed to support clinical development in these populations.

It is not unusual for Sponsors to propose leveraging clinical data from trials conducted in patients with advanced cancer with the same molecule, or a molecule that targets the same pathway. Because it is difficult to interpret toxicities in clinical trials conducted in patients with advanced cancer, and ICH S9 recommends a different drug development program than ICH S6(R1), additional nonclinical data may be needed to support a non-oncology indication that is not life-threatening.

The case study below describes a situation in which a Sponsor proposed to leverage experience from an approved oncology drug to support their proposed dosing with an NME that targeted the same protein.

17.7.2.1 Case Study: Inappropriate Data Extrapolation

Biologic Drug F was an NME proposed to treat rheumatoid arthritis. The opening-IND clinical trial was a FIH study in healthy volunteers. Although the drug was an NME, there were several drugs utilizing the same mechanism of action being developed under different IND applications. In addition, the mechanism of action for Drug F was similar to that of Biologic Drug G, which is approved for treatment of several types of cancer. The Sponsor referred to previous experience from human trials and years of patient experience from prescription use with the approved drug G to support their proposed dosing.

It is generally not possible to extrapolate clinical safety data from one drug to another to support clinical administration. One reason is that biologic drugs that share the same target can have different potencies. In addition, clinical safety profiles obtained in

previous oncology trials are not fully informative of potential clinical toxicities in a healthier population since oncology patients typically have very advanced disease, multiple co-morbidities, and multiple concurrent medications.

In addition to difficulties in extrapolating clinical data, extrapolating nonclinical data can be challenging for a Sponsor who has developed a drug in accordance with ICH S9, which allows for accelerated clinical testing compared to ICH S6(R1). In addition to differences in the timing of studies needed to support clinical development, the level of concern regarding toxicity from novel excipients and impurities may differ based on the indication. For antibody-drug conjugates, which are not covered in this chapter, the level of concern for genotoxicity may change based on the relative benefit-risk assessment for each indication (See Chapter 3.4). In this case, the previous human experience with Drug G was not considered by the Division to adequately address the potential toxicities of Drug F.

FDA did not concur with the Sponsor's approach, and recommended that the clinical doses be determined based on the NOAEL in the submitted a 1-month GLP monkey toxicology study. Unfortunately, the FDA-identified NOAEL did not support the Sponsor's proposed high-dose in the proposed clinical trial. The Sponsor amended the clinical protocol before the 30-day safety date for new INDs. As a result of the protocol change, the trial was allowed to proceed.

17.8 Regulatory Submissions

The goal of this section on regulatory submissions is to provide some historical context for review of biologics at the FDA, and considerations for Sponsors early in drug development.

In 2003, the United States Food and Drug Administration (FDA) transferred[25] review responsibility for some categories of therapeutic biologic products (e.g., monoclonal antibodies, cytokines, and enzymes) from FDA's Center for Biologics Evaluation and Research (CBER) to FDA's Center for Drug Evaluation and Research (CDER). Other categories remained with CBER (e.g., cellular products, gene therapy, vaccines, allergenic extracts, antivenoms, and blood components).

When these products (post-market and pre-market) went from CBER to CDER, review teams and other staff were also transferred to CDER, to share their expertise and to train fellow FDA reviewers. Differences in the approaches for reviewing and regulating biologics versus small molecule drugs sparked robust and spirited discussions about the appropriate level of

---

[24] Chuk MK, et al. *Clinical Cancer Research*. 2017;23(1):9–12.

[25] Letter to Sponsors - Transfer of Therapeutic Products to the Center for Drug Evaluation and Research dated June 20, 2003 from Jesse L. Goodman (M.D., M.P.H., Director, CBER) and Janet Woodcock (M.D., Director, CDER). Accessed from https://www.fda.gov/AboutFDA/CentersOffices/OfficeofMedicalProductsandTobacco/CBER/ucm133463.htm

data needed to support safety for clinical trials. Regulators frequently identified deficiencies and requested more preclinical information to support the safety of the FIH clinical trial. Over time, policy differences were identified, discussed, and refined to minimize regulatory requirements while ensuring safety. Experts from academia and industry provided (and continue to provide) instruction and training at CDER and elsewhere, as do CDER staff, through scientific conferences, and by publishing. ICH S6(R1), which incorporated many of Industry's initial concerns about the dataset needed to support development and approval of novel biologic drugs, was published by ICH in June 2011 and by FDA in May 2012.[26]

The following sections provide considerations for early nonclinical development of a biologic and include recommendations for regulatory submissions.

17.8.1 Applying GLP (21 CFR Part 58) to Biologic Drug Development

The IND-enabling toxicology studies for both biologic drugs and small-molecule drugs should comply with the GLP of each country/region where clinical trials will be conducted. For FDA, GLP is codified in title 21 of the Code of Federal Regulations (CFR) Part 58.[27,28] Regulators expect that the biologic product or test article (TA) used in GLP studies will be adequately characterized for identity, strength, purity, and composition. In addition, the stability of both the TA and vehicle should be determined prior to or during the study per standard operating procedures (SOPs) and confirmed by periodic analysis of the batches used on the study. For biologics, the assays used to characterize the TA and vehicle as well as stability should be conducted under GLP. Assays should also be developed to determine the homogeneity and concentrations of any prepared dose formulations for the study. Many biologics are formulated as solutions, and therefore, an assessment of homogeneity in the context of the GLP studies may not be needed.

For biologic drugs, the dose formulation methods are expected to characterize not only the test article concentration administered, but also to confirm stability of the test article under the conditions of use. Unless a separate stability study has been performed during method validation for the GLP study, the dose formulation analysis should be meet the criteria set forth under 21 CFR Section 58.105. This is particularly important for pivotal toxicology studies, as loss of exposure due to ADA development may sufficiently confound interpretation of the results that could make it difficult to ascertain whether the test article was inactive due to ADA or product instability. GMP stability data for the drug product may be adequate to assure in-use stability of the drug if the product has been formulated prior to use at the GLP testing facility.

Bioanalytical assays to measure the biologic product in serum or plasma, PD markers, and immunogenicity or ADA should also be validated under GLPs; however, when an early exploratory PD marker is evaluated in a toxicology study, a fully validated assay may not always be practical or feasible. In these cases, a GLP exception can be taken for the GLP compliance status of these analyses; however, the data should still be included in the study report.

17.8.1.1 Practical Considerations in Selecting CROs[29]

On a practical level, the development of bioanalytical assays can be extremely time- and resource-intensive, and therefore, a Sponsor should start early. For example, the development and validation of an assay to measure a mAb in serum can take anywhere from 3 to 6 months and approximately cost from \$60,000 to 100,000 in 2018. The bioanalytical costs are multiplied by the number of species being tested in toxicology studies as well as the need for an ADA assay for each species. So, for a standard two-species approach, a total of four assays is possible (measurement of the biologic drug in rodent and nonrodent serum or plasma and ADA in rodent and nonrodent serum or plasma); such a scenario would result in assay costs of approximately \$300,000–400,000 in addition to the cost and time associated with sample analysis (which can take an additional 1–3 months or longer to analyze after the completion of the in-life phase of the study).

If the nonclinical studies are being contracted out to a contract research laboratory, there are several considerations beyond budget that should be explored for the nonclinical development of biologic products.

Selecting a CRO that specialize in developing assays for biologic products is important when assay issues arise during method development or validation. Generally, ELISAs are used for the measurement of the biologic drugs and ADA. Specialized knowledge of the ELISA method is useful when issues such as high background, reproducibility, or lack of sensitivity or specificity are encountered.

Similarly, selecting a CRO with experience in running toxicology studies with biologic products is essential. Biologic-specific toxicities or findings may be observed such as infusion or anaphylactic/anaphylactoid reactions. A laboratory with prior experience with biologics can respond quickly and take action faster than a laboratory experiencing such issues for the first time. In addition, such laboratories usually have already validated in vivo endpoints commonly included in studies with biologics that include flow cytometry/immunophenotyping, cytokine release, complement activation markers, and T-cell-dependent antibody response to a neoantigen (TDAR).

[26] FDA. 2009. S6 (R1) Addendum: Preclinical Safety Evaluation of Biotechnology-Derived Pharmaceuticals. Accessed from https://www.fda.gov/downloads/Drugs/GuidanceComplianceRegulatoryInformation/Guidances/UCM194490.pdf

[27] FDA 21CFR58. Accessed from https://www.accessdata.fda.gov/scripts/cdrh/cfdocs/cfcfr/CFRSearch.cfm?CFRPart=58

[28] Guidance for Industry Good Laboratory Practices Questions and Answers. 1981, 1999, 2007. Accessed from https://www.fda.gov/downloads/ICECI/EnforcementActions/BioresearchMonitoring/UCM133748.pdf

[29] This section was authored by Janice Lansita, PhD, DABT, ToxStrategies.

17.8.2 Pre-IND Meeting and Briefing Package for Biologic Drugs

For biologic products with unique safety issues (e.g., novel construct, difficulty selecting appropriate nonclinical species for testing, entry into pediatric trials early in development, etc.), many Sponsors want feedback from Regulators regarding their nonclinical plans and clinical trial design, prior to formally submitting the IND application. FDA/CDER's pre-IND meeting is comparable to a Scientific Advice meeting with EMA. This section will focus on the FDA/CDER's pre-IND meeting process.[30,31] A Pre-IND meeting may help ensure that the package provided to support initial clinical trials is acceptable to FDA and mitigates the risk of a clinical hold upon submitting the IND. Depending on the data provided in a pre-IND package, the FDA may be able to provide feedback on the proposed nonclinical plan, the IND-enabling study designs, species selection and the FIH dose. If drug-related toxicity with the biologic has been observed, the focus of the Pre-IND could be on the potential need for follow-up studies, and whether a sufficient safety margin has been established to support the proposed clinical trial.

Timing the meeting request and briefing package can be complicated, if the Sponsor is waiting for data from different experiments. In general, FDA feedback is most valuable prior to starting the IND-enabling toxicology studies. If feedback on the IND enabling study design is needed, the Sponsor may want to include the following in the Pre-IND briefing package: the basis for selecting the pharmacologically relevant species, rationale for selecting the proposed dose levels, the overall study design and any additional or specialized endpoints (e.g., PD markers, TDAR, cytokine release, immunophenotyping, cerebrospinal fluid collections, additional tissues or sections for histopathology, as appropriate).

Sponsors may find scheduling difficult (e.g., scheduling the Pre-IND meeting prior to starting the GLP IND-enabling toxicology studies), to allow time to incorporate any FDA feedback into the study. To the extent feasible, Sponsors will want to coordinate timelines with the laboratory or CRO running the GLP toxicology studies, in detail in advance of the Pre-IND meeting. A potential pitfall for biologic drugs is study duration as biologic drugs generally have long elimination half-lives compared to small-molecule drugs. Depending on the PK of the drug product, the mechanism(s) of action, and the clinical indication, regulators may recommend repeat-dosing, interim-sacrifices, or recovery groups to ensure adequate characterization of toxicity. Laboratories may need lead-time to ensure they have the vivarium space and technical staff available to collect all necessary endpoints at necropsy.

17.9 Conclusions

Through case studies of biologic products with differing modalities and different indications, this chapter summarizes key considerations and potential pitfalls to avoid during drug development to ensure a high-quality nonclinical package to support FIH clinical trials and beyond.

For nonclinical deliverables, the key is to provide sufficient *in vitro* and *in vivo* datasets and conduct high-quality GLP-compliant toxicology studies that support the rationale for FIH dosing. These studies should carefully consider the target, the expected MOA, as well as potential on- and off-target effects that may translate to humans. The timing of the nonclinical studies is generally driven by material availability for the GLP toxicology studies, the toxicology reporting timelines, and stage of clinical development.

In conclusion, a pre-IND and subsequent IND submission for a biologic drug require multiple complex elements to come together in a timely fashion.

REFERENCES

Chuk, M. K., Mulugeta, Y., Roth-Cline, M., Mehrotra, N., & Reaman, G. H. (2017). Enrolling adolescents in disease/target-appropriate adult oncology clinical trials of investigational agents. *Clinical Cancer Research*, *23*(1), 9–12.

Federal Register Volume 8, No. 35, 2/21/2020. Definition of the Term "Biological Product". Retrieved from https://www.federalregister.gov/documents/2020/02/21/2020-03505/definition-of-the-term-biological-product

Leach, M. W., Halpern, W. G., Johnson, C. W., Rojko, J. L., MacLachlan, T. K., Chan, C. M., Galbreath, E. J., Ndifor, A. M., Blanset, D. L., Polack, E., & Cavagnaro, J. A. (2010 Dec). Use of tissue cross-reactivity studies in the development of antibody-based biopharmaceuticals: History, experience, methodology, and future directions. *Toxicol Pathol*, *38*(7), 1138–1166. doi: 10.1177/0192623310382559. Epub 2010 Oct 6. PMID: 20926828. https://pubmed.ncbi.nlm.nih.gov/20926828/

Lueking, A., Beator, J., Patz, E., Müllner, S., Mehes, G., & Amersdorfer, P. (2008). Determination and validation of off-target activities of anti-CD44 variant 6 antibodies using protein biochips and tissue microarrays. *Biotechniques*, *45*(4), i–v.

Muller, P. Y., & Brennan, F. R. (2009). Safety assessment and dose selection for first-in-human clinical trials with immunomodulatory monoclonal antibodies. *Clinical Pharmacology & Therapeutics*, *85*(3), 247–258.

Ochoa de Olza, M., Oliva, M., Hierro, C., Matos, I., Martin-Liberal, J., & Garralda, E. (2018). Early-drug development in the era of immuno-oncology: Are we ready to face the challenges? *Annals of Oncology*, *29*(8), 1727–1740.

Pallardy, M. & Hünig, T. (2010 Oct). Primate testing of TGN1412: Right target, wrong cell. *Br J Pharmacol*, *161*(3), 509–511. doi: 10.1111/j.1476-5381.2010.00925.x. PMID: 20880391; PMCID: PMC2990150. https://pubmed.ncbi.nlm.nih.gov/20880391/

---

[30] FDA's webpage "Small Business and Industry Assistance: Frequently Asked Questions on the Pre-Investigational New Drug (IND) Meeting" was accessed from: https://www.fda.gov/Drugs/DevelopmentApprovalProcess/SmallBusinessAssistance/ucm069906.htm

[31] CDER/CBER 2017 Procedural Guidance for Industry and Review Staff. Best Practices for Communication between IND Sponsors and FDA during Drug Development. Accessed from https://www.fda.gov/downloads/Drugs/GuidanceComplianceRegulatoryInformation/Guidances/UCM475586.pdf

Spiess, C., Zhai, Q., & Carter, P. J. (2015 Oct). Alternative molecular formats and therapeutic applications for bispecific antibodies. *Mol Immunol*, *67*(2 Pt A), 95–106. doi: 10.1016/j.molimm.2015.01.003. Epub 2015 Jan 27. PMID: 25637431. https://pubmed.ncbi.nlm.nih.gov/25637431/

U.S. Food and Drug Administration. (2003). Letter to Sponsors - Transfer of Therapeutic Products to the Center for Drug Evaluation and Research. Retrieved from https://www.fda.gov/AboutFDA/CentersOffices/OfficeofMedicalProductsandTobacco/CBER/ucm133463.htm

U.S. Food and Drug Administration. (2005). Guidance for Industry: Estimating the Maximum Safe Starting Dose in Initial Clinical Trials for Therapeutics in Adult Healthy Volunteers. Retrieved from https://www.fda.gov/regulatory-information/search-fda-guidance-documents/estimating-maximum-safe-starting-dose-initial-clinical-trials-therapeutics-adult-healthy-volunteers

U.S. Food and Drug Administration. Guidance for Industry: Good Laboratory Practices Questions and Answers. (1981, 1999, 2007). Retrieved from https://www.fda.gov/downloads/ICECI/EnforcementActions/BioresearchMonitoring/UCM133748.pdf

U.S. Food and Drug Administration. (2009). Guidance for Industry: S6 (R1) Addendum: Preclinical Safety Evaluation of Biotechnology - Derived Pharmaceuticals. Retrieved from: https://www.fda.gov/downloads/Drugs/GuidanceComplianceRegulatoryInformation/Guidances/UCM194490.pdf

U.S. Food and Drug Administration. (2010). Guidance for Industry: S9 Nonclinical Evaluation for Anticancer Pharmaceuticals. Retrieved from https://www.fda.gov/downloads/Drugs/Guidances/ucm085389.pdf

U.S. Food and Drug Administration. (2014). Procedural Guidance for Industry: Expedited Programs for Serious Conditions – Drugs and Biologics. Retrieved from https://www.fda.gov/downloads/Drugs/Guidances/UCM358301.pdf

U.S. Food and Drug Administration. (2016). CY 2016 CDER New Molecular Entity (NME) Drug & Original BLA Calendar Year Approvals as of December 31, 2016. Retrieved from https://www.fda.gov/downloads/Drugs/DevelopmentApprovalProcess/HowDrugsareDevelopedandApproved/DrugandBiologicApprovalReports/NDAandBLAApprovalReports/UCM540569.pdf

Lucentis (ranibizumab) U.S. Package Insert. (2017). Retrieved from https://www.accessdata.fda.gov/drugsatfda_docs/label/2017/125156s114lbl.pdf

Eylea (aflibercept) U.S. Package Insert. (2017). Retrieved from: https://www.accessdata.fda.gov/drugsatfda_docs/label/2017/125387s054lbl.pdf

U.S. Food and Drug Administration. (2018). The Biomarker Qualification Program. Retrieved from https://www.fda.gov/Drugs/DevelopmentApprovalProcess/DrugDevelopmentToolsQualificationProgram/BiomarkerQualificationProgram/default.htm

U.S. Food and Drug Administration. (2020). Compilation of CDER New Molecular Entity (NME) Drug and New Biologic Approvals 1985–2020. Retrieved from https://www.fda.gov/drugs/drug-approvals-and-databases/compilation-cder-new-molecular-entity-nme-drug-and-new-biologic-approvals

U.S. Food and Drug Administration/Center for Drug Evaluation and Research. (2020). New Drugs at FDA: CDER's New Molecular Entities and New Therapeutic Biological Products. Retrieved from https://www.fda.gov/drugs/development-approval-process-drugs/new-drugs-fda-cders-new-molecular-entities-and-new-therapeutic-biological-products

18

Outsourcing and Monitoring Preclinical Studies Including GLP Considerations

P. Mookherjee
Global Blood Therapeutics, Inc.

CONTENTS

18.1 Introduction: Outsourcing as a Strategy

The preclinical safety assessment of biopharmaceuticals to support the conduct of clinical trials and marketing approvals is conducted based on regulations and guidelines outlined by global regulatory agencies while adhering to the principles of the 3Rs. The three Rs are Replacement: developing and utilizing models and tools instead of using animals; Reduction: designing studies to minimize the number of animals used and generate robust data; and Refinement: improving animal welfare and minimizing suffering. The global regulatory agencies have an expectation that the preclinical safety assessment studies to support clinical trials and marketing applications are conducted under good laboratory practice (GLP) regulations and guidelines as much as is feasible. Sponsors may choose to conduct the studies in laboratories within their own facilities or conduct the studies at external facilities such as universities, nonprofit institutes, or contract research organizations (CROs). The test facilities where the GLP studies are conducted need to meet and maintain GLP compliance as well as undergo routine monitoring and inspections. These testing facilities must adhere to GLP regulations in order to prevent from being disqualified as a test facility. It is still the responsibility of the sponsor to ensure that the conduct of any studies placed at a testing facility is GLP-compliant. Because of the additional resources needed to maintain a GLP test facility (e.g., cost for maintaining the facilities, additional dedicated staff with specialized skills, ongoing training), many sponsors opt to outsource the studies to an external laboratory. One benefit for a sponsor conducting the study at a testing facility is the historical database available.

This chapter will provide (1) a high-level overview of the GLP regulations and guidelines, (2) recommended activities to include when identifying CROs for conducting preclinical studies with biopharmaceuticals, (3) some of the main factors used in selecting the test facility for the placement of a study, and (4) recommendations related to sponsor oversight and monitoring studies.

18.2 Overview of GLP Regulations and Guidelines

The GLP regulations and guidelines for pharmaceuticals emerged in the late 1970s in response to needing a standard set of requirements regarding the conduct, documentation, and reporting of data from toxicology studies that were supporting pharmaceutical applications. During this time, there were multiple instances of false data and inaccurate reporting in toxicology studies submitted to the Food and Drug Administration (FDA), the most famous example being the studies conducted at Industrial Bio-Test Laboratories (IBT) [1,2]. In the United States, the Federal Food, Drug, and Cosmetic (FD&C) Act of 1938 is the set of laws that set up the FDA as the authoritative agency to overseeing the safety and efficacy of food, drugs, medical devices, and cosmetics. The FDA establishes regulations that are enforceable by law, along with guidance or guideline documents associated with the regulations that provide the current position of the agency on a specific topic. Specifically, the GLP regulations were published in the Code of Federal Regulations (CFR) under Title 21, Chapter 1, Subchapter A, Part 58 (21 CFR 58) to ensure the quality and integrity of the data submitted to the FDA. The proposed GLP provisions were published in the Federal Registry of November 1976 with the final rule published in December 1978 and effective on July 20, 1979 [3,4]. The US GLP regulations provide a minimum standard for the integrity and quality of the data submitted to the FDA. This also

DOI: 10.1201/9781003124542-20

provides a general outline for industry to follow regarding quality controls and increased confidence in the validity of the data. The US GLP regulations are regularly reviewed, with an amendment published on September 4, 1987, which included the following: (1) the requirement of a quality assurance (QA) department, (2) inclusion of a protocol study plan, (3) the inclusion of characterization of the test and control articles, and (4) the requirement of retentions of samples [5]. The FDA published additional proposed rule to the GLP regulations on August 24, 2016 [6]. The most current version of the US GLP regulations can be found at the website for the US National Archives (www.ecfr.federalregister.gov).

Countries included in the Organisation for Economic Co-operation and Development (OECD) established the OECD Principles of GLP which were approved in May 1981 and revised principles adopted on November 26, 1997 [7]. The revised OECD Principles of GLP, No. 1 (1997) includes guidance on GLP, compliance monitoring, and mutual acceptance of data (MAD) system. The MAD system was established by OECD member countries to enable minimizing the cost and the environmental impact of testing chemicals and pharmaceuticals. Standard requirements for the conduct and oversight of the studies encourage acceptance and sharing of data generated in test facilities fulfilling OECD GLP compliance and conducted following US FDA GLP regulations across the global regulatory agencies, reducing redundancy of testing with animals. A link to the current version of the OECD Principles of GLP is available through the OECD website along with a list of the status of OECD member countries participating in the MAD system (www.oecd.org).

A comparison chart of the US FDA GLP regulations and OECD Principles of GLP was published by the FDA in June 2004 and can be found through the FDA website (www.FDA.gov). This also includes the US Environmental Protection Agency (EPA) GLP regulations for comparison. In general, OECD Principles of GLP provide the recommendations and the US FDA GLP regulations provide the legal standards to ensure preclinical studies produce quality data and the study conduct is documented so that the results could be replicated, if needed.

18.3 Identifying CROs for Conducting Preclinical Studies

To start, one needs to identify the CROs to consider for the studies and establish a confidentiality agreement (CDA) to begin discussions. With a CDA in place, one can submit a request for proposal (RFP) for the scope of work needed for the study(ies) which the CRO will use to generate a price quote. The RFP can facilitate a discussion of the scientific and technical capabilities the CRO has available. Additionally, sponsors should schedule an audit of the specific testing facilities to qualify the site prior to placing a study. The audit of a testing facility is an opportunity for the sponsor to review the technical capabilities, observe the general activities, and evaluate the scientific expertise to determine if the site is suitable for conducting the study(ies). It is important to be sure enough time is available to complete the audit of a test facility prior to awarding the study

to a CRO. There are occasions when an in-person audit cannot be conducted due to study start being available early, travel restrictions, pandemic, etc. In this case, an audit questionnaire can be sent for the test facility to complete. This can be followed up with an additional audit performed via videoconference. Another way to evaluate a CRO that is being considered is conducting a non-GLP study at the facility. At a CRO, the main differences between a non-GLP and a GLP study are the documentation and oversight by QA. Conducting a non-GLP study, such as a dose range-finding or dose escalation study, gives the sponsor an opportunity to see how the staff conducts and reports a study.

A current list of nonclinical contract research laboratory inspections conducted by the FDA is available at the FDA website, and this can be used as a starting point for which CROs to consider using for a study. The website BioPharmGuy includes a comprehensive list of CROs by business type, region, or start-up year categorized under contract research or scientific services (www.biopharmguy.com/biotech-company-directory.php). For compiling a list of CROs to consider for the placement of a study, a sample of some preliminary activities are provided here along with example tables including details of additional activities:

- Preliminary activities to identify a test facility (Table 18.1)
- List of activities to include in a test facility audit (Table 18.2)
- Example test facility audit report (Table 18.3)

18.4 Main Factors in Site Selection: Scientific Expertise, Timelines, and Cost

In order to select a CRO and/or a specific site for the preclinical studies, there are three main factors to consider: (1) scientific capabilities including expertise, (2) timelines, and (3) cost. It is best to consider and compare at least two to three CROs whenever possible, keeping in mind that the balance between these three factors will determine which site is selected. It is important to understand technical capabilities and scientific experience a test facility has in conducting aspects of the study. For example, this includes discussing with the test facility the experience with specific animal species as well as having them provide information about the different types of studies the site can perform. Much of this can be determined

TABLE 18.1

Example Checklist of Preliminary Activities to Identify a Test Facility

Activity
Establish a confidentiality agreement (CDA)
Provide a request for proposal (RFP) for the scope of work
Establish a master service agreement (MSA)
Schedule a test facility qualification audit (coordinated with internal quality assurance (QA) group or a QA consultant)

TABLE 18.2

Example Activities to Include in a Test Facility Site Audit

Activity
Interviews
• Prospective study directors
• Department principal investigators
• Appropriate test site facility staff
○ Area supervisors
○ Husbandry staff
○ Laboratory technicians
• Relevant subject matter experts (SMEs)
Documentation for review during audit
• Study data files (if previous study has been conducted at the site)
• SOPs
• Training records: qualification, experience, and regulatory training documentation
• Equipment calibration and maintenance documentation
• Pharmacy and formulation documentation
• Drug accountability records
• Drug shipment records/chain of custody
Facility tours
• Vivarium (e.g., animal rooms, feed and bedding areas, cage wash areas)
• Laboratories (e.g., clinical chemistry, histology, dosage formulation, bioanalytical, analytical)
• Sample preparation and storage area
• Archives

TABLE 18.3

Example Items Included in an Audit Report for a Test Facility

- Details specific to the audit
  - Date of audit, type of audit, sponsor, auditor (inclusion of consultant if applicable), test facility (address and primary contact), date of audit
- Overall summary of audit observations (critical, major, minor, comments)
- Audit scope and objectives
- Personnel attending audit
- Background information (company overview, recent regulatory inspection history, facility(ies) covered in the audit, services provided at the site)
- List of standard operating procedures (SOPs) documents review prior to and during audit
- List of any equipment calibration and/or maintenance records
- List of IT and/or computer systems reviewed
- List of any other documents rereviewed (e.g., staff training records and CVs, study data and files)
- Detailed description of areas included in the audit and all audit observations (critical, major, minor, comments) and any actions or responses from the test facility

TABLE 18.4

Example List of Study-Specific Expertise and Capabilities Related to Biopharmaceuticals to Review for a Test Facility

- Experience in conducting studies with specific species and strains of animals
  - Request historical data for studies conducted with different rodent strains (e.g., CD-1 mice, Sprague Dawley rats, Wistar Han rats)
  - Request historical data for studies with non-rodents (dogs, rabbits, and NHPs)
- Experience with clinical immunology
  - Check if the test facility has experience with method development and validation of anti-drug antibody (ADA) assays or this will need to be subcontracted to another CRO
- Experience with T-cell-dependent antibody response (TDAR) assay
  - Check which immunogen is used: keyhole limpet hemocyanin (KLH), tetanus toxoid (TT), and/or sheep red blood cells (SRBC)
- Experience conducting studies with intended route of administration
  - Some typically used routes: intravenous, inhalation, intrathecal, intramuscular, intraperitoneal, oral, topical (skin, nasal mucosa, ocular topical), subcutaneous, or depositions
- Experience with safety pharmacology studies
  - Request historical data and the number of safety pharmacology studies conducted in different species (e.g., rodents, dogs, and especially NHPs)
  - Request detailed information related to the experience with different methods for conducting electrocardiography (ECG) collections (e.g., jacket external telemetry (ECG-JET), manual ECG)
- Experience with reproductive and developmental studies with NHPs
- Experience with cytokine assays
- Experience with antibody–drug conjugates (ADCs)
- Experience with quantitative polymerase chain reaction (qPCR) and droplet digital PCR (ddPCR), specifically in relation to biodistribution studies associated with gene therapies
- Clarification on which capabilities the test facility has already qualified and is able to conduct under GLP vs. non-GLP

during the audit of a site. There are technical capabilities that are relevant for the conduct of preclinical studies and additional expertise that need to be included to keep in mind when conducting studies with biologics. Table 18.4 is a list of some study-specific scientific experience and expertise to review for a test facility as factors for consideration in site selection. The relative importance of the items listed will vary based on the specific needs for the biopharmaceutical being developed.

It is usually preferred to have all the components of a study in a single facility or within a single CRO because this makes the oversight of the study easier. However, if the primary test facility does not have the appropriate experience or expertise for a component of the study, that component may need to be conducted elsewhere. In case a test facility does not have all the specific capabilities needed for the study, additional vendors will be needed to conduct that analysis and/or evaluation. Sometimes, a specific assay could be complicated enough that only a select few testing facilities or institutions will have the scientific experience and specific equipment needed to conduct the analysis and/or evaluation. The sponsor may even choose to have a specific analysis conducted in-house. It could also be that the test facility has the capabilities, but it is not qualified yet to be GLP such as a novel assay for a biomarker.

If multiple test facilities or sample analysis sites are being considered for the placement of a study, it is important to keep in mind the logistics and impact of transferring samples. The transfer of samples will add time to the duration of the study. The Convention on International Trade in Endangered Species of Wild Fauna and Flora (CITES) permits are required to transfer nonhuman primate (NHP) samples across international borders. CITES is a treaty that was established to oversee and regulate the international trade of species that are endangered or threatened to become extinct. The process for obtaining a CITES permit takes a minimum of 60 days. Large CROs are accustomed to dealing with CITES permits and include the permit process into the overall study timeline.

The second factor that influences site selection is the timing for conducting the study and generating the final report. Program timelines are critical, especially when conducting safety assessment studies to support the initial clinical trial application. When the RFP is sent to the CRO, it is important to include in the request the target study start date desired and the projected timing for any regulatory submissions that are planned. The study start date is linked to additional activities such as the timing for test article availability (e.g., when will the test article be tested, released, and shipped to the test facility), development and validation supporting assays (e.g., dose formulation analysis, bioanalytical analysis, and biomarker assays), animal availability, and any additional animal acclimation or pre-study activities (specific to the test facility standard operating procedures (SOPs) and institutional animal care and use committee (IACUC) protocols or country regulations). Due to the pre-study activities that are needed to align for a start date, sometimes study slots are reserved 6–8 months in advance. The reporting timeline of a study, including the delivery of key milestones such as the audited draft report and the final report, contributes to which test facility is selected. The study proposal quote from the CRO should include the standard reporting timelines, and one can request options for accelerated reporting (e.g., cost for receiving an expedited audited draft report and/or final report). The timing of the Standard for Exchange of Nonclinical Data (SEND) for specific nonclinical studies is also needed for regulatory submissions to the US FDA for investigational new drugs (INDs), new drug applications (NDAs), abbreviated new drug applications (ANDAs), and biologics license applications (BLAs). The current nonclinical studies requiring the SEND dataset can be found at the FDA website. Some test facilities generate and quality-check (QC) the SEND dataset, whereas others utilize a third-party vendor to provide the SEND dataset. Depending on the regulatory submission strategy for the program, it is important to understand the SEND capabilities when selecting the test facility for a study. The sponsor should also review the internal capabilities to review and QC the SEND dataset for a study. If internal capabilities are not available, one may need to establish a vendor to use and that will add additional time to the submission timeline. Table 18.5 includes some key milestones related to the timeline for a study, both the start and reporting of a study.

TABLE 18.5

Example Milestones Influencing the Timeline of a Study, Including Some Approximate Timing Durations

Activity or Milestone/Questions to Consider	Impact
• Timing of test article availability	Study start
• Animal availability ○ What is the lead time for ordering animals?	Study start
• Bioanalytical assays: method development and/or transfer and validation; time to develop and/or validate a method can be variable, ranging between 4 and 12 weeks (calendar days) ○ Is there enough time for the test facility or laboratory to have the needed bioanalytical assays ready to support the study?	Study start and/or study report

• Pre-study activities: duration is variable and dependent on the specific activity: between 2 and 8 weeks (calendar days)
  ○ How much acclimation time is required for the animals at the test facility prior to being assigned to the study?
  ○ Do the animals need to be trained for any study-specific evaluation activities (e.g., training of the NHPs for dosing or blood collection procedures in restrained dosing chairs; acclimation of NHPs to inhalation devices; NHPs trained for jackets used for ECG-JET)?
  ○ Are there any pre-study collections needed from the animals (e.g., menstrual swabs from female NHPs to confirm sexual maturity, serum clinical chemistry, and/or hematology collections for establishing baseline)?
	Study start

• Unaudited draft report (UDR): timing typically estimated from the end of in-life and is an non-audited version of the report; this is the draft version of a report for non-GLP studies; between 8 and 16 weeks (business days); could be expedited for additional cost
  ○ What is the standard timing for delivery of the UDR after the end of in-life?
  ○ What is the timing for any subreports?
	Final study report; writing regulatory documents

• Audited draft report (ADR): timing typically estimated from the end of in-life and includes an audit of the report by the QA group at a CRO; this is required on GLP studies; between 10 and 16 weeks (business days); could be expedited for additional cost
  ○ What is the standard timing for delivery of the ADR after the end of in-life?
  ○ What is the timing for any subreports?
  ○ Is there an external pathology peer review that will be conducted?
  ○ Are there interim reports for different study phases (i.e., interim report that does not include recovery data)?
	Final study report; writing regulatory documents

• Final report: timing typically estimated from when sponsor provides authorization to finalize the report and includes the final QA audit; between 2 and 6 weeks (business days); could be expedited for additional cost ○ What is the timing to receive the final report after authorization to finalize is provided from the sponsor?	Final study report; writing regulatory documents
• SEND dataset: timing typically estimated from delivery of the final report; between 1 and 26 weeks (business days); could be expedited for additional cost and if CRO is notified of the regulatory filing timing ○ When can the SEND dataset be provided by the CRO?	Depending on the type of study, SEND datasets are required for regulatory submission to the FDA

The third factor to influence site selection is cost. Some sponsors may have a business agreement with a CRO establishing one as a preferred vendor. In these relationships, the sponsor and CRO have agreements in place around the number of studies the sponsor will award to the CRO at a reduced cost. The agreement may include the CRO assigning dedicated staff personnel, sponsor-specific protocol and/or report templates, and modified reporting timelines for studies. Periodic QA reviews along with analysis of specific study metrics may be utilized to determine the cost-benefit of the agreement. Having dedicated staff enables the chance to build the relationship between the sponsor and study team.

If a sponsor does not have a preferred CRO identified or established a relationship with a specific vendor for the conduct of the preclinical studies, it is useful to compare study proposal quotes from 2 to 3 test facilities when possible. Often when considering the placement of a study to support an IND and/or clinical trial application (CTA) regulatory submission, there are additional studies and activities that also need to be placed. Some of the larger CROs can provide a quote for an IND/CTA package of studies, which include method development and/or transfer and validation of bioanalytical assays. The package proposal can result in a discount on the overall cost for the studies supporting the program. If the package of studies is conducted at a single test facility, oversight of the studies becomes easier (i.e., one can monitor multiple activities in a single visit). These three factors determine site selection for preclinical studies. Table 18.6 includes examples of factors that could influence site selection for a study or a package of studies.

18.5 Sponsor Oversight and Monitoring Outsourced Preclinical Studies

Once the test facility is selected and the study is awarded to the CRO, the main work for the study begins. The study director can use the RFP to generate the initial draft of the protocol, although the extent to which it can be done is determined by how much detail the RFP contains. The sponsor should outline and communicate expectations of the study director as soon as possible. This includes preferences in the frequency of updates on the study. Setting up an initial meeting, as a teleconference or a videoconference if available, is a good way to build a good working relationship with the study director. The initial meeting can be an opportunity to share background information about the molecule and any preliminary data from previous studies. Often the sponsor can request to attend the pre-study meeting with the study team to provide an overview of the molecule and program plans. Additionally, it is important to monitor the study, especially if this is the first time the test facility is being used or there are molecule-specific reasons (i.e., need to observe for the occurrence of findings previously noted in another study; a nonstandard activity is planned to be included; and dose formulation preparation is nonstandard). The timing and frequency for monitoring a study can be dictated by multiple factors. Table 18.7 includes a list of reasons for monitoring a study, and Table 18.8 includes an example list of activities to observe during a monitoring visit.

Even though it is preferable to monitor studies in person, sometimes a visit cannot be conducted (e.g., study start is available early; travel restrictions; and pandemic). Current levels of communication technology make it possible to monitor studies remotely. Whenever possible, it is beneficial to utilize videoconferences for meetings with the study director and members of the study team. Secure data exchange portals enable access to data, with the preliminary data in some instances being available in real time. Some sponsors may prefer using their own internal data exchange portals, and the medium of data exchange should be prearranged prior to the start of any study-related discussions and activities. These tools are currently being implemented and are likely to continue to adjust how studies are expected to be monitored in the future. Not only does monitoring virtually reduce the total resources expended

TABLE 18.6

Example Factors to Consider in Site Selection

- Placement of a study may be dependent on a specific scientific expertise and capabilities at a CRO [scientific capabilities and/or expertise]
  - Example: if the route of administration is inhalation, the test facility should have these specific capabilities and staff experienced in conducting those studies
  - Example: if there are concerns for bone effects, the test facility should have specific scientific capabilities (additional bone biomarker measurements validated and capabilities to measure bone density) and either staff with scientific expertise to evaluate the data or established relationships with relevant scientific consultants
- Selection of the CRO may be dependent on the study start available [timing]
- With studies placed at a single test facility can enable one to monitor multiple activities during a single visit [timing/logistics]
- If study activities are split across different test facilities, need to consider timing for transfer of samples between the sites [timing]
  - For NHP studies: need to also consider the need for CITES permits if samples must be transferred across international borders, which requires prior planning; otherwise, it could result in a delay ranging from days to weeks [timing]
- Awarding an IND/CTA package to a single CRO; often the CRO will provide a discount on the total cost for the studies [cost]

TABLE 18.7

Example Reasons to Monitor a Study in Person and Activities to Monitor

- First time using the test facility
  - Observe dose formulation preparation
  - Observe animal handling
  - Review data documentation
  - Observe sample collection and sample processing
  - Meet study team
- Nonstandard event is scheduled (e.g., implant a delivery device)
- Based on findings in previous studies (treatment-related clinical observation), need to be present to provide scientific oversight
- Monitor interim necropsy if issues or special procedures are expected

TABLE 18.8

Example Activities to Observe during a Study Monitoring Visit

- Test article
  - Review storage, handling, and identity (check label for name, expiration, lot number, etc.) for test article and control article
- Dose formulation preparation and analysis
  - Review calculations for dose formulation preparation and compare with most recent body weight data
  - Observe dose formulation and control formulation (if applicable) and compare to protocol or study procedure
- Animal rooms
  - Observe general appearance of room and labels outside study room
  - Observe animals and cage conditions (e.g., food and water availability; enrichment)
- Dose administration
  - Observe and evaluate technical execution
  - Observe dose volume, route, rate of administration, and animal ID
- Blood sample collection
  - Review collection tube labels and animal ID
- Assess sample handling procedures to prevent cross-contamination (e.g., test article sample contamination of control samples)
- Necropsy
  - Observe collection of terminal body weights as per protocol
  - Review necropsy order and tissue fixatives (per protocol)
  - Review data entry procedures for gross observations
- Data
  - Conduct an information review of unaudited data

on studies (saving money as well as time spent associated with travel to a test facility), but this could allow one to select a test facility in another part of the world and monitor it without having to visit in person.

18.6 Conclusions

As most sponsors opt to outsource the conduct of the nonclinical studies supporting clinical trials and marketing applications, the burden to meet and maintain a GLP-compliant facility is shifted to the test facility. Sponsors are still responsible for monitoring that the studies are conducting in compliance with GLP regulations and guidelines. The selection of a test facility or a specific site for the conduct of the safety assessment studies of a biopharmaceutical is influenced by factors falling into these three main categories: (1) scientific capabilities, (2) timelines, and (3) cost. It is a combination of the three factors that influence the final site selection for a study.

REFERENCES

1. Marshall E. The murky world of toxicity testing. *Science* 1983; 220:1130–1132.
2. Schneider K. Faking it: the case against industrial bio-test laboratories. *The Amicus Journal* 1983; Spring:14–26.
3. US FDA. Good Laboratory Practice (GLP) Regulations, Proposed Rule. Federal Register, November 19, 1976. Vol 41:51206–51230.
4. US FDA. Good Laboratory Practice (GLP) Regulations, Final Rule. Federal Register, December 22, 1978. Vol 43: 59985–60025.
5. US FDA. Good Laboratory Practice (GLP) Regulations (Amendment), Final Rule. Federal Register, September 4, 1987. Vol 52:33768–33782.
6. US FDA. Good Laboratory Practice (GLP) Regulations, Proposed Rule. Federal Register, August 24, 1987. Vol 81: 58341–58380.
7. OECD. No. 1: Principles on Good Laboratory Practice, revised 1997.

Part III

Product Attributes

19

Nonclinical Development of Peptides and Therapeutic Proteins

Melanie T. Hartsough
Hartsough Nonclinical Consulting, LLC

CONTENTS

19.1 Introduction

This chapter focuses on the nonclinical development of peptides and therapeutic proteins. United States (US) Food and Drug Administration (FDA) has defined a polymer composed of ≤40 alpha-amino acids, regardless if manufactured by synthetic processes or by recombinant techniques, as a peptide, and a polymer containing 41–99 amino acids, manufactured entirely by chemical synthesis, as a chemically synthesized polypeptide. A protein is a polymer containing greater than 40 alpha-amino acids, produced by recombinant deoxyribonucleic acid (DNA) techniques in cells *in vitro* (e.g., human, animal, insect and bacteria) or in transgenic animals and plants or are purified endogenous proteins.

The classification of the product as a peptide or protein can determine the regulatory licensing pathway. For example, in the US, proteins are considered "biological products", as defined in 351 PHS Act, and are licensed as a Biologics License Application (BLA). Historically, exceptions to this were hormones and enzymes, such as insulin, human growth hormone, pancreas lipase and imiglucerase, which were regulated as drugs under the Federal Food, Drug and Cosmetic Act (FD&C Act). However, with the amended definition of a protein in the Further Consolidation Appropriations (FCA) Act to include chemically synthesized polypeptides, as of March 23, 2020, these products are now considered "biological products" and licensed as a BLA (FDA 2018). In general, peptides (≤40 amino acids) are regulated under the FD&C Act as a New Drug Application (NDA), unless the peptide meets the definition of a biological product (e.g., a peptide vaccine). Examples of peptides are glucagon, nesiritide, plecanatide and teduglutide. While these licensing pathways allow for different legal provisions, such as differing exclusivity rights and avenues for abbreviated drug development for future products (i.e., 505(b)(2), generic or biosimilar pathways), the separate regulatory pathways do not influence the nonclinical development of products as a new molecular entity.

As mentioned above, proteins are considered "biological products", which include blood-derived products; vaccines; *in vivo* diagnostic allergenic products; immunoglobulin products; products containing cells or microorganisms; and most protein products used for the treatment, prevention or cure of disease in humans (351 PHS Act). Initially, all biologics were regulated by the Center of Biologics Evaluation and Research (CBER) in the FDA. However, in 2003, the monoclonal antibodies; therapeutic proteins derived from plants, animals, humans or microorganisms; and recombinant versions of these products (except for purified and recombinant coagulation factors) and proteins used to alter the production of hematopoietic cells *in vivo* were transferred to Center for Drug Evaluation and Research (CDER).

In most instances, peptides are synthetically manufactured, thereby allowing for a well-defined structure and do not have the complexity of a protein product produced in a biological system, i.e., 3-dimensional structure and post-translational modifications (oxidation, glycosylation, methylation, etc.).

DOI: 10.1201/9781003124542-22

While peptides may be thoroughly characterized, proteins are less so due to microheterogeneity, which can provide challenges in establishing comparability of protein products when changes in the manufacturing process are required during clinical development. Regardless of the product quality characterization variances, the development of the nonclinical programs for peptides and proteins uses similar underlying principles.

In the context of this chapter, the term "therapeutic proteins" will be used to represent proteins such as cytokines, plasminogen activators, recombinant plasma factors, growth factors, fusion proteins, enzymes, receptors and hormones that are either purified from natural sources or produced by recombinant biotechnology-derived technologies. The term "peptide" refers to a chemically synthesized protein with <100 amino acids, unless otherwise noted. The intent of the chapter is to discuss the nonclinical programs for unconjugated peptides and proteins. Additional considerations may be required for modified products such as Fc fusion proteins or conjugated proteins (e.g., attached with polymers, glycoproteins, small molecule drugs, or other peptides or proteins). The intended clinical indications encompass therapeutic and prophylactic usages. While the principles discussed for peptides and therapeutic proteins also apply to monoclonal antibodies, this class of biological products are beyond the scope of this chapter but are discussed in **Chapter 20**. Similarly, nonclinical programs to support the development of abbreviated new drug applications (ANDAs) for peptides or a biosimilar for therapeutic proteins are not discussed in this chapter.

19.2 Nonclinical Programs

19.2.1 Regulatory Guidance

The primary regulatory advice available to provide a framework for the development of appropriate and meaningful nonclinical programs for therapeutic proteins is the International Council of Harmonization (ICH) guideline "Preclinical Safety Evaluation of Biotechnology-Derived Pharmaceuticals S6(R1)" (2011), which consists of the original ICHS6 document and addendum. While this document does not specifically pertain to peptides, the principles outlined may be applicable for some peptide safety programs. However, peptide nonclinical programs generally consist of the studies and use the principles outlined in "Nonclinical Safety studies for Conduct of Human Clinical Trials for Pharmaceuticals ICHM3(R2)" (2009), unless otherwise justified. For therapeutic proteins, ICHM3(R2) provides general advice for the timing and duration of the specific study types such as general toxicity and reproductive and developmental toxicity studies. Additionally, there are useful recommendations provided for combination product development, juvenile toxicity studies and exploratory investigational new drug applications (INDs) that may be applicable to therapeutic protein programs. For therapeutic proteins that are being developed as biosimilars, general guidance is available that outlines the nonclinical requirements. Table 19.1 outlines the general guidance available in the US for therapeutic proteins and peptides.

TABLE 19.1

General Information for Nonclinical Programs for Therapeutic Proteins and Peptides

Guidance Title	Applicability
ICHS6(R1): Preclinical Safety Evaluation of Biotechnology-Derived Pharmaceuticals (2011), consisting of original S6 document and addendum	Therapeutic proteins Concepts useful for peptide programs
ICHM3 (R2): Nonclinical Safety Studies for Conduct of Human Clinical Trials for Pharmaceuticals	Peptides Therapeutic proteins—timing of studies and useful discussions on combination products, exploratory INDs and juvenile toxicity studies
Guidance for Industry: "Scientific Considerations in Demonstrating Biosimilarity to a Reference Product" (CDER/CBER, 2015)	Therapeutic proteins Not applicable to peptides

In addition to general regulatory guidelines, there are a variety of documents available to guide sponsors in the development of specific clinical indications. Of particular mention is ICHS9 "Nonclinical Evaluation for Anticancer Pharmaceuticals" (2009), which provides recommendations for peptides and therapeutic proteins that are specifically being developed to treat cancer in patients with serious and life-threatening malignancies. Moreover, there are a variety of guidances published by the FDA that provide advice for nonclinical development of biopharmaceuticals and peptides for specific types of patient populations or diseases (see Table 19.2 for some of the guidance).

Other regulatory agencies may also have specific guidelines, and it is recommended to search the intended authorities' websites for pertinent guidance.

19.2.2 Standard Nonclinical Program

The nonclinical program for peptides and therapeutic proteins consists of a range of *in vitro* and *in vivo* pharmacology, pharmacokinetic and toxicology studies. The pharmacology studies are designed to characterize the mechanism of action and specificity of the product as well as provide some evidence of therapeutic value for the intended clinical indication (i.e., proof-of-concept studies), typically utilizing an animal model of disease or injury. In general, peptides and therapeutic proteins have high specificity and affinity to their intended target. *In vitro* assays may be useful to demonstrate the selectivity of the product to the intended target and not to other related proteins or subtypes of the target, as well as other potential receptors. These types of assays can range from individual binding to closely related receptors using specific enzyme-linked immunosorbent assays (ELISAs) or surface plasmon resonance to microarray screens for general off-target binding using protein-based or genetically-modified-cell-based platforms. Additional *in vitro* studies to evaluate potential safety-related or secondary pharmacology should be considered dependent upon the mode of action of the product. For example, it may be useful to understand the potential for release of cytokines or expansion of immune populations for an immune modulator *in vitro* prior to testing *in vivo*.

TABLE 19.2

FDA Guidances with Nonclinical Development Guidelines for Specific Clinical Indications

Specific Nonclinical Guidance	Date
Nonclinical safety evaluation of pediatric drug products	Feb 2006
Investigational enzyme replacement therapy products: nonclinical assessment	Oct 2019
Reference guide for the nonclinical toxicity studies of antiviral drugs indicated for the treatment of nonlife-threatening diseases: evaluation of drug toxicity prior to Phase 1 clinical studies	Feb 1999
Osteoporosis: nonclinical evaluation of drugs intended for treatment	Aug 2019
Developing medical imaging drug and biological products part 1 conducting safety assessments	July 2005
ICHS9 nonclinical evaluation for anticancer pharmaceuticals	March 2010
Oncology therapeutic radiopharmaceuticals: nonclinical studies and labeling recommendations	Aug 2019
Oncology pharmaceuticals: reproductive toxicity testing and labeling recommendations	May 2019
Severely debilitating or life-threatening hematologic disorders: nonclinical development of pharmaceuticals	March 2019
Other Discipline Guidance with Nonclinical Recommendations	
Drug Products, including Biological Products, that Contain Nanomaterials	Draft Dec 2017
Chronic Hepatitis C Virus Infection: Developing Direct-Acting Antiviral Drugs for Treatment	Nov 2017
Clinical Development Programs for Drugs, Devices, and Biological Products for the Treatment of Rheumatoid Arthritis	Feb 1999
Smallpox (variola) infection: developing drugs for treatment or prevention	Nov 2007
Development of anti-infective drug products for the pediatric population	Draft June 2020

The proof-of-concept studies are typically performed with animal models of disease or injury, specifically chosen to provide the most relevant data to demonstrate a potential therapeutic benefit as well as in some cases to establish a potential therapeutic range in humans. Most often, these are rodent models, e.g., xenograft tumor-bearing animals, BAFF (B cell activation factor of the TNF family) transgenic mice for Sjogren's syndrome and middle cerebral artery transient occlusion to induce stroke. In some instances, the product is not active in rodent models, and higher order animal models of disease in dogs, pigs, monkeys or other large animals are needed to evaluate the *in vivo* biological activity of the clinical intended product. While the intent of the disease model studies is to establish biological activity of the product, there may be instances in which relevant safety information can be extracted from these studies (see Section 19.2.2.2).

The pharmacokinetic programs of peptides and therapeutic proteins consist mainly of studies performed to understand the blood kinetics of the product (i.e., pharmacokinetic assessments). Distribution studies may be performed, but caution should be taken to ensure that the detection method is able to distinguish between full-length product versus inactive degradants or free label. Since peptides and therapeutic proteins are very selective for their target receptor, determining the target receptor tissue expression profile using methods such as immunohistochemistry or *in silico* searches of protein and messenger ribonucleic acid (mRNA) tissue databases may be more informative for determining potential target tissues. Since therapeutic proteins are degraded by normal catabolic pathways, standard metabolism and excretion studies are not required by regulatory authorities. The same principle can be applied to peptides that mimic endogenous proteins, although sometimes these studies are still performed. While peptides and therapeutic proteins may not be metabolized by cytochrome P_{450}s (CYPs), they may be able to induce or inhibit the expression of these enzymes, which, as a result, may indirectly affect the metabolism of other drugs that may be taken by the patient.

For example, Interferon-γ was shown to suppress CYP1A2 and CYP2E1 mRNA levels and ethoxyresorufin-O-deethylase activity, whereas interleukin-4 stimulated CYP2E1 mRNA (Abdel-Razzak 1993). Other cytokines such as interleukin-1α, interleukin-1β, interleukin-6, tumor necrosis factor-α were shown also to be potent depressors of CYP RNA and activity (Abdel-Razzak 1993, Clark et al. 1995). Studies to evaluate this potential drug–drug interaction should be considered during the clinical development of the product.

Safety programs, in general, may consist of safety pharmacology studies, general toxicity studies, reproductive and development studies, genotoxicity assays, carcinogenicity studies and special studies such as immune toxicity studies. The types of toxicology studies and the designs of the studies for a peptide and therapeutic protein are dependent upon the product's innate characteristics. These characteristics can guide the development of unique study designs to generate the most pertinent and appropriate data to inform the clinic. In general, there are key differences in peptides and therapeutic proteins that can result in vastly dissimilar nonclinical programs, even for the same indication. These differences are discussed in the following sections.

19.2.2.1 Pharmacologically Relevant Models

It is expected that the safety program of peptides and therapeutic proteins will incorporate toxicity evaluations in one rodent and one nonrodent species, unless there is a scientific rationale to exclude a species [ICHM3(R2) and ICHS6(R1)]. Additionally, since exaggerated pharmacology of a peptide or therapeutic protein is most often the major source of toxicities associated with these types of molecules, it is extremely important to identify relevant animal species appropriate for toxicology studies. A relevant animal species is one that expresses a responsive orthologous receptor or antigen and responds to the biopharmaceutical similarly to that expected in humans. Ideally, a peptide and therapeutic protein would be tested in an animal species in which it binds to the corresponding receptor with an affinity comparable to that seen with the human receptor and initiates the desired pharmacological response similar to that expected in humans. However, the specificity of a peptide or therapeutic protein to a human target may limit its binding affinity to orthologous substrates and/or hinder the production of the desired pharmacological response in the test species. When the peptide or therapeutic protein does not bind the receptor in the test animal species in a similar manner to humans or when the species does not express the corresponding receptor or its required signaling mechanisms, toxicology studies may result in a false sense of safety. An example is recombinant human interferon-gamma (rhIFN-γ), an immunomodulatory cytokine that has no activity in rodents (Green and Terrel 1992). In early safety assessments, rhIFN-γ produced no toxicities in standard rodent acute, subacute and reproductive and developmental toxicity studies at any dose level. It was not until toxicity studies were conducted in cynomolgus monkeys, a pharmacologically relevant species, that toxicities predictive of dose-limiting toxicities in humans were observed (Green and Terrel 1992, Terrell and Green 1993). Many human endogenous proteins, such as human granulocyte-macrophage colony-stimulating factor (GM-CSF), interferon-α-2b and interferon-β are not conserved across species, having severely reduced activity or no activity that ultimately limits the species that are appropriate for the evaluation of safety (Shanafelt 1991, BLA-99-1488, PLA 98-0261).

While peptides are similar to therapeutic proteins in that they are highly specific for their intended target, peptides tend to have less species restrictions as therapeutic proteins. Regardless, to maximize the utility of animals to identify potentially clinical relevant toxicities and to reduce the potential for irrelevant studies and misuse of animals, it is imperative to determine whether the peptide or protein therapeutic has any species limitations. An in-depth discussion on the assays and a potential process to pursue to identify suitable species is found in **Chapter 2**.

19.2.2.2 Alternative Models

Ideally, toxicity studies will be performed in one or more pharmacologically relevant species; however, there may be instances when the clinically intended peptide or therapeutic protein has no activity in any typical toxicity test species. In these instances, alternative approaches, such as use of a surrogate product, animal model of disease, transgenic animals or knockout animals, can be explored to provide some relevant safety data.

The most common situation is one in which the orthologous target is present in the toxicity species, but the intended clinical product either does not bind to the target or induces low biological activity. In these situations, the safety of the clinical product can be evaluated using a species-specific analogous peptide or therapeutic protein (i.e., surrogate product). In order to generate the most relevant safety data, the surrogate needs to resemble the clinical product as much as possible with respect to activity and impurity content. While it is not uncommon to produce these molecules on the benchtop or at much smaller scales as the clinical product, it is important to mimic the clinical product production process as closely as possible to establish a similar impurity and contaminant profile. The characterization of the surrogate should demonstrate that it has a similar pharmacological response with respect to binding, mechanism of action and biological activity on the test species cells as the intended clinical product on human cells; most often *in vitro* assays are used to establish this similarity. It will also be important to understand whether there needs to be an adjustment in dose to establish a similar pharmacological response to the clinical product for a more accurate interpretation of the toxicity data and selection of clinical doses. Finally, the blood kinetics and immunogenicity of the surrogate in the test species may be different than the clinical product and should be evaluated so the most appropriate doses and dosing regimen can be selected for the toxicity studies. These toxicity studies are performed in compliance with 21CFR Part 58 that prescribes good laboratory practices for nonclinical laboratory studies (GLPs). The use of surrogate proteins has been shown to be acceptable for toxicology programs that have supported licensure of products by regulatory agencies (Green and Terrel 1992, Tracey 2000, Clarke et al. 2004).

In some instances, the intended target is not present in normal animals, but only accessible or expressed during the disease state. Although these models are typically used to allow for an understanding of the mode of action and demonstration of *in vivo* biological activity, they can be sometimes utilized to assess safety. Since many of the disease models are generated at academic institutions, toxicity studies performed in disease models are often not able to be GLP-compliant; however, it is important to conduct the study in such a way to ensure data integrity, such as preparing a prospective study protocol, following defined methods, using appropriately trained personnel, properly collecting and documenting data and generating a study report. Some of the challenges of these types of studies include the lack of characterization of background lesions, which can make identifying test article-related toxicities more difficult. In addition, the duration of the study may be restricted due to the limited life span of the diseased animals and the complexity of generating the diseased animals may result in low numbers of animals per group or staggered allocation of animals and extending the time to complete a study.

In some instances, a transgenic model in which the human target is genetically expressed in the animal (typically mice) can be generated and used to test the safety of the intended clinical product. In order to use these types of models for toxicity purposes, the animals need to produce consistent expression and tissue distribution of the human target in the animal as expected in humans. Similar to animal models of disease, the background pathology associated with gene expression can confound interpretation of the study with respect to the test article and study design and performance can be hindered due to the life span of the animals and difficulty generating the number of animals needed for a well-designed toxicity study. Regardless, this type of models has been successfully used for GLP-compliant chronic toxicity and reproductive and developmental toxicity studies to support licensure (Bugelski et al. 2000).

Finally, if the clinically intended peptide or therapeutic protein does not bind to any toxicity test species and the intent of the product is to inhibit the signaling or activation of the target, some safety information may be gathered from genetically modified animals, typically mice, that have the orthologous target removed (knockout model). One important distinction of this type of model is that it does not mimic the therapeutic setting. There may be spontaneous pathologies associated with knocking out the gene that occur over the lifetime of the animal that do not accurately represent therapeutic inhibition of the target. Additionally, gathering the information may be obstructed by the lack of historical control data, animal availability and length of the life of the animals. Many times knockout models are useful for understanding the potential reproductive and developmental risks.

19.2.2.3 Immunogenicity

One property of peptides and therapeutic proteins is the potential for these products to stimulate the immune system to produce antibodies against the product (referred to as immunogenicity). In some situations, anti-drug antibodies (ADAs) can confound the interpretation of a toxicity study. They can alter the pharmacologic activity by neutralizing the product activity and/or alter the pharmacokinetic profile by binding and increasing the clearance of the product from circulation, thereby reducing the overall systemic exposure of the product, or in some rare cases extend the time present in the systemic circulation and increase the systemic exposure. While it is expected that the duration of the toxicity studies should be equal to or exceed the duration of the clinical trial up to 6 months in rodents for both product types and 9 months in nonrodents for a peptide and 6 months in nonrodents for a therapeutic protein (ICHS6(R1) and ICHM3(R2)); robust immunogenicity clearing or neutralizing the product may be generated with repeat administration, thereby limiting the usefulness of longer duration toxicity studies. The ADAs may also exert toxicities not directly attributed to the product, such as immune complex disease (or serum sickness) or hypersensitivity reactions (Heyen et al. 2014, Rojke et al. 2014). Moreover, if the peptide or therapeutic protein is identical in sequence to an endogenous protein, ADAs may cross-react with the endogenous protein and neutralize its activity (Casadevall 2002, Cases et al. 2003, Rahbar et al. 2017).

In order to understand the consequences of immunogenicity, if it occurs, within the context of the toxicity study, it is important to collect blood at least after the first and last administration of the product in a toxicity study and possibly intermittently throughout the dosing period for longer toxicity studies for evaluation of toxicokinetic profile and presence and neutralizing activity of ADAs. Alternatively, if a pharmacodynamic marker is available, the marker and toxicokinetics can be monitored instead of ADAs. Significant changes in blood levels of the product are usually indicative of the development of ADA even before the ADAs are detected. It is important to note, however, that the sole presence of ADAs may not negatively affect product systemic exposure or activity or cause other toxicities. A more in-depth review of the interpretation of immunogenicity in toxicity studies can be found in Ponce 2009.

The immunogenicity assessments of peptides and therapeutic proteins in animals are performed to interpret the toxicity study and do not predict what may occur in humans. The peptides and therapeutic proteins administered to animals are most often human sequences that are recognized as foreign in animals and will stimulate an immune response, whereas in humans the immune response against a human peptide or therapeutic protein may not be as robust or may be delayed without the same toxicities associated with them. However, in the context of a product with a human sequence identical to an endogenous sequence, the type of antibodies generated, such as cross-reactive antibodies to endogenous protein with the corresponding knockout of the endogenous protein activity, in the animal may aid in the understanding of the risk of a similar type of antibody to be generated in the human patient population. While the toxicity studies are not performed to predict the immunogenicity potential in humans, there are *in silico* and *in vitro* screening assays available that can be used to help understand the risk in humans.

19.2.2.4 Impurities

The impurities in a peptide or therapeutic protein can be product-, host- or process-related. Product-related impurities for peptides and therapeutic proteins are similar and include mismatched disulfide bonds, truncations and oligomers and/or aggregates as well as degradants. Additionally, therapeutic proteins may have variations in post-translational modifications such as glycosylation, and synthetic peptides can have amino acid additions or incomplete deprotection of amino acid side chain protecting groups leading to peptides shorter and non-homologous to the desired amino acid sequence. While aggregation can occur with peptides and/or their product-related impurities, this is more frequent with therapeutic proteins that are greater in size and more complex with post-translational and tertiary structures. Process-related impurities/contaminants are limited for therapeutic proteins, consisting of residuals from the purification columns or viral inactivation steps. For synthetic peptides, process-related impurities include organic (nonpeptide) and inorganic molecules and residual solvents carried over from synthesis (e.g., catalysts or cleavage agents). Host-related impurities are only found in therapeutic proteins or peptides produced using recombinant means and consist of proteins and DNA from the host used to produce the product.

Host-cell proteins and product-related impurities for peptide and therapeutic proteins generally pose minimal safety or efficacy risks; however, consideration should be made to use material for the toxicity studies that is produced either by the same manufacturing train as the clinical material and contains similar impurity content, which would also circumvent the need for formal comparability assessments (see **Chapter 9**), or that overrepresents the impurity profile of the clinical material (i.e., is dirtier). There is no need to do special toxicity assessments, such as *in vitro* genotoxicity studies, for impurities of recombinantly made proteins or peptides. Historically, regulatory authorities have requested genotoxicity studies for synthetic peptides due to the presence of process-related impurities, such as reagents, catalysts, other inorganic impurities (e.g., heavy metals, chloride, or sulfate); however, with the current stringent manufacturing regulations for limits of these types of impurities, a discussion could be had with the regulatory authorities on the necessity of such assays for synthetic peptides that have well-characterized impurity profiles with no identified genotoxic structural alerts.

Finally, adventitious agents may get introduced to peptide or therapeutic protein products inadvertently during their manufacturing. One standard test for purity measures the bacterial endotoxin levels in the product. The current limit for parenteral routes other than intrathecal administration is 5 EU/kg body weight/hour of endotoxin administered to a human per dose; intrathecal limits are currently set at 0.2 EU/kg body weight (USP <85>). While endotoxin levels greater than that can be delivered to animals in toxicity studies, caution should be taken to avoid levels that may induce endotoxin-related toxicities.

19.2.2.5 Safety Pharmacology

Safety pharmacology studies evaluate the effects of a product on vital organs that are crucial for life, such as the cardiovascular, respiratory and central nervous systems. These studies are performed prior to the initiation of the first-in-human studies and are typically stand-alone single-dose studies using relatively standardized protocols evaluating respiratory and central nervous system (CNS) effects in Sprague Dawley rats and cardiovascular effects in Beagle dogs. However, for therapeutic proteins that are highly specific for their target, these endpoints can be incorporated into the general toxicity studies (ICHS7A). While it is not specifically stated in the ICHS7A guidance, the same principles may be applicable to peptides; however, general practice has been to conduct the independent safety pharmacology studies.

The neurobehavioral screening methods, functional observational battery (FOB) or Irwin test, are validated protocols to measure motor, sensory and cognitive function. If the peptide and therapeutic protein are active in rodents, these assessments can be easily incorporated into a repeat-dose general toxicity study, ideally performed at the time blood concentrations are maximal after dose administration, but at a time when there are no other tests or blood collection scheduled. In nonrodent general toxicity studies, an adapted FOB can be performed in dogs; however, in monkeys, the tests are limited to extended clinical observations assessing coordination, motor activity and behavioral changes. Respiratory endpoints (respiratory rate, tidal volume and minute volume) are typically evaluated with rats using plethysmograph chambers with continued pulmonary monitoring for a period of at least 4 hours post-administration. While this method may be able to be incorporated into a rodent repeat-dose toxicity study, depending on the dosing regimen, typical assessments are limited to respiratory rate in a nonrodent species, such as dogs and monkeys. This measurement can be taken at several time points following dose administration throughout the dosing and recovery periods if needed.

Finally, electrocardiograms are routinely performed in repeat-dose toxicity studies in nonrodent species at several time points (e.g., 0.5 and 24 hours) following product administration; however, these assessments are not as robust as the standard cardiovascular safety pharmacology study in which electrocardiograms are performed continuously up to 20 hours subsequent to test article administration. Since the endpoints are incorporated into repeat-dose toxicity studies, the parameters can be performed intermittently throughout the dosing and recovery (if needed) periods.

In addition to the *in vivo* testing, an *in vitro* assessment to determine the potential for delayed ventricular repolarization (i.e., QT interval prolongation) is a standard safety pharmacology assessment (ICH7B) performed for small molecules. The current standard assay is the human ether-a-go-go-related gene (hERG) potassium channel assay. Since therapeutic proteins cannot diffuse into cells and are too big to enter the ion channel, the assay is not performed for these types of products. While there is no regulatory guidance available for the appropriateness of the assay for peptides, using the same basic principles suggests that the assay may not provide a meaningful assessment. With newer technologies being developed, such as human-induced pluripotent stem cell-derived cardiac cell systems, a more relevant and useful assay may be available in the future.

19.2.2.6 General Toxicity Studies

As mentioned previously, regulatory expectations are that general toxicity studies will be performed in two species, a rodent and nonrodent, unless scientifically justified otherwise. The selection of the appropriate toxicity species for therapeutic proteins relies principally on limitations imposed by pharmacological relevancy and/or immunogenicity responses. In contrast, while important principles to consider, peptides tend to be evaluated in both rodents and nonrodents. Rats are regularly the rodent of choice for both peptides and therapeutic proteins. While mice are also used, caution should be taken for highly immunogenic products as some mice strains are more sensitive to ADAs than others, having anaphylactic reactions stimulated through both IgE- and IgG-mediated mechanisms (Finkelman 2007). Dogs are the nonrodent choice more often for peptides than therapeutic proteins, whereas monkeys tend to be the nonrodent of choice for therapeutic proteins, even if the dog is a pharmacologically relevant species. There are a variety of reasons for the difference in nonrodent species preference, for example, reagents needed for more specialized evaluations (such as cytokine assays and immune phenotyping) are more available for monkeys; dogs tend to be more sensitive to ADAs; and dogs are allergic to polysorbate 80 (a typical excipient in the formulation of therapeutic proteins) (Krantz et al. 1949). Other nonrodent species (such as minipigs and rabbits) can also be used as appropriate for either product type.

The duration of the toxicity studies for both peptides and therapeutic proteins follows the intended duration of dosing in the clinic, as outlined in ICHM3(R2), with the exception of chronic toxicity testing. For therapeutic proteins, repeat-dose toxicity studies of 6-month duration in rodents and nonrodents are sufficient to support chronic indications (ICHS6(R1)), whereas 9-month duration studies in nonrodents are required for peptides (ICHM3(R2)). However, specific clinical indications (e.g., advanced cancer malignancies, osteosclerosis), targets of the drug and/or more invasive or novel routes of administration may lead to different duration expectations.

While outlining the specifics of toxicity study designs and endpoints is beyond the scope of this chapter, it is important to note that the expectations for the selection of the high dose for toxicity studies are different between a peptide and a therapeutic protein. The high dose for a therapeutic protein can be limited to a 10-fold exposure multiple greater than the maximum clinical dose (ICHS6(R1)). In contrast, the high-dose selection for a peptide follows the rules laid out in ICHM3(R2)), requiring large exposure multiples, such as 50-fold, or limit doses of 1,000 mg/kg if the exposure multiple is >10-fold or 2,000 mg/kg if the clinical dose exceeds 1 g/day (see ICHM3(R2) for additional guidance on dose selection).

19.2.2.7 Reproductive and Developmental Studies

Reproductive and developmental studies (pre- and post-natal development, embryo-fetal and fertility studies) are performed with peptides and therapeutic proteins as required for the intended clinical population, per ICHS5(R2). In general, embryo-fetal and fertility studies are expected to be completed prior to Phase 3 and the pre-and postnatal development study completed for licensure; however, depending on the intended clinical population, the timing and/or need for certain studies may be delayed or omitted. For small molecules, these studies are performed in rats and rabbits, and these species should be used for peptides and therapeutic proteins if they are pharmacologically relevant species. However, species specificity, mechanism of action, immunogenicity effects or pharmacokinetic profile of the product may require modification of the standard study designs and dosing regimen. For example, if repeat-dose administration results in ADAs that eliminate exposure or neutralize product activity, the duration of dosing may need to be limited (e.g., 7–14 days) and additional groups of animals required with different dosing periods to cover the entire intended period for the study. If there are no pharmacological species, alternative models (as described in **Section 19.2.2.2**) can be considered. Additionally, when there is evidence for adverse effects on fertility, pregnancy or fetal development from the known pharmacological activity and/or literature studies with genetically modified animals, it is recommended to have a discussion with the regulatory authority on the usefulness and need for standard reproductive and developmental studies.

If the biological activity of the peptide or therapeutic protein is limited to the cynomolgus monkey, separate embryo-fetal and pre- and post-natal developmental studies or a combined embryo-fetal and pre- and post-natal development study (referred to as ePPND) can be performed. The ePPND study is a single study in which the product is administered from gestation day 20 to birth. Due to the complications of performing monkey developmental studies, these studies, in most cases, may be conducted in parallel with the Phase 3 clinical trials. Separate fertility studies are not performed with monkeys, instead if there is a concern of fertility effects, fertility endpoints (such as menstrual cyclicity, sperm count, sperm morphology/motility and reproductive hormone levels) can be incorporated into a 3-month repeat-dose toxicity study using sexually mature monkeys.

19.2.2.8 Carcinogenicity

While peptides and therapeutic proteins do not diffuse into the cell nucleus and interact with DNA directly, the biological activity of the product may directly or indirectly support the proliferation of cells that ultimately may result in neoplasia. If the product's dosing regimen satisfies the conditions required for the assessment of carcinogenicity (see ICH S1A: Guideline on the Need for Carcinogenicity Studies of Pharmaceuticals, 1995), additional data may be needed to understand the risks to the patient. For a peptide with low immunogenic risk, regulatory authorities most likely will require the standard carcinogenicity mouse and rat bioassays to be performed. For a therapeutic protein, a risk assessment, including data from transgenic or knockout models, information about the target biology and product's mechanism of action, and relevant *in vitro*, chronic toxicity and clinical data, can be performed. In cases where the tumorigenicity potential is uncertain from the evidence collected, more in-depth studies should be considered. A 2-year rodent carcinogenicity study or a study in a 6-month transgenic model can be considered; however, species specificity and the generation of clearing or neutralizing antibodies usually preclude the utility of such studies for many products. Using a species-specific analogous product to perform the carcinogenicity studies also can be considered; however, these types of studies may be limited to hazard identification. Instead, other product-specific studies designed to understand the biological mechanism related to the particular carcinogenic concern may provide more clinically relevant risk information. If it is clear from the accumulated knowledge from the risk assessment that there is a carcinogenic potential for the product, no follow-up studies are needed.

19.2.3 Dose Translation

Dose extrapolation from animals to humans for a peptide and therapeutic protein can be accomplished in several ways. In the early stages of clinical development when there are no clinical data, animal doses can be extrapolated by body surface area normalization using the conversions described in FDA guidance *Estimating the Maximum Safe Starting Dose in Initial Clinical Trials for Therapeutics in Adult Healthy Volunteers* (July 2005). Alternatively, scaling on an mg/kg basis can be done when the therapeutic protein is ≥100 kDa, administered intravascularly. Additionally, when there is little distribution beyond the application site, normalization to the amount of product at the application site (mg or mg/area of application site) is acceptable. Finally, the pharmacology data such as pharmacodynamic markers and *in vitro* and *in vivo* biological activity and pharmacokinetic data collected in the animal model of disease and/or healthy animals can be used to extrapolate the equivalent human dosages. When there is clinical pharmacokinetic data, a comparison of appropriate exposure parameters (such as C_{max} and/or AUC) from animals to humans can be used to establish equivalent dosages.

REFERENCES

Abdel-Razzak, Z, Loyer P, Fautel A, Gautier JC, Corcos L et al. Cytokines down-regulate expression of major cytochrome P-450 enzymes in adult human hepatocytes in primary culture. *Mol. Pharmacol.* 44: 707–715, 1993.

BLA 99-1488, FDA's Toxicologist's Review, 2000.

Bugelski PJ, Herzyk DJ, Rehm S, Harmsen AR, Gore EV, et al. Preclinical development of keliximab, a primatized anti-CD4 monoclonal antibody in human CD4 transgenic mice: characterization of the model and safety studies. *Human & Exp. Tox.* 19:230–245, 2000.

Casadevall N. Antibodies against rHuEPO: native and recombinant. *Nephrol. Dial. Transplant.* 17 (suppl. 5):42–47, 2002.

Cases A, Esforzado A, Mas M, Ricart MJ and Cruzado JM. Pure red blood aplasia associated with neutralizing antibodies against erythropoietin induced epoetin alfa: a new form of acquired erythroblastopenia in auremic patients. *Nefrologia.* 23(3): 266–270, 2003.

Clark MA, Bing BA, Gottschall PE and Williams JF. Differential effects of cytokines on the phenobarbital or 3-methylcholanthrene induction of P450 mediated mono-oxygenase activity in cultured rat hepatocytes. *Biochem Pharmacol.* 49 (1): 97–104, 1995.

Clarke J, Leach W, Pippig S, Joshi A, Wu B, House R, Beyer J. Evaluation of a surrogate antibody for preclinical safety testing on an anti-CD11a monoclonal antibody. *Regulatory Tox. & Pharm.* 40: 219–22, 2004.

FDA. Implementation of the "deemed to be a license" provision of the biologic price competition and innovation act of 2009, 2018.

Finkelman FD. Anaphylaxis: lessons from mouse models. *J. Allergy Clin. Immunol.* 120:506–525, 2007.

Green JD, Terrel TG. Utilization of homologous proteins to evaluate the safety of recombinant human proteins-case study: recombinant human interferon-gamma (rhIFN-gamma). *Toxicol. Lett.* 64–66, spec No. 321–327, 1992.

Heyen J, Rojko J, Evans M, Brown TP, Bobrowski WF, et al. Characterization, biomarkers, and reversibility of a monoclonal antibody-induced immune complex disease in cynomolgus monkeys (Macaca fascicularis). *Toxicol. Pathol.* 42: 765–773, 2014.

Krantz, J.C., Carr, C.J., Bubert, H.M., et al., Sugar alcohols: XXVII. Drug allergy in the Canine family. *J. Pharm. Exp. Ther.* 97: 125–128,1949.

PLA 98-0261. FDA Toxicologist's Review, 1999.

Rahbar M, Chitsazian Z, Abdoli F, Moeini Taba S-M, Akbari H. Pure red cell aplasia due to antibodies against erythropoietin in hemodialysis patients. *J. Nephropathol.* 6(1): 25–29, 2017.

Rojke JL, Evans MG, Price SA, Han B, Waine G, DeWitte M, Haynes J, Freimark B et al. Formation, clearance, deposition, pathogenicity and identification of biopharmaceutical-related immune complexes: Review and case studies. *Toxicol. Pathol.* 42:725–764, 2014.

Shanafelt AB, Johnson KE and Kastelein RA. Identification of critical amino acid residues in human and mouse granulocyte-macrophage colony-stimulating factor and their involvement in species specificity. *J. Bio. Chem.* 266: 13840–13810, 1991.

Tracey G. Using an analogous monoclonal antibody to evaluate the reproductive and chronic toxicity potential for a humanized anti-TNFα monoclonal antibody. *Human & Exper. Tox.* 19: 226–228, 2000.

Terell TG, Green JD, Comparative pathology of recombinant murine interferon-gamma in mice and recombinant human interferon-gamma in cynomolgus monkeys. *Int. Rev. Exp. Pathol.* 34 pt B: 73–101, 1993.

20

Antibodies (Abs) and Related Products Containing Complementarity-Determining Regions (CDRs)

Michael W. Leach
Pfizer Inc.

CONTENTS

DOI: 10.1201/9781003124542-23

20.1 Introduction/General Considerations

20.1.1 History

In 1890, von Behring and Kitasato showed that graduated doses of sterilized broth cultures of diphtheria or tetanus bacilli caused animals to produce substances in their blood which could neutralize the toxins produced by these bacilli; these were called antitoxins (von Behring and Kitasato 1890, The Nobel Prize. Emil von Behring Biography). Serum from animals actively immunized against diphtheria could be transferred to other animals and cure disease, and the effects were specific in that antitoxin against tetanus did not provide protection. The pharmaceutical company Farbwerke Hoechst began immunizing sheep in 1893 against diphtheria, which was followed by immunization of horses, and by 1894, treatment with antisera from animals had reduced the human diphtheria case mortality in Paris from 52% to 25% (reviewed by Llewelyn et al. 1992). Based on his work, the first Nobel Prize in Physiology or Medicine was awarded to von Behring in 1901 (The Nobel Prize 1901). In 1944, concentrated human immunoglobulins (Igs) were shown to be beneficial in the treatment of measles (Ordman et al. 1944; Stokes Jr et al. 1944). Between 1946 and 1948, the relationship between plasma cells and antibody (Ab) generation was described (Fagraeus 1947, 1948). In 1957, Burnet and Talmage independently developed the clonal selection theory, which stated that each lymphocyte makes a single specific Ab molecule that is determined before it encounters an antigen (Burnet 1957; Talmage 1957, described by Viret and Gurr 2009). The structure of Abs was independently reported by Edelman (1959) and Porter (1959), and in 1972, they were jointly awarded the Nobel Prize in Physiology or Medicine (The Nobel Prize 1972). In 1975, the hybridoma method of producing monoclonal Abs (mAbs) was published (Köhler and Milstein 1975), opening the door for the development of therapeutic mAbs (see Ribatti 2014 for a brief review of their work). The Nobel Prizes in Physiology or Medicine were awarded to Köhler and Milstein in 1984, which they shared with Jerne (The Nobel Prize 1984).

It would be another 20 years from Köhler and Milstein's publication until the United States Food and Drug Administration (US FDA) approved the first mAb for human use, muromonab (Orthoclone OKT3), a mouse IgG2a anti-CD3 for the treatment of acute transplantation rejection. Initial therapeutic mAbs were mouse based and had a number of shortcomings, including induction of anti-drug Abs (ADA), short half-life, reduced effector function, reduced clinical efficacy, and allergic reactions (Shawler et al. 1985; Ribatti 2014; Almagro et al. 2018).

In an effort to reduce and overcome these issues, the humanization of Abs was introduced in the 1980s, first via chimerization and then via CDR grafting (reviewed by Almagro and Fransson 2008). Subsequently, phage display libraries and transgenic animals that could generate human Abs allowed the possibility of fully human therapeutic mAbs (McCafferty et al. 1990; Lonberg et al. 1994; Almagro et al. 2018). Overall, Abs and related products provide the ability to target molecules with high specificity, and depending on their structure, these products may also have certain effector functions as well as bind the neonatal Fc receptor (FcRn, discussed below) and have a long half-life.

20.1.2 Structural and Functional Considerations

For the purposes of this chapter, Abs and related products include those molecules that contain complementarity-determining regions (CDRs). The CDRs are the portion of the molecule that binds the epitope on the target antigen and gives Abs their high degree of specificity (Chiu et al. 2016, 2019). Most of the therapeutic Abs and related products that have been developed, or are currently being developed, are mAbs or based on mAb structures, such that each therapeutic molecule in the product targets the same epitope (or epitopes in the case of multispecific molecules). Ab cocktails contain more than one mAb, and each may target a different epitope; an example is REGN-COV2, a cocktail containing casirivimab and imdevimab, which target non-overlapping epitopes of the severe acute respiratory syndrome coronavirus 2 spike protein for the treatment of COVID-19 (Baum et al. 2020; Weinreich et al. 2020). Polyclonal Abs are a mixture of Abs which target different epitopes.

While different antibody classes (also known as isotypes, including IgA, IgD, IgE, IgG, and IgM) have different basic and functional biology (Schroeder and Cavacini 2010; Beers et al. 2016), the vast majority of Abs and related products developed by the pharmaceutical industry are monoclonal and based on IgG. Within this class are a variety of subclasses (IgG1, IgG2, IgG3, and IgG4 in humans) with somewhat different functional activities (Jefferis 2007; Vidarsson 2014; Almagro et al. 2018). Most mAbs currently approved for use in humans are based on IgG1. Subclasses are not necessarily the same between species (Strohl and Strohl 2012).

A basic understanding of Ab structure and function is necessary in order to understand the rationale behind drug development strategies for these types of molecules, in particular as it relates to systemic exposure, and potential exaggerated pharmacology or toxicity. A standard wild-type mammalian IgG (Figure 20.1) is a glycoprotein composed of two identical light and two identical heavy chains; disulfide bonds join the heavy chains to each other, and additional disulfide bonds join each light chain to a heavy chain. The heavy and light chains form fragment antigen-binding (Fab) regions in each Ab, and the remaining portions of the heavy chains form the fragment crystallizable (Fc) region; the Fab and Fc regions are linked by a flexible "hinge" region (Stanfield and Wilson 2014). In the classic stick diagram of an Ab structure, the molecule is considered to be a Y shaped, with two Fab regions represented by the two arms at the top of the Y, and the Fc region as the single arm at the bottom (Chiu et al. 2019). An IgG is composed of one of these structures, IgA is composed of two, and IgM is composed of five. The area of the Fab region containing the CDRs is called the fragment variable (Fv) region. There are three CDRs on the heavy chain, and three on the light chain in the Fv region that are located in spatial proximity to one another and together form the potential antigen-binding area of about 50–70 amino acids that can bind to an epitope on an antigen (Frank 2002; van Regenmortel 2014; Chiu et al. 2019). It is estimated that only about 15–20 of the amino acids in the potential antigen-binding area actually physically contact the epitope and form the paratope on the Ab that binds the epitope (van Regenmortel 2014). Thus, an antibody has a large number

of potential overlapping 15–20 amino acid paratopes, with each able to bind different epitopes (Frank 2002). The Fv regions in any given wild-type Ab are the same, are mono-specific, and bind the same target epitope. The binding to the target epitope by the CDRs can be considered a direct effect of the test article (Meyer et al. 2014). The Fc region confers a variety of effector functions linking the adaptive and innate arms of the immune system, and functions related to the Fc region can be considered indirect effects of the test article (Meyer et al. 2014). Fc binding to activating and inhibitory Fcγ receptors located on neutrophils, eosinophils, basophils, monocytes, macrophages, dendritic cells, NK cells, B cells, T cells, and platelets can lead to effector activities including antibody-dependent cellular cytotoxicity (ADCC), antibody-dependent cellular phagocytosis (ADCP), and cytokine release (Wang et al. 2018; Bournazos et al. 2020). Fc interactions with complement can lead to effector activities of complement activation and complement-dependent cytotoxicity (CDC) (Meyer et al. 2014; Wang et al. 2018). Ab interactions with Fcγ receptors and C1q are dependent on the hinge and proximal CH2 amino acid sequence as well as glycosylation (Wang et al. 2018). Genetic polymorphisms in Fcγ receptors can impact effector function and are thought to lead to variability in responses between individuals (Nagelkerke et al. 2019). The binding of the hinge region to the FcRn protects Abs from degradation by recycling them following cellular

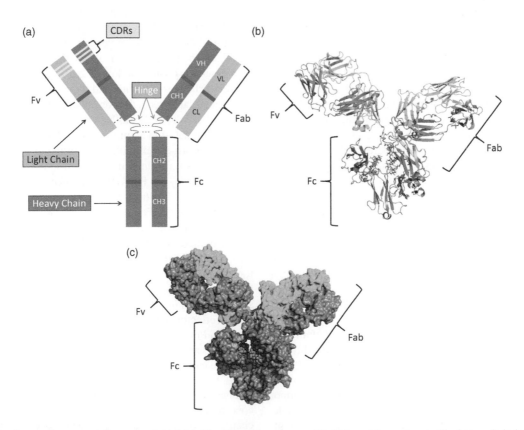

FIGURE 20.1 Structural representations of an IgG. Stick (a), ribbon (b), and space-filled (c) models are shown. The heavy chain is blue, the light chain is green, and glycosylation (shown in b and c) is orange. Disulfide bonds are shown in the stick representation (a) by dashed lines. CDRs = complementarity-determining regions, shown in yellow; CH1, 2, and 3 = constant heavy chain domains 1, 2, and 3; CL = constant light chain domain; Fab = fragment antigen-binding region; Fc = fragment crystallizable; Fv = fragment variable; VH = variable heavy chain domain; VL = variable light chain domain; PDB accession number of the mouse IgG1 shown in b and c is 1IGY.

uptake and allows Abs to often have a long half-life of weeks (Roopenian and Akilesh 2007). Although not identical, antibody Fc functions are generally similar enough between humans and animal species typically used in efficacy and toxicity studies, and thus, these molecules can often be effectively tested in animals if the target is present and can be bound by the Ab.

While the basic wild-type antibody structure is described above, current molecular engineering methods allow the design of a wide variety of structures containing a CDR, from molecules that contain all the elements of normal Abs, to those containing only parts of Abs or components of multiple Abs, and finally to those conjugated to non-Ab biologic elements such as cytokines (Krishnamurthy and Jimeno 2018; Bates and Power 2019; Zhao 2020). Conjugates may also include small molecules such as toxins used in Ab-drug conjugates to increase cytotoxicity (Teicher and Chari 2011; Thomas et al. 2016), or poly(ethylene glycol) used to increase half-life or reduce immunogenicity (Chapman 2002). More information on Ab-drug conjugates is presented in Chapter 22. Another modification is to mask the binding sites on Abs and related products with structures that can be removed by proteases that are highly expressed at disease sites, allowing the therapeutic to be active only at those sites and thereby reducing on-target toxicity in normal tissues (Chen et al. 2017).

The structural elements of the CDR-containing portion(s) of the Ab or related molecule dictate the number of targets/epitopes that can be bound and whether those epitopes are the same or different. As noted above, the antigen-binding region of a normal wild-type Ig is monospecific regardless of isotype, with the Fab regions targeting the same epitope. An IgG has two Fab regions with the antigen-binding Fv regions at the end of each arm, and thus, the wild-type molecule can bind up to two of the same epitopes (it is bivalent and monospecific). In contrast, a wild-type IgM has 10 Fab regions and could bind up to 10 of the same epitopes (it is decavalent and monospecific). However, molecules can be created where the Fab regions do not target the same epitope, and more than one antigen-binding region can be present on each arm. The number of different targets gives these multispecific molecules their name – bispecifics have two different targets, trispecifics have three different targets, etc. (note – some scientists also consider the Fc as another specificity when using this terminology, such that an IgG with Fv regions targeting different epitopes would be called a trispecific, but using the terminology in this manner is not common). Multispecific molecules are usually intended to bring different cell types together, or to block or agonize more than one target to improve efficacy with the simplicity of one therapeutic molecule. For example, one arm of an anti-CD3 bispecific may target an antigen on a tumor cell, while the other arm binds CD3 on T cells (i.e., it is a bispecific and bivalent molecule), thereby bringing the T cell and the tumor cell together, initiating events that lead to the death of the tumor cell (Krishnamurthy and Jimeno 2018). As another example, a trispecific that can bind CD3, CD28, and CD38 (i.e., a trispecific and trivalent molecule) has been created as a therapeutic targeting CD38+ cancer cells, with the goal of bringing CD3+ T cells next to the cancer cells and activating them, as well as supporting T cell survival by also binding CD28 (Wu et al.

2020). Beyond cancer, multispecific multivalent molecules are being used to target multiple cytokines or other components of the immune system in various inflammatory diseases to improve efficacy (Zhao 2020), or to target multiple epitopes on viruses or bacteria to prevent, reduce, or overcome resistance (Palomo et al. 2016). Alternative structures also exist that do not involve only CDRs and antigen binding. For example, one arm might contain a CDR, and another might contain a cytokine or a receptor, thus allowing targeting of the cytokine or receptor to locations/cells with the target epitope. The potential combinations and diverse biology are truly immense.

The other main region of full length Abs is the Fc region, which, as noted above, confers the effector functions and impacts the half-life of the molecule. If a wild-type Fc is present, it permits binding to accessory cells and allows effector functions to occur and additionally permits a long half-life. However, similar to being able to alter the antigen-binding regions of Abs, the Fc can be engineered or even removed to alter Fc-related effector functions and half-life. The most common alterations include (1) removing the Fc to reduce molecular size, shorten the half-life, and remove Fc effector functions; (2) reducing Fc effector functions; (3) enhancing Fc effector functions for potent target cell destruction; and (4) enhancing FcRn binding to increase half-life (Dahlén et al. 2018). For example, the bispecific blinatumomab (Blincyto®) lacks an Fc, has a very short half-life, and relies on bringing CD3+ T cells next to CD19+ tumor cells to form a cytolytic synapse as the mechanism of tumor cell killing in the absence of Fc effector function (Dahlén et al. 2018; Krishnamurthy and Jimeno 2018). The Fab fragment molecules abciximab (ReoPro®) and ranibizumab (Lucentis®) also lack the Fc region and associated functions (Bates and Power 2019). For molecules with an Fc, small changes in amino acid sequence or glycosylation can have remarkable reduction or enhancement of effector functions (Jefferis 2007; Schlothauer et al. 2016; Vafa et al. 2014, reviewed in detail in Saunders 2019). For example, if the goal is to kill a target cell, enhanced immune effector functions might be desired. Three mutations (the AAA mutations) can increase affinity for FcγRIIIa, enhance ADCC, and increase cell killing by 50–100×. Similarly, afucosylation of glycans at site N297 in the Fc can increase ADCC by 50× compared with the wild-type fucosylated form. Modifying three amino acids can increase affinity to C1q by 47× and increase CDC by 6.9× (Moore et al. 2010). Alternatively, if reduced or no effector function is desired, for example, trying to block a receptor without inciting immune reactions or cell killing, similarly small changes in amino acids or glycosylation can be made to impact effector function without removing the Fc region.

Beyond modifying effector functions, the other main area of Fc engineering relates to altering binding to FcRn to increase or decrease half-life and exposure (Mackness et al. 2019; Saunders 2019). In most cases, the goal is to prolong the half-life, which can have the benefits of reduced dosing frequency, higher drug concentrations for a given dose, and improved efficacy. Small changes in the Fc amino acid sequence can increase the affinity/binding and/or slow the off-rate of the Ab for FcRn at low pH, allowing it to be recycled by cells following uptake and not catabolized. The YTE and LS mutations in the Fc are clinically validated for extending half-life, and other potentially superior modifications have been proposed (Mackness et al. 2019). Some of the modifications for enhancing half-life can decrease ADCC (Saunders 2019). It should be noted that human IgG binds very well to mouse FcRn and can have long half-lives in mice, although mouse and rat IgGs do not bind human FcRn very well and thus IgGs from these species tend to have short half-lives in humans (Ober et al. 2001), without considering the impact of ADA.

In addition to the engineering noted above, Abs and related products may undergo various amounts of humanization, in which nonhuman amino acid sequences are replaced with human sequences (Almagro et al. 2018; Chiu et al. 2019). The goal of humanization is to reduce the risk of immunogenicity in humans. Fully human Abs and related products can also be produced, although these molecules can still be immunogenic in humans (van Schouwenburg et al. 2013) and, of course, in animals. In an effort to reduce immunogenicity, potential immunogenic areas of molecules may be replaced with sequences considered to be less immunogenic. All of these manipulations are focused on minimizing immunogenicity in humans, not animals. In fact, it is possible these alterations could make the molecule more immunogenic in animals.

Lastly, while the above discussion has focused on Igs from "standard" species such as humans, monkeys, and rodents, attributes of Abs or Ab-like molecules from other species (e.g., camelids or sharks that have distinct single domain Abs) can also serve as the base structure of Ab-based biotherapeutics (Harmsen and De Haard 2007; Bates and Power 2019; Pothin et al. 2020). Developers of Abs and related products should consider what structures and modifications ought to be employed to optimize the intended therapy. Ultimately, it is critical for scientists to understand the structure of the molecule, the target epitopes and antigen, and know what biological functions are present, enhanced, or reduced to understand what effects are likely in animals and humans following test article administration. This allows the creation of appropriate nonclinical development strategies using a case-by-case approach based on product attributes.

20.1.3 Naming Conventions

Conventions for nonproprietary names of Ab products have changed over the years (World Health Organization [WHO] 2009; Parren et al. 2017; WHO April 2017; WHO May 2017). The "-mab" stem is used to indicate molecules that contain at least one Ig variable domain (i.e., those that include the CDRs) and are monoclonal; "-pab" is used for polyclonal products. A substem preceding the stem was added in 1997 (WHO 1997) to describe the molecule source, with the belief that this would help convey information about immunogenicity. The most widely used of these species source substems were chimeric (-xi-), chimeric/humanized (-xizu-), humanized (-zu-), and fully human (-u-). A substem for the target was also included before the source substem, and a random prefix before that (WHO 1997). However, in 2017, it was decided that the source did not really provide useful information regarding immunogenicity, most Abs and related products were by that time humanized or human, and removing the source stem would allow for easier naming; thus, it was recommended to no longer include the source substem (Parren et al. 2017; WHO April

2017; WHO May 2017). In addition to the base name, a second word may be added to the end for conjugated molecules (e.g., gemtuzumab ozogamicin), or the beginning for radiolabels (e.g., iodine (^{131}I) tositumomab) (WHO 1997). Lastly, the US FDA adds a distinguishing suffix composed of four lowercase letters (e.g., adalimumab-afzb) (US FDA 2017). This was initially related to the company name, but in 2017, it became devoid of meaning. An originator and biosimilar molecule will have the same nonproprietary name, but different suffixes. The suffix allows easier tracking of adverse events or postmarketing safety signals. It is worthwhile to understand the changing naming conventions and understand that Abs developed during different periods will not necessarily have the same rules applied.

20.1.4 General Testing Strategies

The testing strategy for Abs and related products should use a case-by-case approach that considers all applicable regulatory guidelines, the specific characteristics and pharmacology of the test article, and the intended clinical program. The species used and studies conducted should be carefully considered. The pros and cons of selected testing strategies are shown in Table 20.1. Knockout mice can be used to assess the effects of antagonizing a particular pathway, knock-in animals could be used to test agonizing a pathway, and the human target could be inserted into mice. Heterozygous animals may also be useful to look for the equivalent of dose-related effects. A given program may use one or more of these strategies and should overall attempt to maximize information and minimize animal use. For example, general toxicity studies might be conducted in cynomolgus monkeys, and reproductive assessments might be conducted in knockout mice or by using a rodent surrogate molecule to eliminate the need for using more monkeys. When genetically-modified animals are used, it may be useful to include wild-type animals for comparison, and the genotype of all animals should be verified.

20.2 Applicable Regulatory Guidelines

The International Council for Harmonisation of Technical Requirements for Pharmaceuticals for Human Use (ICH) S6(R1) is the primary guideline for understanding international health authority expectations for protein-based biotherapeutics, including Abs and related products, and is the basis for many of the recommendations in this chapter. In addition, a number of other ICH guidelines refer to Abs and related products directly or indirectly in some aspect; these ICH guidelines are shown in Table 20.2. There are some areas of overlap between guidelines, and scientists may need to consult multiple guidelines. Many of the other ICH safety guidelines mention biotherapeutics briefly, and some, such as ICH S9 and ICH S9 Q&A (covering anticancer therapeutics) as well as ICH S11 (covering pediatric support), specifically address both small and large molecules. Other ICH safety guidelines, such as ICH S5(R3) (covering developmental and reproductive toxicity), ICH S7A (covering safety pharmacology), ICH S3A (covering toxicokinetics), and ICH S1A (covering carcinogenicity), mention biotherapeutics as being within their scope, but recognize

TABLE 20.1

Pros and Cons of Selected Testing Strategies for Abs and Related Products

Strategy	Pros	Cons
Standard toxicity species (typically mouse, rat, rabbit, and/or cynomolgus monkey)	• Abundant historical data • Animal availability • Ability to use standard study designs	• Immunogenicity possible • Molecules may have only partial pharmacologic activity • Molecules may have different pharmacologic activity vs humans
Nonstandard toxicity species (e.g., hamster, guinea pig, common marmoset)	• May be only way to conduct in vivo testing for programs that lack pharmacologically-relevant standard species with the clinical candidate	• Lack of historical data • Reagents/assays may not be available • Molecules may have different pharmacologic activity vs humans
Animal models of disease	• Target present/pharmacologically relevant • May more closely mimic effects in human disease state	• Lack of historical data • Animal availability
Genetically-modified animals (e.g., knockout, knock-in, replacement with human target)	• No immunogenicity concerns • Can reduce or eliminate need for certain studies in monkeys (e.g., DART studies) • May be only way to conduct in vivo testing for programs that lack pharmacologically-relevant species with the clinical candidate	• Lack of historical data • Animal availability • Animals impacted from conception • Pathways impacted may not fully mimic human state • Does not replicate exogenous administration of a test article • Genotype may not be accurate (should be tested/confirmed) • Infectious disease concerns if animals come from laboratories with less rigorous disease control standards • Animals may be more prone to health and survival issues
Surrogate molecule pharmacologically active in standard toxicity species	• Reduced risk of immunogenicity • May be only way to conduct in vivo testing for programs that lack pharmacologically-relevant species with the clinical candidate	• Significant effort to generate and characterize surrogate • Not testing clinical candidate, which may have different effects
No in vivo testing (when no pharmacologically-relevant species exists, or for biosimilars)	• Testing in pharmacologically-irrelevant species should not be done and may generate misleading information • Testing biosimilars with adequate analytical and in vitro characterization showing similarity to originator has not proven useful or necessary	• No in vivo assessment of potential toxicity

TABLE 20.2

International Council on Harmonisation[a] Guidelines Applicable to mAbs and Ab-Related Products

ICH S1A – Guideline on the Need for Carcinogenicity Studies of Pharmaceuticals

ICH S3A – Note for Guidance of Toxicokinetics: The Assessment of Systemic Exposure in Toxicity Studies

ICH S5(R3) – Detection of Reproductive and Developmental Toxicity for Human Pharmaceuticals

ICH S6(R1) – Preclinical Safety Evaluation of Biotechnology-Derived Pharmaceuticals

ICH S7A – Safety Pharmacology for Human Pharmaceuticals

ICH S9 and Q&A – Nonclinical Evaluation of Anticancer Pharmaceuticals

ICH S11 – Nonclinical Safety Testing in Support of Development of Paediatric Pharmaceuticals

ICH M3(R2) and Q&A – Guidance on Nonclinical Safety Studies for the Conduct of Human Clinical Trials and Marketing Authorization for Pharmaceuticals

[a] Formerly International Conference on Harmonisation.

that study designs or strategies may differ and/or may need to be altered compared with small molecule paradigms.

In addition to the various ICH guidelines, there is also guidance from regions and countries that may impact development strategies for Abs and related products. The most notable is the US FDA's "Points to Consider in the Manufacture and Testing of Monoclonal Antibody Products for Human Use" (US FDA 1983/1987/1994/1997), which is now over 20 years old. The FDA also released "Guidance for Industry: Developing Medical Imaging Drug and Biological Products" (US FDA 2004), which refers to ICH S6 and the FDA Points to Consider document and

does not provide additional information regarding safety assessment of biologic imaging products. As any of the documents may be updated or superseded, it is recommended that scientists ensure that they are looking at the most recent information. The current chapter will focus on therapeutic molecules.

Beyond reading the various guidelines, early engagement of regulatory authorities is encouraged whenever there are questions regarding the nonclinical development of a given molecule. These interactions may be very useful in designing the nonclinical studies and may prevent sponsors from conducting studies that are not needed.

20.3 Target Characterization/Species Selection

Because the toxicity of Abs and related products is most often an extension of pharmacology, a full understanding of the target and pathway biology is critical in order to conduct toxicity studies in relevant, but not in irrelevant, species (Bussiere 2008; ICH S6(R1) 2011; Leach 2013). ICH S6(R1) defines a relevant species as "[a species] in which the test material is pharmacologically active due to the expression of the receptor or an epitope (in the case of monoclonal antibodies)". Furthermore, ICH S6(R1) indicates that short-term (up to 1-month duration) general toxicity studies should be conducted in one rodent and one nonrodent species (if they are relevant), while chronic general toxicity studies can be conducted in one species if findings from the shorter-term studies are similar or the findings are understood from the mechanism of action standpoint. ICH S6(R1) also states that "Toxicity studies in non-relevant species may be misleading and are discouraged".

Hence, the demonstration of pharmacological relevance (or non-relevance) in the species typically utilized in toxicity studies is a regulatory expectation for any biotherapeutic, including Abs and related products. Species typically used in general toxicity studies with Abs and related products include the mouse, rat, and cynomolgus monkey. The rabbit may be used in developmental and reproductive toxicity studies if pharmacologically relevant and can save substantial time and cost compared with reproductive toxicity studies in monkeys. Other species are sometimes used if pharmacologically relevant, and if there are reasons why more commonly used species are not appropriate. These could include the hamster, dog, common marmoset, and minipig. While chimpanzees were used occasionally in the past, their use is no longer considered acceptable, even if they are the only relevant species identified. There may be times when animal models of disease, including those genetically modified to express the target, may be the most appropriate species to use. In addition, there may be times when modeling might translate better to humans compared with studies using normal animals. The decision on which species/model/procedure to use should be based on pharmacologic and translational relevance balanced with practicality and likely ability to conduct the planned study.

In order to identify appropriate species for in vivo toxicity studies, a variety of analyses, assays, and studies may be conducted, as shown in Table 20.3. While it should be possible to compare at least sequence homology and hopefully target binding in most programs, it may not be possible to conduct all these assays for all programs. There may be no good pharmacology models in vitro or in vivo, or biomarkers may not be available. In some cases, the target might not be present, such as with test articles directed against unique epitopes in a disease state that are not present in normal animals (i.e., exogenous targets including those on infectious agents, or unique tumor antigens). In the final analysis, reasonable efforts should be made to create a strong data set which can be used to select the best species in a data-driven manner. Work demonstrating species relevance should be done in time to support the nonclinical development program; nonclinical toxicity studies should not be initiated without knowing that the species being used are relevant.

The importance of understanding target biology was highlighted with TGN1412, where six human volunteers had severe adverse events related to cytokine release following administration of the anti-CD28 superagonist antibody for the first time with a dose that was believed to be safe based on a nonclinical package that met regulatory requirements (Expert Group on Phase One Clinical Trials 2006; Suntharalingam et al. 2006). Cynomolgus monkeys had been considered to be pharmacologically-relevant toxicology species based on having the identical amino acid sequence homology of the target epitope on the CD28 extracellular domain compared with humans, and in addition having the expected in vivo pharmacology of substantial CD4+ and CD8+ T-cell expansion and activation in vivo (Expert Group on Phase One Clinical Trials 2006). In retrospective analyses investigating the reasons for the failure of nonclinical testing to predict the cytokine storm in the TGN1412 human trial, it was noted that activation of CD4+ effector memory T cells by TGN1412 was likely responsible for the cytokine storm in humans, but the cynomolgus monkeys used in the FIH-enabling good laboratory practice (GLP) toxicity study lacked CD28 expression on CD4+ effector memory T cells (Eastwood et al. 2010; Hünig 2012). Retrospective calculations showed that the FIH dose of 0.1 mg/kg TGN1412 resulted in approximately 45%–91% receptor occupancy in humans (Expert Group on Phase One Clinical Trials 2006; Waibler et al. 2008). This subtle but fundamental difference in biology, which was not understood at the time of the FIH trial, led to serious adverse consequences in the

TABLE 20.3

Analyses, Assays, and Studies Conducted to Determine Relevance of Animal Species for In Vivo Toxicity Testing

Analysis, Assay, or Study	Comments
Sequence homology (comparing animals with humans)	Can be misleading, as targets with relatively lower sequence homology (e.g., 80%) can have test article binding, while others with higher homology (e.g., 99%) may not.
In vitro binding of test article to target	Demonstrates test article binding to the target in the tested species but does not provide evidence of a functional effect. Usually able to compare animal and human data.
Off-target profiling	Tissue cross-reactivity studies or microarray technologies that may identify binding to unwanted targets. Ideally, the nonclinical species selected for toxicity testing have similar off-target binding so that the potential for any effects related to this binding can be assessed. Can be followed up with other in vitro or in vivo studies that determine any functional effects of off-target binding.
In vitro or ex vivo functional assay	Provides evidence of possible pharmacologic activity in vivo in the tested species. Often able to compare animal and human data to more firmly support species relevance.
In vivo pharmacology	Provides the strongest evidence of pharmacologic relevance in the tested species.

volunteers and highlights the importance of understanding target biology. TGN1412 (renamed TAB08) was subsequently safely administered to human volunteers with close clinical monitoring, starting with 0.0001 mg/kg (or 0.1% of dose used in the original trial), followed by several intermediate doses and reaching a maximal dose of 0.007 mg/kg (Tabares et al. 2014). Proinflammatory cytokine concentrations remained at baseline levels, and no evidence of cytokine release syndrome was seen over the full dose range and observation times.

The data on species relevance rarely exactly match across species. Animal assays often have lower binding or activity compared with human tissues or cells; thus, data are not always conclusive regarding whether an animal species is relevant. There are no rules for what % of binding or activity relative to humans is "enough" to consider a species relevant. However, it is useful to note that lower (or higher) binding affinity may not proportionally impact functional activity due to downstream signaling events. For example, 20% binding affinity relative to humans could still result in an equivalent pharmacologic effect in some cases. It is also possible to use higher doses and exposures in animals to overcome lower binding or pharmacologic effects at a given exposure. If a pharmacologic effect cannot be achieved despite higher exposures, it is suggestive that the species might not be useful for in vivo toxicity testing. Alternatively, even when data are suggestive that an animal species is relevant, pharmacologic effects (and toxicity) in normal animals might be reduced or absent relative to humans [e.g., with anti-CTLA-4 and anti-PD-1 mAbs (Keler et al. 2003; Wang et al. 2014)]. It is also possible that studies in disease models might be more informative in some cases, although evaluating toxicity in animals that have underlying disease and assessing the relevance of findings to humans can be challenging. Overall, a full understanding of the biologic pathways involved in the normal and disease states is important when determining species relevance.

For molecules directed at foreign/exogenous targets that have no counterpart in normal animals, such as bacterial or viral targets where it is anticipated that no relevant species will exist, ICH S6(R1) states "…a short-term safety study in one species (choice of species to be justified by the sponsor) can be considered". The value of these studies is questionable. Current manufacturing and assay techniques should be effective in limiting any unknown toxic contaminants. However, because there is a possibility of unexpected cross reactivity to an off-target epitope, and based on historical precedent, these studies are often conducted. Early interactions with regulatory agencies are encouraged to determine whether such studies are needed, and what study design is appropriate in the event a study is required. Under most circumstances, if an in vivo study is conducted in a non-pharmacologically-relevant species, a rodent should be used. If possible, the species selected should have similar off-target profiling results, such as similar staining in tissue cross-reactivity (TCR) studies or binding to the same proteins in microarray profiling assays. It is recommended that studies be 1 to 2 weeks in duration, with dosing ending no later than Day 8 (i.e., two weekly doses) as confounding immunogenicity could develop with longer dosing, although there have been instances where regulatory agencies have requested longer studies (emphasizing the importance of early regulatory interactions). ICH S6(R1) also states that,

when feasible, adding safety endpoints to studies with animal models of disease could be part of the safety assessment strategy for foreign targets, and this may be sufficient to meet regulatory requirements; obtaining regulatory acceptance for such a strategy is important to be sure additional studies are not required that might delay development.

There are additional concerns for anti-infective therapeutic Abs. It is possible that infectious agents could develop resistance by mutating the targeted epitope (or epitopes for multispecifics or cocktails of multiple Abs), thus reducing or eliminating efficacy (DeFrancesco 2020). Antibody-dependent enhancement (ADE) is a term describing the phenomenon by which antiviral Abs promote viral infection of host cells by exploiting the phagocytic Fcγ receptor pathway (Bournazos et al. 2020; DeFrancesco 2020). It has been known for decades and was originally described with dengue virus, which is a flavivirus (Halstead and O'Rourke 1977), but it has occurred with other viruses (including coronaviruses), and there are concerns that this phenomenon could occur with the SARS-CoV-2 coronavirus, which is the cause of COVID-19 (Bournazos et al. 2020; DeFrancesco 2020). In vitro evidence of SARS-CoV-2 causing ADE has been reported (reviewed by Bournazos et al. 2020). It is thought that Fc-engineered mAbs could guide the development of anti-SARS-CoV-2 mAbs to result in superior therapeutic efficacy through selective activation of specific Fcγ receptor pathways on distinct leukocyte types (Bournazos et al. 2020).

20.4 General Toxicity Study Design Considerations

20.4.1 Overview

General testing strategies are discussed above in Section 20.1.4. General toxicity studies may be conducted in standard species (usually mice or rats, and/or cynomolgus monkeys), in animal models of disease, in genetically-modified animals, and/or with surrogate molecules. Selected attributes of general toxicity studies are shown in Table 20.4.

20.4.2 Exploratory (Non-GLP) Studies

Exploratory toxicity studies with Abs and related products (i.e., before GLP studies) should not be conducted as a default strategy. A determination should be made as to whether exploratory studies are necessary based on known biology and existing data. If the biology is well understood, for example if the target has been previously agonized or antagonized and it is unlikely that toxicity will be observed at less than a 10x multiple over the highest clinical exposure based on existing data, then no in vivo study may be necessary and the in vivo nonclinical program may be able to start with GLP studies. In many cases, pharmacokinetics (PK) of standard mAbs can be reasonably estimated based on clearance vs body weight with some exponential scaling, or on modeling from monkey PK data (usually cynomolgus) (Deng et al. 2011; Dong et al. 2011; Oitate et al. 2011). The Tg32 homozygous human FcRn transgenic mouse has also proven very useful for estimating human PK for mAbs (Avery et al. 2016; Fan et al. 2016; Betts et al. 2018); it can be considered

TABLE 20.4

Selected Attributes of General Toxicity Studies

Attribute	Exploratory, Non-GLP Studies	FIH-Enabling Studies, GLP	Post-FIH-Enabling Studies, GLP
Study need	• May not be necessary	• Required	• Usually required unless duration of FIH-enabling study was sufficient
Number of species	• If necessary, only pharmacologically-relevant species	• One rodent and one nonrodent species, if pharmacologically-relevant	• Use only one species if toxicity similar, rodent preferred, even if rodent and nonrodent species are pharmacologically-relevant
Duration	• Variable	• Usually 2 weeks to 3 months	• 6 months (3 months if falling under ICH S9)
Groups	• Variable	• Control + 3 test article-dosed groups	• Control + 2 or 3 test article-dosed groups
Sexes	• Often one	• Two (unless only one will be dosed in humans)	• Two (unless only one will be dosed in humans)
Recovery	• Not as a dedicated group	• Maybe, if included use only control + one test article-dosed group	• Maybe, if included use only control + one test article-dosed group
Number/sex/group	• Up to 5 for rodent • 1–2 nonrodent	• Rodent: 10 for main study, 5 for recovery (if included) • Nonrodent: 3 for main study, 2 for recovery (if included)	• Rodent: 10–15 for main study, 5 for recovery (if included) • Nonrodent: 3 or 4 for main study, 2 for recovery (if included)
Safety pharmacology	• Only if specific cause for concern	• Include as part of general toxicity study if possible	• Only if specific cause for concern remains
Fertility assessments in nonrodent (for programs without activity in rodent)	• No	• If at least 3 months duration, need mature animals; only conduct in FIH-enabling or in chronic study, but not both	• If at least 3 months duration, need mature animals; only conduct in FIH-enabling or in chronic study, but not both

superior to using monkeys on the basis of ethical issues, lower costs, ease of handling, and lower drug material requirements (Avery et al. 2016). In addition, strategies that avoid in vivo monkey studies using small animal numbers that may skew the data may give results that are equal or more predictive of what will occur in humans (Avery et al. 2016; Betts et al. 2018).

If an exploratory study(ies) is deemed necessary, it should be conducted only after the relevant species have been identified. It may be possible to combine exploratory toxicity studies with PK and/or efficacy studies as long as the data generated are sufficient and interpretable for the project needs. In such a scenario, it is suggested that the low dose targets an exposure similar to the anticipated efficacious or maximum anticipated exposure in humans (factoring in differences in affinity and pharmacologic effect) and the high dose provides at least a 10× multiple to aid in the selection of doses for the FIH-enabling study. Regardless of the dosing regimen during the study, it is suggested that a dose be administered at the end of the study, with the necropsy 24–48 hours later; this provides some assessment of effects at a high systemic concentration. It is also possible that repeat doses might be impacted by ADA, if ADA is induced; however, there are many cases where ADA induction is not an issue with this design. Clinical observations and clinical pathology assessments should be done; a necropsy with tissue collection may be done if the data are thought to be necessary, or if animals cannot be reused. Tissues might not be evaluated microscopically unless there is a cause for concern based on the target, or findings during the study. The study duration may be driven by the need to collect a full PK exposure profile. For example, a combined PK/tolerability study in cynomolgus monkeys might dose once on

Day 1 and perhaps again on Day 42 and include only a low- and a high-dose group in one sex, with two animals/group. PK and clinical pathology samples could be collected during the study, and a necropsy on Day 43 may or may not be done at the end of the study. This strategy works best when little or no toxicity is expected. For molecules where toxicity is expected, or sex-related differences are possible, a more standard toxicity study design similar to a GLP study may be necessary (described below), although usually with fewer animals.

There are some additional choices to be made for exploratory studies. Preliminary versions of candidate molecules, such as chimeric mAbs, mAbs that have not been humanized or affinity purified, or mAbs with alternative Fc regions that differ from the final version (i.e., tool molecules), may be used in these studies. However, it is possible that these results may be misleading and not representative of the final candidate molecule. The use of animals in exploratory studies that have been exposed to other test articles may be considered if no residual effects remain that would impact the study, although if previously exposed to a biologic, it is recommended that animals be proven to be negative for ADA prior to dosing or not used for this purpose. Specialized testing may be included if there are areas of specific concern (i.e., immunotoxicity, safety pharmacology). Collection of samples for ADA testing during the study may not be needed, as testing can often be done on residual clinical pathology samples and run only if there is a specific reason for concern (see Section 20.6.3 for more details). Teams need to decide the most appropriate strategy that will provide the necessary information to advance the program most efficiently.

20.4.3 FIH-Enabling Studies

Historically, the test article used in FIH-enabling studies was from the same clone that would be used for the clinical material. This ensured that the material evaluated in the toxicity study(ies) was representative of the clinical material. However, with advances in antibody production, it is now common in the FIH-enabling toxicity studies to use test article from a pool of clones, which allows faster speed to the clinic (Bolisetty et al. 2020). For this strategy to work, it must be shown that the material used in the toxicity studies is representative of the clinical material.

FIH-enabling studies should be conducted in one rodent and one nonrodent species (if they are pharmacologically relevant). Information from exploratory studies (if conducted) can be used to inform the design of the FIH-enabling studies. Induction of ADA alone is not a scientifically valid reason to eliminate considering that species in the toxicology program, as the impacts of ADA can be quite variable, range from nothing to severe, and may not occur at higher doses. If the ADA response is not manageable [e.g., most or all animals lose exposure in all dose groups and/or the ADA results in deleterious effects in most animals (e.g., anaphylaxis)], then discontinuing testing in the species can be considered.

The clinical study plan and strategy should be considered when determining the design of the FIH-enabling toxicity studies. The duration of FIH-enabling toxicity studies should be at least as long as the clinical trial(s) the study is trying to support, but be at least 2 weeks long. If longer toxicity studies will allow additional clinical trials, it may make sense to conduct the longer FIH-enabling toxicity studies to allow uninterrupted clinical development without the need for additional nonclinical studies. For example, some Phase 2 clinical trials are 2 or 3 months in duration, and it may make sense for the initial GLP toxicity studies to cover this duration. This works best when significant toxicity is not expected, and appropriate doses can be selected. If 3-month toxicity studies are done, the monkey study could also include mature animals to meet the requirement for fertility assessments in cases where such evaluations are necessary (see Chapter 12, and Section 20.8). A potential disadvantage of longer-term FIH-enabling toxicity studies can be a potential delay in the FIH study if the toxicity study is rate limiting for filing. Companies should decide what overall strategy makes the most sense for their clinical development program.

Similar to exploratory studies, it is recommended that animals receive a dose of drug one day before the terminal necropsy (e.g., for a 1-month study with once weekly dosing the animals would be administered drug on Days 1, 8, 15, 22, and 29, and necropsy would occur on Day 30). This allows the necropsy to occur at a time when drug exposure will be high. Studies should include the appropriate safety pharmacology endpoints (see Section 20.7 for more details). Specialized assays, such as immunotoxicity assessments, may be added if relevant for the specific test article. It is recommended that ADA samples be collected. Decisions on when and whether to conduct ADA assays are covered in Section 20.6.3, as these assays may or may not need to be conducted.

20.4.4 Post-FIH-Enabling Studies

Under most circumstances, for biotherapeutics that fall outside of ICH S9 for advanced cancer indications, including Abs and related products, 6 months is the longest duration toxicity study that needs to be conducted unless there are specific scientific reasons dictating longer studies [Clarke et al. 2008; ICH S6(R1) 2011]. With proper planning, a 6-month study is the only post-FIH-enabling general toxicity study that should be needed in most cases. Conducting a 1-month, then a 3-month, and finally a 6-month general toxicity study is rarely necessary and usually represents an inappropriate use of resources and animals. Efforts are currently underway to determine whether there are circumstances in which studies 3 months in duration would be the longest needed for non-oncology indications; the outcome of this work may influence the duration of chronic studies in the future. In contrast to the FIH-enabling studies that may have used test article from a pool of clones, the final clone has usually been selected and the material from this clone should usually be used for post-FIH-enabling general toxicity studies.

ICH S6(R1) indicates that if the toxicology profile is similar between rodent and nonrodent species, or if the findings are understood from the mechanism of action of the product, then longer-term general toxicity studies in only one species are usually sufficient. In cases where little or no toxicity was observed in the FIH-enabling study(ies) and there is no expectation that longer dosing will change this, the chronic study can often have only two test article-dosed groups (i.e., only a low- and high-dose groups, without an intermediate-dose group). See Section 20.6.3 for more details on running ADA samples.

20.4.5 Dose Selection

Dose selection should consider all available information on exposure-response relationships, for both pharmacology and toxicity, the latter of which is usually related to exaggerated pharmacology [ICH S6(R1) 2011; Leach 2013]. The PK and efficacious doses of candidate molecules in relevant animal species, the predicted PK in humans, and the predicted efficacious dose in humans should be well understood to allow appropriate dose selection in nonclinical studies. ICH S6(R1) notes that species differences in affinity and potency should also be considered, which may result in adjustments to dose. For example, if a test article has a lower affinity or potency in animals compared with humans, higher doses might be used in animals so that the pharmacologic effect would be adjusted. As discussed in Section 20.3, it is important to consider all available cross-species data, and give more weight to in vivo comparisons, as differences in potency in vitro assays may or may not translate to in vivo differences. It is also important to determine whether higher doses can in fact reach the same pharmacologic effect in animals compared with humans, because higher doses in animals sometimes cannot overcome lower affinity/potency.

Dose selection should usually be based on exposure (area under the curve [AUC], average observed concentration [Cav], and/or cumulative area under the concentration-time curve)-response relationships rather than dose (mg/kg) because the exposure and/or response at a specific dose in one species may not directly translate to a similar exposure/response at the same dose in another animal species or in humans. Because Abs and related products are often dosed weekly, twice a week, or once every other week in animals, while in humans dosing may be less frequent, it is recommended that a composite exposure, such as Cav or cumulative AUC, be used when making exposure comparisons in cases where dosing intervals are not the same (Black et al. 1999).

Doses should be selected so that excessive toxicity will not occur, whenever such information is available. Excessive toxicity can make it challenging to understand whether findings are directly related to the test article or represent effects secondary to debilitation. If toxicity does not drive dose selection, regulatory guidance regarding high dose selection is outlined in ICH S6(R1). The dose that provides the maximum intended pharmacological effect in the nonclinical species and the dose that provides an approximately 10× exposure multiple over the maximum human exposure should be determined. The higher of these two doses should be chosen as the high dose in nonclinical toxicity studies (including general toxicity studies) unless there is a justification for using a lower dose (e.g., maximum feasible dose). From a practical standpoint, it is sometimes difficult to determine the maximum intended pharmacological effect in animals, as PD models may not be available, especially in monkeys. When in vivo efficacy/PD information is not available, the high dose selection can be based on PK data/modeling and in vitro binding and/or pharmacology data. As mentioned earlier, dose adjustments may be needed for differences in affinity/potency, etc.

Because of the potential for partial clinical holds where clinical dosing may be capped at 10× the exposures achieved in animals (M Leach, personal observation), it is suggested that when the highest dose is based on 10× exposure (i.e., when significant/adverse toxicity is not expected), teams consider their confidence in exposure predictions, consider the chance that higher clinical doses/exposures may eventually be desired, and then select doses that ensure the 10× multiple is achieved. From a practical standpoint, this means dosing at >10× multiples, so that if measured exposures result in multiples that are less than predicted, they are still likely to meet the 10× margin. This may lead to doses that target 15–20× of the highest intended clinical exposure when there is more uncertainty about the modeling, predictions, and/or clinical plan. From the standpoint of humane animal care and use, it should be emphasized that doses/exposures should not exceed any known maximum tolerated dose/exposure in that species tested unless there is a clear justification for such a strategy. Finally, if the high dose is based on a maximum feasible dose, the rationale why higher doses are not possible should be clearly articulated. Figure 20.2 shows an algorithm that can be used in high dose selection for any given study based on the most current information available from the program. There is no scientific information to support the concept that high doses of protein in the context of toxicity studies cannot be administered to animals for long periods of time. Therefore, there is currently no rationale to limit the high dose based on concerns about protein overload. One minor finding that may occur at higher mAb doses and exposures is slightly higher total protein and slightly to mildly higher globulins during standard clinical chemistry evaluations. The amount of change is generally similar to the amount of test article that is present in the serum, although an exact match should not be expected.

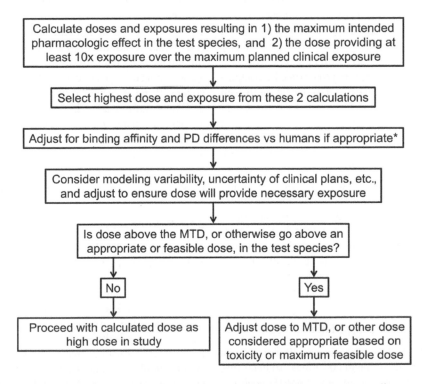

FIGURE 20.2 Selection of high dose for toxicity studies with Abs and related products. *Adjustments are usually not necessary if the highest dose and exposure are derived from the maximum pharmacologic effect in the test species, as higher doses or exposures would not be expected to have any greater PD effect. PD = pharmacodynamic, MTD = maximum tolerated dose.

In general, the low dose should be targeted to match around 1–2× of the highest planned clinical exposure, and the intermediate dose is selected to further characterize the range of toxicity between the high and low doses, usually a geometric mean (e.g., 10, 30, and 100 mg/kg). As with the high dose, adjustments may be needed for differences in affinity/potency. When using different dose routes, it may be appropriate to target the geometric mean of the exposure, not the dose in mg/kg (e.g., 25 SC, 30 IV, and 100 IV in mg/kg might provide a reasonable range or exposures, because the subcutaneous (SC) exposure is likely well below the intravenous (IV) exposure). Input from PK modeling is essential. Although common historically, the same dose or exposure should not be used to test different routes of administration unless there is a clear justification. The involvement of the clinical team is recommended to ensure accurate dose selection. It is likely that the highest planned clinical dose will change over time and that possibility should be considered in study designs; it may be appropriate to use lower doses in a chronic toxicity study compared with earlier studies, for example, if the clinical dose/exposure is lower, or raise them if the clinical dose/exposure is higher. For studies where there is no intermediate dose, as might occur with nontoxic test articles, it is recommended that the high dose be determined as described above, and the low dose be 2–4× the highest planned clinical dose. This provides some exposure multiple if adverse findings are seen in the high-dose group.

20.4.6 Dosing Interval

The dosing interval should usually be the same or more frequent in the nonclinical toxicity studies compared with the clinical trial dosing interval. Because the half-lives of molecules with an Fc that bind the FcRn are typically long (2 weeks or more in humans) due to the recycling of the molecule back into the circulation (Ovacik and Lin 2018), humans are usually dosed once weekly, or less frequently with Fc-containing molecules (although it should be recognized that some Fc containing molecules have shorter half-lives). For molecules with even longer half-lives, such as those with Fc modifications to extend half-life, dosing is even less frequent. Based on this, animals are often dosed weekly or once every other week for a typical Ab or related product with an Fc. In contrast, for molecules that lack the ability to bind the FcRn, such as those lacking an Fc, the half-life is much shorter (e.g., several hours) and more frequent dosing is required. It should be noted that less frequent dosing of animals (less than once a week) has sometimes been associated with increased immunogenicity (Leach et al. 2014), and for that reason, many study designs will dose weekly even if clinical dosing is less frequent. It is also important to recognize that the dosing interval will impact the exposure and therefore the dose that is needed in mg/kg.

20.4.7 Route of Administration, Formulation

Generally, the route of administration in nonclinical toxicity studies should be based on the planned clinical route(s) that will be tested (e.g., IV, SC, intrathecal, etc.). For FIH-enabling toxicity studies, if only one route will be tested in the clinic, then the toxicity study(ies) should use only that route. If more than one route will be tested in the FIH study (e.g., SC and IV), then the low-dose group receiving the test article should receive the drug by the route most likely to be the final commercial route of administration. The high-dose group should receive the drug by the IV route to maximize exposure. The intermediate-dose group can be SC or IV. If CV safety pharmacology endpoints are included in the intermediate-dose group, then the IV route is preferred. In a single control group, individual animals should receive the vehicle by all the routes being tested whenever possible to minimize animal use (e.g., they might receive both SC and IV doses). Post-FIH-enabling studies should also use the planned clinical route(s) that will be tested. When feasible and available, the clinical formulation should be used for nonclinical toxicity studies. However, the clinical formulation is not always available, especially for FIH-enabling studies.

The IV route in particular can be associated with infusion reactions due to various mechanisms (Mease et al. 2017). Moving from an IV bolus to an IV infusion where the dose is given over a longer period of time (e.g., 30 minutes, 1 hour, etc.) can often reduce the reactions and may allow dosing to continue (Mease et al. 2017). This does add some logistical challenges to the study, but it can usually be accomplished.

There is a belief that SC administration may result in greater induction of immunogenicity compared with the IV route, in part because the test article will be delivered to local lymph nodes, which, coupled with the migration of local antigen-presenting dendritic cells to local lymph nodes, is thought to potentially enhance an immune reaction (Fathallah et al. 2013; Hamuro et al. 2017; Turner and Balu-Iyer 2018). In reality, some studies show more immunogenicity by the SC route, others show more immunogenicity by the IV route, and still others suggest no difference (reviewed in Hamuro et al. 2017; and Davda et al. 2019). Thus, there are not clear data at the present time to generalize that SC administration is more likely to result in greater immunogenicity compared with the IV route. That said, if data are available on a given test article that suggests greater immunogenicity by a certain route, it should be considered when designing future studies in that specific species. While almost all Ab and related product therapies developed thus far have evaluated systemic routes of administration, in particular IV and SC, efforts are underway by some companies to develop other routes, such as oral. The success of these efforts remains undetermined at the present time.

20.4.8 Recovery

According to ICH S6(R1), recovery from pharmacological and toxicological effects with potential clinical impact should be understood. Historically, recovery phases were also conducted to assess delayed toxicity or potential immunogenicity; however, ICH S6(R1) clearly states these are not appropriate reasons, and the purpose of the recovery phase is to understand the reversibility of effects seen during the dosing phase. ICH S6(R1) also states that reversibility of clinically-relevant effects should be usually demonstrated in at least one study, evaluating at least one dose, and demonstration of complete reversibility is not essential. In most cases, recovery groups should only be needed in one study or one study duration (if testing in two species). In some cases, recovery groups may not be necessary on any study (e.g., no toxicity suspected, no significant concerns with the target, reversibility of the finding is well understood). A decision on whether to include recovery groups, and on which study or studies, and at what doses should be determined based on program needs and existing data on a case-by-case basis. The default should not be to include recovery groups in all dose groups or on all studies. For many biologics, recovery groups have not usually provided impactful information (Sewell et al. 2014).

Recovery phases are not usually added to exploratory studies, if these studies are conducted. However, if they are conducted, there may be a prolonged period after a dose to assess PK or a prolonged PD effect that may in essence be a recovery phase (at least in the low-dose group). There is an ongoing debate about whether it is better to include recovery phases on FIH-enabling studies, or on chronic studies, if recovery groups are considered necessary (Pandher et al. 2012; Perry et al. 2013; Sewell et al. 2014). There are pros and cons with both approaches, and ultimately, the project team should determine what is most appropriate. From a practical standpoint, one does not know if recovery animals are really needed until the study is underway. Key questions to ask when determining whether recovery is needed on a study include: (1) is the test article predicted to produce an adverse effect at clinically meaningful exposures, (2) has reversibility already been adequately demonstrated in another study, and (3) can an assessment of recovery be made based on knowledge of the finding(s) without using recovery animals (Perry et al. 2013). When included, recovery animals are usually in the control group and high-dose group, but it is also possible to instead assess recovery in the intermediate-dose group if there is concern that toxicity in the high-dose group may be too great (e.g., if toxicity has not yet been well characterized, which is more likely in FIH-enabling studies). Because ICH S6(R1) states that recovery should be understood at clinically-relevant exposures, it is not necessarily a requirement to have recovery in the high-dose group.

The length of the recovery phase should allow enough time for an assessment of reversibility to be made and should consider the half-life of the drug and the expected duration of the PD effects, with longer half-life drugs and/or those with longer-lasting PD effects requiring longer duration recovery phases. A common mistake with Abs and related products with a long half-life is to have a recovery phase that is too short. The recovery duration should be scientifically based on when the expected test article concentration has gone below the concentration at which pharmacology is expected, and then allowing time for recovery of any effects; this may be many months for potent molecules given at high doses. Assessing recovery in the intermediate- or even low-dose group (vs the high-dose group) may reduce the duration of the recovery phase needed, provided these groups have exposures that still meet or exceed clinical exposures. In cases where there is an acceptable biomarker available (e.g., B cells for a B cell-depleting drug), the length of the recovery phase could be based on the recovery of the biomarker using an adaptive type of study design where the recovery phase might end when the biomarker has reached certain values identified in the protocol. In cases where there is

no biomarker, one may consider empirically targeting approximately five half-lives. Conducting a recovery phase that is too short will not provide an assessment of reversibility, could lead to misinterpreting the likelihood of recovery, and does not represent appropriate animal use.

If no toxicity is observed after the dosing phase, it might be possible to reduce data collections or even terminate the recovery phase early (Pandher et al. 2012). However, from a practical standpoint, because dosing phase data are often not available until close to the end of the recovery phase, and it is "better safe than sorry", the recovery phase usually continues up through collection of tissue at necropsy so that all information is potentially available. After the recovery phase, it is only necessary to microscopically examine those target organs identified in the dosing phase in both rodent and nonrodent studies, unless clinical observations, clinical pathology, or necropsy data suggest otherwise. If there are no test article-related microscopic findings at the end of the dosing phase, and no test article-related clinical signs were noted during the recovery phase, then it might not be necessary to microscopically examine any tissues from the recovery phase animals.

20.5 Off-Target Profiling

20.5.1 Overview

Understanding the specificity of Abs and related products is important to appreciate the potential for off-target effects (further discussed in Chapter 11). As noted earlier, it is generally considered that most toxicity associated with biotherapeutics, including Abs and related products, is caused by exaggerated pharmacology, i.e., effects that are the result of binding to the intended target [Bussiere 2008; ICH S6(R1) 2011, Leach 2013]. However, as discussed above (Section 20.1.2), Ab binding regions associated with the CDRs have a number of potential paratopes that could bind specifically to more than one epitope (polyspecificity), or the same paratope could bind more than one epitope (Frank 2002; James and Tawfik 2003; van Regenmortel 2014; Kaur and Salunke 2015). Additionally, the same epitope could be present in more than one molecule (shared epitope). These mechanisms allow specific binding of the Ab to molecules that are not the intended target. Evaluation of binding to 384 different human proteins with the very successful anti-TNF mAb adalimumab showed low-affinity binding to a number of non-target molecules (Feyen et al. 2007), and there have been cases of unintended off-target binding which has occasionally resulted in effects in vivo (Leach et al. 2010; Bumbaca et al. 2011; Rudmann et al. 2012; Santostefano et al. 2012; N Vansell, personal communication 2016; Finlay et al. 2019). Findings can occur even when different mAbs against the same target have not caused that effect and off-target binding is of relatively low affinity (Finlay et al. 2019), can occur via the humanization process (Bumbaca et al. 2011), and can be related to differences in only a few amino acids (Wu et al. 2007; Bumbaca et al. 2011), thus demonstrating that the binding characteristics of each candidate Ab or related product need to be understood. In addition, there are concerns that off-target binding can reduce exposure and efficacy (Bumbaca et al.

2011). Abs produced by current methods lack the in vivo selection and regulatory mechanisms that are designed to limit cross reactivity to unintended targets (Bumbaca et al. 2011). Thus, understanding and limiting cross reactivity related to CDRs is an important factor in creating successful Ab-based therapeutics. Furthermore, off-target binding can also occur via non-CDR-mediated, nonspecific mechanisms. Recent efforts have developed guidelines for optimal physicochemical properties of therapeutic Abs that are analogous to Lipinski's rule of five that is used for small molecules to reduce this type of off-target binding and increase the likelihood of development success (Jain et al. 2017; Avery et al. 2018; Starr and Tessier 2019).

In cases where the target does not exist in nonclinical species, for example, where the test article only binds the human protein or the target is of exogenous origin, such as an infectious agent, profiling human tissues and cells to understand potential on- and off-targets may be one of the most important components of the nonclinical safety package (MacLachlan et al. 2021). This is especially true if the test article has effector functions that may increase the risk of cell and tissue damage.

20.5.2 History

In past decades, screening for potential off-target binding was initially done during the discovery phase by evaluating test article binding a relatively small number of closely related target molecules, which is what technology supported at the time. Later in development, potential off-target binding was assessed via the TCR study, usually by drug safety scientists. Information on the conduct of TCR studies from a regulatory standpoint came primarily from the FDA's "Points to Consider in the Manufacture and Testing of Monoclonal Antibody Products for Human Use", finalized by the FDA in 1983. This guidance was subsequently updated in 1987, 1994, and 1997 (US FDA 1983/1987/1994/1997). TCR studies are screening assays designed to identify binding (i.e., reactivity) of the test article across a broad range of tissues (n = ~35), usually using immunohistochemistry on frozen samples of human and animal tissues (Leach et al. 2010). Binding to the expected target is a desired outcome, and sometimes, these assays will identify previously unknown sites of the target antigen. In some cases, TCR studies also identify binding to unexpected targets (i.e., cross-reactive epitopes), hence the term cross reactivity. It was hoped that the localization of binding in TCR studies would identify potential target organs, allowing greater interrogation during nonclinical and clinical studies.

By the mid-2000s, there were concerns that TCR studies generated many false positives, methods were sometimes difficult or impossible to develop, and there were concerns that scientists in industry and regulatory agencies were not using the data appropriately. Based on these concerns, BioSafe chartered a working group that culminated in a publication that described scientific, strategic, and technical aspects of the assay (Leach et al. 2010). At the same time, a survey on the value of TCR studies was conducted (Bussiere et al. 2011). Together, these efforts showed that TCR studies did generate many false positives, but also on occasion provided useful information on cross reactivity that was not generated via other assays (Leach et al. 2010; Bussiere et al. 2011). In addition, it was noted that the primary goal of TCR studies is to screen for potential off-target,

cross-reactive targets across a wide range of tissues (Leach et al. 2010). In this regard, TCR studies have the ability to evaluate a large number of tissues for binding to unknown epitopes in a relatively rapid manner, and there was no other assay at that time that had the potential to screen across many molecules in a large number of tissues (Leach et al. 2010). Based on the occasional utility and perceived lack of alternatives, TCR studies continued to be used to test for off-target binding.

Since that time, new orthogonal assays evaluating protein–protein interactions have been developed, which can evaluate the potential for off-target binding of Abs and related products, and some are commercially available (MacLachlan et al. 2021). Some can assess the majority of the human proteome using cells transfected with human proteins, and the percent of the proteome that is covered is increasing. The experience thus far with the newer assays has been mixed, with some scientists reporting excellent results and other indicating issues with false positivity, or a lack of identifying the target (MacLachlan et al. 2021). These newer technologies are now being used by many companies, sometimes in conjunction with TCR studies and sometimes in place of TCR studies (MacLachlan et al. 2021). Concerns with the newer technologies include a lack of ability to localize binding within tissues, false positives (which also occurred with TCR studies), and incomplete coverage of the proteome. Some of these issues may be more prevalent with certain platforms/technologies and companies. It is anticipated that these technologies will continue to evolve and improve going forward.

20.5.3 Whether to Conduct

It is recommended that some assessment of off-target binding be incorporated during the discovery and development of Abs and related products. In particular, molecules with Fc functions may have significant impacts after binding to unintended targets, including the killing of bound cells, and these functions can be enhanced via molecular engineering (Almagro et al. 2018; Wang et al. 2018; Saunders 2019). The type of assessment(s) used in any given program should be a case-by-case decision. TCR studies should only be conducted with molecules that contain a CDR (Leach et al. 2010). For molecules that fall under ICH S9 for end-stage cancer indications, TCR studies are not recommended unless there is no relevant animal species (ICH S9 Q&A 2018); alternative methods may also be considered in this situation.

20.5.4 Molecules to Test

A variety of strategies to test for off-target binding can be employed, and where the program is within the discovery and development path dictates which molecule(s) (early candidates vs lead) are tested. Initial assays demonstrating the specificity of binding to the intended target, but not closely related molecules, are usually conducted as part of candidate screening early during discovery. An assessment of favorable physicochemical properties that can reduce interactions with molecules other than the target antigen or various receptors that Abs normally use can also be done at this early time to reduce other avenues of off-target binding (Jain et al. 2017; Avery et al. 2018; Starr et al. 2019). A broader evaluation of CDR-mediated off-target binding can be considered once a few potentially good candidates have been identified to aid in lead selection, potentially using protein arrays and/or immunohistochemical methods (e.g., TCR) as discussed above. These candidates may have different CDRs and target different epitopes, and certain epitopes may prove to be superior in terms of reducing the likelihood of off-target binding. Early assessments provide time to modify or select other molecules in the event of off-target binding or identification of other development liabilities; corrections and decisions made early may reduce the potential for later project delays and resource use on suboptimal molecules. As development progresses and a final lead candidate is chosen/engineered, teams should test the final molecule for off-target interactions if it has not already been tested. If alternative strategies need to be considered for nonclinical toxicity testing (in vitro, alternative species compared with what was originally planned), they can be planned and implemented with less impact on timelines. It should be noted that the test article used at this stage may come from a pool of clones, as the final cell clone that will be used for the clinical product may not yet be determined; however, it should be considered representative material (Bolisetty et al. 2020).

20.5.5 Species to Test

Humans are the primary species of concern with regard to off-target binding of candidate human therapeutics. Thus, the determination of human off-target binding is the information needed to support drug development. In this regard, if no off-target binding is detected in human tissues or cells, then no additional work would be needed in animal tissues unless some unexpected effect is observed in animals that needed to be understood. If off-target binding is seen in humans, then additional work (in vitro and/or in vivo) will likely be needed to determine which animal species are relevant for determining whether there are any effects associated with the off-target binding. It is recommended that only animal species that are pharmacologically relevant for the intended target and planned for use in nonclinical toxicity studies be tested at first. Ideally, similar binding will occur in humans and in these animal species. If these species do not have the off-target binding, then other species could be considered for in vivo toxicity testing.

20.5.6 TCR Strategies

Because TCR studies should usually be conducted with the candidate that is planned for use in the clinic, and because method development is sometimes problematic, it is suggested that method development initiate once the final candidate test article is available, if TCR studies will be conducted. A strategy of only testing for human off-target binding first and then doing animal work on human-positive cells/tissues can sometimes save resources. However, there must be sufficient time to run the assays consecutively. In many drug development programs, there is not time to conduct another round of TCR studies to identify animal species with off-target binding (if any can be found) and then conduct necessary toxicity studies, especially when they involve in vivo animal studies. Additionally, it has been estimated that if five or more animal tissues need to be stained as a consecutive separate study (because five or more human tissues were positive), it is often more expensive compared with running a full panel of human and animal tissues at the same time because controls must be rerun, slides must

be reexamined, etc. Many TCR studies do have more than five positive human tissues (Bussiere et al. 2011). For these reasons, once the final candidate is chosen, some companies choose to conduct human and animal screens at the same time. It is also important to realize that assessments should be conducted on molecules with the final CDRs; earlier molecules that lack the exact same CDRs may give misleading results.

20.5.7 Impact and Regulatory Considerations

If a cross-reactive target is identified, an assessment of the impact in humans, including toxicity, should be made in some manner. This can include efforts to determine whether the binding is via the CDR (for methods using methods such as immunohistochemistry, see Leach et al. 2010), identification of the actual epitope [e.g., using techniques such as immunoprecipitation, sodium dodecyl sulfate polyacrylamide gel electrophoresis, high-performance liquid chromatography, mass spectral sequencing (Bumbaca et al. 2011)], identification of the distribution of the epitope, and determination of whether the target is present in nonclinical species tested in toxicity studies. Ideally, the off-target epitope would be present in at least one species used for toxicity testing and preferably in a species that is also relevant for on-target pharmacology. If not, then testing in species relevant for the off-target binding should be considered; however, this may not be required. The important point is that an appropriate assessment of safety needs to be made in some manner that allows safe clinical dosing.

From a regulatory standpoint, ICH S6(R1) indicates TCR is a recommended component of the safety assessment package supporting FIH trials, but it also acknowledges that sometimes an assay cannot be developed from a technical standpoint. In addition, ICH S6(R1) notes that other technologies can be used. At the present time, there is some movement away from TCR studies for off-target assessment (MacLachlan et al. 2021; and see Chapter 11).

20.6 Immunogenicity

20.6.1 Overview

The issue of immunogenicity of biotherapeutics in nonclinical toxicity studies and underlying immunologic mechanisms has been reviewed (Ponce et al. 2009; Leach et al. 2014; Dingman and Balu-Iyer 2018). Key features associated with immunogenicity in nonclinical studies with Abs and related products are shown in Table 20.5. Immunogenicity is a potential issue in any in vivo toxicity study, as the immune system in animals and humans is fundamentally designed to differentiate self from nonself, thus allowing detection of foreign (nonself) molecules (Jiang and Chess 2009). Abs and related products are usually foreign molecules to the animal being dosed, and it is not surprising that they may be recognized as foreign, resulting in an immune response. Although not common, it is also possible that preexisting Abs may be present (i.e., ADA to the test article prior to dosing), as has been shown in humans (Xue and Rup 2013; van Schie et al. 2015; Gorovits et al. 2016). Preexisting ADA may also occur against molecules that are conjugated to the Ab and related products, such as small molecules, protein toxins, cytokines, etc (see Chapter 22)

TABLE 20.5

Key Features Associated with Immunogenicity in Nonclinical Studies with Abs and Related Products (Adapted from Leach et al. 2014)

- Effects related to immunogenicity often do not appear until after multiple doses and usually not until after approximately 10 to 14 days of dosing. In some cases, the first observed effects may not occur until months after initiation of dosing, despite weekly administration of the test article. However, if animals have preexisting ADAs, or the test article activates the innate immune system, reactions can be seen after the first dose.

- Thrombocytopenia, decreased red cell mass, and neutrophilia can be seen in the peripheral blood.

- There can be significant variability of responses between individual animals in the same study, even at the same dose level.

- The number of animals affected can vary from one to all in each dose group or study.

- Effects can vary in the same animal if dosing is continued and may get worse, improve, or not change.

- There is not always a good association of all the findings that one would associate with immunogenicity in the same animal. For example, ADA titers sometimes correlate with clinical reactions, microscopic findings, loss of PD effect, evidence of complement activation, and so on, but not always. In some animals, all laboratory parameters behave as expected, while in other animals only some or no laboratory parameters seem to correlate well with clinical and/or microscopic observations.

- Dose responses can be bell-shaped or inverse, with greater evidence of immunogenicity and hypersensitivity in intermediate- or low-dose groups, compared with high-dose groups.

- ADA and associated hypersensitivity reactions can occur in animals even when the test articles are immunosuppressive, including those that deplete B cells and plasma cells.

- Administration of antihistamines such as diphenhydramine may be effective or may not ameliorate responses in animals.

- Use of genetically-modified rodents can be helpful in determining whether the immune system is involved in any reactions observed in animals, although pharmacologic mechanisms may also be impacted in genetically-modified rodents depending upon the intended target.

- Less frequent dosing may increase the risk of immunogenicity.

- Immunogenicity in animals is not predictive that immunogenicity will occur in humans. In addition, if immunogenicity does occur in animals and humans, the findings in animals are not necessarily predictive of the findings in humans.

(Gorovits et al. 2016). The fact that detectable immune responses are not observed more frequently in animals administered foreign humanized or human proteins might be considered surprising. However, even if an immune response occurs, it may not preclude using that species in nonclinical toxicity studies.

20.6.2 Effect of Immunogenicity

The effect(s) of immunogenicity can be quite variable, and the extent of this variability between groups, within groups, and even in the same animal at different dosing days cannot be understated (Leach 2013; Leach et al. 2014). The immune responses to Abs and related products can have little or no effect, reduce or eliminate the activity of the test article via neutralization and/or clearance, rarely enhance or prolong the activity by increasing antibody recycling to the circulation and reducing catabolism, and/or result in hypersensitivity reactions. When occurring, hypersensitivity reactions are often immediate (type I) or immune complex-mediated (type III) reactions (Leach et al. 2014; Kronenberg et al. 2017). Clinical pathology assessments may show various cytopenias related to a variety of potential mechanisms (Everds and Tarrant 2013). Unusual manifestations have also occasionally been observed. For example, immunogenicity-related liver necrosis and fibrosis have been described in rats with different mAbs (Leach 2010; Leach et al. 2014; Hu 2021; Leach unpublished observations) and then in cynomolgus monkeys (Zuch de Zafra et al. 2016). Immunogenicity-related effects can sometimes confound interpretation of toxicity studies, as it may be unclear whether effects are pharmacologically mediated or related to immunogenicity. It is possible that both may occur in the same program or study, and even in the same animal. In particular, immune-stimulating agents can mimic immunogenicity-related effects of biotherapeutics, as both can lead to inflammation.

In a review conducted two decades ago, it was noted that immunogenicity in animals is not considered predictive of immunogenicity in humans (Bugelski and Treacy 2004). Since then, many more programs have been evaluated, and the lack of predictivity has been reinforced (Leach et al. 2014; Kronenberg et al. 2017). At the present time, scientists in industry and regulatory agencies generally agree with this concept, and ICH S6(R1) notes this as well. In this regard, it is critically important to determine whether findings seen in nonclinical toxicity studies are related to pharmacology (and are thus more likely predictive and relevant to humans) or whether they are related to immunogenicity (and are thus not predictive and less likely to be relevant to humans). Erroneous decisions can lead to inappropriate impacts on programs (e.g., additional nonclinical studies, additional clinical monitoring, or even project termination), or conversely may represent a failure to recognize potential negative/adverse effects in humans (Leach et al. 2014).

20.6.3 Assessing Immunogenicity

Assessments that may be included in toxicity studies to determine whether findings are related to immunogenicity are shown in Table 20.6 and are also discussed in Chapter 10. Demonstrating that findings in a toxicity study are related to immunogenicity often requires a weight-of-evidence approach across a study or even program, as various assessments in an individual animal often only fulfill some criteria associated with immunogenicity (Leach et al. 2014; Rojko et al. 2014; Mease et al. 2017). It is recommended that standard toxicity study assessments be planned for studies unless there is a cause for concern identified from earlier studies; thus, if there is no cause for concern, additional assessments would not be included in study protocols. If a cause for concern has been identified, additional assessments may be included,

TABLE 20.6

Assessments to Consider in Toxicity Studies to Determine Immunogenicity

Assessment	Findings	Comments
Clinical observations	Infusion reactions following multiple doses, up to anaphylaxis; or evidence of renal failure	Usually occur after 10–14 days of dosing, or longer, to allow the development of ADA
ADA	Evidence of ADA induction	Assays may not detect ADA in the presence of the test article; newer assays are often more tolerant of ADA (i.e., they can detect ADA in the presence of test article)
Pharmacologic effect	Reduced or lack of pharmacology	Rarely can be enhanced pharmacology if exposure is prolonged
Drug clearance	Reduced exposure	Can be a slow or rapid effect beginning after 10–14 days of dosing
Hematology	Various cytopenias	Lower platelet numbers in particular
Complement in peripheral blood	Evidence of complement activation	Measurement of complement components: lower CH50; higher C3a, C5a, SC5b-9
Histamine	Higher concentrations	Can be difficult to measure
CICs	Higher CICs	For IV dosing, suggest measuring 5 minutes after dosing; findings less pronounced or hard to detect with SC dosing
Light microscopy	Immune complex disease (perivascular infiltrates, vasculitis, glomerulopathy), fibrin thrombi, increased size and number of Kupffer cells, evidence of anaphylaxis	Findings may involve only one or a few tissues and may be very sporadic within or between animals; findings in animals with acute death may be minimal or absent, especially in rodents.
Transmission electron microscopy	Immune complexes present	Easiest to detect in renal glomeruli
Immunohistochemistry	Immune complexes present	Often done on kidney, looking for changes in glomeruli. Can also look in various blood vessels if vasculitis present. Typically look for complement components and endogenous Ab deposition. Can also look for the presence of test article.

ADA, anti-drug antibodies; CICs, circulating immune complexes; IV, intravenous; SC, subcutaneous.

usually focusing around collecting additional samples (e.g., for complement measurements, ADA, PK, etc.) around the time of dosing. Methods and technologies may change over time, and some assays may require specialized samples. Scientists should discuss what samples are needed with the laboratories that will be running the assays. It also should be noted that different methods for detecting immunogenicity can give different results, and therefore, comparing results between studies should be viewed with caution (Gorovits et al. 2018). It is recommended that laboratories conducting toxicity studies with Abs and related products be prepared to collect appropriate samples quickly and conduct unscheduled necropsies on short notice even if no immunogenicity-related findings or infusion reactions were previously observed. If immunogenicity takes the form of infusion reactions, these can occur shortly after dosing, or even during dosing, and may require immediate supportive care and/or sample collection (Mease et al. 2017).

ICH S6(R1) notes that immunogenicity assessments should be conducted when needed to assist in the interpretation of the study results and design of subsequent studies. In that regard, ADA should be measured "when there is 1) evidence of altered PD activity; 2) unexpected changes in exposure in the absence of a PD marker; or 3) evidence of immune-mediated reactions (immune complex disease, vasculitis, anaphylaxis, etc.)". Conversely, when potential ADA-mediated effects are not seen, measurement of ADA is not necessary, which can save significant resources. Based on this, it is recommended that decisions on collection of samples for ADA, and running them, be made on a study-by-study basis. If they are conducted, non-GLP exploratory studies may not need to have ADA samples collected or run. If evidence of ADA is seen

in exploratory studies, residual clinical pathology samples can usually be used for the determination of ADA induction. For FIH-enabling studies, it is recommended that specific ADA samples be collected to ensure adequate interpretation of studies is possible. If the study is rate limiting for filing FIH regulatory submissions, it is recommended that samples be run at the end of the study. However, if the study is not rate limiting and there is time to evaluate other data for evidence of ADA-related effects, then it might be possible to wait to determine whether the samples should be run. Finally, for chronic studies, it is also recommended that specific ADA samples be collected. As chronic studies are often not rate limiting, there may be time to assess other study data to determine whether to run the ADA assays.

20.6.4 Managing Immunogenicity in Toxicity Studies

If clinical immunogenicity is encountered during toxicity studies (e.g., infusion reactions including anaphylaxis, evidence of renal disease), decisions need to be made about whether to terminate the study. If large numbers of animals across all test article-dosed groups are affected and findings are moderate or severe, termination may be the best course of action for humane reasons and to try and improve the odds of differentiating test article-related effects from those caused by immunogenicity. However, because immunogenicity-related effects are not necessarily dose related and in some cases are inversely dose related, it may be reasonable to continue dosing in the dose groups not affected. Because of individual animal variability, it may also be reasonable to dose animals that were not significantly affected in groups where other animals were affected. In these cases, study scientists should be prepared to act quickly in the event test article-related effects occur during or shortly after dosing.

If a decision is made to continue dosing, the use of antihistamines such as diphenhydramine, or corticosteroids such as dexamethasone, may be considered (Leach et al. 2014; Mease et al. 2017). These treatments are primarily considered for nonrodent studies. While these drugs may reduce or eliminate infusion reactions, they may also impact test article-related findings. It is also possible that these drugs meant to reduce hypersensitivity reactions may themselves cause various changes, in particular corticosteroids, which can impact the lymphoid system, liver, and other organs systems as well as development (Tanyol and Rehfuss 1955; el Fouhil and Turkall 1993; el Fouhil et al. 1993a, 1993b, Hansen et al. 1999; Papich 2016). Decisions need to be made about whether to treat all animals, just those that previously had reactions, or just those groups in which reactions were observed. It is also possible that these drugs may have little impact on the reactions, i.e., significant reactions including mortality could still occur despite administering these drugs. Overall, scientists need to prioritize getting the most information possible on potential test article-related effects from the study when these situations occur.

If significant immunogenicity was observed in a previous study in many animals, it is likely (although not a given) that similar findings may occur again. If clinical signs were not observed, or were not severe, it may be reasonable and ethical to try and dose higher, which in some cases can overcome or reduce immunogenicity (Leach et al. 2014; Brunn et al. 2016). Consideration might also be given to pretreating all animals with antihistamines or corticosteroids beginning on the first dose. If immunogenicity occurs in a program, it is usually possible to dose for at least a week or two prior to the development of significant reactions and ADA, and at least some data can be collected without being confounded by immunogenicity.

20.6.5 Adversity of Immunogenicity

The topic of whether to consider findings related to immunogenicity adverse is currently contentious. Fundamentally, there are two topics involved. The first is "What is adverse?", and the second is "What is relevant to humans and should impact the no-observed-adverse-effect level (NOAEL) used for human exposure margin calculation and FIH dose selection?". Strategies to address these topics in the context of toxicity studies can be divided into making decisions on adversity in the study report based on suspected relevance to humans, and making decisions on adversity in the study report based on harm to the animal(s) under the conditions of that study. It is also possible to use a hybrid approach and list the NOAEL that is based on adversity in animals in the study, and another that is based on adverse findings considered relevant to humans at the time the study report is written. The pros and cons of each strategy are shown in Table 20.7. Some argue that because the findings are not predictive of humans, they should not be considered adverse. This would include animals that have mortality from what are believed to be immunogenicity-related causes; thus, this test article-related mortality would not be

considered adverse. On the other hand, several position papers from Society of Toxicologic Pathology and European Society of Toxicologic Pathology have suggested that adversity should be based on the specific findings in that animal in the study being conducted, and not on the relevance to humans (Kerlin et al. 2016; Palazzi et al. 2016; Ramaiah et al. 2017). In this regard, findings that are impactful enough (i.e., harmful enough) to animals should be considered adverse, even if they are not relevant to humans. This allows a consistent standard to be applied across studies, regardless of the cause, study location, sponsor, etc. It also allows the incorporation of new information that may impact the interpretation of findings into regulatory documents or investigator's brochures without creating conflict with existing study reports. Regardless of which strategy is chosen, scientists must decide what findings should or should not factor into the calculation of NOAELs, exposure margin calculations, and FIH starting doses, whether this is done in the study report or in other documents (regulatory submissions, investigator's brochures, etc.). In addition, it is recommended that a consistent strategy be used within a given development program.

20.7 Safety Pharmacology Assessments

20.7.1 Overview

In addition to the ICH S6(R1) and ICH S9 guidance, ICH S7A provides supplementary guidance on safety pharmacology studies for human biopharmaceuticals. In accordance with regulatory requirements, assessments of cardiovascular (CV), central nervous system (CNS), and pulmonary function must be performed prior to FIH; this group of assessments is often termed the core battery. It should be noted that there are currently questions about whether respiratory safety pharmacology studies should remain as part of the core battery for all therapeutic modalities (small molecules, biotherapeutics, etc.) based on a perceived lack of value (Paglialunga et al. 2019). In vitro cardiovascular studies, such as hERG assessments, are not considered appropriate as biotherapeutics such as Abs and related products are generally specific in their targeting, and in addition, they are not able to access the inner pore of the hERG channel to exert an effect [Vargas et al. 2008; ICH S6(R1) 2011, Vargas et al. 2013]. Safety pharmacology core battery endpoints can usually be added to general toxicity studies for Abs and related products [Vargas et al. 2013; ICH S6(R1) 2011, ICH S7A 2001], and stand-alone studies are typically not needed and are not an appropriate use of animals. However, if the target is known or suspected to be associated with safety pharmacology risks, stand-alone studies may be appropriate if sufficient information cannot be collected in general toxicity studies (Vargas et al. 2013). Rodents should be used for stand-alone safety pharmacology studies if they are pharmacologically relevant and the necessary assays can be conducted. Beyond the core battery, the gastrointestinal and renal systems are also sometimes evaluated, especially if they are likely targets of the therapeutic effect; these assessments usually require specific, stand-alone studies. Table 20.8 shows some considerations for safety pharmacology core battery assessments for lower- and higher-risk test articles in FIH-enabling general toxicity studies.

TABLE 20.7

Strategies to Address Immunogenicity-Related Adversity in Toxicity Studies

Strategy	Pros	Cons
Make decisions on adversity in the study report based on suspected relevance to humans	• May reduce confusion related to adverse findings that are not relevant to humans • Makes writing regulatory documents and investigator's brochures easier, as study report wording is more likely to exactly match these documents (unless interpretations change)	• Potentially requires that different standards of "what is adverse" be used within the same animal, with in the same studies, between studies, and between laboratories • Study scientists may be pressured into calling findings that are harmful to animals (including mortality) non-adverse, and they may not consider this appropriate • If relevance to humans is changed, the study reports will no longer be accurate • Adding information about relevance to humans may make it challenging to meet study report timelines
Make decisions on adversity in the study report based on harm to the animal(s) under the conditions of that study	• Allows consistent standards of "what is adverse" to be used within the same animal, within the same study, between studies, and between laboratories globally • Study scientists can make consistent, unbiased determinations about the adversity of findings • No impact on study report(s) if the relevance to humans is changed • Allows study reports to be completed without additional challenges of determining the relevance of findings to humans	• There may be confusion about which adverse findings are relevant to humans • Can make writing regulatory documents and investigator's brochures more challenging
Hybrid approach with NOAEL for what is adverse in animals in the study, and another NOAEL (if applicable) based on findings considered relevant to humans at the time the study report is written	• Allows consistent standards of "what is adverse" to be used within the same animal, within the same study, between studies, and between laboratories globally • Study scientists can make consistent, unbiased determinations about the adversity of findings • May reduce confusion related to adverse findings that are not relevant to humans • Makes writing regulatory documents and investigator's brochures easier, as study report wording is more likely to exactly match these documents	• There may be confusion about understanding the use of more than one NOAEL in a study • If relevance to humans is changed, the study reports will no longer be accurate • Adding information about relevance to humans may make it challenging to meet study report timelines

TABLE 20.8

Selected Considerations for In Vivo Safety Pharmacology Assessments with Abs and Related Products[a] in FIH-Enabling Studies to Meet Regulatory Guidelines

Assessment	Lower-Risk Test Articles	Higher-Risk Test Articles (Conduct Studies below in Addition to Assessments for Lower-Risk Test Articles)
Cardiovascular	Surface lead ECG in restrained large animal (usually monkey) at baseline and end of the study. Because of concerns about the impact of ADA, data may also be collected on ~Day 2, prior to the potential development of ADA.	Consider incorporation of implanted telemetry evaluation onto select dose groups as part of a FIH-enabling GLP large animal toxicity study. Stand-alone single-dose telemetry study may be warranted; conduct in rodent if pharmacologically relevant.
Central nervous	Body temperature and appropriately timed standard clinical observations in rodent and large animal studies, if pharmacologically relevant.	Consider detailed clinical neurological examination (for monkeys) or functional observational battery/Irwin test (for rodents).
Respiratory[b]	Clinical signs of respiration in large animal.	Consider whole-body plethysmography assessment in rodent study if pharmacologically relevant.

[a] If a mAb/related product is conjugated to small molecules, these may necessitate a more traditional small molecule safety pharmacology assessment of linkers and payloads.

[b] The need for respiratory assessments is currently being reconsidered by the pharmaceutical industry and regulatory agencies.

20.7.2 Strategy and Timing

It is strongly recommended that appropriate safety pharmacology strategies based upon the perceived level of risk be in place prior to planning the first in vivo toxicity studies. For programs with a high level of concern, for example, where safety pharmacology findings might terminate the program, relevant safety pharmacology assessments may be conducted prior to non-GLP exploratory studies, or as part of these studies. When there is no perceived risk, assessments can be added to the FIH-enabling general toxicity study. If no signals of concern are seen, additional safety pharmacology assessments are not usually needed in chronic studies.

If stand-alone studies are conducted and the duration is longer than 5 days, it is recommended that samples for ADA be collected in case some assessment of immunogenicity is needed. Because of the potential for immunogenicity and long half-lives of mAb and related products, crossover and dose escalation designs are usually not used. In addition, animals should not have been previously administered biotherapeutics unless they are tested and found negative for ADA. Finally, due to the potential development of ADA, it is recommended that safety pharmacology assessments be conducted not only prior to and at the end of the study, but also on ~Day 2 when exposures are likely high and before potential development of ADA.

20.8 Developmental and Reproductive Toxicity (DART) Studies and Juvenile Animal Studies (JAS)

20.8.1 Overview

ICH M3(R2), ICH S5(R3), ICH S6(R1), and ICH S9 all refer in some regard to DART studies, ICH S11 refers to JAS, and more information on these studies is also presented in Chapter 12. While proteins are typically too large to diffuse across the placenta, the binding of molecules with an Fc to the Fc receptors on the placenta, in particular FcRn, allows active transport across the placenta by receptor-mediated transcytosis (Roopenian and Akilesh 2007; DeSesso et al. 2012). This is the same receptor responsible for the long half-life of Fc-containing biotherapeutics, as discussed above. It is known that Fc-containing biotherapeutics can cross the placenta in mice, rats, rabbits, and cynomolgus monkeys, although the timing of exposure (in terms of development) varies between species (Bowman et al. 2013). Differences in exposure based on isotype have also been noted, with a greater transfer of IgG1 in cynomolgus monkeys, compared with IgG2 and IgG4 (Bowman et al. 2013).

A complete DART safety assessment includes evaluation of effects on development (evaluating the potential for maternal toxicity as well as pre- and postnatal developmental toxicity, including juvenile toxicity), and effects on fertility (reproduction) (Denny and Faqi 2017). Developmental toxicity studies typically dose and evaluate animals during pregnancy [an embryo-fetal development (EFD) study] and evaluate offspring in utero and following delivery [a pre- and postnatal development (PPND) study], providing critical information on the potential for drug-induced birth defects. Male and female fertility studies typically dose animals before, during, and after mating to determine potential adverse effects on fertility and early embryonic development.

While these studies are relatively easy to conduct in rodents and rabbits, in monkeys they are time-consuming, expensive, and subject to variable and sometimes high fetal loss that can make interpretation difficult, which has led to modified assessments in monkeys compared with rodents and rabbits (Weinbauer et al. 2011, 2013; Mecklenburg et al. 2019). If monkeys are used, fertility assessments are conducted by evaluating the reproductive tissues in general toxicity studies of at least 3-months duration using sexually-mature monkeys [ICH S5(R3) 2020; ICH S6(R1) 2011], which provides a long enough duration to assess any potential toxic effects. Developmental assessments in monkeys are typically done using an enhanced (e)PPND study (Weinbauer et al. 2011, 2013; Luetjens et al. 2020).

20.8.2 Species to Test and Alternative Models

Details on which species to test based on which are pharmacologically relevant are presented in Section 20.3. General testing strategies are discussed in Section 20.1.4. Generally, if rodents are pharmacologically relevant, they should be used for DART studies, and efforts should be made to minimize the use of large animals (usually monkeys). Rabbits may also be used in EFD studies if they are pharmacologically relevant. Monkeys should only be used for DART studies if they are the only pharmacologically-relevant species. Before using monkeys, alternatives such as testing in genetically-modified animals should be considered (Martin et al. 2009; Wright et al. 2012). Studies in genetically-modified animals have been adequate to support drug development.

20.8.3 Study Design Considerations for Abs and Related Products

For test articles that contain an Fc and have a long half-life, dosing should be infrequent (similar to other in vivo toxicity studies with that test article). If the molecule lacks an Fc, it will likely have a shorter half-life and need more frequent dosing. Dose range finding (DRF) studies are often not necessary unless toxicity is anticipated and reasonable estimates of doses cannot be made; DRF studies are particularly discouraged when monkeys are being used.

Doses should be selected as described for general toxicity studies. It is not necessary to cause maternal toxicity in developmental studies if sufficient (minimum of 10x) exposure multiples are achieved (also considering pharmacology differences as discussed in Section 20.4.5). Loading doses, or two doses close to one another early in a study, may be useful to achieve steady-state concentrations quickly. For molecules that are anticipated to be nontoxic, fewer than three test article-dosed groups may be used. Fewer dose groups should also be considered whenever monkeys are being used.

Similar to other in vivo studies, immunogenicity may be an issue. This is usually less of a concern with studies that dose for less than 14 days (e.g., rodent EFD studies), although ADA can develop in the 7 to 10 day range for highly immunogenic molecules. Thus, it is often possible to complete rodent and rabbit developmental toxicity studies without impact from immunogenicity. For monkey ePPND studies, where dosing is usually from GD20 until birth approximately 140–150 days later, there is a much greater chance for the development of immunogenicity. It is recommended that TK and ADA samples be collected from dams, and possibly from fetuses or infants, depending on the study design.

20.8.4 Strategies and Timing

Scientists should understand the role of the target pathway in development and reproduction, the potential for off-target effects, and the risk tolerance of the patient population. After this assessment, a determination on whether there is sufficient knowledge to inform patient safety about potential risks to reproduction and development should be made. If there is insufficient information, there should be a determination of what toxicity testing is warranted and when it is needed. Alternatively, it has recently been suggested that a weight-of-evidence approach could be used instead of conducting in vivo developmental toxicity study(ies) if there is sufficient information to inform patient risk (Rocca et al. 2018). This approach is supported by ICH S5(R3); however, precedence for this approach is currently limited. Therefore, engagement of regulatory agencies is recommended prior to using this strategy to ensure regulatory acceptance and prevent program delays.

The timing of DART studies will depend on the clinical program (primarily when women of childbearing potential (WOCBP) or pregnant women are enrolled, how many will be enrolled, what species are pharmacologically relevant), and company policy (some companies have guidelines that are more stringent than those of regulatory agencies). For example, if cynomolgus monkeys are the only relevant species and a developmental or ePPND toxicity study in monkeys is deemed necessary, the study is usually conducted during Phase 3 with careful attention to contraception during clinical trials. In contrast, if rodents are pharmacologically relevant and WOCBP are being enrolled in phase 2, then these studies might be conducted in time to support Phase 2 or 3, depending on clinical needs, and the findings might support less stringent contraceptive measures and thus likely aid in clinical study enrollment.

When using monkeys for DART assessments, careful planning well in advance of needing reports is necessary to avoid program delays. Inclusion of fertility assessments in general toxicity studies requires using sexually-mature animals, which at the present time are not easy to obtain. Furthermore, all animals should be tested to ensure they are sexually mature prior to beginning the study (Leach 2013; Mecklenburg et al. 2019). Slots for ePPND studies in monkeys are limited and booked well in advance, and the studies may take over 2 years to complete after dosing has started.

20.8.5 Nonclinical Pediatric Evaluation

If the age of the target pediatric population is younger than the corresponding developmental age that was evaluated in the existing general toxicity study package, a JAS may be warranted. ICH S11 describes when a JAS may be warranted, as well as discusses study design considerations. The design of any studies, if required, should be based on the intended age of the pediatric population, target organs in adult humans and animals (theoretical and identified in clinical and nonclinical studies), and the pharmacological target. JAS should be conducted in rodents if they are pharmacologically relevant, and typically one species is sufficient. The timing of studies is dependent on the clinical pediatric development plan. In general, if a JAS is required, it should be conducted prior to the initiation of clinical trials in pediatric populations. See Chapter 12 for more information on JAS. The use of alternatives such as genetically-modified animals can also be considered; more information on the selection of relevant animal models/species may be found in Chapter 2.

20.9 Genotoxicity

ICH S6(R1) indicates that genotoxicity studies are usually not needed for biotherapeutics, including Abs and related products. However, if small molecule linkers or conjugates are associated with the test article, they will likely need to be assessed in a manner that is similar to standard small molecules [ICH S2(R1) 2012].

20.10 Carcinogenicity Studies

Carcinogenicity testing is not needed for therapeutics that have a limited duration of dosing (<6 months) or are being developed to treat serious disease indications where life expectancy is low (<2–3 years) (ICH S1A 1996). However, for the Abs and related products that fall outside these categories, a thorough product-specific assessment of the carcinogenic potential of the molecule should be conducted. This can include information regarding target biology, data from related molecules or molecules in the same product class, human data involving modulation of the target pharmacologically or via natural gene mutations, in vitro information, data from knockout or knock-in animals, and data from toxicity studies (especially evidence of cell proliferation). An overall weight-of-evidence conclusion around carcinogenic potential should be developed and decisions made about whether additional studies are needed. Additional studies may include in vitro or in vivo assessments of cell proliferation (which may include routine staining or specialized methods), standard rodent carcinogenicity studies, studies with rodent homologues, and studies in genetically-modified animals. While many studies can be done, only studies that will likely provide useful information that will have a meaningful impact on the development of the test article should be conducted. If there is a known hazard, or when nonclinical studies may not be definitive, the hazard may be best dealt with using pharmacovigilance and/or product labeling, and not nonclinical studies. If the weight of evidence suggests carcinogenicity studies are not necessary, a waiver should be requested from regulatory agencies.

It is recommended that the assessment of a biotherapeutic's carcinogenic potential be initiated early in a program and updated throughout development. By end of Phase 2 meetings with regulatory authorities, a firm plan should be in place with agreement from regulatory agencies. It should be noted that is it possible to dose rodents for up to 2 years with biologics, and technical reasons alone are not usually sufficient to claim that a study cannot be conducted (Vahle et al. 2004; Byrd et al. 2015).

20.11 Immunotoxicity

20.11.1 Overview

Immunotoxicity with Abs and related products can be classified in a number of different ways, but at a high level typically includes immunosuppressive or immunostimulatory effects, and those related to immunogenicity (Descotes 2009; Brennan et al. 2010;

Lebrec 2013); immunogenicity can also be considered a cause of immunostimulation (Evans 2014). Immunogenicity is covered in Section 20.6 of this chapter. Immunosuppressive and immunostimulatory effects are often related to the intended pharmacology of the test article. Adverse immunostimulation has also been reported due to impurities in non-Ab biopharmaceuticals (Reijers et al. 2019), and similar events could occur with Abs and related products.

An assessment of potential immunotoxicity should begin with a thorough understanding of the test article biology, including whether the Fc (or parts of the Fc) are present, what modifications have been made to alter effector function or half-life, and what types of effector functions are likely (Brennan et al. 2010). For example, a molecule with enhanced ADCC to more effectively kill tumors cells could also kill normal cells that express the target antigen. In contrast, a test article lacking an Fc that targets a soluble molecule would have a short half-life and lack effector function, making it less likely to directly kill unintended cells expressing the target. After the biology of the molecule is determined, decisions can be made regarding what additional assays are needed, if any.

20.11.2 In Vitro Assays for Assessing Immunotoxicity of Abs and Related Products

Test articles that contain an Fc should be tested for binding to Fcγ receptors and complement. The Fc functions in the test article may be wild-type, or via molecular engineering they may be enhanced, diminished, or eliminated (Wang et al. 2018, see also Section 20.1.2). If there is binding to Fcγ receptors and/or complement, the activity should be further characterized in some manner. These types of analyses are often conducted during the engineering of the molecule in discovery. Additional functional assays for ADCC, ADCP, and/or CDC may be conducted.

Cytokine release assays (CRAs) should be considered for certain molecules but should not be conducted as a default strategy. If the test article binds to immune cells or is designed to stimulate the immune system, then CRAs may be appropriate. Alternatively, if a test article is designed to bind to a soluble mediator not involved in immune stimulation, CRAs are likely not necessary. CRAs are currently best considered as a tool for hazard identification, and not for risk assessment (Grimaldi et al. 2016). There are a variety of assays available, and standardization across the pharmaceutical industry has not occurred (Grimaldi et al. 2016).

More details on specific assays are discussed in Chapter 16.

20.11.3 In Vivo Assays for Assessing Immunotoxicity of Abs and Related Products

A wide range of in vivo assays are possible in rodents and large animals to test for immunotoxicity. Clinical signs, clinical pathology assessments, and microscopic evaluation of tissues in efficacy and toxicity studies should be considered as baseline evaluations. Additional assays or studies should only be included if necessary, and many of these can be included in standard toxicity studies. For example, it is possible to collect peripheral blood for the assessment of complement split products and cytokine concentrations. Immunophenotyping of peripheral blood, lymphoid tissues, or bone marrow can be used to reveal changes in cell surface markers and cell numbers. Assessment of the T-dependent antibody response can be added to general toxicity studies (Lebrec 2013). It is important to note that some assays may require the addition of more animals to the study groups, as some assays may require samples that cannot be collected from main study animals or may require sampling throughout a study. This may be especially true for rodents due to their smaller size. Adding animals will require additional test article.

20.11.4 Immunosuppression

The primary concerns with immunosuppression are increased risk of infections and tumor development, which can occur in animals or humans (Descotes 2009; Brennan et al. 2010; Hutto 2010). A variety of pathogens including bacteria, viruses, and fungi can be involved. Cell proliferation and tumors may be virally induced. Evidence of immunosuppression may be seen in in vivo efficacy or toxicity studies, with clinical, clinicopathologic, and/or microscopic evidence of infection, cell proliferation, or tumors. Alternatively, more subtle effects such as decreased cellularity in tissues such as lymph nodes, spleen, thymus, or bone marrow may be seen (Elmore 2012). Not all animals in a given group may be affected in a similar manner.

20.11.5 Immunostimulation

Immunostimulation can be the direct result of intended pharmacology (e.g., killing of normal cells that express the target antigen by T cells stimulated via T cell-recruiting bispecific molecules), or it can be secondary to more general immune stimulation (e.g., autoimmune-like conditions associated with blockade of checkpoint inhibitors like anti-PD-1 and anti-CTLA4), although normal animals may underpredict toxicities observed in humans, especially if given as monotherapies (Keler et al. 2003; Wang et al. 2014; Selby et al. 2016; Ji et al. 2019). Toxicities related to immunostimulation are particularly common with immuno-oncology molecules, which are designed to stimulate the immune system to respond against cancers (Shimabukuro-Vornhagen et al. 2018; Ji et al. 2019) (also see Chapter 28). Mechanistically, a test article can cause immunostimulation from cytokine release (including cytokine release syndrome or cytokine storm), immune cell proliferation and activation, direct complement activation, and effector activity related to Fc receptor binding (i.e., ADCC, ADCP) or complement activation (CDC) (Brennan et al. 2010; Evans 2014; Ji et al. 2019). One or more mechanisms may be operative at the same time. A wide variety of potential negative effects are possible including infusion reactions, leukocytosis, inflammatory cell infiltrates in tissues (including heart, colon, liver, salivary glands, and endocrine organs), and autoimmune-type syndromes (Descotes 2009; Evans 2014; Ji et al. 2019).

20.11.6 Strategies

From a regulatory standpoint, ICH S6(R1) states that routine tiered testing approaches or standard testing batteries are not recommended for evaluating immunotoxicity. Immunotoxicity can be assessed in standard toxicity studies, evaluating routine assessments of clinical signs, hematology, organ weights and microscopic examination of tissues. If additional assessments or studies are under consideration, scientists should carefully think about whether they will truly add value to the safety assessment, as knowledge of the mechanism of action of the test article often provides such information (e.g., one does not need additional studies with anti-TNF molecules to know they will be immunosuppressive in humans), and it may take studies in large numbers of humans to fully understand the potential risk, making additional nonclinical work unnecessary. If additional in vitro or in vivo assays are needed, they should be carefully selected. It is easy to run a number of assays, but interpreting the data can be difficult due to variability (Lebrec 2013). When considered necessary, it is recommended that in vitro assays including cytokine release assays be conducted before in vivo toxicity studies are conducted, so that they can inform the in vivo study designs.

20.12 Advanced Cancer

The nonclinical toxicity testing requirements for advanced cancer are reduced compared with programs for other diseases and are outlined in ICH S9 and the ICH S9 Q&A. Oncology biotherapeutics in general are discussed in Chapter 28. In cases where follow-on indications are for early-stage cancer or non-oncology indications, they may require additional toxicity studies. A comparison of selected program features in advanced cancer programs falling under ICH S9 is shown in Table 20.9.

20.13 Multispecific Molecules

A discussion of the structural elements of multispecific molecules is in Section 20.1.2. Toxicity programs with multispecifics should follow the same general principles outlined above. Studies should be conducted in pharmacologically-relevant species, which add greater complexity with greater numbers of targets. Ideally, the nonclinical toxicology species and humans will have similar binding and pharmacologic activity across all targets. However, when this is not the case, it may be necessary to test in species where only one target is relevant; regulators have indicated that binding to only one arm of a bispecific can be enough to consider a species relevant in an oncology indication (FDA, personal communication). A variety of alternative models are also present, including using animals that have been genetically-modified to express all targets, use of surrogate molecules, etc., as described in Section 20.1.4. Because of the complexity and potential risks of conducting studies in alternative models, early regulatory engagement is recommended to gain agreement on the nonclinical development strategy. If TCR studies are conducted, it is recommended that the multispecific molecule be tested and not subcomponents. More information on testing multispecific molecules is presented in Chapter 22.

20.14 Biosimilars

Regulators initially required in vivo toxicity studies for biosimilars (Chapman et al. 2016; M Leach, personal observation). However, experience has shown that in vivo nonclinical testing of proposed biosimilar mAbs does not provide any value for molecules that have a strong analytical and in vitro functional data set showing a high degree of similarity (Hurst et al. 2014; Ryan et al. 2014; Chapman et al. 2016; Derzi et al. 2016; Peraza et al. 2018; Derzi et al. 2020). Given that

TABLE 20.9

Comparison of ICH S9 Advanced Cancer vs Non-ICH S9 Nonclinical Toxicology Packages

Program Feature	ICH S9 Programs	Non-ICH S9 Programs
Species	Pharmacologically relevant	Pharmacologically relevant
General Toxicity Study Endpoint	HNSTD, STD10	NOAEL
Longest Duration of General Toxicity Study	3 months	6 months
Recovery in General Toxicity Study(ies)	Not common; only if severe toxicity observed at anticipated clinical exposures and recovery cannot be predicted	Common
Tissue Cross-Reactivity Study	May not be necessary unless no pharmacologically-relevant species identified	Generally done
Safety Pharmacology	Full assessment	Full assessment
DART	Embryo-fetal development study in one species (preferably a rodent if pharmacologically relevant); if only pharmacologically-relevant species is a monkey, consider literature-based weight-of-evidence approach	Full assessment typical
Genotoxicity	Not required	Not required
Carcinogenicity	Not required	Carcinogenicity assessment necessary; in vitro or in vivo studies may be needed if cause for concern

numerous biosimilar molecules have been successfully produced, if a molecule does not show a high degree of analytical and in vitro functional similarity, it should likely not be progressed as a biosimilar. Regulatory agencies globally are now more accepting of nonclinical packages without in vivo toxicity studies when the overall data support such decisions. Thus, in vivo toxicity studies should rarely be conducted for proposed biosimilars. Human clinical efficacy trials with biosimilars have also shown little value when there is a robust understanding of the reference product (i.e., the original molecule) coupled with a strong analytical package showing similarity (Bielsky et al. 2020). More information on biosimilars can be found in Chapter 13.

Acknowledgments

I would like to thank Chris Bowman, Joy Cavagnaro, Mary Ellen Cosenza, Frank Geoly, and Marque Todd for providing helpful information and comments.

REFERENCES

Almagro JC, Daniels-Wells TR, Perez-Tapia SM, Penichet ML. Progress and challenges in the design and clinical development of antibodies for cancer therapy. *Front Immunol*. 2018; 8:1751. doi: 10.3389/fimmu.2017.01751. PMID: 29379493; PMCID: PMC5770808.

Almagro JC, Fransson J. Humanization of antibodies. *Front Biosci*. 2008;13:1619–33. PMID: 17981654.

Avery LB, Wade J, Wang M, Tam A, King A, Piche-Nicholas N, Kavosi MS, Penn S, Cirelli D, Kurz JC, Zhang M, Cunningham O, Jones R, Fennell BJ, McDonnell B, Sakorafas P, Apgar J, Finlay WJ, Lin L, Bloom L, O'Hara DM. Establishing in vitro in vivo correlations to screen monoclonal antibodies for physicochemical properties related to favorable human pharmacokinetics. *MAbs*. 2018;10(2):244–55. doi: 10.1080/19420862.2017.1417718. Epub 2018 Jan 29. PMID: 29271699; PMCID: PMC5825195.

Avery LB, Wang M, Kavosi MS, Joyce A, Kurz JC, Fan YY, Dowty ME, Zhang M, Zhang Y, Cheng A, Hua F, Jones HM, Neubert H, Polzer RJ, O'Hara DM. Utility of a human FcRn transgenic mouse model in drug discovery for early assessment and prediction of human pharmacokinetics of monoclonal antibodies. *MAbs*. 2016;8(6):1064–78. doi: 10.1080/19420862.2016.1193660. Epub 2016 May 27. PMID: 27232760; PMCID: PMC4968115.

Bates A, Power CA. David vs. Goliath: the structure, function, and clinical prospects of antibody fragments. *Antibodies (Basel)*. 2019;8(2):28. doi: 10.3390/antib8020028. PMID: 31544834; PMCID: PMC6640713.

Baum A, Ajithdoss D, Copin R, Zhou A, Lanza K, Negron N, Ni M, Wei Y, Mohammadi K, Musser B, Atwal GS, Oyejide A, Goez-Gazi Y, Dutton J, Clemmons E, Staples HM, Bartley C, Klaffke B, Alfson K, Gazi M, Gonzalez O, Dick E Jr, Carrion R Jr, Pessaint L, Porto M, Cook A, Brown R, Ali V, Greenhouse J, Taylor T, Andersen H, Lewis MG, Stahl N, Murphy AJ, Yancopoulos GD, Kyratsous CA. REGN-COV2 antibodies prevent and treat SARS-CoV-2 infection in rhesus macaques and hamsters. *Science*. 2020;370(6520):1110–15. doi: 10.1126/science.abe2402. Epub 2020 Oct 9. PMID: 33037066.

Beers SA, Glennie MJ, White AL. Influence of immunoglobulin isotype on therapeutic antibody function. *Blood*. 2016;127(9):1097–101. doi: 10.1182/blood-2015-09-625343. Epub 2016 Jan 13. PMID: 26764357; PMCID: PMC4797141.

Betts A, Keunecke A, van Steeg TJ, van der Graaf PH, Avery LB, Jones H, Berkhout J. Linear pharmacokinetic parameters for monoclonal antibodies are similar within a species and across different pharmacological targets: a comparison between human, cynomolgus monkey and hFcRn Tg32 transgenic mouse using a population-modeling approach. *MAbs*. 2018;10(5):751–64. doi: 10.1080/19420862.2018.1462429. Epub 2018 May 14. PMID: 29634430; PMCID: PMC6150614.

Bielsky MC, Cook A, Wallington A, Exley A, Kauser S, Hay JL, Both L, Brown D. Streamlined approval of biosimilars: moving on from the confirmatory efficacy trial. *Drug Discov Today*. 2020;S1359-6446(20)30343-3. doi: 10.1016/j.drudis.2020.09.006. Epub ahead of print. PMID: 32916269.

Black LE, Bendele AM, Bendele RA, Zack PM, Hamilton M. Regulatory decision strategy for entry of a novel biological therapeutic with a clinically unmonitorable toxicity into clinical trials: pre-IND meetings and a case example. *Toxicol Pathol*. 1999;27(1):22–6. doi: 10.1177/019262339902700105. PMID: 10367668.

Bolisetty P, Tremml G, Xu S, Khetan A. Enabling speed to clinic for monoclonal antibody programs using a pool of clones for IND-enabling toxicity studies. *MAbs*. 2020;12(1):1763727. doi: 10.1080/19420862.2020.1763727. PMID: 32449878; PMCID: PMC7531531.

Bournazos S, Gupta A, Ravetch JV. The role of IgG Fc receptors in antibody-dependent enhancement. *Nat Rev Immunol*. 2020;20(10):633–43. doi: 10.1038/s41577-020-00410-0. Epub 2020 Aug 11. PMID: 32782358; PMCID: PMC7418887.

Bowman CJ, Breslin WJ, Connor AV, Martin PL, Moffat GJ, Sivaraman L, Tornesi MB, Chivers S. Placental transfer of Fc-containing biopharmaceuticals across species, an industry survey analysis. *Birth Defects Res B Dev Reprod Toxicol*. 2013;98(6):459–85. doi: 10.1002/bdrb.21089. Epub 2014 Jan 3. PMID: 24391099.

Brennan FR, Morton LD, Spindeldreher S, Kiessling A, Allenspach R, Hey A, Muller PY, Frings W, Sims J. Safety and immunotoxicity assessment of immunomodulatory monoclonal antibodies. *MAbs*. 2010;2(3):233–55. doi: 10.4161/mabs.2.3.11782. Epub 2010 May 23. PMID: 20421713; PMCID: PMC2881251.

Brunn ND, Mauze S, Gu D, Wiswell D, Ueda R, Hodges D, Beebe AM, Zhang S, Escandón E. The role of anti-drug antibodies in the pharmacokinetics, disposition, target engagement, and efficacy of a GITR agonist monoclonal antibody in mice. *J Pharmacol Exp Ther*. 2016;356(3):574–86. doi: 10.1124/jpet.115.229864. Epub 2015 Dec 15. PMID: 26669426.

Bugelski PJ, Treacy G. Predictive power of preclinical studies in animals for the immunogenicity of recombinant therapeutic proteins in humans. *Curr Opin Mol Ther*. 2004;6(1):10–6. PMID: 15011776.

Bumbaca D, Wong A, Drake E, Reyes AE 2nd, Lin BC, Stephan JP, Desnoyers L, Shen BQ, Dennis MS. Highly specific off-target binding identified and eliminated during the humanization of an antibody against FGF receptor 4. *MAbs.* 2011;3(4):376–86. doi: 10.4161/mabs.3.4.15786. Epub 2011 Jul 1. PMID: 21540647; PMCID: PMC3218534.

Burnet FM. A modification of Jerne's theory of antibody production using the concept of clonal selection. *Aust J Sci.* 1957; 20:67–8.

Bussiere JL. Species selection considerations for preclinical toxicology studies for biotherapeutics. *Expert Opin Drug Metab Toxicol.* 2008;4(7):871–7. doi: 10.1517/17425255.4.7.871. PMID: 18624676.

Bussiere JL, Leach MW, Price KD, Mounho BJ, Lightfoot-Dunn R. Survey results on the use of the tissue cross-reactivity immunohistochemistry assay. *Regul Toxicol Pharmacol.* 2011;59(3):493–502. doi: 10.1016/j.yrtph.2010.09.017. Epub 2010 Oct 14. PMID: 20951178.

Byrd RA, Sorden SD, Ryan T, Pienkowski T, LaRock R, Quander R, Wijsman JA, Smith HW, Blackbourne JL, Rosol TJ, Long GG, Martin JA, Vahle JL. Chronic toxicity and carcinogenicity studies of the long-acting GLP-1 receptor agonist dulaglutide in rodents. *Endocrinology.* 2015;156(7):2417–28. doi: 10.1210/en.2014-1722. Epub 2015 Apr 10. PMID: 25860029.

Chapman AP. PEGylated antibodies and antibody fragments for improved therapy: a review. *Adv Drug Deliv Rev.* 2002 17;54(4):531–45. doi: 10.1016/s0169-409x(02)00026-1. PMID: 12052713.

Chapman K, Adjei A, Baldrick P, da Silva A, De Smet K, DiCicco R, Hong SS, Jones D, Leach MW, McBlane J, Ragan I, Reddy P, Stewart DI, Suitters A, Sims J. Waiving in vivo studies for monoclonal antibody biosimilar development: national and global challenges. *MAbs.* 2016;8(3):427–35. doi: 10.1080/19420862.2016.1145331. PMID: 26854177; PMCID: PMC4966840.

Chen IJ, Chuang CH, Hsieh YC, Lu YC, Lin WW, Huang CC, Cheng TC, Cheng YA, Cheng KW, Wang YT, Chen FM, Cheng TL, Tzou SC. Selective antibody activation through protease-activated pro-antibodies that mask binding sites with inhibitory domains. *Sci Rep.* 2017;7(1):11587. doi: 10.1038/s41598-017-11886-7. PMID: 28912497; PMCID: PMC5599682.

Chiu ML, Gilliland GL. Engineering antibody therapeutics. *Curr Opin Struct Biol.* 2016;38:163–73. doi: 10.1016/j.sbi.2016.07.012. Epub 2016 Aug 12. PMID: 27525816.

Chiu ML, Goulet DR, Teplyakov A, Gilliland GL. Antibody structure and function: the basis for engineering therapeutics. *Antibodies (Basel).* 2019;8(4):55. doi: 10.3390/antib8040055. PMID: 31816964; PMCID: PMC6963682.

Clarke J, Hurst C, Martin P, Vahle J, Ponce R, Mounho B, Heidel S, Andrews L, Reynolds T, Cavagnaro J. Duration of chronic toxicity studies for biotechnology-derived pharmaceuticals: is 6 months still appropriate? *Regul Toxicol Pharmacol.* 2008;50(1):2–22. doi: 10.1016/j.yrtph.2007.08.001. Epub 2007 Aug 24. PMID: 17998153.

Dahlén E, Veitonmäki N, Norlén P. Bispecific antibodies in cancer immunotherapy. *Ther Adv Vaccines Immunother.* 2018;6(1):3–17. doi: 10.1177/2515135518763280. Epub 2018 Mar 28. PMID: 29998217; PMCID: PMC5933537.

Davda J, Declerck P, Hu-Lieskovan S, Hickling TP, Jacobs IA, Chou J, Salek-Ardakani S, Kraynov E. Immunogenicity of immunomodulatory, antibody-based, oncology therapeutics. *J Immunother Cancer.* 2019;7(1):105. doi: 10.1186/s40425-019-0586-0. PMID: 30992085; PMCID: PMC6466770.

DeFrancesco L. COVID-19 antibodies on trial. *Nat Biotechnol.* 2020;38(11):1242–52. doi: 10.1038/s41587-020-0732–8. PMID: 33087898; PMCID: PMC7576980.

Deng R, Iyer S, Theil FP, Mortensen DL, Fielder PJ, Prabhu S. Projecting human pharmacokinetics of therapeutic antibodies from nonclinical data: what have we learned? *MAbs.* 2011;3(1):61–6. doi: 10.4161/mabs.3.1.13799. Epub 2011 Jan 1. PMID: 20962582; PMCID: PMC3038012.

Denny KH, Faqi AS. Nonclinical safety assessment of developmental and reproductive toxicology: considerations for conducting fertility, embryo–fetal development, and prenatal and postnatal developmental toxicology studies. In: *Methods in Pharmacology and Toxicology. Developmental and Reproductive Toxicology*, Faqi AS ed, Humana Press, New York, 2017.

Derzi M, Johnson TR, Shoieb AM, Conlon HD, Sharpe P, Saati A, Koob S, Bolt MW, Lorello LG, McNally J, Kirchhoff CF, Smolarek TA, Leach MW. Nonclinical Evaluation of PF-06438179: a potential biosimilar to Remicade® (Infliximab). *Adv Ther.* 2016;33(11):1964–82. doi: 10.1007/s12325-016-0403-9. Epub 2016 Sep 1. PMID: 27585978; PMCID: PMC5083783.

Derzi M, Shoieb AM, Ripp SL, Finch GL, Lorello LG, O'Neil SP, Radi Z, Syed J, Thompson MS, Leach MW. Comparative nonclinical assessments of the biosimilar PF-06410293 and originator adalimumab. *Regul Toxicol Pharmacol.* 2020;112:104587. doi: 10.1016/j.yrtph.2020.104587. Epub 2020 Jan 30. PMID: 32006671.

Descotes J. Immunotoxicity of monoclonal antibodies. *MAbs.* 2009;1(2):104–11. doi: 10.4161/mabs.1.2.7909. Epub 2009 Mar 19. PMID: 20061816; PMCID: PMC2725414.

DeSesso JM, Williams AL, Ahuja A, Bowman CJ, Hurtt ME. The placenta, transfer of immunoglobulins, and safety assessment of biopharmaceuticals in pregnancy. *Crit Rev Toxicol.* 2012;42(3):185–210. doi: 10.3109/10408444.2011.653487. PMID: 22348352.

Dingman R, Balu-Iyer SV. Immunogenicity of protein pharmaceuticals. *J Pharm Sci.* 2019;108(5):1637–54. doi: 10.1016/j.xphs.2018.12.014. Epub 2018 Dec 30. PMID: 30599169; PMCID: PMC6720129.

Dong JQ, Salinger DH, Endres CJ, Gibbs JP, Hsu CP, Stouch BJ, Hurh E, Gibbs MA. Quantitative prediction of human pharmacokinetics for monoclonal antibodies: retrospective analysis of monkey as a single species for first-in-human prediction. *Clin Pharmacokinet.* 2011;50(2):131–42. doi: 10.2165/11537430-000000000-00000. PMID: 21241072.

Eastwood D, Findlay L, Poole S, Bird C, Wadhwa M, Moore M, Burns C, Thorpe R, Stebbings R. Monoclonal antibody TGN1412 trial failure explained by species differences in CD28 expression on CD4+ effector memory T-cells. *Br J Pharmacol.* 2010;161(3):512–26. doi: 10.1111/j.1476-5381.2010.00922.x. PMID: 20880392; PMCID: PMC2990151.

Edelman GM. Dissociation of γ-globulin. *J Am Chem Soc.* 1959;81: 3155–56.

el Fouhil AF, Iskander FA, Turkall RM. Effect of alternate-day hydrocortisone therapy on the immunologically immature rat. II: Changes in T- and B-cell areas in spleen. *Toxicol Pathol.* 1993a;21(4):383–90. doi: 10.1177/019262339302100406. PMID: 8290870.

el Fouhil AF, Iskander FA, Turkall RM. Effect of alternate-day hydrocortisone therapy on the immunologically immature rat. III: changes in T- and B-cell areas in lymph nodes. *Toxicol Pathol.* 1993b;21(4):391–6. doi: 10.1177/019262339302100407. PMID: 8290871.

el Fouhil AF, Turkall RM. Effect of alternate-day hydrocortisone therapy on the immunologically immature rat. I: Effect on blood cell count, immunoglobulin concentrations, and body and organ weights. *Toxicol Pathol.* 1993;21(4):377–82. doi: 10.1177/019262339302100405. PMID: 8290869.

Elmore SA. Enhanced histopathology of the immune system: a review and update. *Toxicol Pathol.* 2012;40(2):148–56. doi: 10.1177/0192623311427571. Epub 2011 Nov 16. PMID: 22089843; PMCID: PMC3465566.

Evans EW. Regulatory forum commentary: is unexpected immunostimulation manageable in pharmaceutical development? *Toxicol Pathol.* 2014 Oct;42(7):1053–7. doi: 10.1177/0192623313513075. Epub 2013 Dec 4. PMID: 24304590.

Everds NE, Tarrant JM. Unexpected hematologic effects of biotherapeutics in nonclinical species and in humans. *Toxicol Pathol.* 2013;41(2):280–302. doi: 10.1177/0192623312467400. PMID: 23471185.

Expert Group on Phase One Clinical Trials (Chairman: Professor Gordon W. Duff): Final Report 2006; TSO (The Stationary Office). https://webarchive.nationalarchives.gov.uk/20130105090249/http://www.dh.gov.uk/en/Publicationsandstatistics/Publications/PublicationsPolicyAndGuidance/DH_063117.

Fagraeus A. Plasma cellular reaction and its relation to the formation of antibodies in vitro. *Nature.* 1947;159(4041):499. doi: 10.1038/159499a0. PMID: 20295228.

Fagraeus A. The plasma cellular reaction and its relation to the formation of antibodies in vitro. *J Immunol.* 1948;58(1):1–13. PMID: 18897986.

Fan YY, Avery LB, Wang M, O'Hara DM, Leung S, Neubert H. Tissue expression profile of human neonatal Fc receptor (FcRn) in Tg32 transgenic mice. *MAbs.* 2016;8(5):848–53. doi: 10.1080/19420862.2016.1178436. Epub 2016 Apr 22. PMID: 27104806; PMCID: PMC4968098.

Fathallah AM, Bankert RB, Balu-Iyer SV. Immunogenicity of subcutaneously administered therapeutic proteins--a mechanistic perspective. *AAPS J.* 2013;15(4):897–900. doi: 10.1208/s12248-013-9510-6. Epub 2013 Jul 16. PMID: 23856740; PMCID: PMC3787214.

Feyen O, Lueking A, Kowald A, Stephan C, Meyer HE, Göbel U, Niehues T. Off-target activity of TNF-alpha inhibitors characterized by protein biochips. *Anal Bioanal Chem.* 2008;391(5):1713–20. doi: 10.1007/s00216-008-1938-7. Epub 2008 Mar 16. PMID: 18344017.

Finlay WJJ, Coleman JE, Edwards JS, Johnson KS. Anti-PD1 'SHR-1210' aberrantly targets pro-angiogenic receptors and this polyspecificity can be ablated by paratope refinement. *MAbs.* 2019;11(1):26–44. doi: 10.1080/19420862.2018.1550321. Epub 2018 Dec 12. PMID: 30541416; PMCID: PMC6343799.

Frank SA. *Immunology and Evolution of Infectious Disease.* Princeton, NJ: Princeton University Press; 2002. Chapter 4, Specificity and Cross-Reactivity. Available from: https://www.ncbi.nlm.nih.gov/books/NBK2396/.

Gorovits B, Baltrukonis DJ, Bhattacharya I, Birchler MA, Finco D, Sikkema D, Vincent MS, Lula S, Marshall L, Hickling TP. Immunoassay methods used in clinical studies for the detection of anti-drug antibodies to adalimumab and infliximab. *Clin Exp Immunol.* 2018;192(3):348–65. doi: 10.1111/cei.13112. Epub 2018 Mar 30. PMID: 29431871; PMCID: PMC5980437.

Gorovits B, Clements-Egan A, Birchler M, Liang M, Myler H, Peng K, Purushothama S, Rajadhyaksha M, Salazar-Fontana L, Sung C, Xue L. Pre-existing antibody: biotherapeutic modality-based review. *AAPS J.* 2016;18(2):311–20. doi: 10.1208/s12248-016-9878-1. Epub 2016 Jan 28. PMID: 26821802; PMCID: PMC4779092.

Grimaldi C, Finco D, Fort MM, Gliddon D, Harper K, Helms WS, Mitchell JA, O'Lone R, Parish ST, Piche MS, Reed DM, Reichmann G, Ryan PC, Stebbings R, Walker M. Cytokine release: a workshop proceedings on the state-of-the-science, current challenges and future directions. *Cytokine.* 2016;85:101–8. doi: 10.1016/j.cyto.2016.06.006. Epub 2016 Jun 13. PMID: 27309676.

Halstead SB, O'Rourke EJ. Dengue viruses and mononuclear phagocytes. I. Infection enhancement by non-neutralizing antibody. *J Exp Med.* 1977;146(1):201–17. doi: 10.1084/jem.146.1.201. PMID: 406347; PMCID: PMC2180729.

Hamuro L, Kijanka G, Kinderman F, Kropshofer H, Bu DX, Zepeda M, Jawa V. Perspectives on subcutaneous route of administration as an immunogenicity risk factor for therapeutic proteins. *J Pharm Sci.* 2017;106(10):2946–54. doi: 10.1016/j.xphs.2017.05.030. Epub 2017 May 31. PMID: 28576695.

Hansen DK, LaBorde JB, Wall KS, Holson RR, Young JF. Pharmacokinetic considerations of dexamethasone-induced developmental toxicity in rats. *Toxicol Sci.* 1999;48(2):230–9. doi: 10.1093/toxsci/48.2.230. PMID: 10353314.

Harmsen MM, De Haard HJ. Properties, production, and applications of camelid single-domain antibody fragments. *Appl Microbiol Biotechnol.* 2007;77(1):13–22. doi: 10.1007/s00253-007-1142-2. Epub 2007 Aug 18. PMID: 17704915; PMCID: PMC2039825.

Hu W, Buetow B, Sachdeva K, Leach MW. Hepatic degeneration, necrosis, and fibrosis in rats associated with administration of ATR-107, a human anti-IL-21 receptor antibody. Manuscript in preparation.

Hünig T. The storm has cleared: lessons from the CD28 superagonist TGN1412 trial. *Nat Rev Immunol.* 2012;12(5):317–8. doi: 10.1038/nri3192. PMID: 22487653.

Hurst S, Ryan AM, Ng CK, McNally JM, Lorello LG, Finch GL, Leach MW, Ploch SA, Fohey JA, Smolarek TA. Comparative nonclinical assessments of the proposed biosimilar PF-05280014 and trastuzumab (Herceptin(®)). *BioDrugs.* 2014;28(5):451–9. doi: 10.1007/s40259-014-0103-4. PMID: 25001079; PMCID: PMC4176567.

Hutto DL. Opportunistic infections in non-human primates exposed to immunomodulatory biotherapeutics: considerations and case examples. *J Immunotoxicol.* 2010;7(2):120–7. doi: 10.3109/15476910903258252. PMID: 19909226.

ICH M3(R2): Guidance on Nonclinical Safety Studies for the Conduct of Human Clinical Trials and Marketing Authorization for Pharmaceuticals. 2009. https://www.ema.

europa.eu/en/documents/scientific-guideline/ich-guide-line-m3r2-non-clinical-safety-studies-conduct-human-clinical-trials-marketing-authorisation_en.pdf.

ICH M3(R2) Q&A: Guidance on Nonclinical Safety Studies for the Conduct of Human Clinical Trials and Marketing Authorization for Pharmaceuticals, Questions and Answers. 2012. https://www.ema.europa.eu/en/documents/other/international-conference-harmonisation-technical-requirements-registration-pharmaceuticals-human-use_en.pdf.

ICH S1A: Guideline on the Need for Carcinogenicity Studies of Pharmaceuticals. 1996. https://www.ema.europa.eu/en/documents/scientific-guideline/ich-s-1-need-carcinogenicity-studies-pharmaceuticals-step-5_en.pdf.

ICH S2(R1): Guidance on Genotoxicity Testing and Data Interpretation for Pharmaceuticals Intended for Human Use. 2012. https://www.ema.europa.eu/en/documents/scientific-guideline/ich-guideline-s2-r1-genotoxicity-testing-data-interpretation-pharmaceuticals-intended-human-use-step_en.pdf.

ICH S3A: Note for Guidance of Toxicokinetics: The Assessment of Systemic Exposure in Toxicity Studies. 1995. https://www.ema.europa.eu/en/documents/scientific-guideline/ich-s-3-toxicokinetics-guidance-assessing-systemic-exposure-toxicology-studies-step-5_en.pdf

ICH S5(R3): Detection of Reproductive and Developmental Toxicity for Human Pharmaceuticals. 2020. https://www.ema.europa.eu/en/documents/scientific-guideline/ich-s5-r3-guideline-reproductive-toxicology-detection-toxicity-reproduction-human-pharmaceuticals_en.pdf.

ICH S6(R1): Preclinical Safety Evaluation of Biotechnology-Derived Pharmaceuticals. 2011. https://www.ema.europa.eu/en/documents/scientific-guideline/ich-s6r1-preclinical-safety-evaluation-biotechnology-derived-pharmaceuticals-step-5_en.pdf

ICH S7A: Safety Pharmacology for Human Pharmaceuticals. 2001. https://www.ema.europa.eu/en/documents/scientific-guideline/ich-s-7-safety-pharmacology-studies-human-pharmaceuticals-step-5_en.pdf.

ICH S9: Nonclinical Evaluation of Anticancer Pharmaceuticals. 2010. https://www.ema.europa.eu/en/documents/scientific-guideline/ich-guideline-s9-non-clinical-evaluation-anticancer-pharmaceuticals-step-5_en.pdf.

ICH S9 Q&A: Nonclinical Evaluation of Anticancer Pharmaceuticals, Questions and Answers. 2018. https://www.ema.europa.eu/en/documents/scientific-guideline/ich-s9-guideline-nonclinical-evaluation-anticancer-pharmaceuticals-questions-answers-step-5_en.pdf.

ICH S11: Nonclinical Safety Testing in Support of Development of Paediatric Pharmaceuticals. 2020. https://www.ema.europa.eu/en/documents/scientific-guideline/ich-guideline-s11-nonclinical-safety-testing-support-development-paediatric-pharmaceuticals-step-5_en.pdf.

Jain T, Sun T, Durand S, Hall A, Houston NR, Nett JH, Sharkey B, Bobrowicz B, Caffry I, Yu Y, Cao Y, Lynaugh H, Brown M, Baruah H, Gray LT, Krauland EM, Xu Y, Vásquez M, Wittrup KD. Biophysical properties of the clinical-stage antibody landscape. *Proc Natl Acad Sci USA*. 2017;114(5):944–49. doi: 10.1073/pnas.1616408114. Epub 2017 Jan 17. PMID: 28096333; PMCID: PMC5293111.

James LC, Tawfik DS. The specificity of cross-reactivity: promiscuous antibody binding involves specific hydrogen bonds rather than nonspecific hydrophobic stickiness. *Protein Sci.* 2003;12(10):2183–93. doi: 10.1110/ps.03172703. PMID: 14500876; PMCID: PMC2366915.

Jefferis R. Antibody therapeutics: isotype and glycoform selection. *Expert Opin Biol Ther.* 2007;7(9):1401–13. doi: 10.1517/14712598.7.9.1401. PMID: 17727329.

Ji C, Roy MD, Golas J, Vitsky A, Ram S, Kumpf SW, Martin M, Barletta F, Meier WA, Hooper AT, Sapra P, Khan NK, Finkelstein M, Guffroy M, Buetow BS. Myocarditis in cynomolgus monkeys following treatment with immune checkpoint inhibitors. *Clin Cancer Res.* 2019;25(15):4735–48. doi: 10.1158/1078-0432.CCR-18-4083. Epub 2019 May 13. PMID: 31085720.

Jiang H, Chess L. How the immune system achieves self-nonself discrimination during adaptive immunity. *Adv Immunol.* 2009;102:95–133. doi: 10.1016/S0065-2776(09)01202-4. PMID: 19477320.

Kaur H, Salunke DM. Antibody promiscuity: understanding the paradigm shift in antigen recognition. *IUBMB Life.* 2015;67(7):498–505. doi: 10.1002/iub.1397. Epub 2015 Jul 15. PMID: 26177714.

Keler T, Halk E, Vitale L, O'Neill T, Blanset D, Lee S, Srinivasan M, Graziano RF, Davis T, Lonberg N, Korman A. Activity and safety of CTLA-4 blockade combined with vaccines in cynomolgus macaques. *J Immunol.* 2003;171(11):6251–9. doi: 10.4049/jimmunol.171.11.6251. PMID: 14634142.

Kerlin R, Bolon B, Burkhardt J, Francke S, Greaves P, Meador V, Popp J. Scientific and regulatory policy committee: recommended ("Best") practices for determining, communicating, and using adverse effect data from nonclinical studies. *Toxicol Pathol.* 2016;44(2):147–62. doi: 10.1177/0192623315623265. Epub 2015 Dec 23. PMID: 26704930.

Köhler G, Milstein C. Continuous cultures of fused cells secreting antibody of predefined specificity. *Nature.* 1975;256(5517):495–7. doi: 10.1038/256495a0. PMID: 1172191.

Krishnamurthy A, Jimeno A. Bispecific antibodies for cancer therapy: a review. *Pharmacol Ther.* 2018;185:122–34. doi: 10.1016/j.pharmthera.2017.12.002. Epub 2017 Dec 18. PMID: 29269044.

Kronenberg S, Husar E, Schubert C, Freichel C, Emrich T, Lechmann M, Giusti AM, Regenass F. Comparative assessment of immune complex-mediated hypersensitivity reactions with biotherapeutics in the non-human primate: Critical parameters, safety and lessons for future studies. *Regul Toxicol Pharmacol.* 2017;88:125–137. doi: 10.1016/j.yrtph.2017.06.004. Epub 2017 Jun 15. PMID: 28624430.

Leach MW. Immunogenicity-related effects in the liver of rats administered a human monoclonal antibody with a bell-shaped dose-response pattern. Presented at BioSafe General Membership Meeting, Cambridge, Massachusetts, April 28–30, 2010.

Leach MW. Regulatory forum opinion piece: differences between protein-based biologic products (biotherapeutics) and chemical entities (small molecules) of relevance to the toxicologic pathologist. *Toxicol Pathol.* 2013;41(1):128–36. doi: 10.1177/0192623312451371. Epub 2012 Jun 28. PMID: 22744226.

Leach MW, Halpern WG, Johnson CW, Rojko JL, MacLachlan TK, Chan CM, Galbreath EJ, Ndifor AM, Blanset DL, Polack E, Cavagnaro JA. Use of tissue cross-reactivity studies in the development of antibody-based biopharmaceuticals: history, experience, methodology, and future directions. *Toxicol Pathol.* 2010;38(7):1138–66. doi: 10.1177/0192623310382559. Epub 2010 Oct 6. PMID: 20926828.

Leach MW, Rottman JB, Hock MB, Finco D, Rojko JL, Beyer JC. Immunogenicity/hypersensitivity of biologics. *Toxicol Pathol.* 2014;42(1):293–300. doi: 10.1177/0192623313510987. Epub 2013 Nov 14. PMID: 24240973.

Lebrec HN. Regulatory forum opinion piece*: immunotoxicology assessments in nonhuman primates–challenges and opportunities. *Toxicol Pathol.* 2013;41(3):548–51. doi: 10.1177/0192623312455526. Epub 2012 Aug 10. PMID: 22886347.

Liu JK. The history of monoclonal antibody development: progress, remaining challenges and future innovations. *Ann Med Surg (Lond).* 2014;3(4):113–6. doi: 10.1016/j.amsu.2014.09.001. PMID: 25568796; PMCID: PMC4284445.

Llewelyn MB, Hawkins RE, Russell SJ. Discovery of antibodies. *BMJ.* 1992;305(6864):1269–72. doi: 10.1136/bmj.305.6864.1269. PMID: 1477573; PMCID: PMC1883762.

Lonberg N, Taylor LD, Harding FA, Trounstine M, Higgins KM, Schramm SR, Kuo CC, Mashayekh R, Wymore K, McCabe JG, et al. Antigen-specific human antibodies from mice comprising four distinct genetic modifications. *Nature.* 1994;368(6474):856–9. doi: 10.1038/368856a0. PMID: 8159246.

Luetjens CM, Fuchs A, Baker A, Weinbauer GF. Group size experiences with enhanced pre- and postnatal development studies in the long-tailed macaque (Macaca fascicularis). *Primate Biol.* 2020;7(1):1–4. doi: 10.5194/pb-7-1-2020. PMID: 32232119; PMCID: PMC7096737.

Mackness BC, Jaworski JA, Boudanova E, Park A, Valente D, Mauriac C, Pasquier O, Schmidt T, Kabiri M, Kandira A, Radošević K, Qiu H. Antibody Fc engineering for enhanced neonatal Fc receptor binding and prolonged circulation half-life. *MAbs.* 2019;11(7):1276–88. doi: 10.1080/19420862.2019.1633883. Epub 2019 Jul 18. PMID: 31216930; PMCID: PMC6748615.

MacLachlan TK, Price S, Cavagnaro J, Andrews L, Blanset D, Cosenza ME, Dempster M, Galbreath E, Giusti AM, Heinz-Taheny KM, Fleurance R, Sutter E, Leach MW. 2020. Classic and evolving approaches to evaluating cross reactivity of mAb and mAb-like molecules – a survey of industry 2008–2019. *Regul Toxicol Pharmacol.* 2021 Apr;121:104872. doi: 10.1016/j.yrtph.2021.104872. Epub 2021 Jan 22. PMID: 33485926.

Martin PL, Breslin W, Rocca M, Wright D, Cavagnaro J. Considerations in assessing the developmental and reproductive toxicity potential of biopharmaceuticals. *Birth Defects Res B Dev Reprod Toxicol.* 2009;86(3):176–203. doi: 10.1002/bdrb.20197. PMID: 19462404.

McCafferty J, Griffiths AD, Winter G, Chiswell DJ. Phage antibodies: filamentous phage displaying antibody variable domains. *Nature.* 1990;348(6301):552–4. doi: 10.1038/348552a0. PMID: 2247164.

Mease KM, Kimzey AL, Lansita JA. Biomarkers for nonclinical infusion reactions in marketed biotherapeutics and considerations for study design. *Curr Opin Toxicol.* 2017;4:1–15. doi: 10.1016/j.cotox.2017.03.005. PMID: 29658009; PMCID: PMC5893855.

Mecklenburg L, Luetjens CM, Weinbauer GF. Toxicologic pathology forum*: opinion on sexual maturity and fertility assessment in long-tailed macaques (Macaca fascicularis) in nonclinical safety studies. *Toxicol Pathol.* 2019;47(4):444–460. doi: 10.1177/0192623319831009. Epub 2019 Mar 21. PMID: 30898082.

Meyer S, Leusen JH, Boross P. Regulation of complement and modulation of its activity in monoclonal antibody therapy of cancer. *MAbs.* 2014;6(5):1133–44. doi: 10.4161/mabs.29670. Epub 2014 Oct 30. PMID: 25517299; PMCID: PMC4622586.

Moore GL, Chen H, Karki S, Lazar GA. Engineered Fc variant antibodies with enhanced ability to recruit complement and mediate effector functions. *MAbs.* 2010;2(2):181–9. doi: 10.4161/mabs.2.2.11158. PMID: 20150767; PMCID: PMC2840237.

Nagelkerke SQ, Schmidt DE, de Haas M, Kuijpers TW. Genetic variation in low-to-medium-affinity Fcγ receptors: functional consequences, disease associations, and opportunities for personalized medicine. *Front Immunol.* 2019;10:2237. doi: 10.3389/fimmu.2019.02237. PMID: 31632391; PMCID: PMC6786274.

Ober RJ, Radu CG, Ghetie V, Ward ES. Differences in promiscuity for antibody-FcRn interactions across species: implications for therapeutic antibodies. *Int Immunol.* 2001;13(12):1551–9. doi: 10.1093/intimm/13.12.1551. PMID: 11717196.

Oitate M, Masubuchi N, Ito T, Yabe Y, Karibe T, Aoki T, Murayama N, Kurihara A, Okudaira N, Izumi T. Prediction of human pharmacokinetics of therapeutic monoclonal antibodies from simple allometry of monkey data. *Drug Metab Pharmacokinet.* 2011;26(4):423–30. doi: 10.2133/dmpk.dmpk-11-rg-011. Epub 2011 May 24. PMID: 21606605.

Ordman CW, Jennings CG, Janeway CA. Chemical, clinical, and immunological studies on the products of human plasma fractionation. XII. The use of concentrated normal human serum gamma globulin (human immune serum globulin) in the prevention and attenuation of measles. *J Clin Invest.* 1944;23(4):541–549. https://doi.org/10.1172/JCI101519.

Ovacik M, Lin K. Tutorial on monoclonal antibody pharmacokinetics and its considerations in early development. *Clin Transl Sci.* 2018;11(6):540–552. doi: 10.1111/cts.12567. Epub 2018 Aug 7. PMID: 29877608; PMCID: PMC6226118.

Paglialunga S, Morimoto BH, Clark M, Friedrichs GS. Translatability of the S7A core battery respiratory safety pharmacology studies: preclinical respiratory and related clinical adverse events. *J Pharmacol Toxicol Methods.* 2019;99:106596. doi: 10.1016/j.vascn.2019.106596. Epub 2019 Jun 5. PMID: 31173885.

Palazzi X, Burkhardt JE, Caplain H, Dellarco V, Fant P, Foster JR, Francke S, Germann P, Gröters S, Harada T, Harleman J, Inui K, Kaufmann W, Lenz B, Nagai H, Pohlmeyer-Esch G, Schulte A, Skydsgaard M, Tomlinson L, Wood CE, Yoshida M. Characterizing "Adversity" of pathology findings in nonclinical toxicity studies: results from the 4th ESTP International Expert Workshop. *Toxicol Pathol.* 2016;44(6):810–24. doi: 10.1177/0192623316642527. Epub 2016 Apr 21. PMID: 27102650.

Palomo C, Mas V, Detalle L, Depla E, Cano O, Vázquez M, Stortelers C, Melero JA. Trivalency of a nanobody specific for the human respiratory syncytial virus fusion glycoprotein drastically enhances virus neutralization and impacts escape mutant selection. *Antimicrob Agents Chemother.* 2016;60(11):6498–509. doi: 10.1128/AAC.00842-16. PMID:27550346; PMCID: PMC5075053.

Pandher K, Leach MW, Burns-Naas LA. Appropriate use of recovery groups in nonclinical toxicity studies: value in a science-driven case-by-case approach. *Vet Pathol.* 2012;49(2):357–61. doi: 10.1177/0300985811415701. Epub 2011 Aug 1. PMID: 21810619.

Papich MG. Dexamethasone. In: *Saunders Handbook of Veterinary Drugs* (4th Ed), Elsevier, Missouri, 2016, pp. 217–19. ISBN: 978-0-323–24485-5. https://doi.org/10.1016/B978-0-323-24485-5.00001-2.

Parren PWHI, Carter PJ, Plückthun A. Changes to International Nonproprietary Names for antibody therapeutics 2017 and beyond: of mice, men and more. *MAbs.* 2017;9(6):898–906. doi: 10.1080/19420862.2017.1341029. Epub 2017 Jun 16. PMID: 28621572; PMCID: PMC5590622.

Peraza MA, Rule KE, Shiue MHI, Finch GL, Thibault S, Brown PR, Clarke DW, Leach MW. Nonclinical assessments of the potential biosimilar PF-06439535 and bevacizumab. *Regul Toxicol Pharmacol.* 2018;95:236–43. doi: 10.1016/j.yrtph.2018.03.020. Epub 2018 Mar 21. PMID: 29574193.

Perry R, Farris G, Bienvenu JG, Dean C Jr, Foley G, Mahrt C, Short B; Society of Toxicologic Pathology. Society of Toxicologic Pathology position paper on best practices on recovery studies: the role of the anatomic pathologist. *Toxicol Pathol.* 2013;41(8):1159–69. doi: 10.1177/0192623313481513. Epub 2013 Mar 26. PMID: 23531793.

Ponce R, Abad L, Amaravadi L, Gelzleichter T, Gore E, Green J, Gupta S, Herzyk D, Hurst C, Ivens IA, Kawabata T, Maier C, Mounho B, Rup B, Shankar G, Smith H, Thomas P, Wierda D. Immunogenicity of biologically-derived therapeutics: assessment and interpretation of nonclinical safety studies. *Regul Toxicol Pharmacol.* 2009;54(2):164–82. doi: 10.1016/j.yrtph.2009.03.012. Epub 2009 Apr 2. PMID: 19345250.

Porter RR. The hydrolysis of rabbit y-globulin and antibodies with crystalline papain. *Biochem J.* 1959; 73, 119–26.

Pothin E, Lesuisse D, Lafaye P. Brain delivery of single-domain antibodies: a focus on VHH and VNAR. *Pharmaceutics.* 2020;12(10):937. doi: 10.3390/pharmaceutics12100937. PMID: 33007904; PMCID: PMC7601373.

Ramaiah L, Tomlinson L, Tripathi NK, Cregar LC, Vitsky A, Beust BV, Barlow VG, Reagan WJ, Ennulat D. Principles for assessing adversity in toxicologic clinical pathology. *Toxicol Pathol.* 2017;45(2):260–6. doi: 10.1177/0192623316681646. Epub 2017 Jan 5. PMID: 28056663.

Reijers JAA, Malone KE, Bajramovic JJ, Verbeek R, Burggraaf J, Moerland M. Adverse immunostimulation caused by impurities: the dark side of biopharmaceuticals. *Br J Clin Pharmacol.* 2019;85(7):1418–26. doi: 10.1111/bcp.13938. Epub 2019 May 29. Erratum in: *Br J Clin Pharmacol.* 2019 Sep;85(9):2182. PMID: 30920013; PMCID: PMC6595286.

Ribatti D. From the discovery of monoclonal antibodies to their therapeutic application: an historical reappraisal. *Immunol Lett.* 2014;161(1):96–9. doi: 10.1016/j.imlet.2014.05.010. Epub 2014 May 27. PMID: 24877873.

Rocca M, Morford LL, Blanset DL, Halpern WG, Cavagnaro J, Bowman CJ. Applying a weight of evidence approach to the evaluation of developmental toxicity of biopharmaceuticals. *Regul Toxicol Pharmacol.* 2018;98:69–79. doi: 10.1016/j.yrtph.2018.07.006. Epub 2018 Jul 24. PMID: 30009863.

Rojko JL, Evans MG, Price SA, Han B, Waine G, DeWitte M, Haynes J, Freimark B, Martin P, Raymond JT, Evering W, Rebelatto MC, Schenck E, Horvath C. Formation, clearance, deposition, pathogenicity, and identification of biopharmaceutical-related immune complexes: review and case studies. *Toxicol Pathol.* 2014;42(4):725–64. doi:10.1177/0192623314526475

Roopenian DC, Akilesh S. FcRn: the neonatal Fc receptor comes of age. *Nat Rev Immunol.* 2007;7(9):715–25. doi: 10.1038/nri2155. Epub 2007 Aug 17. PMID: 17703228.

Rudmann DG, Page TJ, Vahle JL, Chouinard L, Haile S, Poitout F, Baskin G, Lambert AJ, Walker P, Glazier G, Awori M, Bernier L. Rat-specific decreases in platelet count caused by a humanized monoclonal antibody against sclerostin. *Toxicol Sci.* 2012;125(2):586–94. doi: 10.1093/toxsci/kfr318. Epub 2011 Nov 21. PMID: 22106037.

Ryan AM, Sokolowski SA, Ng CK, Shirai N, Collinge M, Shen AC, Arrington J, Radi Z, Cummings TR, Ploch SA, Stephenson SA, Tripathi NK, Hurst SI, Finch GL, Leach MW. Comparative nonclinical assessments of the proposed biosimilar PF-05280586 and rituximab (MabThera®). *Toxicol Pathol.* 2014;42(7):1069–81. doi: 10.1177/0192623313520351. Epub 2014 Mar 6. PMID: 24604381.

Santostefano MJ, Kirchner J, Vissinga C, Fort M, Lear S, Pan WJ, Prince PJ, Hensley KM, Tran D, Rock D, Vargas HM, Narayanan P, Jawando R, Rees W, Reindel JF, Reynhardt K, Everds N. Off-target platelet activation in macaques unique to a therapeutic monoclonal antibody. *Toxicol Pathol.* 2012;40(6):899–917. doi: 10.1177/0192623312444029. Epub 2012 May 2. PMID: 22552394.

Saunders KO. Conceptual approaches to modulating antibody effector functions and circulation half-life. *Front Immunol.* 2019;10:1296. doi: 10.3389/fimmu.2019.01296. PMID: 31231397; PMCID: PMC6568213.

Schlothauer T, Herter S, Koller CF, Grau-Richards S, Steinhart V, Spick C, Kubbies M, Klein C, Umaña P, Mössner E. Novel human IgG1 and IgG4 Fc-engineered antibodies with completely abolished immune effector functions. *Protein Eng Des Sel.* 2016;29(10):457–66. doi: 10.1093/protein/gzw040. Epub 2016 Aug 29. PMID: 27578889.

Schroeder HW Jr, Cavacini L. Structure and function of immunoglobulins. *J Allergy Clin Immunol.* 2010;125(2 Suppl 2):S41–52. doi: 10.1016/j.jaci.2009.09.046. PMID: 20176268; PMCID: PMC3670108.

Selby MJ, Engelhardt JJ, Johnston RJ, Lu LS, Han M, Thudium K, Yao D, Quigley M, Valle J, Wang C, Chen B, Cardarelli PM, Blanset D, Korman AJ. Preclinical development of ipilimumab and nivolumab combination immunotherapy: mouse tumor models, in vitro functional studies, and cynomolgus macaque toxicology. *PLoS One.* 2016;11(9):e0161779. doi: 10.1371/journal.pone.0161779. Erratum in: *PLoS One.* 2016 Nov 18;11(11):e0167251. PMID: 27610613; PMCID: PMC5017747.

Sewell F, Chapman K, Baldrick P, Brewster D, Broadmeadow A, Brown P, Burns-Naas LA, Clarke J, Constan A, Couch J, Czupalla O, Danks A, DeGeorge J, de Haan

L, Hettinger K, Hill M, Festag M, Jacobs A, Jacobson-Kram D, Kopytek S, Lorenz H, Moesgaard SG, Moore E, Pasanen M, Perry R, Ragan I, Robinson S, Schmitt PM, Short B, Lima BS, Smith D, Sparrow S, van Bekkum Y, Jones D. Recommendations from a global cross-company data sharing initiative on the incorporation of recovery phase animals in safety assessment studies to support first-in-human clinical trials. *Regul Toxicol Pharmacol.* 2014;70(1):413–29. doi: 10.1016/j.yrtph.2014.07.018. Epub 2014 Jul 29. PMID: 25078890.

Shawler DL, Bartholomew RM, Smith LM, Dillman RO. Human immune response to multiple injections of murine monoclonal IgG. *J Immunol.* 1985;135(2):1530–5. PMID: 3874237.

Shimabukuro-Vornhagen A, Gödel P, Subklewe M, Stemmler HJ, Schlößer HA, Schlaak M, Kochanek M, Böll B, von Bergwelt-Baildon MS. Cytokine release syndrome. *J Immunother Cancer.* 2018;6(1):56. doi: 10.1186/s40425-018-0343-9. PMID: 29907163; PMCID: PMC6003181.

Stanfield RL, Wilson IA. Antibody structure. *Microbiol Spectr.* 2014;2(2). doi: 10.1128/microbiolspec.AID-0012-2013. PMID: 26105818.

Starr CG, Tessier PM. Selecting and engineering monoclonal antibodies with drug-like specificity. *Curr Opin Biotechnol.* 2019;60:119–27. doi: 10.1016/j.copbio.2019.01.008. Epub 2019 Feb 26. PMID: 30822699; PMCID: PMC6829062.

Stokes Jr J, Maris EP, Gellis SS. Chemical, clinical, and immunological studies on the products of human plasma fractionation. XI. The use of concentrated normal human serum gamma globulin (human immune serum globulin) in the prophylaxis and treatment of measles. *J Clin Invest.* 1944;23(4):531–40. https://doi.org/10.1172/JCI101518.

Strohl WR, Strohl LM. Interactions of human IgGs with non-human systems. In: *Therapeutic Antibody Engineering: Current and Future Advances Driving the Strongest Growth Area in the Pharmaceutical Industry.* Woodhead Publishing, 2012, pp. 405–420.

Suntharalingam G, Perry MR, Ward S, Brett SJ, Castello-Cortes A, Brunner MD, Panoskaltsis N. Cytokine storm in a phase 1 trial of the anti-CD28 monoclonal antibody TGN1412. *N Engl J Med.* 2006;355(10):1018–28. doi: 10.1056/NEJMoa063842. Epub 2006 Aug 14. PMID: 16908486.

Tabares P, Berr S, Römer PS, Chuvpilo S, Matskevich AA, Tyrsin D, Fedotov Y, Einsele H, Tony HP, Hünig T. Human regulatory T cells are selectively activated by low-dose application of the CD28 superagonist TGN1412/TAB08. *Eur J Immunol.* 2014;44(4):1225–36. doi: 10.1002/eji.201343967. Epub 2014 Feb 1. PMID: 24374661.

Talmage DW. Allergy and immunology. *Annu Rev Med.* 1957;8:239–56. doi: 10.1146/annurev.me.08.020157.001323. PMID: 13425332.

Tanyol H, Rehfuss ME. Hepatotoxic effect of cortisone in experimental animals. *Am J Dig Dis.* 1955;22(6):169–73. doi: 10.1007/BF02886003. PMID: 14376366.

Teicher BA, Chari RV. Antibody conjugate therapeutics: challenges and potential. *Clin Cancer Res.* 2011;17(20):6389–97. doi: 10.1158/1078-0432.CCR-11-1417. PMID: 22003066.

The Nobel Prize. Emil von Behring Biography. Accessed 24 Jul 2020. https://www.nobelprize.org/prizes/medicine/1901/behring/biographical/.

The Nobel Prize in Physiology or Medicine 1901. NobelPrize.org. Nobel Media AB 2020. Accessed 24 Jul 2020. https://www.nobelprize.org/prizes/medicine/1901/summary/.

The Nobel Prize in Physiology or Medicine 1972. NobelPrize.org. Nobel Media AB 2020. Accessed 24 Jul 2020. https://www.nobelprize.org/prizes/medicine/1972/summary/.

The Nobel Prize in Physiology or Medicine 1984. NobelPrize.org. Nobel Media AB 2020. Accessed 24 Jul 2020. https://www.nobelprize.org/prizes/medicine/1984/summary/.

Thomas A, Teicher BA, Hassan R. Antibody-drug conjugates for cancer therapy. *Lancet Oncol.* 2016;17(6):e254–62. doi: 10.1016/S1470-2045(16)30030-4. PMID: 27299281; PMCID: PMC6601617.

Turner MR, Balu-Iyer SV. Challenges and opportunities for the subcutaneous delivery of therapeutic proteins. *J Pharm Sci.* 2018;107(5):1247–60. doi: 10.1016/j.xphs.2018.01.007. Epub 2018 Jan 11. PMID: 29336981; PMCID: PMC5915922.

US FDA. Guidance for Industry: Developing Medical Imaging Drug and Biological Products. Part 1: Conducting Safety Assessments. 2004. https://www.fda.gov/media/71237/download.

US FDA. Guidance for Industry: Nonproprietary Naming of Biological Products. 2017. https://www.fda.gov/media/93218/download.

US FDA. Points to Consider in the Manufacture and Testing of Monoclonal Antibody Products. 1983/1987/1994/1997. https://www.fda.gov/media/76798/download.

Vafa O, Gilliland GL, Brezski RJ, Strake B, Wilkinson T, Lacy ER, Scallon B, Teplyakov A, Malia TJ, Strohl WR. An engineered Fc variant of an IgG eliminates all immune effector functions via structural perturbations. *Methods.* 2014;65(1):114–26. doi: 10.1016/j.ymeth.2013.06.035. Epub 2013 Jul 17. PMID: 23872058.

Vahle JL, Long GG, Sandusky G, Westmore M, Ma YL, Sato M. Bone neoplasms in F344 rats given teriparatide [rhPTH(1–34)] are dependent on duration of treatment and dose. *Toxicol Pathol.* 2004;32(4):426–38. doi: 10.1080/01926230490462138. PMID: 15204966.

van Regenmortel MH. Specificity, polyspecificity, and heterospecificity of antibody-antigen recognition. *J Mol Recognit.* 2014;27(11):627–39. doi: 10.1002/jmr.2394. PMID: 25277087.

van Schie KA, Wolbink GJ, Rispens T. Cross-reactive and pre-existing antibodies to therapeutic antibodies–Effects on treatment and immunogenicity. *MAbs.* 2015;7(4):662–71. doi: 10.1080/19420862.2015.1048411. PMID: 25962087; PMCID: PMC4623040.

van Schouwenburg PA, van de Stadt LA, de Jong RN, van Buren EE, Kruithof S, de Groot E, Hart M, van Ham SM, Rispens T, Aarden L, Wolbink GJ, Wouters D. Adalimumab elicits a restricted anti-idiotypic antibody response in autoimmune patients resulting in functional neutralisation. *Ann Rheum Dis.* 2013;72(1):104–9. doi: 10.1136/annrheumdis-2012-201445. Epub 2012 Jul 3. PMID: 22759910.

Vargas HM, Amouzadeh HR, Engwall MJ. Nonclinical strategy considerations for safety pharmacology: evaluation of biopharmaceuticals. *Expert Opin Drug Saf.* 2013;12(1):91–102. doi: 10.1517/14740338.2013.745851. Epub 2012 Nov 21. PMID: 23170873.

Vargas HM, Bass AS, Breidenbach A, Feldman HS, Gintant GA, Harmer AR, Heath B, Hoffmann P, Lagrutta A, Leishman D, McMahon N, Mittelstadt S, Polonchuk L, Pugsley MK, Salata JJ, Valentin JP. Scientific review and recommendations on preclinical cardiovascular safety evaluation of biologics. *J Pharmacol Toxicol Methods.* 2008;58(2):72–6. doi: 10.1016/j.vascn.2008.04.001. Epub 2008 Apr 18. PMID: 18508287.

Vidarsson G, Dekkers G, Rispens T. IgG subclasses and allotypes: from structure to effector functions. *Front Immunol.* 2014;20(5):520. doi: 10.3389/fimmu.2014.00520. PMID: 25368619; PMCID: PMC4202688.

Viret C, Gurr W. The origin of the "one cell-one antibody" rule. *J Immunol.* 2009;182(3):1229–30. doi: 10.4049/jimmunol.182.3.1229. PMID: 19155464.

von Behring E, Kitasato S. (1890). Ueber das Zustandekommen Der Diphtherie-Immunität Und der Tetanus-Immunität Bei Thieren. *Dtsch Med Wochenschr* 49, 1113–4.

Waibler Z, Sender LY, Kamp C, Müller-Berghaus J, Liedert B, Schneider CK, Löwer J, Kalinke U. Toward experimental assessment of receptor occupancy: TGN1412 revisited. *J Allergy Clin Immunol.* 2008;122(5):890–2. doi: 10.1016/j.jaci.2008.07.049. Epub 2008 Sep 20. PMID: 18805577.

Wang C, Thudium KB, Han M, Wang XT, Huang H, Feingersh D, Garcia C, Wu Y, Kuhne M, Srinivasan M, Singh S, Wong S, Garner N, Leblanc H, Bunch RT, Blanset D, Selby MJ, Korman AJ. In vitro characterization of the anti-PD-1 antibody nivolumab, BMS-936558, and in vivo toxicology in non-human primates. *Cancer Immunol Res.* 2014;2(9):846–56. doi: 10.1158/2326-6066.CIR-14-0040. Epub 2014 May 28. PMID: 24872026.

Wang X, Mathieu M, Brezski RJ. IgG Fc engineering to modulate antibody effector functions. *Protein Cell.* 2018;9(1):63–73. doi: 10.1007/s13238-017-0473-8. Epub 2017 Oct 6. PMID: 28986820; PMCID: PMC5777978.

Weinbauer GF, Fuchs A, Niehaus M, Luetjens CM. The enhanced pre- and postnatal study for nonhuman primates: update and perspectives. *Birth Defects Res C Embryo Today.* 2011;93(4):324–33. doi: 10.1002/bdrc.20220. PMID: 2227 1681.

Weinbauer GF, Luft J, Fuchs A. The enhanced pre- and postnatal development study for monoclonal antibodies. *Methods Mol Biol.* 2013;947:185–200. doi: 10.1007/978-1-62703-131-8_15. PMID: 23138905.

Weinreich DM, Sivapalasingam S, Norton T, Ali S, Gao H, Bhore R, Musser BJ, Soo Y, Rofail D, Im J, Perry C, Pan C, Hosain R, Mahmood A, Davis JD, Turner KC, Hooper AT, Hamilton JD, Baum A, Kyratsous CA, Kim Y, Cook A, Kampman W, Kohli A, Sachdeva Y, Graber X, Kowal B, DiCioccio T, Stahl N, Lipsich L, Braunstein N, Herman G, Yancopoulos GD; Trial Investigators. REGN-COV2, a Neutralizing Antibody Cocktail, in Outpatients with Covid-19. *N Engl J Med.* 2020 doi: 10.1056/NEJMoa2035002. Epub ahead of print. PMID: 33332778.

WHO. Guidelines on the Use of International Nonproprietary Names (INNs) for Pharmaceutical Substances. WHO/PHARM S/NOM 1570. 1997. https://apps.who.int/iris/bitstream/handle/10665/63779/WHO_PHARM_S_NOM_1570.pdf?sequence=1&isAllowed=y.

WHO. WHO Drug Information Vol 23, No. 3, 2009. https://www.who.int/medicines/publications/druginformation/issues/DrugInfo09_Vol23-3.pdf.

WHO. 64th Consultation on International Nonproprietary Names for Pharmaceutical Substances, Geneva, 4–7 April 2017. INN Working Doc. 17.469. https://www.who.int/medicines/services/inn/64th_Executive_Summary.pdf?ua=1.

WHO. Revised Monoclonal Antibody (mAb) Nomenclature Scheme. Geneva, 26 May 2017. INN Working Doc. 17.416. https://www.who.int/medicines/services/inn/Revised_mAb_nomenclature_scheme.pdf.

Wright DJ, Adkins KK, Minck DR, Bailey S, Warner G, Leach MW. Reproductive performance and early postnatal development in interleukin (IL)-13-deficient mice. *Birth Defects Res B Dev Reprod Toxicol.* 2012;95(5):346–53. doi: 10.1002/bdrb.21023. Epub 2012 Aug 28. PMID: 22930549.

Wu H, Pfarr DS, Johnson S, Brewah YA, Woods RM, Patel NK, White WI, Young JF, Kiener PA. Development of motavizumab, an ultra-potent antibody for the prevention of respiratory syncytial virus infection in the upper and lower respiratory tract. *J Mol Biol.* 2007;368(3):652–65. doi: 10.1016/j.jmb.2007.02.024. Epub 2007 Feb 20. PMID: 17362988.

Wu L, Seung E, Xu L, Rao E, Lord DM, Wei RR, Cortez-Retamozo V, Ospina B, Posternak V, Ulinski G, Piepenhagen P, Francesconi E, El-Murr N, Beil C, Kirby P, Li A, Fretland J, Vicente R, Deng G, Dabdoubi T, Cameron B, BertrandT, Ferrari P, Pouzieux S, Lemoine C, Prades C, Park A, Qiu H, Song Z, Zhang B, Sun F, Chiron M, Rao S, Radošević K, Yang Z-y, Nabel GJ. Trispecific antibodies enhance the therapeutic efficacy of tumor-directed T cells through T cell receptor co-stimulation. *Nat Cancer.* 2020;1:86–98. https://doi.org/10.1038/s43018-019-0004-z.

Xue L, Rup B. Evaluation of pre-existing antibody presence as a risk factor for posttreatment anti-drug antibody induction: analysis of human clinical study data for multiple biotherapeutics. *AAPS J.* 2013;15(3):893–6. doi: 10.1208/s12248-013-9497-z. Epub 2013 Jun 13. PMID: 23761225; PMCID: PMC3691441.

Zhao Q. Bispecific antibodies for autoimmune and inflammatory diseases: clinical progress to date. *BioDrugs.* 2020; 34(2):111–9. doi: 10.1007/s40259-019-00400-2. PMID: 319 16225.

Zuch de Zafra CL, Ashkenazi A, Darbonne WC, Cheu M, Totpal K, Ortega S, Flores H, Walker MD, Kabakoff B, Lum BL, Mounho-Zamora BJ, Marsters SA, Dybdal NO. Antitherapeutic antibody-mediated hepatotoxicity of recombinant human Apo2L/TRAIL in the cynomolgus monkey. *Cell Death Dis.* 2016;7(8):e2338. doi: 10.1038/cddis.2016.241. PMID: 27512959; PMCID: PMC5108326.

21

Nonclinical Safety Evaluation of Therapies for Rare Diseases

K. McKeever
Ultragenyx Pharmaceutical

T. MacLachlan
Novartis Institutes for Biomedical Research

CONTENTS

21.1 Introduction

With the rapid progress in the fields of genetics and biotechnology, diagnosis and treatment of various genetic and/or other life-threatening diseases affecting very small populations is becoming a reality for an ever-increasing number of indications, many in pediatric patients. The efficiency of genome sequencing and identification of both genetic and protein biomarkers enable clinicians to identify the causes of pediatric maladies even before the development of symptoms. On the treatment side, while small molecule drugs and large molecule protein-based therapies have made a significant impact on symptoms and rate of disease progression in this patient population, an expanding array of alternative modalities such as cell- and gene-based therapies and gene-modified cell-based therapies provide exciting platforms whereby innovation could hopefully lead to cures.

As tends to be the case with any new technology, fitting into established processes/paradigms is challenging. While the principles of preclinical safety evaluation are consistent across the various modalities, the practices have evolved based upon an understanding of the specific product attributes. This customized approach is referred to as the "case-by-case" approach per the International Conference on Harmonisation (ICH) of Technical Requirements for Pharmaceuticals S6 guidance [1]. However, the timing and types of studies to support clinical development are generally similar across modalities and disease indications (ICH M3) [2] with the exception of cancer (ICH S9) [3]. For cancer, based on a risk/benefit consideration for a life-threatening disease, ICH S9 provides sponsors/developers of cancer therapies the opportunity to apply a scientifically justified targeted, sometimes reduced, preclinical package to support initial clinical trials as well as marketing approval.

DOI: 10.1201/9781003124542-24

An explicit intent of ICH S9 was to encourage innovation and an earlier access for the assessment of efficacy and safety in humans. Rare diseases are often chronic, progressive, debilitating and frequently life-threatening. At the very least for genetic diseases, there usually is a certainty of disease progression, which may ultimately lead to blindness, deafness, various levels of physical impairment or in some cases death. As with oncology, there is a critical imperative to optimize and streamline preclinical development programs, including reducing the burden of unnecessary studies, to ensure that innovation continues and cures can more expeditiously be realized.

There has been some discussion in the literature and recent scientific meetings regarding extending the development path similar to the path outlined in ICH S9 for cancer therapeutics for other indications. A review by Prescott et al. [4] highlighted the need to accelerate therapies for indications termed "Severely debilitating or life-threatening" (SDLT) diseases, which in addition to including certain life-threatening rare diseases such as Tay-Sachs disease would also cover more common diseases such as advanced Parkinson's disease, Lupus nephritis and notably severe congenital heart failure. FDA has recently published two draft guidances [5,6] addressing rare disease drug development and enzyme replacement therapy (ERT) in particular. In both, options are provided for sponsors to propose a reduced nonclinical package prior to reaching the clinic, as well as considerations for use of animal models of disease for pivotal nonclinical safety studies. Finally, in April 2018, FDA released a guidance directed at "Severely debilitating life-threatening hematopoietic diseases" or "SDLTHDs" that implemented several of the strategies for nonclinical development of anticancer drugs in ICH S9 as well as others allowing for use of animal models of disease in certain circumstances [7]. As such, the regulatory landscape is changing in favor of accelerating delivery of rare disease therapies to patients.

This chapter will focus on the unique considerations for rare and SDLT disease therapy preclinical safety assessment, with a particular focus on the most fully developed category of rare disease therapies, the ERTs including recombinant protein and gene therapy modalities, and what sponsors could do to accelerate getting their products to first-in-human (FIH) testing.

21.2 Historical Background of Therapies for Rare Diseases

Orphan rare diseases have been characterized in the USA as those populations that affect less than 200,000 patients. There exist more than 6,800 of these diseases, and approximately 35% of infantile deaths worldwide can be attributed to these indications [8]. In the USA, the Orphan Drug Act of 1983 invigorated drug development activity in this area [9]. The Act allows for a designation that, if granted, provides several incentives to sponsors such as tax credits, grants for research, fast track review opportunities and market exclusivity once approved. After the Orphan Drug Act was approved in 1983, the number of drug approvals for these indications skyrocketed, with almost 250 individual drugs on the market by 2010, and about half of those coming in the first 4 years of enactment of the law [10], and has continued to rise in recent years, with 41% of drugs approved in the USA in 2014 (17/41) falling in the orphan category [11]. Similarly, a positive opinion from the Committee for Orphan Medicinal Products in the European Commission led to the approval of 85 orphan drugs by 2015 [12]. While several of the initial approvals were in rare cancer indications such as osteosarcoma, gastrointestinal stromal tumors, renal cell carcinoma and several forms of blood-borne cancers, within the last 10 years, many more non-oncology indications have entered into this paradigm with the lysosomal storage diseases taking the lead (Pompe, mucopolysaccharidosis, Fabry's, Gaucher's, etc.) and other syndromes like pulmonary arterial hypertension, hyperammonemia and idiopathic thrombocytopenia.

Lysosomal storage disorders (LSDs) can be generally characterized as a group of inherited diseases that result from a deficiency in one or more of the 80 metabolic enzymes or transporters that are key components of lysosomes [1–3]. A reduction or loss of one or more of these activities results in the progressive and relentless accumulation of undegraded macromolecules, a consequent derangement of proper lysosomal and autophagosomal functions, and ultimately cellular demise. However, the precise mechanistic links between these altered biochemical and cellular states and disease pathophysiology and pathogenesis remain unclear. Typically, disease severity is correlated with the level of residual activity, with individuals harboring lower levels presenting with more aggressive and severe disease manifestations. Although individually each LSD may be relatively rare, as a group, these disorders have an incidence of approximately 1 per 5,000 live births [8,9].

The first LSD to have a developed therapy is the most common of this class of rare diseases, Gaucher disease. Type 1 Gaucher disease has an incidence of approximately 1 in 20,000 and is characterized by an accumulation of glucocerebroside in several organs including spleen, liver and kidney. The original source for glucocerebrosidase was purification from human placenta, which after treatment with enzymes to expose attached mannose was effective in reducing glucocerebroside in both animals and patients; however, the yield was exceptionally low with only 330 mg enzyme resulting from an input of 1.7 kg placenta. This enzyme has now been withdrawn and replaced with Imiglucerase (Cerezyme™), which is a recombinant glucocerebrosidase produced in CHO cells, approved in 1994. It took several more years for the next ERT to be approved, Agalsidase alfa and beta (Fabrazyme, Replagal) in 2001 and 2003, respectively. Since then, several more ERTs have been approved for the treatment of mucopolysaccharidosis I, II and VI, Pompe disease and lysosomal acid lipase deficiency (see Table 21.1). The production of these enzymes can be very challenging considering the posttranslational modifications that these enzymes undergo. Indeed, Myozyme that was originally approved in 2006 after changing production scales harbored a different glycosylation pattern. While the molecules appeared to have similar efficacy, because of the changes in glycosylation, the new version of alglucosidase was given a new name, Lumizyme.

TABLE 21.1

Approved Enzyme Replacement Therapies

a. Product	b. Enzyme	c. Disorder	d. Regulatory Approval
Ceredase (Alglucerase)	β-Glucocerebrosidase	Gaucher disease	1991-FDA
Cerezyme (Imiglucerase)			1994-FDA; 1997-EMA; 1998-PMDA; 2008-CFDA
VPRIV (Velaglucerase)			2010-FDA, EMA; 2014-PMDA
Elelyso (Taliglucerase)			2012-FDA
Fabrazyme (Agalsidase α)	α-Galactosidase	Fabry disease	2001-EMA
Replagal (Agalsidase β)			2003-FDA, EMA
Aldurazyme (Laronidase)	α-L-iduronidase	MPS I (Hurler syndrome)	2003-FDA, EMA; 2006-PMDA
Naglazyme (Galsulfase)	Arylsulfatase B	MPS VI (Maroteaux-Lamy syndrome)	2005-FDA; 2006-EMA; 2008-PMDA
Myozyme (Alglucosidase)	α-Glucosidase	Pompe disease	2006-FDA, EMA, PMDA
Lumizyme (Alglucosidase)			2010-FDA
Elaprase (Idursulfase)	Iduronate-2-sulfatase	MPS II (Hunter syndrome)	2006-FDA; 2007-EMA, PMDA
Vimizim (Elosulfase α)	N-acetylgalactosamine 6-sulfatase	MPS IV A (Morquio A syndrome)	2014-FDA
Kanuma (Sebelipase α)	Lysosomal acid lipase	Lysosomal acid lipase deficiency	2015-FDA, EMA; 2016-PMDA
Brineura (Cerliponase α)		Batten disease	2017-FDA
Mepsevii (Vestronidase α)	Beta glucuronidase	MPS VII (Sly Syndrome)	2018-FDA

Perhaps the best reason for the success of ERTs in the last two decades is the advent of relevant animal models of disease for LSDs. When Ceredase was first developed, no animal models of Gaucher disease existed, and as such, the protein was moved directly to patients for testing. Nowadays, given more efficient means to modify host genomes in animal models, LSD has been replicated in a wide variety of species including murine, rat, feline, canine and quail models [13]. While the models attempt to genetically match the human condition, sometimes, not surprisingly, the animals manifest the disease in distinct ways from humans. For example, mice modeling Tay-Sachs disease and Sandhoff disease display quite different phenotypes, while the conditions in humans are very similar [14]. A deep understanding of the genetics of the disease is critical as well, since simple knockouts of the enzymes in some cases lead to neonatal death as is the case for b-glucocerebrosidase – this should result in a Gaucher disease phenotype; however, a deletion of the gene results in mice succumbing shortly after birth. Often, disease-specific mutations or truncations of wild-type enzymes must be employed. The utility of these models has proven useful not only for establishing strategies for efficacy, but also for more relevant models for potential human toxicity. During preclinical testing of the enzyme acid sphingomyelinase in type B Niemann–Pick disease (NPD) mice, in an attempt to dose the animals at high levels to reduce substrate in hard to reach organs such as brain, significant toxicity was observed. Given the mechanism of action (MOA) of the enzyme – conversion of sphingomyelin to ceramide and phosphorylcholine – and the known pro-inflammatory properties of ceramide, it is perhaps not surprising that such an adverse event was possible. However, no toxicity was observed in healthy wild-type animals; thus, it is the bulk of accumulated substrate that precisely characterizes this class of diseases that can lead to a rush of potentially harmful by-products of the reaction. Indeed, initial clinical trials found that dose escalation led to acute response protein elevations indicative of inflammation, suggesting that the animal model of Niemann–Pick B was critical in hazard identification. Interestingly, it is also important to note that each LSD patient may have a different level of substrate accumulated, thus differing levels of by-products that could be released into the circulation, meaning that such adverse effects may be induced at very different dose levels of enzyme on a per patient basis. This then emphasizes the need for accurate biomarkers stratifying patients to help guide dosing and reduction in potential toxicity. It also highlights the importance in some cases of using an animal model of disease as the relevant species for preclinical safety evaluation rather than normal healthy animals (see Chapter 2).

In essence, ERT for LSDs has paved the way for other rare disease therapies and approvals for rare diseases other than LSDs can be found at https://rarediseases.info.nih.gov/diseases/fda-orphan-drugs/.

21.3 Available Guidance Relevant to the Development of Therapies for Rare Disease

The preclinical development of therapies for non-oncology indications is guided by two internationally recognized guidances, one addressing multidisciplinary (preclinical and clinical) aspects of development, ICH M3, and another that focuses on the preclinical development of biopharmaceuticals, ICH S6. In both cases, the preclinical development package is advised to consist of a complete toxicology program tested in two species (if relevant) using normal healthy animals, evaluation in juvenile animals if the clinical program enrolls children and a preclinical dosing duration concomitant with the planned clinical dosing length "equal-for-equal". ICH S6 provides an opportunity to use transgenic animals or animal models of disease to support safety provided they are scientifically justified. If long-term dosing (greater than 3 months) is planned in the clinic, preclinical studies up to 9 months for small molecules and up to 6 months for biopharmaceuticals are required to initiate later phase clinical studies. For biotherapeutics, one species may be justified for chronic dosing. Considering the life-threatening nature of rare diseases, especially in children, the duration of dosing for initial clinical trials is similar to a cancer trial, i.e., subjects continue to receive study drug if they are not progressing and there is an adequate safety profile.

21.3.1 FDA Guidance on ERTs and Rare Disease Development – Similarities and Differences from Development of Anticancer Agents

In the mid-2000s, industry sponsors of anticancer therapies and regulators alike recognized that the risk/benefit paradigm for the devastating indication of advanced cancer required a different perspective than that taken with non-life-threatening diseases. Given the poor prognosis in many cancer diagnoses, patients and clinicians are willing to take greater risks related to safety since the options to resolve their cancer are few in number. Getting new options to the oncology clinic needed acceleration and innovation by small enterprises who needed encouragement by reducing the time and resources required for the standard drawn out preclinical investigations characterizing safety prior to entering the clinic. Thus, the ICH formed a working group to produce the ICH S9 guidance document to identify areas where sponsors can shorten the preclinical assessments for this class of drugs. For example, long-term dosing in the clinic could be supported by a variety of different short-term toxicology study dosing strategies, aligned with the schedule planned for the clinic and the modality to be used, while reports from longer-term nonclinical support of 3 months would only be required upon registration of the drug. Defining a no-observed-adverse-effect level (NOAEL) in those studies was deemed unnecessary, and conduct of genotoxicity and carcinogenicity studies is not required. Additionally, it is noted that nonclinical studies evaluating safety in pediatric populations by the use of juvenile animals are not required assuming that enrollment of adults in the clinical trial precedes children. Ethically, this is referred to as the "Prospect of direct benefit" when enrolling pediatric patients in clinical trials. Details on this are outlined in the US Code of Federal Regulations Part 50 Subpart D - Additional Safeguards for Children in Clinical Investigations. In such cases, the use of an animal model of disease could be used to support this.

As outlined in ICH S9, clinical trials for advanced cancer indications are able to begin with preclinical safety support lasting from single doses up to 4 weeks of dosing in duration depending on the planned clinical dosing schedule. In many cases of cytotoxic cancer therapies, particularly small molecules, adverse effects are largely confined to the hematopoietic system and the liver. The characteristics and reversal of these effects are well understood, thus justifying a short-term

preclinical assessment of safety prior to allowing long-term dosing in the clinic. With candidate therapies that target various biological pathways involved in rare diseases, and almost none of these involved in a cytotoxic MOA, it would be in the sponsors interest to understand at least multiple dose effects of the drug and likely longer than 1 month of dosing prior to starting a limitless clinical trial. However, it is unclear what value conducting 6- or 9-month preclinical safety evaluations provides to clinicians interested in getting therapies to initial clinical trials. And after the therapies are in the clinic, as long as the patients are not faring worse over time on the drug, there would be no apparent need to conduct additional nonclinical work to enable longer-term dosing, and increasing dose levels for earlier enrollments to levels identified as safe and efficacious in later cohorts.

A handful of guidances have been published by FDA in the last few years that specifically address options sponsors have when developing therapies to treat rare diseases. The first released as draft in May 2015 "Investigational Enzyme Replacement Therapy Products: Nonclinical Assessment" [6] focuses specifically on animal efficacy and toxicology assessments. This guidance takes significant progressive steps in accelerating the nonclinical portion of ERT development programs by highlighting the following:

- Noting that toxicology "…studies conducted in animal disease models deficient in the targeted enzyme are preferable to using healthy animals in assessing the pharmacodynamic activity – and, in some cases, the toxicology – of ERT products".

- Noting that in the case where a pediatric population is the clinical target, "…juvenile animal toxicity studies potentially may be waived when: (1) clinical development is initiated in adult patients; (2) there are no specific safety concerns from studies in adult animals or adult patients; and (3) target organs with identified toxicity concerns are not undergoing development at the time of treatment".

- Noting that "If the entry criteria define a phenotype that can be expected to rapidly progress to death or substantive irreversible morbidity over the course of 1 year, then repeat-dose toxicology studies in a rodent and a non-rodent species of 1-month dosing duration may be sufficient to initiate clinical trials". In this case, a 3-month toxicology study is required only for registration, potentially in one species only, depending on the outcome of the initial 1-month two species study. In the event that the disease progression is slower, a 3-month toxicology study would be expected to initiate clinical trials.

This guidance provided the most flexible language to date, offering sponsors of ERTs an opportunity for a more rapid entry to the clinic while balancing this with the biology affected by the therapy and the characteristics of the toxicology profile. What is suggested here is a hybrid between the standard biopharmaceutical drug development prescribed by ICH M3 and S6 with the accelerated opportunities offered by the oncology ICH S9. For example, while the guidance states that a toxicology study 3 months in length might be sufficient for registration, studies up to 6 months may be needed to further characterize toxicities that arise in earlier studies.

A second guidance similarly specific to individual indications was published in April 2018 titled "Severely Debilitating or Life-Threatening Hematologic Disorders: Nonclinical Development of Pharmaceuticals". This was the first guidance to borrow from the language used by Prescott et al. [4] on addressing "SDLT" indications and maintains essentially all of the "S9-like" reduced or delayed nonclinical testing discussed above. While this guidance is limited to hematologic disorders identified as SDLTs, it is the first to extend the provisions outlined in the ERT guidance above to small molecules. As such, testing such as genotoxicity, reproductive toxicity, photosafety and carcinogenicity is addressed and provides sponsors options for reduced testing batteries and/or delaying some testing until after drug approval. What will be critical as such guidances specific to organ systems arise such as this one is to identify if a particular indication falls under the scope of these provisions.

These guidances raise the question whether another oncology-specific term used to describe toxicities should be applied to nonclinical safety studies supporting non-oncology life-threatening diseases – the highest non-severely toxic dose (HNSTD). This more "forgiving" term applied to findings from toxicology studies for oncology products allows for a wide range of findings that would be called "adverse" in standard reports to not factor into setting starting doses or capping dose escalation schemes in the clinic. Since patients with life-threatening diseases are likely to accept some adverse effects in hopes that efficacy would be the trade-off, defining those adverse effects as "severe" or not allows for higher dose exploration in the clinic. Thus, based on this differentiation among various adverse reactions observed in earlier toxicology studies, whether a sponsor would actually need to conduct longer-term toxicology studies in addition to an existing 3-month study would need to be evaluated on a case-by-case basis.

Perhaps one of the few gaps in these guidances is that they only apply to a subset of therapies for life-threatening rare diseases. This guidance would not, for example, apply to treatments for spinal muscular atrophy, cystic fibrosis or amyotrophic lateral sclerosis. Enter the more broad draft guidance released by FDA in August 2015 "Rare Diseases: Common Issues in Drug Development Guidance for Industry" [5]. This document acts as more of a "multidisciplinary" guidance akin to the ICH "M" guidance series, offering suggestions on natural history studies, biomarkers, nonclinical studies, clinical endpoints and manufacturing considerations. Given the multitude of topics addressed, the detail offered in the nonclinical section is more general compared to the ERT guidance, lacking any specificity on length of nonclinical studies to support initial clinical trials and registration. However, there is specific mention on the use of animal models of disease, where it is stated "Safety evaluation in an animal model also may be particularly valuable when it is suspected that drug toxicity may be more severe in the presence of disease pathophysiology",

however a preceding statement suggests that while this would be useful in characterizing toxicity in the context of disease, "...will not substitute for all toxicology testing in healthy animals because of concern that the disease pathophysiology may obscure some drug toxicity". This would seem to be at odds with similar statements made in the ERT guidance – it is unclear what circumstances would require evaluation of a therapy in a normal healthy animal in spite of having a well-controlled and conducted study in a well-characterized animal model of disease to initiate clinical trials. It is hoped that further discussion on this more comprehensive guidance will bring a unifying concept on how to accelerate therapeutics through the preclinical space while still providing relevant and valuable nonclinical safety information.

In April 2018, FDA released a new guidance for nonclinical development of SDLTHDs [7], which in large part replicates the provisions for nonclinical development of anticancer therapies in ICH S9. One exception is the suggestion that clinical trials of any length can begin with support from a toxicology study 1 month in length, as opposed to a single-dose clinical trial.

21.3.2 FDA Guidance on Development of Gene and Cell Therapies

Guidance also exists for the modalities of gene and cell therapy that support targeted product-specific approaches. In the USA and Europe, a separate division of the overarching health authority regulates these therapies – the Center for Biologics Evaluation and Research (CBER) in the USA and the Committee for Advanced Therapies (CAT) in Europe. Both have historically taken a more flexible approach to the overall development of novel therapeutic platforms. The specific guidances relevant to advanced therapies incorporate a "case-by-case" approach similar to ICH S6 and more streamlined approach similar to ICH S9. Depending on the type of cell, longer-term nonclinical studies may be required to mitigate the risk for the potential for tumorigenesis, a concern unique to this platform, and as such would necessitate a longer preclinical development phase. However, as more experience is attained with this technology as well as evolving techniques to molecularly characterize cells and relate to potential risks for tumorigenesis, there exists potential to ultimately accelerate this step. Importantly, there is no specific requirement to use two species, and there is an opportunity to combine safety endpoints in an animal model of disease. In vitro assays are also encouraged using patient samples. Since initial clinical trials are conducted in the index population and not normal volunteers, there is also the consideration for extrapolation of not only a safe but also an active dose. Importantly, a safety program that is well justified by the science employs common sense and is discussed and agreed with regulators in advance of the studies.

In July 2018, FDA/CBER released a suite of guidances that, like the April 2018 FDA/CDER guidance on hematology SDLTs, addressed organ system and disease type-specific guidance on the development of gene therapies for retinal, hemophilia and rare diseases [15–17]. As has already been discussed, these guidances maintain many of the core concepts described above for more limited nonclinical safety packages, but also address issues specific to indications, such as the potential need for large animals in retinal gene therapy programs owing to the more similar size of the eye compared to humans.

21.3.3 Proposals for Severely Debilitating or Life-Threatening (SDLT) Illnesses

As mentioned above, recent publications and guidance from FDA have suggested that an expedited route for nonclinical safety testing, like what is available for life-threatening cancer indications, should be made available also for diseases where a similar non-oncologic life-threatening illness is involved. This can certainly apply to the LSDs where life expectancy is significantly decreased, sometimes to the point of affected individuals not progressing past infancy. Prescott et al. [4] proposed the following considerations when structuring a nonclinical safety program supporting an SDLT:

- Safety pharmacology should be included in general toxicology studies, which would be in accordance with ICH S6 for any other protein therapeutic.
- Toxicology studies of 1 month in length to support FIH studies, with studies no longer than 3 months supporting market authorization, with recovery groups only needed in the 3-month studies
- Dedicated combination toxicology studies should not be required, and safety of the combination can be obtained from efficacy studies.
- A streamlined embryo-fetal development assessment (pilot studies, in vitro assessments and/or a written rationale for the predicted risks) may be acceptable. Fertility assessments can be obtained from histopathology of reproductive organs in the general toxicology studies.
- Genotoxicity and carcinogenicity testing done as appropriate as per the modality; however, it is worth noting that carcinogenicity assessments could be made after registration and that the FDA has recently stated in its 2018 Hematology SDLT guidance that more limited genotoxicity assessments can be made for these indications. In any event, a communication of risk assessment of the compound could be made using the existing literature on the product/target.

We believe there are additional considerations that can be made for the treatment of rare diseases:

- An emphasis placed on identifying a clinical starting dose from preclinical data that balances the risk of potential adverse effects with the prospect of benefit for the patient that has no or limited therapeutic alternatives. A similar risk/benefit ratio is offered in interpreting preclinical safety studies for advanced cancer therapeutics, whereas the key metric used to determine a starting dose is the HNSTD rather than a NOAEL.
- In the event that clinical data already exist for the compound being developed for the rare life-threatening disorder, such data can be leveraged to either reduce or eliminate additional preclinical safety data requirements.
- For therapies targeted for pediatric populations, but which initiated clinical studies in adults first with the supporting toxicology program in adult animals, a preclinical program conducted in juvenile animals would only be performed in the event that the pharmacology of the drug is specifically known to target organ systems still under development in the age range proposed for the clinic. However, if the first clinical trial starts in pediatrics, then the supporting preclinical program may be conducted with juvenile animals. In most cases, the age that would trigger a concern is a clinical population less than 2 years of age.
- As many rare diseases arise from genetic anomalies and as such are typically modeled in animals for purposes of evaluating efficacy, a primary safety evaluation obtained in efficacy studies could be sufficient for the initiation of clinical trials. Studies conducted in healthy normal animals when such data are available may not be relevant to humans.

21.4 Nonclinical Strategies for Efficiently Enabling First-in-Human (FIH) Studies

21.4.1 Animal Models

A highlight of the recently adopted guidance from FDA addressing gene and cell therapies is the encouragement of applying safety endpoints to animal models of disease, sometimes in lieu of conducting a formal safety assessment in normal healthy animals [18]. This provides sponsors a valuable opportunity to perform "integrated pharmacology" studies, where safety endpoints obtained within the efficacy studies already planned could suffice for the toxicology needs prior to entering the clinic. This also helps reduce the number of animals used in the nonclinical program and the financial burden, particularly on small companies. While this advice is presently only applying to gene and cell therapies and perhaps ERTs, it should also be noted that similar guidance exists in ICH S6. But beyond these practical benefits, recently published examples of nonclinical safety studies have suggested that sometimes testing in disease models and not healthy animals makes good scientific sense [19]. Particularly in syndromes where substrates accumulate in the body as a result of a malfunctioning enzyme, the introduction of an active enzyme can result in a bolus release of the enzymatic products, which in some cases could be toxic. In a healthy animal possessing no defects in that pathway, toxicities would be missed and/or other findings may crop up that are irrelevant to the disease state. Of course, leveraging safety information from a genetically modified animal model requires careful evaluation and characterization of the model prior to basing any conclusions on safety, which does burden the sponsor with significant front-loaded work. However, in the long run, that diligence pays off with the most relevant safety information coupled with often shorter timelines getting to the clinic.

21.4.1.1 Special Considerations with Animal Models of Disease for Safety Evaluation

The potential limitations of using animal models of disease for safety evaluation are highlighted in a publication by Morgan et al. [20] and the draft guidance on ERTs (REF). To justify the relevance of use, consideration must be given to the disease pathophysiology and phenotype in the animal model versus the human condition, the potential enhanced toxicity in the disease model versus healthy animals, and the possible exacerbation of the disease resulting from the administration of the potential therapeutic drug. If planning to incorporate safety endpoints into a study with an animal model of disease, the protocol should particularly include standard toxicology endpoints and histopathology evaluation. Often, these types of studies may be conducted under non-good laboratory practice (GLP) conditions in-house or with an investigator. An option to elevate the quality of the safety evaluation from such a study is to conduct the histopathologic evaluation at a Contract Research Organization (CRO) where they can employ more standard GLP assessments. Incorporating appropriate numbers of animals per sex and appropriate control groups aids in the safety evaluation from disease models, given that a large historical control database is likely unavailable and the assessment of any effects of the drug needs to be determined in conjunction with age- and gender-matched controls. While complete reports of pharmacology and proof of concept (POC) studies are generally not required for an investigational new drug, in the case where safety endpoints have been included to overall support the safety of the investigational drug, complete study reports are indeed necessary. While not required, the author has found benefit in a more hands-on approach to these types of studies through close collaboration with the investigator beginning with protocol design, study monitoring, study documentation and support for report writing.

21.4.2 When No Relevant Animal Models Exist

The definition of a relevant species is defined within multiple regulatory guidances [1–3]. However, this needs to be assessed for each molecule under evaluation. For example, for ERTs, additional consideration must include whether the animal species has the appropriate homology for uptake of the enzyme into the cell and potential immune response to the human enzyme in the animal. While the advent of CRISPR and other gene-editing technology may reduce this concern in the future, there are currently still diseases where there is no existing animal model (either naturally occurring or genetically modified). In this situation, the ideal path forward should be discussed with regulatory agencies in a prospective manner. There may still be a requirement for some demonstration of safety in an animal prior to a FIH study, but the design may be of limited nature.

21.4.3 Nonclinical Approaches for Specific Clinical Populations

21.4.3.1 Healthy Volunteers

Generally, therapies for rare and SDLT diseases are not often tested first in healthy volunteers.

21.4.3.2 Pediatric Patient Populations

Because rare diseases are most often genetic in origin, they disproportionately effect children. The consequences of an inborn genetic anomaly, due to an altered pathway, be it metabolic, differentiation, growth or something else, typically manifest early in life, often in the first few years. Some of these rare syndromes may have a spectrum of severities that results in patient populations falling into a wide range of ages, such as the LSDs Pompe and Gaucher's. This variability has its roots in the genetics of the disease, where some mutations just reduce the activity of an enzyme where in others deletions and key mutations will eliminate activity entirely. This clinical layout would allow sponsors to initiate clinical trials in adults and then proceed in progressively younger ages testing the safety in those populations slowly in the clinic. However, some disorders arise from mutations in gene products whose importance in pre- and postnatal development and well-functioning organ systems is so critical that patients rarely pass the first decade of life. In these cases, there are no adult populations to test efficacy and evaluation of safety in a normal adult population would not be informative. In both of these scenarios of moving into pediatric clinical populations, a standard drug development paradigm driven by ICH S6 and M3 guidances would dictate that nonclinical testing in juvenile animals is needed prior to enrolling children. Comparing again to the ICH S9 anticancer therapies guidance, it is stated that nonclinical studies in juvenile animals are typically not required prior to moving trials into a pediatric population; however, it is assumed that most if not all cancer treatments to be ultimately tested in children would have been applied to adults in the clinic first. It is important to point out here that the ICH, noting that with increasing drug development activities ongoing for indications that would be appropriate, if not exclusively, for pediatric populations, has initiated a working group to develop an internationally agreed-upon guidance for nonclinical testing supporting pediatric clinical trials – thus, more clarity on the what, when and how to conduct juvenile toxicology studies will be forthcoming in the next few years. We want to highlight, however, that juvenile toxicology studies for protein drugs would need to be conducted in non-human primates, where obtaining appropriately aged animals is an exceptionally difficult proposition. It is also unclear, in the absence of an obvious safety risk specifically in a juvenile population, based on the known biology of therapy and the pathways it affects, what results testing in juvenile animals will yield to help design pediatric trials. In many cases of biopharmaceutical toxicity testing, non-sexually mature primates are used, usually in the range of 2–4 years of age. Extrapolation of this age to similar human ages is approximately in the 6–12 years of age range already; thus, the rationale for testing in an even younger population of primates would seem to require a very specific concern around an organ system development that is vulnerable during the first few years of life.

21.4.4 Case Studies for Nonclinical Strategies for the Development of Rare Disease Therapeutics

21.4.4.1 Rare (ERT)

Mepsevii (Vestronidase alfa; recombinant human glucuronidase α; rhGUS) is an example of an ERT that was recently approved in 2018 for MPS VII. The nonclinical program was conducted prior to the draft guidance on ERTs; thus, the approach was a hybrid of a traditional protein drug and the streamlined approach as outlined in the 2015 guidance. The Biologics License Application (BLA)-enabling package primarily consisted of referenced literature for the assessment of pharmacology and pharmacokinetics. The toxicology assessment included the following: a single-dose GLP toxicity study in normal rats, a non-GLP repeat-dose (8-week) study in a mouse model of disease and a 26-week GLP chronic toxicology study in normal juvenile cynomolgus monkeys. Additionally, standard safety pharmacology studies were conducted in rats (CNS and respiratory) and cardiovascular (CV) safety pharmacology endpoints were included within the chronic toxicology study in juvenile cynomolgus monkeys. For BLA filing, standard rat (Segment I/II combined) and rabbit (Segment II) GLP developmental and reproductive toxicity (DART) studies were conducted. A pre- and postnatal development (PPND; Segment III) rat study was requested as a postmarketing requirement (PMR) by the FDA. The typical limitation around immunogenicity did present a challenge in the rat DART studies; however, this was mitigated through the confirmation of adequate exposure at the mid- and high-dose groups and did not deter the FDA from requesting the PPND study as a PMR. Standard genotoxicity and carcinogenicity studies were waived due to the nature of the molecule.

As mentioned previously, these studies were conducted prior to the draft guidance on ERTs; therefore, some consideration of what might have been done differently is warranted. The biggest difference would likely have been in the conduct of the 26-week cynomolgus monkey study. The guidance allows for a 1-month study to be supportive of a FIH study and 3-month studies as being likely sufficient for approval if the disease is rapidly progressing; therefore, this study could have been shortened. Additionally, all of the DART studies could potentially have been delayed to postmarketing versus just the Segment III study; however, this would have warranted a discussion with the FDA for confirmation. Otherwise, the nonclinical safety evaluation was conducted similarly to what is described in the guidance (e.g., inclusion of toxicology endpoints and histopathology evaluation by a CRO in the POC study in the MPS VII mouse model).

21.4.4.2 Rare (Non-ERT)

Spinal muscular atrophy is a monogenic disorder that results from the loss of expression of the SMN1 gene leading to loss of motor neuron function. In the SMA1 disease phenotype, where almost no residual expression is obtained from the tandem but defective gene SMN2, patients lose muscular function very early on in life and have a life expectancy of only 2–3 years. LMI070 (branaplam) is a low-molecular-weight drug in development that targets the transcriptional deficiency in SMN2 in an attempt to boost levels of wild-type SMN protein in SMA1 patients. While a full general toxicology program was conducted for LMI070 in rats and dogs, it was only conducted in juvenile animals owing to the patient population of the indication. Additionally, based on this age difference, no reproductive toxicology has yet been performed. The more significant provisions for this program came in setting the starting clinical dose, as the top dose in both the rat and dog studies, while not technically a NOAEL, had findings that were not severe and were reversible. This qualifies this dose as a rat "STD10" and a dog "HNSTD", which under ICH S9 provisions would allow clinical trials to start as high as 1/10th of these dose levels. Indeed, the LMI070 clinical trial used these dose levels, which were accepted by health authorities and enabled the generation of efficacy data without proceeding through multiple dose cohorts.

21.4.4.3 Severely Debilitating or Life-Threatening

One of the examples provided by Prescott et al. in their SDLT publication [4] is the development of pharmaceuticals for the treatment of heart failure, an indication that is far from rare with over 20 million patients worldwide and accounting for almost 2% of all healthcare spending. Of particular focus is a subset of patients with reduced ejection fraction (HFrEF), where there exists a clear need to accelerate more therapies to the clinic. Like with gene and cell therapies, and with advanced cancer, Prescott et al. [4] outlined a preclinical and clinical scenario where a reduced nonclinical package and the ability to proceed directly to patients in the SAD and MAD phases of clinical development provide significant time and cost benefits to prospective programs. With a reduction in 20 months to POC, 33 months to registration filing, 1,800 animals used in the nonclinical program and an overall savings of more than $41 million dollars, the advantages for these diseases where the risk of accelerating a product would be tolerated at much higher levels than a standard drug development programs are clear.

21.5 Nonclinical and Clinical Immunogenicity Concerns and Mitigations

One of the biggest challenges that sponsors face as they develop biologic molecules is the development of antidrug antibodies (ADAs). It is well-accepted that an immunogenic response in animals is not predictive of an immunogenic response in patients; however, immunogenicity in nonclinical studies still often presents a challenge. This is typically centered around the ability to maintain exposure to demonstrate adequate safety margins or the ability to differentiate between ADA-induced toxicity and drug-induced toxicity. Clinically, the development of ADA is often thought of in terms of any potential impact on safety or diminished therapeutic response over time.

Immunogenic responses to gene therapy are particularly challenging and limit both patient enrollment into clinical trials (i.e., exclusion criteria often include screening for anti-adeno-associated virus (AAV) capsid antibodies) and subsequently the ability to re-dose patients.

21.6 New Modalities for Rare Diseases and Implications for Nonclinical Development

The foundation of treatment of LSDs has clearly been biologic therapies consisting of the wild-type enzyme that is lost of mutant in the patient population. Indeed, this approach played a key role in the biopharmaceutical and biotechnology industry in general, with companies like Genzyme (now a subsidiary of Sanofi), BioMarin and Transkaryotic Therapies (purchased by Shire in 2008) founded on the development of enzyme replacement treatments. While administration of purified and recombinant proteins is the most advanced strategy for the treatment of LSDs, other modalities are making progress as alternatives. As noted above, the first ERT, Ceredase, was purified from human placenta, using a process that highly enriched for the enzyme, however, yielded only a small fraction of the initial amount. This led to recombinant production of various enzymes which has proven successful, however issues with manufacturing, potential for immunogenicity upon repeated dosing into patients, the exorbitant cost of repeated administration (which could last decades if successful) and the need to decorate the protein with the appropriate glycosylation moieties in order to get efficient transcytosis and access to lysosomes begs for the development of more robust and less labor-intensive modalities.

Low-molecular-weight approaches, such as substrate inhibitors, chemical chaperones and cytosolic molecule modulators, could have advantages over protein treatment owing to the ability to access the brain and not result in immunogenicity. One strategy involves reduction in the production of the accumulating substrate in the first place, including the approved therapies Zavesca and Cerdelga, both of which inhibit glucosylceramide synthase for the treatment of Gaucher's disease. Naturally however, issues with specificity and metabolism can cause problems with this approach.

The fact that these disorders are monogenic makes these diseases ideal candidates for classic approaches to gene therapy. Theoretically, the transfer of the wild-type form of the gene to the appropriate tissue should correct the defect in clearance of the substrate. In some cases, the transduction of the liver via a systemic route, as this potentially can be transformed into an ERT production factory for systemic exposure of an ERT, would be ideal. Clinical trials are underway for mucopolysaccharidosis, Fabry and Pompe diseases. In others, individual tissues need to be transformed, which may require challenging routes of administration or difficult-to-transduce cell types. Nevertheless, evidence of clinical benefit can sometimes be obtained with even very small levels of correction. On occasion, the transduction of hematopoietic stem cells using an ex vivo approach is performed so that the entirety of the hematopoietic system is corrected, notably the reticuloendothelial system that is often the most dramatically affected. This has been attempted with arylsulfatase A and B deficiencies as well as various forms of mucopolysaccharidosis. Other forms of LSDs are most prominent in the brain, where systemically administered proteins are unlikely to have any access. While proteins can be administered intrathecally or intracranially, this is not a long-term option as ports allowing for routine administration in these areas are at risk for infection. Alternatively, one-time administration via these routes is possible and has been explored for the treatment of Batten disease and Sanfilippo syndrome, and AAV vectors that are more proficient at the transduction of neural tissues and potentially have the ability to cross the blood–brain barrier are being investigated for mucopolysaccharidosis as well. Similar to the HSC approach for mucopolysaccharidosis, induced pluripotent neural stem cells engineered ex vivo to treat metachromatic leukodystrophy, MPS VII and Batten disease and then implanted in nonclinical models have been successful, with hopes that a more CNS-specific approach to these diseases can be taken.

Finally, the new technologies of "genome editing" have taken hold in this field, in attempts to directly modify the host genome to introduce a wild-type gene at a safe harbor locus or modify an existing gene to correct the causative mutation. Platforms using zinc finger nucleases (ZFN) and CRISPR/Cas9 have been described in the nonclinical space to be successful in treating LSDs, with at least one program using the ZFN approach reaching the clinic.

These new modalities of gene, cell and genome editing come with their own challenges with respect to safety, including immune system recognition and sometimes rejection of viral vectors and modified cells and genotoxicity from viral vector integration or off-target genome editing, sharing some concerns with other modalities while bringing to light some new ones. However, the field of biopharmaceutical safety assessment is rapidly developing the appropriate tools to determine the risk of these new modalities, so that such new approaches can be added to the armamentarium of the treating physicians for these challenging diseases.

21.7 Summary

The prognosis of many rare non-oncology life-threatening diseases is often no better than advanced cancer indications. Several advances have been made to inspire developers of cancer therapies to proceed to clinical trials, including a guidance outlining the preclinical strategy which reduces the time and expense to proceed to filing investigative proposals. Similarly, the development of the challenging and complex field of gene- and cell-based therapies would likely be stifled in the absence of clear guidance allowing sponsors to take a case-by-case and science-driven approach to moving their products to the clinical stage. We propose here that the same guidance should be applied to non-oncologic rare life-threatening diseases as well. While many incentives are already applied to sponsors of orphan diseases, many of these are realized only after a program has proceeded to the clinic. The same principles used for cancer and gene/cell therapies could make up this gap where some programs are being held up in the nonclinical space. Targeted guidance for this, including the key points outlined above, would assist in moving promising therapies to patients and recruit new developers into this arena.

REFERENCES

1. ICH Harmonised Tripartite Guideline Preclinical Safety Evaluation of Biotechnology-Derived Pharmaceuticals S 6(R1). https://database.ich.org/sites/default/files/S6_R1_Guideline_0.pdf
2. ICH Harmonised Tripartite Guideline Guidance on Nonclinical Safety Studies for the Conduct of Human Clinical Trials and Marketing Authorization For Pharmaceuticals M</A>3(R2). https://database.ich.org/sites/default/files/M3_R2__Guideline.pdf
3. ICH Harmonised Tripartite Guideline Nonclinical Evaluation for Anticancer Pharmaceuticals S9. https://database.ich.org/sites/default/files/S9_Guideline.pdf
4. Prescott JS, Andrews PA, Baker RW, Bogdanffy MS, Fields FO, Keller DA, Lapadula DM, Mahoney NM, Paul DE, Platz SJ, Reese DM, Stoch SA, DeGeorge JJ (2017). Evaluation of therapeutics for advanced-stage heart failure and other severely-debilitating or life-threatening diseases. *Clin Pharmacol Ther.* 102: 219–227.
5. Rare Diseases: Common Issues in Drug Development Guidance for Industry, U.S. Department of Health and Human Services Food and Drug Administration, Center for Drug Evaluation and Research (CDER), Center for Biologics Evaluation and Research (CBER), August 2015.
6. Investigational Enzyme Replacement Therapy Products: Nonclinical Assessment Guidance for Industry, U.S. Department of Health and Human Services, Food and Drug Administration Center for Drug Evaluation and Research (CDER), May 2015.
7. Severely Debilitating or Life-Threatening Hematologic Disorders: Nonclinical Development of Pharmaceuticals, U.S. Department of Health and Human Services, Food and Drug Administration Center for Drug Evaluation and Research (CDER), April 2018.
8. Braun MM, Farag-El-Massah S, Xu K, Coté TR (2010). Emergence of orphan drugs in the United States: a quantitative assessment of the first 25 years. *Nat Rev Drug Discov.* 9: 519–522.
9. Orphan Drug Act, H.R. 5238, Public Law No. 97–414, 97th Congress (1983).
10. Fagnan DE, Yang NN, McKew JC, Lo AW (2015). Financing translation: analysis of the NCATS rare-diseases portfolio. *Sci Transl Med.* 7: 276.
11. Lists of Medicinal Products for Rare Diseases in Europe. OrphaNet Report Series, October 2015. http://www.orpha.net/consor/cgi-bin/Education_Home.php
12. CY 2014 CDER Rare Disease and Orphan Drug Designated Approvals. http://www.fda.gov/Drugs/DevelopmentApprovalProcess/HowDrugsareDevelopedandApproved/DrugandBiologicApprovalReports/NDAandBLAApprovalReports/ucm373419.htm
13. Haskins ME, Giger U, Patterson DF (2006). Animal models of lysosomal storage diseases: their development and clinical relevance. In: Mehta A, Beck M, Sunder-Plassmann G, editors. *Fabry Disease: Perspectives from 5 Years of FOS.* Oxford: Oxford PharmaGenesis.
14. Sango K, Yamanaka S, Hoffmann A, Okuda Y, Grinberg A, Westphal H, McDonald MP, Crawley JN, Sandhoff K, Suzuki K, Proia RL (1995). Mouse models of Tay-Sachs and Sandhoff diseases differ in neurologic phenotype and ganglioside metabolism. *Nat Genet.* 11: 170–176.
15. Human Gene Therapy for Retinal Disorders, U.S. Department of Health and Human Services, Food and Drug Administration Center for Biologics Evaluation and Research (CBER), July 2018.
16. Human Gene Therapy for Rare Diseases, U.S. Department of Health and Human Services, Food and Drug Administration Center for Biologics Evaluation and Research (CBER), July 2018.
17. Human Gene Therapy for Hemophilia, U.S. Department of Health and Human Services, Food and Drug Administration Center for Biologics Evaluation and Research (CBER), July 2018.
18. Guidance for Industry - Preclinical Assessment of Investigational Cellular and Gene Therapy Products, U.S. Department of Health and Human Services Food and Drug Administration, Center for Biologics Evaluation and Research, November 2013.
19. Murray JM, Thompson AM, Vitsky A, Hawes M, Chuang WL, Pacheco J, Wilson S, McPherson JM, Thurberg BL, Karey KP, Andrews L (2015). Nonclinical safety assessment of recombinant human acid sphingomyelinase (rhASM) for the treatment of acid sphingomyelinase deficiency: the utility of animal models of disease in the toxicological evaluation of potential therapeutics. *Mol Genet Metab.* 114: 217–225.
20. Morgan SJ, Elangbam CS, Berens S, Janovitz E, Vitsky A, Zabka T, Conour L. (2013). Use of animal models of human disease for nonclinical safety assessment of novel pharmaceuticals. *Toxicol Pathol.* 41(3): 508–518. doi: 10.1177/0192623312457273. Epub 2012 Sep 11. PMID: 22968286.

22

Development of Antibody-Drug Conjugates[1]

Stanley A. Roberts
SAR Safety Assessment

Simon Chivers
Integrated Biologix GmbH

Anu Connor
Novartis

Hadi Falahatpisheh and Magali Guffroy
AbbVie Inc.

Anthony J. Lee
Seagen Inc.

Lise I. Loberg, Colin Phipps, and Sherry L. Ralston
AbbVie Inc.

Melissa M. Schutten and Nicola J. Stagg
Genentech, Inc.

Jay Tibbitts
Surrozen Inc.

CONTENTS

---

[1] These authors are members of the Biotechnology Innovation Organization's (BIO) ADC Task Force. This Task Force is a group within the BioSafe Preclinical Safety Committee, comprised of BIO members working to serve as a resource for BIO members and BIO staff by identifying and responding to key scientific and regulatory issues related to the preclinical safety evaluation of biopharmaceuticals products.

DOI: 10.1201/9781003124542-25

22.1 Introduction

Historically, therapeutic approaches in oncology have been limited by poor efficacy or unacceptable toxicity. For small molecule agents, this typically is associated with poor tumor specificity, affecting both healthy and diseased tissue, resulting in toxicity (both acute and long term) and often limited therapeutic benefit. For antibodies and other biotherapeutic molecules, tumor or target specificity is generally very high, thus avoiding on-target toxicity; however, potency can be limited. A similar case can be made for therapeutic areas outside oncology where specific delivery of a potent agent directly to the target cells could substantially improve clinical outcomes and patients' therapeutic experience. Antibody-drug conjugates (ADCs) provide a unique opportunity to deliver on this promise by virtue of their structural amalgamation of an antibody and small molecule agent (Figure 22.1). The tumor/target specificity is afforded by the antibody component of the

ADC, typically resulting in tumor/target specific uptake and/or localization to the diseased microenvironment, with the small molecule component of the ADC providing a therapeutically relevant pharmacologic effect upon release within the target cell.

Despite the great promise of targeted delivery, the pharmacology and toxicology of ADCs have been found to be considerably more complex and posed challenges to developing clinically successful drugs. Some of these challenges, and strategies to overcome them, will be described in the following pages. To fully appreciate these challenges, it is important to understand the mechanisms by which ADCs can exert their activity—beyond the specific targeting described above. Figures 22.2 and 22.3 show four distinct mechanistic pathways that have been described for ADCs. In Figure 22.2, the commonly accepted mechanism is shown by which the ADC binds to its intended target on a cell, is internalized by the cell as part of the trafficking of the ADC target, followed by drug release

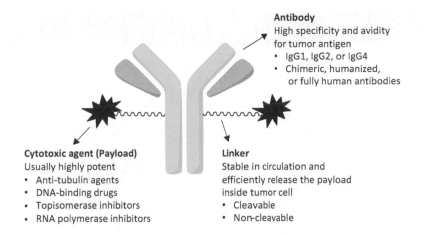

Antibody
High specificity and avidity
for tumor antigen
- IgG1, IgG2, or IgG4
- Chimeric, humanized,
  or fully human antibodies

Cytotoxic agent (Payload)
Usually highly potent
- Anti-tubulin agents
- DNA-binding drugs
- Topisomerase inhibitors
- RNA polymerase inhibitors

Linker
Stable in circulation and
efficiently release the payload
inside tumor cell
- Cleavable
- Non-cleavable

FIGURE 22.1 Schematic diagram of an antibody-drug conjugate (ADC) for the treatment of cancer.

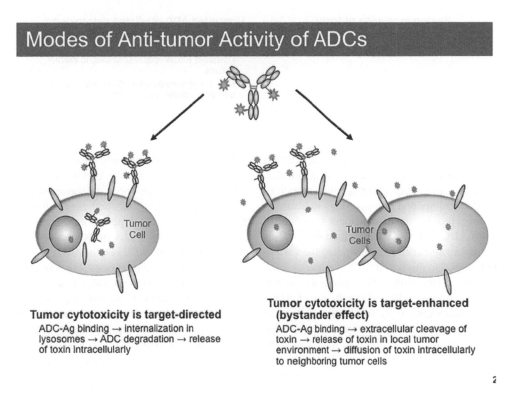

Modes of Anti-tumor Activity of ADCs

Tumor cytotoxicity is target-directed
ADC-Ag binding → internalization in
lysosomes → ADC degradation → release
of toxin intracellularly

**Tumor cytotoxicity is target-enhanced
(bystander effect)**
ADC-Ag binding → extracellular cleavage of
toxin → release of toxin in local tumor
environment → diffusion of toxin intracellularly
to neighboring tumor cells

FIGURE 22.2 Modes of Anti-Tumor Activity of ADC's.

and cellular effects consistent with the ADC payload (illustrated below as cell death). Cells, both target-bearing and non-target, are capable of nonspecifically internalizing proteins and other macromolecules, including ADCs, from the extracellular fluid (Figures 22.2 and 22.3). The result of this internalization can be the release of the ADC payload and either desired or undesired effects on the internalizing cells, perhaps leading to toxicity. Upon release of the payload within cells, either via target-mediated uptake (upper left) or nonspecific uptake (lower left), the payload can diffuse out of the cell and into neighboring cells resulting in effects on those 'bystander' cells. Finally, the attachment of the payload to the antibody can have varying levels of stability resulting in the potential for release of the payload either in circulation or in the extracellular fluid (Figures 22.2 and 22.3). This process can result

in pharmacologically active levels of payload in tissues or circulation with the potential for efficacious or toxic effects. The successful design and implementation of ADCs must consider all of these mechanisms to appreciate their relevance and contributions to the observed efficacy and toxicity, and seek to balance them to achieve the optimal therapeutic index.

22.2 Special Considerations for ADCs in Development

The objectives of this chapter are to introduce the structure and various formats of antibody-drug conjugates (ADCs), to discuss the importance of target antigen and species selection, to evaluate what is known about the class and species-specific

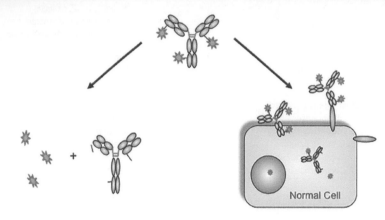

Modes of Toxicity of ADCs

Systemic release of toxin
- Instability of linker
- Catabolism of ADC

Unwanted ADC-mediated cytotoxicity
- Targeted binding to normal tissues expressing antigen
- Off-target (cross-reactive) binding to normal tissues
- Non-antigen-mediated ADC uptake (e.g., Fc-mediated uptake, pinocytosis)

FIGURE 22.3 Modes of Toxicity of ADC's

effects of the available linker payloads and the opportunities/challenges associated with each of these. The nonclinical development of ADCs is thoroughly addressed with numerous case studies, for both oncology and non-oncology indications, along with some insights into the management of off-target safety liabilities with ADCs. The ADME evaluation of ADCs, complex due to the nature and chemistry including the various components of ADCs, is also discussed.

This chapter's aims differ from other publications that review ADC development as we will address the use of ADCs in both oncology (post-publication of the ICH S9 Q&A document) and non-oncology indications. Examples are provided that provide industry-wide input and actual examples of ADC nonclinical development approaches. Since ADCs include both a small molecule cytotoxin and an antibody, an ADC nonclinical program overlaps both small and large molecule nonclinical development paradigms.

22.3 Anatomy of ADCs—Linker, mAb, Payload

22.3.1 Introduction

ADCs are targeted therapeutics that are composed of monoclonal antibodies and small molecule agents (payloads) covalently conjugated through chemical linkers (Figure 22.1). The monoclonal antibody component of an ADC selectively binds a cell surface antigen, resulting in the internalization of the ADC-antigen complex. The ADC-antigen complex then traffics to the endolysosomal system and is degraded, releasing the cytotoxic payloads inside the cell. The majority of ADCs in development today are anticancer therapeutics that utilize tumor antigens for tumor targeting while incorporating payloads that cause

cell death through cytotoxic mechanisms of action (MOAs). However, numerous advancements have led to the broadening use of ADCs in non-oncology therapeutic indications, which include the use of payloads with novel MOAs; current strategies for the nonclinical development of these molecules are underway and will be discussed later in the non-oncology indication section. There are nine ADCs on the market as of August 2020, and numerous ADCs are in various stages of clinical development. Gemtuzumab ozogamicin (Mylotarg®), an anti-CD33 ADC bearing a calicheamicin derivative payload, was first approved by the US Food and Drug Administration (FDA) in 2000 but was later withdrawn from the market in 2010 only to re-enter in 2017. It was followed by brentuximab vedotin (Adcetris®), a CD30-directed ADC containing monomethyl auristatin E (MMAE) payload, trastuzumab emtansine (Kadcyla®), a HER2-targeted ADC that contains a maytansine derivative payload, inotuzumab ozogamicin (Besponsa®), a CD22-directed ADC bearing the same linker-payload as Mylotarg, and polatuzumab vedotin-piiq (Polivy™), a CD79b-directed ADC containing MMAE payload, enfortumab vedotin-ejfv (Padcev™), a nectin-4-directed ADC containing MMAE payload, famtrastuzumab deruxtecan-nxki (Enhertu®), a HER2-directed ADC containing topoisomerase inhibitor DXd payload, sacituzumab govitecan-hziy (Trodelvy™), a Trop-2-directed ADC containing topoisomerase inhibitor SN-38 payload, and belantamab mafodotin-blmf (Blenrep), a B-cell maturation antigen (BCMA)-directed antibody conjugated with a microtubule inhibitor monomethyl auristatin F (MMAF). ADCs and the contribution of each component to toxicity and efficacy have been extensively reviewed in a number of review articles (Carter and Senter 2008, Panowski et al. 2014, Peters and Brown 2015, Polakis 2016, Thomas et al. 2016, Tolcher 2016, Beck et al. 2017, Dan et al. 2018, Khera and Thurber 2018).

22.3.2 Antibody

The antibody component of an ADC is desired to have high specificity for its target. Whether the affinity is high or low affinity needs to be balanced based on need for uptake and release within the tumor cell, and the distribution of antibody within the tumor depends on on- and off-rates. The ideal antibody is minimally immunogenic, in both nonclinical species and humans, and shows PK properties consistent with typical well-behaved antibodies (Dirks and Meibohm 2010). And, consistent with the evaluation of other biotherapeutic agents, cross-reactivity of binding to the desired target should be evaluated for the mAb portion of the ADC. Confirmation that the binding affinity is comparable between humans and the nonclinical species proposed for use in preclinical development is an important element of the justification for the relevance of the species used in the preclinical program. Most mAbs are selected from three human IgG isotypes (IgG1, IgG2, or IgG4) with the large majority of ADCs being the IgG1 subtype. These antibodies may be chimeric, humanized, or fully human. Humanized or fully human monoclonal antibodies are usually the first choice in an attempt on increasing the probability for improving high cell target specificity, increasing the circulating half-life in humans, and minimizing immunogenicity. Historically, the immunogenicity seen with murine or chimeric mAbs has been countered by converting them to humanized or fully human mAbs.

The Fab region of the antibody is responsible for antigen recognition and binding and can lead to ADC internalization, which, therefore, drives the intended specificity or specific uptake to the target cells. The Fc region of the antibody can trigger antibody effector functions such as antibody-dependent cellular cytotoxicity (ADCC) and complement-dependent cytotoxicity (CDC) through binding to Fcγ receptors (FcγR). Fc-mediated antibody effector functions are typically secondary in terms of MOA for most ADCs; however, FcγR binding of ADCs could mediate nonspecific uptake to normal cells, causing off-target cytotoxicity (Uppal et al. 2015). Neonatal Fc receptor (FcRn) binds to the Fc region of IgG in the acidic environment of an endosome, which can then recycle and release the bound IgG at the cell surface. Therefore, FcRn binding plays an important role not only in pharmacokinetics of ADCs but also in safety by reducing ADC accumulation and release of cytotoxic payloads in normal cells. Understanding expression patterns and species differences of FcγR and FcRn as well as physicochemical aspects of ADCs contributing Fc-mediated binding is important for understanding nonspecific uptake and toxicity of ADCs. Modulation of FcγR or FcRn binding can provide potential opportunities to overcome undesired adverse events related to nonspecific uptake (Schroeder and Cavacini 2010, Pyzik et al. 2015, Hamblett et al. 2016).

22.3.3 Linkers

Linker design and selection is an essential element of creating the optimal ADC. The ideal linker is one that finds the best balance between stability in plasma and effective release of active payload in the tumor. The design/selection of the linker should be tumor- and/or payload-dependent with the objective of optimizing the therapeutic index. Research should be conducted on this optimization as it cannot be assumed that the theoretical or actual stability (i.e., non-cleavable or cleavable) of the linkers will be predictive of the safety of the ADCs. Premature release of toxin in circulation could result in toxicity, and ineffective release of active payload in tumors could compromise efficacy (Jain et al. 2015, Tsuchikama and An 2018). However, complete stability may not be necessarily beneficial and a degree of instability may be advantageous in some cases (Ab et al. 2015, Cardillo et al. 2015). Since premature release of payload presents a perceived safety risk, demonstration of the ADC linker stability in the plasma of both the nonclinical test species and humans is required to support first-in-human (FIH) trials (ICH S6, S9, S9 Q&A). Based on chemistry of the release mechanism, linkers are generally classified as cleavable or non-cleavable. Upon internalization, the ADC is trafficked to the lysosomes, an acidic environment rich in proteolytic enzymes; therefore, cleavable linkers are typically designed to be activated or metabolized in this environment. Structures of representative cleavable and non-cleavable linkers described in this chapter are shown in Figure 22.4.

22.3.3.1 Cleavable Linkers

Cleavable linkers include motifs that are sensitive to lysosomal proteases, acidic pH, redox potential, or other conditions that may be preferentially found within cells. For example, the valine-citrulline linker used in brentuximab vedotin (Figure 22.4a) and the valine-alanine linker used in rovalpituzumab tesirine (Figure 22.4f) are rapidly hydrolyzed by proteases including cathepsins present in the lysosomal compartment of cells. The acid-labile linkers are relatively stable at the neutral pH of plasma but hydrolyzed in the acidic environment of lysosomes (pH 4.5–5). Gemtuzumab ozogamicin and inotuzumab ozogamicin use an acid-cleavable linker composed of the condensation product of 4-(4′-acethyphenoxy)-butanoic acid and 3-methyl-3-mercaptobutane hydrazide (known as dimethyl hydrazide) (Figure 22.4b). Sacituzumab govitecan also uses a pH-triggered linker, CL2A (Figure 22.4c). The disulfide linkers (Figure 22.4d) that have been used for DM1 and DM4 maytansinoids take advantage of the reducing environment of the endolysosomal pathway for the release of active drug (Kellogg et al. 2011).

22.3.3.2 Non-cleavable Linkers

Non-cleavable linkers are designed without an engineered cleavage mechanism and are generally highly stable in circulation. This class of linkers includes the thioether linker SMCC (succinimidyl-4-(N-maleimidomethyl) cyclohexane-1-carboxylate), which is used for ado-trastuzumab emtansine (Figure 22.4h), or mc (maleimidocaproic acid) in monomethyl auristatin F (MMAF) ADCs, which is used for belantamab mafodotin (Figure 22.4g). For such linkers, the payload is generally released from the ADC upon complete proteolytic degradation (often termed catabolism) of the antibody backbone. The released payload-bearing catabolic products will still include the linker and the amino acid (often cysteine or lysine)

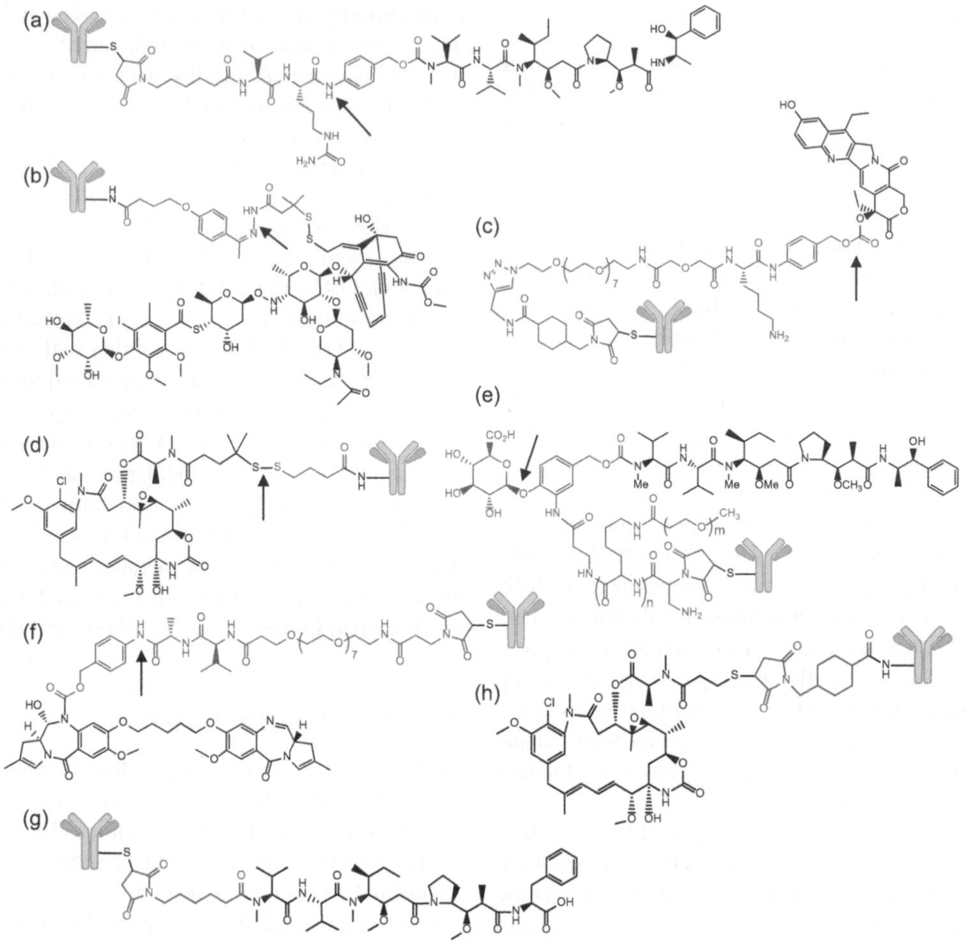

FIGURE 22.4 Representative cleavable (a–f) and non-cleavable (g and h) linker-payloads in ADCs. (a) mc-vc (maleimidocaproyl valine-citrulline)-PABC (p-aminobenzyloxycarbonyl) MMAE ADC; (b) AcBut (4-(4-acetylphenoxy) butanoic acid)-hydrazone N-acetyl-gamma-calicheamicin ADC; (c) CL2A SN-38 ADC; (d) SPDB (N-succinimidyl-4-(2-pyridyldithio) butanoate) DM4 ADC; (e) mDPR (maleimide diaminopropionic acid)-PEGx-glucuronide MMAE ADC; (f) maleimidopropionyl-PEG$_8$-valine-alanine-tesirine; (g) mc (maleimidocaproyl) MMAF ADC; (h) SMCC (succinimidyl-4-(N-maleimidomethyl) cyclohexane-1-carboxylate) DM1 ADC. Structures of linkers were highlighted in red, and cleavage sites of cleavable linkers were marked by arrows.

of antibody to which they were conjugated; for example, the released payload moiety for the ADC shown in Figure 22.2g is Cys-mc-MMAF. Because of their large molecular weight and hydrophilic nature, they are generally less membrane permeable than payloads released from the cleavable linkers and can be less capable of killing neighboring cells through the bystander effect (to be discussed later).

22.3.4 Next-Generation Linkers

Earlier generation linkers such as those described above have been used successfully in marketed and clinically tested ADCs, but they still provide opportunities for improvements, such as chemical stability and linker hydrophobicity. A number of commonly used linkers contain a maleimide moiety that facilitates attachment to the antibody (Figure 22.4). This maleimide, depending on its configuration, can undergo a chemical reaction (referred to as retro-Michael addition) that results in the payload, and possibly part of the linker, being transferred to endogenous thiol-containing molecules such as albumin, cysteine, and glutathione in plasma resulting in measurable

ADC loss and the generation of new payload-bearing molecules. The pharmacological consequences are unclear but may include diminished antitumor activity and greater toxicity (Alley et al. 2008, Shen et al. 2012a, Lyon et al. 2014, Szijj et al. 2018). It has been proposed that post-conjugation hydrolysis increases the stability of thiol-maleimide conjugates (Shen et al. 2012a) and that modifications of the linker by using diaminopropionic acid (DPR), which can facilitate rapid in vivo hydrolysis, have been shown to stabilize linker and prevent nonspecific deconjugation related to the maleimide (Lyon et al. 2014). Conjugation of a linker-drug to an antibody can have substantial effects on its physicochemical characteristics. In particular, the addition of hydrophobic linker-drugs can result in ADC aggregation, reduced ADC exposure, and increased immunogenicity (Joubert et al. 2012, Adem et al. 2014, Guo et al. 2016). To mitigate such effects, numerous linker modifications have been proposed. One such strategy is the incorporation of a hydrophilic β-glucuronide moiety into the linker (Jeffrey et al. 2006, 2010) (Figure 22.4e). Another approach to decreasing hydrophobicity of the vc-MMAE linker-drug, which may also facilitate higher DAR, is the incorporation of a PEG side chain into a glucuronidase cleavable linker. A PEG chain of 8–24 units has resulted in ADCs with improved pharmacokinetics that showed greater tolerability in a rodent model (Lyon et al. 2015, Burke et al. 2017). Additional new linkers in clinical, preclinical, and early-stage development are reviewed in recent publications (Frigerio and Kyle 2017, Tsuchikama and An 2018).

22.3.5 Conjugation

22.3.5.1 Conventional or Heterogeneous Conjugation

In earlier generation ADCs, linker-payloads were conjugated to amino acid residues, typically via the side chain amine or thiol on lysines or cysteines, respectively. Depending on the method, this process affords a mixture of ADC species with variable drug-antibody ratios (DARs) and conjugation sites. Lysine conjugation generally results in a mixture of molecular species with a DAR of 1 to 8 that are conjugated at about 20 different lysine residues, which could potentially generate a large number of different ADC species (Kim et al. 2014). For cysteine conjugation, four interchain disulfide bonds in the IgG1 antibody can be reduced to generate 2, 4, 6, or 8 free thiols, with resulting ADCs with different DARs. These multiple ADC species can have distinct properties, differential physical stability and may exhibit different pharmacokinetic and pharmacodynamics properties (Hamblett et al. 2004). This heterogeneous conjugation increased the risk of conjugation at sites on the antibody that can affect target binding, particularly if there is a lysine or cysteine in or near the complementarity-determining regions (CDRs). While the presence of lysine or cysteine residues can increase this risk, it may still be possible to achieve successful conjugation even under these circumstances.

22.3.5.2 Site-Specific or Homogeneous Conjugation

Among the improvements in the next generation, ADCs were a transition from conventional methods of conjugation to a site-specific approach in order to overcome the liabilities of heterogeneity (e.g., clearance and toxicity). Site-specific conjugation enables the attachment of a specific number of payloads at defined sites on the antibody, leading to a more homogeneous product with a defined and uniform drug loading (Panowski et al. 2014, Schumacher et al. 2016). The methodologies can be categorized as (1) genetic engineering of cysteine: engineering additional cysteine residues to the antibody leaving the interchain disulfides untouched (Junutula et al. 2008); (2) incorporation of non-natural amino acids possessing reactive handles such as p-acetyl phenylalanine (Axup et al. 2012); and (3) enzymatic modification: the use of engineered glycotransferases (Zhou et al. 2014), transglutaminases (Dennler et al. 2014), and the transpeptidase sortase A (Beerli et al. 2015). The advantage of site-specific conjugation has been noted in a number of publications with the efficacy of site-specific conjugates being comparable to conventional conjugates in both in vitro and in vivo studies despite having a lower DAR; engineered site-specific conjugates were also better tolerated in

nonclinical species compared with traditional ADC (Junutula et al. 2008, 2010). In addition, ADC with site-specific conjugation showed slower clearance than traditional ADC (Boswell et al. 2011), and coupling relatively stable sites with optimized linkers may provide optimal stability and reduction of payloads metabolism in circulation (Junutula et al. 2008, Strop et al. 2013, Su et al. 2018).

22.3.6 Drug-Antibody Ratio (DAR)

As described above, ADCs can have varying amounts of conjugated payload per unit of antibody, the stoichiometry of which is typically referred to as the DAR and is another key design parameter for ADCs. The amount of drug conjugated to the antibody can have a substantial effect on the stability, PK, and safety of an ADC. In the case of Kadcyla®, where the drug DM1 is conjugated through the side chain lysine residues, the average DAR is approximately 3.5 with a range from 1 to 8, whereas Adcetris, where MMAE is conjugated through side chain cysteine residue, leads to an average of four molecules of MMAE with a distribution from 2 to 8. The average number of calicheamicin derivative molecules conjugated to each inotuzumab molecule in Besponsa is approximately 6 with a range from 2 to 8. A high DAR can increase potency but may also the risk of aggregation and faster clearance rates. Hydrophobic vc-MMAE conjugates using interchain cysteines with higher DAR were found to be physically unstable and resulted in faster clearance, while reducing the DAR resulted in an improved therapeutic window of vc-MMAE ADC (Hamblett et al. 2004, Adem et al. 2014). In a report studying effects of drug loading on the antitumor activity (Hamblett et al. 2004), in vitro potency was shown to be directly dependent on drug loading; however, the in vivo antitumor activities of ADC with a DAR 4 were comparable with DAR 8 at equal mAb doses. Similarly, in another study (Sun et al. 2017) with maytansinoid-conjugated ADCs that were targeting the folate receptor α or epidermal growth factor receptor, the in vitro potency consistently increased with increasing DAR; however, in vivo results suggested that maytansinoid conjugates with DAR 2 to 6 provided a more desirable and higher therapeutic index than conjugates with higher DAR (9 to 10). It was suggested that the faster clearance of high DAR ADCs was the likely reason for the decreased efficacy. Although decreasing DAR was associated with better outcomes for hydrophobic payloads, recently developed hydrophilic and polyvalent polymer-based platform allowing much higher DAR (>10) not only showed promising activity in xenograft tumor models, but also demonstrated good PK properties in nonclinical animal models (Yurkovetskiy et al. 2015).

22.3.7 Payloads

The selection of the optimal payload can depend on a number of important factors including payload potency, MOA, target indication, potential for organ toxicity, and the suitability for potential combinations with standard of care co-medicants. In principle, the cytotoxic potency of the payload should be high enough to effectively kill target cells at low intracellular concentrations. However, high potency payloads may also worsen dose-limiting toxicities (DLTs) of ADCs, and it may be possible to overcome low potency of the payload with high DAR if appropriate linker-conjugation can solve potential stability and hydrophobicity problems. The cytotoxic payloads currently in clinical development can be categorized into three general types of mechanisms: the majority of them being anti-microtubule agents (auristatins, maytansinoids, tubulysins) or DNA targeting drugs (pyrrolobenzodiazepines, calicheamicins, duocarmycins) with a smaller number using topoisomerase inhibitors (camptothecin analogues) or other mechanisms (amanitin). Class effects of linker payloads are further discussed in a later section.

In addition to the direct killing of antigen-positive tumor cells, some ADCs also have the capacity to kill adjacent antigen-negative tumor cells, referred to as a bystander killing effect (Sahin et al. 1990). For these examples, the payload is either released from the target cell following ADC internalization and degradation or by release within the extracellular space, followed by entering and killing surrounding cells that presumably do not express the target antigen. Payload selection can even be influenced by the desire for bystander effect, using a careful selection of the payload type, amount of released payloads, and physicochemical properties (Li et al. 2016). This can be beneficial in solid tumors with heterogeneous target expression, but can also be yield complications by increasing toxicity.

Intrinsic or acquired drug resistance is a common problem in cancer chemotherapy. A prominent mechanism by which cancer cells can exhibit resistance is by efflux transporters including P-glycoprotein (P-gp), breast cancer resistance protein (BCRP), and multidrug resistance protein 1 (MRP1), which are efflux pumps of the ATP-binding cassette (ABC) superfamily transmembrane proteins. Their substrates include not only commonly used chemotherapeutic agents such as vinca alkaloids, anthracyclines, epipodophyllotoxins, taxanes, SN-38, and tyrosine kinase inhibitors, but also cytotoxic agents and drug-linker conjugates such as MMAE and N-acetyl-γ-calicheamicin dimethyl hydrazide. Efflux pumps have been shown to be able to reduce the in vitro potency of ADCs by reducing intracellular concentrations of cytotoxin. Several investigators have conducted nonclinical studies demonstrating strategies for overcoming this problem: (1) the use of MDR inhibitors PSC833 and MS209 to restore the cytotoxic effect of inotuzumab ozogamicin in P-gp expressing cell lines (Takeshita et al. 2009); (2) the use of maleimidyl-based hydrophilic linker for DM1 to evade the MDR-mediated resistance (Kovtun et al. 2010); and (3) the combination of a BCRP inhibitor, YHO-13351 with sacituzumab govitecan to restore cytotoxicity of SN-38 in ABC transporter expressing cell lines and in mouse xenograft model (Chang et al. 2016). However, the translatability of these nonclinical strategies has yet to be proven to be successful in human patients.

22.4 Target Selection

22.4.1 Fictionalized Strategies and Principles: Heat Map and Clinical Liabilities

The holy grail of target selection lies in identifying a target antigen that is solely expressed on the surface of the target cancer cell with limited or no normal tissue expression. Other than known B-cell targets (CD19, CD20, CD22, etc.), which also result in normal B-cell depletion, target antigens are invariably expressed on other non-tumor normal tissues. This normal tissue expression can be in various tissues and with varying expression levels, depending on the target, the disease, the individual, and prior therapies. The level of target expression (up and down) can be modulated, by numerous factors, including prior therapies, disease and inflammation status. As such, choosing suitable selection criteria for targets is complex, balancing normal tissue expression and tumor expression.

However, the expression on tumor cells is not in itself a guarantee of success. A poorly internalizing target may not deliver sufficient toxin to the target cell, and nonspecific toxicity may be more likely to occur at sub-therapeutic doses. The density of expression is also key, with a certain threshold needed to see a response. It is not really possible to define what an appropriate target expression level looks like, as this will be very dependent on the nature of the target (internalization rate, for example), antibody affinity, and ultimately the potency of the cytotoxin used. Ultimately, a cell needs to be exposed to a sufficient amount of toxin to result in cell death, and the amount of toxin required will depend on the potency of the toxin. Low-density expression targets may therefore be more sensitive to highly potent toxins, assuming appropriate delivery via the ADC. The presence of abundant normal tissue expression may also present a significant antigen sink that needs to be overcome before targeting to the tumor can take place—this can have a marked impact on PK/PD, efficacy, and, in general, the therapeutic index.

In terms of normal tissue expression, careful consideration needs to be given to both the cell types and organs involved as well as the number of organs involved. For example, an attractive target antigen may have high expression in tumor cells, but low expression on cardiomyocytes in the heart. In this case, target-dependent toxicity in the heart could potentially result in life-threatening toxicities, whereas targeting a tumor antigen with low levels of expression on B cells may not result in serious, DLTs and could be more clinically manageable and reversible than cardiac pathology. In addition to understanding the extent and level of antigen expression in normal tissues, knowledge of the biology, especially in terms of a relationship to tissue homeostasis and repair, is also critical in the antigen selection. This is highlighted in the case of an ADC targeting Lgr5, a marker of intestinal stem cells. In this case, a Lgr5 monoclonal antibody conjugated to a PBD dimer through a cleavable peptide linker caused significant small intestinal damage after a single intravenous dose in rats (Junttila et al. 2015). Similar intestinal pathology was not identified in rats with a control (non-Lgr5+)-PBD ADC (data not published), suggesting that the finding is antigen-dependent. In addition, understanding the target antigen biology is informative to the payload selection. For example, using the same Lgr5 antibody as in the previous example but conjugating it instead to a microtubule inhibitor resulted in minimal single-cell necrosis and arrested mitotic figures in the intestinal epithelium. Although there are potency differences between the PBD and MMAE payloads in this example, the intestinal pathology from the PBD ADC study was consistent with a stem cell-related effect causing significant disruption and/or abnormal villous repair compared to the much less severe MMAE-ADC intestinal toxicity. It may be possible to overcome the normal tissue expression challenge by using technologies to mask the antibody-antigen recognition site (such as the Probody®) in normal tissues, with the ADC only recognizing the tumor antigen within the specific milieu of the tumor microenvironment.

Normal tissues expression is clearly an important factor, but we also need to be mindful that a significant number of clinical DLTs with ADCs are antigen-independent, and not predictable based on target expression in normal cells.

22.5 Class Effects of Linker Payloads

Several reviews of ADC-related toxicity have concluded that toxicity profiles are consistent within payload classes and are related to the MOA of the payload (Donaghy 2016, Hinrichs 2015, Guffroy 2018). Toxicity profiles of selected payload classes are discussed below.

22.5.1 Microtubule Inhibitors

Maytansine (i.e., DM1 and DM4) and auristatins (monomethyl auristatin E [MMAE] and monomethyl auristatin F [MMAF]) are microtubule inhibitors (or anti-microtubule) payloads and still the most common class of cytotoxic agents used in ADC development. They are used in two of the approved ADCs, Adcetris® and Kadcyla®. They cause cytotoxicity to tumor cells by disrupting microtubules, structures critical for intracellular transport within cells and required for cell division during mitosis (Lambert and Morris 2017, Chen et al. 2018).

The benefits of microtubule inhibitor payloads are that they have good activity against many tumors, and the safety is mostly monitorable, manageable, and consistent with microtubule inhibitor small molecules (i.e., chemotherapy; vinca alkaloids and taxanes) that have been used as a treatment for cancer patients for decades. In addition, the toxicities are mainly attributed to the payload and not antigen-dependent; therefore, antigen targets that are widely expressed in normal tissue are not excluded when developing microtubule inhibitor ADCs.

The primary toxicities observed with microtubule inhibitor payloads are bone marrow toxicity, peripheral neuropathy (PN), and/or ocular toxicity. Bone marrow toxicity consisting of neutropenia, thrombocytopenia, and/or anemia is mostly consistent between nonclinical species (rats and monkeys) and patients, although differences in severity have been observed (Saber and Leighton 2015, Lin et al. 2015, Li et al. 2013, Dieras et al. 2014). PN is a significant limitation with anti-tubulin ADCs in patients, particularly MMAE, but it is not consistently observed in nonclinical species (rats and monkeys) (Stagg et al. 2016, Saber and Leighton 2015). This is thought to be due to several factors, which will be discussed in the translatability section. Ocular toxicity is most frequently observed with the MMAF and DM4 and, to a lesser extent, MMAE containing ADCs in patients, and the symptoms include dry eye, blurred vision, keratitis, and corneal epitheliopathy (Eaton et al. 2015). Some of these ophthalmic observations in the cornea have been reported in cynomolgus monkey and rabbit toxicology studies (Matulonis et al. 2019, Bialucha et al. 2017, Zhao et al. 2018).

22.5.2 DNA Binding

22.5.2.1 Calicheamicin

Calicheamicin is a highly potent cytotoxic natural product from the enediyne class of DNA-damaging agents. It binds to the minor groove of DNA and induces DNA double-strand breaks with ensuing cell apoptosis independent of cell cycle status. Mylotarg® and Besponsa® are 2 approved drugs that contain the same calicheamicin derivative, N-acetyl-γ-calicheamicin, linked to the targeting antibodies, CD33 and CD22, respectively, via an acid-labile linker. Similar to PBDs, the major benefit of calicheamicin is related to both its potency and cell cycle-independent MOA that allow it to target a broader range of antigens and expand the potential target space.

Major non-hematological adverse events in patients treated with Mylotarg® or Besponsa® include liver toxicity, in particular hepatic veno-occlusive disease (VOD), that resulted in a FDA black box warning for both drugs. VOD is a serious medical condition that is characterized clinically by jaundice, painful hepatomegaly, weight gain, and ascites, and that is thought to be initiated by injury to sinusoidal endothelial cells. The risk of VOD is higher among patients treated with Mylotarg or Besponsa who undergo hematopoietic stem cell transplantation (HSCT). In Phase 2 trials of Mylotarg as a single agent at 9 mg/m^2/dose for two doses separated by 2 weeks in first-relapse patients with acute myeloid leukemia, VOD was diagnosed in 0.9% of patients in the absence of associated HSCT, while the VOD rates rose to 19% and 15% in patients who underwent HSCT prior to or after Mylotarg treatment, respectively. Other common adverse events with these conjugates include thrombocytopenia, fever, sepsis, infection, bleeding, mucositis, and rash. Liver microvascular injury consistent with VOD was similarly reported in monkeys dosed with Mylotarg and was characterized by increases in liver enzymes associated with microscopic findings of sinusoidal dilation and/or hepatocyte atrophy and of SEC alterations.

22.5.2.2 Pyrrolobenzodiazepines

Pyrrolobenzodiazepine (PBD) dimers (e.g., Tesirine or Talirine) are DNA interactors that are active by specific cross-linking of base pairs in the minor groove of DNA. The cross-linking does not distort the DNA structure so it is relatively insensitive to DNA repair mechanisms, resulting in a stalled replication fork and apoptosis when the cell attempts to undergo mitosis.

The advantage of PBDs that are active in the picomolar range of potency for cell killing is their potential for activity in access to targets with low levels of expression. PBD-based ADCs could also have potential utility in the treatment of tumors with known sensitivities to DNA-damaging agents. Typically, PBD ADCs will have a maximum of DAR2.

In terms of clinical toxicity, PBD dimers (including both PBD ADCs and the small molecule SJG-136) are associated with reversible 'third-space' fluid accumulation, resulting in effusions in the pleural, pericardial, and/or abdominal cavities. Skin toxicity and hematological toxicities (evidenced as reductions in most peripheral blood cell populations) have also been observed. A similar toxicity profile has also been observed nonclinically in the rat and cynomolgus monkeys. Renal toxicity, characterized by tubular degeneration in the medullary rays and collecting ducts, has been observed in cynomolgus monkeys dosed with PBD ADCs. The PN (clinically and nonclinically) observed with some other ADC payloads (maytansinoids and auristatins, for example) has not been observed with PBD dimers or PBD ADCs. Although there have been many PBD ADCs in preclinical studies, the clinical efficacy and toxicity data are currently being generated and the translatability of organ toxicities from animals to humans remains yet to be clearly established in the published literature.

22.5.3 RNA Pol II Inhibitors

Alpha amanitin is a toxin found in several species of the amanita mushroom (e.g., Amanita phalloides) that inhibits RNA polymerases (Lindell et al. 1970). IC50 information on amanitins dates back to the 1960s, with limited publication on the safety of this class within the last several years. Amanitin ADCs are currently being pursued by a few companies with the outcome of development still pending. The primary toxicity with amanitins is noted in the liver, with renal toxicity also noted due to the filtration of the toxin by the glomerulus (Fiume et al. 1969). A species sensitivity difference exists with amanitin toxicity, where mice are far less sensitive than higher-order species such as nonhuman primate. For novel payloads such as the amanitins, the potential for wide species variation in toxicity should be considered. These differences should be evaluated as much as possible before assuming triage results from early toxicity studies in rodents are predictive (Connor BAPTG Meeting Fall 2016).

22.5.4 Topoisomerase Inhibitors

Topoisomerases are enzymes involved in DNA replication, transcription, and recombination and play an essential role in DNA binding and catalysis of these essential functions to repair DNA strand breaks. In general, topoisomerase I inhibitors stabilize the complex between topo I and DNA, which collide with moving DNA replication forks, eventually leading to double-stranded DNA damage (Yu and Gao 2019). Topoisomerase inhibitors are validated anticancer therapeutics. Currently, available topoisomerase I inhibitors are derivatives of the parent compound, camptothecin.

Topoisomerase inhibitors are highly potent, but comparatively not as potent as the PBDs; this is believed to be potential advantage in terms of decreasing the severity of toxicities (Seiter 2005). The primary toxicities of the topoisomerase inhibitors alone (i.e., unconjugated to an antibody) have been primarily hematologic and gastrointestinal (Seiter 2005).

Topoisomerase I inhibitors have been explored as payloads for ADCs for many years. Two such ADCs have recently been approved or are in late-stage clinical trials. Trodelvy™ (sacituzumab govitecan) is an ADC that contains SN-38, the active metabolite of irinotecan, conjugated to an anti-TROP-2 antibody and has been FDA approved for the treatment of patients with triple-negative breast cancer (TNBC) who have failed prior therapies for metastatic disease (Goldenberg and Sharkey 2020). Based on clinical experience, the primary toxicities are primarily bone marrow- and gastrointestinal-related. The other topoisomerase-containing ADC DS-8201a is a HER2-targeting ADC. Structurally, this molecule is composed of a humanized anti-HER2 antibody (trastuzumab) conjugated by an enzymatically cleavable peptide linker to a small molecule topoisomerase I inhibitor (Tamura et al. 2019). Toxicities associated with this drug are similar to those described with Trodelvy™. However, lung toxicity has also been described in both cynomolgus monkeys and patients. Lung toxicity (pneumonitis) has been deemed likely on target and related to HER2-expression in the lung epithelial cells.

22.6 ADC Current Guidance (ICH S9 Q & A) and Regulatory Pubs

Historically, there has been minimal regulatory guidance for the development of ADCs. In the ICH S9 guidance, there is a brief description of conjugated products. In general, it states that the conjugated material is the primary concern; however, toxicokinetic evaluation of both the conjugated and unconjugated materials is still recommended. In ICH S9 Q&A, there is further clarification about recommendations for ADC development, which includes expectations for characterization of the ADC, the payload or linker payload, toxicokinetics, and stability. In general, the ADC is the main focus, limited characterization of the payload is needed, and the expectation for which species to test the ADC is similar to that of any biologic consistent with ICH S6. ICH S6 guidance also has minimal direction on ADC development and addresses expectations for species selection and payload safety evaluation.

Because an ADC is a combination between a biologic and a small molecule, one of the clarifying questions in the ICH S9 Q&A focused on the selection of the FIH starting dose. Basically, the starting dose calculation for an ADC is consistent with ICH S9 and can be determined by using either 1/10th the Severely Toxic Dose in 10% of animals (STD10) in rodents or 1/6th the Highest Non Severely Toxic Dose (HNSTD) in nonrodents, both using the BSA approach. Further discussion of oncology ADCs and starting dose calculation can also be found in the publication by Saber and Leighton (2015).

In general, treatments with ADCs are limited by toxicity and ADCs are dosed on an intermittent schedule with a common schedule being once every 3 weeks. One clarification in ICH S9 Q&A included that a clinical dosing schedule of once every 3 weeks could be supported by a single-dose animal toxicity study. Given the extended half-life of an ADC and the potential for cumulative toxicity as compared to a cytotoxic small molecule, at least two doses should be administered in animals in the toxicology studies to support initial clinical dosing regimens of once every 3 or 4 weeks.

As with any guidance, one needs to consider each ADC program on a case-by-case basis and complete the studies or assays that are rational and scientifically based for the program and would provide patient safety information. As new or novel classes of ADCs are developed, other studies may be warranted that have not been specifically listed in a regulatory guidance.

In 2015, the US Food and Drug Administration published an article that reviewed 20 separate oncology investigational new drug (IND) applications for ADCs (2 approved and 18 in development) and provided an analysis on FIH dose selection, plasma stability, toxicities in animals, and toxicology study designs (Saber and Leighton 2015). The INDs examined were from December 2012 to August 2013 and were within the scope of ICH S9 for those projects that had completed Phase 1 clinical trials. This review was prior to ICH S9 Q&A and was informative and provided insight into the FDA's thinking about certain aspects of ADC development, particularly with respect to the calculating starting dose for Phase 1. The ADCs reviewed contained payloads that were commonly being developed at that time, which were genotoxic agents that targeted rapidly dividing cells and did not include data from some of the more novel payloads presently being developed. In addition, the linkers used were disulfide-based linkers, peptidic linkers (e.g., protease-cleavable valine-citrulline linker), or protease-resistant linkers (e.g., maleimidocaproyl linker). Overall, their conclusion revealed that there was little consistency in toxicology study designs and the approaches being used for FIH dose selection. There was a good correlation between the HNSTD and the human maximum tolerated dose (MTD), suggesting this was a reasonable approach for calculating the starting dose. However, as more ADCs are being developed with novel payloads, a different approach may be appropriate.

22.6.1 Considerations for Novel Payloads

Thorough characterization of the toxicity profile of the payload alone is essential for ADC development. One objective of this characterization is to understand the potential toxicity profile associated with the release of the payload from the ADC (Hinrichs and Dixit (2015). Before initiating the characterization of the payload, it is important to confirm the identity of the released payload (or payload-related products) as it may differ from what was conjugated to the antibody due to unanticipated chemical or enzymatic processes. This topic is discussed in more detail in the section of this chapter describing ADME strategies for ADCs. In addition, characterization of the toxicity, genotoxicity, reproductive and developmental toxicity of the released payload will contribute toward a weight-of-evidence approach for reproductive and developmental characterization of the ADC.

A novel payload calls for an approach to species selection similar to that used for a new chemical entity on a case-by-case approach (e.g., for anticancer products in accordance with ICH S9 Guideline); in these cases, a rodent is preferred unless the payload is not active in the rodent [Note 2, ICH S6(R1)]. Minimally, a single-dose non-GLP study in appropriate species will be required; depending on MOA, the sponsor should consider a GLP repeat-dose study.

In vitro genotoxicity studies of the released payload will be required. These studies may not be required to support FIH. If the released payload is positive in an in vitro genotoxicity study, an in vivo genotoxicity study may not be required; furthermore, positive genotoxicity result of the released payload may preclude the necessity for an embryo-fetal developmental toxicity study with the ADC. The sponsor may consider

whether to conduct an in vitro hERG assay prior to FIH, although this may not be required.

In addition to characterization that is required for the development of candidate ADCs, there are options for better understanding the PK and toxicity profile of the released payload.

22.7 Non-oncology Indications

22.7.1 Considerations for Target and Payload Characterization for Non-oncology Indications

Although most ADCs currently in development are for oncology indications, there are a growing number of ADCs being evaluated for non-oncology indications such as autoimmune conditions or antibody-antibiotic conjugates for infectious diseases.

There is currently minimal regulatory guidance specific to non-oncology ADCs. ICH S9 and ICH S9 Q&A provide some guidance for oncology; however, non-oncology ADC programs will likely follow ICH S6 and ICH M3. Therefore, it would be best if sponsors seek early interactions with regulatory agencies to ensure the adequacy of their planned nonclinical testing strategy.

22.7.2 General Toxicology

Both the ADC and the payload (or linker-payload) alone will need to be characterized in toxicology studies. The FIH dose will be calculated from the toxicity study of the ADC, and not from toxicity studies conducted with the mAb or the payload. For the ADC, toxicity studies in the relevant species for the appropriate duration (typically dictated by the clinical development plan) will follow ICHS6 and ICHM3 guidance on species selection and appropriate study timing and duration.

In addition to ADC toxicity, the toxicity profile of the payload component will need to be evaluated. To determine the precise molecule to be investigated, the physicochemical properties of the linker and conjugation chemistry need to be understood. This includes attachment stability and whether the linker is cleavable or not cleavable. The released payload moiety is what should be evaluated in nonclinical toxicity studies.

One could consider adding an arm in the general GLP toxicity study for the ADC as a way to characterize the payload; however, for practical purposes, a stand-alone repeat-dose GLP study might be desired if the same payload will be used for multiple ADCs. For a well-characterized payload, the conduct of a bridging non-GLP repeat-dose study could be addressed with regulatory agencies.

Toxicity studies with the naked antibody (i.e., no payload) may or may not be needed, depending on the extent of prior characterization and/or pharmacological activity of the antibody. If the antibody component is intended to have activity of its own, it is possible that the characterization of the mAb will need to be provided. If the mAb has activity, but the doses of the ADC will be lower than pharmacologically relevant, minimal characterization of the mAb is likely to be sufficient. Antibody-only studies may provide information regarding antigen-dependent toxicities, but such studies may not be necessary from a regulatory perspective.

Toxicity studies with the linker are not likely to be required at any phase of development unless there is something unique about the linker that causes concern from a regulatory perspective.

22.7.2.1 Pharmacokinetics

Generally, the predominant mechanisms that govern the pharmacokinetics of non-oncology ADCs are similar to those discussed for oncology ADCs elsewhere in this chapter. However, non-oncology indications require some additional considerations, including potential non-intravenous administration routes and altered pharmacological MOAs that can impact absorption, biodistribution, and pharmacokinetics.

Subcutaneous administration may be desirable for many non-oncology ADCs, including those under development for infectious diseases and immunology indications. The structure of the subcutaneous space limits the possible dose volume and thus the maximum drug level from a single administration. While intravenous administration, typically used in oncology, tends to utilize lyophilized drug product that once dissolved provides flexible dosing options based on the patient's weight or body surface area, very limited dose adjustment is possible for subcutaneously administered drugs, which are typically administered as a fixed dose with a single or a few simultaneous injections. Thus, formulation development will require focus on stability, including high concentrations in liquid formulation, especially if retaining the self-administration capabilities that many therapeutic antibodies possess in this disease area are desired. Subcutaneous injection results in a slow absorption phase as antibody likely traverses the lymphatic system before appearing in the systemic circulation. This results in significantly lower maximum plasma concentrations than those exhibited after IV bolus or short-term infusion. The residence time in the subcutaneous space may preclude the consideration of payloads that cause skin toxicities and require stable linkers that prevent payload release in the injection site. Engineering extended half-life ADCs enables less frequent injections, which may improve the convenience of administration and patient compliance. These extended half-lives come with the additional requirement that these sustained ADC and payload exposures are tolerated.

Current oncology ADCs typically rely on antibody-antigen binding to membrane targets expressed on tumor cells. The relative accessibility of hematological malignant cells and the enhanced permeability and retention effect in solid tumors can result in preferential delivery to the site of action (Iyer et al. 2006). Although many distributional barriers, such as tortuous, leaky vasculature and elevated hydrodynamic pressure, impede the delivery of large molecules to solid tumors (Jain 1990), the potential benefit of selective distribution may not be present in non-oncology diseases where the site of action resides in tissues with less compromised physiology.

The payloads for oncology ADCs have thus far been cytotoxic agents, so minimizing systemic exposure of the released drug is highly desirable to avoid off-target effects that could reduce the therapeutic index. However, for non-oncology indications and drug classes for which payload-associated side effects are better tolerated, ADCs that exhibit some payload release and sustained systemic exposure may be more acceptable. These ADCs could couple the mechanisms of targeted payload delivery with slow systemic payload release, resulting in higher tolerated payload exposures than those observed in oncology. In addition, the antibodies utilized in oncology ADCs typically facilitate targeted delivery without eliciting a direct anti-tumor effect; however, ADCs that leverage antibodies that elicit a pharmacological effect may seek to optimize pharmacokinetic profiles to synergize with payload effects.

Oncology patients are commonly immunocompromised, which can temper their immune response after ADC administration. However, the potential for immunogenicity is especially concerning for indications where patients are not immunocompromised, or that require chronic dosing for disease management. The formation of antidrug antibodies (ADAs) may accelerate drug clearance or neutralize target engagement, both of which may have an impact on resulting ADC and payload exposures. Therefore, as with other biologics, the formation of ADAs for these therapies and their impact on pharmacokinetics remains a key consideration. In addition, the potential use of subcutaneous administration may increase the probability of ADA formation due to the presence of antigen-presenting cells around the site of injection and the increased residence time prior to ADC absorption. Therefore, patient convenience will have to be carefully balanced with the potential drawbacks during the development of ADCs in non-oncology indications.

22.7.2.2 Genetic Toxicology

Genotoxicity of the small molecule payload should be evaluated consistent with principles outlined in ICH M3 and ICH S2(R1).

22.7.2.3 Reproductive and Embryo-Fetal Toxicity

In contrast to an advanced cancer patient population as described in ICH S9 and ICH S9 Q&A, for non-S9 indications, a full reproductive toxicity package including fertility, embryo-fetal developmental (EFD) toxicity, and peri- and post-natal developmental (PPND) toxicity may be required (per ICH S6, ICH M3, and ICH S5(R3)) depending on patient population. As with other aspects of development, the sponsor should consider seeking regulatory scientific advice to ensure agreement with the reproductive and embryo-fetal developmental toxicity strategy.

In some cases, the characterization of the small molecule or the small molecule conjugated to a non-targeting antibody with respect to reproductive and embryo-fetal developmental toxicity could be considered in lieu of testing the ADC. When the toxicity of the ADC is clearly related to the MOA of the payload and if this is consistent across multiple ADCs with different antibody targets, then evaluation of the payload alone for reproductive and developmental toxicity may be supported, particularly if NHP is the only relevant species. Alternatively, one might consider the use of the payload conjugated to a non-targeting antibody for assessment. If the characterization of the payload alone is sufficient, it is likely that this characterization can be conducted in standard species (i.e., rat, mouse, and rabbit). Once these evaluations are conducted, they can be used to support multiple ADCs carrying the same payload.

22.7.2.4 Juvenile Toxicity

Evaluation of the ADC toxicity profile in juvenile animals will need to be considered, particularly if the intended indication of the ADC includes pediatric patients. As with general toxicity studies, a toxicity study in juvenile animals will be conducted in a relevant species (preferably rodent) and will focus on the assessment deemed appropriate based upon the toxicity profile in adult animals and/or other information about the mechanism. Toxicity studies in juvenile animals may not be needed when the target and payload are already well characterized with respect to juvenile toxicity.

22.7.2.5 Carcinogenicity

Whether an evaluation of carcinogenicity potential is required should be determined based on the intended clinical population and treatment duration (per ICH S1A guidance). Considerations supporting the decision to conduct a study include relevant species and knowledge of the target and payload. If the relevant species for the ADC includes both a rodent and nonrodent species, versus NHP only, then the sponsor would be more likely to conduct in vivo carcinogenicity studies in the rodent species. If the relevant species for the ADC is NHP only, carcinogenicity studies with the payload may not be needed. On the other hand, if the target and payload are well characterized with regard to carcinogenicity potential, then a scientific justification for not conducting in vivo studies may be warranted.

22.7.2.6 Phototoxicity

Phototoxicity of the payload should be evaluated consistent with principles outlined in ICH M3 and ICH S10. Consistent with ICH S6 principles, phototoxicity evaluation of a mAb is not relevant. However, for risk assessment of an ADC with a potentially phototoxic small molecule payload, distribution of the ADC to the skin and eye should be considered; therefore, an understanding of the pharmacokinetic properties of the mAb and/or ADC could be informative.

22.7.3 Case Examples for ADCs in Non-oncology Indications

22.7.3.1 Adcetris® for Autoimmune Disorders

Adcetris®, which targets the CD30 cell surface receptor that is upregulated in hematological malignancies, is approved for the treatment of different lymphomas highlighted in as discussed elsewhere. CD30 is also upregulated in leukocytes in patients with chronic inflammatory diseases, including lupus erythematosus, asthma, rheumatoid arthritis, and atopic dermatitis (AD) (Vachhani et al. 2014, Nakazato et al. 2018), and there have been several case examples of lymphoma patients treated with Adcetris that reported improvement of other concomitant autoimmune diseases, including lupus and rheumatoid arthritis (Vachhani et al. 2014, Nakazato et al. 2018). In a press release in 2015, Seattle Genetics announced that it initiated a Phase 2 clinical trial evaluating Adcetris® in systemic lupus erythematosus (SLE, or lupus). The nonclinical toxicology package that was used to support registration of Adcetris® in oncology was likely adequate to enable dosing patients in a non-oncology indication, but continued clinical development and registration in lupus patients may have required more toxicity testing or waivers to justify no additional testing. However, the Phase 2 clinical trial evaluating Adcetris® in lupus patients was terminated in 2017 (for reasons unknown).

22.7.3.2 Antibiotic Conjugate for *Staphylococcus aureus* Infections

DSTA4637A is a novel THIOMAB™ antibody antibiotic conjugate (TAC), which is currently being investigated as a potential therapy against *Staphylococcus aureus* infections (Lehar et al. 2015). *S. aureus* is able to invade and survive inside cells, and intracellular *S. aureus* in tissues is associated with chronic or recurrent infections including osteomyelitis, recurrent rhinosinusitis, pulmonary infections, and endocarditis. Most antibiotics are ineffective at killing intracellular bacteria, but DSTA4637A consists of an anti-*S. aureus* antibody conjugated to a highly efficacious antibiotic that is activated only after it is released in the proteolytic environment of the phagolysosome. DSTA4637A effectively kills intracellular *S. aureus* (Lehar et al. 2015).

The toxicology program was designed to evaluate the nonclinical safety profile of TAC and the unconjugated antibiotic payload, dmDNA31, to support the proposed Phase 1 trials (Stagg 2019). A series of single- and repeat-dose intravenous (IV) administration studies in rats and monkeys were conducted. The pivotal toxicity studies additionally integrated genotoxicity (rat), male fertility (sperm analysis), and safety pharmacology endpoints. To characterize the contribution of dmDNA31 to the toxicity profile of TAC, dmDNA31 was evaluated in a repeat-dose rat toxicity study and in a series of in vitro assays for genotoxicity, cardiovascular toxicity, secondary pharmacodynamic activity, and phototoxicity. The no-observed-adverse-effect levels (NOAELs) with TAC were identified as the highest doses tested of 500 mg/kg in Sprague Dawley rat and 250 mg/kg in cynomolgus monkey following 8 weekly doses (Stagg 2019). In addition, there was no evidence of genotoxicity, cardiovascular toxicity, or neurotoxicity with TAC or dmDNA31 (Stagg 2019). The selection of the Phase 1 starting dose (5 mg/kg) was based on data from nonclinical studies with adequate safety margins. DSTA4637S was safe and well tolerated in healthy volunteers and is undergoing continued clinical development as a novel therapeutic for *S. aureus* infections. While there was no clear evidence of toxicity in rats or monkeys, there was evidence of discoloration of body fluids that was transient and attributed to the antibiotic portion of the molecule, which is blue in color. Similar effects have been seen with rifampicin and other compounds in this class (red discoloration of tears, urine, etc.) that are monitorable and not associated with adverse clinical effects (RIFADIN® [rifampin], package insert 2010).

TAC was evaluated in healthy male and female volunteers in a Phase 1, randomized, double-blind, placebo-controlled, single-ascending dose study (Peck et al. 2019). The patients were dosed at 5, 15, 50, 100, and 150 mg/kg. TAC was safe and well tolerated in healthy volunteers with observations of a moderate infusion-related reaction in one patient and non-adverse blue discoloration (as observed in the nonclinical studies). A Phase 1b multiple ascending dose study in patients is ongoing. To support the ongoing clinical development of TAC, developmental and reproductive toxicology studies in rat and rabbit and a longer-term (6-month) repeat-dose toxicology study in rat will be conducted.

22.8 Impurities

The manner in which impurities are assessed is likely to be different for non-oncology ADCs compared to ADCs developed for oncology indications. For oncology compounds, the ICH S9 guidance allows for impurities to be greater than ICH Q3A/Q3B limits, providing that adequate controls are in place; furthermore, ICH M7 (potentially mutagenic impurities) does not strictly apply for products developed under ICH S9. This is not the case for compounds outside of ICH S9, and the developer will need to consider all available guidance when assessing impurities. An impurity risk assessment will be staged during the course of development, with controls needed in early development and full assessment in late development and for marketing application.

Regardless of indication, ADCs have four moieties to assess for impurities, residual solvents, and/or degradation products: mAb drug substance, small molecule drug substance (e.g., drug-linker or linker and payload separately depending on manufacturing method), ADC drug substance, and ADC drug product. In addition, extractables and leachables assessment is required for packaging materials. Manufacturing method and identification of regulatory intermediates will be the determining factors in whether the drug-linker can be considered as a single entity or whether the linker and payload will be evaluated separately. In most cases, the drug and linker are manufactured as a single entity that is then conjugated to the antibody; in this case, the drug-linker is the intermediate. However, there are other manufacturing strategies, in which the linker is attached to the antibody first, followed by conjugation of the small molecule; in this case, both the linker and small molecule will be considered intermediates. Gong et al. (2018) provided a control strategy for small molecule impurities in ADCs; although this white paper focuses on the assessment of impurities for oncology indications, it reflects industry consortium practices and viewpoints and provides aspects to consider for non-oncology indications as well.

Impurity assessments for the mAb drug substance follow ICH Q6B and consider levels of aggregates, charge variants, or other aspects for biotherapeutic quality. Drug-linker drug substance impurity assessments may consider conjugatable vs. non-conjugatable impurities separately, as non-conjugatable impurities are most likely removed or controlled to very low levels in the purification process. In addition, residual solvents are evaluated in the impurity assessment for drug-linker drug substance. For ADC drug substance and drug product,

purification methods limit impurities in final drug substance. Therefore, the focus of impurity assessment and controls occurs with the small molecule drug-linker intermediate.

22.9 ADME Strategy for Development of Next-Generation ADCs

A thorough appreciation of the absorption, distribution, metabolism, and elimination (ADME) behavior of an ADC can provide useful insights at all stages of development. For example, in the early stages of ADC discovery, in vitro and in vivo evaluation of linker stability can help guide optimization of linker chemistry, which may modulate the effects of free payload on toxicity (Shen et al. 2012a). Pharmacokinetic studies can provide insights into the effects of conjugation on ADC elimination and tissue distribution that may lead to modifications in ADC design (Boswell et al. 2011). As the development of the ADC proceeds, it may also be important to understand the catabolic fate of the ADC and its payload-containing products to assess the potential for deleterious drug–drug interactions (DDIs) between the ADC and other drugs a patient may be taking. These are but a few, of many, possible examples of the valuable ADME information. However, it is important to generate only relevant and useful information for the development of the ADC. In any event, a diverse set of analytical tools and experimental systems will be required to support a rational and focused ADME strategy for ADCs to support molecule discovery and development.

22.9.1 Bioanalysis of ADCs—What to Measure and Why

An important first step in investigating the ADME of an ADC is determining analytes should be quantitated. A robust and diverse bioanalysis strategy for an ADC is essential for understanding not only the exposure of the ADC as a correlate to pharmacologic activity, but also important aspects of the in vivo behavior of ADCs (Kaur et al. 2013). This information can guide ADC design and development not only for nonclinical studies but may also be of value providing insights into optimizing clinical study design.

Bioanalysis of ADCs can be quite complex due to the potential limits of quantitation and the existence of multiple relevant analytes with the potential for pharmacologic or mechanistic importance. The bioanalysis strategy for therapeutic agents is typically focused on the determination of the concentrations of active, or potentially active, pharmacologic species in blood, plasma, or serum. This information supports the typical pharmacokinetic and toxicokinetic analyses conducted during discovery and development and also can provide insights into ADC behaviors that may inform new ADC technology. Measurement of ADCs and other relevant ADC-related analytes in tissues is less frequently conducted, but may be done to support specific investigations of biodistribution or elimination of ADC, as elsewhere in this chapter.

In contrast to the bioanalysis of other classes of therapeutic agents where a single active molecular species is measured, the bioanalysis of ADCs often includes multiple analytes. This can be explained in part by the appreciation that there are at least three potentially active components of the ADC—the complete ADC bearing the targeting antibody and the active small molecule payload, the unconjugated antibody (existing either as a component of the drug product, or formed as a result of payload being cleaved or released from the ADC), and any unconjugated (free) payload released from the ADC. The drug product (or what might be considered the parent drug) is the ADC, and this is generally the species that would be providing the bulk of the desired pharmacologic effect. Thus, the measurement of ADC (or a surrogate) is an essential part of the bioanalytical strategy.

The potential for heterogeneity of ADCs can complicate the bioanalytical strategy. An example would be ado-trastuzumab emtansine, which consists of an antibody conjugated to DM1 via linkers attached to lysine residues on the antibody (Kim and Kim 2015). The conjugation process leads can lead to a DAR range of 1–8 conjugated DM1 molecules located at several lysines at various locations on the antibody. This heterogeneity is not unique and can be found in other ADCs (Chen et al. 2016). However, many companies are now using conjugation technologies that allow specific and homogeneous conjugation of a payload to the antibody resulting in a more consistent drug product (Chudusama et al. 2016). The heterogeneity in the number and location of payloads can also be further complicated by the loss of the payload over time, which can lead to a constantly evolving mixture of ADC species (Xu et al. 2011, Wei et al. 2016). The pharmacologic relevance of this heterogeneity can be difficult to accurately determine, but it is possible that different catabolites of ADCs could have different potencies. There is clear evidence that ADC potency, pharmacokinetics, and toxicity can not only be a function of the DAR, but extensive analyses of the potency of individual DAR species generated over time have shown while the circulating profile of potentially active compounds can be different than those in the drug product, this concern has not resulted in substantial differences of activity (Hamblett et al. 2004, Sun 2017). Furthermore, one could question the relevance of such an exercise as the pharmacologic effects of the ADC can be considered the aggregate effect of all circulating species.

Sponsors have generally approached quantitation of ADC concentrations in one of two ways (Wang 2017, Gorovits et al. 2013). One is an immunoassay that relies on the presence of the two pharmacologically relevant parts of an intact ADC, the antibody and the cytotoxic drug. In general, this type of assay uses reagents that cause the ADC to form a bridge between reagents to capture the antibody via the CDR while detecting the bound ADC using a labeled antibody against the payload. This bridging assay would therefore produce a signal only when both antibody and payload are present on the ADC. ADC immunoassays have some limitations that can affect their interpretation. In general, such assays are developed and conducted using the drug product as a standard, which, as described above, can differ substantially from the circulating drug. And, depending on their design and performance, ADC immunoassays can vary in their sensitivity of detection of ADCs with higher or lower amounts of conjugated toxin (Kumar et al. 2015). Thus, it can be difficult in a blood sample to link the measured concentration value to a specific payload species, or specific mixture of species. It is important to understand these limitations when using such assays to understand ADC behavior. Despite these limitations, a robust ADC immunoassay can provide the necessary information to support an ADC development program. A second bioanalytical method commonly applied for the measurement of ADC concentrations relies on the presence of a specific enzymatic cleavage site that may be part of the linker (Sanderson et al. 2016). The purpose of this cleavage site is to facilitate the release of the payload in the enzyme-rich endocytic and lysosomal vesicles in tumor cells, but this cleavage site can also be used to exogenously release the payload from the ADC during the analytical process, followed by analysis of the released payload using LC-MS/MS. The resulting plasma concentration, often referred to as 'antibody conjugated drug', can provide an accurate measure of the circulating payload bound to the ADC. However, this assay does not provide a direct measure of the ADC concentration nor does it provide information on the number of payloads conjugated to each ADC. To obtain an estimate of the ADC concentrations, one can apply a simple mathematical transformation of the antibody-conjugated payload concentrations and the total antibody concentrations.

The second pharmacologic activity of an ADC is associated with the binding and activity of the antibody to its target, which is independent of the delivered payload. Under certain circumstances, the unconjugated antibody may have pharmacologic activity (e.g., trastuzumab is an approved biotherapeutic for the treatment of HER2-positive breast cancer and is also the antibody component of ado-trastuzumab emtansine). It could be argued that it may be relevant to measure concentrations of total antibody (unconjugated plus conjugated) to provide improved understanding of the pharmacologic effects of the ADC, but in practice, this argument is not usually applied as it is generally assumed that the bulk of the pharmacologic activity of the ADC is provided by the payload and the concentration of ADC can be considered a surrogate for both ADC and antibody pharmacologic effect. The utility of total antibody concentrations is typically related to understanding linker stability (the rate and extent of release of payload from the ADC), which can be accomplished by integrating total antibody PK with ADC PK, which will be explained further below. Therefore, an assay to measure total antibody is often developed. This is typically an immunoassay (but can be an LC-MS/MS assay) that quantifies all of the ADC-related antibody concentrations in plasma or serum, irrespective of whether the ADC bears a payload.

The remaining pharmacologic activity associated with an ADC can be attributed to unconjugated (free) payload released from the ADC following administration or formed as a consequence of catabolism of the ADC. These processes, and their implications, are discussed at length in other parts of this chapter, but for the purposes of bioanalysis, an assay, usually based on LC-MS/MS, is performed using plasma or serum samples. An important consideration for this assay is ensuring that the assay is capable of measuring the appropriate molecular species. The identity of the payload-related products generated by either linker cleavage, ADC catabolism, or other processes can be difficult to predict a priori (Shen et al. 2012a, Shen et al. 2012b). As some or all of these products may be pharmacologically active or may contribute to drug-drug interactions, thorough investigation to identify these products prior to assay development is critical to ensuring the appropriate measurement of relevant analytes, particularly for novel linker-drugs.

22.9.2 Integration and Interpretation of ADC PK

The interpretation of bioanalytical data can provide information essential for understanding ADC behavior. There are several key elements of ADC behavior that can be determined from an integrated evaluation of the assays described above. Conjugation of an antibody with one or more payload molecules can result in changes in the physicochemical characteristics of the antibody or affect binding interactions (e.g., FcRn) and thus adversely affect the PK behavior of an ADC resulting in accelerated clearance and enhanced elimination by tissues such as the liver (Hamblett et al. 2004, Sun 2017, Lyon et al. 2015). In effect, under ideal circumstances, the ADC should have a similar PK as the unconjugated antibody. Careful analysis of the total antibody PK, and comparison with the PK of an unconjugated antibody (either the same antibody as the ADC, or a similar molecule), can reveal differences that can suggest that conjugation is affecting PK behavior, and can guide the development of ADCs with acceptable product qualities.

The stability of the linker is a critical ADC characteristic and of keen interest to regulators. Rapid release of the payload upon ADC administration could lead to unanticipated toxicity and reduced efficacy (Phillips et al. 2008, Strop et al. 2013), so for most ADCs, it is desirable to minimize this process. Unfortunately, no single assay can provide specific information on the rate at which the payload is released from the ADC. However, this rate can be inferred by integrating the elimination rate of the total antibody and the rate of elimination of either the ADC (using immunoassay) or the antibody conjugated drug. In this type of analysis, the smaller the difference between these elimination rates, the lower will be the rate of payload release. Free payload (or payload-related species) concentrations can provide insights into the rate and extent of release of the payload from the ADC, but need to be carefully integrated with data from other assays and studies (e.g., PK studies with the payload or payload-related species) to provide this information. Free payload concentrations can also be used in conjunction with potency data to understand the potential toxicologic risks that may be associated with the free payload in plasma.

22.9.3 ADC Disposition

An appreciation of the ADME properties of an ADC can provide insights crucial to optimizing its design and development and the resulting impact on clinical efficacy and toxicity. The primary physicochemical attribute of an ADC is the antibody backbone; thus, much of the ADME of an ADC is determined by its mAb (Boswell et al. 2011, Erickson and Lambert 2012). However, the presence of an active small molecule payload conjugated to the ADC could introduce unique and important considerations that could lead to pronounced differences from an unconjugated mAb.

The evaluation of biotherapeutic ADME, particularly mAbs, is not a typical part of their development in part due to the fact that these characteristics are well understood with a large body of existing data (Vugmeyster et al. 2012, Tibbitts

et al. 2016, Zhou and Theil 2015, Lee 2013). Conjugation of a payload to a mAb can cause changes in the underlying ADME of both the mAb and payload with potentially substantial implications on pharmacokinetics and toxicity. And, the presence of the small molecule payload requires the evaluation of ADME characteristics normally associated with small molecule drugs.

22.9.4 ADC Distribution

Distribution is typically defined as the processes by which drugs move into and out of tissues. For drugs that can bind to, and subsequently be cleared in, tissues (including ADCs), the elimination that occurs as a result of these processes is discussed in more detail in that subsequent section. The tissue distribution of an ADC is typically governed by its antibody; specifically, distribution is limited to the plasma and the extracellular fluid in tissues (Glassman et al. 2015). Concentrations in tissue are generally below those in plasma, unless there is appreciable target expression in tissue that can facilitate binding and uptake. Tissue distribution is generally rather slow, with peak concentrations in tissue (including tumors) achieved in hours to days, depending on tissue characteristics such as perfusion and vascular structure (Glassman et al. 2015, Tabrizi et al. 2010). Under certain circumstances, the distribution of an ADC can differ from its component antibody. This is most commonly seen for ADCs that have been affected by conjugation with payload. In particular, conjugation of antibodies with payloads that are large and lipophilic—particularly with a large number per antibody—can alter the physicochemical characteristics of the ADC and affect its distribution. Two commonly cited examples are the effects of MMAE conjugation on an anti-STEAP1 antibody, which resulted in increased hepatic uptake relative to unconjugated antibody, and a similar observation following high DAR maytansinoid conjugation of an antibody to the folate receptor (Boswell et al 2011, Sun 2017). Of course, depending on the nature and degree of the perturbation, the amount and location of the distribution can vary. Nevertheless, increased distribution of an ADC to a non-target normal tissue can result in the elimination of the ADC in that tissue and contribute to increased toxicity or reduced efficacy.

The distribution of the cytotoxic drug is closely linked to the distribution of the ADC, largely due to the fact that for most ADCs the vast majority of payload in the body is in the conjugated state. Studies of ADC distribution have confirmed that a very high fraction of the payload in tissues is bound to ADC, with a much smaller fraction as unconjugated (free) drug (Erickson and Lambert 2012, Cohen et al. 2014, Alley et al. 2009).

22.9.5 ADC Elimination

The elimination of an ADC, like its distribution, is strongly associated with processes that govern antibody elimination. For mAbs and most protein-based biotherapeutics, elimination and metabolism are synonymous. To distinguish the processes that govern biotherapeutic elimination from small molecule elimination, the word catabolism rather than metabolism is commonly used to describe these processes for protein therapeutics.

The predominant mechanism by which mAbs and ADCs are eliminated is via nonspecific uptake by cells, followed by protein catabolism (Tibbitts et al. 2016, Zhou and Theil 2015). This process occurs in many cells and tissues of the body and is generally independent of target binding and Fc-mediated binding. The role of the neonatal Fc receptor (FcRn) in recycling ADCs is similar to that of mAbs, resulting in slow elimination rates and long half-lives (Lin and Tibbitts 2012). Upon the degradation of the ADC in cells, the amino acids of the mAb are recycled for use by cells while the payload-related catabolic products can be released by the cell into the extracellular fluid and ultimately into the circulation. These nonspecific uptake and elimination processes are particularly important in the context of an ADC. For biotherapeutics consisting solely of amino acids, the catabolism that occurs is not likely to have toxicologic consequences. However, nonspecific uptake of an ADC bearing a pharmacologically active payload can result in substantial toxicity. This toxicity may be due to the direct effect on the cells that catabolize the ADC, or due to toxicity to other cells locally or distantly as a result of active payload released from cells. While the rate of catabolism of the ADC is generally very low, and the clearance of the cytotoxic drugs (and its related catabolic products) is comparatively high, the concentrations of payload-related catabolic products in plasma are usually very low relative to ADC concentrations (Han et al. 2013, Doi 2017, Younes et al. 2012). Nevertheless, the concentrations of payload (and active payload-containing catabolites) can be sufficiently high to have pharmacologic effect.

Another process that could be considered ADC elimination is the release of the payload from the ADC without ADC catabolism (often referred to as deconjugation). This process, and the products formed, is dependent on the nature of the linker and drug. It is important to recognize that the payload-containing products formed by the release of payload from the intact ADC can differ from those produced by catabolism, and developers of ADCs should conduct thorough investigations of their ADCs to understand the identity of these products to allow a rational determination of whether further characterization (e.g., measurement in plasma, ADME studies) is warranted (Shen et al. 2012a, Shen et al. 2012b, Tumey and Han 2017, Wei et al. 2016, Tumey et al. 2015). An excellent review of these considerations provides a useful guide to investigators managing ADC ADME (Kraynov et al. 2016). ADCs with cleavable linkers may have higher rates of deconjugation than ADCs with non-cleavable linkers, but this generalization is not absolute. As described previously, the rate and extent of payload release are usually determined by integrating total antibody and ADC concentration data. The rate of deconjugation is generally quite low relative to the rate of clearance of the antibody and the elimination rate of the released payload-containing product; thus, plasma concentrations of these products are typically much lower than ADC concentrations.

Despite their low levels, these payload-containing catabolic products or release products can be extremely potent, especially for cytotoxic payloads, and low concentrations can still have pharmacologic effects that can manifest themselves in in vivo studies. Thus, circulating concentrations of these products need to be put into the context of their pharmacologic potency to fully appreciate the potential safety risks.

The fate of payload-containing catabolic or released products can vary depending on their structure. As would be expected for low-molecular-weight drug products, they are subject to the well-described metabolic and elimination processes of the liver, kidney, and other organs and such processes may make them subject to pharmacokinetic interactions with other co-administered drugs. Such DDIs can take the form of a perpetrator interaction whereby the payload-containing product reduces or increases the elimination of the co-administered drug. Such interactions may be unlikely due to the very low concentrations of payload-containing product. A more likely scenario may be that the payload-containing product is a victim of an interaction with a co-administered drug (which, for example, inhibits the metabolism or excretion of the payload) resulting in higher concentrations of the payload product. The potential for such interactions will need to be addressed during drug development for ADCs. Currently, there are no regulatory guidances specific for ADC DDIs, but investigators can refer to an extensive guidance literature for small molecule DDI (Prueksaritanont et al. 2013).

Understanding the ADME of an ADC can provide valuable information to guide discovery and development. As discussed above, distribution studies can help explain unexpected pharmacokinetic or toxicologic findings, providing knowledge about where an ADC has distributed leading to changes in the ADC molecule or development strategy to mitigate potential risks. Investigation of the identity and concentrations of payload-bearing catabolic products, or other released payload-bearing products, allows the design and conduct of a rational bioanalysis, catabolite assessment, and DDI strategy.

22.10 Translatability of Nonclinical to Clinical Safety

22.10.1 Approved ADCs: Lessons Learned about Translatability

22.10.1.1 Kadcyla®

Trastuzumab emtansine (T-DM1), also known as Kadcyla®, is approved for the treatment of HER2-positive metastatic breast cancer for patients who have received prior treatment with trastuzumab and a taxane, either combined or separately. Kadcyla® is composed of a monoclonal antibody, trastuzumab, targeting HER2 conjugated with DM1 (maytansine class of microtubule inhibitors) through a non-cleavable thioether linker. The clinical safety and efficacy of Kadcyla®, as well as the nonclinical development program, have been previously described (Poon et al. 2013, Burris et al. 2011, Martinez et al. 2016).

In general, the spectrum of Kadcyla®-related toxicities in nonclinical animal species and in humans is very similar. The major toxicities in both cynomolgus monkeys and humans include the bone marrow, namely thrombocytopenia (TCP), and liver toxicities. There was evidence of axonal degeneration of the sciatic nerve and spinal cord in monkeys administered T-DM1 that was not reversible after 6 weeks of recovery.

Thrombocytopenia was the most common grade ≥3 adverse event observed in patients treated with the single-agent

Kadcyla®. Kadcyla®-induced thrombocytopenia often began ~24 hours post-dose, with a nadir at ~day 8, and was generally reversible before the next dose (21 days). The majority of patients experiencing thrombocytopenia did not have spontaneous bleeding events, but cases of fatal hemorrhagic events have been reported. Thrombocytopenia was also described in the repeat administration toxicity studies in cynomolgus monkeys but was minimal to mild in severity and not a DLT, unlike in humans. Hepatic toxicity in patients has typically manifested as transient, asymptomatic transaminase elevations that may include either AST, ALT, or both. However, in a small subset of patients ($n=4$), multifocal nodular regenerative hyperplasia of the liver has occurred (Kadcyla® Label). Nodular regenerative hyperplasia is a rare liver condition that may result in portal hypertension and/or a cirrhosis-like architecture. Similar liver pathology was not identified in monkeys.

In the peripheral and central nervous system of cynomolgus monkeys given multiple doses of Kadcyla®, axonal degeneration and hyperplasia or hypertrophy of Schwann cells in the sciatic nerve and axonal degeneration of the dorsal funiculus of the spinal cord were present. These histologic findings did not result in clinically evident neurologic deficits in animals. Low-level HER2 expression on Schwann cells and glial cells is believed to have potentially been a driver of this toxicity (Poon et al. 2013). However, evidence of axonal degeneration in nonclinical studies in monkeys with DM1 conjugated to a different target (i.e., CD22) that is not expressed in peripheral nerves was observed at a similar incidence and severity (Stagg et al. 2016). This suggests that target expression in Schwann cells has little or no impact on PN observed in cynomolgus monkeys administered DM1 ADC conjugates, and the PN observed with Kadcyla® in monkeys is more likely due to the nonspecific uptake of the ADC in the peripheral nerves and release of lys-MCC-DM1. PN has been reported in patients dosed at the established clinical dose, 3.6 mg/kg; the incidence and severity have been relatively low and managed by dose reduction.

Although HER2 is widely expressed on epithelial cells of numerous organs, including gastrointestinal tract and skin, the majority of the toxicities described in human patients are largely target-independent and payload-driven. Despite the fact that there are differences in the DLTs in patients versus nonclinical species, the majority of the toxicities had been previously identified in the safety assessment of this molecule. The reasons for differences in sensitivity between nonclinical species and clinical patients remain unclear (Poon et al. 2013).

22.10.1.2 Adcetris®

Adcetris® is approved for the treatment of Hodgkin's lymphoma (HL), anaplastic large cell lymphoma (ALCL), and certain types of peripheral T-cell lymphoma (PTCL). It employs a monoclonal Ab targeting CD30 conjugated to the MMAE cytotoxic agent via a protease-cleavable linker. The safety and efficacy of Adcetris® have been evaluated in several clinical trials and summarized in Deng et al. (2012).

Two of the primary clinical toxicities reported with Adcetris® in HL and ALCL patients are neutropenia and PN (Deng et al. 2012) and are attributed to the MMAE payload

and independent of the antigen. Neutropenia (grades 1 and 2) was a frequently observed AE, and grade 3 or higher incidences were also reported in these patients. Neutropenia has been consistently observed in nonclinical toxicology studies (primarily cynomolgus monkeys) administered vc-MMAE ADCs (Lin et al. 2015, Li et al. 2013, Donaghy 2016). PN, primarily sensory PN, was another frequently reported AE, and the only non-hematologic toxicity of grade 3 or higher was reported in these patients (Deng et al. 2012). Mariotto et al. (2015) reported a patient with Adcetris®-induced PN that had a sural nerve biopsy that demonstrated axonal degeneration, a loss of microtubules, and findings suggestive of an impairment of fast anterograde transport. PN, however, has not been reported in nonclinical toxicology studies with vc-MMAE ADCs (Stagg et al. 2016).

Other factors found to impact the safety of patients that received Adcetris® were dosing schedule and patient age. Adcetris® was dosed every 3 weeks and weekly (for 3 weeks in a 4-week cycle) in different clinical studies (Younes et al. 2012, Younes et al. 2010, Fanale et al. 2012), and the MTDs were determined to be 1.8 and 1.2 mg/kg, respectively. The Phase 1 results showed similar overall tumor response between the two regimens, with the suggestion of a higher complete response rate for the weekly regimen. However, a greater incidence of PN was observed for 1.2 mg/kg administered weekly compared to 1.8 mg/kg every 3 weeks (75% vs. 33% for any grade PN, respectively). The median time to onset of neuropathy-related events was also shorter with the weekly regimen.

A retrospective analysis of the safety and efficacy of Adcetris® in adults ≥60 years with relapsed CD30-positive lymphomas was conducted: similar exposure, but older patients had more preexisting conditions (median 11 vs. 6) and were receiving more concomitant medications (median 7.5 vs. 4) (Gopal et al. 2014). Higher rates of anemia (30% vs. 10%), peripheral sensory neuropathy (60% vs. 46%), fatigue (58% vs. 43%), and adverse events ≥grade 3 (70% vs. 56%) occurred in older patients.

22.10.1.3 Mylotarg® and Besponsa®

Mylotarg® is approved for the treatment of patients with newly diagnosed and relapsed or refractory CD33-positive AML. Besponsa is approved for the treatment of patients with relapsed or refractory B-cell precursor acute lymphoblastic leukemia (ALL). Mylotarg® and Besponsa® are composed of humanized monoclonal antibodies against CD33 and CD22, respectively, conjugated to a calicheamicin derivative via an acid-labile linker.

Two of the primary adverse reactions reported with Mylotarg® and Besponsa® include thrombocytopenia and hepatic injury. Thrombocytopenia with Mylotarg®, although in part expected from the targeting of CD33-positive hematopoietic progenitor cells, showed prolonged duration in some AML patients despite complete bone marrow remission. Thrombocytopenia was also one of the main side effects of Besponsa® and one of the most common reasons for dose delay, dose reduction, or treatment discontinuation. Liver effects reported with both drugs include increases in aminotransferases, hyperbilirubinemia, and hepatic VOD.

In a dedicated investigative study in monkeys, Guffroy et al. (2017) have reported that thrombocytopenia and microscopic liver injury consistent with early VOD were similarly seen in monkeys dosed with a non-binding ADC containing the same linker and cytotoxic agent as Mylotarg® and Besponsa®. Briefly, the study has shown that target-independent damage to liver SECs is likely responsible for the development of VOD and is associated with thrombocytopenia through platelet sequestration in liver sinusoids. Results of the repeat-dose 3-month toxicity study in monkeys with Mylotarg further demonstrated the relevance of the cynomolgus monkey for characterization of these target-independent toxicities.

A meta-analysis across dose schedules of Mylotarg® in patients with relapsed or refractory AML showed that a lower-dose 'fractionated' schedule of 3 mg/m^2 on Days 1, 4, and 7 (as compared to the initial recommended dose of 9 mg/m^2) was associated with lower rates of early mortality, hemorrhage, and VOD that occurred without an apparent decrease in complete remission (CR) rate (FDA Briefing Document, Oncology Drugs Advisory Committee Meeting. July 11, 2017). Common adverse reactions were fever, infections, nausea, vomiting, constipation, bleeding, increased liver enzymes, and mucositis. There were no cases of VOD. Similarly, in the case of Besponsa®, the modified fractionated weekly dose schedule in patients with ALL resulted in less frequent fever, hypotension, and liver function abnormalities than were previously observed with the more intense q3w/q4w schedule. Bilirubin or liver enzyme elevations were all reversible within 1 or 2 weeks. VOD was observed only in 1 of 14 patients who underwent allogeneic SCT after weekly ADC treatment (Kantarjian et al. 2013). These results suggest that dose fractionation can mitigate the liver toxicity associated with calicheamicin conjugates.

Overall, based on review of the nonclinical and clinical toxicities, one can generally conclude that there is often good translatability between findings in nonclinical species and patients. There may be differences in the DLTs noted between nonclinical species and patients, likely reflecting species-specific sensitivity to certain target organ toxicities. Importantly, a significant difference between nonclinical species and patients is that cancer patients will have received and/or are undergoing chemotherapy and may have also concurrent or preexisting clinical conditions that may impact the types of toxicities, the timing of their onset, and the dose at which toxicities develop. However, toxicity studies in nonclinical species remain an essential part of the safety assessment of ADCs for patients.

22.11 On-target Toxicities with ADCs

On-target toxicities are those toxicities that are related to interaction with the target antigen, either in the desired location (tumor) or in normal tissue (when the target is expressed in normal tissue). The nature of such toxicities is typically target location expression- and payload-dependent. On-target toxicities due to interactions with target in the desired location are usually due to tumor-lysis syndrome, in the case of significant tumor burden, or due to bystander killing. Bystander killing is very payload and drug-linker dependent, with the more lipophilic warheads having a greater effect. Bystander killing can be advantageous in the setting of heterogeneous target expression in the tumor, but can also result in local toxicity around the tumor site. On-target, but off-tumor toxicity can be a real problem for target antigens that are expressed on normal tissue. The normal tissue expression can act like an 'antigen-sink', making it difficult to target the tumor, impacting on efficacy with payload-dependent toxicity at the normal tissue sites having a marked impact on therapeutic index.

Additional examples of on-target toxicity with ADCs include pharmacologically relevant antibody-mediated toxicity. This on-target toxicity is related to signaling through the target antigen resulting in downstream functional consequences. This would occur with antibodies that have pharmacologic activity both as an unconjugated antibody and as a conjugated antibody. An example of this would be B-cell depletion occurring with the naked antibody as well as the conjugated antibody (Walles et al. 2018, Zheng et al. 2009). An additional example of on-target ADC toxicity is discussed below.

22.11.1 Case Example 1: Immunologic Target

LOP628 is an ADC that targets c-KIT, which is amplified and overexpressed in multiple cancer types. It utilizes a maytansinoid cytotoxic payload conjugated to a c-KIT-directed IgG antibody via a non-cleavable linker (Abrams et al. 2018). Cynomolgus monkey was selected as the relevant toxicology species based on the sequence homology of c-KIT binding epitope of LOP628 across cynomolgus monkey and human and binding affinity assessments (Abrams 2018).

As discussed previously, an important element to a successful ADC target is having a clear differential between tumor antigen expression and normal tissue expression. c-KIT in general has low normal tissue expression; however, it is expressed on hematopoietic stem cells. Specifically, KIT is expressed on mast cells, which contain granules that are primarily responsible for cytokine and histamine release and subsequent inflammatory and hypersensitivity reactions (Metcalfe 2008). ADCs with normal tissue expression on immunologic cells would require additional examinations for potential effects on the immune system. Specifically, immunophenotyping (IPT), cytokine release, and Fc-mediated functions (i.e., ADCC and CDC) are assessed both in vivo and in vitro for this class of target antigen. Based on the normal tissue expression profile, potential effects due to mast cell degranulation were expected. Initial in vitro experiments to further understand the risk of normal tissue expression on mast cells demonstrated that LOP628 alone did not induce mast cell degranulation unless LOP628 was cross-linked with human IgG (World ADC Summit, October 2017a, San Diego, CA).

The repeat administration cynomolgus monkey toxicity study utilized a clinically relevant dosing regimen, which has been used for similar maytansinoid ADCs (Q3-week) with dose levels that were known to be tolerated for the DM1 platform-based ADCs (Abrams 2018). The monkey study included an isotype control ADC (non-c-KIT cross-reactive DM1 ADC) was included as part of the evaluation to understand the contribution of the maytansinoid payload (DM1) to the overall ADC toxicity profile. LOP628 was dosed every 3 weeks with terminal necropsy occurring 1 week after the last dose administration or 6 weeks after the last dose administration to understand the potential for recovery or exacerbation of toxicity after an extended non-dosing period.

The overall toxicity profile was consistent with hematopoietic toxicity and infusion reactions, which occurred acutely after IV bolus injection. Transient neutropenia was observed in which the nadir generally occurred 3 weeks after dose administration (i.e., immediately before the next dose administration), followed by recovery during the week after that next dose administration. Neutropenia was determined to be a pharmacodynamic effect of c-KIT targeting due to the presence of c-KIT on hematopoietic stem cells (Abrams 2018). The infusion reactions after initial dose administration presented within 5 minutes of dosing and were characterized as transient (resolving within 20 minutes) hypoactivity, scratching, and incoordination. Similar clinical signs were noted after repeat dosing but differed slightly with additional clinical signs of emesis, facial reddening, and decreased blood pressure observed with no scratching. These observations were persistent for up to 2 hours after each LOP628 administration. An important parameter that was also measured as part of the in vivo monkey studies was immunogenicity of the ADC. The emergence of ADAs (approximately 21 days after first dose administration) resulted in rapid clearance of LOP628. However, despite rapid clearance, neutropenia continued to be seen after every dose administration occurring in the same time interval as that which was noted after the first dose administration with a similar magnitude of response with each subsequent dose administration.

To understand the infusion reaction mechanism observed after LOP628 dosing in the GLP monkey study, a subsequent investigative single-dose monkey study was conducted. Serum histamine and tryptase were included at several collection time points (up to 24 hours post-dose) to determine whether infusion reactions were related to mast cell degranulation (Abrams 2018). Based on these analyses, LOP628 did not cause elevations in serum tryptase and histamine above baseline values. Therefore, it was concluded that infusion reactions observed in monkeys were likely not due to mast cell degranulation.

The information from the GLP monkey study (HNSTD) along with additional safety margins was used to support the FIH dose estimation for the LOP628 Phase 1 clinical trial. Upon clinical dosing of LOP628, acute clinical hypersensitivity reactions were noted that were consistent with mast cell degranulation (L'Italien et al. 2018). From a translatability perspective, the studies in monkeys did not predict the clinical acute hypersensitivity reactions noted at the clinical starting dose, which were presumably due to mast cell degranulation. These hypersensitivity reactions ultimately led to cessation of Phase 1 clinical trial. Additional investigations were conducted to understand the mechanism of mast cell degranulation in humans and concluded that these reactions were potentially Fcγ-related (L'Italien et al. 2018).

22.11.2 Case Example 2: Species-Specific Toxicity

ADC 'X' contains an antibody against a receptor tyrosine kinase that is highly expressed in cancer with low normal tissue expression (Connor 2017a). ADC 'X' had a similar binding affinity in rats, monkeys, and humans, and normal tissue expression of target antigen 'X' is overall similar in all three species. Based on this, both rats and cynomolgus monkeys were used as relevant toxicology species for the development of ADC 'X'. The linker payload utilized for ADC 'X' was a non-cleavable clinically validated cytotoxic payload.

The IND-enabling program was performed in rats and monkeys and was dosed on a clinically relevant dosing regimen (Q3-week×3). In order to identify potential target organs of toxicity, related to ADC 'X', the study incorporated a terminal necropsy, which was 1 week after last dose administration and a recovery necropsy occurring 6 weeks later to understand reversibility or exacerbation of toxicity after a non-dosing period. Dose levels were based on known target organ toxicities with the payload, which has been well studied clinically, with the high dose providing multiple safety factors above anticipated clinical exposures.

Although there was an overlap in the toxicity profile across rat and monkey studies, there were also distinct differences when comparing toxicity profiles across the two species. Payload-related toxicity was noted in both rats and monkeys, where target organs in both species included bone marrow, liver, and multiple tissues with payload-related effects consistent with cell cycle inhibition due to the anti-mitotic nature of the MOA of the cytotoxic payload. However, there were distinct findings in rats that were not present in monkeys exposed to ADC 'X'. Proliferative lung lesions were noted in the rat study at all dose levels with ADC 'X' at both terminal and recovery necropsy (Connor 2017b). This was a single species observation and could represent the activation of an internal signaling cascade related to the target antigen or other mechanism. For example, in instances of damage, the target for ADC 'X' could be upregulated and result in further tissue damage upon repeated exposure to ADC 'X'. Molecular localization revealed the presence of the target for ADC 'X', supporting this was likely an on-target effect. The mechanism and translatability to humans of the lung finding in rats were unclear, but an understanding of the pathogenesis, species specificity, and human relevance was deemed necessary prior to progressing forward with the therapeutic ADC 'X' candidate.

The first steps in the investigative effort into this species-specific toxicity were the determination of signaling cascade activation by ADC 'X' in rats as well as the assessment of the comparative biology and translational relevance across species. In order to address these questions, a follow-up repeat-dose rat investigative study was conducted inclusive of several different biomarker collections to understand on a molecular level the mechanistic basis for the progression of the proliferative lesion in the lung. Replication of the lung lesion with the appropriate rat study dosing regimen and necropsy time points allowed samples to be collected to determine whether specific pathway markers downstream of the target for ADC 'X' were upregulated and, if so, the potential role of agonism of the target antigen as a possible explanation of the proliferative lung lesions.

Overall, the data from the investigative study did not support the agonism of the target antigen for ADC 'X', but did support the presence of a specific lung marker consistent with an increase in type II pneumocytes (World ADC Summit 2017a,

San Diego, CA). Based on this, a similar marker was assessed retrospectively in monkey toxicology studies. The results of these additional analyses demonstrated that molecular markers consistent with the proliferative lung lesion were identified in rats, while similar proliferation does not occur in monkeys. Knowledge of the specific mechanism driving toxic phenotypes may shed further understanding into the risk-benefit ratio for patients when marked differences in toxicity profiles exist across species.

22.11.3 Off-target Toxicities with ADCs

Target-independent toxicities are those toxicities that are unrelated to interaction with the target antigen, in normal tissues. The nature of such toxicities is typically payload driven, but the location may be a function of both the payload and antibody components. For example, one hypothesis around the skin toxicity observed PBD ADCs may be due to the skin being a major site of antibody catabolism (Wright et al. 2000) with subsequent release of the ADC payload resulting in toxicity.

22.11.4 Hematologic Toxicities with MMAE and DM1

Hematologic toxicities are one of the major toxicities noted in microtubule inhibitor-bearing ADCs (i.e., MMAE, MMAF, DM4, and DM1 ADCs). The spectrum of hematologic toxicities described in nonclinical species and in the clinical setting has generally been similar and is primarily neutropenia and/or thrombocytopenia. These toxicities are understood to be antigen-independent and driven by the free payload, as similar cytopenias have been described with single-dose-free MMAE and DM1 studies as with their respective conjugates in both rats and cynomolgus monkeys. Modifications of antibody format by the generation of engineered cysteine residues to enable site-specific conjugation of the payload (MMAE) have resulted in the improvement of hematologic toxicities (decreased severity) as compared to conjugation through native amino acid residues(i.e., conjugation of payload through interchain disulfide bonds) (Junutula et al. 2008, Nature Biotech). These antibodies, named THIOMABs, have also allowed for uniform stoichiometry of payload conjugation, site-specific conjugation, and consistent manufacturing.

In cynomolgus monkeys, the most common DLT with MMAE ADCs has been neutropenia; this is consistent with what has been observed in clinical trials with neutropenia as the primarily DLT (however, longer-term dosing in patients receiving MMAE ADCs has been PN, which is discussed elsewhere in this chapter. In the case of DM1 conjugates, the DLT in humans has been thrombocytopenia (as described elsewhere in this chapter). Thrombocytopenia was also described in the cynomolgus monkey studies, but was decreased in severity (minimal to mild) as compared to humans (Poon et al. 2013, Uppal et al. 2015).

22.11.5 Ocular Toxicity

Ocular toxicities have been reported in clinical trials with ADCs, primarily ADCs carrying maytansinoid or auristatin payloads (Eaton 2015, Donaghy 2016). These ocular toxicities have most often corneal in nature, with adverse events described as keratitis, dry eye, corneal microcysts, corneal deposits, and/or conjunctivitis. Patients with these ocular toxicities experience symptoms such as blurred vision. Corneal toxicity associated with ADCs has been shown to be reversible.

Based on the totality of data available from clinical trials, the corneal toxicity associated with ADCs is considered to result from off-target uptake of ADCs into corneal epithelium, although on-target mechanisms of toxicity must also be considered (Eaton 2015). ADCs with MMAF and DM4 payloads are most often associated with corneal toxicity, regardless of mAb target or expression of the target in the cornea, therefore providing strong evidence for association of the payload with ocular toxicity and therefore would be an apparent off-target mechanism of toxicity (Eaton 2015, Donaghy 2016). Furthermore, corneal effects have been observed with unconjugated tubulin-binding drugs (i.e., docetaxel and paclitaxel), adding to the weight of evidence for an off-target mechanism of corneal toxicity with ADCs.

Several factors may contribute to the susceptibility of the cornea to toxicity: the eye has robust blood supply, populations of rapidly dividing cells, and a role as a barrier tissue in the innate immune system with abundant expression of cell surface receptors. Despite the clinical reports of ADC-mediated ocular toxicity, there are few published nonclinical reports of this toxicity (Zhao et al. 2018, Bialucha et al. 2017) or of clinical investigations into the potential mechanism of this toxicity (Eaton et al. 2015, Matulonis et al. 2019). In toxicity studies in nonclinical species, the microscopic evaluation revealed increased mitotic figures and single-cell necrosis in the corneal epithelium; these changes were dose-related and reversible (Bialucha et al. 2017). Zhao et al. (2018) presented investigative in vitro studies demonstrating that biophysical properties of the ADC, e.g., hydrophobicity and/or presence of positive charges, may drive non-target receptor-mediated uptake and subsequent cytotoxicity in normal cells such as corneal epithelial cells and that cytotoxicity to normal cells can be reduced, without loss of efficacy, by reducing hydrophobicity and/or modifying positive charges on the antibody component of the ADC. The data presented to date support the role of non-target receptor-mediated uptake of ADCs into normal corneal epithelial cells via mechanisms such as micropinocytosis and that this off-target toxicity is independent of target expression in cornea and can occur with any of the anti-tubulin payloads currently in development (e.g., maytansinoid or auristatin).

22.11.6 Liver

Hepatic disturbances have been reported clinically with diverse ADC constructs and are not specific of a single cytotoxic agent. They are mainly observed with more stable ADCs containing non-cleavable linkers (e.g., maleimide linkers mc and SMCC) or with more potent ADCs containing DNA-damaging cytotoxic agents (e.g., calicheamicin).

Liver injury may manifest as asymptomatic liver function abnormalities (elevations of transaminases and/or bilirubin) and/or may be characterized by the development of more serious specific liver diseases, such as nodular regenerative hyperplasia (NRH) or sinusoidal obstruction syndrome (SOS). In a pivotal Phase 3 T-DM1 trial, hepatic disturbances in T-DM1-treated patients were characterized by elevations in AST and ALT (22% and 17% of patients, respectively), with low rates of grade ≥3 elevations (4% and 3% of patients for AST and ALT, respectively) (Verma, NEJM, 2012). In addition, rare cases of biopsy-confirmed NRH have been reported in patients receiving a T-DM1-based regimen, and temporal association and absence of competing etiologies suggested a direct contribution of T-DM1 (Force *J Clin Oncol* 2016, Prochaska *Cancer Treat Comm* 2016). In a pivotal Phase 3 inotuzumab ozogamicin trial, liver-related laboratory abnormalities in inotuzumab ozogamicin-treated patients consisted mainly of increases in AST (23% of patients), ALT (15%), γ-glutamyltransferase (21%), bilirubin (21%), and alkaline phosphatase (13%), with grade ≥3 elevations noted in ≤5% of patients (except for increases in γ-glutamyltransferase grade ≥3 noted in 10% of patients) (Kantarjian et al. 2017). In addition, in the same Phase 3 inotuzumab ozogamicin trial, SOS was reported overall in 13% of patients and was more frequent in the subset of patients that proceeded to hematopoietic stem cell transplantation (HSCT) (22%).

NRH and SOS are both liver vascular disorders that are thought to result from initial insults to liver sinusoidal endothelial cells (SECs) (Wanless 2012, Rubbia-Brandt Histopath 2010). Nonclinical investigations in monkeys with a non-cross-reactive antibody-calicheamicin conjugate demonstrated an initial and selective injury to liver SECs associated with increases in liver transaminases and recovery or progression to microscopic changes consistent with subclinical SOS (Guffroy *Clin Cancer Res* 2017), providing evidence for the relevance of the monkey model for characterization and assessment of the liver toxicity.

Noteworthy also are the significant platelet effects reported clinically with these hepatotoxic ADCs, which may be related to the liver endothelial injury with associated intrasinusoidal platelet sequestration as investigated and demonstrated in monkeys for calicheamicin conjugates.

Challenges in the translatability between nonclinical and clinical data are multifold and include:

- Liver microvascular injuries (i.e., SOS and NRH) are uncommon pathologies that represent diagnostic challenges both clinically (absence of validated diagnostic blood test) and nonclinically (histochemical and/or immunohistochemical stains mandatory for accurate histopathological diagnosis)
- Liver endothelial injury may recover very efficiently in young healthy monkeys as compared to advanced cancer patients
- Peripheral thrombocytopenic events are rapidly obscured by bone marrow response in healthy monkeys as compared to patients with compromised hematopoiesis.

22.11.7 Peripheral Neuropathy

PN is a common and challenging toxicity observed in patients with anti-tubulin-containing ADCs, particularly MMAE

ADCs. Anti-tubulin ADCs cause predominantly sensory PN, which is characterized as paresthesia, pain or burning, allodynia, hyperesthesia or numbness in the hands or feet.

The PN observed in patients is attributed primarily to nonspecific uptake of the ADC in the peripheral nerves and release of the anti-tubulin payload (Stagg et al. 2016). Unlike the highly proliferative cells that anti-tubulin agents tend to mainly target, the high rates of PN observed in the patients are due to the susceptibility of the peripheral nerves. The peripheral nerves are made up of long projections of axons, and the microtubule network plays a critical role in the nerve cell for axonal transport (Almedia-Souza et al. 2011).

PN has not been consistently observed in IND-enabling nonclinical studies with anti-tubulin ADCs, but it is more difficult to assess in animals than in patients. Patients are able to report PN symptoms (starting in the most distal regions of the fingers and toes), whereas nonclinical assessments are based primarily on histopathology changes of peripheral nerves, primarily sciatic nerve (i.e., degeneration), and gross neurobehavioral effects.

Four hypotheses have been evaluated for the lack of translatability between nonclinical and clinical studies: (1) species differences in exposure; (2) insensitivity of animal models; (3) species differences in target biology and other vc-MMAE ADC properties in peripheral nerves; and (4) increased susceptibility of patient population (Stagg et al. 2016). The result of this hypothesis-based approach, particularly with vc-MMAE ADCs, identified key challenges with trying to model the PN observed in late-stage oncology patients in nonclinical toxicology studies with microtubule inhibitor-containing ADCs. Two key learnings were that the duration of exposure needs to be increased in nonclinical species since this is a delayed onset toxicity in the clinic and also that an expanded neurohistopathology assessment of distal peripheral nerves in study animals should be included, as these tissues may better represent the anatomic region most commonly affected in patients (Stagg et al. 2016).

The lack of translatability of PN from ADCs is thought to be result of several factors: (1) the delayed onset is not captured in the typical dosing duration of nonclinical studies; (2) the nature of the toxicity in that it is reported as discomfort by patients that can only be assessed as physical damage in animals by invasive techniques that may not be sensitive enough to detect changes; and (3) patients are at an increased risk of developing PN because of prior chemotherapy, comorbidities and age and disease-related factors.

22.12 Management of Off-target Toxicities

In general, early recognition of the symptoms, drug administration vacations, and dosage reductions are used to manage most off-target toxicities (i.e., bone marrow toxicity, PN, ocular toxicity, vascular leak syndrome, and liver toxicity). Prior to initiating drug administration, it is important to obtain patient baseline data (i.e., complete blood counts, any symptoms of PN, and ocular examinations) in order to recognize symptoms early after ADC treatment has begun. In many cases, delaying dosing or reducing the dose level can reverse the toxicities.

Some ADC-induced toxicities can be managed with additional medications. Neutropenia is a common toxicity in patients that receive vc-MMAE ADCs, and it can be treated with hematopoietic growth factors to regenerate neutrophils to enable higher doses and continuous treatment, which could include granulocyte-macrophage colony-stimulating factor (GM-CSF) or granulocyte colony-stimulating factor (G-CSF) PB (Pallanca-Wessels et al. 2015). Ocular toxicity occurs with MTI ADCs, particularly MMAF and DM4, and can be somewhat managed with steroid or regular eye drops (Matulonis et al. 2019). Peripheral edema occurs with the PBD containing ADCs as part of vascular leak syndrome (VLS) or capillary leak syndrome (CLS) and has been managed effectively with diuretics, steroids, and non-steroidal anti-inflammatory drugs (Rudin et al. 2017).

22.13 Conclusions

ADCs are promising new modalities for the treatment of cancer because they offer a method for delivering potent cytotoxic molecules directly to tumors. Over the past few years, advances have been made in the understanding, the technologies, and the clinical application of ADCs. To date, nine oncology ADCs have been approved (Adcetris, Kadcyla®, Besponsa, Mylotarg, Polivy, Padcev, Enhertu, Trodelvy, and Blenrep) and are currently on the market (as of August 2020) for the treatment of liquid tumors. Emerging areas of focus for ADCs are the development of ADCs for solid tumors and for non-oncology indications such as anti-inflammatory, antimicrobials, and antivirals. ADC technology has been subject to many challenges, in part arising from target-independent toxicity to normal tissues, and has resulted in the termination of many ADCs from the development due to insufficient benefit. Toxicity of oncology ADCs has been shown to primarily result from MOA of the cytotoxic payload, and it is reasonable to assume that the same will be true for non-cytotoxic payloads as well as ADCs for non-oncology indications. Current optimization of ADCs includes improving targeting and delivery to the tumor or other site of interest, improving conjugation methods and linker technology, and developing better payloads. Nonclinical safety and pharmacokinetic evaluation of ADCs must consider the biological and small molecule components of ADCs. Bioanalytical assay development for PK evaluation of ADCs can be challenging; however, the insights derived from these assays are essential to designing and developing an effective and safe ADC. In recent years, the nonclinical regulatory expectations for developing ADCs for oncology are better understood based on experience, publications, and guidances. The regulatory landscape for non-oncology ADCs is less well understood but expected to evolve as more and more non-oncology ADCs are developed. The ADC platform continues to provide an opportunity for selective delivery of potent therapeutic molecules for clinical application.

REFERENCES

Ab, O., et al. (2015). "IMGN853, a folate receptor-a (FRα)–targeting antibody–drug conjugate, exhibits potent targeted antitumor activity against FRα expressing tumors." *Mol Cancer Ther* 14(7): 1605–1613.

Abrams, T. J., et al. (2018). "Preclinical antitumor activity of a novel anti-c-KIT antibody drug conjugate against mutant and wild type c-KIT positive solid tumors." *Clin Cancer Res*. DOI: 10.1158/1078-0432.CCR-17-3795

Adem, Y. T., et al. (2014). "Auristatin antibody drug conjugate physical instability and the role of drug payload." *Bioconjug Chem* 25(4): 656–664.

Alley, S. C., et al. (2008). "Contribution of linker stability to the activities of anticancer immunoconjugates." *Bioconjug Chem* 19(3): 759–765.

Alley, S. C., et al. (2009). "The pharmacologic basis for antibody-auristatin conjugate activity." *J Pharmacol Exp Ther* 330(3): 932–938.

Almedia-Souza, L. et al (2011). Microtubule dynamics in the peripheral nervous system. A matter of balance. Bioarchitecture 1e6, 267e270. http://dx.doi.org/10.4161/bioa.1.6.19198.

Anami, Y., et al. (2017). "Enzymatic conjugation using branched linkers for constructing homogeneous antibody-drug conjugates with high potency." *Org Biomol Chem* 15(26): 5635–5642.

Axup, J. Y., et al. (2012). "Synthesis of site-specific antibody-drug conjugates using unnatural amino acids." Proc Natl Acad Sci USA, 109: 16101–16106.

Bander, N. H. (2013). "Antibody-drug conjugate target selection: critical factors." *Methods Mol Biol* 1045: 29–40.

Beck, A., L. Goetsch, C. Dumontet and N. Corvaia (2017). "Strategies and challenges for the next generation of antibody-drug conjugates." *Nat Rev Drug Discov* 16(5): 315–337.

Beerli, R. R., T. Hell, A. S. Merkel and U. Grawunder. (2015). "Sortase enzyme-mediated generation of site-specifically conjugated antibody drug conjugates with high in vitro and in vivo potency." PLoS One 10: e0131177.

Bhatnagar, S., et al. (2018). "Oral administration and detection of a near-infrared molecular imaging agent in an orthotopic mouse model for breast cancer screening." *Mol Pharm* 15(5): 1746–1754.

Bialucha, C. U., et al. (2017). "Discovery and optimization of HKT288, a cadherin-6–targeting ADC for the treatment of ovarian and renal cancers." *Bioconjug Chem* 25: 1223–1232.

Boswell, C. A., et al. (2011). "Impact of drug conjugation on pharmacokinetics and tissue distribution of anti-STEAP1 antibody-drug conjugates in rats." *Bioconjug Chem* 22(10): 1994–2004.

Bot, I., et al. (2017). "A novel CCR2 antagonist inhibits atherogenesis in apoE deficient mice by achieving high receptor occupancy." *Sci Rep* 7(1): 52.

Burke, P. J., et al. (2017). "Optimization of a PEGylated glucuronide-monomethylauristatin E linker for antibody-drug conjugates." *Mol Cancer Ther* 16(1): 116–123.

Burris III HA, et al. (2011). "Phase II study of the antibody drug conjugate trastuzumab-DM1 for the treatment of human epidermal growth factor receptor 2 (HER2)-positive breast cancer after prior HER2-directed therapy." *J Clin Oncol* 29: 398–405.

Campagne, O., et al. (2018). "Integrated pharmacokinetic/pharmacodynamic model of a bispecific CD3xCD123 DART molecule in nonhuman primates: evaluation of activity and impact of immunogenicity." *Clin Cancer Res*. 24 (11): 2631-2641

Cardillo, T. M., et al. (2015). "Sacituzumab Govitecan (IMMU-132), an anti-trop-2/SN-38 antibody-drug conjugate: characterization and efficacy in pancreatic, gastric, and other cancers." Bioconjug Chem 26: 919–931.

Carter, P. J. and P. D. Senter (2008). "Antibody-drug conjugates for cancer therapy." *Cancer J* 14(3): 154–169.

Chang, C. H., et al. (2016). "Combining ABCG2 inhibitors with IMMU-132, an anti-trop-2 antibody conjugate of SN-38, overcomes resistance to SN-38 in breast and gastric cancers." *Mol Cancer Ther* 15(8): 1910–1919.

Chen, T., et al. (2016). "Antibody-drug conjugate characterization by chromatographic and electrophoretic techniques." *J Chromatogr B* 1032: 39–50.

Chen, B., et al. (2018). "Design, synthesis, and in vitro evaluation of multivalent drug linkers for high-drug-load antibody-drug conjugates." *Chem Med Chem* 13(8): 790–794. doi: 10.1002/cmdc.201700722. Epub 2018 Mar 8. PMID: 29517131.

Chudusama, V., et al. (2016). "Recent advances in the construction of antibody–drug conjugates." *Nat Chem* 8(2): 114–119. Doi: 10.1038/nchem.2415

Cohen, R., et al. (2014). "Development of novel ADCs: conjugation of tubulysin analogs to trastuzumab monitored by dual radiolabeling." *Cancer Res* 1141: 5700-57010.

Connor, A. (2016). Considerations for novel ADC development, Boston Area Pharmaceutical Toxicology Group Meeting (BAPTG), October 2016, Cambridge, MA.

Connor, A. (2017a). On-Target Toxicity with ADCs: (1) Species-Specific Toxicity and (2) Preclinical to Clinical Translation. Presented at the World ADC Summit, San Diego, CA.

Connor, A. (2017b). Platform Presentation at World ADC Summit, October 2017, San Diego, CA.

Chudasama, V., A. Maruani and S. Caddick. (2016). "Recent advances in the construction of antibody–drug conjugates." Nature Chem 8: 114–119. doi: 10.1038/nchem.2415.

Dan, N., et al. (2018). "Antibody-drug conjugates for cancer therapy: chemistry to clinical implications." *Pharmaceuticals (Basel)* 11(2).

de Lange, E. C. M., et al. (2017). "Novel CNS drug discovery and development approach: model-based integration to predict neuro-pharmacokinetics and pharmacodynamics." *Exp Opin Drug Discov* 12(12): 1207–1218.

de Witte, W. E. A., et al. (2016a). "In vivo target residence time and kinetic selectivity: the association rate constant as determinant." *Trends Pharmacol Sci* 37(10): 831–842.

de Witte, W. E. A., et al. (2016b). "Mechanistic models enable the rational use of in vitro drug-target binding kinetics for better drug effects in patients." *Expert Opin Drug Discov* 11(1): 45–63.

de Witte, W. E. A., et al. (2017). "The influence of drug distribution and drug-target binding on target occupancy: The rate-limiting step approximation." *Eur J Pharm Sci* 109S: S83–S89.

de Witte, W. E. A., et al. (2018a). "Correction to: modelling the delay between pharmacokinetics and EEG effects of morphine in rats: binding kinetic versus effect compartment models." *J Pharmacokinet Pharmacodyn* 45(5): 763.

de Witte, W. E. A., et al. (2018b). "In vitro and in silico analysis of the effects of D2 receptor antagonist target binding kinetics on the cellular response to fluctuating dopamine concentrations." *Br J Pharmacol* 175(21): 4121–4136.

de Witte, W. E. A., et al. (2018c). "Modelling the delay between pharmacokinetics and EEG effects of morphine in rats: binding kinetic versus effect compartment models." *J Pharmacokinet Pharmacodyn* 45(4): 621–635.

Deng, C., B. Pan and O. A. O'Connor (2012). "Brentuximab vedotin." *Clin Cancer Res* 19(1): 22–27.

Dieras, V., et al. (2014). "Trastuzumab emtansine in human epidermal growth factor receptor 2- positive metastatic breast cancer: an integrated safety analysis." *J Clin Onc* 25: 2750–2757.

Dirks, N. L. and B. Meibohm. 2010. "Population pharmacokinetics of therapeutic monoclonal antibodies." Clin Pharmacokinet 49: 633–659.

Dubois, V. F., et al. (2016). "Assessment of interspecies differences in drug-induced QTc interval prolongation in cynomolgus monkeys, dogs and humans." *Pharm Res* 33(1): 40–51.

Dennler, P., et al. (2014). "Transglutaminase-based chemoenzymatic conjugation approach yields homogeneous antibody-drug conjugates." Bioconjug Chem 25: 569–578.

Donaghy, H. (2016). "Effects of antibody, drug and linker on the preclinical and clinical toxicities of antibody-drug conjugates." *MAbs* 8(4): 659–671. doi: 10.1080/19420862.2016.1156829. Epub 2016 Apr 5. PMID: 27045800; PMCID: PMC4966843.

Eaton, J. S., et al. (2015). "Ocular adverse events associated with antibody–drug conjugates in human clinical trials." *J Ocul Pharmacol Ther* 31(10): 589–604.

Erickson, H. K. and J. M. Lambert (2012). "ADME of antibody–maytansinoid conjugates." *AAPS J* 14(4): 799–805.

Fanale, M. A., et al. (2012). "A phase I weekly dosing study of brentuximab vedotin in patients with relapsed/refractory CD30-positive hematologic malignancies." *Clin Cancer Res* 18(1): 248–255.

FDA Briefing Document, Oncology Drugs Advisory Committee Meeting. (July 11, 2017).

Fiume, L., V. Marinozzi and F. Nardi (1969). "The effects of amanitin poisoning on mouse kidney." *Brit J Exptl Pathol* 50: 270.

Frigerio, M. and A. F. Kyle (2017). "The chemical design and synthesis of linkers used in antibody drug conjugates." *Curr Top Med Chem* 17(32): 3393–3424.

Gao, H., et al. (2016). "Immobilization of multi-biocatalysts in alginate beads for cofactor regeneration and improved reusability." *J Vis Exp* (110): 53944.

Glassman, P. M., et al. (2015). "Assessments of antibody biodistribution." *J Clin Pharmacol* 55(S3): S29–S38.

Goldenberg, D. M. and R. M. Sharkey (2020). "Sacituzumab govitecan, a novel, third-generation, antibody-drug conjugate (ADC) for cancer therapy". *Expert Opin Biol Ther.* DOI: 10.1080/14712598.2020.1757067

Gong, H. H., et al. (2018). "Control strategy for small molecule impurities in antibody-drug conjugates." *AAPS PharmSciTech* 19(3): 971–977.

Gopal, A. K., et al. (2014). "Brentuximab vedotin in patients aged 60 years or older with relapsed or refractory CD30-positive lymphomas: a retrospective evaluation of safety and efficacy." *Leuk Lymphoma* 55(10): 2328–2334.

Gorovits, B., et al. (2013). "Bioanalysis of antibody–drug conjugates: American association of pharmaceutical scientists antibody–drug conjugate working group position paper." *Bioanalysis* 5(9): 997–1006.

Guffroy, M., et al. (2017). "Liver microvascular injury and thrombocytopenia of antibody-calicheamicin conjugates in Cynomolgus monkeys-mechanism and monitoring." *Clin Cancer Res* 23(7): 1760–1770. doi: 10.1158/1078-0432.CCR-16-0939. Epub 2016 Sep 28. PMID: 27683177.

Guffroy M, et al. (2018). Improving the safety profile of ADCs. In: M. Damelin (ed.), Innovations for Next-Generation Antibody-Drug Conjugates, Cancer Drug Discovery and Development. Springer International Publishing AG. https://doi.org/10.1007/978-3-319-78154-9_3

Guo, J., et al. (2016). "Characterization and higher-order structure assessment of an interchain cysteine-based ADC: impact of drug loading and distribution on the mechanism of aggregation." *Bioconjug Chem* 27(3): 604–615.

Hamblett, K. J., et al. (2004). "Effects of drug loading on the antitumor activity of a monoclonal antibody drug conjugate." *Clin Cancer Res* 10(20): 7063–7070.

Hamblett, K. J., et al. (2016). "Altering antibody-drug conjugate binding to the neonatal FC receptor impacts efficacy and tolerability." Mol Pharm 13: 2387–2396.

Han, T. H., et al. (2013). "CYP3A-mediated drug–drug interaction potential and excretion of brentuximab vedotin, an antibody– drug conjugate, in patients with CD30-positive hematologic malignancies." *J Clin Pharmacol* 53(8): 866–877.

Hengel, S. M., et al. (2014). "Measurement of in vivo drug load distribution of cysteine-linked antibody–drug conjugates using microscale liquid chromatography mass spectrometry." *Anal Chem* 86(7): 3420–3425.

Hinrichs, M. J. and R. Dixit. (2015). "Antibody drug conjugates: nonclinical safety considerations." AAPS J 17(5): 1055–1064.

Hill, B. D., et al. (2018). "Engineering virus-like particles for antigen and drug delivery." *Curr Protein Pept Sci* 19(1): 112–127.

ICH M3 (R2) Nonclinical Safety Studies for the Conduct of Human Clinical Trials and Marketing Authorization for Pharmaceuticals January 2010

ICH M7 (R1) Assessment and control of DNA reactive (mutagenic) impurities in pharmaceuticals to limit potential carcinogenic risk February 2018

ICH Q6B Specifications: Test Procedures and Acceptance Criteria for Biotechnological/Biological Products August 1999

ICH S2 (R1) Genotoxicity Testing and Data Interpretation for Pharmaceuticals Inteded for Human Use June 2012

ICH S5 (R3) Guideline on reproductive toxicology: Detection of Toxicity to Reproduction for Human Pharmaceuticals June 2020

ICH Guideline S6 (R1) Preclinical Safety Evaluation of Biotechnology-Derived Pharmaceuticals December 2011

ICH Guideline S9 Nonclinical Evaluation of Anticancer Pharmaceuticals March 2010

ICH Guideline S9 Nonclinical Evaluation of Anticancer Pharmaceuticals. Questions and Answers. June 2018

ICH S10 Photosafety Evaluation of Pharmaceuticals January 2015

Iyer, A. K., G. Khaled, J. Fang and H. Maeda (2006). "Exploiting the enhanced permeability and retention effect for tumor targeting." *Drug Discov Today* 11(17–18): 812–818.

Jain, N., S. W. Smith, S. Ghone and B. Tomczuk (2015). "Current ADC linker chemistry." *Pharm Res* 32(11): 3526–3540.

Jain, R. K. (1990). "Physiological barriers to delivery of monoclonal antibodies and other macromolecules in tumors." *Cancer Res* 50(3 Suppl): 814s–819s.

Jeffrey, S. C., et al. (2006). "Development and properties of beta-glucuronide linkers for monoclonal antibody-drug conjugates." *Bioconjug Chem* 17(3): 831–840.

Jeffrey, S. C., J. De Brabander, J. Miyamoto and P. D. Senter (2010). "Expanded utility of the beta-glucuronide linker: ADCs that deliver phenolic cytotoxic agents." *ACS Med Chem Lett* 1(6): 277–280.

Joubert, M. K., et al. (2012). "Highly aggregated antibody therapeutics can enhance the in vitro innate and late-stage T-cell immune responses." *J Biol Chem* 287(30): 25266–25279.

Junttila, M. R., et al. (2015). "Targeting Lgr5+ stem cells with antibody-drug conjugates for the treatment for colon cancer." *Sci Trans Med* 7(314): 1–12.

Junutula, J. R., et al. (2008). "Site-specific conjugation of a cytotoxic drug to an antibody improves the therapeutic index." *Nat Biotechnol* 26: 925–932.

Junutula, J. R., et al. (2010). Engineered thio-trastuzumab-DM1 conjugate with an improved therapeutic index to target human epidermal growth factor receptor 2-positive breast cancer. *Clin Cancer Res* 16(19): 4769–4778. doi: 10.1158/1078-0432.CCR-10-0987. Epub 2010 Aug 30. PMID: 20805300.

Kantarjian, H., et al. (2013). Results of inotuzumab ozogamicin, a CD22 monoclonal antibody, in refractory and relapsed acute lymphocytic leukemia. *Cancer* 119(15): 2728–2736. doi: 10.1002/cncr.28136. Epub 2013 Apr 30. PMID: 23633004; PMCID: PMC3720844.

Kantarjian H, et al. (2017). Hepatic adverse event profile of inotuzumab ozogamicin in adult patients with relapsed or refractory acute lymphoblastic leukaemia: results from the open-label, randomised, phase 3 INO-VATE study. Lancet Haematol 4(8):e387-e398. DOI: "https://doi.org/10.1016/s2352-3026(17)30103-5"10.1016/S2352-3026(17)30103-5 PMID: 28687420

Kaur, S., et al. (2013). "Bioanalytical assay strategies for the development of antibody–drug conjugate biotherapeutics." *Bioanalysis* 5(2): 201–226.

Kellogg, B. A., et al. (2011). "Disulfide-linked antibody-maytansinoid conjugates: optimization of in vivo activity by varying the steric hindrance at carbon atoms adjacent to the disulfide linkage." *Bioconjug Chem* 22(4): 717–727.

Khera, E. and G. M. Thurber (2018). "Pharmacokinetic and immunological considerations for expanding the therapeutic window of next-generation antibody-drug conjugates." *BioDrugs* 32(5): 465–480.

Kim, M. T., et al. (2014). "Statistical modeling of the drug load distribution on trastuzumab emtansine (Kadcyla), a lysine-linked antibody drug conjugate." *Bioconjug Chem* 25(7): 1223–1232.

Kim, E. G. and K. M. Kim. (2015). "Strategies and advancement in antibody-drug conjugate optimization for targeted cancer therapeutics." *Biomol Ther (Seoul)* 23(6): 493–509.

Kovtun, Y. V., et al. (2010). "Antibody-maytansinoid conjugates designed to bypass multidrug resistance." *Cancer Res* 70(6): 2528–2537.

Kraynov, E., et al. (2016). "Current approaches for absorption, distribution, metabolism, and excretion characterization of antibody-drug conjugates: an industry white paper." *Drug Metab Dispos* 44(5): 617–623.

Kumar, S., et al. (2015). "Antibody–drug conjugates nonclinical support: from early to late nonclinical bioanalysis using ligand-binding assays." *Bioanalysis* 7(13): 1605–1617.

Lambert, J. A. and C. Q. Morris (2017) "Antibody-drug conjugates (ADCs) for personalized treatment of solid tumors: a review." *Adv Ther* 34(5): 1015–1103.

Lee, J. W. (2013). "ADME of monoclonal antibody biotherapeutics: knowledge gaps and emerging tools." *Bioanalysis* 5(16): 2003–2014.

Lehar, S. M., et al. (2015). "Novel antibody-antibiotic conjugate eliminates intracellular S. aureus." *Nature* 527(7578): 323–328. doi: 10.1038/nature16057. Epub 2015 Nov 4. PMID: 26536114.

Levengood, M. R., et al. (2017). "Orthogonal cysteine protection enables homogeneous multi-drug antibody-drug conjugates." *Angew Chem Int Ed Engl* 56(3): 733–737.

Li, D., et al. (2013). "DCDT2980S, an anti-CD22-monomethyl auristatin E antibody–drug conjugate, is a potential treatment for non-Hodgkin lymphoma." *Mol Cancer Ther* 12: 1255–1265.

Li, F., et al. (2016). Intracellular released payload influences potency and bystander-killing effects of antibody-drug conjugates in preclinical models. Cancer Res 76: 2710–2719.

Lin, K. and J. Tibbitts (2012). "Pharmacokinetic considerations for antibody drug conjugates." *Pharm Res* 29(9): 2354–2366.

Lin, K., et al. (2015). "Preclinical development of an anti-NaPi2b (SLC34A2) antibody drug conjugate as a therapeutic for non-small cell lung and ovarian cancers." *Clin Cancer Res* 21: 5139–5150.

Lin, K., et al. (2015). "Preclinical development of an anti-NaPi2b (SLC34A2) antibody-drug conjugate as a therapeutic for non-small cell lung and ovarian cancers." *Clin Cancer Res* 21(22): 5139–5150. doi: 10.1158/1078-0432.CCR-14-3383. Epub 2015 Jul 8. PMID: 26156394.

Lindell, T. J., F. Weinberg, P. W. Morris, R. G. Roeder and W. J. Rutter (1970). "Specific inhibition of nuclear RNA polymerase II by α-amanitin." *Science* 170(3956): 447.

L'Italien, L., et al. 2018. Mechanistic insights of an immunological adverse event induced by an anti-KIT antibody drug conjugate and mitigation strategies. *Clin Cancer Res* 24: 3465–3474.

Lucas, A., et al. (2018). "Factors affecting the pharmacology of antibody–drug conjugates." *Antibodies* 7(1): 10.

Lyon, R. P., et al. (2014). "Self-hydrolyzing maleimides improve the stability and pharmacological properties of antibody-drug conjugates." *Nat Biotechnol* 32(10): 1059–1062.

Lyon, R. P., et al. (2015). "Reducing hydrophobicity of homogeneous antibody-drug conjugates improves pharmacokinetics and therapeutic index." *Nat Biotechnol* 33(7): 733–735.

Mariotto, S., et al. (2015). "Brentuximab vedotin: axonal microtubule's Apollyon." *Blood Cancer J* 5(8): e343.

Martinez, M. T., et al. (2016). Treatment of HER2 positive advanced breast cancer with T-DM1: a review of the literature. *Crit Rev Oncol Hematol* 97: 96–106.

Matulonis, U. A., et al. (2019). "Evaluation of prophylactic corticosteroid eye drop use in the management of corneal abnormalities induced by the antibody-drug conjugate mirvetuximab soravtansine." *Clin Cancer Res* 25(6): 1727–1736.

Metcalfe, D. M. (2008). "Mast cells and mastocytosis." *Blood* 112: 946–956.

Nakazato, T., et al. (2018). "Brentuximab vedotin is effective for rheumatoid arthritis in a patient with relapsed methotrexate-associated Hodgkin lymphoma." *Annals Hematol* 97(8): 1489–1491.

Nederpelt, I., et al. (2017). "From receptor binding kinetics to signal transduction; a missing link in predicting in vivo drug-action." *Sci Rep* 7(1): 14169.

Nessler, I., et al. (2018). "Quantitative pharmacology in antibody-drug conjugate development: armed antibodies or targeted small molecules?" *Oncoscience* 5(5–6): 161–163.

Palanca-Wessels M et al. (2015). Safety and activity of the anti-CD79B antibody-drug conjugate polatuzumab vedotin in relapsed or refractory B-cell non-Hodgkin lymphoma and chronic lymphocytic leukaemia: a phase 1 study. Lancet Oncol. Jun;16(6):704-15. doi: 10.1016/S1470-2045(15)70128-2. Epub 2015 Apr 27. PMID: 25925619.

Panowski, S., S. Bhakta, H. Raab, P. Polakis and J. R. Junutula (2014). "Site-specific antibody drug conjugates for cancer therapy." *MAbs* 6(1): 34–45.

Peck, M., et al. (2019). "A phase 1, randomized, single ascending-dose study to investigate the safety, tolerability, and pharmacokinetics of DSTA4637S, an anti-*Staphylococcus aureus* THIOMAB™ antibody antibiotic conjugate, in healthy volunteers." *Antimicrob Agents Chemother*. pii: AAC.02588-18. DOI: 10.1128/AAC.02588-18. [Epub ahead of print].

Perrino, E., et al. (2014). "Curative properties of noninternalizing antibody-drug conjugates based on maytansinoids." *Cancer Res* 74(9): 2569–2578.

Peters, C. and S. Brown (2015). "Antibody-drug conjugates as novel anti-cancer chemotherapeutics." *Biosci Rep* 35(4).

Phillips, G. D. L., et al. (2008). "Targeting HER2-positive breast cancer with trastuzumab-DM1, an antibody–cytotoxic drug conjugate." *Cancer Res* 68(22): 9280–9290.

Polakis, P. (2016). "Antibody drug conjugates for cancer therapy." *Pharmacol Rev* 68(1): 3–19.

Poon, K., et al. (2013). "Preclinical safety profile of trastuzumab emtansine (T-DM1): mechanism of action of its cytotoxic component retained with improved tolerability." *Tox Appl Pharmacol* 273: 298–313.

Prueksaritanont, T., et al. (2013). "Drug–drug interaction studies: regulatory guidance and an industry perspective." *AAPS J* 15(3): 629–645.

Pyzik, M., et al. (2015). "FcRn: the architect behind the immune and nonimmune functions of IgG and albumin." *J Immunol* 194: 4595–4603.

RIFADIN® (rifampin), package insert. (2010). Sanofi Aventis U.S. LLC; Bridgewater, NJ.

Rossin, R., et al. (2018). "Chemically triggered drug release from an antibody-drug conjugate leads to potent antitumour activity in mice." *Nat Commun* 9(1): 1484.

Rudin, C. M., et al. (2017). "Rovalpituzumab teserine, a DLL3-targeted antibody-drug conjugate, in recurrent small-cell lung cancer: a first-in-human, first-in-class, open-label, phase 1 study." *Lancet Oncol* 18: 42–51.

Saber, H. and J. K. Leighton (2015). "An FDA oncology analysis of antibody-drug conjugates." *Reg Tox Pharm* 71(3): 444–452.

Sahin, U., F. et al. (1990). "Specific activation of the prodrug mitomycin phosphate by a bispecific anti-CD30/anti-alkaline phosphatase monoclonal antibody." *Cancer Res* 50(21): 6944–6948.

Samineni, D., S. Girish and C. Li (2016). "Impact of Shed/Soluble targets on the PK/PD of approved therapeutic monoclonal antibodies." *Expert Rev Clin Pharmacol* 9(12): 1557–1569.

Sanderson, R. J., et al. (2016). "Antibody-conjugated drug assay for protease-cleavable antibody–drug conjugates." *Bioanalysis* 8(1): 55–63.

Schuetz, D. A., et al. (2017). "Kinetics for drug discovery: an industry-driven effort to target drug residence time." *Drug Discov Today* 22(6): 896–911.

Schroeder, H. W. JR. and L. Cavacini. (2010). "Structure and function of immunoglobulins." J Allergy Clin Immunol 125: S41–S52.

Schumacher, D., C. P. Hackenberger, H. Leonhardt and J. Helma (2016). "Current status: site-specific antibody drug conjugates." *J Clin Immunol* 36(Suppl 1): 100–107.

Seiter, K. (2005). "Toxicity of topoisomerase inhibitors." *Expert Opin Drug Saf* 4(1): 45–53.

Shen, B. Q., et al. (2012a). "Conjugation site modulates the in vivo stability and therapeutic activity of antibody-drug conjugates." *Nat Biotechnol* 30(2): 184–189.

Shen, B.-Q., et al. (2012b). "Catabolic fate and pharmacokinetic characterization of trastuzumab emtansine (T-DM1): an emphasis on preclinical and clinical catabolism." *Curr Drug Metab* 13(7): 901–910.

Smith, M. R., et al. (2015). "Engineering novel and improved biocatalysts by cell surface display." *Ind Eng Chem Res* 54(16): 4021–4032.

Stagg, N. J., et al. (2016). "Peripheral neuropathy with microtubule inhibitor containing antibody drug conjugates: challenges and perspectives in translatability from nonclinical toxicology studies to the clinic." *Regul Toxicol Pharmacol* 82: 1–13. doi: 10.1016/j.yrtph.2016.10.012. Epub 2016 Oct 20. PMID: 27773754.

Stagg, N. (2019) "A novel antibody antibiotic conjugate for treating invasive *S. aureus*: a window into the nonclinical development." Charles River Biotech Symposium. September 2019.

Stein, E. M., et al. (2017). "A phase 1 trial of vadastuximab talirine as monotherapy in patients with CD33." *Blood* 131(4): 387–396.

Strop, P., et al. (2013). "Location matters: site of conjugation modulates stability and pharmacokinetics of antibody drug conjugates." *Chem Biol* 20(2): 161–167.

Su, D., et al. (2018). "Modulating antibody-drug conjugate payload metabolism by conjugation site and linker modification." *Bioconjug Chem* 29(4): 1155–1167.

Sun, X., et al. (2017). "Effects of drug–antibody ratio on pharmacokinetics, biodistribution, efficacy, and tolerability of antibody-maytansinoid conjugates." *Bioconjug Chem* 28(5): 1371–1381.

Szijj, P. A., C. Bahou and V. Chudasama. (2018). "Minireview: Addressing the retro-Michael instability of maleimide bioconjugates." Drug Discov Today Technol 30: 27–34.

Tabrizi, M., et al. (2010). "Biodistribution mechanisms of therapeutic monoclonal antibodies in health and disease." *AAPS J* 12(1): 33–43.

Takeshita, A., et al. (2009). "CMC-544 (inotuzumab ozogamicin) shows less effect on multidrug resistant cells: analyses in cell lines and cells from patients with B-cell chronic lymphocytic leukaemia and lymphoma." Br J Haematol 146: 34–43.

Tamura, K., et al. (2019). "Trastuzumab deruxtecan (DS-8201a) in patients with advanced HER2-positive breast cancer previously treated with trastuzumab emtansine: a dose-expansion, phase 1 study". *Lancet Oncol* 20(6): 816–826.

Thomas, A., B. A. Teicher and R. Hassan (2016). "Antibody-drug conjugates for cancer therapy." *Lancet Oncol* 17(6): e254–e262.

Tibbitts, J., et al. (2016). *Key factors influencing ADME properties of therapeutic proteins: a need for ADME characterization in drug discovery and development.* MAbs, Taylor & Francis.

Tolcher, A. W. (2016). "Antibody drug conjugates: lessons from 20 years of clinical experience." *Ann Oncol* 27(12): 2168–2172.

Tolcher, A. W., et al. (1999). "Randomized phase II study of BR96-doxorubicin conjugate in patients with metastatic breast cancer." *J Clin Oncol* 17(2): 478–484.

Tsuchikama, K. and Z. An (2018). "Antibody-drug conjugates: recent advances in conjugation and linker chemistries." *Protein Cell* 9(1): 33–46.

Tumey, L. N. and S. Han (2017). "ADME considerations for the development of biopharmaceutical conjugates using cleavable linkers." *Curr Topics Med Chem* 17(32): 3444–3462.

Tumey, L. N., et al. (2015). "In vivo biotransformations of antibody–drug conjugates." *Bioanalysis* 7(13): 1649–1664.

Uppal, H., et al. (2015). "Potential mechanisms for thrombocytopenia development with trastuzumab emtansine (T-DM1)." *Clin Cancer Res* 21(1): 123–133. DOI: 10.1158/1078-0432. CCR-14-2093

Vlot, A. H. C., et al. (2017). "Target and tissue selectivity prediction by integrated mechanistic pharmacokinetic-target binding and quantitative structure activity modeling." *AAPS J* 20(1): 11.

Vugmeyster, Y., et al. (2012). "Absorption, distribution, metabolism, and excretion (ADME) studies of biotherapeutics for autoimmune and inflammatory conditions." *AAPS J* 14(4): 714–727.

Walles, M., A. Connor and D. Hainzl (2018). "ADME and safety aspects of non-cleavable linkers in drug discovery and development." *Curr Topics Med Chem* 18: 1–13.

Walter, R. B., et al. (2007). "CD33 expression and P-glycoprotein-mediated drug efflux inversely correlate and predict clinical outcome in patients with acute myeloid leukemia treated with gemtuzumab ozogamicin monotherapy." *Blood* 109(10): 4168–4170.

Walvoort, M. T., et al. (2011). "Mannopyranosyl uronic acid donor reactivity." *Org Lett* 13(16): 4360–4363.

Wang, J. (2017). "Current status of antibody-drug conjugate bioanalysis." *J Appl Bioanal* 3(2): 26–30.

Wei, C., et al. (2016). "Where did the linker-payload go? A quantitative investigation on the destination of the released linker-payload from an antibody-drug conjugate with a maleimide linker in plasma." *Anal Chem* 88(9): 4979–4986.

Wright, A., et al. (2000). "In vivo traffick- ing and catabolism of IgG1 antibodies with Fc associated carbohydrates of differing structure." *Glycobiology* 10: 1347–1355.

Xu, K., et al. (2011). "Characterization of intact antibody–drug conjugates from plasma/serum in vivo by affinity capture capillary liquid chromatography–mass spectrometry." *Anal Biochem* 412(1): 56–66.

Younes, A., et al. (2010). "Brentuximab vedotin (SGN-35) for relapsed CD30-positive lymphomas." *N Engl J Med* 363(19): 1812–1821.

Younes, A., et al. (2012). "Results of a pivotal phase 2 study of brentuximab vedotin for patients with relapsed or refractory Hodgkin's lymphoma." *J Clin Oncol* 30: 2183–2189.

Yu, F. and Gao, C. (2019). "Topoisomerase inhibitors and targeted delivery in cancer therapy". *Curr Topics Med Chem* 19: 713–729.

Yurkovetskiy, A. V., et al. (2015). "A polymer-based antibody-vinca drug conjugate platform: characterization and preclinical efficacy." *Cancer Res* 75(16): 3365–3372.

Zhao, H., et al. (2018). "Modulation of macropinocytosis-mediated internalization decreases ocular toxicity of antibody–drug conjugates." *Cancer Res* 78(8): 2115–2126.

Zheng, B., et al. (2009). "In vivo effects of targeting CD79b with antibodies and antibody-drug conjugates." *Mol Cancer Ther* 8: 2937–2946.

Zhou, H. and F.-P. Theil (2015). *ADME and translational pharmacokinetics/pharmacodynamics of therapeutic proteins: applications in drug discovery and development*. John Wiley & Sons, Hoboken NJ USA.

23

Preventive and Therapeutic Vaccines

D.L. Novicki
DL Novicki Toxicology Consulting LLC

Sheri D. Klas
Klas Act Consulting, LLC

CONTENTS

23.1 Introduction and Background

Vaccinology has been defined as "a new field of microbiology and immunology" that has evolved, "that comprises not only vaccine development but also the use of vaccines and their effects on public health" (Plotkin, 2003) and as "the science of vaccines, and historically includes basic science, immunogens, the host immune response, delivery strategies and technologies, manufacturing, and clinical evaluation" (Barrett, 2016). The field crosses so many disciplines and diseases that

DOI: 10.1201/9781003124542-26

comprehensive vaccinology training for healthcare providers has been identified as an educational gap in medical and biological sciences curricula at university and postgraduate levels that has direct impacts on global health. To begin to deal with the knowledge gap, specialized courses of short duration, for example, the Vaccine Safety Basics E-learning Course offered by the World Health Organization (WHO) to Master's programs, have been created and are offered by many institutions and agencies (Lambert and Podda, 2018 and Google Search #1). So given that it is impossible to cover the complex field of vaccinology in a single chapter, or to cite all pertinent publications, we have attempted to provide select reviews and references and touch upon important concepts that go across the disciplines that exploit the host immune system to impact disease outcomes.

The term immunotherapy broadly covers treatments that use the body's own immune system to combat diseases. As such, preventive (prophylactic) and therapeutic vaccines, as well as allergen-specific treatments, are all immunotherapies because each modality exploits the immune response to induce the desired outcome: protection from infection/disease (preventive), treatment of a chronic infectious disease (therapeutic), treatment of a non-infectious disease (therapeutic), or modification of the immune responses to allergens (therapeutic).

Each of these modalities has a surprisingly long history. Early "active immunotherapy" for cancer was practiced more than 4000 years ago by the Egyptian physician Imhotep who described inducing an infection at a poulticed incised tumor and the infection causing tumor regression (Jessy, 2011).

Around 429 BCE, Thucydides observed that people who survived smallpox were not re-infected upon direct exposure, which is thought to be the earliest written record of the concept of acquired immunity. The first intentional vaccinations are thought to be in the 900s in China where Buddhist monks would drink snake venom to become immune to snakebites, and as early as the 1000s, also in China, when smallpox variolation (the use of material from lesions of smallpox-infected people to protect the uninfected) was performed. Variolation became popular in many parts of the world between the 14th and 17th centuries, and the word vaccine, coined by Jenner, comes from the Latin for cow (vacca), from the cowpox (vaccinia) that he used to protect against smallpox in the 1790s (Boylston, 2012).

The history of passive immunization began around 1890 with the work of von Behring, Wernicke, and Kitasato on tetanus and diphtheria showing that sera from infected rabbits could protect naïve mice from infection with the organism used to infect the rabbits (Kaufmann, 2017). Based on their work in animals, von Behring began clinical testing of "antitoxins" in 1892. The work with antitoxins also paved the way for the first vaccine for diphtheria, a diphtheria toxin:antitoxin mixture used to vaccinate humans until replaced with diphtheria toxoid-based vaccines (Park and Zinger, 1915). Concurrently, Erlich's work demonstrated that inoculation with increasing sublethal doses of bacterial toxins could provide immunity against lethal doses and that the induced immunity was the basis for the serum therapy findings. The work led to the concepts of active and passive immunization (Graham and Ambrosino, 2015). There are too many luminaries in the timeline of important achievements in immunology, so intimately tied to vaccine successes (see detailed sections on preventive and therapeutic vaccines below), to do the immunologists justice here. But the article by Greenberg provides a nice summary through 1997 (Greenberg, 2003) as does a more recent review by Kaufmann (2019).

Side by side with the evolution of human vaccines, and by nature of the animal models that were utilized in vaccine research and the close relationship between human and animal health and the food chain, veterinary vaccines evolved, the first being for chicken cholera in 1879 by Pasteur (see https://americanhistory.si.edu/collections/object-groups/antibody-initiative/veterinary for a historical timeline). Veterinary vaccines are not discussed further in this chapter, so the interested reader is referred to reviews by Jorge and Dellagostin (2017), Roth (2011), Heldens et al. (2008), the US Department of Agriculture Center for Veterinary Biologics website (https://www.aphis.usda.gov/aphis/ourfocus/animalhealth/veterinary-biologics/sa_about_vb/ct_vb_about), and the European Medicines Agency website (https://www.ema.europa.eu/en/veterinary-medicines-regulatory-information).

Lastly, allergy immunotherapies are essentially vaccines, but instead of eliciting an immune response, they tamp down immune responses. Human allergies and asthma were recognized as early as 3000 BC, and treatments were developed throughout history. However, the first allergen-specific immunotherapy (ASIT) study, which was conducted with aqueous grass pollen extracts, was not published until 1911 (Noon). ASITs are mentioned only briefly below, so readers are referred to reviews of its history (Ring and Gutermuth, 2011), the basis of disease and treatments (Globinska et al., 2018), regulatory considerations (Bonini, 2012), and future prospects (Pfaar et al., 2019).

23.2 Vaccine Development in a Nutshell

To set the stage for the remainder of the chapter, which focuses primarily on nonclinical aspects of vaccine development, a generalized overview of preventive vaccine development is provided in Table 23.1 and consulting the in-depth review article on the regulation and testing of vaccines by Gruber and Marshall (2018) is highly recommended.

As opposed to therapeutics, which have a different benefit:risk ratio, preventive vaccines are administered to millions of healthy individuals, including children and infants, who do not have but just might get the disease, so the safety bar is set exceedingly high. Almost all of us are familiar with the common side effects of vaccination that are considered minor: pain, swelling, or redness at the injection site, mild fever, chills, headache, fatigue, myalgia, and arthralgia. The United States Food and Drug Administration (FDA) Guidance for Industry: Toxicity Grading Scale for Healthy Adult and Adolescent Volunteers Enrolled in Preventive Vaccine Clinical Trials (2007) provides the grading tables for clinical and laboratory abnormalities. Parallels between clinical toxicity grading and the parameters that are monitored in nonclinical studies will be discussed later in the chapter.

TABLE 23.1

Synopsis of Development of a Preventive Vaccine

Discovery	Develop the vaccine rationale based on how the infectious agent causes disease, develop assays, select antigens, determine the need for adjuvant, test dose levels, number of doses, dosing interval, formulations, etc., defining the desired immune responses.
Preclinical	In vitro and in vivo testing for induced immune responses (immunogenicity), protection against infection (challenge), local tolerability and systemic toxicity (compliant with GLP), and special studies that may be needed (e.g., biodistribution, neurovirulence, others related to the vaccine type).
Phase 1	Testing of increasing doses of vaccine candidate(s) in generally healthy naïve volunteers at low risk of acquiring the disease to assess safety (reactogenicity – local and systemic reactions) and immunogenicity. Age de-escalation if vaccine is only for pediatric population.
Phase 2	Safety testing in volunteers of broader health status, at low risk of acquiring the disease, and wider demographic groups with subjects randomized to vaccine candidate(s) and control groups. Goals include defining short-term side effects and risks, refining the dose/immune response relationship, exploring dose intervals, obtaining preliminary efficacy data usually using validated assays. The control group may receive an approved vaccine, a placebo, or other comparators.
Phase 3	Continuation of safety data monitoring including longer-term follow-up using the dose/formulation intended for commercialization. The studies are powered to show reduction in infection rates or protection from severe disease in vaccinated compared with control (unvaccinated) subjects. These studies are also intended to identify less common side or adverse effects.
	If the vaccine is intended for women of childbearing potential, a GLP-compliant reproductive and developmental toxicity study in a relevant animal model is required and is usually performed in parallel with Phase 3 trials using vaccine Phase 3/commercial drug product (see later discussion on timing for vaccines indicated for use in pregnancy).
	Manufacturers submit data to support the processes, facilities, product characterization, and lot-to-lot consistency. A lot release protocol is developed, and release tests for commercial vaccine lots are agreed upon with Health Authority.
	Filing of Biologics License Application, Marketing Authorisation Application (or geographic equivalent)
Post-approval/ Phase 4	Postmarketing safety surveillance to identify uncommon/rare adverse events. As opposed to use in clinical trials, the vaccine is being used in the real world and an effectiveness assessment may be requested.
	Real-time continuous product quality monitoring using lot release protocols and tests is performed by the manufacturer. The manufacturer also submits vaccine samples from the lot in question to an applicable Health Authority to perform confirmatory testing. The manufacturer cannot distribute a specific lot of vaccine until released by the Health Authority.

Source: Adapted from FDA Vaccine Development 101 (https://www.fda.gov/vaccines-blood-biologics/development-approval-process-cber/vaccine-development-101).

23.3 Challenges in the Development of Vaccines and the Valley(s) of Death

From January 2000 to January 2020, private sector development programs succeeded in bringing a candidate vaccine to the market 39.6% of the time (MIT News, 2020). Though there are varying percentages reported in many other publications over the years, there is agreement that vaccines do have a better record of success than any other drug development area. But a ±40% success rate also illustrates that, like the other drug development areas discussed in this book, vaccine programs are also subject to so-called valleys of death where candidates fail or stall during development. The failure to advance can be due to lack of efficacy, funding, recommendation/reimbursement, or sustainability, hurdles that exist on the basis of science, economics, and policy.

A group of MIT researchers analyzed 406,038 clinical trials and more than 21,000 drugs and vaccines from 1 January 2000 to 31 October 2015 to determine probabilities of success (POS) of clinical phase transitions (Wong et al. 2019), and Gouglas et al. (2018) summarized the POS of preclinical, Phase 1, and Phase 2 in the process of deriving costs

associated with developing vaccines to Phase 2b/3 readiness for a portfolio of 11 infectious diseases that can cause epidemics. The POS at each phase of vaccine development are summarized in Table 23.2.

The first valley of death is between the preclinical stage of a candidate vaccine developed in the research laboratory and proof-of-concept (POC, Phases 1 and 2) clinical trials. The new antigen/s, adjuvant/s, and/or formulations created in the research laboratory must then be produced under increasing levels of quality for testing in pivotal preclinical efficacy, safety, toxicology, and vaccine class-specific special studies, to enable the initiation of clinical trials. The Bill & Melinda Gates Medical Research Institute calls this stage "translational product development…defined as preclinical candidate selection to human/clinical proof of concept (POC) in the target population" (https://www.gatesmri.org/user/themes/quark/assets/GatesMRI_FAQ.pdf).

Reasons for failure at this interface can be manifold: On the preclinical side, failures in translating research findings to the clinic can be related to biological factors and/or research practices. Regarding biology, inbred and even outbred strains of small animals used in research POC studies do not reflect the variability in human populations. Differences in pathogen recognition

TABLE 23.2

Probabilities of Success at Development Phase Transitions

Preclinical to Phase 1	Phase 1 to 2	Phase 2 to 3	Phase 3 to approval	Overall POS Phase 1 to approval
40%–57%	76.8%	58.2%	85.4%	33.4%
Gouglas et al. (2018)	Wong et al. (2019)			

systems, dose, regimen, and route of administration can vary between animals and humans, as can B- and T-cell repertoires and the context of presentation of dominant antigen epitopes to T cells. Because of these limitations, additional studies may be conducted in other animal species, often non-human primates (NHPs), which may be more translatable to humans, but for ethical (and supply and cost issues), are usually limited to relatively small numbers per group. The selection of animal models for vaccine studies is discussed further in the chapter.

Regarding research practices, lack of reproducibility of research results has recently been highlighted as a contributor to a lack of translatability to humans. A poor hypothesis and/or experimental design, low statistical power or incorrect analyses, not repeating experiments at all or not in the same way, insufficient oversight/quality control (QC), unavailability of study raw data/methods/code, difficulties with peer review, and overt fraud have been identified as roots of irreproducibility of preclinical results (Samsa and Samsa, 2019). The authors described improving reproducibility by having prospective data analysis plans (to decrease selective reporting); clear and detailed data management, analysis, and experimental protocols (enable repeatability); holding senior investigators responsible for the details of their research (e.g., active laboratory management practices like random QC audits of raw data, less focus on data summaries, hands-on supervision of experiments); and encouraging contributors to challenge results, essentials of good research practice (Kabitzke et al., 2019). Compliance with good laboratory practice (GLP) for clinical trial- and license-enabling toxicity studies mitigates several of the issues raised above for research studies that are generally non-GLP, but the same issues with the relevance of the toxicology animal model to humans, and what safety issues for humans can be predicted, still apply.

Financial issues also play a clear role in the ability to execute clinical phase transitions. The Gouglas et al. study (Ibid.) found that the cost of developing one epidemic infectious disease vaccine from preclinical testing through the end of Phase 2a, and assuming no risk of failure, was 31–68 million US$ (range 14–159 million US$). The costs were substantially higher when the POS were factored in. So, in the last 10+ years, bridging this research to early clinical gap has been tackled by the creation of many academic vaccine translational sciences centers (Google Search #2) and public–private partnerships (PPPs) that have been established. PPPs include the Bill & Melinda Gates Foundation and its Medical Research Institute, Wellcome Trust, European Commission, US Department of Health and Human Services, GlaxoSmithKline (GSK) Vaccines' Institute for Global Health, Hilleman Laboratories, Program for Appropriate Technology in Health (PATH), International Vaccine Institute, the Jenner Institute, the Human Vaccines Project, and CEPI, the Coalition for Epidemic Preparedness Innovations (Rappuoli et al., 2019) as well as smaller entities.

The "second valley of death" comes between Phase1/2 and the large and very expensive Phase 3 efficacy trials that are required for a novel vaccine for a disease that does not have an established correlate/surrogate of immunity or protection (see WHO https://apps.who.int/iris/bitstream/handle/10665/84288/WHO_IVB_13.01_eng.pdf for definitions). Because preventive vaccines are intended for healthy people, the clinical trials tend to require testing of higher numbers of subjects vs.

therapeutics for people with a disease. For example, the total number of subjects in Phase 2 trials for a vaccine ranged from N = 361 for inactivated poliovirus vaccine to N = 7,471 for Daptacel (Weinberg et al., 2012). Phase 3 is the most resource-intensive stage of vaccine development, often requiring clinical trials in several countries, potentially new manufacturing facilities, and an investment as high as hundreds of millions of dollars due, in part, to the number of subjects required, which ranged from N = 2,358 for inactivated poliovirus vaccine to N = 80,427 for Rotarix (Ibid.). In general, only big pharma/big biotech companies and large foundations or public institutions have the financial wherewithal to run these programs. For vaccine candidates without a high-income market to ensure the return on investment, or if the potential market is limited to only low- and middle-income countries, the challenge can be insurmountable without philanthropic and public funding. Additional resource-intensive commitments are required for Phase 4 clinical trials consisting of postmarketing surveillance studies for continued monitoring of safety and the determination of effectiveness under "real-world use".

Despite these many challenges, the global response to the COVID-19 crisis is an inspiring example of what partnerships can yield. The Access to COVID-19 Tools (ACT) Accelerator partnership, launched by the WHO and partners in April 2020, with the COVID-19 Vaccine Facility (COVAX) has supported the fastest, most coordinated, and successful global vaccine effort in history (https://www.who.int/initiatives/act-accelerator/about). Even rival vaccines and pharmaceutical companies have come together in unprecedented cooperation. But humans tend to forget what is not right in our faces: COVID-19 is the third coronavirus outbreak in just 20 years, and the list of agents with pandemic (WHO Emergencies – Disease outbreaks https://openwho.org/courses/pandemic-epidemic-diseases) or biowarfare (Centers for Disease Control and Prevention Bioterrorism Agents/Diseases https://emergency.cdc.gov/agent/agentlist-category.asp) potential is long. The case has been made that now is the time to structure a standing global mechanism of financing that can act quickly to help finance the "end-to-end components of the R&D ecosystem and ensure global equitable access to these [pandemic] products. Determining what scientific advances are required, as well as how these elements will be mobilized, funded, and orchestrated, is work that must and can be done now, before the world moves on to its next crisis, still suffering from the impacts of COVID-19" (Lurie et al., 2021). One can also imagine that the principles that allowed for the COVID-19 rapid response could be applied to accelerate other globally important diseases for which there is currently no vaccine, i.e., increasing resources, working in parallel, starting and working at risk, and improving processes (Hanney et al., 2020).

23.4 Preventive Vaccines

Preventive vaccination, next to the availability of clean water, is considered by many experts to have had the greatest historical and ongoing impact on improving human and animal health, with some debate that decreased infectious disease was also associated with improvements in housing, nutrition, and sanitation that reduced child mortality prior to the wide availability of vaccines (Greenwood, 2014). Regardless of any debate, it is undeniable that vaccines have had an enormous global societal impact. Ehreth (2003) estimated that vaccines had prevented 6 million annual deaths from vaccine-preventable diseases, and the WHO estimated that at least 10 million lives were saved between 2010 and 2015 and that many millions more were protected from disease (https://www.who.int/publications/10-year-review/chapter-vaccines.pdf).

Despite the previous statistics, proven effectiveness, and quite rare occurrences of serious adverse effects documented historically and currently by the Institute of Medicine (IOM, 2012) and updated by Dudley et al. (2020), many people avoid(ed) immunizations for themselves and their families. According to the WHO, this phenomenon of "vaccine hesitancy" has been identified as one of ten major threats to global health (https://www.who.int/news-room/spotlight/ten-threats-to-global-health-in-2019). Vaccine hesitancy in a "post-truth" era, within the context of some citizens more focused on individual choice versus societal responsibility, has made combating hesitancy a challenge of very high priority. Measles outbreaks in the US, where the disease was considered eliminated, along with COVID-19, serve as a current examples where notable portions of society are choosing not to vaccinate for non-scientific reasons. The Sabin-Aspen Vaccines Science & Policy Group report (May 2020) provides an excellent overview for the interested reader.

Timelines, with important milestones, have been created by the College of Physicians of Philadelphia and the Immunization Action Coalition (see references) to track key historical and current advances in vaccinology and are summarized in generally chronological order in Table 23.3:

In general terms, vaccines work by appearing to the immune system as "non-self" or "abnormal self", like an invading organism or abnormal cell. First, the innate (non-specific) immune system, the well-conserved, germline-encoded system of defenses (Table 23.4), is triggered within minutes to hours.

The triggering of innate responses post-vaccination can give rise to the common post-administration symptoms often associated with vaccines (pain, swelling, or redness at the injection site, mild fever/chills, fatigue, headache, myalgia/arthralgia), commonly referred to as "reactogenicity". Overlapping with and subsequent to the innate responses, adaptive immune responses are initiated, which recognize non-self in the context of self, are antigen-dependent, are antigen-specific, and have the capacity for immunological memory. The adaptive response requires complex interactions between antigen-presenting dendritic cells (DCs), macrophages, and B cells, the main antigen-presenting cells (APCs) for T cells, or lymphoid follicular DCs, the main APCs for B cells. In general terms, the process is as follows:

- Vaccine antigen is phagocytosed by APCs
- APCs travel to lymphoid tissue containing immature T and B cells
- Antigen is processed and bound to major histocompatibility complex class II (MHC II) receptors and

TABLE 23.3

Preventive Vaccines Over the Centuries[a]

1800s	Widespread to mandatory smallpox vaccination, Pasteur's development of the first attenuated bacterial (chicken cholera) and live-attenuated rabies vaccines, and the first cholera, typhoid, and plague vaccines
1900–1950	Rabies and pertussis vaccines licensed in the US, Bacillus Calmette–Guérin (BCG) vaccine for tuberculosis used in infants, 17D yellow fever, diphtheria toxoid, adsorbed tetanus toxoid, inactivated influenza; diphtheria/tetanus (DT), and diphtheria-tetanus-whole-cell pertussis (DTwP) vaccines
1950–2000	Typhoid, yellow fever, polio (inactivated – IPV and oral – OPV); live, attenuated, and inactivated measles (M), rubella (R), and mumps (M), MM, MR, and MMR; polysaccharide meningitis (C, A, AC, ACYW-135); pneumococcal 14- then 23-valent; hepatitis B (HepB, from human serum then recombinant); improved rabies; Haemophilus influenzae B (Hib, polysaccharide then conjugate); live oral typhoid; acellular pertussis (aP) with DT; Japanese encephalitis; Vi injectable typhoid; live Varicella; inactivated hepatitis A (HepA); variations of D, T, aP including adsorbed; combinations (Hib/DTwP and D/T/aP/Hib/IPV); live oral rotavirus (withdrawn because of intussusception); Lyme disease (withdrawn for poor sales); and Men-C conjugate vaccine
2000 to 2019	Pneumococcal conjugates; intranasal, seasonal, pandemic, intradermal, high-dose, quadrivalent, adjuvanted, and cell culture-derived flu; human papillomavirus (HPV); smallpox for high-risk personnel; rotavirus; pre-/post-exposure anthrax; meningitis B; cholera; live-attenuated and recombinant adjuvanted shingles; CpG-adjuvanted HepB; Ebola; and combination vaccines (T/D, HepAB, DTaP/IPV, DTaP/IPV/Hib, DTaP/IPV/Hib/HepB, Hib/MenCY; CRM-, DT-, and TT-conjugated MenACYW-135)
2020 (US)[b]	Adjuvanted quadrivalent influenza for adults 65+ MenACWY conjugate for children 2+ Emergency Use Authorizations (EUA) for two mRNA/lipid nanoparticle COVID-19 vaccines
2021 (US; 1 Jan to 3 Mar)	EUA recombinant, replication-incompetent adenovirus serotype 26 (Ad26) vector COVID-19 vaccine Quadrivalent (cell-based) influenza vaccine for US persons 2+

[a] Adapted from https://www.immunize.org/timeline/; vaccine brand names/companies not shown above but currently approved US vaccines are shown in the FDA listing of Vaccines Licensed for Use in the US (current as of 10 February 2021; https://www.fda.gov/vaccines-blood-biologics/vaccines/vaccines-licensed-use-united-states).

[b] For updated global COVID-19 vaccines in development, approved for emergency use, or fully authorized, see, for example, https://extranet.who.int/pqweb/sites/default/files/documents/Status_COVID_VAX_17March2021.pdf, https://www.ema.europa.eu/en/human-regulatory/overview/public-health-threats/coronavirus-disease-covid-19/covid-19-latest-updates, and https://www.raps.org/news-and-articles/news-articles/2020/3/covid-19-vaccine-tracker.

Note: The approved HPV (Merck's Gardasil® and Gardasil9®, and GSK's Cervarix®) and HepB vaccines (several manufacturers) are preventive on two fronts: They prevent viral infection, and by preventing infection, prevent cancer.

TABLE 23.4

Simplified Overview of Components of the Innate Immune System[a]

Skin and mucosal surfaces	Physical/anatomical barriers and resident cells can secrete sweat/mucus, express pattern recognition receptors (PRRs, see below), and produce cytokines (inflammatory responses) and antimicrobial peptides (pathogen killing).
Effector cells	Granulocytes, monocytes/macrophages (phagocytosis, cytokine production, protein and enzyme secretion, destruction of pathogens)
	Mast cells (cytokines and inflammatory mediators)
	Natural killer (NK) cells (lyse infected and cancer cells, activate macrophages via secreted cytokines)
	Innate lymphoid cells (mediate immune response and regulate tissue homeostasis and inflammation)
	Endothelial/epithelial cells (microbial recognition, cytokine production)
Epithelial and phagocyte antimicrobial enzymes and peptides	Proteases, cationic proteins, lysozyme, elastases, cathepsin G, defensins, cathelicidins (and phagocyte generation of reactive oxygen species/intermediates and nitric oxide production)
Serum proteins	Complement system (opsonization, destroys pathogens, activates T cells)
	Collectins and C-reactive protein (opsonize pathogens and activate complement)
	Coagulation system (limits the extent of damaged/infected tissue)
	Lectins (e.g., mannose-binding lectin, and ficolins)
Cytokines	TNF-α, IL-1, chemokines (immune response and inflammation)
	IFN-α (resistance to viral infection)
	IFN-γ (resistance to intracellular pathogen infection and activation of macrophages)
	IL-12 (stimulates NK cells and T cells to produce IFN-γ)
	IL-15 (stimulates NK cell proliferation)
	IL-10 and TGF-β (regulate inflammation)
Pathogen-associated molecular patterns (PAMPs)	Proteins that recognize molecules common in pathogens (PAMPs) or molecules released from damaged cells (DAMPs) that bind to PRRs that are generally divided into five families:
Damage-associated molecular patterns (DAMPs)	Toll-like receptors (TLRs) in plasma or endosomal membranes recognize various microbial components
	NOD-like receptors (NLRs) in the cytoplasm that sense bacterial components in the cytoplasm
	C-type lectin receptors (CLRs) in cell membranes that sense bacterial and fungal sugar structures
	RIG-like receptors (RLRs) in the cytoplasm that sense viral RNA
	Cytosolic double-stranded DNA sensors (CDSs)
	Note: This is an extremely active area of research and numbers of receptors and the ligands they detect, including host-derived ligands, are being continually expanded.

[a] Adapted from Aristizábal B, González Á. Innate immune system. In: Anaya JM, Shoenfeld Y, Rojas-Villarraga A, et al., editors. Autoimmunity: From Bench to Bedside [Internet]. Bogota (Colombia): El Rosario University Press; 2013 Jul 18. Chapter 2. Available from: https://www.ncbi.nlm.nih.gov/books/NBK459455/.

MHC I receptors on the cell membrane of the APC and presented to immature T helper cells and cytotoxic T cells through binding the MHC II (helper T) or MHC I (cytotoxic T) to the T-cell receptor (TCR)

- The T cells mature and proliferate, helper T cells activate B cells to proliferate and produce antibodies specific to the antigen, and cytotoxic T cells destroy pathogens that bear the antigen presented to them by the APCs
- Memory B and T cells are formed

If one looks at first-generation vaccines like those from the 1800s to the 1950s (and used even to this day), many were based on killed (inactivated) or live-attenuated whole organisms, or toxoids, and it is clear that they possess attributes of their infectious correlate organisms that can engage innate and adaptive immunity to elicit robust immune responses. As second-generation more refined vaccines based on subunits, polysaccharides, or antigens derived from reverse or structural vaccinology were developed, a trade-off was often decreased immune responses (immunogenicity) to the antigens alone. The decreased immunogenicity could be increased by repeated administrations, conjugation to toxoids

(polysaccharides), presenting protein antigens as virus-like particles (VLPs), and/or the use of adjuvants to provide additional pathogen-associated molecular patterns (PAMPs)/damage-associated molecular patterns (DAMPs) stimuli needed for the engagement of the innate and adaptive immune mechanisms. A third generation of mRNA and adenoviral-vectored vaccines are approaching full licensure, spurred by the need for a rapid response to the ongoing severe acute respiratory syndrome coronavirus (SARS-CoV-2) pandemic, do not rely on the direct administration of antigens but use the host intracellular machinery to synthesize the protein antigen of interest. In simplistic terms, the nucleic acid or vector not only expresses the antigen but is recognized as PAMPs and DAMPs, so also promulgates the immune response to the antigen. Other novel vaccine technologies in various stages of development for COVID-19 include vaccines based on various viral vectors, self-replicating RNA vaccines, gene-encoded antibody vaccines, self-assembling vaccines, cellular vaccines, and mucosal vaccines (Milken Institute COVID-19 Treatment and Vaccine Tracker: https://covid-19tracker.milkeninstitute.org/-vaccines_intro and Regulatory Affairs Professional Society COVID-19 Vaccine Tracker https://www.raps.org/news-and-articles/news-articles/2020/3/covid-19-vaccine-tracker). The plethora of COVID-19 vaccines and technologies in preclinical and clinical testing have leveraged knowledge from efforts to develop vaccines for other infectious and non-infectious diseases.

23.5 "One Bug, One Vaccine" vs. "Plug and Play" Platforms for Vaccines – Antigens

The technologies used to produce the different generations of vaccines are as diverse as the vaccines themselves and, like other biologics, the manufacturing process is intimately tied to the product, leading some to describe the approach as "one bug, one drug" with an average time of 10–12 years for the development of a new vaccine, but acknowledging that many have taken much longer (e.g., Ebola). Once a new vaccine is approved, product quality testing can comprise up to 70% of the production timeline (Vaccines Europe and Sanofi, 2017). Such long-duration timelines have led to the concept of "plug and play" wherein the same technology is used repeatedly to manufacture different vaccines, with the primary difference being the antigen(s) expressed, also referred to as a "platform".

The Johns Hopkins Center for Health Security explores the platform concept in their report entitled *Vaccine Platforms: State of the Field and Looming Challenges* (2019) and defines a platform as follows: "a technology was defined as a platform if an underlying, nearly identical mechanism, device, delivery vector, or cell line was employed for multiple target vaccines". Late 20th- and 21st-century seasonal influenza vaccines, and their pandemic derivatives, are straightforward examples of a platform approach: The same egg- or cell-based manufacturing processes, with minor variations, are used to manufacture the vaccines. For example, the European Medicines Agency (EMA) developed the concept of a pandemic preparedness vaccine (formerly mock-up) that can serve as the basis for an actual pandemic vaccine allowing for accelerated timelines (see https://www.ema.europa.eu/en/documents/scientific-guideline/influenza-vaccines-non-clinical-clinical-module_en.pdf for the non-clinical and clinical module). There are currently four EU pandemic preparedness vaccines that can be modified into pandemic vaccines: Foclivia (Seqirus), Adjupanrix (GlaxoSmithKline Biologicals), pandemic influenza vaccine H5N1 (Baxter AG), and pandemic influenza vaccine H5N1 AstraZeneca. Information on the EMA influenza pre-pandemic, emergency, seasonal modification, and zoonotic processes is provided at https://www.ema.europa.eu/en/human-regulatory/overview/public-health-threats/pandemic-influenza/vaccines-pandemic-influenza. As of 10 February 2021 (https://www.fda.gov/vaccines-blood-biologics/vaccines/vaccines-licensed-use-united-states), the US has three licensed vaccines for A(H5N1) and five for A(H1N1). The 2011 Fifty-eighth Report of the WHO Expert Committee on Biological Standardization: WHO Technical Report Series 963 (https://apps.who.int/iris/bitstream/handle/10665/44677/WHO_TRS_963_eng.pdf;jsessionid=31BE2B65AE409320EC610ECF3ABE66FC?sequence=1) captures an international view on the current

considerations for diverse biologics and vaccines, with Annex 2 providing guidelines on regulatory preparedness for human pandemic influenza vaccines, including nonclinical considerations.

Current examples of other vaccine platforms include nucleic acid and viral-vectored vaccines in which the backbone/construct remains the same while antigen sequence swaps can be inserted into the same region of the construct. Exploiting platform approaches allowed for the remarkably expedited COVID-19 vaccines to address current and emerging variant SARS-CoV-2 viruses. But there were also previous nonclinical and clinical virology, immunology, and safety learnings from the 2002-2004 SARS-CoV outbreak and the MERS-CoV outbreak that began in 2012. Numerous experimental vaccines were tested in animal models, then clinically, for both (Jiang et al., 2005; Lanying et al., 2016; Li et al., 2020).

The current SARS-CoV-2 pandemic, the earlier coronavirus outbreaks, and the 2013–2016 Ebola outbreak have highlighted the ever-increasing need for global cooperation and streamlining and harmonizing of regulatory requirements and advancements. For example, Merck's Ervebo®, one of two recently approved Ebola vaccines, took over two decades to develop for many reasons including insufficient investment, the inability to demonstrate efficacy in the absence of an outbreak, and no potential to recoup development costs (Branswell, 2020 and Wolf et al., 2020). For one of Merck's two COVID-19 vaccine candidates, they leveraged the Ervebo recombinant vesicular stomatitis virus (VSV) backbone, substituting their SARS-CoV-2 spike sequence for the sequence of the Zaire Ebola envelope glycoprotein. Unfortunately, clinical immune responses were insufficient and Merck discontinued development to focus on COVID-19 therapeutics and other potential vaccines using the technology (https://www.merck.com/news/merck-discontinues-development-of-sars-cov-2-covid-19-vaccine-candidates-continues-development-of-two-investigational-therapeutic-candidates/), highlighting the fact that the same platform may not work for all antigens. In contrast, Janssen/Johnson & Johnson's efficacious COVID-19 vaccine (Ad26.COV2.S), which is approved for emergency use as of April 2021, is based on the same platform as one component of their licensed two-dose Ebola vaccine regimen, Zabdeno® (Ad26.ZEBOV) and Mvabea® (MVA-BN-Filo), which leveraged Janssen's AdVac® vaccine technology and Bavarian Nordic's established MVA-BN® technology, an approved smallpox vaccine in Canada (IMVAMUNE®) and the EU IMVANEX®. AdVac technology is also being used for the development of candidate vaccines for Zika, RSV, and HIV (https://www.janssen.com/belgium/janssen-vaccine-technology).

As mentioned above, many other diseases with pandemic potential have been identified by diverse agencies also including The Global Alliance for Vaccines and Immunizations (https://www.gavi.org/vaccineswork/10-infectious-diseases-could-be-next-pandemic), National Institute of Aids and Infectious Diseases (https://www.niaid.nih.gov/research/emerging-infectious-diseases-pathogens), and the WHO (Ibid.) and could be amenable to platform approaches. Later in the chapter, examples of how select COVID-19 vaccine nonclinical development programs were expedited, based on studies performed with other vaccines using the same platform technology, will be reviewed.

23.6 "Plug and Play" Platforms for Vaccines – Adjuvants

Another aspect of vaccinology that has applied platform approaches is adjuvants research and development. Adjuvants are not approved on their own, the vaccines they are part of are the products, and adjuvants are used in both preventive and especially therapeutic vaccines for infectious and non-infectious diseases.

Historically, and in parallel with vaccine antigens research, investigators sought ways to improve immune responses to antigens beginning in 1925 with Gaston Ramon, who observed that horses' immune responses to diphtheria toxoid (for the production of antitoxin) were stronger in those that developed abscesses at the injection site. He mixed toxoid with tapioca, starch, agar, lecithin, an emulsion of oil, or breadcrumbs (Ramon, 1925), paving the way for the use of adjuvants (from Latin adjuvare, to help or aid), to make existing vaccines more effective. Approximately a year later, Glenny showed that aluminum salts significantly increased the effectiveness of diphtheria toxoid, the vaccine antigens used to protect against diphtheria in challenged guinea pigs (Glenny et al., 1926). *Aluminum-based adjuvants remained the only type used in approved vaccines for upwards of 70 years.*

The next non-aluminum-based adjuvant used in an approved vaccine was Epaxal hepatitis A vaccine, licensed in the EU/ US in 1991/1995 but discontinued with the Crucell-Janssen merger in 2014. Epaxal contained spherical immunopotentiating reconstituted influenza virosomes (IRIVs, D'Acremont et al., 2006). Since then, GlaxoSmithKline adjuvants systems (AS) AS01b (Monophosphoryl Lipid "MPL"/QS21/liposome-based in Shingrix, 2017), AS03 (α-tocopherol/squalene/polysorbate 80 emulsion in Q-Pan H5N1, 2013), AS04 (MPL/ Aluminum salt in Cervarix, 2009); Dynavax CpG 1018 (synthetic oligodeoxynucleotide in Heplisav, 2017); and Novartis/ Seqirus MF59 (squalene/Tween 80/Span 85 oil-in-water emulsion in Fluad trivalent, 2015, and Fluad quadrivalent, 2020) are used in FDA-approved human vaccines (Nanishi, et al., 2020). In the EU, Fluad (MF59) was approved in twelve countries from 1997 to2000 and Fendrix (AS04) hepatitis vaccine was approved in the EU in 2017. (https://www.ema.europa.eu/ en/medicines/human/EPAR/fendrix).

Based on physicochemical properties and mechanisms of action, adjuvants have been broadly categorized, by too many authors to cite, into delivery systems and immunopotentiators (Table 23.5).

In addition to the adjuvants used in approved vaccines, there are experimental adjuvants that are quite well-characterized and used in clinically tested experimental vaccines including liposomes, lipid nanoparticles, and particulate systems such as ISCOMATRIX/Matrix M (spherical, hollow, and cage-like self-assembled particles containing Quil A saponin, phospholipids, and cholesterol in Novavax COVID-19 vaccine). An excellent review article on adjuvants by O'Hagan et al. (2020) provides an up-to-date overview of the state of the field, adjuvant mechanisms of action, and cautions that, with the profusion of newer/novel adjuvants included in COVID-19 vaccines under accelerated programs and timelines, and in novel non-COVID-19 vaccines, "the accumulated lessons of the last decade will be sufficient to avoid any unfortunate missteps, so that the established adjuvants will not be in any way jeopardized by issues that may emerge for newer ones". Another current review (Nanishi et al., 2020) also provides current perspectives on adjuvanticity vs. reactogenicity and how striking the proper balance is key. As mentioned above, it took 70+ years for new adjuvants to be included in approved vaccines, and with the almost zero-risk tolerance of the public, it is extremely important not to have setbacks in the field.

A challenge for academic or smaller vaccine companies is that the newer adjuvants that are in approved vaccines (e.g., GSK adjuvant systems, MF59, CpG 1018) are not generally available to researchers or other companies unless material transfer agreements, licenses, or collaborations are in force. Therefore, "clones" of proprietary adjuvants have been developed by several companies. The major companies in the vaccine adjuvants business   (https://www.marketsandmarkets.com/Market-Reports/ vaccine-adjuvants-market-152603894.html)   are   Brenntag Biosector (aluminum-based), CSL Limited (MF59), SEPPIC (Montanide), Agenus, Inc. (QS-21), Novavax, Inc. (Matrix M), SPI Pharma, Inc. (aluminum-based), InvivoGen (wide portfolio), Avanti Polar Lipids, Inc. (MPL and related), MVP Laboratories, Inc. (Emulsigen), and OZ Biosciences (wide portfolio).

A database of pattern recognition receptors (PRRs) (see Table 23.4, DAMPs and PAMPs) in different organisms/ species, PRRDB 2.0, has been created by Kaur et al. (2019) as a resource for researchers in relevant fields. Together with the PRRs that are exploitable as targets, novel adjuvants that can target them are being actively investigated in academia,

TABLE 23.5

Broad Categories and Examples of Vaccine Adjuvants[a]

Particulate vaccine delivery systems that target antigen to antigen-presenting cells	Aluminum salts/alum, calcium phosphate, incomplete Freund's adjuvant, MF59, cochleates, virus-like particles, virosomes, polylactic acid, poly lactide-co-glycolide
Immunostimulatory adjuvants that directly activate cells through specific receptors, e.g., TLRs, that induce inflammation and engage innate, followed by adaptive immune responses	Double-stranded RNA: poly-I:C, poly-IC:LC, monophosphoryl lipid A, lipopolysaccharide, flagellin, imiquimod/R837, resiquimod/848, CpG oligodeoxynucleotides, muramyl dipeptide, saponins/QS-21

[a] Adapted from Singh, M., O'Hagan, D.T. Recent Advances in Vaccine Adjuvants. *Pharm Res* 19, 715–728 2002: https://doi.org/10.1023/A:1016104910582 and J de Souza Apostólico, VAS Lunardelli, FC Coirada, SB Boscardin, DS Rosa, Adjuvants: Classification, Modus Operandi, and Licensing, *Journal of Immunology Research*, vol. 2016, Article ID 1459394, 16 pages, 2016: https://doi.org/10.1155/2016/1459394.

government, and biotech/pharma, and one functional database has been developed so far (Sayers et al., 2012). As of April 2021, the database, VIOLIN (Vaccines Investigation and Online Information Network (http://www.violinet.org/), contains 4,168 vaccines or vaccine candidates for 218 pathogens by manual curation from 4,396 peer-reviewed papers, 24,345 vaccine-related abstracts, and 10,317 full-text documents. Japan has an ongoing Adjuvant Database Project https://adjuvantdb.nibiohn.go.jp/about_en.html, and it is likely there are others we may have missed or that are under development.

Adjuvant research has advanced to the point that vaccine developers can select single or multiple adjuvants to "tailor" the immune response toward antibody, cell-mediated, or balanced immune responses. This immune response tailoring is, of course, relevant to preventive vaccines but especially so for therapeutic vaccines for chronic infectious and non-infectious diseases as will be highlighted in the section on this topic below.

23.7 Vaccine Excipients

In addition to antigens, vaccines contain small amounts of formulation-related excipients including buffers, adjuvants, stabilizers, and possibly preservatives, to maintain potency during transport and storage. Trace amounts of residual materials used during the manufacturing process and removed can include cell culture reagents, inactivating agents, and antibiotics used during production. The Centers for Disease Control and Prevention (CDC) maintains a listing of these compounds in US vaccines (Vaccine Excipient Summary: Excipients Included in U.S. Vaccines, by Vaccine https://www.cdc.gov/vaccines/pubs/pinkbook/downloads/appendices/b/excipient-table-2.pdf), and the Johns Hopkins Institute for Vaccine Safety maintains a list by excipient showing the amount per dose when available (Excipients in Vaccines per 0.5 mL dose (https://www.vaccinesafety.edu/components-Excipients.htm). The FDA Inactive Ingredients Database is also a resource as formulation components are being considered. Note that it is important to make sure that formulation researchers realize that, just because a compound is "generally recognized as safe" (GRAS, https://www.fda.gov/food/food-ingredients-packaging/generally-recognized-safe-gras), it does not mean it is safe for inclusion in parenteral vaccines. The qualification of novel excipients for vaccines needs to be assessed in the context of applicable Health Authority guidelines for excipients. Also,

though it may be further out in a company's development plans, if an excipient is not contained in a product that is approved in Japan, a toxicity assessment would be needed, and additional testing could be required.

23.8 Therapeutic Vaccines

The introductory statement by Boukhebza et al. (2012) in their publication on therapeutic vaccines (and the Modified Vaccinia Ankara virus platform) is the following: "Therapeutic vaccination is a field still in its infancy when compared with the two worlds from which it originates: prophylactic vaccination and immune-therapeutics...Therapeutic vaccines combine features from both of these worlds while also displaying specific ones". Considering this premise, the antigen and adjuvant approaches and platforms exploited for preventive vaccines cross over into therapeutic vaccines, as do many of the principles of nonclinical assessment of efficacy and safety. Targets of therapeutic vaccines include chronic infectious diseases (e.g., HBV, HCV, HIV, herpes simplex), metabolic diseases (e.g., diabetes, dyslipidemia/cholesterol, hypertension, obesity), addiction (nicotine, cocaine, heroin), autoimmune diseases (e.g., systemic lupus erythematosus, rheumatoid arthritis, multiple sclerosis, myasthenia gravis), allergies (ASIT), and cancer (Wyman, 2012 and Pharmaceutical Research and Manufacturers of America, PhRMA, 2020a). The platforms exploited are as diverse as the disease targets and, like preventive vaccines, include whole-cell vaccines, tumor cell lysates, gene-modified cells, protein- or peptide-based vaccines, RNA and DNA vaccines, viral vectors expressing antigens, and DC vaccines loaded with DNA, RNA, or peptides. Too many therapeutic candidate vaccines to review here have progressed through preclinical development into clinical trials, but very few have been approved (Table 23.6). Because of the variety of disease targets, the mechanisms by which the therapeutic outcome is achieved can vary from antibody production, to cell-mediated immunity, or both. Readers can search publications on their disease of interest, but because of renewed excitement for cancer vaccines with the advent of approved checkpoint inhibitors (Vaddepally et al., 2020), this category of vaccines will be explored in some detail in the next section. DC vaccines will also be highlighted below because one of the few currently approved therapeutic cancer vaccines (Provenge, Table 23.6) is based on DC technology. The

TABLE 23.6

Currently Approved Therapeutic Vaccines/Immunotherapies

1990 TheraCys® (Sanofi Pasteur)	TheraCys was discontinued due to supply issues and replaced with TICE® (Merck) in 1998. Indicated for intravesical use in the treatment and prophylaxis of urothelial carcinoma in situ of the urinary bladder and for prophylaxis of primary or recurrent stage Ta and/or T1 urothelial carcinoma following transurethral resection (https://www.fda.gov/media/76396/download)
2010 Sipuleucel-T (Provenge; Dendreon Corporation)	Provenge is an autologous cellular immunotherapy indicated for the treatment of asymptomatic or minimally symptomatic metastatic castrate-resistant (hormone-refractory) prostate cancer (https://www.fda.gov/media/78511/download).
2015 IMLYGIC (talimogene laherparepvec; Amgen), or T-VEC	T-VEC is a genetically modified oncolytic viral therapy considered a type of therapeutic cancer vaccine that is indicated for the local treatment of unresectable cutaneous, subcutaneous, and nodal lesions in patients with melanoma recurrent after initial surgery (https://www.fda.gov/vaccines-blood-biologics/cellular-gene-therapy-products/imlygic-talimogene-laherparepvec).

nonclinical program of studies that enabled the clinical testing and licensing of Provenge is presented in the Case Studies section below. The technology also holds promise for therapeutic vaccines for infectious and other non-cancer chronic diseases (Tel et al., 2016).

23.9 Cancer Vaccines

Earlier in the chapter, we touched on the very ancient roots of cancer "immunotherapy", but concepts that led to clinical testing began in earnest with the 1813 observation of tumor inhibition in cancer patients with gas gangrene and erysipelas (reviewed by Carlson et al. 2020 and Felgner et al., 2016). The first "clinical trial" was performed in 1863 by W. Busch and colleagues in Berlin who intentionally infected a female cancer patient by putting her into the bed of a patient who had died from erysipelas, a recurrent disease caused by a bacterial infection defined by large, raised red patches on the skin, fever, and severe illness. The patient became infected, the tumor regressed, but she died from the infection. The next advancements began when William Coley, a bone surgeon, lost an osteosarcoma patient on whom he had successfully operated. In his research on her disease, he read an account of a patient with an inoperable sarcoma who experienced complete regression after developing erysipelas. Friedrich Fehleisen, a colleague of Busch, had identified Streptococcus pyogenes as the bacterium responsible for erysipelas a few years earlier, so Coley began to test what would later be named Coley's toxins by injecting sarcoma patients with Streptococcus pyogenes. From 1888 to 1933, he tested many preparations, some of which lacked efficacy and others that worked but were highly infectious and killed patients. Coley eventually settled on a combination of heat-killed Streptococcus pyogenes and Serratia marcescens. Coley himself injected more than 1,000 cancer patients and published over 150 papers on the therapy. In the years following Coley's 1936 death, the approach was generally out of favor until the 1960s and 1970s when small clinical trials were performed with formulations similar to Coley's toxins (e.g., Vaccineurin and others) with variable results (Hobohm, 2001). But this work led to the first approved cancer immunotherapy. In 1929, it was noted that there was a lower incidence of bladder cancer in patients with tuberculosis (Pearl R. Cancer and tuberculosis. American Journal of Hygiene; 9: 97–159 1929). Animal studies in the 1950s showed that Bacillus Calmette–Guérin (BCG) decreased cancer rates, but it took a generation until intravesical BCG was tested clinically (Morales et al., 1976). Since the late 1980s, oncologists used intravesical BCG after primary tumor surgery to prevent relapses of bladder cancer, ultimately leading to approval of the treatment, TheraCys®, in 1990.

To date, the only FDA-approved therapeutic "vaccines" are for cancer (Table 23.6), or are oral immunotherapeutic products (four, to date) approved for pollen allergy (https://www.fda.gov/vaccines-blood-biologics/allergenics/allergen-extract-sublingual-tablets) or for peanut allergy (Palforzia https://www.fda.gov/news-events/press-announcements/fda-approves-first-drug-treatment-peanut-allergy-children).

Current cancer vaccine candidates can be based on tumor-associated antigens (TAAs), which are preferentially or abnormally expressed self-antigens in tumor cells or tumor-specific antigens (TSAs) that include antigens expressed by oncoviruses or neoantigens created by mutations in tumor cells (Buonaguro and Tagliamonte, 2020). TAAs are also expressed on normal cells, albeit at lower levels, so vaccines based on TAAs have an autoimmunity risk and have not been as successful as hoped, many experimental vaccines having induced weak and/or short-lived immune responses in clinical trials (Ibid. see Table 1 in reference).

TSAs are unique to the tumor, so tend to be more immunogenic than TAAs, and can activate CD4+ (helper) and CD8+ T (cytotoxic) cells to generate an anti-tumor response. Oncoviral TSAs are expressed in select tumor types in many patients (e.g., HPV E6 and E7 antigens in cervical cancer). Mutational neoantigens can be unique to an individual patient's tumor or shared, i.e., found across different patients and tumor types. Unique neoantigen vaccines require the creation of a personalized (autologous) product and can be based on different platforms including nucleic acid, DC, tumor cell, or synthetic long peptide platforms that deliver the neoantigen(s) to prime the patient's immune system to attack the tumor (Peng et al., 2019). Autologous vaccines can be manufactured in different ways including resecting tumor, genetically modifying the tumor cells *ex vivo* to increase their immunogenicity then injecting them back into the same subject or by genetically modifying tumor cells *in situ* if the tumor is accessible (Nößner and Schendel, 1999). As of mid-2019, Hundal and Mardis (2019) counted more than 24 ongoing personalized autologous vaccines in clinical trials and provided a great overview of the subject.

In contrast to unique neoantigen vaccines, shared neoantigen vaccines could theoretically be "off the shelf" (L Li et al., 2020).

Despite the approved products listed in Table 23.6, the promise of cancer vaccines has not been fulfilled in humans, to date, because although immunization could elicit immune responses, the relevant tumors tended not to respond. But there is renewed interest because of the potential to turn "cold" tumors (microenvironment has myeloid-derived suppressor cells and T regulatory cells that inhibit reactive T-cell infiltration) into "hot" tumors (those with inflammation/T-cell infiltration) by combining vaccination with checkpoint inhibitors that block inhibitory CTL-4 and PD-1 pathways (Mougel et al., 2019 and Chen and Flies, 2013). Igarashi and Sasada (2020) reviewed the state of the art of cancer vaccines and touched on related immunotherapies including tumor-infiltrating lymphocyte (TIL) therapy, TCR-T therapy (T cells transduced with antigen-specific TCRs), CAR-T therapy (cancer antigen-recognizing antibody gene, gene fragments from intracellular TCR domains, and other T-cell costimulatory molecules) that are covered in other chapters in the book.

23.10 Dendritic Cell Vaccines

DCs, professional antigen-presenting cells, are bone marrow-derived cells that migrate through the blood to populate peripheral tissues/organs where they are resident immature cells with high phagocytic capacity. Once DCs phagocytize antigens, they migrate to the draining lymph node. Phagocytized antigens are processed to peptides, loaded onto MHC II molecules to be recognized by antigen-specific CD4+ T helper cells to enhance B cell expansion and antibody production, or onto MHC I molecules to be recognized by antigen-specific CD8+ T cells, that then proliferate and are activated to be cytotoxic (Steinman, 2008 and Cohn and Delamarre, 2014). In addition, DCs interact with B lymphocytes, as well as with natural killer (NK) cells to augment cytolytic activity and interferon-γ (IFN-γ) production. DC vaccines are being explored for cancer (Perez and De Palma, 2019) and infectious diseases (Freitas-Silva et al., 2014), but they are also involved in tolerogenesis, so have the potential to treat allergies (Jutel et al., 2016) and autoimmune diseases (Gross and Wiendl, 2013).

In order to make DC vaccines, the patient's DCs are extracted and immune growth stimuli are used to expand the cells ex vivo. The DCs are then exposed to antigens from the patient's cancer (or other antigens depending upon the therapeutic target). The combination of DCs and antigens is then injected back into the patient and the DCs can then program T cells. See the Provenge case study below for an example of a nonclinical program for a DC vaccine.

23.11 Nonclinical Development of Vaccines

Aspects of vaccines nonclinical development are also mentioned in Chapter 31 (Nonclinical Development of Biologics for Infectious Diseases) by B. Birkestrand-Smith. The overarching international guidelines that currently provide direction for the nonclinical development of vaccines and adjuvants are the 2003 WHO guidelines on nonclinical evaluation of vaccines (WHO Technical Report Series No. 927, Annex 1) and the 2013 Guidelines on the nonclinical evaluation of vaccine adjuvants and adjuvanted vaccines (WHO Technical Report Series, TRS 987, Annex 2). These and select other generally applicable guidelines/guidance are listed in Table 23.7. Guidelines and topics specific to COVID-19 vaccines are discussed in the relevant section below.

23.12 Animal Models

It is widely recognized that animal models have inherent limitations when used as surrogates for humans. However, these limitations can be managed if they are well understood and studies are well controlled. The nature of the vaccine candidate and the experimental purpose dictates the best animal model for testing. Species used in early development (e.g., antigen selection, efficacy/POC testing) may or may not be best for toxicology studies.

23.13 Common Animal Models for Vaccines – Immunogenicity and Challenge (Efficacy/POC) Studies

Considerations in the selection of animal models for vaccine immunogenicity and challenge studies are concisely reviewed by Herati and Wherry (2018). As a basic premise, they divide predictive factors into those that are intrinsic (pathophysiology of infection, intrinsic genetic differences, pathogen–host interaction, host susceptibility) and those that can be controlled experimentally (mixed genders, coinfections, genetic diversity, microbiome diversity, human gene knock-ins, individual immune history). They conclude that although the success of an intervention in "humans may be difficult to accurately estimate from animal models because of the variety of differences described…careful study of animal models can yield insights into the likelihood of success of a vaccine candidate. Animal models may be most useful in stratifying vaccine candidates to facilitate more careful evaluation in an efficient manner for later studies in humans". The authors also highlighted the importance of developing suitable biomarkers and robust correlates of protection to increase the translatability of findings from animal models to humans (Plotkin, 2010). Golding et al. (2018) also explored the value of animal challenge models for predicting vaccine effectiveness in humans using HIV and Ebola as examples.

Mice are by far the most commonly used animal model for vaccine immunogenicity and POC studies. The mouse and NHP immune systems are very well characterized, so have the most reagents available to study immune responses. Hamsters (Miao et al., 2019), various standard rat strains (Wilson et al. 2020), cotton rats (Kolappaswamy, 2015), guinea pigs (Padilla-Carlin et al., 2008 and Hickey, 2011), ferrets (Albrecht et al., 2018), and rabbits (Estevez et al., 2018) are smaller models commonly used in vaccines research, and the availability of immunological reagents for these models is constantly evolving. Larger, less common models include dogs, pigs (influenza), sheep, cows, and horses, depending upon the pathogen of interest. For some diseases, there is an animal equivalent of the human disease, which can play a valuable role in vaccine development when other species are non-permissive for the human pathogen (Gerdts et al., 2015). Species selection, whether for efficacy or toxicity testing, may also depend upon the route of vaccine administration, e.g., intranasal (or other mucosal surfaces), oral, inhalation, or intradermal versus the more standard subcutaneous or intramuscular routes.

23.14 Common Animal Models for Vaccine Studies – Toxicology

Common (and less common) toxicology animal models are presented by species in the comprehensive book edited by Gad (2016). Vaccine toxicology studies are usually carried out in a single species, but an additional species may be required if species-specific differences in immune responses or adverse effects are detected. The animal model chosen for toxicology studies should have immune responses that are qualitatively similar to what is expected in humans. There should be a large database of historical values for the selected species at the laboratory conducting the toxicology study in case an unexpected/unusual finding requires contextualization. According to WHO vaccine guidelines: "It is highly recommended that the animal species chosen is one for which relevant and sufficient historical control data exist. Analysis and interpretation of data from the toxicity studies commonly include a

TABLE 23.7

Select Guidelines[a] Relevant to Vaccines and Adjuvants

Vaccine Type	Geography	Guideline
All	International	WHO guidelines on nonclinical evaluation of vaccines (2005) World Health Organization Technical Report Series, No. 927, Annex 1: https://www.who.int/publications/m/item/annex1-nonclinical.p31-63
DNA	USA	FDA Guidance for industry: considerations for plasmid DNA vaccines for infectious disease indications: https://www.fda.gov/regulatory-information/search-fda-guidance-documents/considerations-plasmid-dna-vaccines-infectious-disease-indications
	International	WHO Guidelines for assuring the quality, safety, and efficacy of plasmid DNA vaccines - Post ECBS version/1 September 2020: https://www.who.int/publications/m/item/DNA-post-ECBS-1-sept-2020
Viral vector and cell-based vaccines	US	FDA Guidance for industry: guidance for human somatic cell therapy and gene therapy: https://www.fda.gov/regulatory-information/search-fda-guidance-documents/guidance-human-somatic-cell-therapy-and-gene-therapy
	EMA	EMA Guideline on quality, nonclinical and clinical aspects of live recombinant viral vectored vaccines: https://www.ema.europa.eu/en/quality-non-clinical-clinical-aspects-live-recombinant-viral-vectored-vaccines
		EMA Note for guidance on the quality, preclinical and clinical aspects of gene transfer medicinal products: https://www.ema.europa.eu/en/quality-preclinical-clinical-aspects-gene-therapy-medicinal-products
		EMA Guideline on Human Cell-based Medicinal Products: https://www.ema.europa.eu/en/documents/scientific-guideline/guideline-human-cell-based-medicinal-products_en.pdf
Recombinant protein/peptide	USA	FDA Points to consider in the production and testing of new drugs and biologicals produced by recombinant DNA technology and Supplement to the points to consider in the production and testing of new drugs and biologics produced by recombinant DNA technology: Nucleic acid characterization and genetic stability: https://www.fda.gov/vaccines-blood-biologics/guidance-compliance-regulatory-information-biologics/other-recommendations-biologics-manufacturers
	International	ICH Preclinical safety evaluation of biotechnology-derived pharmaceuticals: https://database.ich.org/sites/default/files/S6_R1_Guideline_0.pdf
Viral vaccines	USA	FDA Characterization and qualification of cell substrates and other biological materials used in the production of viral vaccines for infectious disease indications: https://www.fda.gov/regulatory-information/search-fda-guidance-documents/characterization-and-qualification-cell-substrates-and-other-biological-materials-used-production
	International	WHO Recommendations for the evaluation of animal cell cultures as substrates for the manufacture of biological medicinal products and for the characterization of cell banks: https://www.who.int/biologicals/vaccines/TRS_978_Annex_3.pdf
	USA	FDA Viral safety evaluation of biotechnology products derived from cell lines of human or animal origin: https://www.fda.gov/regulatory-information/search-fda-guidance-documents/q5a-viral-safety-evaluation-biotechnology-products-derived-cell-lines-human-or-animal-origin
Vaccines for women of childbearing potential or use in pregnancy	USA	FDA Guidance for industry: considerations for developmental toxicity studies for preventative and therapeutic vaccines for infectious disease indications: https://www.fda.gov/regulatory-information/search-fda-guidance-documents/considerations-developmental-toxicity-studies-preventive-and-therapeutic-vaccines-infectious-disease
Therapeutic cancer vaccines	USA	FDA Guidance for industry: clinical considerations for therapeutic cancer vaccines: https://www.fda.gov/media/82312/download
Adjuvants	Europe	EMA Guideline on adjuvants in vaccines for human use: https://www.ema.europa.eu/en/adjuvants-vaccines-human-use
	International	Guidelines on the nonclinical evaluation of vaccine adjuvants and adjuvanted vaccines: https://www.who.int/biologicals/areas/vaccines/ADJUVANTS_Post_ECBS_edited_clean_Guidelines_NCE_Adjuvant_Final_17122013_WEB.pdf

[a]   Adapted and updated from Wolf and Plitnick (2013).

Note: There are many disease-specific vaccines (e.g., influenza, country-specific, and CMC-related guidelines that are not captured in this table that should be consulted by researchers and developers).

comparison with the inactive control (e.g., saline control) in the same study. However, historical control data from the same laboratory in which the study was conducted and for animals of comparable age and from the same species and/or strain may provide additional information".

As discussed above, mice are the most common species used in early evaluations of vaccine candidates but they are less convenient for use in toxicology studies because of volume constraints for dosing and for blood sampling. In most cases, mice cannot receive the full human dose of vaccine by the intended clinical route of administration; therefore, the toxicology study designs in mice are often limited to scaled-down doses. Because multiple blood samples cannot be collected from a single mouse, the statistical unit for evaluation is typically a group, often 5–10, using either pooled sera or different cohorts per parameter per time point. For example, if immune responses, hematology, clinical chemistry, and coagulation are all study endpoints, a cohort of five males and five females each for immunogenicity assessment, for hematology, for clinical chemistry, and for coagulation, then 10 per gender for histopathology at the main necropsy, and 5 to 10 per gender at the recovery necropsy requires 70–80 mice in both the control and vaccinated groups for a total of 140–160 mice in a two-group study. The same principles apply to an immunogenicity and/or efficacy study with multiple samplings, depending upon volumes needed for the various assays, or if there are terminal endpoints such as spleen or lymph node assessments.

Rats, obviously, are larger than mice, but volume constraints are still an issue so the intended human dose may have to be scaled down or administered by an alternate route. If an alternate route is used, e.g., subcutaneous in rat vs. intramuscular in humans, comparability of the immune responses should be demonstrated. Limits on blood collection volumes and frequency are less challenging than for mice, but cohorts for different parameters, or population approaches, may be needed in terms of the statistical unit. Rats are more commonly used in toxicology studies so there is vast historical experience with rats, which can be helpful when evaluating toxicology data. Rats (and rabbits discussed below) are preferred models for reproductive and developmental toxicology studies. It may be important to conduct a pilot (non-pivotal) study prior to initiating the very large pivotal GLP study to understand vaccine-related effects and aid in pivotal study dose selection.

Rabbits have been used to evaluate vaccines for decades and have been a commonly used animal model for repeat-dose vaccine toxicology studies for many years in the US, EU, and for WHO qualification. However, some countries may challenge the use of the model and have country-specific expectations, so it is important to take this into consideration in species selection. Rabbits have several advantages over rodents: They can receive the human dose and volume (usually 0.5 mL but up to 1 mL intramuscularly) and can tolerate the required multiple blood collections from a single individual. Because of their larger size, data from an individual animal can be evaluated throughout a study. They are also a favored species in reproductive and developmental toxicology studies, but there are inherent challenges of which investigators should be aware. Rabbits occasionally abort fetuses

if stressed or abandon their neonates more readily than do rodents. In addition, behavioral assessments on rabbit kits are more limited compared to rodent pups.

NHPs can be used for vaccine toxicology studies, but the majority of vaccines are immunogenic in lower species. If NHPs are selected, their use must be justified on both scientific and ethical bases, and most health authorities suggest that NHP be considered only if they are the only model to show immune responses that are relevant to humans. Needless to say, there are many inherent challenges if NHPs are used for reproductive and developmental toxicity testing (see below), so all efforts to find an alternative model must be exhausted.

23.15 Less Common Animal Models for Vaccine Toxicology Studies

Certain vaccine targets may not exist in any animal model and, therefore, an available genetically modified model may need to be used or developed. Transgenic (TG), knock-out/knock-in (KO/KI), and humanized models are commonly used in vaccine POC studies and can be very useful for understanding disease mechanisms and evaluating the efficacy of a vaccine. However, these models are not widely used in toxicology studies and can have limitations including scant historical data available on clinical pathology, organ weights, background incidences of spontaneous histopathological changes, neoplasms, etc. While potential limitations of engineered animals are acknowledged, their use in nonclinical development has gained more acceptance in recent years, especially in the absence of a relevant standard animal model (Schuh, 2016), and the International Conference on Harmonisation (ICH) S6(R1) guideline (2011) suggests that genetically modified animal models can be viable alternatives for safety testing when appropriate.

Eliciting a measurable immune response can present a challenge during the early stages of product development for some viral vaccines if standard models are not growth-permissive. Using dengue virus models as an example (reviewed by Muhammed Azami et al., 2020), the virus cannot readily establish infections in animals with fully functional interferon responses, which makes evaluating new treatments or vaccines very challenging. To address the challenge, three KO mouse strains were developed: The G129 mouse has the IFN-γ receptor knocked out, has normal CTL and T helper responses, but shows poor resistance to Listeria monocytogenes infection (Huang et al., 1993). The A129 mouse has an IFN-α/β receptor KO that is unable to resist some viral injections (e.g., vaccinia, lymphocytic choriomeningitis, and vesicular stomatitis viruses) (Muller et al., 1994) but has normal resistance to Listeria monocytogenes. The AG129 mouse, which completely lacks an interferon response, was developed from G129 and A129 mice. AG129 mice lack both the IFN-α/β and IFN-γ receptors that play an important role in preventing viral replication and in protecting against viral disease, so are immunocompromised, but are an important tool for evaluating viral vaccine efficacy (Rossi et al., 2016). AG129 mice are healthy and have normal lymphocyte counts and MHC expression, so are well suited to study dengue vaccine efficacy because they allow for in-depth assessment of permissiveness and lethality of an attenuated vaccine virus and may also display exaggerated pharmacology and toxicity (Johnson and Roehrig, 1999 and Brewoo et al., 2012). AG129 mice inoculated with DENV-2 virus exhibited neurological symptoms, suggesting that the virus was able to establish an infection. In contrast, in A129 mice, the parental strain only lacking IFN-α/β receptor does not show neurological symptoms, indicating the possibility that IFN-γ may provide protection against virus infection in neurological tissues (Prestwood et al., 2012 and Mustafa et al., 2019).

The AG129 mouse has also been used as a permissive model for other viral infections including Zika (Bradley et al., 2017), chikungunya (Gardner et al., 2012), enterovirus D68 (Evans et al., 2019), Heartland virus (Bosco-Lauth et al., 2016, and yellow fever (Thibodeaux et al., 2012). The creation and use of transgenic animal models increase the ability to study diseases and treatments or vaccines in ways that cannot be done in humans unless a human challenge model is ethical and feasible (see discussion later in the chapter). However, a clear understanding of the limitations of these models must be carefully considered.

Obtaining consensus on the utility of transgenic animal data to enable human clinical trials is still in progress. For example, transgenic mice were used to support clinical trials with a primatized CD4 monoclonal antibody, keliximab (Bugelski et al., 2000), and Alzheimer's disease-related pathologies (Elder et al., 2010). Instead of using NHPs for the pivotal repeat-dose toxicology studies as was done by Sanofi Pasteur Inc. for Dengvaxia (FDA, 2019), Takeda Vaccines used AG129 mice for testing vaccine efficacy in the POC stages of development and for vaccine toxicity testing to support the clinical development of the dengue vaccine candidate TAK-003 (SD Klas personal knowledge, communication approved by Takeda). One aspect of risk that Takeda considered when choosing the model for toxicity testing was that testicular teratomas, a rare abnormality in mice in general, had been reported in some substrains of the 129 inbred mouse (the parent line of the AG129) over 60 years ago (Stevens and Little, 1954). The authors suggested that the highest incidence rate of the tumors (1.8%) was in mice that were 0–20 days old. The tumor incidence rate declined slightly to approximately 0.7% as the mice aged. The teratomas contained undifferentiated embryonic cells, nervous tissue, and cysts but did not develop into progressively growing transplantable tumors. A more recent online poster reported two cases of testicular teratoma in AG129 mice, but no denominator was provided so the incidence in the test facility is not known (Bethur and Rahim, no date provided). This is an example of how a background incidence of an unusual congenital abnormality, and a lack of historical data on other potential abnormalities, presents a high hurdle for using the model in reproductive and developmental toxicology studies even if more permissive than standard models.

Mice with humanized immune systems have also been developed as models for products targeting the immune system (Shultz et al., 2012). However, like transgenic mice, the lack of historical control data on humanized mice has hindered their use in toxicology studies.

The same species discussed above in the section on animal models for immunogenicity/efficacy may under certain circumstances be selected as the toxicology species, but the caveats regarding test facility experience with the species and the availability of historical data assumes greater significance if there are unexpected findings that can compromise and delay development.

23.16 Animal Models for COVID-19

The angiotensin-converting enzyme 2 (ACE2) was implicated as the receptor for SARS-CoV and was also confirmed to be the receptor for SARS-CoV-2 (Luan et al., 2020). Coronaviruses do not bind to mouse ACE2 receptor (ACE2R), so a transgenic mouse model expressed the humanized ACE2R to study SARS-CoV (McCray et al., 2007 and Yang et al., 2007) and SARS-CoV-2. Syrian hamsters, ferrets, and NHPs have all been used in SARS-CoV-2 vaccine studies, and these, and other species that can be infected (minks, cats), have been reviewed by Muñoz-Fontela et al. (2020).

NHPs are a common animal model for SARS-CoV and MERS and now SARS-CoV-2. A recent report compared rhesus and cynomolgus macaques and determined that the rhesus monkey is a good animal model for the evaluation of vaccines against SARS-CoV-2 because they had increases in body temperatures and had abnormal chest radiographs after COVID-19 infections (Lu et al., 2020). The Moderna vaccine, mRNA-1273, that is currently approved under EUA was also tested in rhesus monkeys and protected upper and lower airways from COVID-19 infection-related damage (Corbett et al., 2020). In a separate study, another group evaluated SARS-CoV-2 infectious outcomes in cynomolgus monkeys and found that while older monkeys are more susceptible, they did not progress into symptomatic disease (Rockx et al., 2020).

The search for the ideal animal model to evaluate SARS-CoV-2 infections and treatments continues. This is an emerging field so information will continue to change over time as more data are generated. The bottom line: The animal model chosen for nonclinical studies should produce a measurable immune response and that response should be similar to what is desired in humans.

23.17 Toxicology Program and Study Designs

When properly designed, conducted, and interpreted, and when no major safety signals are revealed in the study results, one GLP repeat-dose toxicity study in one relevant species should be sufficient to support an investigational new drug (IND) for the administration of the vaccine candidate to healthy adult males and non-pregnant females using birth control measures. If pregnant females will be included in a clinical trial, then a completed reproductive and developmental toxicity study will be required prior to trial initiation.

The GLP repeat-dose toxicology study should be conducted using the clinical route of administration and the highest anticipated clinical dose and volume of vaccine, when feasible, and a clinically relevant formulation including any intended adjuvant(s) and excipients. In addition, if good manufacturing practice (GMP) drug product (the clinical lot) will not be used, comparability of the lot used in toxicity testing to the clinical lot must be demonstrated. The feasibility of using the clinical route, dose, volume, and formulation is not an issue if a large animal species is relevant. However, if a small animal model is selected, one option is not to use the clinical route or precise clinical formulation. The other option is to administer the highest feasible based on animal welfare considerations.

The number of doses administered to the animals in repeat-dose toxicity studies should minimally equal the number of doses proposed in humans (N). However, in many cases, studies are designed to include one dose more (N+1) than is planned for the clinical trial to allow for the possible inclusion of an additional dose in the clinical trial, or to support subsequent "boosts".

Although the "ideal" may be to mimic the clinical dosing schedule, the dosing interval used in the toxicity study is usually compressed, e.g., dosing every two to three weeks, compared to the proposed clinical dosing, which is often 1–6 months apart. The toxicity study dosing interval should ensure that robust immune responses are elicited but need not be identical to intervals in nonclinical immunogenicity studies. A compressed schedule can represent a worst-case scenario from a tolerability/toxicity standpoint, but also accelerate project timelines if toxicity studies are rate-limiting for regulatory filings based on the grade (research, tox lot, pre-GMP engineering run, or GMP) of vaccine to be used in the IND-enabling study.

A sample design of a typical repeat-dose vaccine toxicology study of a vaccine containing a novel adjuvant in New Zealand White rabbits is shown in Table 23.8.

The following parameters are typically evaluated:

TABLE 23.8

Typical Repeat-Dose Rabbit Study Design

Treatment	Dose (µg/mL)	Number of Animals (N)			
		Main Necropsy (M/F)		Recovery Necropsy (M/F)[a]	
Control article	0	5	5	5	5
Antigen alone[b]	Highest anticipated clinical dose	5	5	5	5
Adjuvant alone[b]	Highest anticipated clinical dose	5	5	5	5
Vaccine	Highest anticipated clinical dose	5	5	5	5

[a] Typically performed 2-4 weeks post-last dose.

[b] The antigen alone group may not be necessary if the vaccine requires adjuvant for stability, and the adjuvant alone group may not be required if the adjuvant has been well characterized alone and/or with a sponsor's other similar vaccines.

Viability and clinical observations	General health, morbidity, and mortality assessed on a daily basis throughout the study. Clinical observations pre-dose, each day post-dose, and at each necropsy.
Body weights	Pretest, 1 and 2 days after each dose, then weekly, and at each necropsy.
Food consumption	Daily.
Body temperature	Pre-dose, 3–8 h, and 24 h after each dose. If there is an increase in temperature, additional measurements should be taken every 24 hours until the values return to baseline.
Route-specific local reactions	For intradermal or intramuscular, scored using a prospectively defined system, e.g., the modified Draize test (Draize et al.,1944) along with an assessment of any vesiculation, ulceration, severe eschar formation, or other manifestations of significant toxicity (e.g., limb impairment). For alternative routes, any site that comes in contact with vaccine (e.g., eye exposure during aerosol administration, digestive tract after oral administration, and intranasal tissues) should also be evaluated histopathologically. In addition, a description of cellular infiltrates based on routine histological staining, if present, should be reported as part of the postmortem evaluation, as well as any manifestation of tissue reactions in surrounding anatomic structures (e.g., sciatic nerves, nasal cavities, or olfactory bulb).
Clinical pathology	Pre-dose, 1–3 days following the first and last dose (main necropsy), and at the end of the recovery period. Hematology – cellular morphology, erythrocyte count, hematocrit, hemoglobin, mean cell hemoglobin, mean cell hemoglobin concentration, mean cell volume, reticulocytes, leukocytes, leukocyte differential, mean platelet volume, platelet count. Clinical chemistry – liver and kidney function, creatine kinase, serum proteins, electrolytes, glucose, lipids. Coagulation – prothrombin time, activated partial thromboplastin time, and fibrinogen. Urinalysis usually not done.
Marker for acute-phase reactions	C-reactive protein in rabbits (also monkeys, and humans, other markers in rodents (see Green, 2015, and Kushner and Mackiewicz, 2019). Reactants should be measured pretest, at time points following administration (commonly 1–2 days post-dose), and after ~7 days (WHO, 2013).
Immunogenicity	Binding (ELISA) and/or neutralizing antibody assays (effector T cells can be assessed in other species/studies if cell-mediated mechanism). Data demonstrate that control group(s) do not seroconvert and vaccinated animals responded with the desired pharmacology
Ophthalmic examination	Typically evaluated during the pretest phase and again just prior to necropsy.
Necropsy	Main necropsy 2 or 3 days after last dose and recovery necropsy (14 up to 28 days after last dose). Examine major organs for macroscopic abnormalities or lesions, take organ weights, and collect tissues for preservation and histopathology
Histopathology	Tissues evaluated per WHO (2013) and Bregman et al. (2003)
Special endpoints	Case-by-case

23.18 Developmental and Reproductive Toxicology (DART) Studies

Generally, DART studies are not warranted for vaccines being developed for neonates, pre-pubertal children, geriatric populations, or if the target population does not include pregnant women or women of childbearing potential. However, if the target population will include women of childbearing potential, a DART study will be needed prior to product approval. If the indication will include use in pregnancy, the DART study must be completed prior to exposing pregnant women (also see section on timing of studies during development). According to the ICH S5(R3) Detection of Reproductive and Developmental Toxicity for Human Pharmaceuticals guideline, the animal species used for DART studies should demonstrate a measurable immune response. Mice, rats, and rabbits are commonly used animal models for DART studies, and testing in one species is usually sufficient to support product licensure for a vaccine. As with repeat-dose toxicology studies, NHPs should be used only if no other relevant animal species demonstrates an immune response, and there is more latitude in defining an "acceptable" immune response in such cases.

Even if there is not an appropriate animal model identified, an early fetal development study in rodents or rabbits may be useful to provide information on the potential for risk from the components of the vaccine.

23.19 General Considerations for DART Studies

It is usually sufficient to assess a single dose level that elicits a measurable immune response, and this is usually the highest anticipated clinical dose. The vaccine should be administered using the clinical route of administration. If the full human dose cannot be delivered to a single animal because of volume constraints or dose-limiting toxicity, then the dose could be scaled such that it exceeds the human dose on a mg/kg body weight basis. The control group receives a relevant negative control article under the same conditions. The most common design for vaccines is the pre- and postnatal development (PPND) study.

The goal of the vaccination regimen is to maximize the maternal immune response (e.g., antibody titers and cellular responses) throughout the gestation period and into the postnatal period. Pre-mating administration of the vaccine to maternal animals is usually necessary to ensure that the embryo/fetus is exposed to the vaccine itself and the immune responses to the vaccine. Usually, two doses are administered: one during organogenesis and one at the time of hard palate closure. It is critical to understand the characteristics of the vaccine in terms of the pharmacology and the potential for embryo/fetal exposure relative to patient exposure (Martin et al., 2009). Please see Table 23.9 for study design details.

TABLE 23.9

GLP DART Study Design Examples

Parameter	Species		
	Rat	Rabbit	NHP[a]
Minimum number of pregnant females per ICH	N=16 generally, but see https://www.fda.gov/regulatory-information/search-fda-guidance-documents/considerations-developmental-toxicity-studies-preventive-and-therapeutic-vaccines-infectious-disease.		
Administration days	GD6/7-17 (6/7-15)	GD6/7-19	Approximately GD20- to at least GD50
Clinical observations	Once daily	Once daily	Once daily
Body weight	Twice weekly	Twice weekly	Once weekly
Food consumption	Once weekly	Once weekly	Optional
Cesarean section[b]	GD20/21 (17/18)	GD28/29	GD100
Macroscopic examination	Yes	Yes	Optional
Gravid uterine weight	Optional	Optional	NA
Corpora lutea	Yes	Yes	NA
Implant sites	Yes	Yes	NA
Live and dead conceptuses	Yes	Yes	Yes
Early and late resorptions	Yes	Yes	NA
Macroscopic evaluation of placenta	Yes	Yes	Yes
Weight of placenta	Optional	Optional	Optional
Fetal body weight	Yes	Yes	Yes
Fetal sex	Yes	Yes	Yes
Fetal external evaluations	Yes	Yes	Yes
Fetal soft tissue evaluations	Yes	Yes	Yes
Fetal skeletal evaluations	Yes	Yes	Yes

[a] Information in the NHP column pertains to cynomolgus macaques and may need to be adapted as appropriate for other NHPs.

[b] Cesarean sections (C-section) for rodents and rabbits should be conducted approximately one day prior to expected parturition. Cynomolgus macaques should be C-sectioned on approximately GD100.

23.20 Timing of Studies During Development

Repeat-dose toxicology studies should follow GLP guidelines and be conducted prior to filing an IND or equivalent for a first-in-human (FIH) clinical trial. The reproductive and developmental toxicity study is typically conducted concurrent with Phase 3 clinical trials and prior to licensure. The exception to this is if the product is specifically targeted for pregnant women, which would require a completed study prior to the clinical trial.

Maternal immunization is a strategy for protecting the mother during pregnancy and the infant postnatally. The CDC (August 24, 2020) recommends that pregnant women get MMR vaccine at least a month before becoming pregnant to protect against rubella during pregnancy. The injected inactivated flu vaccine (not the live nasal flu version) and the Tdap vaccine are recommended during pregnancy to protect against influenza and pertussis, respectively. HPV, MMR, Varicella (chicken pox) vaccine, and the yellow fever, typhoid fever, and Japanese encephalitis travel vaccines are contraindicated during pregnancy unless the healthcare provider determines that the benefits outweigh the risks. There are other vaccines that are being considered for use in pregnancy that are explored in the FDA presentation "Vaccines for Use in Pregnancy to Protect Young Infants from Disease" (https://www.fda.gov/media/98997/download), and this topic is further discussed in Section 23.29.

23.21 Studies Generally Not Performed with Vaccines

Safety pharmacology studies (specific assessments of central nervous, respiratory, and cardiovascular systems) are not usually required in most countries unless there are known effects of the target disease that suggest a vaccine targeting the disease could affect those systems (e.g., toxoids derived from toxins). If indicated based on biology, or there are country-specific requirements, safety pharmacology endpoints can often be built into the repeat-dose toxicology study.

Classic absorption, distribution, metabolism, and excretion (ADME) studies are not required for vaccines. The characterization of the immune response serves as a "surrogate" for pharmacokinetics. For certain types of vaccines, e.g., nucleic acid or vectored vaccines, a biodistribution study will be required (Green and Humadi, 2017) if there is insufficient experience with the platform.

Traditional genotoxicity or carcinogenicity studies are not typically required for vaccines. Exceptions that could trigger concerns include the use of novel adjuvants or excipients, if there are vaccine components that could elevate the risk of tumorigenicity, or if the vaccine is produced using a cell-based manufacturing platform that could increase the risk of tumorigenicity or oncogenicity (Dempster and Haworth, 2007). Early communication with Health Authorities can obviate unforeseen testing requirements and subsequent delays in clinical trial initiation (ICH, 2012).

Although vaccines are often indicated for pediatric populations, juvenile toxicology studies are not usually required unless there is evidence that there is an age-related difference in the safety profile (FDA, 2006).

23.22 Test Material Considerations Including Cold Chain Issues

As biologics, most vaccines have quite complex manufacturing processes, so it is critical that comparability of the vaccine lots used in research, toxicology, early- and late-stage clinical development, and commercial manufacturing is demonstrated. This is accomplished through vaccine characterization and release testing. All quality-indicating tests do not need to be done on all lots, but having defined test panels, even at the research stage (albeit with "research assays"), will help the continual bridging across product development. Project timelines often drive the grade of material selected for use in pivotal nonclinical studies, and there is often pressure not to wait for the GMP clinical trial vaccine. When GMP material will not be available to meet timelines, strategies in order of decreasing risk for clinical trial enabling toxicology, or other GLP-compliant (or critical non-GLP) nonclinical studies include using a pre-GMP "engineering" lot, a "tox lot" produced at smaller scale but using the same process, a tox lot produced with a similar process, or a well-characterized research lot (least favored). The further from the GMP process, the higher the risk for demonstration of comparability. Assays that can provide bridging may include in vivo assays (e.g., potency) early in development, but the focus should be on developing biochemical/biophysical methodologies that allow moving away from animal tests for ethical and practical reasons. For example, in vivo tests for vaccine potency rely upon the induction of an immune response, usually in mice, and this can take 1–3 months depending upon the number of doses needed, potentially one to three months of lost development time or commercial sales.

In the process of developing a vaccine formulation, product stability at different temperatures is an important consideration, especially if the vaccine will be deployed to geographies that are less able to maintain the cold chain. As complex biologics, many vaccines are not ambient-temperature stable. Therefore, vaccines may require lyophilization (costly and requires manipulation and diluent in the vaccine kit), refrigeration, or freezing at anywhere from −20 to −80°C. Temperature considerations have played out in the public eye with the different COVID-19 vaccines now being broadly used or still being developed. Clear global vaccine inequities have emerged based on where ultralow temperatures can be maintained and vaccine doses with short room temperature or refrigerated stability may be wasted. The publication by Kumru et al. (2014) introduces the reader to the topic of vaccine instability and strategies for improvement.

23.23 Actual Safety of Vaccines and Adjuvants vs. Myths and Misinformation

Earlier in the chapter, we mentioned the global threat posed by vaccine hesitancy and rejection. Vaccine avoidance based on safety concerns is driven by myths and misinformation that circulate primarily online with the most common being fear of aluminum (and other) adjuvants, preservatives and mercury, formaldehyde used to inactivate organisms, impurities/residuals like DNA, and that the number of vaccines could overwhelm, weaken, or otherwise perturb the immune system. Autism, diabetes, developmental delays, hyperactivity, and attention-deficit disorders, and other diseases are feared results of vaccinations that are unfounded. These myths persist despite overwhelming data to the contrary (IOM, 2012 and Geoghegan et al., 2020). Dudley et al. (2020) updated the 2012 IOM report and the subsequent Agency for Healthcare Research and Quality report (2014) and their results on adverse events following immunization are summarized as follows:

Strength of evidence (SOE) "was high for the following associations in nonpregnant adults: seasonal influenza vaccine and arthralgia, myalgia, malaise, fever, pain at the injection site; 2009 monovalent H1N1 vaccine and Guillain-Barré syndrome (GBS); and a lack of association between influenza and pneumococcal vaccines and cardiovascular events in the elderly. The risk of GBS was estimated at 1.6 excess cases per million persons vaccinated. SOE was high for the following associations in children and adolescents: measles, mumps, rubella (MMR) vaccine and febrile seizures in children under age 5; lack of association between MMR vaccine and autism spectrum disorders; and varicella vaccine and disseminated Oka strain varicella zoster virus with associated complications (i.e., meningitis, encephalitis) in individuals with demonstrated immunodeficiencies. There is moderate SOE that vaccines against rotavirus are associated with intussusception in children; the risk was estimated as 1–5 cases per 100,000 vaccine doses, depending on the brand. Moderate SOE exists regarding the human papillomavirus vaccine and a lack of association with the onset of juvenile rheumatoid arthritis, type 1 diabetes, and GBS. Moderate SOE shows no association between inactivated influenza vaccine and serious AEs in pregnant women.

Evidence was insufficient to make conclusions regarding whether several routinely recommended vaccines are associated with serious conditions such as multiple sclerosis, transverse myelitis, and acute disseminated encephalomyelitis".

The authors concluded that vaccines can be associated with serious adverse events (SAEs) but pointed out that SAEs are extremely rare and must be weighed against the protective benefits that vaccines provide. If data suggest that future studies are needed, it is key that they are powered for investigating rare to very rare events and that the severity and frequency of the AE being studied are collected in standardized ways. The Johns Hopkins Institute for Vaccine Safety maintains a "What's New on the IVS Website" that is regularly updated (https://www.vaccinesafety.edu/), which is a good resource for current, vetted safety information.

Related to myths and misinformation regarding vaccines, adjuvants are subject to similar public mistrust and controversy, much of which was (and is still) precipitated by the now-discredited UK doctor, Andrew Wakefield, who published on autism and MMR vaccine in 1998 (Lancet paper retracted) but who still influences subsets of the public (see https://www.theguardian.com/society/2018/jul/18/how-disgraced-anti-vaxxer-andrew-wakefield-was-embraced-by-trumps-america) with unfounded theories. Another controversy surrounds the highly debated existence of a syndrome, Autoimmune/ Autoinflammatory Syndrome Induced by Adjuvants (ASIA), coined by Shoenfeld and Agmon-Levin in 2011. Since 2011, and reviewed by Ameratunga et al. (2017), there have been other publications on the topic, from different groups, with many having Schoenfeld as co-author, attributing diverse diseases including several autoimmune disorders, macrophagic myofasciitis syndrome, Gulf war syndrome, sick building syndrome, silicosis, and chronic fatigue syndrome to ASIA, and suggesting the aluminum-containing adjuvants in the HepB and the HPV vaccines as major causes of ASIA. To examine the controversy, a group of global academic, industry, and government experts convened a 2-day International Life Sciences Institute (ILSI) Health and Environmental Sciences Institute (HESI) workshop on adjuvants and autoimmunity (van der Laan et al., 2015) and concluded that there was no compelling evidence supporting the association of the reviewed emulsion-based or TLR agonist vaccine adjuvants with autoimmunity signals. Similarly, the publication by Ameratunga et al. (Ibid., 2017) presents evidence against the existence of the syndrome based on a large pharmacoepidemiological study (in contrast to the small N in case series of ASIA) in patients receiving aluminum-containing allergen immunotherapy (IT) preparations. Subjects in the trial had a lower incidence of autoimmune disease despite receiving 100–500 times more aluminum over 3–5 years vs. recipients of HepB and HPV vaccines, and in another clinical trial, there were no increases in exacerbations of systemic lupus erythematosus in a cohort of patients immunized with HepB vaccine. The authors concluded that "current data do not support the causation of ASIA by vaccine adjuvants containing aluminum, which should be of reassurance to patients undergoing routine immunizations as well as to those undergoing allergen-specific IT".

23.24 Theoretical Safety Considerations for Vaccines – Vaccine-Enhanced Disease and Molecular Mimicry

In the case of a few infectious diseases, the enhancement of disease has been noted in vaccine recipients that subsequently became infected. Munoz et al. (2021) described a case definition developed by a CEPI-organized group of experts for vaccines for SARS-CoV-2 and other emerging pathogens, and their article and the publication by Graham (2020) are the basis for the following text. Vaccine-associated enhanced respiratory disease (VAERD) was reported in macaques infected with measles after receiving an inactivated measles vaccine and in infants infected with RSV after receiving inactivated RSV vaccines, which led to deaths. There is evidence of a role for humoral (non-neutralizing antibodies) and cellular (Th2-biased) immune responses in VAERD. Antibody-mediated disease enhancement (ADE) was demonstrated in cats given an alum-adjuvanted inactivated vaccine that was subsequently infected with feline infectious peritonitis virus (FIPV), a coronavirus with tropism for macrophages that causes a systemic vasculitis-like disease and has been reported with dengue flavivirus. The mechanism is thought to involve increased binding efficiency of virus-non-neutralizing antibody complexes to cells with Fc receptors, which can enhance the viral entry. Antibodies that do not neutralize can be caused by an insufficient concentration, low affinity, or wrong specificity.

Although there were concerns stemming from some SARS and MERS experimental vaccine candidates in animal models, vaccine-associated enhanced disease (VAED) has not been reported, to date, with millions vaccinated against SARS-CoV-2, or with SARS or MERS vaccines given to humans (but only small numbers of people received SARS or MERS experimental vaccines). The VAED concern has been addressed by vaccine developers by evaluating parameters that could indicate risk: ratio of non-neutralizing antibodies, IgG subtypes, Th2 vs. Th1 bias of responses, and lung pathology in vaccinated then challenged animal models, for example. The Brighton Collaboration Webinar on Tools for COVID-19 Vaccine Safety Assessment (2020) is a valuable resource that addresses several COVID-19 vaccine human safety topics as well as VAED.

Autoimmunity due to molecular mimicry, i.e., the vaccine antigen mimics a human moiety such that the immune response to the vaccine results in immune reactions to the self-antigen, is another theoretical safety concern with vaccines in general, and some cancer vaccines in particular based on TAAs that are expressed highly on tumors but at some low level on normal tissues. Because there are no accepted predictive models, autoimmunity risk is monitored primarily in clinical trials and postmarketing surveillance. Similar to the situation with vaccine adverse effects discussed in the previous section on myths and misinformation, there is a similar controversy on the role of mimicry in exacerbation or induction of autoimmunity, and the Schoenfeld Lab has publications on the topic (Segal and Schoenfeld, 2018). Offit and Hackett (2003) suggested that large well-controlled epidemiologic studies they reviewed did not support the hypothesis that vaccines cause chronic diseases. They further suggested that infections would be more likely to expose self-antigens and induce levels of cytokines more that vaccines based on attenuated or non-infectious pathogens and that some vaccines could likely prevent or modify autoimmune diseases (e.g., Lyme vaccine for genetically susceptible individuals, or influenza vaccine for patients with multiple sclerosis). From a nonclinical perspective, some de-risking can be achieved by assessing any associations between the target disease and autoimmunity and by comparing vaccine antigen sequences or structures to human sequences/structures. It is uncommon, but depending upon the target antigen and the related level of concern (e.g., group A streptococcus and cardiac effects), developers of novel vaccines may be requested to perform tissue cross-reactivity studies using immune sera tested on a panel of human tissues (FDA, 1997).

23.25 How SARS CoV-2, and Emerging Variants, Are Changing the "standard" Path of Nonclinical Vaccine Development

Global Health Authorities have published COVID-19-specific guidance for product developers of various classes, including vaccines. It is yet to be seen how the strategies for expediting vaccines for COVID-19 will impact the development of non-pandemic or next-pandemic vaccines. But many of the principles applied in this emergency setting could also enable more streamlined vaccine development programs in the future.

The USFDA provided guidance for COVID-19 vaccine developers (FDA, June 2020) where expectations and requirements to move into FIH clinical trials, and eventually to licensure, stating "There are currently no accepted surrogate endpoints that are likely to predict clinical benefit of a COVID-19 vaccine". Therefore, they recommended that vaccine development should take the traditional approval pathway of demonstrating vaccine safety and efficacy in protecting humans from infection or disease. However, the document also recognizes the challenges of being in the middle of a public health emergency, which is why this guidance will be replaced 60 days following the termination of the public health emergency. The guidance describes that traditional vaccine toxicology studies may not be needed prior to FIH clinical trials if there are adequate data to support product safety using other sources, e.g., if the manufacturer is using a platform from a previously licensed or a previously studied investigational vaccine. The guidance goes on to discuss the theoretical risk of COVID-19 VAED (discussed above) and that vaccine candidates with novel components and without any previous nonclinical data will require nonclinical safety assessment prior to FIII clinical trials as per 21 CFR 312.23(a)(8). Biodistribution studies may also be required prior to FIH studies, but it will depend on the product class. The case study of Moderna's mRNA vaccine is presented below to illustrate these points.

EMA developed a guideline outlining the acceleration process for reviewing applications for COVID-19 treatments and vaccines (EMA, Revision 1, March 2021). Their requirements and processes have not changed, but they have committed to review applications in a significantly faster time frame.

WHO wrote a document that describes acceptable target product profiles (TPPs) for vaccines for people at high ongoing risk of COVID-19, such as healthcare workers, and for reactive use in outbreak settings with rapid onset of immunity (WHO, 29 April 2020). A review by Funk et al. (2021) presents a detailed analysis of twelve late-stage candidate vaccines based on four platforms and ranked how they conformed to the TPP. The rankings (of 100) were 82 for mRNA, 80 for protein, 74 for vectored, and 71 for inactivated viral vaccines.

Most authorities are showing flexibility during the pandemic, and the timing of studies and/or expectations for non-clinical safety programs have been temporarily modified. The case studies include vaccine programs that illustrate the concepts outlined in the COVID-19-specific guidance documents.

The CDC (as of 2 April 2021) listed five variants of concern (VOCs) in the US: UK B.1.1.7 (identified in the US in December 2020), South Africa B.1.351 (identified in the US end of January 2021), Brazil P.1 (identified in the US in early January 2021), and California B.1.427 and B.1.429 (identified in February 2021). Focusing on the US, FDA (2021) has provided updated guidance for COVID-19 vaccine developers including expectations for nonclinical information needed for an amended EUA to address VOCs, which includes the following points:

- The nonclinical studies done with the prototype vaccine made by the same manufacturer that enabled the initial EUA are the basis for the VOC program
- An additional GLP repeat-dose toxicology or DART study with the VOC may not be needed based on data with the same vaccine platform or prototype vaccine
- Vaccination/challenge studies in a relevant model with the prototype and the VOC(s) vaccines and clinically relevant circulating wild-type viruses are encouraged as contributory to the evidence supporting a variant vaccine (especially in the case that clinical immunogenicity data are "ambiguous")
- Challenge studies with VOC(s) can be performed concurrently with clinical immunogenicity studies described in the guidance
- FDA review of the protocols should be sought

Developers of variant vaccines without an existing EUA for a prototype will be expected to provide a full program of nonclinical studies expected for a novel COVID-19 vaccine.

23.26 Case Studies

The nonclinical programs summarized in the following sections were selected to highlight the application of pertinent guidelines to support clinical development and market authorization.

23.26.1 Bexsero Preventive Meningitis B Vaccine

The information on Bexsero is taken from the European Public Assessment Report (EPAR) located at https://www.ema.europa.eu/en/documents/overview/bexsero-epar-summary-public_en.pd, and the approach is considered standard for a vaccine. The vaccine was designed using reverse vaccinology (expressed genomic sequences used to find new antigens) and is a mixture of two protein-protein fusion antigens (287–953 and 936–741, where 287 and 741 are the primary antigen components and 953 and 936 are present as accessory protein), one single antigen (961c), and OMV NZ (the basis of MeNZB™ vaccine https://www.health.govt.nz/our-work/preventative-health-wellness/immunisation/immunisation-programme-decisions/meningococcal-b-immunisation-programme-and-menzbtm-vaccine), formulated with aluminum hydroxide adjuvant.

Immunogenicity was demonstrated in mice, guinea pigs, rabbits, and NHPs using non-GLP ELISA and serum bactericidal assays, and passive protection was demonstrated in mice given immune antisera and challenged with various serogroup B strains of N. meningitidis. In addition, a GLP repeat-dose toxicity study in rabbits (similar in approach as in Tables 23.8 and 23.9), a non-GLP dose range-finding rabbit fetal development study, and pivotal GLP PPND study in rabbits were conducted. No safety pharmacology, PK/ADME, or other toxicity studies were performed. One of the many challenges to the

program was the demonstration of cross-bacterial strain protection and the establishment of a clinical surrogate of protection. In contrast to the assay challenges, the nonclinical animal studies for Bexsero were fairly typical, and the history of and science behind the vaccine is reviewed by Pizza et al. (2019).

23.26.2 Provenge Therapeutic Cancer Vaccine

The following information is taken from the EPAR for Provenge (sipuleucel-T) located at https://www.ema.europa.eu/en/documents/assessment-report/provenge-epar-public-assessment-report_en.pdf). The product "consists of autologous peripheral blood mononuclear cells (PBMCs), including antigen-presenting cells (APCs) that have been activated ex vivo with a recombinant fusion protein, PA2024, composed of prostatic acid phosphatase (PAP) and granulocyte-macrophage colony-stimulating factor (GM-CSF). The aim of sipuleucel-T is to break immunological tolerance toward PAP, a self-antigen that is primarily expressed in prostate epithelial cells and prostate cancer cells, and to induce an immune response that translates into clinical efficacy". The product is no longer authorized in the EU but is still available in the US.

The nonclinical data package included the non-GLP POC studies summarized in Table 23.10, and detailed descriptions of the designs, methods, and results can be found in the EPAR. An additional study (TR30548) defined non-prostate tissues that express PAP to predict cross-reactivity and other potential therapeutic uses. Immunohistochemistry (IHC) study of human tissue samples, quantitative polymerase chain reaction (qPCR) study of an array of human tissue RNA samples, and in silico analysis of PAP mRNA distribution in human tissues were performed.

Because of the nature of the product, no safety pharmacology, PK/ADME, or toxicology studies of any kind were performed.

23.26.3 Moderna COVID-19 mRNA Vaccine (Spikevax)

The following information is abstracted from the EPAR located at https://www.ema.europa.eu/en/documents/assessment-report/spikevax-previously-covid-19-vaccine-moderna-epar-public-assessment-report_en.pdf. The program supporting the Moderna EUA leveraged nonclinical, as well as clinical data, with COVID-19 mRNA-1273 vaccine (product-specific), as well as other vaccine candidates based on the mRNA/LNP platform intended for other disease indications, and includes the following studies:

- Product-specific pharmacology studies were conducted in mice (immunogenicity, protection from challenge), hamsters (immunogenicity and protection), and rhesus macaques (immunogenicity, protection). Potential for VAED was also evaluated.
- Biodistribution of the "vaccine platform" was evaluated in a non-GLP single-dose rat study (males only) with mRNA-1647 vaccine (a Cytomegalovirus candidate) with tissues sampled pre-dose, 2, 8, 24, 48, 72, and 120 hours post-dose.

TABLE 23.10

Provenge Nonclinical Primary Pharmacodynamic Studies

Study Type	Study No.	Objective	Species/Strain	Product(s) Tested	Route
POC	TR 30511	Assess rat immune responses to recombinant PAP derived from human or from rat	Rat/Copenhagen or Wistar	hPAP: 200 µg or 7.5 µg rPAP: 200 µg or 10 µg rPAP + hPAP: 100 µg each Ovalbumin: 200 µg or 20 µg hPAP•mGM-CSF: unknown rPAP•rGM-CSF: crude cell lysate	Subcutaneous Footpad Intraperitoneal
POC	TR 30508	Determine whether fusion of hPAP to mGM-CSF would enhance immune responses to hPAP	Mouse/DBA/2	hPAP•mGM-CSF: 220 µg or 50 µg hPAP: 40 µg or 50 µg	Intraperitoneal Intravenous
POC and characterization	TR 30509	Establish PAP-specific, HLA-DR1-restricted murine T-cell hybridomas and determine the PAP epitopes to which they respond	Mouse/C57Bl/6, B10.M/J [TG] Dr1N3	hPAP•hGM-CSF: 20 µg	Subcutaneous
POC and immunopathology	TR 30507	Define conditions under which immunity results in prostate-specific inflammation Determine the degree to which inflammation is restricted to the prostate	Rats/ Copenhagen or Wistar	hPAP: 7.5 µg rPAP: 10 µg rPAP•rGM-CSF: 200 µg Ovalbumin: 20 µg or 200 µg rPAP•rGM-CSF-loaded spleen-derived APCs: various ovalbumin-loaded spleen-derived APCs	Intraperitoneal Subcutaneous Intravenous
POC	TR 30510	Determine whether immunizations with hPAP•hGM-CSF-loaded APCs protect against challenge with PAP expressing tumor	C57Bl/6 Mouse	hPAP•hGM-CSF-loaded spleen-derived mouse APCs 2.5×10^5 cells/mouse	Intraperitoneal

- Genotoxicity was assessed in a bacterial reverse mutation study with the novel LNP excipient, SM102, in *S. typhimurium* and *E. coli*, an in vitro human peripheral blood lymphocyte micronucleus test with SM102, and two in vivo rat erythrocyte micronucleus studies (one with a luciferase-coding and one with a Zika antigen-coding mRNA/LNP.

- Product-specific repeat-dose toxicity was assessed in a non-GLP rat toxicology study and toxicity to reproduction was assessed in a repeat-dose GLP rat DART study. The company also leveraged additional toxicology support provided by six GLP repeat-dose rat studies conducted with five other mRNA/LNP-based products.

As is appropriate for a vaccine for which no notable concerns arose in nonclinical testing, no secondary pharmacodynamics, safety pharmacology, or pharmacodynamic drug interaction studies were performed. Moderna's approach illustrates very well the concept of leveraging data from similar products produced on the same platform.

The reader is encouraged to also look at the EPAR for the EUA-approved Pfizer-BioNTech mRNA COVID-19 vaccine, BNT162b2 (Comirnaty), which can be found at https://www.ema.europa.eu/en/documents/assessment-report/comirnaty-epar-public-assessment-report_en.pdf, to compare the approaches taken with the two nonclinical programs.

23.26.4 Janssen/Johnson & Johnson COVID-19 Ad26.COV2.S Vaccine

The following information is abstracted from the EPAR located at https://www.ema.europa.eu/en/documents/assessment-report/covid-19-vaccine-janssen-epar-public-assessment-report_en.pdf. Similar to Moderna's approach, the program supporting the Janssen/J&J EUA referenced nonclinical, as well as clinical data, with Ad26.COV2.S vaccine (product-specific), as well as other vaccine candidates based on the Ad26 platform intended for other disease indications, and includes the following studies:

- Pharmacology studies with Ad26.COV2.S vaccine in mice (antibody and cellular responses including Th polarization and Th1/Th2 balance), hamsters (two immunogenicity/challenge studies including evaluation for VAED/VAERD), rabbits (immunogenicity dose comparison to validate species for toxicity studies), and rhesus macaques (immunogenicity/ challenge studies with Ad26.COV2.S and other Ad26 COVID-19 vaccine candidates, correlate of protection analyses, Th bias/VAERD assessments, passive protection, aged animals) were conducted.

- Biodistribution and persistence of the Ad26 "vector platform" was evaluated in two single-dose rabbit studies with other Ad26-based vaccines with the identical backbone but encoding non-SARS COV-2 antigens. No product-specific biodistribution study was performed.

- Repeat-dose toxicity and local tolerance of Ad26. COV2.S vaccine were evaluated in a GLP rabbit study.

- A GLP DART study in rabbits that combined maternal, embryo-fetal, and pre- and postnatal evaluations was conducted.

- Genotoxicity assessments were not performed because adenoviruses are generally regarded as non-integrating. In addition, there are no novel excipients or adjuvants in the formulation that warranted testing.

Secondary pharmacodynamics, safety pharmacology, or pharmacodynamic drug interaction studies were not deemed necessary based on the nonclinical results.

For comparison, the EPAR for the AstraZeneca COVID-19 vaccine, Vaxzevria, which is not currently approved for use in the US and is based on a different adenoviral vector (ChAdOx1-S), can be found at https://www.ema.europa.eu/en/documents/assessment-report/vaxzevria-previously-covid-19-vaccine-astrazeneca-epar-public-assessment-report_en.pdf.

23.27 The Animal Rule: When Human Clinical Trials Are Impossible or Unethical

The FDA passed the Animal Efficacy Rule ("Animal Rule") in 2002, which is located in 21 CFR 314.600–314.650 for drugs and 21 CFR 601.90–601.95 for biological products. The Rule allows for the approval of products for "serious or life-threatening conditions caused by exposure to lethal or permanently disabling toxic biological, chemical, radiological, or nuclear substances" based on efficacy studies in animals and safety testing in humans. Substances designed for weaponized exposures, like nerve or microbiological agents, or accidental exposures, like emerging infectious diseases, snake bites, and industrial chemicals, are covered. The Rule is applicable when the threat exists, but clinical efficacy testing is not feasible or ethical. To date, only a handful of compounds have been approved under the Rule. From 2003 to 2021, the FDA Center for Drug Evaluation and Research (CDER) has approved 12 products and the FDA Center for Biologics Evaluation and Research (CBER) has approved three (CDER Drug and Biologic Animal Rule Approvals https://www.fda.gov/media/145827/download): one antitoxin (Botulinum anti-toxin heptavalent), one immune globulin (Anthrasil for anthrax), and one vaccine (BioThrax for anthrax).

FDA issued the Guidance for Industry entitled Product Development Under the Animal Rule (2015a). The guidance is applicable to drugs and biologics, including vaccines and cellular and gene therapy products, but cancer vaccines and therapeutic vaccines for non-infectious diseases are not in scope. Products developed under the Rule still require safety assessment under existing requirements for establishing the safety of the type of new product. To be eligible for development under the Rule, the following four criteria must all be met:

- "There is a reasonably well-understood pathophysiological mechanism of the toxicity of the substance and its prevention or substantial reduction by the product
- The effect is demonstrated in more than one animal species expected to react with a response predictive for humans, unless the effect is demonstrated in a single animal species that represents a sufficiently well-characterized animal model for predicting the response in humans

- The animal study endpoint is clearly related to the desired benefit in humans, generally the enhancement of survival or prevention of major morbidity; and
- The data or information on the kinetics and pharmacodynamics of the product or other relevant data or information, in animals and humans, allows the selection of an effective dose in humans".

The following statements are synopsized directly from the guidance: The study endpoint in the animal model(s) must be clearly related to the desired human endpoint, usually survival or prevention of major morbidity. The vaccine dose chosen for the adequately designed and well-controlled animal efficacy studies should elicit an immune response in animals that reflects the desired human response. Prior to definitive studies, pilot and POC studies should establish a relationship between the vaccine dose and the desired immune response. The dose, route of administration, and frequency of administration may be different in animal and human studies if the relevant immune response is similar and there is adequate justification.

Bridging of animal responses to humans should be based on careful selection of relevant immune markers and as much immune response data as possible should be obtained from the animal model(s) such that the immune response that results in disease prevention, and its duration, is sufficiently well characterized that it can be used to select the dose and schedule in humans that will induce analogous immune responses. The sponsors' choice of species (ideally, the animal model(s) should show pathophysiology, progression of disease, symptoms, and host immune response similar to that observed in humans), challenge agent, route of exposure, and immune marker(s) should be agreed upon with FDA. The optimal vaccine dose, schedule, and time to and duration of protection may differ depending upon the indication: Pre- or post-exposure prophylaxis, or both, may be needed depending upon public health needs.

Post-exposure animal studies should utilize immune response kinetics data from related pre-exposure studies to vaccinate at a time post-challenge that is relevant to human exposure and induces an immune response that is extrapolable to clinical benefit in humans. The sponsor must also consider the possible concomitant use and influence of post-exposure therapeutic and antimicrobial drugs on vaccine efficacy that may have to be evaluated.

The guidance is 50 pages long and very detailed. In addition to the vaccine-specific recommendations above, the guidance addresses many additional nonclinical considerations applicable to all in-scope products, provides guidance for cell and gene therapies, includes checklists (Essential Elements of an Animal Model; Elements of an Adequate and Well-Controlled Animal Efficacy Study Protocol), expectations for natural history studies, animal care, use, and interventions, highlights communications with FDA, regulatory, and human safety considerations, and briefly discusses Ebola as a case where the infeasibility of a clinical trial shifted over time. The guidance is relevant from a scientific/study design perspective from the standpoint of nonclinical vaccine efficacy studies even if the reader's product will not be developed under the Animal Rule. The risks and benefits of using the Animal Rule are explored in a 2018 article by Allio (2018) and a case study for BioThrax (Anthrax Vaccine Adsorbed) is presented in the next section.

Similar to the Animal Rule, the National Regulatory Authority, Health Canada, can approve vaccines and other products under the Extraordinary Use New Drugs regulations (updated 2021-02-03). EMA does not have a comparable process, but states "the possibility that animal models data in principle could have a critical role in the assessment" for the approval of a product via their conditional marketing authorization or marketing authorization under exceptional circumstances pathways (http://www.ema.europa.eu/docs/en_GB/document_library/Regulatory_and_procedural_guideline/2009/10/WC500004883.pdf).

23.27.1 Case Study – BioThrax Anthrax Vaccine

BioThrax (Anthrax Vaccine Adsorbed) was the first vaccine to receive approval for a new indication, post-exposure prophylaxis (PostEP), using the Animal Rule. Because the approval of the vaccine under the rule was groundbreaking, this case is presented in greater detail than the other case studies. In addition, the case more generally illustrates the importance of nonclinical models and immunological assays (in this case neutralization) in the prediction of efficacy in humans.

The vaccine is made from a cell-free filtrate of a *Bacillus anthracis* strain that is avirulent and non-encapsulated. The final product contains the 83 kDa protective antigen (PA) protein as well as other proteins and is adsorbed to aluminum hydroxide. Anthrax bacteria produce PA, lethal factor (LF), and edema factor (EF). If PA interacts with LF or EF on the surface of human or animal cells, the toxins formed can be lethal. BioThrax stimulates the immune system to produce antibodies against PA, and when PA is blocked, LF and EF are not able to interact with PA, and the toxins are neutralized.

BioThrax (subcutaneous) was first approved in 1970 for pre-exposure prophylaxis (PreEP) of disease in persons at high risk of exposure based on early animal studies (see references in Brachman et al, 1962), chemistry and manufacturing controls (CMC), a 1950s field efficacy study in U.S. woolen mill workers by Brachman et al. (Ibid.) conducted with a Merck anthrax vaccine (Institute of Medicine, 2002), a CDC open-label safety study in the 1960s, and disease surveillance data compiled by the CDC (FDA, 2012). In 2002, the intramuscular (IM) route and an alternate regimen was approved for PreEP, which was followed in 2012 by approval of a PreEP primary vaccination series of three IM doses of BioThrax at Months 0, 1, and 6 followed with boosts at 12 and 18 months after initiation of the series, and then at 1-year intervals for at-risk people (Ibid.).

The post-exposure prophylaxis (PostEP) indication is for subcutaneous vaccination following suspected or confirmed *B. anthracis* exposure administered with recommended antibacterial drugs (Emergent BioSolutions Product Monograph; https://www.emergentbiosolutions.com/sites/default/files/inline-files/Product%20Monograph%20BioThrax%20%28EN%29.pdf). The program of nonclinical and clinical studies leading to approval of the Post-EP indication is described

by Beasley et al. (2016), in which it is stated that "Products approved under the Animal Rule are subject to requirements for post-licensure studies to demonstrate clinical efficacy, when such studies become feasible; restrictions to ensure safe use of the product; and requirements for labeling to clearly indicate that approval of the product was based on efficacy studies in animals". The author also points out the importance of robust and validated assays to bridge immune responses from animals to humans.

Because the basis of protection against anthrax is the elicitation of anti-PA antibodies and toxin neutralization, correlating animal and human immune response data was an absolute requirement. CBER stated that the "vaccine dose in humans elicit an immune response comparable to that of animals protected by the vaccine" (FDA, 2016). Therefore, the key measure of the protective immune response used to bridge animal and human data was the anthrax toxin-neutralizing antibody (TNA) assay, considered the most appropriate indicator of protection against anthrax. Per the Summary Basis of Regulatory Action, "The FDA concluded that protective TNA thresholds corresponding to a 70% probability of survival in animal models of inhalational anthrax predict a reasonable survival benefit. Vaccine protection in humans was determined by the percentage of clinical study subjects that achieve a TNA level that corresponds to a 70% probability of survival in the animal models" (FDA, 2015b).

Based on the rule and FDA feedback in various meetings, the nonclinical program for BioThrax (Emergent BioSolutions Product Monograph) focused on TNA levels vs. protection in animal challenge studies, and included toxicity studies, as summarized below:

- A GLP rabbit and a non-GLP NHP post-vaccination challenge study with inhaled aerosolized *B. anthracis* spores were conducted to correlate post-vaccination protection against challenge with analysis of anthrax TNA titers to support the pre-exposure indication (logistic regression analysis).

- Two rabbit studies with challenge by inhalation of aerosolized *B. anthracis* spores, with daily levofloxacin by oral gavage given 6–12 hours post-exposure for 1 week, with or without two IM BioThrax injections 1 week apart, were conducted to support the post-exposure indication.

- A single-dose GLP toxicity study in rats and a four-dose GLP toxicity study in rabbits were conducted.

- A pre- and postnatal reproductive and developmental toxicity study in rabbits (two doses premating and one dose during pregnancy on either day 7 or day 17) was also performed to fulfill the toxicology requirements for any vaccine for use in women of childbearing potential.

- Supportive animal passive immunization protection studies served as proof-of-concept that antibodies alone can protect against anthrax.

- A supportive (limited) non-GLP rabbit toxicology study was conducted with BioThrax administered with a second compound (redacted from the FDA

Summary Basis for Regulatory Action). Based on the publication by Malkevich et al., the compound was likely human anthrax immunoglobulin (AIGIV), which blunted the immune response to vaccination.

The importance of the TNA assays to the program is highlighted in the Summary Basis of Approval (2015b) as is the importance of the assay reference sera.

23.28 The Role of Human Challenge Studies in Vaccine Development

Controlled human infection models (CHIM) have been developed for many diseases and utilized to investigate interventions for treating and preventing infection. CHIM can streamline vaccine development in several ways including elucidating disease pathogenesis, selecting candidates, evaluating the ability of the vaccine to protect from infection/disease, establishing the durability of protection, and identifying correlates or surrogates of protection. The checkered history prior to ethical, regulatory, and clinical standards being instituted and the important roles that controlled human challenge studies have played in vaccine development to date are reviewed by Sekhar and Kang (2020). Challenge trials have been carried out with more than 20 infectious diseases (viruses, bacteria, and parasites) and have played an important role in new vaccines for malaria, typhoid, and cholera. As of 2020, there were more than 200 CHIM trials on http://clinicaltrials.gov/. Although there has been vigorous debate on the ethics of COVID-19 human challenge trials, the UK has created The Human Challenge Program, funded by the Department of Business, Energy, and Industrial Strategy (BEIS) through the Vaccines Taskforce, which is a partnership between government, hVIVO, Imperial College London, and The Royal Free London NHS Foundation Trust (https://hvivo.com/the-human-challenge-programme/). The stated goal of the partnership is to "explore the use of human challenge studies to improve and accelerate the development of vaccines and treatments against COVID-19 and will create a UK-based infrastructure for future human challenge trials supporting the world's biotech and pharmaceutical industries. The first stage of this project will explore the feasibility of exposing healthy volunteers to COVID-19. In this initial phase, called the Virus Characterisation Study, the aim will be to discover the smallest amount of virus it takes to cause a person to develop COVID-19. Imperial College London is the study sponsor, and the study will be conducted by hVIVO at the Royal Free Hospital's specialist research unit in London, under the scrutiny of hVIVO's highly trained scientists and medics. The study received ethics approval from a specially convened Research Ethics Committee in February 2021, and the study will commence in H1 2021".

The FDA Guidance for Industry: General Principles for the Development of Vaccines to Protect Against Global Infectious Diseases (2011) briefly touches on human challenge trials and recommends that sponsors discuss their development plan with CBER prior to initiation of such studies for either POC or efficacy. The WHO document entitled "Key criteria for the ethical acceptability of COVID-19 human challenge studies" (6 May 2020) provides a multifaceted perspective on expectations for human challenge studies as does the WHO R&D Blueprint on the topic (7 December 2020).

23.29 General Comments and Future Directions

From ancient to more recent roots of active and passive immunotherapies, the tree of vaccinology has grown, its trunk dividing into the many branches of the field that have yielded life-altering approaches and products. A recent PhRMA tabular summary of medicines in development only for infectious diseases lists approximately 130 vaccines (novel, improved, or combined) in clinical phases of development (PhRMA, 2020b). Adding these infectious disease vaccines to the vaccines and immunotherapies in development for non-infectious diseases, and the emergence of novel technologies and platforms, suggest that the future holds great promise for individual and public health.

One of the 17 United Nations Sustainable Development Goals, Goal 3 – Health and Wellbeing, currently shows an image with "VACCINATE YOUR FAMILY" as the gateway to the detailed Goal 3 targets (https://www.un.org/sustainabledevelopment/sustainable-development-goals/). Pregnant women and neonates/infants are uniquely susceptible to some infectious diseases and can have a higher risk of severe disease or death, so interest in maternal immunization has been growing globally and is being viewed in the context of "life course immunization" (Bergin et al., 2018) that includes women (before, during, and after pregnancy), newborns, children, adolescents, and the aged. Some of these populations are more vulnerable to infection and disease because they are not covered by current immunization recommendations or strategies. Focusing on maternal immunization because of its impact on both mothers and babies, a publication by Engmann et al. (2020) reviews the vaccines recommended during pregnancy (diphtheria, pertussis, tetanus, and influenza), several others vaccines that may be recommended under special circumstances, how physicians can manage the "antenatal care visit", some vaccines in development for preventing maternal and/or newborn infections (RSV, HepE, Group B strep, CMV, VSV, Zika, and Ebola), considerations for introduction of a new maternal vaccines, available guidance, and opportunities for maternal vaccines for non-infectious diseases.

Beyond vaccines for new diseases, improved existing vaccines, new combinations, new adjuvants, and vaccines for life-course immunization, opportunities exist for new vaccine manufacturing and adjuvant technologies, vaccine delivery techniques, cold-chain solutions, safety data reporting, data mining, regulatory science, and perhaps most importantly, ways to combat misinformation and vaccine hesitancy. Those of us engaged in the myriad aspects of vaccinology have their work cut out for them!

REFERENCES

Albrecht RA, Liu W-C, Sant AJ, Tompkins SM, Pekosz A, Meliopoulos V, Cherry S, Thomas PG, Schultz-Cherry S. (2018). Moving forward: recent developments for the ferret biomedical research model. *mBio* 9:e01113-18. https://doi.org/10.1128/mBio.01113-18.

Allio T. (2018). The FDA Animal Rule and its role in protecting human safety, *Expert Opinion on Drug Safety*, 17:10, 971–973. https://doi.org/10.1080/14740338.2018.1518429.

Ameratunga R, Gillis D, Gold M, Linneberg A, Elwood JM. (2017). Evidence refuting the existence of autoimmune/auto-inflammatory syndrome induced by adjuvants (ASIA). *The Journal of Allergy and Clinical Immunology: In Practice*, 5(6): 1551–1555.e1. https://doi.org/10.1016/j.jaip.2017.06.033.

Barrett A. (2016). Vaccinology in the twenty-first century. *Vaccines* 1: 16009. https://doi.org/10.1038/npjvaccines.2016.9.

Beasley D, Brasel T and Comer J. (2016). First vaccine approval under the FDA Animal Rule. *Vaccines* 1: 16013. https://doi.org/10.1038/npjvaccines.2016.13.

Bergin N, Murtagh J, Philip RK. (2018). Maternal vaccination as an essential component of life-course immunization and its contribution to preventive neonatology. *Int J Environ Res Public Health*, 15: 847. https://www.mdpi.com/1660-4601/15/5/847.

Bethur N and Rahim N. *A Case of Spontaneous Testicular Teratoma Observed in Genetically Modified AG129 Mice*. Dept. Vet Services, InVivos Pte Ltd, Singapore. https://www.invivos.com.sg/wp-content/uploads/2017/11/Poster-Vet-final.pdf.

Bonini S. 2012 Regulatory aspects of allergen-specific immunotherapy: Europe sets the scene for a global approach. *The World Allergy Organization Journal*, 5(10): 120–123. https://doi.org/10.1097/WOX.0b013e318272484e.

Bosco-Lauth AM, Calvert AE, Root JJ, Gidlewski T, Bird BH, Bowen RA, Muehlenbachs A, Zaki SR, and Brault AC. (2016). Vertebrate host susceptibility to heartland virus. *Emerging Infectious Diseases*, 22(12): 2070–2077 https://doi.org/10.3201/eid2212.160472.

Boukhebza H, Bellon N, Limacher JM, and Inchauspé G. (2012). Therapeutic vaccination to treat chronic infectious diseases: Current clinical developments using MVA-based vaccines. *Human Vaccines & Immunotherapeutics*, 8(12): 1746–1757. https://doi.org/10.4161/hv.21689.

Boylston A. (2012). The origins of inoculation. *Journal of the Royal Society of Medicine*, 105(7): 309–313. https://doi.org/10.1258/jrsm.2012.12k044.

Brachman PS, Gold H, Plotkin SA, et al. (1962). Field evaluation of a human anthrax vaccine. *American Journal of Public Health*, 52: 632–645.

Bradley MP, Nagamine CM. (2017). Animal models of Zika virus. *CompMed*, 67(3):242–252. PMID: 28662753; PMCID: PMC5482516).

Branswell H. (2020). Against all odds: The inside story of how scientists across three continents produced an Ebola vaccine. STAT Jan. 7, 2020. https://www.statnews.com/2020/01/07/inside-story-scientists-produced-world-first-ebola-vaccine/.

Bregman CL, Adler RR, Morton DG, Regan KS, and Yano BL. (2003). Recommended tissue list for histopathologic examination in repeat-dose toxicity and carcinogenicity studies: A proposal of the society of toxicologic pathology (STP). *Toxicologic Pathology*, 31(2): 252–253. https://doi.org/10.1080/01926230390183751.

Brewoo JN, Kinney RM, Powell TD, Arguello JJ, Silengo SJ, Partidos CD, Huang C, Stinchcomb DT, and Osorio JE. (2012). Immunogenicity and efficacy of chimeric dengue vaccine (DENVax) formulations in interferon-deficient AG129 mice. *Vaccine*, 30(8): 1513–1520. https://doi.org/10.1016/j.vaccine.2011.11.072

Brighton Collaboration Webinar on Tools for COVID-19 Vaccine Safety Assessment. 27 August 2020. Brighton Collaboration Webinar on Tools for COVID-19 Vaccine Safety Assessment Thursday 27th August 2020.

Bugelski PJ, Herzyk DJ, Rehm S, Harmsen AG, Gore EV, Williams DM, Maleeff BE, et al. (2000). Preclinical development of keliximab, a PRIMATIZED anti-CD4 monoclonal antibody, in human CD4 transgenic mice: Characterization of the model and safety studies. *Human & Experimental Toxicology* 19:230–243.

Buonaguro L, Tagliamonte M. (2020). Selecting target antigens for cancer vaccine development. *Vaccines*, 8(4):615. https://doi.org/10.3390/vaccines8040615.

Carlson RD, Flickinger JC, Jr, and Snook AE. (2020). Talkin' toxins: From Coley's to modern cancer immunotherapy. *Toxins*, 12(4): 241. https://doi.org/10.3390/toxins12040241).

CDC. (August 24, 2020). Vaccines During Pregnancy FAQs. https://www.cdc.gov/vaccinesafety/concerns/vaccines-during-pregnancy.html.

CDC. (April 2, 2021). About Variants of the Virus that Causes COVID-19 https://www.cdc.gov/coronavirus/2019-ncov/transmission/variant.html.

Chen L, Flies D. (2013). Molecular mechanisms of T cell co-stimulation and co-inhibition. *Nature Reviews Immunology* 13: 227–242. https://doi.org/10.1038/nri3405.

Cohn L, Delamarre L. (2014). Dendritic cell-targeted vaccines. *Frontiers in Immunology*, 5: 1–11. https://www.frontiersin.org/article/10.3389/fimmu.2014.00255.

College of Physicians of Philadelphia. The History of Vaccines – An educational resource by the College of Physicians of Philadelphia. https://www.historyofvaccines.org/timeline#EVT_100741.

Corbett KS, et al. (2020). Evaluation of the mRNA-1273 vaccine against SARS-CoV-2 in nonhuman primates. *New England Journal of Medicine*. https://www.nejm.org/doi/full/10.1056/NEJMoa2024671.

D'Acremont V, Herzog C, Genton B. (2006). Immunogenicity and safety of a virosomal hepatitis A vaccine (Epaxal®) in the elderly. *Journal of Travel Medicine*, 13(2):78–83, https://doi.org/10.1111/j.1708-8305.2006.00001.x.

Dempster AM, Haworth R. (2007). Preclinical safety evaluation of viral vaccines. In: *Preclinical Safety Evaluation of Biopharmaceuticals*, J.A. Cavagnaro (Ed.). https://doi.org/10.1002/9780470292549.ch31.

Depil S, Bonaventura P, and Alcazer V. (2019). Cancer vaccines: what's next? *Oncotarget*, 10(40): 3985–3987. https://doi.org/10.18632/oncotarget.27006.

Draize JH, Woodard G, and Calvery HO. Methods for the study of irritation and toxicity of substances applied topically to the skin and mucous membranes. *Journal of Pharmacology and Experimental Therapeutics*, 1944, 82:377–390.

Dudley MZ, Halsey NA, Omer SB, Orenstein WA, O'Leary ST, Limaye RJ, and Salmon DA. (2020). The state of vaccine safety science: Systematic reviews of the evidence. *The Lancet Infectious Diseases*, 20(5): e80–e89. https://doi.org/10.1016/S1473-3099(20)30130-4.

Ehreth J. (2003). The global value of vaccination. *Vaccine*, 21(7–8):596–600. https://dx.doi.org/10.1016/S0264-410X(02)00623-0.

Elder GA, Gama Sosa MA, and De Gasperi R. (2010). Transgenic mouse models of Alzheimer's disease. *The Mount Sinai Journal of Medicine*, 77(1): 69–81. https://doi.org/10.1002/msj.20159.

Engmann C, Fleming, JA, Khan, S. et al. (2020). *Closer and closer? Maternal immunization: current promise, future horizons. Journal of Perinatology* 40: 844–857. https://doi.org/10.1038/s41372-020-0668-3.

Esteves PJ, Abrantes J, Baldauf HM., et al. (2018). The wide utility of rabbits as models of human diseases. *Experimental & Molecular Medicine* 50: 1–10. https://doi.org/10.1038/s12276-018-0094-1.

Evans WJ, Hurst BL, Peterson CJ, Van Wettere AJ, Day CW, Smee DF, and Tarbet EB. (2019). Development of a respiratory disease model for enterovirus D68 in 4-week-old mice for evaluation of antiviral therapies. *Antiviral Research*, 162: 61–70 https://doi.org/10.1016/j.antiviral.2018.11.012.

FDA. (1997). Points to Consider in the Manufacture and Testing of Monoclonal Antibody Products for Human Use. Points to Consider in the Manufacture and Testing of Monoclonal Antibody Products for Human Use.

FDA. (2006). Guidance for Industry: Nonclinical Safety Evaluation of Pediatric Drug Products https://www.fda.gov/regulatory-information/search-fda-guidance-documents/nonclinical-safety-evaluation-pediatric-drug-products.

FDA. (2011). Guidance for Industry: General Principles for the Development of Vaccines to Protect Against Global Infectious Diseases https://www.fda.gov/regulatory-information/search-fda-guidance-documents/general-principles-development-vaccines-protect-against-global-infectious-diseases.

FDA. (2012). Summary Basis for Regulatory Action - BioThrax, May 17, 2012. https://wayback.archive-it.org/7993/20170723023408/https://www.fda.gov/downloads/BiologicsBloodVaccines/Vaccines/ApprovedProducts/UCM308410.pdf

FDA. (2015a). Guidance for Industry entitled Product Development Under the Animal Rule https://www.fda.gov/media/88625/download.

FDA. (2015b). Summary Basis for Regulatory Action Template – BioThrax https://wayback.archive-it.org/7993/20170723023407/https://www.fda.gov/downloads/BiologicsBloodVaccines/Vaccines/ApprovedProducts/UCM474886.pdf

FDA. (2016). Pathway to Licensure for Protective Antigen-based Anthrax Vaccines for a Postexposure Prophylaxis Indication Using the Animal Rule. Briefing Document for the Vaccines and Related Biological Products Advisory Committee Meeting, November 16, 2010. https://wayback.archive-it.org/7993/20170405194315/https://www.fda.gov/downloads/AdvisoryCommittees/CommitteesMeetingMaterials/BloodVaccinesandOtherBiologics/VaccinesandRelatedBiologicalProductsAdvisoryCommittee/ UCM232400.pdf

FDA. (2019). Dengvaxia Summary Basis of Regulatory Action. https://www.fda.gov/media/125157/download.

FDA. (2020). Development and Licensure of Vaccines to Prevent COVID-19: Guidance for Industry https://www.fda.gov/regulatory-information/search-fda-guidance-documents/development-and-licensure-vaccines-prevent-covid-19.

FDA. (2021). Emergency Use Authorization for Vaccines to Prevent COVID-19: Guidance for Industry (supersedes the guidance of the same title issued on October 2020) https://www.fda.gov/regulatory-information/search-fda-guidance-documents/emergency-use-authorization-vaccines-prevent-covid-19.

Felgner S, Kocijancic D, Frahm M, and Weiss S. (2016). Bacteria in cancer therapy: renaissance of an old concept. *International Journal of Microbiology*, 2016: 8451728. https://doi.org/10.1155/2016/8451728.

Freitas-Silva R, Brelaz-de-Castro MC, and Pereira VR. (2014). Dendritic cell-based approaches in the fight against diseases. *Frontiers in Immunology*, 5:78. https://doi.org/10.3389/fimmu.2014.00078.

Gad SC. (2016). *Animal Models in Toxicology*, 3rd edition, Taylor & Francis Group, LLC, pp. 935–956. https://doi.org/10.1201/b18705.

Gardner CL, Burke CW, Higgs ST, Klimstra WB, and Ryman KD. (2012). Interferon-alpha/beta deficiency greatly exacerbates arthritogenic disease in mice infected with wild-type chikungunya virus but not with the cell culture-adapted live-attenuated 181/25 vaccine candidate. *Virology*, 425(2): 103–112, ISSN 0042-6822, https://doi.org/10.1016/j.virol.2011.12.020.

Geoghegan S, O'Callaghan KP, and Offit PA. (2020). Vaccine safety: Myths and misinformation. *Frontiers in Microbiology*, 11, 372. https://doi.org/10.3389/fmicb.2020.00372.

Gerdts V, Wilson HL, Meurens F, van Drunen Littel - van den Hurk S, Wilson D, Walker S, Wheler C, Townsend H, Potter AA. (2015). Large animal models for vaccine development and testing. *ILAR Journal*, 56(1): 53–62. https://doi.org/10.1093/ilar/ilv009.

Glenny A, Pope C, Waddington H, Falacce U. (1926). The antigenic value of toxoid precipitated by potassium alum. *The Journal of Pathology and Bacteriology* 29:31–40. https://doi.org/10.1002/path.1700290106.

Globinska A, et al. (2018). Mechanisms of allergen-specific immunotherapy: Diverse mechanisms of immune tolerance to allergens. *Allergy, Asthma & Immunology Research* 121: 306–312 https://doi.org/10.1016/j.anai.2018.06.026.

Golding H, Khurana S, and Zaitseva M. (2018). What is the predictive value of animal models for vaccine efficacy in humans? The importance of bridging studies and species-independent correlates of protection. *Cold Spring Harbor Perspectives in Biology*, 10(4): a028902. https://doi.org/10.1101/cshperspect.a028902.

Google search #1 on vaccine training programs. https://www.google.com/search?q=education+in+vaccinology+2021&rlz=1C5CHFA_enUS723US729&oq=education+in+vaccinology+2021&aqs=chrome.69i57.7002j1j7&sourceid=chrome&ie=UTF-8.

Google search #2 on academic vaccine translational sciences centers. https://www.google.com/search?q=academic+vaccine+research+and+development+centers&rlz=1C5CHFA_enUS723US729&sxsrf=ALeKk01YpFX1XKZF0AiA5qYdAtY7EzYARg%3A1618152341

953&ei=1QtzYPewOd_15NoP6P-84AM&oq=academ
ic+vaccine+research+and+development+centers&gs_
lcp=Cgdnd3Mtd2l6EAMyCAghEBYQHRAeMggIIRA-
WEB0QHjoHCAAQRxCwAzoECCMQJzoGCAAQFh
AeOggIABAIEA0QHjoFCCEQoAE6BQghEKsCULf
pAVifxwJggtQCaAFwAngAgAFviAGLG5IBBDM1Lj
WYAQCgAQGqAQdnd3Mtd2l6yAEIwAEB&sclient=
gws-wiz&ved=0ahUKEwi3z6Kct_bvAhXfMlkFHeg_
DzwQ4dUDCA0&uact=5.

Gouglas D, Le TT, Henderson K, Kaloudis A, Danielsen T,
Hammersland NC, Robinson JM, Heaton PM, Røttingen
J-A. (2018). Estimating the cost of vaccine develop-
ment against epidemic infectious diseases: A cost mini-
misation study. *Lancet Global Health*, 6: e1386–e1396
Published Online October 17, 2018 http://dx.doi.org/10.1016/
S2214-109X(18)30346-2.

Graham BS. (2020). Rapid COVID-19 vaccine development.
Science, 2020: 945–946. https://www.science.org/doi/
full/10.1126/science.abb8923.

Graham BS, Ambrosino DM. (2015). History of passive antibody
administration for prevention and treatment of infectious
diseases. *Current Opinion in HIV and AIDS*, 10(3): 129–
134. https://doi.org/10.1097/COH.0000000000000154.

Green MD. (2015). Acute phase responses to novel, investigational vaccines in toxicology studies: The relationship
between C-reactive protein and other acute phase proteins. *International Journal of Toxicology*, 34(5): 379–383.
https://doi.org/10.1177/1091581815598750.

Green MD, Al-Humadi NH. (2017). Preclinical Toxicology
of Vaccines. A Comprehensive Guide to Toxicology
in Nonclinical Drug Development, 709–735.
https://doi.org/10.1016/B978-0-12-803620-4.00027-X.

Greenberg S. (2003). A Concise History of Immunology, 1–15.
http://www.columbia.edu/itc/hs/medical/pathophys/immu-
nology/readings/ConciseHistoryImmunology.pdf.

Greenwood B. (2014). The contribution of vaccination to global
health: Past, present and future. *Philosophical Transactions
of the Royal Society B*, 369(1645):20130433. 10.1098/
rstb.2013.0433. PMID: 24821919.

Gross CC, Wiendl H. (2013). Dendritic cell vaccina-
tion in autoimmune disease. *Current Opinion in
Rheumatology*, 25(2): 268–274. https://doi.org/10.1097/
BOR.0b013e32835cb9f2.

Gruber MF, Marshall VB. (2018). Regulation and testing of vaccines. *Plotkin's Vaccines*, 1547–1565.e2.
https://doi.org/10.1016/B978-0-323-35761-6.00079-1.

Hanney SR, Wooding S, Sussex J., et al. (2020). From
COVID-19 research to vaccine application: why might
it take 17 months not 17 years and what are the wider
lessons? *Health Research Policy and Systems* 18: 61.
https://doi.org/10.1186/s12961-020-00571-3.

Health Canada Extraordinary Use New Drugs regulations. (2021).
https://www.canada.ca/en/health-canada/services/drugs-
health-products/biologics-radiopharmaceuticals-genetic-
therapies/applications-submissions/guidance-documents/
submission-information-requirements-extraordinary-drugs-
eunds.html.

Heldens JG, Patel JR, Chanter N, Ten Thij GJ, Gravendijck M,
Schijns VE, Langen A, Schetters TP. (2008). Veterinary
vaccine development from an industrial perspective.
Veterinary Journal (London, England: 1997), 178(1): 7–20.
https://doi.org/10.1016/j.tvjl.2007.11.009.

Herati RS, Wherry, EJ. (2018). What is the predictive value of animal models for vaccine efficacy in humans? Consideration
of strategies to improve the value of animal models. *Cold
Spring Harbor Perspectives in Biology*, 10(4): a031583.
https://doi.org/10.1101/cshperspect.a031583.

Hickey AJ. (2011). Guinea pig model of infectious disease -
viral infections. *Current Drug Targets*, 12: 1018.
https://doi.org/10.2174/138945011795677827.

Hobohm U. (2001). Fever and cancer in perspective.
Cancer Immunology, Immunotherapy 50, 391–396
https://doi.org/10.1007/s002620100216.

Huang S, Hendricks W, Althage A, Hemmi S, Bluethmann H,
Kamijo R, Vilcek J, Zinkernagel RM, and Aguet M. (1993).
Immune response in mice that lack the interferon-gamma
receptor. *Science*, 1993: 1742–1745.

Hundal J, Mardis ER. (2019). The Scientist: Personalized
Cancer Vaccines in Clinical Trials. https://www.the-
scientist.com/features/personalized-cancer-vaccines-
in-clinical-trials-66075.

International Conference on Harmonisation Guidance for Industry:
S2(R1) Genotoxicity Testing and Data Interpretation for
Pharmaceuticals Intended for Human Use. Jun 2012.

Immunization Action Coalition. Historic Dates and Events
Related to Vaccines and Immunization. https://www.
immunize.org/timeline/

Institute of Medicine (US) Committee to Assess the Safety
and Efficacy of the Anthrax Vaccine; Joellenbeck LM,
Zwanziger LL, Durch JS, et al., editors. (2002). The Anthrax
Vaccine: Is It Safe? Does It Work? Washington, DC: National
Academies Press, 7, Anthrax Vaccine Manufacture. https://
www.ncbi.nlm.nih.gov/books/NBK220526/

Institute of Medicine. (2012). *Adverse Effects of Vaccines:
Evidence and Causality*. Washington, DC: The National
Academies Press https://www.nap.edu/catalog/13164/
adverse-effects-of-vaccines-evidence-and-causality.

International Conference on Harmonisation S6(R1) Guideline
Preclinical Safety Evaluation of Biotechnology-derived
Pharmaceuticals https://database.ich.org/sites/dcfault/files/
S6_R1_Guideline_0.pdf

Jessy T. (2011). Immunity over inability: The spontaneous regression
of cancer. *Journal of Natural Science, Biology, and Medicine*,
2(1): 43–49. https://doi.org/10.4103/0976-9668.82318).

Jiang S, He Y, and Liu S. (2005). SARS vaccine development.
Emerging Infectious Diseases, 11(7):1016–1020. 10.3201/
eid1107.050219.

Johns Hopkins Center for Health Security. (2019). Vaccine
Platforms: State of the Field and Looming Challenges
https://www.centerforhealthsecurity.org/our-work/
pubs_archive/pubs-pdfs/2019/190423-OPP-platform-
report.pdf.

Johnson AJ., Roehrig JT. (1999). New mouse model for dengue
virus vaccine testing. *Journal of Virology*, 73(1): 783–786.
https://doi.org/10.1128/JVI.73.1.783-786.1999.

Jorge S, Odir and Dellagostin A. (2017). The development of
veterinary vaccines: A review of traditional methods
and modern biotechnology approaches, *Biotechnology
Research and Innovation*, 1(1): 6–13. ISSN 2452-0721
https://doi.org/10.1016/j.biori.2017.10.001.

Jutel M, Kosowska A, and Smolinska S. (2016). Allergen
immunotherapy: Past, present, and future. *Allergy,
Asthma & Immunology Research*, 8(3): 191–197.
https://doi.org/10.4168/aair.2016.8.3.191.

Kabitzke P, Cheng KM, Altevogt B. (2019). Guidelines and initiatives for good research practice. In: Bespalov A., Michel M., Steckler T. (eds) *Good Research Practice in Non-Clinical Pharmacology and Biomedicine. Handbook of Experimental Pharmacology*, vol 257. Springer, Cham. https://doi.org/10.1007/164_2019_275.

Kaufmann SHE. (2017). Remembering Emil von Behring: from tetanus treatment to antibody cooperation with phagocytes. *mBio* 8:e00117-17. https://doi.org/10.1128/mBio.00117-17.

Kaufman SHE (2019). Immunology's coming of age. *Frontiers in Immunology*, 10:1–13. https://www.frontiersin.org/article/10.3389/fimmu.2019.00684.

Kaur D, Patiyal S, Sharma N, Usmani SS, Raghava GPS. (2019). PRRDB 2.0: a comprehensive database of pattern-recognition receptors and their ligands, Database, 2019, baz076, https://doi.org/10.1093/database/baz076.

Kim Y-I, Kim S-G, Kim S-M, Webby RJ, Jung JU, Choi YK. (2020). Infection and Rapid Transmission of SARS-CoV-2 in Ferrets. *Cell Host & Microbe*, V27(5): 704–709.e2, ISSN 1931-3128. https://doi.org/10.1016/j.chom.2020.03.023.

Kolappaswamy K. (2015). Susceptibility of Sigmodon hispidus. *Lab Animal*, 44(6): 199. https://doi.org/10.1038/laban.767.

Kumru OS, Sangeeta B. Joshi, DE, Smith, C, Russell M, Ted P, Volkin DB. (2014). Vaccine instability in the cold chain: Mechanisms, analysis and formulation strategies. *Biologicals*, 42(5): 237–259. https://doi.org/10.1016/j.biologicals.2014.05.007.

Kushner I and Mackiewicz A. (2019). The acute phase response: an overview. In: Mackiewicz A, Kushner I, Baumann H, eds. (2019). *Acute Phase Proteins: Molecular Biology, Biochemistry, and Clinical Applications*. Boca Raton, FL: CRC Press, 1993: 3–19.

Lambert PH, Podda A. (2018). Education in vaccinology: An important tool for strengthening global health. *Frontiers in Immunology*, 9: 1134. https://doi.org/10.3389/fimmu.2018.01134.

Lanying D, Wanbo T, Yusen Z & Shibo J. (2016). Vaccines for the prevention against the threat of MERS-CoV. *Expert Review of Vaccines*, 15(9): 1123–1134. https://doi.org/10.1586/14760584.2016.1167603

Li L, Goedegebuure SP & Gillanders W. (2020). Cancer vaccines: Shared tumor antigens return to the spotlight. *Signal Transduction and Targeted Therapy* 5: 251. https://doi.org/10.1038/s41392-020-00364-8.

Li YD, Chi WY, Su, JH et al. (2020). Coronavirus vaccine development: From SARS and MERS to COVID-19. *Journal of Biomedical Science* 27: 104. https://doi.org/10.1186/s12929-020-00695-2.

Luan J, Lu Y, Jin X, Zhang L. (2020). Spike protein recognition of mammalian ACE2 predicts the host range and optimized ACE2 for SARS-CoV-2 infection. *Biochemical and Biophysical Research Communications*, 2020.

Lurie N, Keusch GT, and Dzau VJ. (2021). Urgent lessons from COVID-19: Why the world needs a standing, coordinated system and sustainable financing for global research and development. *Lancet*, 397: 1229–1236. https://doi.org/10.1016/ S0140-6736(21)00503-1.

Maglione MA, Gidengil C, Das L, et al. (2014). *Safety of Vaccines Used for Routine Immunization in the United States*. Rockville, MD: Agency for Healthcare Research and Quality (US); (Evidence Reports/Technology Assessments, No. 215.) https://www.ncbi.nlm.nih.gov/books/NBK230053/.

Malkevich NV, Basu S, Rudge Jr TL, Clement KH, Chakrabarti AC, Aimes RT, Nabors GS, Skiadopoulos MH, and Ionin B. (2013). Effect of anthrax immune globulin on response to BioThrax (anthrax vaccine adsorbed) in New Zealand White Rabbits. *Antimicrobial Agents and Chemotherapy*, 57(11). https://journals.asm.org/doi/full/10.1128/AAC.00460-13.

McCray PB, Jr, Pewe L, Wohlford-Lenane C, Hickey M, Manzel L, Shi L, Netland J, Jia HP, Halabi C, Sigmund CD, Meyerholz DK, Kirby P, Look DC, & Perlman S. (2007). Lethal infection of K18-hACE2 mice infected with severe acute respiratory syndrome coronavirus. *Journal of Virology*, 81(2), 813–821. https://doi.org/10.1128/JVI.02012-06.

Miao J, Chard LS, Wang Z, & Wang Y. (2019). Syrian hamster as an animal model for the study on infectious diseases. *Frontiers in Immunology*, 10, 2329. https://doi.org/10.3389/fimmu.2019.02329.

MIT News. How often do vaccine trials hit paydirt? https://news.mit.edu/2020/how-often-vaccine-trials-succeed-0527.

Morales A, Eidinger D, Bruce AW. (1976). Intracavitary Bacillus Calmette-Guerin in the treatment of superficial bladder tumors. *The Journal of Urology*, 116(2):180–183 https://doi.org/10.1016/S0022-5347(17)58737-6.

Mougel A, Terme M, & Tanchot C. (2019). Therapeutic cancer vaccine and combinations with antiangiogenic therapies and immune checkpoint blockade. *Frontiers in Immunology*, 10: 467. https://doi.org/10.3389/fimmu.2019.00467.

Muhammad Azami NA, Takasaki T, Kurane I, & Moi ML. (2020). Non-human primate models of dengue virus infection: A comparison of viremia levels and antibody responses during primary and secondary infection among old world and new world monkeys. *Pathogens (Basel, Switzerland)*, 9(4): 247. https://doi.org/10.3390/pathogens9040247.

Muller U, Steinhoff U, Reis LF, Hemmi S, Pavlovic J, Zinkernagel RM, & Aguet M. (1994). Functional role of type I and type II interferons in antiviral defense. *Science*, 1994: 1918–1921.

Muñoz-Fontela C, Dowling WE, Funnell SGP. et al. (2020). Animal models for COVID-19. *Nature*, 586: 509–515. https://doi.org/10.1038/s41586-020-2787-6.

Munoz FM, Cramer JP, Dekker CL, Dudley MZ, Graham BS, Gurwith M, Law B, Perlman S, Polack FP, Spergel JM, Van Braeckel E, Ward BJ, Didierlaurent AM, Lambert PH, & Brighton Collaboration Vaccine-associated Enhanced Disease Working Group (2021). Vaccine-associated enhanced disease: Case definition and guidelines for data collection, analysis, and presentation of immunization safety data. *Vaccine*, S0264-410X(21)00094-3. Advance online publication. https://doi.org/10.1016/j.vaccine.2021.01.055.

Mustafá YM, Meuren LM, Coelho SVA and de Arruda LB (2019). Pathways exploited by flaviviruses to counteract the blood-brain barrier and invade the central nervous system. *Frontiers in Microbiology*, 10:525.

Nanishi A, Pope C, Waddington H, Falacce U. (1926). The antigenic value of toxoid precipitated by potassium alum. *The Journal of Pathology and Bacteriology*, 29:31–40. https://doi.org/10.1002/path.1700290106.

Nanishi E, Dowling DJ, Levy O. (2020). Toward precision adjuvants: Optimizing science and safety. *Current Opinion in Pediatrics*, 32(1):125–138. https://journals.lww.com/co-pediatrics/fulltext/2020/02000/toward_precision_adjuvants_optimizing_science_and.18.aspx.

Noon, L. (1911). Prophylactic inoculation against hay fever. *The Lancet*, 177(4580): 1572–1573, ISSN 0140-6736. https://doi.org/10.1016/S0140-6736(00)78276-6.

Nößner E, Schendel DJ. (1999). Autologous and allogeneic tumor cell vaccines. In: Blankenstein T. (eds) *Gene Therapy*. Birkhäuser, Basel. https://doi.org/10.1007/978-3-0348-7011-5_19.

Offit PA, Hackett CJ. (2003). Addressing parents' concerns: Do vaccines cause allergic or autoimmune diseases? *Pediatrics*, 111(3): 653–659. https://doi.org/10.1542/peds.111.3.653.

O'Hagan DT, Lodaya RN, and Lofano G. (2020). The continued advance of vaccine adjuvants - 'we can work it out'. *Seminars Immunology*, 50:101426 https://doi.org/10.1016/j.smim.2020.101426.

Padilla-Carlin DJ, McMurray DN, and Hickey AJ. (2008). The guinea pig as a model of infectious diseases. *Comparative Medicine*, 58(4): 324–340. https://www.ncbi.nlm.nih.gov/pmc/articles/PMC2706043/pdf/cm2008000324.pdf.

Park WH, Zingher A. (1915). Active immunization with diphtheria toxin-antitoxin: And with toxin-antitoxin combined with diphtheria bacilli – Second paper: Late results. *JAMA*, LXV(26):2216–2220. https://jamanetwork.com/journals/jama/article-abstract/447678

Peng M, Mo Y, Wang Y. et al. (2019). Neoantigen vaccine: An emerging tumor immunotherapy. *Molecular Cancer*, 18: 128. https://doi.org/10.1186/s12943-019-1055-6.

Perez CR, De Palma, M. (2019). Engineering dendritic cell vaccines to improve cancer immunotherapy. *Nature Communication*, 10:5408. https://doi.org/10.1038/s41467-019-13368-y.

Pfaar O, Agache I, de Blay F, et al. (2019). Perspectives in allergen immunotherapy: 2019 and beyond. *Allergy*, 74 (Suppl. 108): 3–25. https://doi.org/10.1111/all.1407.

Pharmaceutical Research and Manufacturers of America, (PhRMA, 2020a) https://www.phrma.org/en/Media/New-Era-of-Medicine-Vaccines.

Pharmaceutical Research and Manufacturers of America (PhRMA). (2020b) https://www.phrma.org/-/media/Project/PhRMA/PhRMA-Org/PhRMA-Org/PDF/M-O/MID_2020_InfectiousDiseases_DrugList.pdf

Plotkin SA. (2010). Correlates of protection induced by vaccination. *Clinical and Vaccine Immunology: CVI*, 17(7): 1055–1065. https://doi.org/10.1128/CVI.00131-10.

Prestwood TR, Morar MM, Zellweger RM, Miller R, May MM, Yauch LE, Lada SM, Shresta S. (2012). Gamma interferon (IFN-γ) receptor restricts systemic dengue virus replication and prevents paralysis in IFN-α/β receptor-deficient mice. *Journal of Virology,* 86(23):12561–12570. 10.1128/JVI.06743-11. Epub 2012 Sep 12. PMID: 22973027; PMCID: PMC3497655.

Ramon G. (1925). Sur la production de antitoxins. *Comptes rendus de l'Académie des Sciences,* 181:157–159.

Rappuoli R, Black S, and Bloom DE. (2019). Vaccines and global health: In search of a sustainable model for vaccine development and delivery. *Science Translational Medicine*, 11(497): eeaw2888. https://doi.org/10.1126/scitranslmed.aaw2888.

Ring J and Gutermuth J. (2011). 100 years of hyposensitization: History of allergen-specific immunotherapy (ASIT). *Allergy*, 66: 713–724. https://doi.org/10.1111/j.1398-9995.2010.02541.x.

Rockx B, Kuiken T, Herfst S, Bestebroer T, Lamers MM, Oude Munnink BB, de Meulder D, van Amerongen G, van den Brand J, Okba N, Schipper D, van Run P, Leijten L,

Sikkema R, Verschoor E, Verstrepen B, Bogers W, Langermans J, Drosten C, Fentener van Vlissingen, M, … Haagmans BL. (2020). Comparative pathogenesis of COVID-19, MERS, and SARS in a nonhuman primate model. *Science (New York, N.Y.)*, 368(6494): 1012–1015. https://doi.org/10.1126/science.abb7314.

Rossi SL, Tesh RB, Azar SR, Muruato, AE, Hanley KA, Auguste AJ, Langsjoen RM, Paessler S, Vasilakis N, Weaver SC. (2016). Characterization of a novel murine model to study Zika virus. *The American Society of Tropical Medicine and Hygiene,* 94(6): 1362–1369.

Roth JA. (2011). Veterinary vaccines and their importance to animal health and public health. *Procedia in Vaccinology*, 5: 127–136, ISSN 1877-282X. https://doi.org/10.1016/j.provac.2011.10.009.

Sabin-Aspen Vaccines Science & Policy Group Report. (2020). https://www.sabin.org/sites/sabin.org/files/sabin-aspen-report-2020_meeting_the_challenge_of_vaccine_hesitancy.pdf.

Sakurai A, Ogawa T, Matsumoto J, Kihira T, Fukushima S, Miyata I, Shimizu H, Itamura S, Ouchi K, Hamada A, Tani K, Okabe N, Yamaguchi T. (2019). Regulatory aspects of quality and safety for live recombinant viral vaccines against infectious diseases in Japan. *Vaccine* 37(43): 6573–6579. https://doi.org/10.1016/j.vaccine.2019.08.031.

Samsa G, Samsa L. (2019). A guide to reproducibility in preclinical research. *Academic Medicine: Journal of the Association of American Medical Colleges*, 94(1), 47–52. https://doi.org/10.1097/ACM.0000000000002351.

Sanofi Article. (2017). https://www.sanofi.com/en/media-room/articles/2017/understanding-the-complexity-of-vaccine-manufacturing.

Sasaki E, Momose H, Hiradate Y, Furuhata K, Mizukami T, Hamaguchi I. (2018). Development of a preclinical humanized mouse model to evaluate acute toxicity of an influenza vaccine. *Oncotarget*, 9(40):25751–25763. https://doi.org/10.18632/oncotarget.25399.

Sayers S, Ulysse G, Xiang Z, He Y. (2012). Vaxjo: A web-based vaccine adjuvant database and its application for analysis of vaccine adjuvants and their uses in vaccine development. *BioMed Research International*, 2012: 13 Article ID 831486. https://doi.org/10.1155/2012/831486.

Schuh J. (2016). *Animal Models in Toxicology*, 3rd edition, by Shane Gad, Taylor & Francis Group, LLC, pp. 935–956. https://doi.org/10.1201/b18705.

Sekhar A, Kang G. (2020). Human challenge trials in vaccine development, *Seminars in Immunology*, 50: 101429, ISSN 1044-5323. https://doi.org/10.1016/j.smim.2020.101429.

Shultz L, Brehm M, Garcia-Martinez J. et al. (2012). Humanized mice for immune system investigation: progress, promise and challenges. *Nature Reviews Immunology*, 12: 786–798. https://doi.org/10.1038/nri3311.

Steinman, R. (2008). Dendritic cells and vaccines. *Proceedings (Baylor University. Medical Center)*, 21(1): 3–8. https://doi.org/10.1080/08998280.2008.11928346.

Stevens LC, Little CC. (1954). Spontaneous testicular teratomas in an inbred strain of mice. *Proceedings of the National Academy of Sciences of the United States of America*, 40(11):1080–1087. 10.1073/pnas.40.11.1080.

Thibodeaux BA, Garbino NC, Liss NM, Piper J, Blair CD, Roehrig JT. (2012). A small animal peripheral challenge model of yellow fever using interferon-receptor deficient mice and the 17D-204 vaccine strain. *Vaccine*, 30(21): 3180–3187 https://doi.org/10.1016/j.vaccine.2012.03.003.

U.S. Department of Health and Human Services Food and Drug Administration Center for Biologics Evaluation and Research. (2007). FDA Guidance for Industry: Toxicity Grading Scale for Healthy Adult and Adolescent Volunteers Enrolled in Preventive Vaccine Clinical Trials. https://www.fda.gov/media/73679/download.

Vaccines Europe and Sanofi. (2017). https://www.vaccineseurope.eu/about-vaccines/how-are-vaccines-produced.

Vaddepally RK, Kharel P, Pandey R, Garje R, Chandra AB. (2020). Review of indications of FDA-approved immune checkpoint inhibitors per NCCN guidelines with the level of evidence. *Cancers*, 12(3): 738. https://doi.org/10.3390/cancers12030738.

van der Laan, JW, Gould, S, Tanir JY. (2015). Safety of vaccine adjuvants: Focus on autoimmunity. *Vaccine*, 33(13): 1507–1514. https://doi.org/10.1016/j.vaccine.2015.01.073.

Weinberg SH, Butchart AT, Davis MM. (2012). Size of clinical trials and introductory prices of prophylactic vaccine series. *Human Vaccines & Immunotherapeutics*, 8(8): 1066–1070. https://doi.org/10.4161/hv.20506.

WHO. (2003). Guidelines on Nonclinical Evaluation of Vaccines (WHO Technical Report Series No. 927, Annex 1). https://www.who.int/publications/m/item/nonclinical-evaluation-of-vaccines-annex-1-trs-no-927.

WHO. (2013). Guidelines on the Nonclinical Evaluation of Vaccine Adjuvants and Adjuvanted Vaccines. (WHO Technical Report Series, TRS 987, Annex 2). https://www.who.int/biologicals/areas/vaccines/ADJUVANTS_Post_ECBS_edited_clean_Guidelines_NCE_Adjuvant_Final_17122013_WEB.pdf.

WHO. (2020). Key criteria for the ethical acceptability of COVID-19 human challenge studies. https://apps.who.int/iris/bitstream/handle/10665/331976/WHO-2019-nCoV-Ethics_criteria-2020.1-eng.pdf?ua=1.

WHO R&D Blueprint. (2020). WHO Advisory Group Tasked to Consider the Feasibility, Potential Value, and Limitations of Establishing a Closely Monitored Challenge Model

Experimental COVID-19 in Healthy Young Adult Volunteers as does the 7 December 2020. https://cdn.who.int/media/docs/default-source/blue-print/hcs-who-ag_meeting-report_09feb2021.pdf?sfvrsn=fb65ebff_5&download=true.

WHO Vaccine Safety Basics e-Learning Course. (2021). https://vaccine-safety-training.org/home.html.

Wilson JM, Makidon PE, Bergin IL. (2020). Chapter 31: Rat models of infectious disease. In: Mark A. Suckow, F. Claire Hankenson, Ronald P. Wilson, Patricia L. Foley. (eds.) *American College of Laboratory Animal Medicine: The Laboratory Rat* (Third Edition), Academic Press, pp. 1107–1134. https://doi.org/10.1016/B978-0-12-814338-4.00031-3.

Wolf J, Bruno S, Eichberg, M et al. (2020). Applying lessons from the Ebola vaccine experience for SARS-CoV-2 and other epidemic pathogens. *Vaccines* 5(51): https://doi.org/10.1038/s41541-020-0204-7).

Wolf JJ, Plitnick LM, Herzyk DJ. (2013). Strategies for the Nonclinical Safety Assessment of Vaccines. In: Singh M. (eds). *Novel Immune Potentiators and Delivery Technologies for Next Generation Vaccines*. Springer, Boston, MA. https://doi.org/10.1007/978-1-4614-5380-2_16.

Wong CH, Siah KW, Lo AW. (2019). Estimation of clinical trial success rates and related parameters. *Biostatistics*, 20(2): 273–286. https://doi.org/10.1093/biostatistics/kxx069.

Wyman O. (2012). Therapeutic Vaccines. Health and Life Sciences https://www.oliverwyman.com/content/dam/oliver-wyman/global/en/files/archive/2011/OW_EN_HLS_Publ_2012_Therapeutic_Vaccines_Portfolio_Decisions.pdf).

Yang XH, Deng W, Tong Z, et al. (2007). Mice transgenic for human angiotensin-converting enzyme 2 provide a model for SARS coronavirus infection. *Comp Med*, 57(5):450–459 PMID: 17974127.

Yuka I, Sasada, T. (2020). Cancer vaccines: Toward the next breakthrough in cancer immunotherapy. *Journal of Immunology Research*, 2020: 13. Article ID 5825401. https://doi.org/10.1155/2020/5825401.

24

Understanding the Nonclinical Safety Considerations for Therapeutic Oligonucleotides

Cathaline den Besten
ProQR Therapeutics BV

Scott P. Henry
Ionis Pharmaceuticals, Inc.

Arthur A. Levin
Avidity Biosciences

CONTENTS

DOI: 10.1201/9781003124542-27

24.1 Introduction

Synthetic oligonucleotide drugs (ONDs) continue to make steady progress on their journey to a mature and clinically validated therapeutic platform (Crooke et al., 2018b). The genomic revolution has rapidly increased our understanding of the genetic basis of health and disease and fueled the innovation of RNA-modulating therapies. A key advantage is the rational sequence design to their cognate RNA target, driven by highly selective complementary Watson–Crick base pairing. This avoids the need to identify compounds with complex ligand-protein binding sites, interactions that are critical to small molecule drugs. Another key advantage is the high degree of selectivity without being restricted to extracellular epitopes, as is the case for most antibody drugs. An important advantage allowing a rational drug discovery approach is that oligonucleotides of a given chemistry and design demonstrate a consistent and predictive "class" behavior in terms of drug metabolism and pharmacokinetics (DMPK) and target organs for toxicity.

The DMPK and toxicological properties of single-stranded phosphorothioate (PS) backbone ONDs and 2′MOE-modified gapmers have been comprehensively summarized (Henry et al., 2008a; Levin, 1999; Levin et al., 2001, 2008), and these reviews shaped the concept of oligonucleotide class effects. Since then, the field has progressed considerably with an expanding toolbox of chemical modifications and therapeutic OND approaches. We have increased our understanding of the molecular mechanisms critical to efficacy, distribution and toxicity, and how these are affected by OND sequence, chemical modifications and design. Moreover, preclinical and clinical safety databases covering subchronic and chronic treatments are now becoming large enough for meaningful analyses across multiple targets and sequences (Crooke et al., 2016, 2017a, 2018a; Henry et al., 2017), providing a body of data to confirm or disprove clinical translation of preclinical observations.

The current overview summarizes key DMPK and toxicological aspects of OND therapeutics and how these properties are influenced by design and chemistry, with a focus on new learnings in the last decade. In scope are OND classes acting *via* hybridization-dependent mechanisms, such as single-stranded antisense ONDs (ASOs) acting *via* RNase H degradation, splice interference or anti-microRNA mechanisms, and double-stranded ONDs directed at RNA interference (miRNA, siRNA). Out of scope are other promising oligonucleotide modalities acting *via* other mechanisms than Watson–Crick hybridization, e.g., protein-coding mRNA (Sahin et al., 2014) and aptamers (Nimjee et al., 2017; Zhou and Rossi, 2017) designed to act at the protein level rather than RNA. However, some of the principles described for hybridization-targeting ONDs may also apply to the non-hybridization ONDs.

24.2 Oligonucleotide Chemistries and Mode of Action (MOA)

24.2.1 Chemistry and Design Considerations of Therapeutic ONDs

The DMPK and safety profile of OND therapeutics are highly impacted by design and chemical modification of the oligonucleotide. Significant progress has been made to optimize these parameters for a balanced improvement of affinity, nuclease resistance, distribution, pharmacokinetics (PK), cellular uptake and safety. The design and chemistry requirements of the various oligo classes have been described in excellent recent review articles (Khvorova and Watts, 2017; Seth and Swayze, 2014; Wan and Seth, 2016). Key features are summarized below to facilitate the understanding of the complex interplay between chemical design and RNA-modulating mechanism on the one hand, and DMPK and safety properties on the other hand.

24.2.2 OND Chemistry

Chemical optimization strategies have been implemented since the late 1990s to improve drug-like properties of naturally occurring oligonucleotides. Incorporation of PS linkages in the OND backbone provided resistance against nuclease degradation, improved tissue uptake and drug retention and increased plasma protein binding resulting in reduced renal excretion (Eckstein, 2000; Freier and Altmann, 1997; Miller et al., 2016). The protein binding associated with the PS backbone is what has enabled the uptake and distribution of these modified ONDs into tissues. As an alternative to negatively charged PS backbone ASOs, phosphorodiamidate morpholinos (PMOs) and peptide nucleic acids (PNA) have neutral OND backbones with excellent nuclease resistance, but they have high renal clearance and relatively low cellular uptake due to their low degree of protein binding (Wan and Seth, 2016). To improve delivery, tissue-targeting approaches are increasingly being explored to advance this chemistry to clinical meaningful potential (Hammond et al., 2016).

A variety of modifications at the 2′ ribose position increased hybridization affinity (Egli et al., 2005; Manoharan, 1999). Commonly used 2′ ribose modifications include 2′-fluoro (2′F), 2′-O-methyl (2′OMe) and 2′-O-methoxyethyl (2′MOE) (Khvorova and Watts, 2017; Swayze and Bhat, 2007; Wan and Seth, 2016). The newer 2′-O-4′-C-bridged ribose modifications locked nucleic acid (LNA) and constrained ethyl (cEt) have been implemented in single-stranded ASOs to achieve even higher binding affinity to the RNA targets. The most common chemistries used for double-stranded RNA ONDs are 2′F and 2′OMe as well as some PS linkages for stability (Khvorova and Watts, 2017; Swayze and Bhat, 2007; Wan and Seth, 2016).

24.2.2.1 OND Design

ONDs acting *via* hybridization-dependent mechanisms are single- or double-stranded stretches of generally 12–30 nucleotides, depending on the intended mechanism. The shorter ONDs (12–16 nucleotides) generally carry higher-affinity 2′ ribose modifications such as LNA or cEt. The clinically most advanced OND classes are ASOs acting *via* RNase H (Bennett et al., 2017; Crooke, 2017) or splice-modifying (Disterer et al., 2014; Havens and Hastings, 2016; Rigo et al., 2014b) mechanisms, and siRNAs acting *via* mechanism(s) dependent on the RNA-induced silencing complex (RISC) (Bobbin and Rossi, 2016; Titze-de-Almeida et al., 2017). Although nucleobase sequence is absolutely key for hybridization specificity, the chemistry and design determine most other properties (Figure 24.1). The degrees of freedom of OND chemistry

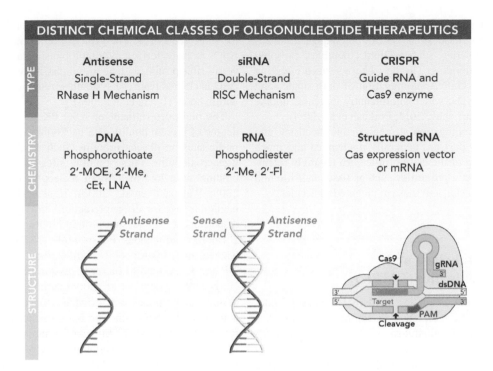

FIGURE 24.1 Common types of therapeutic oligonucleotides. There are several distinct classes of oligonucleotides which are designed to produce pharmacologic effects at the level of RNA or DNA. Antisense and siRNA oligonucleotides are designed to interact with RNA and to alter its function. CRISPR uses a guide RNA to interact with bacterial enzymes to interact with and to edit the DNA in a sequence-specific manner. Each of these classes have different structures and will employ distinct chemical modifications design to optimize hybridization affinity and nonspecific tolerability.

and design are dictated by the intended mechanism of action, with some RNA-modulating approaches being more tolerant to variations than others. Thus, for a given RNA-modulating mechanism, only certain designs and combinations of chemical modifications are accepted. For example, RNase H-mediated RNA knockdown tolerates a fully modified PS backbone, but does not tolerate neutral PMO or PNA backbones (Wan and Seth, 2016). The RNase H mechanism also requires a central stretch of DNA, allowing ribose modification only in the wings, a so-called gapmer design (Agrawal et al., 1990; Monia et al., 1993). Splice-correcting and anti-miR ASOs act *via* a steric blocking mechanism and can carry PS and ribose modifications throughout the full sequence of the OND (Sazani et al., 2008). These mechanisms allow neutral backbones such as PMO and PNA (Alter et al., 2006; Cirak et al., 2011; Sazani et al., 2002). For double-stranded ONDs acting *via* RISC, full PS modification is not tolerated and the higher-affinity LNA and cEt ribose modifications negatively affect the separation of the antisense and sense strands of a duplex (Manoharan and Rajeev, 2008).

Within each of these OND classes, the chemistry and design variations are kept relatively constant with only the nucleobase sequence being varied to match the target transcript. Some chemistry and design variations are more dominant than others, resulting in certain common properties across the OND classes. For example, the prominent polyanionic nature of PS-modified ASOs results in a relatively consistent protein binding and PK profile regardless of mechanism, although sequence-specific exceptions have been described (Hagedorn et al., 2018; Vickers and Crooke, 2016). GalNAc conjugation results in enhanced hepatocyte uptake of both single- and double-stranded ONDs regardless of whether they have a full PS

backbone or not (Nair et al., 2014; Prakash et al., 2014). On the other hand, other seemingly subtle changes such as various 2′ ribose modifications and their position in the oligo can have significant impact on a given property. This also includes the chirality of the PS linkages, which is known to impact affinity, RNase H activity and nuclease resistance (Eckstein, 2014; Koziolkiewicz et al., 1995, 1997; Levin et al., 2008; Wan et al., 2014). In recent years, more evidence has been generated on PS backbone stereochemistry also impacting efficacy and safety (Hagedorn et al., 2018). Given such variability, extrapolation of DMPK and safety properties between different oligonucleotide classes and chemistries should therefore be carried out with caution, supported by robust experimental data.

Safety findings referred to as "oligonucleotide class effects" are mainly based on findings with single-stranded PS backbone ASOs with or without 2′MOE and 2′OMe modifications (Henry et al., 2008a; Levin, 1999). Although many of these safety effects are still observed at higher doses with newer ASO classes, the combination of a better mechanistic understanding leading to improved OND chemistry, design and screening cascades has resulted in successful mitigation of many of these "oligonucleotide class effects" for more recent clinical candidates.

24.2.3 Delivery Approaches

Complex formulation strategies, such as lipid nanoparticles (LNP), need to be applied for non-stabilized siRNA and miR mimetics to avoid rapid degradation and excretion (Czauderna et al., 2003; Gao et al., 2009; Layzer et al., 2004; Morrissey et al., 2005). Due to the uncharged backbone of PMO- and PNA-based ONDs, protein binding is low resulting in low tissue distribution and rapid excretion. To improve uptake and distribution to target tissues, ONDs can be conjugated to different targeting moieties, such as lipids, peptides, carbohydrates and even antibodies. The best characterized targeting approach to date is GalNAc conjugation of both single- and double-stranded ONDs, which significantly increases uptake into hepatocytes (Nair et al., 2014; Prakash et al., 2014).

When applying conjugation strategies, the chemistry and design of the OND part are generally unchanged and much of the understanding of the class profile with regard to intrinsic potency and kinetic properties such as tissue half-life and metabolism also translates to these conjugated molecules.

24.3 Drug, Metabolism and Pharmacokinetics (DMPK)

The DMPK properties of ONDs are largely sequence independent and driven by their physicochemical characteristics as determined by the chemical design. Most of the knowledge on pharmacokinetics (PK) and toxicity of ONDs is based on a relatively limited number of chemical modifications. Overall, the concept of a consistent and predictive DMPK behavior driven by the plasma protein-binding properties of PS backbone ASOs as described 10 years ago still stands (Levin et al., 2008), but we now know that multiple additional protein interactions have a significant impact on cellular uptake and intracellular trafficking, and thereby efficacy (Crooke et al., 2017b; Juliano, 2016; Miller et al., 2018). Compared to ASOs with an anionic PS ribose backbone, ASOs with a neutral morpholino backbone have different PK and cellular uptake properties that follow from their different physicochemical characteristics. This includes primarily their weak binding affinity for proteins and as a result their rapid excretion from plasma by glomerular filtration (Iversen, 2008).

The preclinical and clinical DMPK properties of PS, 2'MOE and 2'OMe ASOs have been comprehensively described elsewhere (Geary, 2009; Levin et al., 2008). Most of this understanding is applicable also for newer, high-affinity chemistry PS backbone ASOs. The section below therefore focuses on new learnings, such as productive uptake and targeted delivery, and only briefly summarizes the established DMPK understanding to support the subsequent discussions of OND toxicity.

24.3.1 DMPK Properties of ONDs

24.3.1.1 Plasma and Tissue Pharmacokinetics

One of the main challenges to the OND platforms has been to achieve sufficient productive uptake into the target tissue (Dowdy, 2017; Juliano, 2016). In contrast to most small molecule drugs, ONDs are poorly absorbed from the GI tract (Tillman et al., 2008). More similar to antibodies and therapeutic peptides and proteins, ONDs are therefore administered *via* subcutaneous (SC) or intravenous (IV) injection to obtain clinically meaningful systemic exposures. Alternatively, they can be administered *via* local delivery to, e.g., CNS or the eyes. Bioavailability after SC injection is generally complete,

although low bioavailability has occasionally been observed for some sequences. The typical PK profile of PS backbone ASOs is characterized by a multiphasic plasma concentration versus time profile, with an initial distribution phase where the ASO is cleared from the systemic circulation by tissue uptake within hours (Levin et al., 2008).

The main determinant of ASO PK properties is the high degree of protein binding. PS backbone ASOs bind to hydrophilic sites on plasma proteins, such as albumin and alpha-2-macroglobulin. These binding sites are distinct from the binding sites, to which small molecules bind (Levin et al., 2008; Watanabe et al., 2006). Hence, ONDs demonstrate negligible risk for drug interactions through protein binding displacement. The plasma protein binding can be affected by 2' ribose modifications. For example, 2'MOE tends to reduce, whereas more hydrophobic modifications, such as 2'O-methyl, 2'F and LNA, tend to increase plasma protein binding (generally >99%) (Levin et al., 2008). Scaling exposure between animals and humans is somewhat dependent on species, but generally does not align with body surface area scaling used for small molecules. The kinetics for monkeys, the most representative species, scale to humans directly on the basis of body weight dosing (Yu et al., 2014). Mice are the common rodent species for ASOs, and their plasma kinetics are 5- to 8-fold lower than humans on clearance or plasma AUC (Yu et al., 2014). The best practice is to use plasma AUC when available to scale between species, but these allometric relationships are generally applicable for use in early development.

Because of relatively less PS linkages in the backbone, siRNA shows less plasma protein binding than single-stranded PS ASOs resulting in higher renal clearance and lower tissue exposure (Gao et al., 2009). Non-formulated, chemically unmodified siRNA is cleared within 1–2 minutes from plasma of mice dosed intravenously (Gao et al., 2009; Morrissey et al., 2005). In addition, unmodified siRNA was rapidly degraded in human plasma (Layzer et al., 2004) or calf serum (Czauderna et al., 2003), indicating that the rapid clearance of unmodified siRNA may be the result of both kidney clearance and nuclease degradation. Modification of the siRNA with 2'O-methyl or phosphorothioate linkages can help to stabilize the duplex against metabolic degradation, but the siRNA are still readily excreted in urine following systemic administration. For this reason, siRNA needs to be either formulated in a cationic lipid nanoparticle or conjugated to a ligand, such as GalNAc, to further increase plasma half-life (Gao et al., 2009) and achieve significant tissue uptake and pharmacology. Chemical modifications like 2'F, 2'OMe, some PS linkages and cholesterol conjugation increase plasma stability and tissue exposure of non-formulated siRNA (Foster et al., 2018; Gao et al., 2009; Layzer et al., 2004; Morrissey et al., 2005; Nair et al., 2017; Thompson et al., 2012).

Pharmacokinetics of uncharged PMOs reflect their different physicochemical properties, resulting in low protein binding and rapid clearance from plasma. Their plasma concentration versus time profile for unformulated siRNA is therefore primarily dependent on glomerular filtration, rather than on tissue distribution and may be more variable with sequence than a PS ASO (Iversen, 2008).

24.3.1.2 Tissue Distribution

Due to their molecular size and charge, formulated and non-formulated ONDs are primarily taken up by phagocytically active cells or tissues with fenestrated endothelium (Juliano, 2016). The PS ASOs have the broadest tissue distribution profile because of the high degree of binding to plasma proteins, which keeps them in circulation and binding to cell surface proteins, and this facilitates cellular uptake (Levin et al., 2008). The highest concentrations are found in the kidney and liver (Butler et al., 1997; Geary, 2009; Levin et al., 2008). To a lesser extent, ASOs are also taken up in other organs such as spleen, lymph nodes, adipocytes, bone marrow and vascular endothelial cells (Geary, 2009). There is minimal uptake of systemically administered PS ASOs into organs such as CNS and across the placenta (Geary, 2009; Henry et al., 2004a, 2004b; Hung et al., 2013; Soucy et al., 2006).

The uptake of PS backbone ONDs within a given organ is strikingly non-homogenous. Although the hepatocyte parenchymal cells show good uptake and pharmacology in the liver, sinusoidal endothelial and Kupffer cells show the highest concentration of non-conjugated ASOs (Butler et al., 1997; Hung et al., 2013). Targeting strategies are now applied successfully to increase hepatocellular uptake. In the kidney, the proximal tubular epithelial cells of the convoluted tubule show the highest uptake with very little OND in distal and collecting tubules (Butler et al., 1997; Hung et al., 2013). Despite significant research, the molecular basis for this remarkable cell specificity in uptake is still incompletely understood.

Chemically stabilized but unformulated and unconjugated[32]P-labelled siRNA was found in several tissues 30 minutes after intravenous administration. The pattern differed between type of modification but included lung, heart, kidney, spleen and liver. No intact siRNA was found after 24 hours after administration (Gao et al., 2009). The distribution pattern for LNP-formulated siRNA is quite similar to that observed for non-formulated ASOs. Autoradiographic detection of[3]H-labelled guide strand and MALDI-MS imaging of the cationic lipid in the LNP showed a similar distribution pattern after IV administration to mice. Highest concentrations were observed in the spleen, followed by liver, kidney and adrenals (Christensen et al., 2014; Marlowe et al., 2017).

Uncharged ONDs (such as PMO) accumulate to a much lower extent in tissue, due to their low degree of protein binding and rapid glomerular filtration. This results in the kidney having by far the highest PMO concentration (FDA, Accessed March 2018). To achieve clinically meaningful doses in other tissues, frequent intravenous administration of high doses is required, as illustrated with eteplirsen, an FDA-approved therapy in Duchenne muscular dystrophy (DMD) patients at a weekly IV infusion of 30 mg/kg. Of note, once PMOs are taken up in cells, they have a long tissue residence time due to their nuclease-resistant backbone (Hudziak et al., 1996).

The non-homogenous tissue uptake properties for ONDs have important implications for both pharmacodynamics and safety. To have the desired pharmacodynamic effect, the drug needs to have access to the target cell type. For safety assessment, one needs to be aware of the cells in tissues that possess the highest concentrations of drug.

24.3.1.3 Metabolism

ONDs are degraded by endo- and exonucleases that are ubiquitously present in plasma and tissues. Both single-stranded and double-stranded therapeutics are often chemically modified to reduce degradation. Replacing phosphodiester (PO) with PS linkages in the ASO backbone significantly reduces nuclease activity, and most 2′ ribose modifications confer additional nuclease resistance. ASOs acting *via* a RNase H mechanism require a design with a central DNA "gap", and therefore, 2′ ribose modifications are only present on 3′ and 5′-terminal residues. Such chemical modifications blunted exonuclease metabolism but allow cleavage in the deoxy gap region by endonucleases. This is followed by exonuclease degradation of the unprotected ends (Baek et al., 2010).

The neutral PMO backbone resists nuclease-mediated degradation and is excreted unchanged (Iversen, 2008). The ultimate fate of an internalized PMO has not been established.

The stereochemistry of PS backbone linkages has a major impact on nuclease resistance, with the Sp configuration being more stable than the Rp configuration (Eckstein, 2014; Koziolkiewicz et al., 1997; Levin et al., 2008). However, the Sp isomer has lower hybridization affinity leading to reduced RNase H activity (Koziolkiewicz et al., 1995; Wan et al., 2014), and a stereo-random mixture is regarded to provide the best balance of these properties for ASO gapmers (Wan et al., 2014).

Unformulated and unmodified siRNA is rapidly degraded in plasma and tissues (Czauderna et al., 2003; Gao et al., 2009; Layzer et al., 2004; Morrissey et al., 2005); therefore, many of the siRNAs currently in clinical trials have some degree of modification at the ends to limit degradation by nucleases. For example, the introduction of PS linkages at the 5′-end of GalNAc-conjugated siRNA (Nair et al., 2014, 2017) or an increase in the proportion of the more nuclease-resistant ribose modification 2′OMe over 2′F (Foster et al., 2018) resulted in significantly improved resistance to exonuclease degradation plasma and tissues (Nair et al., 2017).

ONDs are not substrates for Phase I (Cytochrome P450) or Phase II metabolizing enzymes (glucuronyl and sulfotransferases) or drug transporters (such as PgP), nor do they inhibit or induce these enzymes that are critical for small molecule metabolism, uptake and excretion (Shemesh et al., 2017; Yu et al., 2009b, 2016b). Hence, drug–drug interaction potential of ONDs is negligible as confirmed by clinical experience to date (Geary et al., 2002, 2006; Laskin et al., 2012; Yu et al., 2009a). Dedicated studies to address metabolism or transporter interactions are typically not done to support early development. However, these studies have been done for several programs to support final registration.

24.3.1.4 Excretion

ONDs are primarily excreted *via* urine. Mass-balance studies indicate that for a typical 2′MOE gapmer, approximately 80% of the total dose is excreted into the urine after 90 days, only a few percent is found in feces and the remaining fraction can be found in the carcass (Levin et al., 2008). The renal excretion rate is inversely proportional to plasma protein binding, with lower protein binding resulting in higher degree of glomerular filtration and excretion (Dirin and Winkler, 2013; Levin et al., 2008). Plasma protein binding can be saturated at high doses in toxicity studies (particularly in mice) resulting in an increased excretion of the parent ASO in urine (Yu et al., 2007).

24.3.2 Delivery Strategies

Most therapeutic ONDs are administered *via* parenteral administration to reach adequate systemic exposures. However, reaching effective local concentrations in a broader range of tissues and cell types has been an ongoing challenge from the early days of these platforms, due to inefficient membrane passage (Dowdy, 2017; Juliano et al., 1999, 2008; Juliano, 2016; Khvorova and Watts, 2017; Wan and Seth, 2016). Moreover, unstable ONDs such as siRNA need protection against nuclease degradation to facilitate cellular uptake. Successful strategies to overcome these hurdles have been the use of local administration, advanced formulations (LNP) or conjugation for targeted delivery (e.g., GalNAc). Specific considerations for DMPK and safety are briefly discussed below.

24.3.2.1 Local Delivery

To overcome the poor uptake of oligonucleotides in some tissues, direct administration to target organs has been proven successful to obtain clinically relevant tissue levels. Local application, for example, intravitreal (Danis et al., 2001; Henry et al., 2001; Leeds et al., 1998; Solano et al., 2014), inhalation (Fey et al., 2014; Jackson et al., 2017) or CNS (Khorkova and Wahlestedt, 2017; Querbes et al., 2009; Rigo et al., 2014a), resulted in extensive local distribution and accumulation. The ease of rapidly achieving therapeutically relevant concentrations after local administration combined with slow tissue clearance provides the advantage of a low dosing frequency. The first OND approved for local administration was the fully 2'MOE-modified ASO designed to modulate splicing of the SMN2 transcript in patients with spinal muscular atrophy. This program demonstrated the ability to distribute an ASO to the cell type of interest and to exert the desired antisense effect with good duration of action. The proof of concept for local pharmacology in the eye and in CNS tissues will enable additional applications, and pulmonary delivery trials are in progress.

The low doses used in local applications combined with slow clearance to the circulation minimize systemic exposure for many local administration routes (Fey et al., 2014; Leeds et al., 1997, 1998). Side effects, if any, are therefore limited to locally administered tissues, with negligible risk of systemic toxicity. Nonetheless, local tolerability can be an issue. The nature and the mechanisms for local toxicities, however, are likely to be related to those associated with systemic administration. Specifically, the safety evaluation should focus on the potential for local inflammation, cellular activation and accumulation-related effects. Of note, systemic exposure following direct CNS application is more pronounced than with other local application routes, due to the turnover of CSF resulting in more OND leaking out of the CNS into the systemic circulation.

Clinical validation of local administration has been achieved for ocular injection (fomivirsen) and, more recently, for CNS administration (nusinersen). Fueled by the latter success, the exploration of therapeutic opportunities of ONDs in other CNS indications is currently an active area of R&D (Khorkova and Wahlestedt, 2017).

24.3.2.2 Advanced Formulation Approaches

OND designs with nuclease-resistant chemical modifications normally do not require protective formulations. However, compared to single-stranded ASOs that are highly protein bound, the physicochemical properties including lower flexibility of double-stranded siRNA make them less prone to plasma protein binding (Schmidt et al., 2017) with rapid filtering through the kidney glomerulus as a result. Thus, effective delivery of siRNA requires either receptor-mediated transport into the cell or a lipid formulation. The most common approaches in clinical practice are conjugation to GalNAc or encapsulation in LNP, often containing cationic lipids (Juliano, 2016). LNP formulations improve the potency of siRNA (Prakash et al., 2013), but need to be administered intravenously together with steroids and anti-histamines to suppress hypersensitivity immune responses elicited by the LNP (Coelho et al., 2013), and is therefore normally avoided unless required.

24.3.2.3 Targeted Delivery

Successful productive uptake into target cells is recognized as a key hurdle for full clinical optimization and maturation of ONDs. One way to overcome this is to conjugate the OND or OND carrier system to various ligands (Juliano, 2016). Early examples included conjugation to lipids, such as cholesterol and alpha-tocopherol, with improved activity in animal studies. Rather than binding to a specific receptor on the cell surface, the improved PD was attributed to the enhanced hydrophobicity which increases association with serum lipoproteins facilitating the delivery of the polar OND across the plasma membrane (Juliano, 2016; Wan and Seth, 2016).

A more specific approach is conjugation to a ligand that specifically binds to an internalizing receptor, allowing the OND to "hitchhike" into the cell. The most successful example is the conjugation of siRNA and ASO gapmers to N-acetyl galactosamine (GalNAc). This carbohydrate binds to the asialoglycoprotein receptor (ASGR), which is a high capacity, rapidly recycling cell surface receptor that is almost exclusively expressed in high density on hepatocytes (Juliano, 2016; Schwartz et al., 1980). The efficient liver targeting of GalNAc conjugates has enabled siRNA delivery to move away from complex LNP formulations in favor of simple SC injections in saline (Nair et al., 2014). This approach has also significantly reduced doses for single-stranded ASOs (Prakash et al., 2014), illustrated in a clinical study demonstrating a 30-fold potency improvement of GalNAc-conjugated compared to non-conjugated gapmers of the same sequence (Viney et al., 2016).

The chemistry and design of the OND part are generally unchanged in conjugates. After tissue uptake, most of the understanding of what affects, e.g., intrinsic potency and kinetic properties, such as tissue half-life and metabolism of the oligonucleotide moiety, also translates to conjugated molecules. The overall liver exposure is only slightly increased with GalNAc conjugates, where the biggest improvement is the larger fraction of total liver exposure that is taken up by hepatocytes versus non-parenchymal cells (Prakash et al., 2014). It is important to note that the main benefit of these targeted delivery examples is to increase delivery to the target cell, leading to significantly lower dose levels required for efficacy. This contrasts with many other targeting approaches, such as antibody-drug conjugates (ADCs), which are frequently used in oncology and mainly aim to avoid exposure of the (often cytotoxic) cargo in other tissues than the tumor (Hinrichs and Dixit, 2015). In fact, uptake of ASO gapmers is observed in other tissues such as the kidney, also when conjugated to GalNAc (Yu et al., 2016a, 2016b), most likely *via* the PS backbone-dependent mechanism(s). However, since the doses required for hepatocyte pharmacology are 10- to 30-fold lower for GalNAc conjugates, the net uptake and exposure in cells other than hepatocytes become proportionally much lower.

Interestingly, many of the early experiments that evaluate different conjugates utilized cargo that was only partially modified. When comparing fully modified siRNA conjugated to cholesterol, GalNAc or docosahexaenoic acid (DHA), Hassler and colleagues achieved significantly improved uptake and target gene knockdown in several tissues compared to partially modified siRNA cargo of the same sequence (Hassler et al., 2018). It has also been demonstrated that GalNAc binding affinity to the receptor ASGR was significantly affected by the chemistry of the conjugated ASO (Schmidt et al., 2017). Hence, not only the choice of targeting ligand, but also the chemistry of the cargo affects the overall properties of conjugated ONDs.

Targeted delivery is directed at changing the relative tissue distribution to favor productive uptake in target cells, and this could be associated with a novel pattern of toxicity when cell types are exposed to concentrations and activity at levels much higher than previously possible to achieve. Also, distribution, expression levels, capacity and even function of the internalization receptor could differ between species, and between states of health and disease. These factors may introduce more variability in uptake than previously observed for unconjugated ONDs, so careful characterization of pharmacodynamics, DMPK and toxicity behavior is warranted for each of the new targeting approaches.

24.4 Class Profile of Toxicity

Based on early experience with PS and 2′MOE ASOs, a common profile of "class toxicities" was identified, which highly correlated with the PK properties of these large, hydrophilic poly-anionic molecules (Henry et al., 2008a; Levin, 1999). Toxicities were largely considered to be independent of antisense hybridization and more related to tissue accumulation, proinflammatory mechanisms or aptameric effects (Frazier, 2015; Henry et al., 2008a). Chemical modifications modulated these toxicities to some extent, likely *via* changing the degree of protein binding (Henry et al., 2002, 2008a; Levin et al., 2001).

In the last decade, the rapidly expanding experience beyond PS and 2′MOE ASOs has provided more nuance to the concept of class toxicity. The significant efforts using sophisticated bioinformatic analytics on large safety data sets of defined sequences and chemical design have improved our mechanistic understanding (Burel et al., 2016; Hagedorn et al., 2013, 2017). We now see a more composite toxicity profile where the class fingerprint of potential target organs has not changed from earlier days, but the manifestations and underlying mechanisms causing toxicity might be different.

Apart from sporadic cases of thrombocytopenia (TCP) recently being reported (Chi et al., 2017), no other "new" toxicities or target organs of clinical relevance have been added to the list of potential liabilities that can be observed with ONDs. Thus, even with today's increased knowledge, we can still recognize a consistent pattern of potential safety liabilities related to ONDs as modality. However, some of the class toxicities are primarily observed for a given chemistry (e.g., PS backbone, 2′OMe), a specific OND mechanism (e.g., ASO gapmer or siRNA RNA degradation) or sequence (e.g., unmethylated CpG motifs).

24.5 Hybridization-Dependent Toxicities

As with any pharmaceutical modality, concerns with on-target safety (exaggerated pharmacology) and off-target interactions need to be considered. For ONDs, this translates to Watson–Crick hybridization to the target RNA and to non-target RNA species. By virtue of their RNA-modulating mechanism, ASO gapmers and siRNAs are more liable to hybridization-dependent off-target toxicities than fully 2′ ribose-modified splice-modulating ASOs.

If carefully designed and evaluated, ASOs usually provide excellent selectivity for a specific sequence within the intended target mRNA, minimizing the risk for off-target hybridization-dependent toxicities. Preclinical activities carried out to understand and manage potential hybridization-dependent on- and off-target risk should consider both parent compound and potentially active shortened metabolites sometimes observed after exonuclease metabolism of non-gapmer ASOs. These analyses should ideally start early during the discovery and screening stage, with continued awareness during the development process to de-risk for hybridization-dependent toxicities.

24.5.1 On-target Safety/Exaggerated Pharmacology

As with any drug platform, exaggerated on-target pharmacology of ONDs, by excessive or prolonged activity in the intended or non-intended organ, could potentially lead to toxicity. De-risking on-target toxicities for any drug modality starts with a thorough understanding of the biology of the pharmacological target and the patient population to identify and assess the likelihood and potential impact of potential on-target toxicities. Valuable information for this assessment includes expression levels and tissue distribution of the target RNA, phenotypes associated with known human mutations and polymorphisms, and genetically modified animal models as well as data from other compounds modulating the same target. The next steps are to confirm experimentally or refute the risks of concern, establish safety margins and, if needed, identify biomarkers for either desired pharmacology or safety concerns that can be used to monitor for the specific toxicity in preclinical and clinical studies.

For OND drugs, this on-target safety assessment can be performed using the human drug candidate if there is sufficient homology and cross-reactivity to animals but is often done using a surrogate OND that has been shown to be active in the animal species of choice, usually mice or rats. This is practical for species-specific surrogate ONDs of the same chemistry and design, since they have the same plasma kinetics, distribution and pharmacological mechanism of action as the human candidate. Importantly, any surrogate OND to be used to assess potential exaggerated on-target pharmacology should be selected with similar stringency as the human candidate to minimize the variability in "class effect"-related changes that could complicate the final interpretation.

For splice-correcting ONDs, the intended pharmacology is often patient (mutation) specific and addressing potential consequences of exaggerated pharmacology in preclinical species would not be meaningful, obviating the need for inclusion of a surrogate OND in the preclinical development program.

Risk assessment of exaggerated pharmacology of miRNA modulation is challenging. In contrast to ASO gapmers and siRNA that are intended to degrade a single transcript, miRNAs have subtle effects on the expression of several targets in multiple signaling pathways, affecting the expression of different set of genes depending on species and cell type (Jackson and Levin, 2012). Broad omics analyses with refined statistical analyses should be used to provide insight into the downstream consequences of exaggerated pharmacology of anti-miRs and miR mimics to inform on potential on-target toxicities.

24.5.2 Off-target Pharmacology

In earlier years of ASO development, the potential for off-target effects was of little concern for optimized clinical candidates. In fact, the authors are not aware of any reports on clinically meaningful off-target toxicities with optimized gapmers or splice-switching ASOs of 20–25 nucleobases in length. Off-target hybridization effects were regarded to be well managed in terms of the rational in silico design process. ONDs are designed to minimize the number of homologous sequences in non-target RNA, and it is well known that simple homology does not necessarily mean the compound will be active. Thus, the off-target activity assessment is often made on the collective information related to the informatic assessment of potential hybridization, cell expression profile, the temporal expression of the transcript and the biology of the gene. If possible homologous RNA is identified that is of concern, in vitro experiments in human cell lines can be done to compare the relative activity between the intended on-target and potential off-target activity. Moreover, and in contrast to small molecule therapeutics, the relatively few cell types being amenable to sufficient productive uptake also limit the number of organs and cell types where hybridization-dependent off-target effects can occur.

SiRNA-induced liver toxicity caused by RISC-dependent off-target activity has been described in multiple preclinical publications (Birmingham et al., 2006; Fedorov et al., 2006;

Jackson et al., 2003, 2006; Janas et al., 2018). Using different approaches, Janas and colleagues elegantly demonstrated that RISC loading and the sequence and affinity of the seed region (i.e., nucleotides 2–8) were key determinants of off-target activity causing liver toxicity (Janas et al., 2018). This could be reduced by the introduction of lower-affinity chemistry in the seed region. Other chemical modifications such as 2'OMe (Swayze and Bhat, 2007) abasic spacers in the so-called pivot region (Lee et al., 2015) or placing unnatural triazolyl nucleotide at position 1 (Suter et al., 2016) have been reported to reduce off-target effects for siRNA.

Off-target effects that lead to unintended degradation of many non-target transcripts have not been observed with splice-modulating ASOs. For these ASOs, the target site of binding in the pre-mRNA is critical for hybridization-dependent splicing interference. Splice-modulating ASOs non-specifically bound to unintended mRNAs have been shown to be removed by helicase activity of ribosomes, indicating avoidance of off-target pharmacodynamic or toxicological effect (Takyar et al., 2005).

Importantly, unintended reduction of non-target transcripts is not unique to RNA targeting therapeutics. Analysis of publicly available transcriptomics data from 315 FDA-approved small molecules and 25 ASO gapmers revealed that the median number of affected transcripts was around 60 for both modalities (Hagedorn et al., 2017).

In 2012, the Oligonucleotide Safety Working Group (OSWG) subcommittee on off-target analysis published recommendations on how to assess and manage potential hybridization-dependent off-target activities (Lindow et al., 2012). Although progress in the field has led to increased insights and understanding, and an OSWG update has been initiated, the basic steps in the risk assessment of hybridization-dependent off-target effects described in the 2012 recommendations remain valid (Lindow et al., 2012).

Several different approaches can be used for the *in silico* analysis. Character-based searches like BLAST and FASTA are relatively rapid but are less precise than more demanding search algorithms based on hybridization energy (Hagedorn et al., 2017). For ONDs such as ASO gapmers or splice-switching ASOs that (mainly) exert their activity in the nucleus, off-target sequence analysis needs to cover also introns of the unspliced pre-mRNA (Kamola et al., 2015). Defining the stringency in search criteria regarding tolerated mismatches and gaps is also critical and should ideally be informed by experience from the given OND design and chemical modifications used (Hagedorn et al., 2017). There is currently no *in silico* model that can reliably predict whether a given gapmer or siRNA sequence, with or without mismatches, will lead to RNase H- or RISC-mediated degradation or not, so experimental confirmation is important. In fact, many gapmers with perfect sequence match can be totally inactive, possibly due to inaccessibility of the target site due to protein binding or secondary structures of the transcript (Hagedorn et al., 2017). Moreover, with the high-affinity LNA or cEt modifications, minor changes in gapmer design and number or positions of modified nucleotides in the wings can have a dramatic impact on knockdown potency of both on- and off-target transcripts (Hagedorn et al., 2018).

The examples above describe some of the challenges for off-target analyses and risk assessment for RNase H-dependent gapmers and siRNA aimed at targeting one single transcript. For oligonucleotide approaches aimed at simultaneously affecting multiple transcripts such as anti-microRNA and miR mimics, the off-target detection and subsequent risk assessment become even more complex. Interestingly, when downstream effects of two anti-miRs targeting miR-122 of 8 or 15 nucleobases in length were compared using transcriptomics, there were surprisingly few differences in the number of affected transcripts, despite the anticipated lower specificity of the short "tinymer" (Obad et al., 2011).

24.6 Hybridization-Independent Toxicities

As has been reviewed many times, the majority of the OND-induced toxicities are not caused by Watson–Crick base pairing to RNA, but are instead due to accumulation, proinflammatory potential and/or protein binding (Henry et al., 2008b; Levin and Henry, 2008). Although sequence can have an impact, these toxicities are largely driven by the OND chemistry and design. Hybridization-independent effects make up a highly consistent and predictive class profile of toxicities, which has been summarized comprehensively by others (Frazier, 2015; Henry et al., 2008a; Levin, 1999). Some of the common observations are well understood in terms of mechanisms and species translatability. This includes coagulation prolongation and complement activation effects related to binding to specific proteins. Molecular mechanisms of other class effects are, however, less well understood, such as the mechanism for severe TCP. It is also possible that some target organ effects may have mechanisms that are dependent on chemical class. Such is the case with liver toxicity of gapmer ASOs in mice, which can lead to increased ALT either secondary to accumulation or proinflammatory effect (i.e., as reported for PS OND and 2'MOE ASOs), or *via* off-target mechanisms for those with higher-affinity modifications such as LNA and cEt. This underscores the need to provide more nuance to the OND class profile concept for novel OND classes with different properties.

24.6.1 Effects Related to Transient Protein Binding

24.6.1.1 Inhibition of the Coagulation Cascade

Prolongation of the clotting time is a well-characterized effect of PS ASOs (Henry et al., 1997d; Sheehan and Lan, 1998; Wallace et al., 1996) directly correlated with the PS content and extrapolating well across all species and different sequences (Advani et al., 2005; Braendli-Baiocco et al., 2017; Chen et al., 2000; Henry et al., 1997d, 2008a). The effect results from transient binding and inhibition of the intrinsic tenase complex, a key activator of the intrinsic coagulation cascade, resulting in prolongation of the coagulation time of the intrinsic pathway (Sheehan and Lan, 1998; Sheehan and Phan, 2001). Prolongation of coagulation is a highly predictable, plasma C_{max}-related class toxicity (Levin et al., 2001), but has little clinical significance as it is usually not associated with increased bleeding risk or other symptoms of coagulation

disorders at clinically relevant exposure levels. It can be well managed by dosing regimens avoiding high plasma levels (e.g., SC administration or longer IV infusions instead of bolus IV), or by reducing the degree of protein binding through shorter oligonucleotide length, chemical ribose and/or backbone modifications. This effect is clearly linked to the overall PS backbone content and is therefore not observed with siRNA or ONDs with neutral backbones, e.g., morpholinos or PNA.

24.6.1.2 Complement System Activation

Another well-characterized protein-binding feature of PS ASOs is the activation of the alternative complement pathway (Henry et al., 1997c, 2008a, 2016), a complex system of proteolytic cascades contributing to innate immunity. NHPs are particularly sensitive to this effect (Henry et al., 2014b), but at high bolus IV doses, it may also be seen in other species (Braendli-Baiocco et al., 2017) or man when given as prolonged infusion (Advani et al., 2005; Kwoh, 2008; Rudin et al., 2001). Aggressive IV dose regimens in NHPs may lead to pronounced complement-related clinical symptoms and/or mortality (Henry et al., 2002), but lower dose IV infusions or SC administration is usually without acute symptoms. Complement activation is generally not seen in the clinic with SC injection at doses up to 1,000 mg/kg, even when circulating drug levels were similar to or exceeded those associated with complement activation in monkeys (Crooke et al., 2016; Shen et al., 2014). Thus, although complement activation is a dose-dependent toxicity in NHPs, it appears to have little clinical relevance (Shen et al., 2016).

The mechanism of complement activation for PS backbone ASOs is well established. They inhibit complement factor H (CFH) (Henry et al., 1997a, 2014a), an endogenous inhibitor of the alternative pathway of complement activation, resulting in a transient increase in complement split factors (Bb, C3a) at the cost of complement C3 protein. The particular sensitivity of NHP does not seem to lie in a higher binding affinity to CFH, but rather in the lower intrinsic inhibitory activity of monkey CFH compared to human CFH (Henry et al., 2014b; Shen et al., 2014). Whether binding to other complement factors, such as identified for C3 (Henry et al., 2014b), also plays a role in OND-induced complement activation and potential species differences awaits further investigations.

Decreased circulating levels of complement factors may have detrimental effects on the overall function of the complement system and its role in innate immune surveillance, including clearance of immune complexes. Chronic complement activation following repeat dosing in NHP led to increased basal levels of split products and sustained complement C3 depletion, with secondary increased inflammation, particularly in the vascular beds of organs like heart, liver and kidneys (Engelhardt et al., 2015). As a consequence, vasculitis is a commonly encountered complement-related pathology in NHP studies (Engelhardt et al., 2015). However, the clinical experience to date has not shown evidence of vascular inflammation or sustained complement activation in humans (Crooke et al., 2016), confirming that complement activation and downstream pathologies are a NHP specific concern with limited relevance to humans.

Complement activation is generally not observed with neutral backbone PMO or unformulated ONDs such as siRNA and microRNA-mimics containing only a limited number of backbone PS linkages. However, lipid-formulated ONDs can induce complement activation in several species, including humans although the pattern and likely also the mechanism are different than observed for unformulated PS backbone ASOs (Marlowe et al., 2017).

24.6.2 Immune-Mediated Effects

24.6.2.1 Proinflammatory Effects

Immune-stimulatory effects have long been a prominent feature of oligonucleotides, where responses may vary widely between species and depend on oligonucleotide design and sequence, as well as chemical modifications of the base, ribose or backbone. The immunomodulatory potential can be used deliberately to design nucleotide-based immunotherapies and vaccine adjuvants, often harboring so-called CpG motifs (Holtick et al., 2011; Jackson et al., 2017; Krieg, 2006; Vollmer and Krieg, 2009), but in most other cases, these effects are unwanted.

24.6.2.2 Manifestations of Immune Stimulation

The manifestations of immune stimulation by DNA- and RNA-based ONDs have been described in detail elsewhere (Bridge et al., 2003; Frazier, 2015; Henry et al., 2008a; Hornung et al., 2005; Judge et al., 2005, 2006; Kariko et al., 2004a, 2004b; Krieg, 2000, 2002; Monteith and Levin, 1999; Paz et al., 2017; Robbins et al., 2009). Rodents are particularly sensitive to the immunostimulatory effects of ONDs, with a typical Th-1 like response illustrated by a dose-dependent lymphoid hyperplasia and enlargement of spleen and lymph nodes. Lymphohistiocytic cell infiltration is often seen in multiple tissues, and when it occurs in liver, it is sometimes associated with mild to moderate elevations in liver enzymes. Variable increases can be detected in cytokines (e.g., IL-1, IL-6, IL10, IL-12, IFNγ) and/or chemokines (particularly MCP-1), as well as increased serum immunoglobulin levels related to polyclonal B-cell stimulation (Frazier, 2015; Monteith and Levin, 1999). Upon chronic exposure (generally >3 months), unresolved inflammatory processes associated with those ASOs with stronger inflammatory effects may become associated with cell degeneration and ultimately fibrosis in affected tissues. A rather extreme example is the irreversible glomerulonephritis in mice, reported for some ONDs (Frazier, 2015). However, for 2′MOE ASOs designed to minimize the inflammatory effects, there is typically no progression of the inflammation to degenerative or fibrotic changes (Zanardi et al., 2018). Compared to rodents, inflammatory responses in NHP (Henry et al., 1997b, 2008a; Monteith et al., 1998), minipig (Braendli-Baiocco et al., 2017) and man are usually milder and less pronounced. However, prominent inflammatory responses including vasculitis have occasionally been seen in NHP (EMA, Accessed March 2018b; Engelhardt et al., 2015; Frazier, 2015), particularly with sequences that also show pronounced complement activation. The underlying mechanisms for the rodent sensitivity are not fully understood, but are thought to include differences in expression patterns of pattern recognition receptors (PRRs) of the innate immune system, ligand specificity and signaling pathways (Barchet et al., 2008; Jurk et al., 2006).

Although PS DNA ONDs, and to a lesser extent 2′MOE gapmers or non-gapmer ASOs at high doses, have been associated with injection site reactions and systemic flu-like symptoms of fever, chills and fatigue (Kwoh, 2008; Mustonen et al., 2017), other proinflammatory effects observed in rodents are not prominent in man. Tolerability was improved when administration regimens were adapted to avoid high circulating drug levels (Kwoh, 2008) or by lower clinical doses of more potent ONDs. Stricter screening criteria to minimize the inflammatory effects have also contributed to improve the overall tolerability (Monia et al., 2008). Local injection site reactions following SC administration have been described as erythema, induration, itching, pain, and sometimes ulceration or necrosis (Kwoh, 2008; Mustonen et al., 2017; van Meer et al., 2016). These local responses were dose limiting with early candidates (PS backbone DNA), but better tolerated with the 2′MOE gapmers. However, more recent reports on long-term clinical experience with a 2′OMe-modified ASO (drisapersen) revealed how the initial mild responses of erythema and hyperpigmentation developed with chronic dosing into a severe presentation including sclerosis and lipoatrophy, with the appearance of sclerodermic scars or morphea-like skin changes that were poorly reversible (Goemans et al., 2016; Nguyen et al., 2016). The pathophysiology underlying these local skin reactions likely involves the high local concentration of the proinflammatory OND (EMA, Accessed March 2018b; Kwoh, 2008).

ONDs administered in lipid formulations have been shown to induce inflammatory responses. Humans seem to be more sensitive to these effects than both rodents and NHP (Marlowe et al., 2017). TKM-080301 is an LNP-formulated siRNA that triggered flu-like infusion-related reactions, which were associated with cytokine increases and dyspnea at the top dose (Ramanathan et al., 2014). Despite pretreatment with anti-inflammatory steroids and anti-histamine, intravenous administration of the LNP-formulated siRNAs patisiran and ALN-VSP triggered some cases of infusion-related reactions in clinical studies, including erythema, tachycardia and breathing difficulties and activation of complement. This was associated with cytokine increases (Suhr et al., 2015; Tabernero et al., 2013).

24.6.2.3 Mitigating Proinflammatory Effects

Chemical modifications can modify the immune-stimulatory potential of ONDs of a given sequence. PS modification of the backbone has long been known to increase the immune-stimulatory properties of ONDs (Jeske et al., 2013; Liang et al., 1996; Zhao et al., 1996), but some PO backbone ONDs have been reported to be more inflammatory than the same sequence on a PS backbone (Jeske et al., 2013; Jurk et al., 2011; Tluk et al., 2009). The neutral backbone in PMOs does not evoke an immune response, which contributes to their good tolerability (Iversen, 2008). Methylation and other posttranscriptional modifications are more abundant in mammalian DNA and RNA than in pathogenic nucleic acids and help the immune system to distinguish between self and non-self (Kariko et al., 2005; Krieg et al., 1995). 5′-Methylation of cytosine is frequently used to suppress the immune-stimulatory effect of CpG DNA sequences (Henry et al., 2000; Krieg, 2002). 2′OMe modification of ssRNA or siRNA sequences inhibit immune stimulation *via* suppressing recognition by TLR7 or TLR8 (Hamm et al., 2010; Robbins et al., 2007) or RIG-I (Hornung et al., 2006), whereby even single modifications can significantly reduce the cytokine upregulation of inflammatory siRNA motifs (Judge et al., 2005; Tluk et al., 2009). Other 2′ ribose modifications (2′F, 2′H, 2′MOE, LNA) have also been described to reduce proinflammatory effects (Henry et al., 2000; Sioud, 2006).

For most disease indications, unintended immunostimulation of OND sequence or delivery vehicle remains a liability that warrants a careful design strategy and screening process. The increased awareness and understanding of immune-stimulatory sequence motifs and immunosuppressive chemical modifications have helped the design of safer ASO and siRNA sequences. Moreover, the increased pharmacological potency leading to lower doses and injection volumes has significantly reduced the proinflammatory risk. Nevertheless, dedicated screening remains warranted, and in early drug development, this is often done *in vitro* using human-derived cells or whole blood (Coch et al., 2013).

24.6.2.4 Immunogenicity – Antidrug Antibodies (ADAs)

PS backbone ONDs were long considered to be devoid of antigenic properties based on the available literature that DNA/RNA are poor antigens and the difficulty to generate an acute antibody response without using the stimulatory carrier protein keyhole limpet hemocyanin. However, the growing clinical experience with PS ONDs has revealed that antidrug antibodies (ADAs) can be detected in NHPs and patients upon longer-term dosing. Primary publications in this area are still pending, but unpublished data show that ADAs emerge with a relatively late onset, between 3 and 6 months of repeated administration (Yu et al., 2020). ADAs have been reported in 65% of the patients receiving mipomersen (EMA, Accessed March 2018a) and 30% of the patients receiving drisapersen, generally with low median titers (EMA, Accessed March 2018b). The occurrence of ADAs correlated with significantly higher drug trough levels in plasma, indicating ADA-induced increase in plasma half-life of the ASOs. However, there is no indication of adversely affected pharmacokinetic (C_{max}, AUC or tissue concentration), efficacy or safety outcomes in ADA-positive patients. These antibodies are generally directed against the chemically modified portions such as PS backbone or 2′ ribose modifications (Henry, Unpublished data) and generally do not react with dsDNA alleviating concerns for an increased autoimmune potential. Since animal studies are poorly predictive for the potential to develop ADAs in humans, this risk should be characterized in patients when ONDs are progressing to larger-scale clinical testing. The mechanism for the ADA response is not clear but is likely associated with the proinflammatory properties described above. With the trend toward lower (systemic) doses and exposures, and infrequent administration regimens, the risk to induce ADAs is expected to be reduced.

Many lipid formulations contain conjugates of polyethylene glycol (PEG). The development of anti-PEG antibodies is fairly common but has not been reported to constitute a safety concern in the context of lipid-formulated ONDs (Marlowe et al., 2017). The summary basis of approval for patisiran does indicate an ADA response to the LNP occurred in rat, resulting in increased drug clearance by 6 months of treatment.

24.6.2.5 Thrombocytopenia

TCP is a common side effect of many pharmaceuticals (Aster and Bougie, 2007; Visentin and Liu, 2007) and has also been observed with PS ONDs. Dose-dependent reductions in platelet counts have been reported in mice and NHP following repeated dosing of PS ASOs, but it is not clear whether the mechanism is the same between the species. In rodents, this effect is often accompanied by splenomegaly and seems to be associated with the proinflammatory effect of ASOs common in rodents.

Based on the broad nonclinical NHP and clinical human experience with PS gapmer and non-gapmer ASOs, two distinct phenotypic presentations of platelet reductions are now recognized, each with a different clinical implication. The more common phenotype presents as a mild to moderate, gradual and dose-dependent decline in platelet count, which is non-progressive upon continued treatment (Henry et al., 2017). This reproducible profile of platelet reduction normally does not fall below the lower limit of normal (150,000 platelets/μL in humans). Recent evaluations using large proprietary safety databases on 2′MOE gapmers showed that 40% of the 102 independent sequences induced mild to moderate platelet reductions in NHPs (Henry et al., 2017) vs. <20% of 16 independent sequences in clinical trials (Crooke et al., 2017a), indicating sequence dependency of the effect. Since PLT counts generally remain within the normal range and do not further decline with longer treatment duration and are not associated with any evidence of clotting impairment or increased bleeding risk (Crooke et al., 2017a; Goemans et al., 2016), this mild PLT reduction is considered to be of limited safety concern.

The second phenotype is a low incidence of severe TCP. In the database of 2′MOE gapmer studies in NHP, sporadic decreases (2%–4%) to <50,000/μL were observed above a threshold dose of ≥5 mg/kg/week (Henry et al., 2017). These events increase in frequency with higher doses and are not seen with all sequences or even between studies using the same sequence and dose levels. Several observations, including recurring platelet count reductions after re-dosing of affected monkeys and responsiveness to steroids, suggest an immune-mediated mechanism. Severe TCP in NHP has also been reported for the splice-switching ASO, drisapersen (EMA, Accessed March 2018b).

Although not observed in the majority of the clinical trials of 2′MOE ASOs (Crooke et al., 2017a), this type of sporadic and severe TCP has been reported in a few studies. For example, there are cases of TCP reported for early PS DNA ASOs in oncology trials where the doses were relatively high (2–6 mg/kg/day) and patients had prior exposure to multiple chemotherapeutics (Adjei et al., 2003; Advani et al., 2005; Tolcher et al., 2011; Waters et al., 2000; Yuen and Sikic, 2000). In addition, recent experience in longer duration clinical programs has revealed incidental grade 3 or 4 TCP with three, unrelated single-stranded 2′ribose-modified PS ASOs at high SC doses ≥5 mg/kg/week SC – the two 2′MOE gapmers volanesorsen and inotersen, and the 2′OMe PS ASO drisapersen (Chi et al., 2017; EMA, Accessed March 2018b; FDA, Accessed May 2018; Goemans et al., 2016).

Subjects treated chronically with drisapersen had platelet counts generally within the normal range, but after treatment for at least 9 months, some experienced a rapid decline in platelet count over 1–2 weeks. For the 2′MOE gapmers, the time to onset of severe TCP was 3–9 months of treatment (FDA, Accessed May 2018). The decline in platelet counts to <50,000/μL is seen over the course of some weeks. When treatment is withdrawn, platelet counts recover to normal values over a similar time course (one to several weeks), although sometimes requiring supportive treatment. Clinical symptoms of clotting impairment, such as ecchymosis, bleeding gums, bruises and petechiae, were apparent when platelet counts dropped very low (generally <10,000/μL), and a single fatality due to intracranial bleeding has been reported in the inotersen program. It should be noted that the cases of severe TCP occurred in patients that received relatively high doses of ASOs (200 mg/week SC drisapersen or 300 mg/week SC of volanesorsen and inotersen), and where the disease background may have increased the sensitivity to platelet clearance. In particular, the FCS patient population treated with volanesorsen are reported to have low baseline levels of platelets and a high degree of fluctuation in platelet count (Akcea, Accessed May 2018). Of note, although TCP has occasionally been reported as a dose-limiting side effect in Phase 1/2 clinical trials with formulated siRNA (Tabernero et al., 2013), severe TCP has not appeared to be a clinical risk for this class of ONDs based on the available experience to date.

ASO-induced TCP is not associated with general bone marrow toxicity, impaired platelet production or presence of ADAs (Geary, 2017; Narayanan et al., in press). Several different mechanisms have been proposed for drug-induced TCP, both immune-mediated and non-immune-mediated, and it is possible that more than one mechanism is involved. Recent investigations have started to provide some understanding of the interaction between ASOs and platelets. Heparin-induced TCP (HIT) is caused by the induction of IgG antibodies formed to a complex of heparin binding to platelet factor 4 (PF4), with subsequent clearance of platelets. Binding to PF4 was demonstrated for unmodified DNA and RNA structures (Jaax et al., 2013) and PS ASOs without ribose modifications (Sewing et al., 2017). However, this interaction was blunted by the introduction of ribose modification (Sewing et al., 2017). Other findings contradicting a HIT-like mechanism for ASO-induced TCP include non-HIT-like *in vivo* manifestations of severe TCP in patients and monkeys, such as an apparent dose dependency, lack of thrombosis and very low platelet nadir counts. Moreover, anti-PF4 IgG antibodies were not detected in a monkey with severe TCP (Henry, 2017), but this monkey did have increased levels of anti-platelet IgG antibodies that were independent of the presence of drug (Narayanan et al., in press). Similarly, the presence of antiplatelet IgG antibodies was also confirmed in five out of the eight patients that developed severe TCP on drisapersen (EMA, Accessed March 2018b). The collective evidence points toward an immune-mediated, PF4-independent mechanism for severe TCP that involves anti-platelet IgG antibodies.

Other studies addressed the direct and indirect effects of PS backbone ONDs on platelet functionality, using an immunostimulatory tool sequence containing a CpG motif (Flierl et al., 2015), or a series of 5–11 AC-dinucleotide repeats (Sewing et al., 2017). Both studies demonstrated that PS-modified ONDs are bound to the glycoprotein VI receptor (GPVI) on the platelet surface, and activated platelets in a PS (length)- and dose-dependent manner. Similar to the PF4 binding, this effect was attenuated when ribose modifications were introduced in a gapmer design (Sewing et al., 2017), suggesting that other mechanisms than agonist-independent platelet activation are involved in the platelet decline with ribose-modified ASOs. Recent *in vitro* data show that both PS ONDs and 2′MOE gapmers lower the threshold of platelet activation of known platelet activators like ADP in a sequence-dependent manner (Italiano, 2017). Similar experiments using the fully modified 2′OMe PS ASO, drisapersen, showed little effect on platelet activation in the presence of ADP, but a reproducible sensitization was observed for ribose-modified ASOs in the presence of collagen-related peptide (CRP). This is a different PLT activator that signals through the GP-VI receptor to which PS ASOs have been shown to bind (Flierl et al., 2015). Thus, depending on sequence and chemical modification, ASOs may differentially impact platelet activation, but it remains to be established if and to what extent this contributes to platelet declines seen in the clinic.

It cannot be excluded that other, more general mechanisms contribute to the platelet reductions seen in animal species and man. A chronic, low level of inflammatory cytokines and macrophage activation could potentially contribute to the observed platelet declines through several mechanisms, including increased rate of clearance through phagocytosis. Moreover, recent data provide support for the involvement of an innate immune-mediated polyclonal IgM antibody response in the mild to moderate platelet reductions, whereas drug-independent anti-platelet IgG antibodies may contribute to the severe TCP (Chi et al., 2017; Henry, 2017; Narayanan et al., 2018). Altered pre-study baseline levels of inflammation-related cytokines like BAFF and IL-23 were observed in the FCS and TTR patient populations treated with the TCP-inducing ASOs volanesorsen and inotersen, respectively (Geary, 2017; Narayanan et al., 2020), suggesting a possible disease-related predisposition. Lastly, although no clear correlation has been observed for 2′MOE gapmers (Geary, 2017), it is not known whether complement activation in any way contributes to the observed platelet effects, particularly in monkeys, considering their high sensitivity toward ASO-induced complement activation.

In conclusion, grade 3 or 4 TCP is now recognized as a rare, but serious clinical risk of single-stranded ASOs, which requires a well-defined monitoring strategy that is informed by the dose response and safety margins. Improved mechanistic insights will contribute to the optimization and selection of safer ASO candidates and could ultimately facilitate the early identification of patients at risk. Given that the few clinical cases of severe TCP known to date were observed at relatively high doses, the improved potency of next-generation ASO candidates should translate to a reduced risk for this effect.

24.6.3 Class Effects in High Exposure Organs

As discussed in Section 24.2.2.1, ONDs within a class show consistent tissue distribution and PK characteristics across sequences with the highest OND concentrations in liver and kidney. Due to their first-order kinetics, once steady state is reached, there is no further increase in tissue concentration resulting from subsequent administrations. This understanding is important when considering potential accumulation-related toxicities.

Highly concentrated ASOs can be observed as basophilic granules in tissue sections stained with hematoxylin and eosin, in cells of high uptake like the Kupffer cells of the liver and in proximal tubular cells of the kidney and resident macrophages in many other tissues. Since these granules disappear with dosing cessation and do not lead to degenerative changes *per se*, they are regarded as non-adverse, adaptive changes.

24.6.3.1 *Liver Accumulation and Toxicity*

Although the liver can achieve high local concentrations of ONDs, hepatotoxicity observed in animals is more dependent on sequence and the sensitivity of various species than absolute concentration. Mice and rats tend to be the most sensitive species with regard to increased ALT and hepatocyte degeneration, even though tissue concentrations are lower than in monkeys. Through careful screening and selection of sequences (Monia et al., 2008), hepatotoxicity has not been a general feature of most PS and 2′OMe and 2′MOE ASOs in the clinic (Henry et al., 2008a; Kwoh, 2008), with the exception of toxicity secondary to exaggerated pharmacologic inhibition of apoB-100 as described for mipomersen (Hashemi et al., 2014). Another clinical case is the GalNAc-conjugated siRNA ALN-AAT, which was terminated after increased liver enzymes in a Phase 1 study, described to be caused by microRNA-like off-target activity.

The overall lack of hepatic toxicity in the clinic is consistent with the absence of hepatotoxicity in monkeys, where findings are usually confined to hypertrophy and basophilic granules in Kupffer cells, regarded to be non-adverse (Henry et al., 2008a). Liver toxicity in rodents has been more common, partly due to their particular sensitivity to the proinflammatory effects, with increased lymphohistiocytic cell infiltrates as a key pathology feature. This is usually associated with slow onset, mild to moderate liver enzyme elevations (<5 fold) that do not progress with chronic treatment, and single-cell necrosis, hepatocellular hypertrophy, and occasionally increased mitoses and karyomegaly, particularly in studies of longer duration (Henry et al., 2008a). Overall, monkeys are considered to better predict clinically relevant hepatotoxic liability related to tissue accumulation.

With the introduction of ASO gapmers with high-affinity 2′ ribose modifications such as LNA and cEt, a distinct and more severe type of liver toxicity has emerged that is not caused by ASO accumulation or proinflammatory effects *per se*. This type of hepatotoxicity can be observed as early as after a single or a few doses in mice (Burdick et al., 2014; Burel et al., 2016; Hagedorn et al., 2013; Seth et al., 2012; Swayze et al., 2007). Mild pathologies at low doses or early time points may be similar to those described above. However, hepatic inflammation is not common, and, if present, is more secondary to degenerative

changes (Burdick et al., 2014). In more severe cases, changes are more profound with larger areas of overt necrosis (Hagedorn et al., 2013; Swayze et al., 2007), reflected by pronounced liver enzyme elevations, morbidity and mortality. Rodent studies have proven effective in filtering out these hepatotoxic candidates before progressing into the clinic, indicated by only one known clinical example of LNA gapmer-induced liver toxicity to date (Tolcher et al., 2011), despite the increasing clinical use of LNA- and cEt-modified gapmer ASOs.

24.6.3.1.1 *GalNAc Conjugation*

The field of OND development has been transformed by the advent of conjugates that can increase uptake in specific cell types. The most advanced of these is the GalNAc conjugate that was first demonstrated for siRNA delivery to hepatocytes, but also effectively facilitated uptake of 2′MOE gapmers in this cell type. At a given dose, GalNAc conjugation significantly increases hepatocyte uptake of both single-stranded and double-stranded ONDs (Nair et al., 2014; Prakash et al., 2014). As a consequence, effective concentrations in hepatocytes are achieved without complex LNP formulations for siRNA or are reached at more than ten times lower dose of the conjugate compared to the unconjugated OND. Hence, for a given degree of hepatocyte pharmacology, much lower administered doses are required with correspondingly reduced exposure in non-hepatocyte cells. There is no evidence to date that GalNAc conjugates induce liver toxicity *per se*. Mice lacking the GalNAc receptor ASGR1 are phenotypically normal (Tozawa et al., 2001), and no adverse effects have been observed with multiple GalNAc-conjugated siRNAs and ASO gapmers in the clinic (Fitzgerald et al., 2017; Graham et al., 2017; Ray et al., 2017; Viney et al., 2016) or in preclinical toxicity studies even after administration of high doses of GalNAc oligonucleotides (Keirstead, 2015; Prakash et al., 2016).

Taken together with the low clinical doses of GalNAc-conjugated ONDs and the high capacity of this receptor system (Schwartz et al., 1980), it is unlikely that the transient utilization of the receptor for the delivery of GalNAc-conjugated ONDs will impact the physiological function(s) of ASGR. As indicated above, the greatly reduced dose of GalNAc conjugates required to achieve desired hepatocyte pharmacology leads to a significantly improved therapeutic index. However, GalNAc conjugation of hepatotoxic OND sequences will reach critical hepatocyte threshold concentrations and induce liver toxicity at lower administered doses compared to unconjugated versions of the same sequences. In a recent publication, candidate GalNAc-conjugated siRNAs were reported to have an attrition rate of about 40%, due to liver toxicity in repeat-dose screening studies in rats (Janas et al., 2018), further described below. Although most GalNAc-conjugated ONDs in clinical trials have been reported as safe, there have been a few isolated clinical examples of liver safety findings with GalNAc-conjugated siRNA (Alnylam_Press_Release, Accessed March 2018; Garber, 2016) and an anti-miR ASO (Regulus_Press_Release, Accessed March 2018).

24.6.3.1.2 *Toxic Sequence Motifs*

Important efforts have been made to better understand the sequence component and define particular sequence motifs that are associated with hepatotoxic liabilities. Applying machine learning on *in vivo* data from a large number of LNA gap-mers, two groups identified motifs comprising two or three nucleotides that correlated fairly well with the toxic potential of sequences (Burdick et al., 2014; Hagedorn et al., 2013). The position of the toxic sequence in the gapmer (gap vs. wings), the position of the LNAs in the wings and the size of the gap all impacted the toxicity profile (Burdick et al., 2014; Hagedorn et al., 2013; Swayze et al., 2007).

24.6.3.1.3 Mechanistic Hypotheses

The understanding of the mechanism involved in the high-affinity gapmer hepatotoxicity has greatly evolved in the last decade, facilitating today's screening efforts to advance safer candidates. We know that hepatotoxicity is seen in different strains of mice (Burdick et al., 2014; Hagedorn et al., 2013; Swayze et al., 2007) and in rats (Swayze et al., 2007), but there is a clear knowledge gap as to the translation to monkey or man, because these toxic candidates are usually not taken further in development. Toxicity is not caused by metabolites or impurities (Swayze et al., 2007) and appears unrelated to local concentration or knockdown of the primary target mRNA (Burel et al., 2016; Hagedorn et al., 2013; Swayze et al., 2007).

Current evidence points toward a critical contribution of RNase H in gapmer-induced hepatotoxicity. Several potential mechanistic hypotheses have been put forward, including promiscuous off-target antisense activity or aptameric mechanisms. Although sequences are carefully designed to minimize hybridization to RNA other than the target transcript, transcriptomic analysis revealed that hepatotoxic sequences are often associated with downregulation of a significantly higher number of non-target transcripts than non-hepatotoxic sequences. For example, Burel and colleagues analyzed transcriptional profile in mouse livers of several 3-10-3 LNA gapmers with varying degrees of liver toxicity (Burel et al., 2016). Although no ALT increase was observed at 24 hours post-dose for any of these sequences, transcriptomics analysis showed downregulation of up to 1,300 unique transcripts, whereas the number of downregulated transcripts for safe sequences administered at higher doses did not exceed 121 (Burel et al., 2016). Similar effects have been observed with cEt-modified gapmers. Knocking down RNase H1 dramatically reduced the toxicity of the toxic gapmers (Burel et al., 2016; Dieckmann et al., 2018; Kakiuchi-Kiyota et al., 2014), clearly indicating that this severe hepatotoxicity is RNase H-dependent.

A very similar pattern of liver toxicity caused by primary mechanism-dependent off-target activity has been described also for GalNAc-conjugated siRNA (Janas et al., 2018). Transcriptomics analysis of rat hepatocytes and rat livers demonstrated an enrichment of perfect seed region matches in the genes that are downregulated by liver toxic sequences. Janas and colleagues used multiple approaches to show the importance of RISC activity for causing the liver toxicity. Keeping sequence and chemical modifications the same, capping of the siRNA to prevent RISC-loading or blocking downstream RISC activity by administrating REVERSIR™ antagonists 24 hours before or after the siRNA abrogated liver toxicity. Further support for an off-target mechanism was demonstrated by the reduced liver toxicity when replacing the seed region of a toxic with seed region from a safe siRNA (Janas et al., 2018).

While off-target activity is one potential mechanism, a chemistry- and sequence-dependent aptameric mechanism for hepatotoxicity has also been proposed. The binding of certain sequences with high affinity to important intracellular proteins, resulting in perturbation of critical pathways, might also explain the observed toxicity (Burdick et al., 2014; Kakiuchi-Kiyota et al., 2016). More than 50 intracellular proteins have been identified to which gapmer ASOs bind, where some interactions show a clear sequence and chemistry dependence (Crooke et al., 2017b; Vickers and Crooke, 2016). For a given gapmer sequence, protein binding affinity is dependent on the 2′ ribose modification with the rank order 2′F>2′cEt>2′MOE (Crooke et al., 2017b). In a recent study using 2′F-substituted 5-10-5 gapmers in mice, hepatotoxicity was linked to binding to and degradation of Drosophila behavior human splicing proteins. Gapmers with the same sequence with MOE modifications were non-toxic, whereas LNA and cEt modifications resulted in an intermediate degree of toxicity (Shen et al., 2018). An aptameric mechanism, dependent on RNase H-dependent delocalization of paraspeckle proteins to the nucleolus with specific toxic cEt ASOs, was followed by nucleolar stress, P53 activation and apoptosis.

Taken together, the available evidence suggests that the high-affinity gapmer (LNA, cEt) liver toxicity observed with some sequences is RNase H-dependent leading to cleaved transcripts and/or protein interactions that lead to apoptosis. Identification and removal of liver toxic sequences from progression into the clinic have so far relied on rodent studies (Henry et al., 2008a; Sewing et al., 2016). Although further refinement may be needed before replacing *in vivo* studies, the emerging examples of reasonably predictive *in silico* (Burdick et al., 2014; Hagedorn et al., 2013) and *in vitro* models (Dieckmann et al., 2018; Sewing et al., 2016) indicate that alternative methods for filtering out liver toxic ASO gapmers can be established, reducing the use of animals for screening for liver toxicity. Cellular toxicity by this mechanism can also be abrogated by incorporation of a 2′-O-methyl modification at gap position #2 with minimal impairment of antisense activity.

24.6.3.2 Kidney Accumulation

High local concentrations of oligonucleotide make the kidney one of the common organs for toxicity of all OND modalities, including the charge-neutral backbone PMOs (Carver et al., 2016; Sazani et al., 2011a, 2011b). Changes at the proximal tubule are more common than in other tubular sections or in the glomeruli. Renal effects of PS backbone ASOs have been summarized in reviews (Engelhardt, 2016; Frazier, 2015; Henry et al., 2008a), and a brief overview of current knowledge is presented below.

24.6.3.2.1 Tubular Effects

The morphological and functional tubular changes in animal studies follow a predictive course, whereby initial microscopic changes of cytoplasmic basophilic granules at low doses become associated with tubular atrophy, regeneration and degeneration at high doses and tissue concentrations (Henry et al., 2008a, 2012; Monteith et al., 1999). In addition, it is not uncommon to see cytoplasmic vacuolation that is associated with the basophilic granules. These vacuoles have been shown to be lysosomal structures that likely reflect either swelling or extraction of oligonucleotide from this subcellular organelle upon fixation and staining of tissues. Functional tubular changes in monkeys are usually only seen at doses that are high multiples of the clinically relevant dose, as reported for 2′ MOE gapmers (Henry et al., 2008a, 2012). NHPs appear to predict well for the tubular toxicity risk in man, since there was no evidence of clinically significant renal dysfunction following evaluation of a large safety database on >2,400 subjects involving up to 52 weeks of treatment data from multiple clinical trials of different 2′MOE gapmer sequences (Crooke et al., 2018a).

Proteinuria was reported in most DMD patients upon chronic treatment with the splice-switching uniform PS 2′OMe ASO, drisapersen (Goemans et al., 2016). This proteinuria was mostly mild in severity, primarily affecting low-molecular-weight proteins, reversible with temporary treatment interruptions and not progressive over time or associated with other signs of renal dysfunction (Goemans et al., 2016, 2018). A similar, reversible low-molecular-weight proteinuria was observed in monkeys treated with drisapersen at and above clinically relevant doses (Den Besten, Unpublished data), confirming good monkey-to-man translation of this effect. The mechanism for this mild, reversible tubular dysfunction is not entirely clear, but could be related to transient and competitive interference with proximal tubular reabsorption of solutes including proteins from the glomerular filtrate, since both ASOs and proteins are known to be reabsorbed from the glomerular filtrate *via* scavenging receptor-mediated endocytic processes (such as the megalin–cubilin receptor). This would result in increased excretion of low-molecular-weight proteins and, to a lesser extent, albumin and is readily reversed when treatment is interrupted (Engelhardt, 2016; Goemans et al., 2016).

Of note, acute tubular dysfunction as illustrated by a dose-dependent increase in serum creatinine and increased urinary excretion of beta-2 microglobulin and KIM1 was reported in human volunteers treated with an unusually short (12-mer) 2′MOE gapmer designed to accumulate in the kidney and target the renal SGLT2 transporter. Although a direct tubular effect could not be excluded (van Meer et al., 2017), the intended pharmacology is likely to be the main contributor (Zanardi et al., 2012). In monkeys, the increased creatinine was correlated with the increased glucosuria rather than renal pathology and attributed to tubular-glomerular feedback.

For ASOs with higher-affinity modifications, a different pattern of tubular toxicity has been observed (Frazier et al., 2015), where sequence appears to be more important than tubular accumulation above a critical concentration threshold. This can be exemplified by overt kidney toxicity in mice after only 2 weeks of dosing of 3-8-3 LNA gapmers that were also toxic to the liver (Stanton et al., 2012). A clinical example of a highly sequence-dependent renal toxicity is the acute tubular necrosis after three administrations (5 mg/kg) of the LNA gapmer SPC5001 (van Poelgeest et al., 2013). There were no indications of renal changes in the pivotal mouse and monkey toxicity studies, but a retrospective high dose study in rats confirmed the tubular toxicity for this sequence (Moisan et al., 2017). Similar to the sequence-dependent liver toxicity of high-affinity gapmers, similar mechanisms of excessive

accumulation of RNase H-dependent off-target transcripts (Burel et al., 2016; Dieckmann et al., 2018) and/or aberrant protein binding (Shen et al., 2018) may be involved in the sequence-dependent renal toxicity of selected ASOs with high-affinity modifications.

24.6.3.2.2 Glomerular Effects

Glomerular lesions are not commonly observed with PS ONDs and 2′MOE gapmers and are not considered a class effect (Engelhardt, 2016; Frazier and Obert, 2018). The only reported glomerulopathies occurred in mouse and monkey toxicity studies of ≥3 months duration using uniform 2′OMe ASOs in the development for the treatment of DMD (Frazier, 2015; Frazier et al., 2014). These glomerular lesions were generally seen at or below the clinical doses and exposures, and not associated with glomerular accumulation. They were characterized by profound species differences where local inflammatory activity and mouse-specific conditions appeared to be important determinants in the progressive and irreversible murine pathology. The reversible monkey lesions indicated an underlying chronic complement activation (Frazier et al., 2014), which is known to be caused by ASOs when administered to monkeys above a certain dose threshold (Engelhardt et al., 2015; Henry et al., 2014b; Shen et al., 2016). Since glomerular pathology following OND treatment has only been observed rarely and in the context of background inflammation or complement activation, these are not considered to be related directly to the accumulation of OND in kidney (Frazier and Obert, 2018).

The use of OND in human clinical trials has generally been associated with good renal and glomerular tolerability; however, there are a couple of notable exceptions. The first was manifested as acute tubular nephropathy in a human Phase 1 trial with an LNA-modified ASO. This effect was dose-dependent and reversible and has not been observed in other LNA- or cEt-modified ASOs that are in clinical trials, suggesting this was a sequence-specific effect. Another example is the cases of glomerular nephritis observed in the Tegsedi Phase 3 study (TTR MOE ASO). This study was conducted at 300 mg/wk SC in patients with renal amyloid deposits and was associated with cases of glomerular nephritis (3% incidence) that lead to severe adverse events and discontinuation of treatment. While this has not been seen in other patient populations to date, such as diabetic patients, caution should be taken in treating patients with underlying renal disease with higher doses of OND.

24.6.4 Regulatory Considerations for Preclinical Development

The existing regulatory guidances do not directly address OND therapeutics, but the general principles do apply. Being chemically synthesized, ONDs are formally regulated as new chemical entities (NCEs) by most regulatory authorities, and their nonclinical development should therefore follow small molecule guideline recommendations (ICH M3 [R2]). This includes the assessment of repeat-dose toxicity in two species for up to 6 months in one rodent and 9 months in one non-rodent species, as well as the assessment of safety pharmacology, genotoxicity, carcinogenicity and reproductive toxicity, normally *via* the intended route of administration. However, some OND characteristics, such as their larger size, species specificity, predictive degradation pathways and selected tissue distribution, are more like that of biological therapeutics, and therefore, principles from ICH S6 should also be considered when designing a non-clinical testing strategy for ONDs. Strict application of ICH S6 is not appropriate, however. For example, rodent active surrogates can be applied much more easily in the case of OND therapeutics for the purpose of assessing the safety of pharmacologic activity (see Section 24.5.1), and there are generally no issues with regard to species-specific drug-neutralizing antibodies. This said, although rodents are generally more useful for OND safety assessment than stated in the ICH S6 guidance, the monkey is considered the preferred species.

24.7 Conclusions

During the last 10 years, the area of therapeutic ONDs has undergone a remarkable evolution and maturation that has resulted in several regulatory approvals for both single-stranded ASOs and double-stranded siRNA ONDs and a large number of ongoing clinical trials. Meanwhile, our understanding of how chemistry and sequence impact safety and DMPK properties has greatly evolved, opening up new therapeutic opportunities. The GalNAc conjugation of siRNA and ASOs is a promising showcase of a major increase in productive uptake into target cells, demonstrating that the big hurdle of delivering ONDs to target cells can be overcome. Higher-affinity ribose modifications for ASOs and enhanced designs for siRNA have led to a great reduction in the doses needed for desired PD effects in the liver and enabled siRNA to be delivered *via* SC injection in saline without the need for complex formulations. The use of more robust screening cascades has resulted in the ability to filter out unsafe candidates, leading, for example, to a significantly reduced incidence and severity of SC injection site reactions and other proinflammatory responses in clinical trials. Neutral backbone PMOs appear to have an advantage over PS backbone ONDs in terms of tolerability, but the true assessment of safety of this class needs confirmation once next-generation PMOs achieve higher tissue concentrations.

Compared to earlier OND generations, today's high-affinity OND designs that significantly increase potency are also more prone to sequence-dependent liver and kidney toxicity, due to increased RNase H- and RISC-dependent degradation of off-target transcripts. This may become increasingly relevant also for other organs, when higher uptake in other tissues is achieved. The broader clinical experience with higher patient numbers and longer duration of treatment for multiple clinical candidates has revealed a sporadic, serious side effect of severe TCP for three PS ASOs to date, but the improved potency of next-generation ASO candidates is expected to reduce this risk in future programs.

In the coming decade, further elucidation of OND delivery mechanisms will broaden the therapeutic opportunities of ONDs. The success of GalNAc conjugation has paved the way for the development of novel targeting approaches that will increase productive uptake in cell types other than

hepatocytes, expanding the range of tissues amenable to therapeutic OND approaches. This will require new PK/PD relationships to be established and may unfold novel safety issues in tissues previously not in focus for OND studies due to low uptake. The coming decade will also witness a much deeper understanding of the mechanisms behind the sequence-dependent OND toxicities with a significant improvement of predictive *in silico* and *in vitro* models to filter out toxic sequences at an early stage. The growing databases containing both clinical and preclinical safety information will provide critical information about the translational value between preclinical and clinical observations. Taken together, this will further improve the efficient and rational design process to identify potent and safe OND clinical candidate compounds. This will be a necessary step for ONDs to be the first platform that is truly adapted for the exciting era of personalized medicine.

REFERENCES

Adjei, A.A., Dy, G.K., Erlichman, C., Reid, J.M., Sloan, J.A., Pitot, H.C., Alberts, S.R., Goldberg, R.M., Hanson, L.J., Atherton, P.J. (2003). A phase I trial of ISIS 2503, an antisense inhibitor of H-ras, in combination with gemcitabine in patients with advanced cancer. *Clin Cancer Res 9*, 115–123.

Advani, R., Lum, B.L., Fisher, G.A., Halsey, J., Geary, R.S., Holmlund, J.T., Kwoh, T.J., Dorr, F.A., and Sikic, B.I. (2005). A phase I trial of aprinocarsen (ISIS 3521/LY900003), an antisense inhibitor of protein kinase C-alpha administered as a 24-hour weekly infusion schedule in patients with advanced cancer. *Invest New Drugs 23*, 467–477.

Agrawal, S., Mayrand, S.H., Zamecnik, P.C., and Pederson, T. (1990). Site-specific excision from RNA by RNase H and mixed-phosphate-backbone oligodeoxynucleotides. *Proc Natl Acad Sci U S A 87*, 1401–1405.

Akcea (Accessed May 2018). https://www.ema.europa.eu/en/documents/overview/waylivra-epar-medicine-overview_en.pdf

Alter, J., Lou, F., Rabinowitz, A., Yin, H., Rosenfeld, J., Wilton, S.D., Partridge, T.A., and Lu, Q.L. (2006). Systemic delivery of morpholino oligonucleotide restores dystrophin expression bodywide and improves dystrophic pathology. *Nat Med 12*, 175–177.

Aster, R.H., and Bougie, D.W. (2007). Drug-induced immune thrombocytopenia. *N Engl J Med 357*, 580–587.

Baek, M.S., Yu, R.Z., Gaus, H., Grundy, J.S., and Geary, R.S. (2010). In vitro metabolic stabilities and metabolism of 2′-O-(methoxyethyl) partially modified phosphorothioate antisense oligonucleotides in preincubated rat or human whole liver homogenates. *Oligonucleotides 20*, 309–316.

Barchet, W., Wimmenauer, V., Schlee, M., and Hartmann, G. (2008). Accessing the therapeutic potential of immunostimulatory nucleic acids. *Curr Opin Immunol 20*, 389–395.

Bennett, C.F., Baker, B.F., Pham, N., Swayze, E., and Geary, R.S. (2017). Pharmacology of Antisense Drugs. *Annu Rev Pharmacol Toxicol 57*, 81–105.

Birmingham, A., Anderson, E.M., Reynolds, A., Ilsley-Tyree, D., Leake, D., Fedorov, Y., Baskerville, S., Maksimova, E., Robinson, K., Karpilow, J., *et al.* (2006). 3′ UTR seed matches, but not overall identity, are associated with RNAi off-targets. *Nat Methods 3*, 199–204.

Bobbin, M.L., and Rossi, J.J. (2016). RNA interference (RNAi)-based therapeutics: delivering on the promise? *Annu Rev Pharmacol Toxicol 56*, 103–122.

Braendli-Baiocco, A., Festag, M., Dumong Erichsen, K., Persson, R., Mihatsch, M.J., Fisker, N., Funk, J., Mohr, S., Constien, R., Ploix, C., *et al.* (2017). From the cover: the minipig is a suitable non-rodent model in the safety assessment of single stranded oligonucleotides. *Toxicol Sci 157*, 112–128.

Bridge, A.J., Pebernard, S., Ducraux, A., Nicoulaz, A.L., and Iggo, R. (2003). Induction of an interferon response by RNAi vectors in mammalian cells. *Nat Genet 34*, 263–264.

Burdick, A.D., Sciabola, S., Mantena, S.R., Hollingshead, B.D., Stanton, R., Warneke, J.A., Zeng, M., Martsen, E., Medvedev, A., Makarov, S.S., *et al.* (2014). Sequence motifs associated with hepatotoxicity of locked nucleic acid – modified antisense oligonucleotides. *Nucleic Acids Res 42*, 4882–4891.

Burel, S.A., Hart, C.E., Cauntay, P., Hsiao, J., Machemer, T., Katz, M., Watt, A., Bui, H.H., Younis, H., Sabripour, M., *et al.* (2016). Hepatotoxicity of high affinity gapmer antisense oligonucleotides is mediated by RNase H1 dependent promiscuous reduction of very long pre-mRNA transcripts. *Nucleic Acids Res 44*, 2093–2109.

Butler, M., Stecker, K., and Bennett, C.F. (1997). Cellular distribution of phosphorothioate oligodeoxynucleotides in normal rodent tissues. *Lab Invest 77*, 379–388.

Carver, M.P., Charleston, J.S., Shanks, C., Zhang, J., Mense, M., Sharma, A.K., Kaur, H., and Sazani, P. (2016). Toxicological characterization of exon skipping phosphorodiamidate morpholino oligomers (PMOs) in non-human primates. *J Neuromusc Dis 3*, 381–393.

Chen, H.X., Marshall, J.L., Ness, E., Martin, R.R., Dvorchik, B., Rizvi, N., Marquis, J., McKinlay, M., Dahut, W., and Hawkins, M.J. (2000). A safety and pharmacokinetic study of a mixed-backbone oligonucleotide (GEM231) targeting the type I protein kinase A by two-hour infusions in patients with refractory solid tumors. *Clin Cancer Res 6*, 1259–1266.

Chi, X., Gatti, P., and Papoian, T. (2017). Safety of antisense oligonucleotide and siRNA-based therapeutics. *Drug Discov Today 22*, 823–833.

Christensen, J., Litherland, K., Faller, T., van de Kerkhof, E., Natt, F., Hunziker, J., Boos, J., Beuvink, I., Bowman, K., Baryza, J., *et al.* (2014). Biodistribution and metabolism studies of lipid nanoparticle-formulated internally [3H]-labeled siRNA in mice. *Drug Metab Dispos 42*, 431–440.

Cirak, S., Arechavala-Gomeza, V., Guglieri, M., Feng, L., Torelli, S., Anthony, K., Abbs, S., Garralda, M.E., Bourke, J., Wells, D.J., *et al.* (2011). Exon skipping and dystrophin restoration in patients with Duchenne muscular dystrophy after systemic phosphorodiamidate morpholino oligomer treatment: an open-label, phase 2, dose-escalation study. *Lancet 378*, 595–605.

Coch, C., Luck, C., Schwickart, A., Putschli, B., Renn, M., Holler, T., Barchet, W., Hartmann, G., and Schlee, M. (2013). A human in vitro whole blood assay to predict the systemic cytokine response to therapeutic oligonucleotides including siRNA. *PLoS One 8*, e71057.

Coelho, T., Adams, D., Silva, A., Lozeron, P., Hawkins, P.N., Mant, T., Perez, J., Chiesa, J., Warrington, S., Tranter, E., *et al.* (2013). Safety and efficacy of RNAi therapy for transthyretin amyloidosis. *N Engl J Med 369*, 819–829.

Crooke, S.T. (2017). Molecular mechanisms of antisense oligonucleotides. *Nucleic Acid Ther 27*, 70–77.

Crooke, S.T., Baker, B.F., Kwoh, T.J., Cheng, W., Schulz, D.J., Xia, S., Salgado, N., Bui, H.H., Hart, C.E., Burel, S.A., *et al.* (2016). Integrated safety assessment of 2′-O-methoxyethyl chimeric antisense oligonucleotides in nonhuman primates and healthy human volunteers. *Mol Ther J Am Soc Gene Ther 24*, 1771–1782.

Crooke, S.T., Baker, B.F., Pham, N.C., Hughes, S.G., Kwoh, T.J., Cai, D., Tsimikas, S., Geary, R.S., and Bhanot, S. (2018a). The effects of 2′-O-methoxyethyl oligonucleotides on renal function in humans. *Nucleic Acid Ther 28*, 10–22.

Crooke, S.T., Baker, B.F., Witztum, J.L., Kwoh, T.J., Pham, N.C., Salgado, N., McEvoy, B.W., Cheng, W., Hughes, S.G., Bhanot, S., *et al.* (2017a). The effects of 2′-O-methoxyethyl containing antisense oligonucleotides on platelets in human clinical trials. *Nucleic Acid Ther 27*, 121–129.

Crooke, S.T., Wang, S., Vickers, T.A., Shen, W., and Liang, X.H. (2017b). Cellular uptake and trafficking of antisense oligonucleotides. *Nat Biotechnol 35*, 230–237.

Crooke, S.T., Witztum, J.L., Bennett, C.F., and Baker, B.F. (2018b). RNA-targeted therapeutics. *Cell Metab 27*, 714–739.

Czauderna, F., Fechtner, M., Dames, S., Aygun, H., Klippel, A., Pronk, G.J., Giese, K., and Kaufmann, J. (2003). Structural variations and stabilising modifications of synthetic siRNAs in mammalian cells. *Nucleic Acids Res 31*, 2705–2716.

Danis, R.P., Henry, S.P., and Ciulla, T.A. (2001). Potential therapeutic application of antisense oligonucleotides in the treatment of ocular diseases. *Expert Opin Pharmacother 2*, 277–291.

Dieckmann, A., Hagedorn, P.H., Burki, Y., Brugmann, C., Berrera, M., Ebeling, M., Singer, T., and Schuler, F. (2018). A sensitive in vitro approach to assess the hybridization-dependent toxic potential of high affinity gapmer oligonucleotides. *Mol Ther Nucleic Acids 10*, 45–54.

Dirin, M., and Winkler, J. (2013). Influence of diverse chemical modifications on the ADME characteristics and toxicology of antisense oligonucleotides. *Expert Opin Biol Ther 13*, 875–888.

Disterer, P., Kryczka, A., Liu, Y., Badi, Y.E., Wong, J.J., Owen, J.S., and Khoo, B. (2014). Development of therapeutic splice-switching oligonucleotides. *Hum Gene Ther 25*, 587–598.

Dowdy, S.F. (2017). Overcoming cellular barriers for RNA therapeutics. *Nat Biotechnol 35*, 222–229.

Eckstein, F. (2000). Phosphorothioate oligodeoxynucleotides: what is their origin and what is unique about them? *Antisense Nucleic Acid Drug Dev 10*, 117–121.

Eckstein, F. (2014). Phosphorothioates, essential components of therapeutic oligonucleotides. *Nucleic Acid Ther 24*, 374–387.

Egli, M., Minasov, G., Tereshko, V., Pallan, P.S., Teplova, M., Inamati, G.B., Lesnik, E.A., Owens, S.R., Ross, B.S., Prakash, T.P., *et al.* (2005). Probing the influence of stereoelectronic effects on the biophysical properties of oligonucleotides: comprehensive analysis of the RNA affinity, nuclease resistance, and crystal structure of ten 2′-O-ribonucleic acid modifications. *Biochemistry 44*, 9045–9057.

EMA (Accessed March 2018a). Kynamro Assessment Report. http://www.ema.europa.eu/docs/en_GB/document_library/ EPAR_-_Public_assessment_report/human/002429/ WC500144511.pdf

EMA (Accessed March 2018b). Kyndrisa Assessment Report. http://www.ema.europa.eu/docs/en_GB/document_library/Application_withdrawal_assessment_report/2016/09/WC500212619.pdf

Engelhardt, J.A. (2016). Comparative renal toxicopathology of antisense oligonucleotides. *Nucleic Acid Ther 26*, 199–209.

Engelhardt, J.A., Fant, P., Guionaud, S., Henry, S.P., Leach, M.W., Louden, C., Scicchitano, M.S., Weaver, J.L., Zabka, T.S., Frazier, K.S., *et al.* (2015). Scientific and regulatory policy committee points-to-consider paper: drug-induced vascular injury associated with nonsmall molecule therapeutics in preclinical development: part 2. Antisense oligonucleotides. *Toxicol Pathol 43*, 935–944.

FDA (Accessed March 2018). FDA PharmTox Review. https://www.accessdata.fda.gov/drugsatfda_docs/nda/2016/206488Orig1s000PharmR.pdf

FDA (Accessed May 2018). Volanesorsen FDA Briefing Document Endocrinologic and Metabolic Drugs Advisory Committee Meeting, https://www.fda.gov/downloads/Advisory Committees/CommitteesMeetingMaterials/Drugs/EndocrinologicandMetabolicDrugsAdvisoryCommittee/UCM606857.pdf

Fedorov, Y., Anderson, E.M., Birmingham, A., Reynolds, A., Karpilow, J., Robinson, K., Leake, D., Marshall, W.S., and Khvorova, A. (2006). Off-target effects by siRNA can induce toxic phenotype. *RNA 12*, 1188–1196.

Fey, R.A., Templin, M.V., McDonald, J.D., Yu, R.Z., Hutt, J.A., Gigliotti, A.P., Henry, S.P., and Reed, M.D. (2014). Local and systemic tolerability of a 2′O-methoxyethyl antisense oligonucleotide targeting interleukin-4 receptor-alpha delivery by inhalation in mouse and monkey. *Inhal Toxicol 26*, 452–463.

Fitzgerald, K., White, S., Borodovsky, A., Bettencourt, B.R., Strahs, A., Clausen, V., Wijngaard, P., Horton, J.D., Taubel, J., Brooks, A., *et al.* (2017). A Highly Durable RNAi Therapeutic Inhibitor of PCSK9. *N Engl J Med 376*, 41–51.

Flierl, U., Nero, T.L., Lim, B., Arthur, J.F., Yao, Y., Jung, S.M., Gitz, E., Pollitt, A.Y., Zaldivia, M.T., Jandrot-Perrus, M., *et al.* (2015). Phosphorothioate backbone modifications of nucleotide-based drugs are potent platelet activators. *J Exp Med 212*, 129–137.

Foster, D.J., Brown, C.R., Shaikh, S., Trapp, C., Schlegel, M.K., Qian, K., Sehgal, A., Rajeev, K.G., Jadhav, V., Manoharan, M., *et al.* (2018). Advanced siRNA designs further improve in vivo performance of GalNAc-siRNA conjugates. *Mol Ther 26*, 708–717.

Frazier, K.S. (2015). Antisense oligonucleotide therapies: the promise and the challenges from a toxicologic pathologist's perspective. *Toxicol Pathol 43*, 78–89.

Frazier, K.S., Engelhardt, J.A., Fant, P., Guionaud, S., Henry, S.P., Leach, M.W., Louden, C., Scicchitano, M.S., Weaver, J.L., Zabka, T.S., *et al.* (2015). Scientific and regulatory policy committee points-to-consider paper: drug-induced vascular injury associated with nonsmall molecule therapeutics in preclinical development: part I. Biotherapeutics. *Toxicol Pathol 43*, 915–934.

Frazier, K.S., and Obert, L.A. (2018). Drug-induced glomerulonephritis: the spectre of biotherapeutic and antisense oligonucleotide immune activation in the kidney. *Toxicol Pathol 46*, 904–917.

Frazier, K.S., Sobry, C., Derr, V., Adams, M.J., Besten, C.D., De Kimpe, S., Francis, I., Gales, T.L., Haworth, R., Maguire, S.R., *et al.* (2014). Species-specific inflammatory responses as a primary component for the development of glomerular lesions in mice and monkeys following chronic administration of a second-generation antisense oligonucleotide. *Toxicol Pathol 42*, 923–935.

Freier, S.M., and Altmann, K.H. (1997). The ups and downs of nucleic acid duplex stability: structure-stability studies on chemically-modified DNA:RNA duplexes. *Nucleic Acids Res 25*, 4429–4443.

Gao, S., Dagnaes-Hansen, F., Nielsen, E.J., Wengel, J., Besenbacher, F., Howard, K.A., and Kjems, J. (2009). The effect of chemical modification and nanoparticle formulation on stability and biodistribution of siRNA in mice. *Mol Ther 17*, 1225–1233.

Garber, K. (2016). Alnylam terminates revusiran program, stock plunges. *Nat Biotechnol 34*, 1213–1214.

Geary, R.S. (2009). Antisense oligonucleotide pharmacokinetics and metabolism. *Expert Opin Drug Metab Toxicol 5*, 381–391.

Geary, R.S. (2017). Conference Presentation (Presented in part at the DIA Oligonucleotide Conference, North Bethesda, MD October).

Geary, R.S., Bradley, J.D., Watanabe, T., Kwon, Y., Wedel, M., van Lier, J.J., and VanVliet, A.A. (2006). Lack of pharmacokinetic interaction for ISIS 113715, a 2′-O-methoxyethyl modified antisense oligonucleotide targeting protein tyrosine phosphatase 1B messenger RNA, with oral antidiabetic compounds metformin, glipizide or rosiglitazone. *Clin Pharmacokinet 45*, 789–801.

Geary, R.S., Henry, S.P., and Grillone, L.R. (2002). Fomivirsen: clinical pharmacology and potential drug interactions. *Clin Pharmacokinet 41*, 255–260.

Goemans, N., Mercuri, E., Belousova, E., Komaki, H., Dubrovsky, A., McDonald, C.M., Kraus, J.E., Lourbakos, A., Lin, Z., Campion, G., *et al.* (2018). A randomized placebo-controlled phase 3 trial of an antisense oligonucleotide, drisapersen, in Duchenne muscular dystrophy. *Neuromuscul Disord 28*, 4–15.

Goemans, N.M., Tulinius, M., van den Hauwe, M., Kroksmark, A.K., Buyse, G., Wilson, R.J., van Deutekom, J.C., de Kimpe, S.J., Lourbakos, A., and Campion, G. (2016). Long-term efficacy, safety, and pharmacokinetics of drisapersen in Duchenne muscular dystrophy: results from an open-label extension study. *PLoS One 11*, e0161955.

Graham, M.J., Lee, R.G., Brandt, T.A., Tai, L.J., Fu, W., Peralta, R., Yu, R., Hurh, E., Paz, E., McEvoy, B.W., *et al.* (2017). Cardiovascular and metabolic effects of ANGPTL3 antisense oligonucleotides. *N Engl J Med 377*, 222–232.

Hagedorn, P.H., Hansen, B.R., Koch, T., and Lindow, M. (2017). Managing the sequence-specificity of antisense oligonucleotides in drug discovery. *Nucleic Acids Res 45*, 2262–2282.

Hagedorn, P.H., Persson, R., Funder, E.D., Albaek, N., Diemer, S.L., Hansen, D.J., Moller, M.R., Papargyri, N., Christiansen, H., Hansen, B.R., *et al.* (2018). Locked nucleic acid: modality, diversity, and drug discovery. *Drug Discov Today 23*, 101–114.

Hagedorn, P.H., Yakimov, V., Ottosen, S., Kammler, S., Nielsen, N.F., Hog, A.M., Hedtjarn, M., Meldgaard, M., Moller, M.R., Orum, H., *et al.* (2013). Hepatotoxic potential of therapeutic oligonucleotides can be predicted from their sequence and modification pattern. *Nucleic Acid Ther 23*, 302–310.

Hamm, S., Latz, E., Hangel, D., Muller, T., Yu, P., Golenbock, D., Sparwasser, T., Wagner, H., and Bauer, S. (2010). Alternating 2′-O-ribose methylation is a universal approach for generating non-stimulatory siRNA by acting as TLR7 antagonist. *Immunobiology 215*, 559–569.

Hammond, S.M., Hazell, G., Shabanpoor, F., Saleh, A.F., Bowerman, M., Sleigh, J.N., Meijboom, K.E., Zhou, H., Muntoni, F., Talbot, K., *et al.* (2016). Systemic peptide-mediated oligonucleotide therapy improves long-term survival in spinal muscular atrophy. *Proc Natl Acad Sci U S A 113*, 10962–10967.

Hashemi, N., Odze, R.D., McGowan, M.P., Santos, R.D., Stroes, E.S., and Cohen, D.E. (2014). Liver histology during Mipomersen therapy for severe hypercholesterolemia. *J Clin Lipidol 8*, 606–611.

Hassler, M.R., Turanov, A.A., Alterman, J.F., Haraszti, R.A., Coles, A.H., Osborn, M.F., Echeverria, D., Nikan, M., Salomon, W.E., Roux, L., *et al.* (2018). Comparison of partially and fully chemically-modified siRNA in conjugate-mediated delivery in vivo. *Nucleic Acids Res 46*, 2185–2196.

Havens, M.A., and Hastings, M.L. (2016). Splice-switching antisense oligonucleotides as therapeutic drugs. *Nucleic Acids Res 44*, 6549–6563.

Henry, S., Giclas, P., Leeds, J., Pangburn, M., Auletta, C., Levin, A., and Kornbrust, D. (1997a). Activation of the alternative pathway of complement by a phosphorothioate oligonucleotide: potential mechanism of action. *J Pharmacol Exp Ther 281*(282):810–286.

Henry, S., Jagels, M., Hugli, T., Manalili, S., Geary, R., Giclas, P., and Levin, A. (2014a). Mechanism of alternative complement pathway dysregulation by a phosphorothioate oligonucleotide in monkey and human serum. *Nucleic Acid Ther 24*(25):326–335.

Henry, S., Stecker, K., Brooks, D., Monteith, D., Conklin, B., and Bennett, C.F. (2000). Chemically modified oligonucleotides exhibit decreased immune stimulation in mice. *J Pharmacol Exp Ther 292*, 468–479.

Henry, S.P. (2017). Conference Presentation (Presented in part at the DIA Oligonucleotide Conference, North Bethesda, MD October).

Henry, S.P., Beattie, G., Yeh, G., Chappel, A., Giclas, P., Mortari, A., Jagels, M.A., Kornbrust, D.J., and Levin, A.A. (2002). Complement activation is responsible for acute toxicities in rhesus monkeys treated with a phosphorothioate oligodeoxynucleotide. *Int Immunopharmacol 2*, 1657–1666.

Henry, S.P., Bolte, H., Auletta, C., and Kornbrust, D.J. (1997b). Evaluation of the toxicity of ISIS 2302, a phosphorothioate oligonucleotide, in a four-week study in cynomolgus monkeys. *Toxicology 120*, 145–155.

Henry, S.P., Denny, K.H., Templin, M.V., Yu, R.Z., and Levin, A.A. (2004a). Effects of an antisense oligonucleotide inhibitor of human ICAM-1 on fetal development in rabbits. *Birth Defects Res B Dev Reprod Toxicol 71*, 368–373.

Henry, S.P., Denny, K.H., Templin, M.V., Yu, R.Z., and Levin, A.A. (2004b). Effects of human and murine antisense oligonucleotide inhibitors of ICAM-1 on reproductive performance, fetal development, and post-natal development in mice. *Birth Defects Res B Dev Reprod Toxicol 71*, 359–367.

Henry, S.P., Giclas, P.C., Leeds, J., Pangburn, M., Auletta, C., Levin, A.A., and Kornbrust, D.J. (1997c). Activation of the alternative pathway of complement by a phosphorothioate oligonucleotide: potential mechanism of action. *J Pharmacol Exp Ther 281*, 810–816.

Henry, S.P., Jagels, M.A., Hugli, T.E., Manalili, S., Geary, R.S., Giclas, P.C., and Levin, A.A. (2014b). Mechanism of alternative complement pathway dysregulation by a phosphorothioate oligonucleotide in monkey and human serum. *Nucleic Acid Ther 24*, 326–335.

Henry, S.P., Johnson, M., Zanardi, T.A., Fey, R., Auyeung, D., Lappin, P.B., and Levin, A.A. (2012). Renal uptake and tolerability of a 2′-O-methoxyethyl modified antisense oligonucleotide (ISIS 113715) in monkey. *Toxicology 301*, 13–20.

Henry, S.P., Kim, T.-W., Kramer-Stickland, K., Zanardi, T.A., Fey, R.A., and Levin, A.A. (2008a). Toxicologic properties of 2′-methoxyethyl chimeric antisense inhibitors in animals and man. In *Antisense Drug Technology: Principles, Strategies and Applications*, S.T. Crooke, ed. (Carlsbad, CA: CRC Press), pp. 327–363.

Henry, S.P., Kim, T.-W., Kramer-Stickland, K., Zanardi, T.A., Fey, R.A., and Levin, A.A. (2008b). Toxicologic properties of 2′-O-methoxyethyl chimeric antisense inhibitors in animals and man. In *Antisense Drug Technology, Principles, Strategies and Applications*, S.T. Crooke, ed. (Boca Raton, FL: Taylor & Francis Group), pp. 327–364.

Henry, S.P., Miner, R.C., Drew, W.L., Fitchett, J., York-Defalco, C., Rapp, L.M., and Levin, A.A. (2001). Antiviral activity and ocular kinetics of antisense oligonucleotides designed to inhibit CMV replication. *Invest Ophthalmol Vis Sci 42*, 2646–2651.

Henry, S.P., Narayanan, P., Shen, L., Bhanot, S., Younis, H.S., and Burel, S.A. (2017). Assessment of the effects of 2′-methoxyethyl antisense oligonucleotides on platelet count in cynomolgus nonhuman primates. *Nucleic Acid Ther 27*, 197–208.

Henry, S.P., Novotny, W., Leeds, J., Auletta, C., and Kornbrust, D.J. (1997d). Inhibition of coagulation by a phosphorothioate oligonucleotide. *Antisense Nucleic Acid Drug Dev 7*, 503–510.

Henry, S.P., Seguin, R., Cavagnaro, J., Berman, C., Tepper, J., and Kornbrust, D. (2016). Considerations for the characterization and interpretation of results related to alternative complement activation in monkeys associated with oligonucleotide-based therapeutics. *Nucleic Acid Ther 26*, 210–215.

Hinrichs, M.J., and Dixit, R. (2015). Antibody drug conjugates: nonclinical safety considerations. *AAPS J 17*, 1055–1064.

Holtick, U., Scheulen, M.E., von Bergwelt-Baildon, M.S., and Weihrauch, M.R. (2011). Toll-like receptor 9 agonists as cancer therapeutics. *Expert Opin Investig Drugs 20*, 361–372.

Hornung, V., Ellegast, J., Kim, S., Brzozka, K., Jung, A., Kato, H., Poeck, H., Akira, S., Conzelmann, K.K., Schlee, M., *et al.* (2006). 5′-Triphosphate RNA is the ligand for RIG-I. *Science 314*, 994–997.

Hornung, V., Guenthner-Biller, M., Bourquin, C., Ablasser, A., Schlee, M., Uematsu, S., Noronha, A., Manoharan, M., Akira, S., de Fougerolles, A., *et al.* (2005). Sequence-specific potent induction of IFN-alpha by short interfering RNA in plasmacytoid dendritic cells through TLR7. *Nat Med 11*, 263–270.

Hudziak, R.M., Barofsky, E., Barofsky, D.F., Weller, D.L., Huang, S.B., and Weller, D.D. (1996). Resistance of morpholino phosphorodiamidate oligomers to enzymatic degradation. *Antisense Nucleic Acid Drug Dev 6*, 267–272.

Hung, G., Xiao, X., Peralta, R., Bhattacharjee, G., Murray, S., Norris, D., Guo, S., and Monia, B.P. (2013). Characterization of target mRNA reduction through in situ RNA hybridization in multiple organ systems following systemic antisense treatment in animals. *Nucleic Acid Ther 23*, 369–378.

Italiano, J.E. (2017). Conference presentation (Presented in part at the DIA Oligonucleotide Conference, North Bethesda, MD October).

Iversen, P.L. (2008). Morpholinos. In *Antisense Drug Technology: Principles, Strategies and Applications*, S.T. Crooke, ed. (Carlsbad, CA: CRC Press), pp. 565–582.

Jaax, M.E., Krauel, K., Marschall, T., Brandt, S., Gansler, J., Furll, B., Appel, B., Fischer, S., Block, S., Helm, C.A., *et al.* (2013). Complex formation with nucleic acids and aptamers alters the antigenic properties of platelet factor 4. *Blood 122*, 272–281.

Jackson, A.L., Bartz, S.R., Schelter, J., Kobayashi, S.V., Burchard, J., Mao, M., Li, B., Cavet, G., and Linsley, P.S. (2003). Expression profiling reveals off-target gene regulation by RNAi. *Nat Biotechnol 21*, 635–637.

Jackson, A.L., Burchard, J., Schelter, J., Chau, B.N., Cleary, M., Lim, L., and Linsley, P.S. (2006). Widespread siRNA "off-target" transcript silencing mediated by seed region sequence complementarity. *RNA 12*, 1179–1187.

Jackson, A.L., and Levin, A.A. (2012). Developing microRNA therapeutics: approaching the unique complexities. *Nucleic Acid Ther 22*, 213–225.

Jackson, S., Candia, A.F., Delaney, S., Floettmann, S., Wong, C., Campbell, J.D., Kell, S., Lum, J., Hessel, E.M., Traquina, P., *et al.* (2017). First-in-human study with the inhaled TLR9 oligonucleotide agonist AZD1419 results in interferon responses in the lung, and is safe and well-tolerated. *Clin Pharmacol Ther*.

Janas, M.M., Schlegel, M.K., Harbison, C.E., Yilmaz, V.O., Jiang, Y., Parmar, R., Zlatev, I., Castoreno, A., Xu, H., Shulga-Morskaya, S., *et al.* (2018). Selection of GalNAc-conjugated siRNAs with limited off-target-driven rat hepatotoxicity. *Nat Commun 9*, 723.

Jeske, S., Pries, R., and Wollenberg, B. (2013). CpG-Induced IFN-alpha production of plasmacytoid dendritic cells: time and dosage dependence and the effect of structural modifications to the CpG backbone. *Nucleic Acid Ther 23*, 118–124.

Judge, A.D., Bola, G., Lee, A.C., and MacLachlan, I. (2006). Design of noninflammatory synthetic siRNA mediating potent gene silencing in vivo. *Mol Ther 13*, 494–505.

Judge, A.D., Sood, V., Shaw, J.R., Fang, D., McClintock, K., and MacLachlan, I. (2005). Sequence-dependent stimulation of the mammalian innate immune response by synthetic siRNA. *Nat Biotechnol 23*, 457–462.

Juliano, R., Alam, M.R., Dixit, V., and Kang, H. (2008). Mechanisms and strategies for effective delivery of antisense and siRNA oligonucleotides. *Nucleic Acids Res 36*, 4158–4171.

Juliano, R.L. (2016). The delivery of therapeutic oligonucleotides. *Nucleic Acids Res 44*, 6518–6548.

Juliano, R.L., Alahari, S., Yoo, H., Kole, R., and Cho, M. (1999). Antisense pharmacodynamics: critical issues in the transport and delivery of antisense oligonucleotides. *Pharm Res 16*, 494–502.

Jurk, M., Chikh, G., Schulte, B., Kritzler, A., Richardt-Pargmann, D., Lampron, C., Luu, R., Krieg, A.M., Vicari, A.P., and Vollmer, J. (2011). Immunostimulatory potential of silencing RNAs can be mediated by a non-uridine-rich toll-like receptor 7 motif. *Nucleic Acid Ther 21*, 201–214.

Jurk, M., Kritzler, A., Schulte, B., Tluk, S., Schetter, C., Krieg, A.M., and Vollmer, J. (2006). Modulating responsiveness of human TLR7 and 8 to small molecule ligands with T-rich phosphorothiate oligodeoxynucleotides. *Eur J Immunol 36*, 1815–1826.

Kakiuchi-Kiyota, S., Koza-Taylor, P.H., Mantena, S.R., Nelms, L.F., Enayetallah, A.E., Hollingshead, B.D., Burdick, A.D., Reed, L.A., Warneke, J.A., Whiteley, L.O., *et al.* (2014). Comparison of hepatic transcription profiles of locked ribonucleic acid antisense oligonucleotides: evidence of distinct pathways contributing to non-target mediated toxicity in mice. *Toxicol Sci 138*, 234–248.

Kakiuchi-Kiyota, S., Whiteley, L.O., Ryan, A.M., and Mathialagan, N. (2016). Development of a method for profiling protein interactions with LNA-modified antisense oligonucleotides using protein microarrays. *Nucleic Acid Ther 26*, 93–101.

Kamola, P.J., Kitson, J.D., Turner, G., Maratou, K., Eriksson, S., Panjwani, A., Warnock, L.C., Douillard Guilloux, G.A., Moores, K., Koppe, E.L., *et al.* (2015). In silico and in vitro evaluation of exonic and intronic off-target effects form a critical element of therapeutic ASO gapmer optimization. *Nucleic Acids Res 43*, 8638–8650.

Kariko, K., Bhuyan, P., Capodici, J., and Weissman, D. (2004a). Small interfering RNAs mediate sequence-independent gene suppression and induce immune activation by signaling through toll-like receptor 3. *J Immunol 172*, 6545–6549.

Kariko, K., Buckstein, M., Ni, H., and Weissman, D. (2005). Suppression of RNA recognition by Toll-like receptors: the impact of nucleoside modification and the evolutionary origin of RNA. *Immunity 23*, 165–175.

Kariko, K., Ni, H., Capodici, J., Lamphier, M., and Weissman, D. (2004b). mRNA is an endogenous ligand for Toll-like receptor 3. *J Biol Chem 279*, 12542–12550.

Keirstead, N.D. (2015). Toxicity, Pathology and Safety Profiles of siRNA GalNAc Conjugates. Paper presented at: DIA/FDA Oligonucleotide-Based Therapeutic Conference.

Khorkova, O., and Wahlestedt, C. (2017). Oligonucleotide therapies for disorders of the nervous system. *Nat Biotechnol 35*, 249–263.

Khvorova, A., and Watts, J.K. (2017). The chemical evolution of oligonucleotide therapies of clinical utility. *Nat Biotechnol 35*, 238–248.

Koziolkiewicz, M., Krakowiak, A., Kwinkowski, M., Boczkowska, M., and Stec, W.J. (1995). Stereodifferentiation – the effect of P chirality of oligo (nucleoside phosphorothioates) on the activity of bacterial RNase H. *Nucleic Acids Res 23*, 5000–5005.

Koziolkiewicz, M., Wojcik, M., Kobylanska, A., Karwowski, B., Rebowska, B., Guga, P., and Stec, W.J. (1997). Stability of stereoregular oligo(nucleoside phosphorothioate)s in human plasma: diastereoselectivity of plasma 3′-exonuclease. *Antisense Nucleic Acid Drug Dev 7*, 43–48.

Krieg, A.M. (2000). DNA-based immune enhancers. *Curr Opin Drug Discov Devel 3*, 214–221.

Krieg, A.M. (2002). CpG motifs in bacterial DNA and their immune effects. *Annu Rev Immunol 20*, 709–760.

Krieg, A.M. (2006). Therapeutic potential of Toll-like receptor 9 activation. *Nat Rev Drug Discov 5*, 471–484.

Krieg, A.M., Yi, A.K., Matson, S., Waldschmidt, T.J., Bishop, G.A., Teasdale, R., Koretzky, G.A., and Klinman, D.M. (1995). CpG motifs in bacterial DNA trigger direct B-cell activation. *Nature 374*, 546–549.

Kwoh, T.J. (2008). An overview of the clinical safety experience of first-and second-generation antisense oligonucleotides. In *Antisense Drug Technology: Principles, Strategies and Applications*, S.T. Crooke, ed. (Carlsbad, CA: CRC Press), pp. 365–399.

Laskin, J.J., Nicholas, G., Lee, C., Gitlitz, B., Vincent, M., Cormier, Y., Stephenson, J., Ung, Y., Sanborn, R., Pressnail, B., *et al.* (2012). Phase I/II trial of custirsen (OGX-011), an inhibitor of clusterin, in combination with a gemcitabine and platinum regimen in patients with previously untreated advanced non-small cell lung cancer. *J Thorac Oncol 7*, 579–586.

Layzer, J.M., McCaffrey, A.P., Tanner, A.K., Huang, Z., Kay, M.A., and Sullenger, B.A. (2004). In vivo activity of nuclease-resistant siRNAs. *RNA 10*, 766–771.

Lee, H.S., Seok, H., Lee, D.H., Ham, J., Lee, W., Youm, E.M., Yoo, J.S., Lee, Y.S., Jang, E.S., and Chi, S.W. (2015). Abasic pivot substitution harnesses target specificity of RNA interference. *Nat Commun 6*, 10154.

Leeds, J.M., Henry, S.P., Bistner, S., Scherrill, S., Williams, K., and Levin, A.A. (1998). Pharmacokinetics of an antisense oligonucleotide injected intravitreally in monkeys. *Drug Metab Dispos 26*, 670–675.

Leeds, J.M., Henry, S.P., Truong, L., Zutshi, A., Levin, A.A., and Kornbrust, D. (1997). Pharmacokinetics of a potential human cytomegalovirus therapeutic, a phosphorothioate oligonucleotide, after intravitreal injection in the rabbit. *Drug Metab Dispos 25*, 921–926.

Levin, A.A. (1999). A review of the issues in the pharmacokinetics and toxicology of phosphorothioate antisense oligonucleotides. *Biochim Biophys Acta 1489*, 69–84.

Levin, A.A., Henry, S.P., Monteith, D., and Templin, V.T. (2001). Toxicity of antisense oligonucleotides. In *Antisense Drug Technology - Principles, Strategies, and Applications*, S.T. Crooke, ed. (New York, USA: Marcel Dekker, Inc.), pp. 201–267.

Levin, A.A., Yu, R.Z., and Geary, R.S. (2008). Basic principles of the pharmacokinetics of antisense oligonucleotide drugs. In *Antisense Drug Technology - Principles, Strategies, and Applications*, S.T. Crooke, ed. (Boca Raton, FL: CRC Press, Taylor and Francis group), pp. 183–215.

Levin, A.L., and Henry, S.P. (2008). Toxicology of oligonucleotide therapeutics and understanding the relevance of the toxicities. In *Preclinical Safety Evaluation of Biopharmaceuticals: A Science-Based Approach to Facilitating Clinical Trials*, J.A. Cavagnaro, ed. (Hoboken, NJ: John Wiley & Son), pp. 537–574.

Liang, H., Nishioka, Y., Reich, C.F., Pisetsky, D.S., and Lipsky, P.E. (1996). Activation of human B cells by phosphorothioate oligodeoxynucleotides. *J Clin Invest 98*, 1119–1129.

Lindow, M., Vornlocher, H.P., Riley, D., Kornbrust, D.J., Burchard, J., Whiteley, L.O., Kamens, J., Thompson, J.D., Nochur, S., Younis, H., *et al.* (2012). Assessing unintended hybridization-induced biological effects of oligonucleotides. *Nat Biotechnol 30*, 920–923.

Manoharan, M. (1999). 2′-Carbohydrate modifications in antisense oligonucleotide therapy: importance of conformation, configuration and conjugation. *Biochim Biophys Acta 1489*, 117–130.

Manoharan, M., and Rajeev, K.G. (2008). Utilizing chemistry to harness RNA interference pathways for therapeutics; chemically modified siRNAs and antagomirs. In *Antisense Drug Technology - Principles, Strategies, and Applications*, S.T. Crooke, ed. (Boca Raton, FL: CRC Press, Taylor and Francis group), pp. 437–464.

Marlowe, J.L., Akopian, V., Karmali, P., Kornbrust, D., Lockridge, J., and Semple, S. (2017). Recommendations of the oligonucleotide safety working group's formulated oligonucleotide subcommittee for the safety assessment of formulated oligonucleotide-based therapeutics. *Nucleic Acid Ther 27*, 183–196.

Miller, C.M., Donner, A.J., Blank, E.E., Egger, A.W., Kellar, B.M., Ostergaard, M.E., Seth, P.P., and Harris, E.N. (2016). Stabilin-1 and Stabilin-2 are specific receptors for the cellular internalization of phosphorothioate-modified antisense oligonucleotides (ASOs) in the liver. *Nucleic Acids Res 44*, 2782–2794.

Miller, C.M., Tanowitz, M., Donner, A.J., Prakash, T.P., Swayze, E.E., Harris, E.N., and Seth, P.P. (2018). Receptor-mediated uptake of phosphorothioate antisense oligonucleotides in different cell types of the liver. *Nucleic Acid Ther 28*, 119–127.

Moisan, A., Gubler, M., Zhang, J.D., Tessier, Y., Dumong Erichsen, K., Sewing, S., Gerard, R., Avignon, B., Huber, S., Benmansour, F., *et al.* (2017). Inhibition of EGF uptake by nephrotoxic antisense drugs in vitro and implications for preclinical safety profiling. *Mol Ther Nucl Acids 6*, 89–105.

Monia, B.P., Lesnik, E.A., Gonzalez, C., Lima, W.F., McGee, D., Guinosso, C.J., Kawasaki, A.M., Cook, P.D., and Freier, S.M. (1993). Evaluation of 2′-modified oligonucleotides containing 2′-deoxy gaps as antisense inhibitors of gene expression. *J Biol Chem 268*, 14514–14522.

Monia, B.P., Yu, R.S., Lima, W., and Siwkowski, A. (2008). Optimization of second-generation antisense drugs: going beyond generation 2.0. In *Antisense Drug Technology - Principles, Strategies, and Applications*, S.T. Crooke, ed. (Boca Raton, FL: CRC Press, Taylor and Francis group), pp. 487–506.

Monteith, D.K., Geary, R.S., Leeds, J.M., Johnston, J., Monia, B.P., and Levin, A.A. (1998). Preclinical evaluation of the effects of a novel antisense compound targeting C-raf kinase in mice and monkeys. *Toxicol Sci 46*, 365–375.

Monteith, D.K., Horner, M.J., Gillett, N.A., Butler, M., Geary, R., Burckin, T., Ushiro-Watanabe, T., and Levin, A.A. (1999). Evaluation of the renal effects of an antisense phosphorothioate oligodeoxynucleotide in monkeys. *Toxicol Pathol 27*, 307–317.

Monteith, D.K., and Levin, A.A. (1999). Synthetic oligonucleotides: the development of antisense therapeutics. *Toxicol Pathol 27*, 8–13.

Morrissey, D.V., Lockridge, J.A., Shaw, L., Blanchard, K., Jensen, K., Breen, W., Hartsough, K., Machemer, L., Radka, S., Jadhav, V., *et al.* (2005). Potent and persistent in vivo anti-HBV activity of chemically modified siRNAs. *Nat Biotechnol 23*, 1002–1007.

Mustonen, E.K., Palomaki, T., and Pasanen, M. (2017). Oligonucleotide-based pharmaceuticals: Non-clinical and clinical safety signals and non-clinical testing strategies. *Regul Toxicol Pharmacol 90*, 328–341.

Nair, J.K., Attarwala, H., Sehgal, A., Wang, Q., Aluri, K., Zhang, X., Gao, M., Liu, J., Indrakanti, R., Schofield, S., *et al.* (2017). Impact of enhanced metabolic stability on pharmacokinetics and pharmacodynamics of GalNAc-siRNA conjugates. *Nucleic Acids Res 45*, 10969–10977.

Nair, J.K., Willoughby, J.L., Chan, A., Charisse, K., Alam, M.R., Wang, Q., Hoekstra, M., Kandasamy, P., Kel'in, A.V., Milstein, S. (2014). Multivalent N-acetylgalactosamine-conjugated siRNA localizes in hepatocytes and elicits robust RNAi-mediated gene silencing. *J Am Chem Soc 136*, 16958–16961.

Narayanan, P., *et al.* (2018). Investigation into the mechanism(s) that leads to platelet decreases in cynomolgus monkeys during administration of ISIS-104838, a 2′-MOE-modified antisense oligonucleotide. *Toxicol Sci 164*, 613–626.

Narayanan, P., Curtis, B.R., Shen, L., Schneider, E., Tami, J.A., Paz, S., Burel, S.A., Tai, L.J., Machemer, T., Kwoh, T.J. and Xia, S. (2020). Underlying immune disorder may predispose some transthyretin amyloidosis subjects to inotersen-mediated thrombocytopenia. *Nucleic Acid Ther 30*(2), 94–103. doi:10.1089/nat.2019.0829..

Nguyen, A.L., Niks, E.H., van Zuuren, E.J., and van Doorn, R. (2016). Lipoatrofie ten gevolge van subcutane injecties met antisense oligonucleotiden als behandeling voor de ziekte van Duchenne. *Ned Tijdschr voor Dermatologie en Venereol 26*, 670–673.

Nimjee, S.M., White, R.R., Becker, R.C., and Sullenger, B.A. (2017). Aptamers as therapeutics. *Annu Rev Pharmacol Toxicol 57*, 61–79.

Obad, S., dos Santos, C.O., Petri, A., Heidenblad, M., Broom, O., Ruse, C., Fu, C., Lindow, M., Stenvang, J., Straarup, E.M. (2011). Silencing of microRNA families by seed-targeting tiny LNAs. *Nat Genet 43*, 371–378.

Paz, S., Hsiao, J., Cauntay, P., Soriano, A., Bai, L., Machemer, T., Xiao, X., Guo, S., Hung, G., Younis, H., *et al.* (2017). The distinct and cooperative roles of toll-like receptor 9 and receptor for advanced glycation end products in modulating in vivo inflammatory responses to select CpG and non-CpG oligonucleotides. *Nucleic Acid Ther 27*, 272–284.

Prakash, T.P., Graham, M.J., Yu, J., Carty, R., Low, A., Chappell, A., Schmidt, K., Zhao, C., Aghajan, M., Murray, H.F., *et al.* (2014). Targeted delivery of antisense oligonucleotides to hepatocytes using triantennary N-acetyl galactosamine improves potency 10-fold in mice. *Nucleic Acids Res 42*, 8796–8807.

Prakash, T.P., Lima, W.F., Murray, H.M., Elbashir, S., Cantley, W., Foster, D., Jayaraman, M., Chappell, A.E., Manoharan, M., Swayze, E.E., *et al.* (2013). Lipid nanoparticles improve activity of single-stranded siRNA and gapmer antisense oligonucleotides in animals. *ACS Chem Biol 8*, 1402–1406.

Prakash, T.P., Yu, J., Migawa, M.T., Kinberger, G.A., Wan, W.B., Ostergaard, M.E., Carty, R.L., Vasquez, G., Low, A., Chappell, A., *et al.* (2016). Comprehensive structure-activity relationship of triantennary N-acetylgalactosamine conjugated antisense oligonucleotides for targeted delivery to hepatocytes. *J Med Chem 59*, 2718–2733.

Querbes, W., Ge, P., Zhang, W., Fan, Y., Costigan, J., Charisse, K., Maier, M., Nechev, L., Manoharan, M., Kotelianski, V., *et al.* (2009). Direct CNS delivery of siRNA mediates robust silencing in oligodendrocytes. *Oligonucleotides 19*, 23–29.

Ramanathan, R.K., Hamburg, S.I., Borad, M.J., Seetharam, M., Kundranda, M.N., Lee, P., Fredlund, P., Gilbert, M., Mast, C., Semple, S.C., *et al.* (2014). Abstract LB-289: a phase I dose escalation study of TKM-080301, a RNAi therapeutic directed against PLK1, in patients with advanced solid tumors. *Cancer Res 73*, LB-289.

Ray, K.K., Landmesser, U., Leiter, L.A., Kallend, D., Dufour, R., Karakas, M., Hall, T., Troquay, R.P., Turner, T., Visseren, F.L., *et al.* (2017). Inclisiran in patients at high cardiovascular risk with elevated LDL cholesterol. *N Engl J Med 376*, 1430–1440.

Regulus_Press_Release (Accessed March 2018). Regulus Announces Pipeline Updates and Advancements. http://ir.regulusrx.com/news-releases/news-release-details/regulus-announces-pipeline-updates-and-advancements

Rigo, F., Chun, S.J., Norris, D.A., Hung, G., Lee, S., Matson, J., Fey, R.A., Gaus, H., Hua, Y., Grundy, J.S., *et al.* (2014a). Pharmacology of a central nervous system delivered 2′-O-methoxyethyl-modified survival of motor neuron splicing oligonucleotide in mice and nonhuman primates. *J Pharmacol Exp Ther 350*, 46–55.

Rigo, F., Seth, P.P., and Bennett, C.F. (2014b). Antisense oligonucleotide-based therapies for diseases caused by pre-mRNA processing defects. *Adv Exp Med Biol 825*, 303–352.

Robbins, M., Judge, A., Liang, L., McClintock, K., Yaworski, E., and MacLachlan, I. (2007). 2′-O-methyl-modified RNAs act as TLR7 antagonists. *Mol Ther J Am Soc Gene Ther 15*, 1663–1669.

Robbins, M., Judge, A., and MacLachlan, I. (2009). siRNA and innate immunity. *Oligonucleotides 19*, 89–102.

Rudin, C.M., Holmlund, J., Fleming, G.F., Mani, S., Stadler, W.M., Schumm, P., Monia, B.P., Johnston, J.F., Geary, R., Yu, R.Z., *et al.* (2001). Phase I trial of ISIS 5132, an antisense oligonucleotide inhibitor of c-raf-1, administered by 24-hour weekly infusion to patients with advanced cancer. *Clin Cancer Res 7*, 1214–1220.

Sahin, U., Kariko, K., and Tureci, O. (2014). mRNA-based therapeutics – developing a new class of drugs. *Nat Rev Drug Discov 13*, 759–780.

Sazani, P., Gemignani, F., Kang, S.H., Maier, M.A., Manoharan, M., Persmark, M., Bortner, D., and Kole, R. (2002). Systemically delivered antisense oligomers upregulate gene expression in mouse tissues. *Nat Biotechnol 20*, 1228–1233.

Sazani, P., Graziewicz, M.A., and Kole, R. (2008). Splice switching oligonucleotides as potential therapeutics. In *Antisense Drug Technology - Principles, Strategies, and Applications*, S.T. Crooke, ed. (Boca Raton, FL: CRC Press, Taylor and Francis group), pp. 89–114.

Sazani, P., Ness, K.P., Weller, D.L., Poage, D., Nelson, K., and Shrewsbury, A.S. (2011a). Chemical and mechanistic toxicology evaluation of exon skipping phosphorodiamidate morpholino oligomers in mdx mice. *Int J Toxicol 30*, 322–333.

Sazani, P., Ness, K.P., Weller, D.L., Poage, D.W., Palyada, K., and Shrewsbury, S.B. (2011b). Repeat-dose toxicology evaluation in cynomolgus monkeys of AVI-4658, a phosphorodiamidate morpholino oligomer (PMO) drug for the treatment of duchenne muscular dystrophy. *Int J Toxicol 30*, 313–321.

Schmidt, K., Prakash, T.P., Donner, A.J., Kinberger, G.A., Gaus, H.J., Low, A., Ostergaard, M.E., Bell, M., Swayze, E.E., and Seth, P.P. (2017). Characterizing the effect of GalNAc and phosphorothioate backbone on binding of antisense oligonucleotides to the asialoglycoprotein receptor. *Nucleic Acids Res 45*, 2294–2306.

Schwartz, A.L., Rup, D., and Lodish, H.F. (1980). Difficulties in the quantification of asialoglycoprotein receptors on the rat hepatocyte. *J Biol Chem 255*, 9033–9036.

Seth, P.P., Jazayeri, A., Yu, J., Allerson, C.R., Bhat, B., and Swayze, E.E. (2012). Structure activity relationships of alpha-L-LNA modified phosphorothioate gapmer antisense oligonucleotides in animals. *Mol Ther Nucleic Acids 1*, e47.

Seth, P.P., and Swayze, E.E. (2014). Unnatural nucleoside analoges for antisense therapy. In *Natural Products in Medicinal Chemistry*, S. Hanessian, ed. (Wiley-VCH Verlag), pp. 403–439.

Sewing, S., Boess, F., Moisan, A., Bertinetti-Lapatki, C., Minz, T., Hedtjaern, M., Tessier, Y., Schuler, F., Singer, T., and Roth, A.B. (2016). Establishment of a predictive in vitro assay for assessment of the hepatotoxic potential of oligonucleotide drugs. *PLoS One 11*, e0159431.

Sewing, S., Roth, A.B., Winter, M., Dieckmann, A., Bertinetti-Lapatki, C., Tessier, Y., McGinnis, C., Huber, S., Koller, E., Ploix, C., *et al.* (2017). Assessing single-stranded oligonucleotide drug-induced effects in vitro reveals key risk factors for thrombocytopenia. *PLoS One 12*, e0187574.

Sheehan, J.P., and Lan, H.C. (1998). Phosphorothioate oligonucleotides inhibit the intrinsic tenase complex. *Blood 92*, 1617–1625.

Sheehan, J.P., and Phan, T.M. (2001). Phosphorothioate oligonucleotides inhibit the intrinsic tenase complex by an allosteric mechanism. *Biochemistry 40*, 4980–4989.

Shemesh, C.S., Yu, R.Z., Warren, M.S., Liu, M., Jahic, M., Nichols, B., Post, N., Lin, S., Norris, D.A., Hurh, E., *et al.* (2017). Assessment of the drug interaction potential of unconjugated and GalNAc3-conjugated 2′-MOE-ASOs. *Mol Ther Nucl Acids 9*, 34–47.

Shen, L., Engelhardt, J.A., Hung, G., Yee, J., Kikkawa, R., Matson, J., Tayefeh, B., Machemer, T., Giclas, P.C., and Henry, S.P. (2016). Effects of repeated complement activation associated with chronic treatment of cynomolgus monkeys with 2′-O-methoxyethyl modified antisense oligonucleotide. *Nucleic Acid Ther 26*, 236–249.

Shen, L., Frazer-Abel, A., Reynolds, P.R., Giclas, P.C., Chappell, A., Pangburn, M.K., Younis, H., and Henry, S.P. (2014). Mechanistic understanding for the greater sensitivity of monkeys to antisense oligonucleotide-mediated complement activation compared with humans. *J Pharmacol Exp Ther 351*, 709–717.

Shen, W., De Hoyos, C.L., Sun, H., Vickers, T.A., Liang, X.H., and Crooke, S.T. (2018). Acute hepatotoxicity of 2′ fluoro-modified 5-10-5 gapmer phosphorothioate oligonucleotides in mice correlates with intracellular protein binding and the loss of DBHS proteins. *Nucleic Acids Res 46*, 2204–2217.

Sioud, M. (2006). Single-stranded small interfering RNA are more immunostimulatory than their double-stranded counterparts: a central role for 2′-hydroxyl uridines in immune responses. *Eur J Immunol 36*, 1222–1230.

Solano, E.C., Kornbrust, D.J., Beaudry, A., Foy, J.W., Schneider, D.J., and Thompson, J.D. (2014). Toxicological and pharmacokinetic properties of QPI-1007, a chemically modified synthetic siRNA targeting caspase 2 mRNA, following intravitreal injection. *Nucleic Acid Ther 24*, 258–266.

Soucy, N.V., Riley, J.P., Templin, M.V., Geary, R., de Peyster, A., and Levin, A.A. (2006). Maternal and fetal distribution of a phosphorothioate oligonucleotide in rats after intravenous infusion. *Birth Defects Res B Dev Reprod Toxicol 77*, 22–28.

Stanton, R., Sciabola, S., Salatto, C., Weng, Y., Moshinsky, D., Little, J., Walters, E., Kreeger, J., DiMattia, D., Chen, T., *et al.* (2012). Chemical modification study of antisense gapmers. *Nucleic Acid Ther 22*, 344–359.

Suhr, O.B., Coelho, T., Buades, J., Pouget, J., Conceicao, I., Berk, J., Schmidt, H., Waddington-Cruz, M., Campistol, J.M., Bettencourt, B.R., *et al.* (2015). Efficacy and safety of patisiran for familial amyloidotic polyneuropathy: a phase II multi-dose study. *Orphanet J Rare Dis 10*, 109.

Suter, S.R., Sheu-Gruttadauria, J., Schirle, N.T., Valenzuela, R., Ball-Jones, A.A., Onizuka, K., MacRae, I.J., and Beal, P.A. (2016). Structure-guided control of siRNA off-target effects. *J Am Chem Soc 138*, 8667–8669.

Swayze, E.E., and Bhat, B. (2007). The medicinal chemistry of oligonucleotides. In *Antisense Drug Technology - Principles, Strategies, and Applications*, S.T. Crooke, ed. (Boca Raton, FL: CRC Press, Taylor & Francis), pp. 143–182.

Swayze, E.E., Siwkowski, A.M., Wancewicz, E.V., Migawa, M.T., Wyrzykiewicz, T.K., Hung, G., Monia, B.P., and Bennett, C.F. (2007). Antisense oligonucleotides containing locked nucleic acid improve potency but cause significant hepatotoxicity in animals. *Nucleic Acids Res 35*, 687–700.

Tabernero, J., Shapiro, G.I., LoRusso, P.M., Cervantes, A., Schwartz, G.K., Weiss, G.J., Paz-Ares, L., Cho, D.C., Infante, J.R., Alsina, M., *et al.* (2013). First-in-humans trial of an RNA interference therapeutic targeting VEGF and KSP in cancer patients with liver involvement. *Cancer Discov 3*, 406–417.

Takyar, S., Hickerson, R.P., and Noller, H.F. (2005). mRNA helicase activity of the ribosome. *Cell 120*, 49–58.

Thompson, J.D., Kornbrust, D.J., Foy, J.W., Solano, E.C., Schneider, D.J., Feinstein, E., Molitoris, B.A., and Erlich, S. (2012). Toxicological and pharmacokinetic properties of chemically modified siRNAs targeting p53 RNA following intravenous administration. *Nucleic Acid Ther 22*, 255–264.

Tillman, L.G., Geary, R.S., and Hardee, G.E. (2008). Oral delivery of antisense oligonucleotides in man. *J Pharm Sci 97*, 225–236.

Titze-de-Almeida, R., David, C., and Titze-de-Almeida, S.S. (2017). The race of 10 synthetic RNAi-based drugs to the pharmaceutical market. *Pharm Res 34*, 1339–1363.

Tluk, S., Jurk, M., Forsbach, A., Weeratna, R., Samulowitz, U., Krieg, A.M., Bauer, S., and Vollmer, J. (2009). Sequences derived from self-RNA containing certain natural modifications act as suppressors of RNA-mediated inflammatory immune responses. *Int Immunol 21*, 607–619.

Tolcher, A.W., Patnaik, A., Papadopoulos, K.P., Agnew, J., Lokiec, F.M., Rezai, K., Kalambakas, S., and Buchbinder, A. (2011). Abstract A216: Results of a phase 1, open-label, dose-escalation study evaluating the safety and tolerability of EZN-3042, a survivin mRNA antagonist, administered with docetaxel (D) in adult patients (Pts) with advanced solid tumors. *Mol Cancer Ther 10*, A216–A216.

Tozawa, R., Ishibashi, S., Osuga, J., Yamamoto, K., Yagyu, H., Ohashi, K., Tamura, Y., Yahagi, N., Iizuka, Y., Okazaki, H., *et al.* (2001). Asialoglycoprotein receptor deficiency in mice lacking the major receptor subunit. Its obligate requirement for the stable expression of oligomeric receptor. *J Biol Chem 276*, 12624–12628.

van Meer, L., Moerland, M., Gallagher, J., van Doorn, M.B., Prens, E.P., Cohen, A.F., Rissmann, R., and Burggraaf, J. (2016). Injection site reactions after subcutaneous oligonucleotide therapy. *Br J Clin Pharmacol 82*, 340–351.

van Meer, L., van Dongen, M., Moerland, M., de Kam, M., Cohen, A., and Burggraaf, J. (2017). Novel SGLT2 inhibitor: first-in-man studies of antisense compound is associated with unexpected renal effects. *Pharmacol Res Perspect 5*, e00292.

van Poelgeest, E.P., Swart, R.M., Betjes, M.G., Moerland, M., Weening, J.J., Tessier, Y., Hodges, M.R., Levin, A.A., and Burggraaf, J. (2013). Acute kidney injury during therapy with an antisense oligonucleotide directed against PCSK9. *Am J Kidney Dis 62*, 796–800.

Vickers, T.A., and Crooke, S.T. (2016). Development of a quantitative BRET affinity assay for nucleic acid-protein interactions. *PLoS One 11*, e0161930.

Viney, N.J., van Capelleveen, J.C., Geary, R.S., Xia, S., Tami, J.A., Yu, R.Z., Marcovina, S.M., Hughes, S.G., Graham, M.J., Crooke, R.M., *et al.* (2016). Antisense oligonucleotides targeting apolipoprotein(a) in people with raised lipoprotein(a): two randomised, double-blind, placebo-controlled, dose-ranging trials. *Lancet 388*, 2239–2253.

Visentin, G.P., and Liu, C.Y. (2007). Drug-induced thrombocytopenia. *Hematol Oncol Clin North Am 21*, 685–696, vi.

Vollmer, J., and Krieg, A.M. (2009). Immunotherapeutic applications of CpG oligodeoxynucleotide TLR9 agonists. *Adv Drug Deliv Rev 61*, 195–204.

Wallace, T.L., Bazemore, S.A., Kornbrust, D.J., and Cossum, P.A. (1996). Repeat-dose toxicity and pharmacokinetics of a partial phosphorothioate anti-HIV oligonucleotide (AR177) after bolus intravenous administration to cynomolgus monkeys. *J Pharmacol Exp Ther 278*, 1313–1317.

Wan, W.B., Migawa, M.T., Vasquez, G., Murray, H.M., Nichols, J.G., Gaus, H., Berdeja, A., Lee, S., Hart, C.E., Lima, W.F., *et al.* (2014). Synthesis, biophysical properties and biological activity of second generation antisense oligonucleotides containing chiral phosphorothioate linkages. *Nucleic Acids Res 42*, 13456–13468.

Wan, W.B., and Seth, P.P. (2016). The medicinal chemistry of therapeutic oligonucleotides. *J Med Chem 59*, 9645–9667.

Watanabe, T.A., Geary, R.S., and Levin, A.A. (2006). Plasma protein binding of an antisense oligonucleotide targeting human ICAM-1 (ISIS 2302). *Oligonucleotides 16*, 169–180.

Waters, J.S., Webb, A., Cunningham, D., Clarke, P.A., Raynaud, F., di Stefano, F., and Cotter, F.E. (2000). Phase I clinical and pharmacokinetic study of bcl-2 antisense oligonucleotide therapy in patients with non-Hodgkin's lymphoma. *J Clin Oncol 18*, 1812–1823.

Yu, R.Z., Geary, R.S., Flaim, J.D., Riley, G.C., Tribble, D.L., van-Vliet, A.A., and Wedel, M.K. (2009a). Lack of pharmacokinetic interaction of mipomersen sodium (ISIS 301012), a 2′-O-methoxyethyl modified antisense oligonucleotide targeting apolipoprotein B-100 messenger RNA, with simvastatin and ezetimibe. *Clin Pharmacokinet 48*, 39–50.

Yu, R.Z., Graham, M.J., Post, N., Riney, S., Zanardi, T., Hall, S., Burkey, J., Shemesh, C.S., Prakash, T.P., Seth, P.P., *et al.* (2016a). Disposition and pharmacology of a GalNAc3-conjugated ASO targeting human lipoprotein (a) in mice. *Mol Ther Nucl Acids 5*, e317.

Yu, R.Z., Grundy, J.S., Henry, S.P., Kim, T.W., Norris, D.A., Burkey, J., Wang, Y., Vick, A., and Geary, R.S. (2015). Predictive dose-based estimation of systemic exposure multiples in mouse and monkey relative to human for antisense oligonucleotides with 2′-o-(2-methoxyethyl) modifications. *Mol Ther Nucl Acids 4*, e218. doi:10.1038/mtna.2014.69.

Yu, R.Z., Gunawan, R., Post, N., Zanardi, T., Hall, S., Burkey, J., Kim, T.W., Graham, M.J., Prakash, T.P., Seth, P.P., *et al.* (2016b). Disposition and pharmacokinetics of a GalNAc3-conjugated antisense oligonucleotide targeting human lipoprotein (a) in monkeys. *Nucl Acid Ther 26*, 372–380.

Yu, R.Z., Kim, T.W., Hong, A., Watanabe, T.A., Gaus, H.J., and Geary, R.S. (2007). Cross-species pharmacokinetic comparison from mouse to man of a second-generation antisense oligonucleotide, ISIS 301012, targeting human apolipoprotein B-100. *Drug Metab Dispos 35*, 460–468.

Yu, R.Z., Lemonidis, K.M., Graham, M.J., Matson, J.E., Crooke, R.M., Tribble, D.L., Wedel, M.K., Levin, A.A., and Geary, R.S. (2009b). Cross-species comparison of in vivo PK/PD relationships for second-generation antisense oligonucleotides targeting apolipoprotein B-100. *Biochem Pharmacol 77*, 910–919.

Yu, R.Z., Wang, Y., Norris, D.A., Kim, T.W., Narayanan, P., Geary, R.S., Monia, B.P., and Henry, S.P. (2020). Immunogenicity assessment of inotersen, a 2′-O-(2-methoxyethyl) antisense oligonucleotide in animals and humans: Effect on pharmacokinetics, pharmacodynamics, and safety. *Nucleic Acid Ther 30*(5), 265–275. doi:10.1089/nat.2020.0867.

Yuen, A.R., and Sikic, B.I. (2000). Clinical studies of antisense therapy in cancer. *Front Biosci 5*, D588–593.

Zanardi, T.A., Han, S.C., Jeong, E.J., Rime, S., Yu, R.Z., Chakravarty, K., and Henry, S.P. (2012). Pharmacodynamics and subchronic toxicity in mice and monkeys of ISIS 388626, a second-generation antisense oligonucleotide that targets human sodium glucose cotransporter 2. *J Pharmacol Exp Ther 343*, 489–496.

Zanardi, T.A., Kim, T.W., Shen, L., Serota, D., Papagiannis, C., Park, S.Y., Kim, Y., and Henry, S.P. (2018). Chronic toxicity assessment of 2′-O-methoxyethyl antisense oligonucleotides in mice. *Nucleic Acid Ther 28*, 233–241.

Zhao, Q., Temsamani, J., Iadarola, P.L., Jiang, Z., and Agrawal, S. (1996). Effect of different chemically modified oligodeoxynucleotides on immune stimulation. *Biochem Pharmacol 51*, 173–182.

Zhou, J., and Rossi, J. (2017). Aptamers as targeted therapeutics: current potential and challenges. *Nat Rev Drug Discov 16*, 181–202.

25

Cellular-Based Therapies

Ellen G. Feigal
NDA Partners LLC

Mary Ellen Cosenza
MEC Regulatory & Toxicology Consulting, LLC

CONTENTS

25.1 Introduction

Biologics encompass a broad spectrum of diverse products. In the USA, as amended by the Biologic Price Competition and Innovation (BPCI) Act[1] and the Further Consolidated Appropriations (FCA) Act,[2] a "biological product" is defined as "a virus, therapeutic serum, toxin, antitoxin, vaccine, blood, blood component or derivative, allergenic product, protein, or analogous product, or arsphenamine or derivative of arsphenamine (or any other trivalent organic arsenic compound), applicable to the prevention, treatment, or cure of a disease or condition of human beings" (see section 351(i)(1) of the PHS Act).[3] Biologics subject to the PHS Act also meet the definition of drugs under the Food Drug and Cosmetic Act and are subject to applicable provisions of that law.[4] Section 361 of the PHS Act

---

[1] Biologic Price Competition and Innovation Act of 2009 amended the definition of "biologic product" in section 351(i) of the PHS Act to include a "protein (except any chemically synthesized polypeptide)."

[2] Further Consolidated Appropriations Act of 2020, section 605 further amended the definition of "biological product" in section 351(i) of the PHS Act to remove the parenthetical "(except any chemically synthesized polypeptide)" from the statutory category of "protein."

[3] Final Rule Effective date March 23, 2020 https://www.federal-register.gov/documents/2020/02/21/2020-03505/definition-of-the-term-biological-product

[4] Federal Food, Drug and Cosmetic Act, 21 U.S.C. 321(g), section 201(g).

DOI: 10.1201/9781003124542-28

gives FDA the authority to make and enforce regulations that are necessary to prevent the introduction, transmission, and spread of communicable diseases. In 1993, pursuant to section 361, FDA published an interim rule regarding human tissue intended for transplantation, which required testing for communicable diseases, donor screening, and record keeping. FDA then issued a final rule on human tissue intended for transplantation in 1997 that created Part 21 CFR 1270, and announced plans for a more comprehensive system of regulation for human cells, tissues, and cellular and tissue-based products (HCT/Ps). The first of three final rules to implement various aspects of FDA's plans for a more comprehensive system of regulation was published in 2001 and created 21 CFR Part 1271. Subpart A of Part 1271 contains definitions and general provisions regarding the scope and purpose of the HCT/P regulations, and set out criteria that formed the foundation of a tiered, risk-based approach to regulating HCT/Ps. On May 25, 2004, FDA published the second final rule entitled "Eligibility Determination for Donors of Human Cells, Tissues, and Cellular and Tissue-Based Products" (69 FR 29786) (the donor eligibility final rule). On November 24, 2004, FDA published the third final rule entitled "Current Good Tissue Practice for manufacturers of Human Cells, Tissues, and Cellular and Tissue-Based Products; Inspection and Enforcement" (69 FR 68612). As of May 25, 2005, all three final rules were in effect.

Regulation focuses on three general areas: (1) limiting the risk of transmission of communicable disease from donors to recipients, (2) establishing manufacturing practices that minimize the risk of contamination, and (3) requiring an appropriate demonstration of safety and effectiveness for cells and tissues that present greater risks due to their processing or their use. Examples of HCT/Ps include bone, skin, corneas, ligaments, tendons, dura mater, heart valves, hematopoietic stem/progenitor cells derived from bone marrow and peripheral blood, and oocytes and semen. FDA does not regulate the transplantation of vascularized human organ transplants such as kidney, liver, heart, lung, or pancreas. The Health Resources Services Administration (HRSA) oversees the transplantation of vascularized human organs.

25.1.1 Where Biologics Are Regulated at the FDA

Center for Biologics Evaluation and Research (CBER) regulates most biologics which includes allergenics, blood and blood products, cellular and gene therapies, tissue and tissue-based products, vaccines, and xenotransplantation products, distributed among three product review offices. The Office of Tissues and Advanced Therapies (OTAT) regulates cell, tissue, and gene therapies as well as therapeutic vaccines for various disease indications. The Center for Devices and Radiological Health (CDRH) historically regulated some acellular tissue-"engineered" products and some are still CDRH products. The most commonly used product are the dermis products, some of which are regulated under the tissue framework, but others are in CDRH. However, all new human (not animal) acellular tissue-engineered products will be regulated in CBER.

The focus of this chapter is on cell therapies, which is regulated under the jurisdiction of OTAT, CBER, FDA. There are a growing number of these products advancing to the marketplace. From 2017 through 2019, the numbers of BLAs approved in CBER ranged from 21 to 22 per year, of which four have been for cell therapies/genetically modified cell therapies. In 2020, there were eight BLAs approved in CBER[5], of which one was for a genetically modified T-cell therapy. As of March 2021, there have been two genetically modified T-cell therapies approved in CBER. During this same time, there has been a tremendous amount of focus within CBER on the development of effective vaccines and therapies for COVID-19, a pandemic sweeping the world. From a search of ClinicalTrials.gov, there are hundreds of cell therapy approaches being evaluated in patients with COVID-19 across the world, with approximately 85 studies in the USA being investigated, with the majority being cell therapy with mesenchymal stem/stromal cells (MSCs), T regulatory cells, and natural killer (NK) cells.

25.1.2 What Are Cell-Based Therapies?

Science and technology continue to evolve and expand in this field, and includes explorations and development of gene-edited cells, combinations of different cells, cell patches for cardiovascular indications, gene-modified T cells for noncancer indications, and 3D printed organs, to mention only a few. However, all the technologies either are using or will be using case-by-case approaches as they advance through the product development and regulatory interactions to the clinic, and eventually the marketplace.

Cell-based therapies are the transfer of intact, live cells into a patient with the goal of preventing, treating, or curing a disease or condition. The source of the cells may come from the patient who will also be the recipient, in which case the source is termed autologous, or the cells may be obtained from a donor, in which case the source is termed allogeneic. The cells can be categorized by their potential to self-renew and/or generate several different cell types.

Pluripotent cells can self-renew as well as give rise to cells from all three germ layers of the body; multipotent cells can give rise to multiple, but not all cells in the body, and unipotent cells are fixed and produce one type of lineage and not other cell types.

Examples of pluripotent cells include human embryonic stem cells (hESCs) and induced pluripotent stem cells (iPSCs). Pluripotent cells can give rise to cells from all three embryonic germ layers, namely, the ectoderm, mesoderm, and endoderm. The ectoderm layer gives rise to brain, spinal cord, nerve, hair skin, teeth, sensory cells of the eyes, ears, nose and mouth, and pigment epithelial cells. The mesoderm layer gives rise to muscles, blood, blood vessels, connective tissues, and the heart. The endoderm layer gives rise to the pancreas, stomach, liver (and other organs of the gut), lungs, bladder, and germ cells.

---

[5] https://www.fda.gov/vaccines-blood-biologics-development-approval-process-cber

hESCs are pluripotent cells derived from the inner cell mass of an approximately 4-to-5-day old blastocyst of a fertilized embryo. In cell therapies their source has been derived from unused unimplanted embryos generated from in vitro fertilization for assisted reproduction. Within a developing human, the key abilities of these undifferentiated cells are proliferation by the formation of the next generation of stem cells and differentiation into specialized cells under certain physiological conditions. The stem cell differentiation process is influenced by external signals such as physical contact between cells or chemical secretion by surrounding tissue, and internal signals, which are controlled by genes in DNA. Stem cells also act as internal repair systems of the body. The replacement and formation of new cells are unlimited if an organism remains alive; however, the stem cell activity depends on the organ in which they reside. Division may be constant within bone marrow, but quiescent in organs such as the pancreas unless triggered by special physiological conditions (Zakrzewski et al. 2019).

iPSCs are artificially generated from somatic cells, a type of reverse engineering in proceeding from a differentiated to an undifferentiated state, and they function similarly to hESCs, in terms of being pluripotent. The technology was pioneered by Shinya Yamanaka of Kyoto University, Japan, initially making embryonic-like cells derived from adult cells in the mouse, avoiding the need for embryonic cells, and called these new cells "induced pluripotent stem cells". Subsequently Yamanaka and Thomson independently derived human iPSCs, utilizing skin cells that had four genes inserted into them with viruses, resulting in skin cells acquiring properties similar to embryonic stem cells. Once these cells are undifferentiated, they can then be treated with transcription factors or other types of growth factors to differentiate into specific types of cells, such as beating heart cells and nerve cells.

Multipotent cells can give rise to multiple lineages of cells, but not all lineages of the body, and thus are not pluripotent. Examples of multipotent cells include MSCs and hematopoietic stem cells (HSCs).

- MSCs are present in many tissues, such as the umbilical cord, bone marrow, and fat. In bone marrow, these cells differentiate primarily into bone, cartilage, and fat cells.
- HSCs form all the blood cell lineages of erythrocytes, leukocytes, and platelets. HSCs are found in umbilical cord blood, adult bone marrow, and peripheral blood, the most comprehensively characterized tissue-specific stem cell – studied for more than five decades and is the most commonly used stem cell therapy.

Unipotent cells produce only one lineage of cell; thus, they are neither multipotent nor pluripotent. Examples include T cells and NK cells. Recently developed are cell therapies that involve self-renewing T lymphocytes which have been genetically engineered to weaponize their immune potency to target and kill disease-causing cells, with FDA approvals in cancer indications; investigational uses are being explored in noncancer indications, such as in infectious diseases. Figure 25.1 provides a graphic representing the broad spectrum of clinical applications being pursued with the cell therapy approaches.

Cell therapies as a potentially viable approach to treat diseases began in the 1950s with pioneering work in bone marrow transplantation in hematologic malignancies by Dr. Donnall Thomas, which led to his receiving the Nobel Prize in 1990 (Thomas et al. 1957, Appelbaum 2007). The identification of human leukocyte antigens (HLA) by Dr. Jean Dausset in 1958, and the elucidation of its role in immune reactions and the need for HLA compatibility between a donor and recipient for successful transplantation subsequently led to his Nobel Prize in 1980. The first unequivocally successful bone marrow cell transplantation in humans was recorded in 1968 by

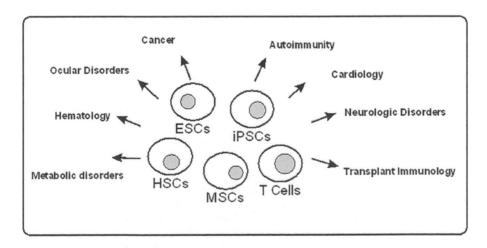

FIGURE 25.1 The broad spectrum of clinical approaches.

the University of Minnesota team of Robert A. Good (Gatti et al. 1968). The patient was an 8-year-old child with severe combined immunodeficiency (SCID) and the donor was his HLA-compatible sister. This achievement was a direct extension of mouse models of acquired immunologic tolerance that were established 15 years earlier. Human umbilical cord blood was identified as a source of HSCs, with the first transplant performed in 1988. Cord blood banks have been established worldwide for the collection and cryopreservation of cord blood for allogeneic HSC transplant (Gluckman 2009).

The preparation of bone marrow for transplantation is considered minimum manipulation if the processing does not alter the relevant biological characteristics of cells or tissues. For structural tissue, minimal manipulation would involve processing that does not alter the original relevant characteristics of the tissue relating to the tissue's utility for reconstruction, repair, or replacement. When transplanted for homologous use, it means the repair, reconstruction, replacement, or supplementation of a recipient's cells or tissues with an HCT/P that performs the same basic function or functions in the recipient as in the donor. Autologous use means the implantation, transplantation, infusion, or transfer of human cells or tissue back into the individual from whom the cells or tissues were recovered. On the other hand, FDA decided that allogeneic unrelated cord blood is a 351 product as they considered the product to have a systemic effect and therefore should be regulated as biological products and drugs under the PHS Act and the Federal FDC Act and required a BLA, even if minimally manipulated. The process is very different than for a conventional BLA. Because there was a large amount of clinical data from existing cord blood centers, the FDA created a docket to which the data were submitted.[6]

Since the 1990s, there has been an explosion of innovative approaches with various types of cell therapies for a wide scale of pathologies and disorders, such as cancer, hematologic disorders, diabetes, neurodegenerative disease, and cardiovascular and musculoskeletal disorders. Stem cell research has been an enabling technology for tissue/cell replacement, gene therapy and drug delivery, models of disease, drug screening and drug development, toxicity testing, cancer screening and therapy, and to enhance our basic knowledge of human development.

25.2 Regulation of Cell Therapy in the USA

There are two major regulatory categories of cell therapies in the USA, those which are substantially manipulated or intended for nonhomologous use are regulated under PHS 351(a), and those which are minimally manipulated and intended for homologous use are regulated under PHS 361. Minimally manipulated products have included blood products, bone marrow, and *in vitro* fertilization. An HCT/P is regulated solely under section 361 of the PHS Act if it meets all of the following criteria:

> The HCT/P is minimally manipulated; the HCT/P is intended for homologous use only; the manufacture of the HCT/P does not involve the combination of the cells or tissues with another article, except for water, crystalloids, or a sterilizing, preserving, or storage, and either i) the HCT/P does not have a systemic effect and is not dependent upon the metabolic activity of living cells for its primary function, or ii) the HCT/P has a systemic effect or is dependent upon the metabolic activity of living cells for its primary function, and a) is for autologous use; b) is for allogeneic use in a first-degree or second-degree blood relative; or c) is for reproductive use. Another exception to the 351 process is same day surgical procedure.

Processing that alters the original characteristics of the HCT/P raises increased safety and effectiveness concerns as there would be less basis on which to predict the product's function after transplantation. The determination of whether an HCT/P is minimally manipulated is based on the effect of manufacturing on the original relevant characteristics of the HCT/P as the HCT/P exists in the donor, and not based on the intended use in the recipient.

Over the past 30 years, the FDA has published a series of guidance documents regarding the regulatory oversight of cell therapy products, and FDA's perspectives on oversight has evolved over time based on expanding scientific discoveries and increasingly sophisticated technology advancements as well as taking into consideration public perspectives from stakeholders including product developers, patients and professional organizations. The decade of the 1990s saw the emergence of the increase in FDA publications and guidances related to cell therapy oversight, and the need for evolution of perspectives continues as more innovative approaches develop (FDA 1991, 1996, Kessler et al. 1993).

Carticel[7] was the first cell therapy to be approved by the FDA in August 1997 after the FDA had instituted specific cell therapy guidelines (FDA 1997a, 1997b). As FDA noted in the summary basis of approval for Carticel, "a variety of mechanisms have been used in the past to regulate somatic cell products. Depending on the make-up and the intended use of the product, some were regulated as biologics, others as devices, others not at all. With the rapid growth of interest in and development of such therapies in recent years, the regulatory approaches have been under careful consideration and evolution. Genzyme Tissue Repair (GTR) began marketing Carticel in 1995 based upon indications from the agency that, being an autologous cell therapy, Carticel would not be regulated. Later that year, CBER notified GTR that CBER considered Carticel to be a somatic cell therapy product as defined in the

---

[6] https://www.federalregister.gov/documents/2009/10/20/E9-25135/guidance-for-industry-minimally-manipulated-unrelated-allogeneic-placentalumbilical-cord-blood#:~:text=The%20Food%20and%20Drug%20Administration%20(FDA)%20is%20announcing,Hematopoietic%20Reconstitution%20for%20Specified%20Indications,%E2%80%9D%20dated%20October%202009

https://www.fda.gov/regulatory-information/search-fda-guidance-documents/bla-minimally-manipulated-unrelated-allogeneic-placentalumbilical-cord-blood-intended-hematopoietic; https://www.fda.gov/media/86387/download

[7] http://wayback.archive-it.org/7993/20170112211215/http://www.fda.gov/downloads/BiologicsBloodVaccines/CellularGeneTherapyProducts/ApprovedProducts/UCM109339.pdf

October 14, 1993, Federal Register notice concerning human somatic cell and gene therapy products and advised GTR that marketing approval would be required. After substantial public consultation, on May 28, 1996, the agency issued a document entitled *Guidance on Applications for Products Comprised of Living Autologous Cells Manipulated Ex Vivo and Intended for Structural Repair or Reconstitution* (these cells are referred to as MAS cells), which notified GTR and other sponsors of MAS cell products that they were involved in the manufacture of biological products and that, effective November 1997, those products could be used only under approved licensed application or IND exemption." The product, autologous cultured chondrocytes, was approved under an accelerated pathway for the indication of repair of clinically significant, symptomatic, cartilaginous defects of the femoral condyle (medial, lateral or trochlear) caused by acute or repetitive trauma. The post-marketing commitments for accelerated approval were met in 2007.

Assessments on cell products utilize a risk-based approach. HCT/Ps are defined in 21 CFR 1271.3(d) as articles containing or consisting of human cells or tissues that are intended for implantation, transplantation, infusion, or transfer into a human recipient. Because of the unique nature of HCT/Ps, FDA proposed, and in 2005 implemented, a tiered, risk-based approach to the regulation of HCT/Ps. Under this tiered, risk-based approach, those HCT/Ps that meet specific criteria or fall within detailed exceptions do not require premarket review and approval.[8] General considerations consider varying regulatory pathways and requirements, and outside of the specific regulatory issues, there are legal and political realities, costs, and reimbursement.

Chemistry, Manufacturing, and Controls (CMC) requirements include donor testing and assessing risk for transmissible diseases; Preclinical considerations include the assessment of appropriate animal models for human cell-based products, and clinical considerations include drug administration, clinical outcome measurement, monitoring, and pharmacovigilance.

25.3 Development Outside of the USA

Compliance with national and international regulations is important in the development of high-risk drugs obtained from engineered cells that are promising for the treatment of chronic or debilitating diseases. Manufacturing these products within a pharmaceutical quality assurance system during development stages is a critical step toward faster transition from research and development to the clinic. This requires multidisciplinary research teams and the establishment of infrastructure with GMP conditions that meet the legal requirements of pharmaceutical quality systems.

The European Medicines Agency (EMA) is an agency of the European Union (EU) responsible for the scientific evaluation, supervision, and safety monitoring of medicines in the EU. The Committee for Medicinal Products for Human Use (CHMP) is the EMA committee responsible for human medicines. In the centralized procedure, the CHMP is responsible for conducting the initial assessment of EU-wide Marketing Authorization Applications (MAAs); assessing modifications or extensions to an existing marketing authorization; considering the recommendations of the Agency's pharmacovigilance risk assessment committee on the safety of medicines on the market and when necessary, recommending to the European Commission changes to a medicine's marketing authorization, or its suspension or withdrawal from the market. The CHMP also evaluates medicines authorized at national level referred to EMA for a harmonized position across the EU. In addition, the CHMP and its working groups provide scientific advice to companies researching and developing new medicines; prepare scientific guidelines and regulatory guidance to help pharmaceutical companies prepare MAAs for human medicines and cooperate with international partners on the harmonization of regulatory requirements.

In the EU, there is a special category of products considered Advanced Therapy Medicinal Products (ATMPs). Products included in this ATMP category are gene therapy medicinal products, somatic cell therapy medicinal products, tissue-engineered medicinal products, and combined ATMPs. The Committee for Advanced Therapies (CAT) is the primary evaluation committee for the CHMP, and the CAT considers applications, presents opinions, and performs classification and certification procedures. A centralized procedure is required for a MAA for these types of products. Clinical trials require a clinical trial application (CTA) through National Competent Authorities (NCA), and Notified Bodies are engaged to review the device part of combination products. There is a requirement for the registration of test facilities and donor screening test kits (e.g., CE mark), and there is the role of the designated responsible person for releasing an ATMP in Europe.

In Japan, the Ministry of Health, Labor and Welfare (MHLW) is the regulatory body that oversees food and drugs in Japan, which includes creating and implementing safety standards for medical devices and drugs. In conjunction with the MHLW, the Pharmaceutical and Medical Device Agency (PMDA) is an independent agency that is responsible for reviewing drug and medical device applications. Market approval for drugs and medical devices has been governed by the PMD Act, which set forth criteria necessary for market approval issued by the PMDA (i.e., safety and efficacy) and detailed rules required for applicant compliance at both the pre- and post-marketing stage. After Dr. Shinya Yamanaka won a Nobel Prize for his work on induced pluripotent stem cells in 2012, Japan substantially increased its commitment to regenerative medicine, and in May 2013, the Japanese legislature passed the Regenerative Medicine Promotion Act to implement changes to facilitate the more rapid development of regenerative medicine. The government passed the Safety of Regenerative Medicine (RM) Act and amended the PMD Act in November 2013. Japan implemented this novel regulatory framework unique for regenerative medicine/cell therapies in November 2014, with adaptive licensing to allow earlier introduction into the marketplace, based on small confirmatory trials of probable benefit and safety (Asahara 2019). Regenerative medical products approved for marketing, including through

---

[8] FDA Guidance Regulatory Considerations for Human Cells, Tissues, and Cellular and Tissue-Based Products: Minimal Manipulation and Homologous Use, 2020

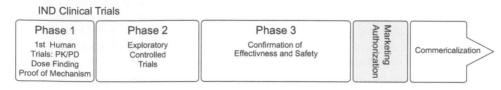

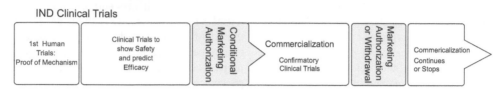

FIGURE 25.2 Traditional vs. development paradigm for regenerative medicine in Japan.

expedited conditional market approval, are guaranteed coverage by Japanese health insurance. Expedited conditional approvals can be based on very small numbers of patients and surrogate endpoints. The expedited approvals, however, must have post-marketing plans in place for a more comprehensive evaluation of safety and efficacy. As of November 2018, approximately five products were approved through this expedited conditional pathway. Figure 25.2 is a schematic representing the traditional drug development pathway vs the expedited, conditional pathway available for regenerative medicine products.

25.4 Regulation Requires a Case-By-Case Approach

There are many FDA Guidances addressing cell therapy products due to the diverse spectrum of such products. The case-by-case approach is governed by the product attributes. The following are some of the diverse categories of issues to consider: source of cells/donor tissue; heterogeneity of cell cultures; varying degree of potency in the different cell products; degree of foreignness, whether autologous or allogeneic; reactivity to environment within organs/tissues of interest; degree of disease specificity; whether the function of the cells depends on their continued survival, and the potential of uncontrolled proliferation. Among many questions needed to be addressed prior to clinical entry are the following: What is the test article? What are the best assays to characterize the cellular product? What is the best route of delivery? What is the fate of the cells? What is the "off-target" and "on-target" toxicity of the cells? What is the impact of other drugs on safety and efficacy? What are the specific risks/benefits in the intended population?

Specific challenges include establishing the dose and regimen: dose administration, i.e., concentration, volume, optimal site of delivery (location of injection), number of injections,

i.e., whether there is a need for repeat dosing, cell stability; dose extrapolation, i.e., number of cells delivered expanded; encapsulated, scaffold, sheet; scaling factors (e.g., body weight, body surface area, target organ); there may not be an opportunity for cross-species selection and validation; need for the use of an immunoincompetent animal or immune-suppressed animal since by necessity many of these products would be xenogeneic in an animal.

25.5 Relevant FDA Guidance Documents for Cell-based Therapeutics

FDA Guidance documents, which provide the Agency's current thinking of regulatory requirements and how to meet them, creates a framework to guide developers as they design and develop gene and cell therapy products. The Guidances cover elements of the manufacturing and quality controls sections of gene therapy INDs, retroviral safety testing, and guidelines specific to the development of treatments for rare diseases, retinal disorders, and hemophilia, and acknowledge that the durability of the treatment response cannot be fully answered in clinical trials, and that there will be a level of uncertainty around long-term responses. FDA issues Guidances regarding blood and blood component requirements for donors in terms of travel history and exposure, and infectious disease laboratory testing. The list of key FDA Guidances and their dates published are provided in Table 25.1.

FDA is planning the following additional Guidance documents from OTAT in 2021: Considerations for the Development of Chimeric Antigen Receptor (CAR) T Cell Therapies; Considerations for the Development of Human Gene Therapy Products Incorporating Genome Editing; Studying Multiple Versions of a Cellular or Gene Therapy Product in a Clinical Trial; and Regulation of Human Cells, Tissues, and Cellular and Tissue-Based Products (HCT/Ps) – Small Entity Compliance Guide.

TABLE 25.1

Relevant FDA Guidance Documents for Cell-based Therapeutics (Chronological Order)

Date Issued	FDA Guidance Document
01/2021	Manufacturing Considerations for Licensed and Investigational Cellular and Gene Therapy Products During COVID-19 Public Health Emergency; Guidance for Industry
07/2020	Regulatory Considerations for Human Cells, Tissues, and Cellular and Tissue-Based Products: Minimal Manipulation and Homologous Use; Guidance for Industry and Food and Drug Administration Staff
02/2019	Evaluation of Devices Used with Regenerative Medicine Advanced Therapies; Guidance for Industry
02/2019	Expedited Programs for Regenerative Medicine Therapies for Serious Conditions; Guidance for Industry
11/2017	Same Surgical Procedure Exception under 21 CFR 1271.15(b): Questions and Answers Regarding the Scope of the Exception; Guidance for Industry
09/2017	Deviation Reporting for Human Cells, Tissues, and Cellular and Tissue-Based Products Regulated Solely Under Section 361 of the Public Health Service Act and 21 CFR Part 1271; Guidance for Industry
12/2017 (updated)	Regulatory Considerations for Human Cells, Tissues, and Cellular and Tissue-Based Products: Minimal Manipulation and Homologous Use; Guidance for Industry and Food and Drug Administration Staff
06/2015	Considerations for the Design of Early-Phase Clinical Trials of Cellular and Gene Therapy Products; Guidance for Industry
03/2014	Guidance for Industry: BLA for Minimally Manipulated, Unrelated Allogeneic Placental/Umbilical Cord Blood Intended for Hematopoietic and Immunologic Reconstitution in Patients with Disorders Affecting the Hematopoietic System Note: This guidance finalizes the draft guidance of the same title dated June 2013.
03/2014	IND Applications for Minimally Manipulated, Unrelated Allogeneic Placental/Umbilical Cord Blood Intended for Hematopoietic and Immunologic Reconstitution in Patients with Disorders Affecting the Hematopoietic System - Guidance for Industry and FDA Staff Note: This guidance finalizes the draft guidance of the same title dated June 2013.
11/2013	Guidance for Industry: Preclinical Assessment of Investigational Cellular and Gene Therapy Products Note: This guidance finalizes the draft guidance entitled "Guidance for Industry: Preclinical Assessment of Investigational Cellular and Gene Therapy Products" dated November 2012.
12/2011	Guidance for Industry: Preparation of IDEs and INDs for Products Intended to Repair or Replace Knee Cartilage Note: This guidance finalizes the draft guidance of the same title dated July 2007.
01/2011	Guidance for Industry: Potency Tests for Cellular and Gene Therapy Products Note: This guidance finalizes the draft document of the same name, dated October 2008.
10/2010	Guidance for Industry: Cellular Therapy for Cardiac Disease Note: This guidance finalizes the draft guidance entitled "Guidance for Industry: Somatic Cell Therapy for Cardiac Disease" dated March 2009 (April 2, 2009, 74 FR 14992).
09/2009	Guidance for Industry: Considerations for Allogeneic Pancreatic Islet Cell Products
04/2008	Guidance for FDA Reviewers and Sponsors: Content and Review of Chemistry, Manufacturing, and Control (CMC) Information for Human Somatic Cell Therapy Investigational New Drug Applications (INDs)
08/2007	Eligibility Determination for Donors of Human Cells, Tissues, and Cellular and Tissue-Based Products; Guidance for Industry
3/1998	Guidance for Industry: Guidance for Human Somatic Cell Therapy and Gene Therapy

25.6 CMC Considerations

Challenges for emerging cell therapies include differences in donor and tissue sources, heterogeneity in cellular phenotypes, differences in the gene delivery systems, differences in scale of manufacturing, and the need for cryopreservation. Many of these may impact on product characteristics and critical quality attributes (CQAs) of a product, which are the physical, chemical, biological, or microbiological property or characteristic that should be within an appropriate limit, range, or distribution to ensure the desired product quality and are important for assessing product comparability. Assessment of potency and bioactivity and functionality can be challenging but are critical in the development process.

For early-phase clinical trials, a sponsor should be able to evaluate the identity, purity, quality, dose/potency, and safety of the product. Potency is defined as "the specific ability or capacity of the product, as indicated by appropriate laboratory tests or by adequately controlled clinical data obtained through the administration of the product in the manner intended, to effect a given result" (21 CFR 600.3(s)). Tests for potency can consist of either *in vitro* or *in vivo* tests, or both, which have been specifically designed for each product so as to indicate its potency in a manner adequate to satisfy the interpretation of potency given by the definition. Potency measurements are used to demonstrate that only product lots that meet defined specifications or acceptance criteria are administered during all phases of clinical investigation and following market approval. FDA regulations allow for considerable flexibility in determining the appropriate measurement(s) of potency for each product. Potency is determined based on individual product attributes; therefore, the adequacy of potency tests is evaluated on a case-by-case basis. However, all potency assays used for release testing of licensed biological drug products (DPs) must comply with applicable biologics and current GMP regulations. Ideally, the potency assay will represent the product's mechanism of action (MOA), i.e., relevant therapeutic activity or intended biological effect. The proposed MOA may be dependent on more than one active ingredient, e.g., multiple cell types and/or multiple vectors. If the product contains more than one active ingredient, more than one assay to measure potency of the product may be needed: in addition, considerations for potential non-additive effects between active ingredients, such as interference or synergy. A potency assay to assess the biological activity of the final product, with relevant lot release specifications, should be developed early in development and established prior to the initiation of clinical trials intended to provide substantial evidence of effectiveness for a marketing application. Tests for potency, sterility, purity, and identity apply to all biological products, including autologous and single patient allogeneic products, where a lot may be defined as a single dose. To support licensure of the product, manufacturing processes and all testing methods for product release must be validated (21 CFR 211.165(e)) by the end of Phase 3 studies. The earlier the manufacturing process and analytical assays are decided upon and validated, the more likely that the data obtained from these studies will be applicable to pivotal trials.

The sponsor will need to set a target or range of target values for those CQAs designated for product acceptability and release. The CQAs apply to both drug substances (DS) and DP as well as to excipients and in-process materials. Justification in support of a CQA should provide results from specific studies or published literature. As product development progresses, CQAs may be used to define DS and DP specifications. FDA recommends that a sponsor evaluate a number of product characteristics during early clinical development to help the sponsor identify and understand the CQAs of the product. This will also help ensure the sponsor's ability to assess manufacturing process controls, manufacturing consistency, and product stability as product development advances. FDA also notes that establishing and being able to evaluate CQAs is especially important if there are plans to pursue any of the available expedited product development programs.

Importantly, as the early-phase studies may provide evidence of safety and effectiveness, the characterization of product CQAs should be implemented during early clinical development. Demonstrating process control to ensure a consistent product with predefined CQAs for potency, identity, and purity is required to demonstrate compliance with licensure and regulatory requirements.

25.7 Preclinical Considerations

There are several unique challenges with preclinical development programs for cell therapies. The case-by-case approach (Cavagnaro 2008) is key as each project is unique in its product attributes, indications, and patient population. While examining the clinical relevance of preclinical models is not new, the concern is even more relevant when considering the many and varied cell therapy products which may have multiple mechanisms of action. Some cell therapies are designed for long-term or even permanent host engraftment – so preclinical data needs to support a long "in-life" phase to fully elucidate the product's potential benefit and safety concerns. In addition, many of these therapies may include a novel delivery device which may require additional preclinical evaluation.

As with other innovative therapies, selecting the right preclinical model can be especially challenging. Ideally, the model would accurately reflect/predict critical elements of the cell therapy product's intended clinical use. The key product attributes that can help design the sponsor's preclinical program include the source of the cells (autologous vs allogeneic); how well differentiated the cells are (iPSC vs mature cells); the amount of manipulation (minimal to genetically modified) of the cells before transfer to a patient; the expected life span and reproducibility of the cells once they have been transferred to the patient; and the route or delivery methodology, i.e., the need to use genetically or chemically immune-suppressed models as the cells will all be xenogeneic unless using analogous products, if an analogous animal product is used to prevent rejection and allow interpretability of the study, a comparability study will need to be conducted with the clinical candidate; and other factors include the indication and patient status.

25.7.1 Pharmacology

Pharmacology for cell-based products refers to the biologic activity of the cells at their target (and off-target) sites. *In vitro* and *in vivo* pharmacology and proof-of-concept studies can be helpful for planning the human clinical trials. The biggest challenge for conducting pharmacology studies with cell therapies is the identification and availability of appropriate animal models. Different animal models may have advantages or disadvantages for particular cell therapy products, and a combination of *in vitro* and *in vivo* assays/studies may best address these limitations. The FDA Guidance: Preclinical Assessment of Investigational Cellular and Gene Therapy Products (November 2013) recommends that studies be conducted with the actual clinical investigational product. For cell therapies, this can be challenging as human cells are often rejected by normal animals and few disease models exist in immune-altered/suppressed animals. In addition, the feasibility of using the clinical dosing route or delivery system can be challenging. Test species that have been genetically modified or nonstandard test species such as sheep can be acceptable. *In vitro* studies can be useful in determining whether an animal model or species is relevant for testing of the clinical product. Multiple models may be necessary to investigate different aspects of a new cell therapy, and some information about activity can be obtained even if by a different clinical route of administration. Larger animal models may be needed to mimic the disease or surgical intervention, including the use of a medical device if relevant for the product.

25.7.2 Pharmacokinetics/ Biodistribution/Cell Fate

Pharmacokinetics for cell therapies refers to the time course and strength of the biologic effects of the cells after dosing and determining the biodistribution and cell fate, i.e., are the cells destroyed, or do they multiply. The tracking of cells in preclinical species can hold additional challenges, assuming you can find a model that does not completely reject the cells upon initial administration. Immunosuppression, chemically or genetically induced, is necessary when human cells are used to support long-term persistence or engraftment in animals. The goal is to assess exposure in either pharmacology or toxicity studies in order to predict safe and effective doses in patients. Labeling of cells is one method that can be used to track distribution. Immunohistochemistry is most frequently used to identify the cell product. This can confirm whether the product reaches the target tissues or organ(s) and help determine the optimal dosing regimen. Route of delivery should be as similar as possible to the intended clinical route but may not always be feasible in the animals. If the intended route is unique, then associated risks of the procedure may also need to be investigated. The use of devices needs to be addressed as well and may involve cross-referencing of device master files (MF) or Investigational Device Exemptions (IDEs) as well. The risks associated with these devices (e.g., scaffolds) also need to be evaluated. See discussion of approved products later in this chapter for examples.

25.7.3 Toxicology/Safety Studies

As with the pharmacology (POC) and cell fate (PK/distribution) studies, animals have significant limitations in testing human cell-based products. Understanding the product attributes and potential clinical use and clinical trial plans is key to developing a preclinical toxicology plan. A combination of *in vitro* and *in vivo* studies is often necessary to fully investigate potential concerns. Depending on the indication, specialty studies such as local tolerance, safety pharmacology, and reproductive and developmental toxicity may need to be conducted, or these concerns may need to be addressed using other investigative methods such as cytotoxicity in target or nontarget cells.

For autologous products, the amount of preclinical investigation is usually dependent on the amount of "manipulation" or the type(s) of treatments the cells have undergone before being re-administered back into the patients. The source and types of cells (e.g., iPSC, T cells, NK cells) are one factor. If the cells are just purified and stimulated to differentiate and/or be responsive to tumor antigens (such as with dendritic cells), there may be little that can be done in animal models to help identify potential toxicities that are not already identified as "on-target." On the other hand, if the cells are altered genetically and then expected to proliferate or remain active in the patient for years, then there are certain categories of concerns that should be addressed. Additional information on how to address concerns with genetic manipulation can be found in Chapters 26 (Myer) and 27 (Cavagnaro) of this book. CAR T cells are addressed in Chapter 28 (Todd). These concerns can range from risks associated with the delivery procedures, inappropriate cell proliferation or differentiation, and cell migration to nontarget tissues.

Human cells are xenogeneic to animal species; thus, immunosuppression, genetically immunodeficient, or humanization of animals are strategies used to prevent rejection. The creation of analogous cells (the animal-derived equivalent of the human product) has also been used to investigate some of these products. This may eliminate the species difference but may raise questions about the comparability of the products. All of these models carry their own unique challenges in extrapolation of this preclinical data to predict potential clinical concerns. These models may also mask or confound their interpretation and so need to be evaluated in this context.

As with other modalities, there is often a wealth of information that can be gained by conducting a liability assessment of the cell targets. What are the consequences of binding, stimulating, or blocking the intended target with a CAR T-cell product? Often this information can be investigated in a combination of literature searches, public data on molecules or therapies with the same or similar targets, genetic or protein analysis, and other *in vitro* assays or arrays. A common challenge with cell therapies is how to track cell fate. Tagging of the cells and the use of imaging have been used for some tumor models.

If animal studies are to be conducted, it is important that unbiased preclinical study designs (number of test animals and groups, use of controls) be used and Good Laboratory Practice (GLP) regulations be adhered to where possible. The collection of multiple study parameters should be considered to make the best use of the animals, even if this means collecting samples for future potential analysis. The FDA will expect detailed complete reports for any toxicology studies being conducted even if they are not the standard GLP studies generally conducted for standard biologics (e.g., proteins and monoclonal antibodies).

Another challenge for pluripotent, undifferentiated or certain genetically altered cells is the assessment of tumorigenicity or inappropriate cell differentiation. There may also be concern for unintended contamination of other cell products with these cell types. Assessment of this risk will be required before entering clinical trials and usually requires evaluation with the intended clinical product in which case efforts to minimize contamination with undifferentiated cells are critical. *In vitro* assays include cell proliferation or soft agar colony formation assays. It is also critical to have assays that can monitor for unwarranted cell types and genetic instability of the product cells. *In vivo* models generally involve the use of severe combined immunodeficient (SCID) mice for engraftment studies. Other models include athymic nude rats where a larger rodent may be required. The appropriate assay for a particular cell therapy type is usually a case-by-case decision based on the product attributes. There have been some recent cross-industry and regulatory agency efforts to collect data that may provide additional insight and guidance on investigating this risk (Sato et al. 2019).

An important consideration is how best to extrapolate dose from the various animal studies for first-in-human (FIH) dose. Standard algorithms used for small molecules, protein therapeutics, or monoclonal antibodies or their derivatives are not applicable for cell therapies. It is important to provide data and information to support the intended human starting dose and dose escalation scheme. References to other similar products and literature can be used to make these extrapolations. Dose administration such as concentration of cells, total volume, rate of delivery, site of injection, and number of injections are all factors to consider. Advice needs to be provided on what parameters can be monitored to identify potential toxicities.

The unique issues with cell therapies underscore the importance of early regulatory feedback. In the USA, FDA's

CBER has the OTAT, which has established the process of INTERACT (INitial Targeted Engagement for Regulatory Advice on CBER producTs) and Pre-IND meetings. The INTERACT meetings are informal non-binding, scientific discussions to help address specific issues. In Europe, early scientific advice is encouraged for unique and challenging ATMPs.

25.8 Regulatory Challenges – IND Stage

Common deficiencies in manufacturing at the IND stage include incomplete information regarding the quality of the materials used to make the product; manufacturing process development (e.g., no process development runs); safety, quality, and stability testing (e.g., inappropriate testing, sampling); cross-referenced information (e.g., wrong cross reference, or the cross reference was deficient), and manufacturing facility, QA/QC, and shipping. In addition, the submission may be poorly organized, and there is a lack of alignment of CMC development with the clinical timeline, and inadequate comparability plans (FDA November 2019).

Recommendations for improvement include planning ahead, communicating with FDA, following FDA guidance, organizing submissions according to eCTD, resolving CMC issues early in product development, identifying CQAs, and validating assays early (crucial for establishing comparability; FDA November 2019).

Common pharmacology/toxicology deficiencies include preclinical testing programs that have insufficient information to assess patient risk, i.e., lack of preclinical safety data with incomplete safety study reports, route of administration/ anatomic site of delivery; differences between the preclinical and clinical product; inadequate preclinical study designs, i.e., in terms of safety monitoring for safety/activity endpoints, animal number, study dose, i.e., extrapolation to clinical dose, and study duration; study conduct issues; safety concerns based on toxicity profile, and insufficient data to establish the prospect of direct benefit for pediatric subjects (FDA November 2019).

Recommendations for improvement include using opportunities for early communication with FDA; read the guidance documents – Preclinical Assessment of Investigator Cellular and Gene Therapy Products (Nov 2013); use biologically relevant test systems; use available tools, e.g., *in silico*, *in vitro*, *in vivo*) to thoroughly assess safety; conduct toxicology studies in accordance with GLP; and submit complete study reports.

In order to facilitate an efficient clinical development in the setting of rare diseases, it is important for the sponsor to have robust natural history data as early as possible for the intended indication and ideally collaborate precompetitively; even in the FIH study design, consider a randomized, concurrent controlled trial, blinded if possible; otherwise blinded evaluators to reduce bias; evaluate effects on clinically meaningful endpoints, in addition to safety and biomarkers; and get early buy-in from patient groups, FDA, and other regulatory agencies (FDA November 2019). Investigational studies are in progress in a multitude of rare diseases, including retinitis pigmentosa (i.e., with retinal progenitor cells), Duchenne muscular dystrophy (i.e., stem cell-based, which utilize myoblasts, satellite cells, bone marrow cells, mesoangioblasts, and CD133+ cells,

in addition to hESC-derived to a myogenic lineage) (Sun et al. 2020), rare forms of rheumatologic disorders and mitochondrial diseases.

25.9 Clinical Considerations

Preclinical studies are conducted to establish the feasibility and rationale for clinical use, as well as to characterize the product's safety profile, and also provide the scientific basis to support the conduct of the proposed clinical studies. Unlike small-molecule development, the preclinical data generated for cell therapy products may not always be as informative, as it may not be feasible to conduct traditional preclinical pharmacokinetic studies; i.e., many of the cell-based therapies are delivered into tissue compartments intended to engraft and are not available for measurement systemically, or the appropriate assays for measurement may be lacking. If available, previous clinical experience with the product or related products, even if for a different indication, might help to justify the clinical starting dose. In some cell therapy products, the potential for prolonged biologic activity after a single administration, a high potential for immunogenicity, or the need for relatively invasive procedures to deliver the product may pose increased risks for the patient. In the preceding section of this chapter, we referred to the FDA Guidance documents for general considerations in the design of early-phase clinical trials of cellular and gene therapy products, in specific indications (i.e., for repair or replacement of knee cartilage; for cardiovascular disease) and utilizing specific technology (i.e., allogeneic pancreatic islet cell products) and technologies that will be discussed in other chapters (gene therapy approaches).

At a December 2020 2nd NCI Workshop on Cell-based Immunotherapy for Solid Tumors, the FDA presentation focused on critical elements in FIH study design, which cannot be conducted in normal healthy volunteers, study population, treatment plan, safety monitoring, dose-limiting toxicity criteria, and potential clinical hold issues. Potential clinical hold issues for the early studies included deficits in trial design, i.e., study enrollment was not staggered, the dose-escalation was too aggressive, there was intra-patient dose escalation; deficits in eligibility, i.e., excessive risk for patients with early-stage disease or with newly diagnosed disease without prior therapy, lack of a diagnostic to select for the cell therapy target of interest; deficits in the treatment plan, i.e., irrational dosing regimen, inappropriate route of administration; and deficits in safety monitoring, i.e., inadequate toxicity grading, problems with the dose-limiting toxicity criteria, or lack of stopping rules.

The designs for cell therapy products differ from the design for conventional pharmaceutical products due to the unique features of these products and may also reflect previous clinical experience. The nature of the risks depends on the cell type used and could include the potential risk of uncontrolled growth of the cells and development of tumors, contamination of the product with or reversion of the product to an undifferentiated state although such risks have not been documented in cell therapies with regulatory oversight; however, there have been documented instances outside of regulatory oversight or in "stem cell clinics," in which the development of tumors in the brain and spinal cord of a patient who received intrathecal allogeneic stem cells for ataxia telangiectasia occurred (Amariglio et al. 2009), consecutive case series of serious adverse events associated with intravitreal stem cell injections performed in the USA with blinding visual outcomes in three patients after they received bilateral intravitreal injection of autologous adipose tissue–derived stem cells at the same stem cell clinic (Kuriyan et al. 2017), and potential risks with cells with the characteristics of cardiomyocytes generating a focus of electrical activity uncoordinated with the rest of the heart (Zhang et al. 2002).

Product characteristics can influence the clinical trial design. Some products may persist for an extended period after administration or have an extended or permanent effect even after the product itself is no longer present. The effects might evolve over time as the stem cells proliferate and differentiate. This may necessitate a prolonged duration of clinical follow-up to evaluate safety, although this may also provide an opportunity to evaluate continued pharmacologic activity. For pluripotent derived cells or those involving genetically modified cells, the duration of follow-up may be up to 15 years. The need for such extended follow-up may change as further experience with such products is gained.

Some products may require an invasive procedure for delivery to the target, and the procedure itself may add substantial risk. Specialized training is always conducted for novel routes of administration and/or novel delivery devices.

Allogeneic products or proteins that might be produced may be immunogenic, which can be desired in the case of vaccines but pose a potential risk for other types of therapeutics by reducing or neutralizing the beneficial effect or by causing an adverse reaction such as an autoimmune syndrome.

Some indications, i.e., the use of genetically engineered T cells in patients with hematologic malignancies, may require the recipient be treated with lymphocyte depletion or other conditioning regimens to facilitate cell survival, and these also add risks to be considered in the overall benefit-risk assessment.

The manufacturing of the cells may set practical limits on the dose, concentration, or volume of the product that can be delivered, as well as the timing for delivery, due to the length of the manufacturing process itself. This is particularly relevant for autologous approaches, and cryopreservation is a key enabling technology that has been used to provide stable and secure extended cell storage for primary tissue isolates and constructs and cell preparations. Provenge (sipuleucel T) was a distribution challenge in which fresh cells manufactured from the patient needed to be initially delivered within a very restricted time frame. With many of the autologous CAR T therapies, the manufacturing process itself leads to limitations on when the product can be delivered, which is a very different issue than what is possible with an "off-the-shelf" type of product which would not have the similar challenges of a lag time for manufacturing.

In addition to general tests and monitoring for safety issues, evaluations may include assessments targeting specific safety issues that might be expected, such as acute or delayed infusion reactions, autoimmunity, graft failure, graft vs. host disease (GVHD), new malignancies, or transmission of infectious agents from a donor, the latter of which can only be assessed at the time of infection unless one of the donor tests came back positive and may prompt the need for particular vigilance. Elements of the trial design such as efficacy endpoints and methods for statistical analysis are generally the same for cell therapy products and other types of products.

25.10 FDA-Approved Cell Products

While there have been hundreds of INDs for cell-based therapies, many of them from small academic investigators and not sponsored by commercial entities, it is illustrative to look back at the preclinical studies that were conducted for products that have been approved by FDA. While not all of the studies may have been required, in hindsight, or may have been conducted for scientific exploration, rather than as regulatory IND enabling requirements, these studies do reflect the nonclinical research and development for these products.

Twenty cell and gene therapy products have received FDA approval, with the first approval in April 2010, and the most recent in March 2021. Of these 20 products, 17[9] were cell therapies. Of the 17 cell therapies, eight were placental/umbilical cord blood products and nine were more complex cell products, including genetically modified cell therapies. The placental/umbilical cord products required a BLA as the FDA determined these products derived their MOA through a systemic effect and put in place a process in which if the manufacturers met specific standards for specific types of indications, they could provide safety and CMC information, including the establishment selection and description, but not be required to provide preclinical data. If the manufacturing involved more than minimally manipulated, or included other indications, the manufacturer would need to submit an IND or other premarketing application appropriate for that product. If the manufacturing included cell selections and incubation of the selected cells with culture media and growth factors to achieve large numbers of cells capable of long-term repopulation of the bone marrow, the HCT/Ps would generally be considered more than minimally manipulated because the processing affects the production of intracellular or cell surface proteins and other markers of cell lineage, activation state, and proliferation, thereby altering the cells' relevant biological characteristics of multipotency and capacity for self-renewal. Table 25.2 provides a summary of the FDA-approved products.

25.10.1 Hematopoietic Progenitor Cell Cord Blood Products

In October 2009, FDA announced that manufacturers of cord blood would be required to have an approved BLA or IND in effect for unrelated cord blood shipped after October 20, 2011. FDA developed and finalized guidance for industry entitled Minimally Manipulated, Unrelated Allogeneic Placental/Umbilical Cord Blood Intended for Hematopoietic Reconstitution for Specified Indications (October 2009),

---

[9] The Summary Basis of Approval and related key documents for each of the products was accessed and reviewed from the OTAT website, FDA.

TABLE 25.2

List of FDA Approved Cell-Therapy Products 2010–March 2021

Product	FDA Approval Date
Class: Hemato-Progenitor Cell, Cord Blood	
HEMACORD; New York Blood Center	November 2011
HPC; Clinimmune Labs, University of Colorado Cord Blood Bank	May 2012
Ducord; Duke University School of Medicine	October 2012
ALLOCORD; SSM Cardinal Glennon Children's Medical Center	May 2013
HPC; LifeSouth Community Blood Centers, Inc.	June 2013
HPC; Bloodworks	January 2016
CLEVECORD; Cleveland Cord Blood Center	September 2016
HPC; MD Anderson Cord Blood Bank	June 2018
Class: Cell Therapy	
PROVENGE (sipuleucel-T)	April 2010
LAVIV (azficel-T)	June 2011
GINTUIT (Allogeneic Cultured Keratinocytes and Fibroblasts in Bovine Collagen)	March 2012
MACI (Autologous Cultured Chondrocytes on a Porcine Collagen Membrane)	December 2016
Class: Genetically-Modified Chimeric Antigen Receptor-T Cell Therapy (CAR-T T)	
KYMRIAH (tisagenlecleucel) with Lentiviral vector	
Relapsed/refractory B-cell precursor Acute Lymphoblastic Leukemia	August 2017
Relapsed/refractory diffuse large B-cell lymphoma	May 2018
YESCARTA (axicabtagene ciloleucel) with gamma retroviral vector	October 2017
Relapsed/refractory diffuse large B-cell lymphoma	
TECARTUS (brexucabtagene autoleucel) with gamma retroviral vector	July 2020
Relapsed/refractory mantle cell lymphoma	
BREYANZI (lisocabtagene maraleucel) with lentiviral vector	February 2021
Relapsed/refractory diffuse large B-cell lymphoma	
ABECMA (idecabtagene vicleucel) with lentiviral vector	March 2021
Relapsed/refractory multiple myeloma	

which was updated in March 2014 and further clarified in the July 2020 FDA Guidance.[10]

---

[10] In addition, the November 2017 version of the guidance informed manufacturers, healthcare providers, and other interested persons that over the next 36 months (through November 2020), FDA intended to exercise enforcement discretion under limited conditions with respect to the investigational new drug (IND) application and premarket approval (biologics license application (BLA)) requirements, for certain HCT/Ps. The July 2020 version of the guidance explained that FDA intended to exercise such enforcement discretion for a longer period of time through May 2021. The November 2017 version of the guidance finalized the document entitled "Minimal Manipulation of Human Cells, Tissues, and Cellular and Tissue-Based Products (HCT/Ps); Draft Guidance for Industry and Food Administration Staff" dated December 2014, and "Homologous Use of Human Cells, Tissues, and Cellular and Tissue-Based Products (HCT/Ps); Draft Guidance for Industry and FDA Staff" dated October 2015. It also finalized certain material related to adipose tissue that was included in draft guidance entitled "Human Cells, Tissues, and Cellular and Tissue-Based Products (HCT/Ps) from Adipose Tissue: Regulatory Considerations; Draft Guidance for Industry" dated December 2014 (Adipose Draft Guidance). This material, together with the material related to adipose tissue included in the final guidance entitled "Same Surgical Procedure Exception under 21 CFR 1271.15(b); Questions and Answers Regarding the Scope of the Exception" dated November 2017, superseded the Adipose Draft Guidance. FDA did finalize the Adipose Draft Guidance, and that draft guidance was withdrawn in November 2017. Finally, the November 2017 version of the guidance superseded the document entitled "Minimal Manipulation of Structural Tissue (Jurisdictional Update); Guidance for Industry and FDA Staff" dated September 2006 (2006 Guidance).

An FDA Advisory Committee for HEMACORD, the first of the products to come in under the mandate requiring a BLA, was held on September 22, 2011. Topics discussed included HEMACORD's indications for hematologic malignancies, bone marrow failure, primary immunodeficiency diseases, beta thalassemia, and metabolic disorders. HEMACORD, as well as all of the subsequent allogeneic cord blood hematopoietic progenitor cell therapy products to follow, have the same indication, i.e., for use in unrelated donor hematopoietic progenitor cell transplantation procedures in conjunction with an appropriate preparative regimen for hematopoietic and immunologic reconstitution in patients with disorders affecting the hematopoietic system that are inherited, acquired, or result from myeloablative treatment.

None of the products required the conduct of preclinical pharmacology/toxicology studies based on consideration of the extent of the manipulation of the product and the previous human experience with the products.

25.10.2 Cell Therapy Products

PROVENGE (sipuleucel-T) from Dendreon Corp. is an autologous cellular immunotherapy indicated for the treatment of asymptomatic or minimally symptomatic metastatic castrate resistant (hormone refractory) prostate cancer. The product contains a minimum of 50 million autologous CD54$^+$ cells activated with PAP-GM-CSF. PAP-GM-CSF consists of human prostatic acid phosphatase (PAP), an antigen expressed in prostate cancer tissue, linked to human granulocyte-macrophage colony-stimulating factor (GM-CSF), an immune cell activator.

To manufacture sipuleucel-T, patient cells are collected by standard leukapheresis, and then the recombinant protein, human PAP linked to human GM-CSF, is added to the cells. The GM-CSF portion of the protein helps to target the PAP protein to antigen-presenting cells (APCs) and activate those cells. PAP provides the tumor-specific antigen that is intended to direct the immune system to target prostate cancer. The cells are cultured, then washed, and suspended for infusion back into the patient. The cellular composition of sipuleucel-T will vary, depending on the cells obtained from the individual patient during leukapheresis. In addition to the autologous APCs, the product also contains T cells, B cells, NK cells, and other cells. Each dose is shipped and administered fresh (without cryopreservation) within 18 hours of manufacture.

Due to the autologous nature of sipuleucel-T, limited pre-clinical studies were conducted. Pharmacology studies demonstrated that PAP is a potential immune target for prostate cancer active immunotherapy. *In vitro* studies showed that two murine T-cell hybridoma cell lines that responded to both murine and human HLA-DR1+ APCs and recognized two HLA-DR1 restricted PAP-specific epitopes could be established, indicating that human PAP can be taken up, processed, and presented in the context of human MHC. Immunization of mice or rats with hPAP, rPAP, or hPAP-mGM-CSF resulted in both humoral and cellular immune responses to PAP antigen. While immunization of rat with rPAP-rGM-CSF could induce prostate-specific inflammation in rats, no inflammation was observed in a limited set of normal non-prostate tissues examined, thus breaking of tolerance to autologous prostate tissue was shown to be possible, providing a rationale to support clinical development of sipuleucel-T. Mice immunized with hPAP-hGM-CSF-loaded APCs prior to challenge with murine EL4 lymphoma transfected with the human PAP gene showed a prolonged survival compared to the control groups; however, the rationale for selection of the dose level of the hPAP-hGM-CSF-loaded APCs used, as well as the immunization regimen, was not provided. In a tumor challenge model, immunological endpoints associated with an antitumor response mediated by hPAP-hGM-CSF-loaded APCs were not determined. In addition, the antitumor response in mice bearing established tumors prior to immunization was not evaluated with the rodent equivalent of sipuleucel-T. *In vitro* analysis of PAP protein or PAP gene expression in human tissues demonstrated high expression of the PAP protein or gene in normal and malignant prostate tissue, with significantly lower expression in a limited set of nonprostate normal tissues. Toxicology studies were not conducted due to the autologous nature of sipuleucel-T and the patient population of focus, those with prostate cancer.

The preclinical data supported the proposed MOA that CD54 up-regulation was a good indicator of APC activation and provided evidence that the therapy had the potential to improve antigen presentation to tumor-specific T cells. Information was deficient to (1) determine the function of APCs in the product in stimulating T- and B-cell responses, (2) determine the role of PAP antigen in eliciting an immune response, and (3) evaluate host T-cell activation and suppression in product function, and how that will or will not correlate with survival.

Dendreon submitted a BLA on November 9, 2006, and an AC was held. FDA issued a Complete Response Letter (CRL) on May 8, 2007. The ongoing Phase 3 study was subsequently completed and confirmed the clinical effectiveness of the product, the CMC issues were resolved, and FDA approved the product in 2010.

LAVIV (azficel-T) from Fibrocell Technologies is an autologous cellular product indicated for the improvement of the appearance of moderate to severe nasolabial fold wrinkles in adults. The product had been previously marketed in the USA between December 1995 and February 1999 without pre-market approval, and in compliance with FDA's regulation of somatic cell therapies the company removed the product from the US market in 1999 and subsequently submitted an IND for clinical testing in 2003. Azficel-T contains a minimum of 18 million autologous fibroblasts. The fibroblasts are cultured, using standard methodologies, from punch biopsies (dermal and epidermal layers), and following *in vitro* expansion, the fibroblasts are harvested, quality control tests are performed, and the cell suspension is cryopreserved. A dose of cells is thawed, washed, formulated, and shipped to the clinical site at 2°C–8°C by overnight delivery for use within 24 hours of final formulation. The cells are injected intradermally into the nasolabial folds.

Approximately 1,100 subjects had received azficel-T at 110 clinics during the 4-year period when the product was marketed in the USA and no serious adverse events were reported during this time. Considering the previous commercial experience in humans, and due to the lack of an appropriate animal model for wrinkles, no preclinical studies using azficel-T were required.

Fibrocell Technologies, Inc submitted a BLA on March 6, 2009. An AC was held, focused on tumorigenicity potential of the fibroblast cell suspension; potential risk for hypertrophic scarring, keloid formation, or abnormal pigmentation, in the non-White population; potential safety risks in patients over 65 years of age and in males; and a post-marketing training program for practitioners. The AC commented on the lack of sufficient data related to the processing, characterization, and collagen production of the injected cells; concerns regarding the underlying changes in the dermis, the fate of the cells, and tumor risks from cell transformation, and suggested that additional safety and mechanistic data be obtained by conducting a clinical study in which azficel-T is injected into a less visible area on the body, followed by taking serial biopsies for analysis.

The FDA determined that the safety data presented for azficel-T in the original application were not sufficient to support approval and issued a CRL. Fibrocell conducted a 29-subject, double-blind, intrasubject controlled study of the histology of cutaneous tissue of the upper arms injected with azficel-T, compared to tissue injected with saline, and compared to untreated tissue. On December 22, 2010, the applicant resubmitted the BLA with responses to all FDA information requests in the CRL, and these responses and subsequent amendments addressed adequately all of the outstanding issues from the FDA CRL, and the product was approved. A post-marketing registry study was required to assess the risk of skin cancer in the area of azficel-T injections and the risk of immune-mediated hypersensitivity reactions in 2,700 patients.

GINTUIT (allogeneic cultured keratinocytes and fibroblasts in bovine collagen) from Organogenesis Inc. is an allogeneic cellularized scaffold product indicated for topical application to a surgically created vascular wound bed in the treatment of mucogingival conditions in adults. The product is a cellular sheet that consists of two layers: an upper cornified layer that is made of living human keratinocytes (the primary cell type in the skin's outer layer) and a lower layer constructed of bovine-derived collagen, human extracellular matrix proteins, and living human dermal fibroblasts (skin cells that generate connective tissue). The cells are isolated from donated human newborn foreskin tissue and are multiplied into cell banks used in large-scale manufacturing. The cell banks are tested for microbiological and cytogenetic safety.

The MOA by which GINTUIT increases keratinized tissue at the treated site was not identified; however, *in vitro* studies demonstrated that GINTUIT secretes human growth factors and cytokines and contains extracellular matrix proteins that are known to be involved in wound repair and regeneration. In addition to the nonclinical studies submitted to the Apligraf PMA, two nonclinical studies were also submitted to this BLA. In nonclinical pharmacology studies for the cutaneous wound indication, the data suggested that Apligraf functions similar to a skin graft when transplanted onto nude mice. *In vitro* studies suggested that following physical injury, the keratinocytes within Apligraf migrate, re-epithelialize, and keratinize. In addition, Apligraf secreted growth factors. *In vivo* transplantation of Apligraf onto full-thickness cutaneous wounds in nude mice resulted in graft integration with the host tissue and persistence of the human keratinocytes and fibroblasts for 1 year. GINTUIT transplants on cutaneous wounds in nude mice suggested compatibility with periodontal dressings and with chlorhexidine solution (an antimicrobial agent). The allogeneic human keratinocytes and dermal fibroblasts in Apligraf did not appear to induce an alloimmune response when evaluated by assay. The potential for Apligraf to induce an alloimmune response by indirect allorecognition was not evaluated. Biocompatibility testing of Apligraf was conducted in conformance to ISO-10993 standards. Tests performed included: (1) general safety test; (2) cytotoxicity; (3) sensitization; (4) intracutaneous reactivity/irritation; (5) systemic toxicity (acute and subacute); (6) subchronic toxicity; and (7) hemocompatibility. This testing paradigm did not reveal any findings of significant biological concern. Subcutaneous administration of Apligraf into rabbits resulted in implantation site reactions, likely due to the xenogeneic immune response. Additional toxicology studies were not conducted due to the nature of GINTUIT and the extensive clinical experience with Apligraf.

The product used in clinical studies submitted to the BLA was manufactured in the same way as Apligraf, a product that had been approved under a PMA. Apligraf was approved by FDA for the treatment of venous leg ulcers (VLU) on May 22, 1998, and for the treatment of diabetic foot ulcers (DFU) that had not healed with conventional therapies on June 20, 2000. While the regulatory experience of the approved PMA was considered, this application was reviewed according to the regulatory requirements for a BLA.

MACI (autologous cultured chondrocytes on porcine collagen membrane) from Vericel Corp. is an autologous cellularized scaffold biologic-device combination product indicated for the repair of single or multiple symptomatic, full-thickness cartilage defects of the knee with or without bone involvement in adults. MACI consists of autologous cultured chondrocytes (biologic constituent) seeded onto a resorbable porcine Type I/III collagen membrane (device constituent). The cells are isolated from patient's cartilage biopsy taken from non-load-bearing regions of the knee, expanded in culture, and seeded onto the ACI-Maix Collagen membrane manufactured by Matricel GmbH. The assembled construct yielded the DP, MACI, which was released based on predefined criteria for safety and quality.

Implantation of ACI-Maix porcine membrane seeded with homologous (animal-derived) cultured chondrocytes and secured with a commercially available fibrin sealant resulted in an improved repair of critical-sized defects in the knee/stifle of rabbits and horses, compared to implanted membrane alone or empty defect. There were no significant local or systemic safety signals identified in the animals. Mild inflammation was observed in the knees of both species, which resolved over time. The ACI-Maix membrane was still present in both species at 6 months post-implant, and microscopic fibers from the membrane were noted out to 53 weeks in the horses. In the 53-week horse study, any observed lameness was mild in nature and occurred early (12 weeks) in approximately 50% of all animals in each group, with full gait recovery by 53 weeks in all animals. A trend toward improved cartilage repair for the defects implanted with chondrocyte-seeded ACI-Maix compared to the ACI-Maix-implanted defects and the empty defects was observed at 12 and 53 weeks. Improved biomechanical testing outcomes were observed in some of the defects implanted with chondrocyte-seeded ACI-Maix compared to defects implanted with ACI-Maix membrane alone or empty defects. However, the biomechanical properties of the cartilage defects implanted with chondrocyte-seeded ACI-Maix were not identical to native cartilage. Studies to evaluate the carcinogenicity, developmental/reproductive toxicity, or impairment of fertility potential of MACI were not performed. However, biocompatibility testing of the ACI-Maix porcine membrane showed that the collagen membrane was not toxic or incompatible with biological tissue. In addition, the expansion process for chondrocytes did not induce changes to the cellular karyotype.

There were multiple post-marketing commitments relating to quantitation and appropriate validation of the methods on the ACI-Maix collagen membrane quality.

25.10.3 Genetically Modified Chimeric Antigen Receptor T-Cell Products

The key take-home for these five products for indications in hematologic malignancies is that there is little translational value in the preclinical studies with respect to the translation of dose. The preclinical studies are conducted as hybrid pharmacology/toxicology studies generally in tumor-bearing NSG mice and duration is limited to avoid GVHD. For this class of product, the off-target binding to human cells is the most relevant preclinical assessment for safety. Post-approval, all five products were required to implement a Risk Evaluation Mitigation Strategy (REMS) with Elements To Assure Safe Use (ETASU) for the management of cytokine release syndrome and neurologic toxicity, training and assessment of sites and the use of tocilizumab and a 15-year observational study to assess the short- and long-term toxicities.

KYMRIAH (tisagenlecleucel) from Novartis Pharmaceuticals Corp. is a CD19-directed genetically modified autologous T-cell immunotherapy intended for two indications: (1) patients up to 25 years of age with B-cell precursor acute lymphoblastic leukemia (ALL) that is refractory or in second or later relapse and (2) adult patients with relapsed or refractory (r/r) large B-cell lymphoma after two or more lines of systemic therapy, including diffuse large B-cell lymphoma (DLBCL) not otherwise specified, high grade B-cell lymphoma, and DLBCL arising from follicular lymphoma. The product is comprised of genetically modified antigen-specific autologous T cells reprogrammed to target cells that express CD19. CD19 is an antigen expressed on the surface of B cells and tumors derived from B cells. The CAR protein has a murine anti-CD19 single-chain antibody fragment (scFv) and signaling domains (CD3-ζ) and 4-1BB. These intracellular signaling domains play critical roles in KYMRIAH functions, including T-cell activation, persistence *in vivo*, and antitumor activity. The autologous T cells are genetically modified with a lentiviral vector encoding a CAR. The CAR specifically recognizes the CD19 protein present on CD19+ B lineage tumor cells as well as normal B cells. The presumed MOA is direct cytolytic killing of tumor cells. Activation of the CAR T cells also promotes cell expansion and differentiation.

Manufacturing risks included manufacturing failures, the theoretical concern for replication-competent lentivirus (RCL) as well as the potential risk for insertional mutagenesis. In the clinical study, there was an approximately 9% failure rate due to either termination of manufacturing or out-of-specification results. At the time of review, no RCL had been detected in any clinical trials using a lentiviral vector-transduced cell product, as tested on the vector product with a sensitive co-culture RCL assay or on the final transduced cell product with the same RCL assay or a PCR-based RCL assay. Insertional mutagenesis due to vector integration is a potential risk for inducing secondary malignancies. Integration of the vector into the patient's cells might inadvertently activate a cellular proto-oncogene or disrupt a tumor suppressor gene, leading to malignant transformation events. To mitigate the risk of insertional mutagenesis, the vector used for KYMRIAH manufacturing was designed to remove any known viral enhancer elements (self-inactivating design). In addition, the average vector copy number per cell was limited.

The nonclinical studies included (1) evaluation of the specificity of the CD19-binding domain using a human plasma membrane protein array, (2) assessment of *in vivo* antitumor activity of KYMRIAH in mouse xenograft tumor models, (3) evaluation of selected toxicology parameters, cell distribution, and persistence of KYMRIAH in tumor-bearing mice, and (4) genomic insertion site analysis of lentiviral integration into the human genome. The genomic insertion site analysis was performed from 14 individual donors (two healthy donors and 12 patients with pediatric ALL or DLBCL). The transduced samples exhibited conventional lentivirus integration site patterns with no preferential insertion sites near genes of concern or clonality observed. Genotoxicity assays, *in vivo* carcinogenicity studies, and developmental and reproductive toxicity (DART) studies were not conducted. No safety concerns were identified in the resulting data from the nonclinical studies. No new nonclinical pharmacology/toxicology information was included in the supplement to support the indication of relapsed/refractory DLBCL.

There was no apparent relationship between preexisting or treatment-induced anti-mCAR19 antibodies on the cellular kinetics or impact on response or relapse.

A meeting of FDA's AC was held on July 12, 2017. The AC agreed that the risk-mitigation measures in the study were reasonable, did not express concern about testing for RCL; however, they considered insertional mutagenesis to be a potential risk, and discussion centered on the planned 15-year follow-up post-marketing observational trial. The BLA was approved with post-marketing requirements.

YESCARTA (axicabtagene ciloleucel) from Kite Pharma, Inc. is a CD19-directed genetically modified autologous T-cell immunotherapy indicated for the treatment of adult patients with relapsed or refractory large B-cell lymphoma after two or more lines of systemic therapy, including DLBCL not otherwise specified, primary mediastinal large B-cell lymphoma, high-grade B-cell lymphoma, and DLBCL arising from follicular lymphoma. The product is comprised of genetically modified, antigen-specific autologous T cells reprogrammed to target cells that express CD19. CD19 is an antigen expressed on the surface of B cells and tumors derived from B cells. The YESCARTA CAR protein has a murine single-chain variable fragment (scFv) with specificity for CD19 linked to two signaling domains derived from human CD3-ζ and CD28 genes. The CAR protein plays a critical role in YESCARTA function, including T-cell activation and antitumor activity. The autologous T cells were transduced with a retroviral vector containing a CAR directed against human CD19, an antigen expressed by most B-cell malignancies as well as all normal B lymphocytes in peripheral blood and spleen. For the production of YESCARTA, a patient's own T cells are harvested and genetically modified ex vivo by transduction using a γ-retroviral construct encoding an anti-CD19 CAR. The anti-CD19 CAR consists of a single-chain variable region fragment (scFv) derived from a CD19-specific monoclonal antibody, CD28 elements (i.e., and CD3 ζ.)

The manufacturing process begins by enriching the patient's apheresis material for lymphocytes and activating the patient's T cells during a defined culture period in the presence of human IL-2 IL-2) and anti-CD3 antibody (anti-CD3 Ab). The patient's T cells are then transduced with a retroviral vector expressing an anti-CD19 CAR and expanded. YESCARTA is cryopreserved and stored at not greater than −150°C. It is shipped in a vapor phase liquid nitrogen dry shipper (dewar) to the clinical infusion center by a qualified courier. The chain-of-identity of the entire process from leukapheresis to infusion and throughout all manufacturing steps is controlled by a computer-based system to ensure the product's identity and product traceability. Generation of replication-competent retrovirus (RCR) during the manufacturing process for YESCARTA is a theoretical safety concern. To date, no RCR has been detected.

Co-culture of anti-CD19 CAR T cells derived from peripheral blood mononuclear cells obtained from patients with NHL demonstrated CD19-specific induction of multiple cytokines, chemokines, and effector molecules. To evaluate CD19-specific antitumor activity *in vivo*, an analogous murine CAR construct recognizing the murine CD19 molecule was evaluated in a lymphodepleted syngeneic mouse model of CD19+ B-cell lymphoma. Following intravenous injection of murine T cells expressing the anti-murine CD19 CAR into the mice, tumors were eliminated (i.e., lymphoma cells were undetectable) and animal survival was extended. However, the depletion of normal B cells (i.e., B-cell aplasia) also occurred, but no effect on overall animal health was observed (Kochenderfer et al. 2010). No *in vitro* or *in vivo* genotoxicity and carcinogenicity assessments for YESCARTA were conducted. To address the risk of retroviral vector insertional mutagenesis and potential carcinogenicity/tumorigenicity, the sponsor performed a review of published nonclinical and clinical information reported for T cells transduced with retroviral vectors. The data suggested that T cells are relatively resistant to malignant transformation by retroviral vectors. No animal DART studies were conducted with YESCARTA to assess whether the product can cause embryo or fetal harm when administered to women of childbearing potential.

The product was approved with similar warnings and post-marketing requirements as KYMRIAH.

TECARTUS (brexucabtagene autoleucel) from Kite Pharma, Inc. is a CD19-directed genetically modified autologous T-cell immunotherapy indicated for the treatment of adult patients with relapsed/refractory mantle cell lymphoma (r/r MCL). The TECARTUS CAR protein has a murine single-chain variable fragment (scFv) specific to human CD19 linked to two signaling domains derived from human CD28 and CD3ζ. The CAR protein plays a critical role in TECARTUS function, mediating T-cell activation and antitumor effector function following binding of the scFv to CD19. The CAR expressed in TECARTUS is identical to that in YESCARTA (axicabtagene ciloleucel), but differs from YESCARTA in that T cells are enriched during the TECARTUS manufacturing process; T-cell enrichment is not performed during YESCARTA manufacture.

The TECARTUS manufacturing process begins with the collection of apheresis material from patients at qualified apheresis centers. The apheresis material is shipped to the Kite Pharma manufacturing facility, where it is processed via washing, followed by the enrichment of T cells. Enriched T cells are then activated using anti-CD3 and anti-CD28 mAbs in the presence of IL-2. Activated T cells are then transduced with the vector and expanded in culture until sufficient anti-CD19 CAR-T cells are available to meet dose requirements. The culture is then harvested and washed. The DP is formulated in saline/human serum albumin (HSA)/CryoStor® infusible cryopreservation solution. Each dose is comprised of a fixed number of anti-CD19 CAR-T cells calculated based on viable cell count (determined by CAR expression) and patient body weight. Formulated DP is filled into cryopreservation bags, with each bag containing one dose in a 68 ml nominal volume.

Doses of TECARTUS are produced from each manufacturing run. Filled DP bags are cryopreserved and stored at ≤ −150°C in vapor-phase liquid nitrogen until lot release testing is complete. Released DP is then shipped frozen to qualified treatment sites for administration back to the same patient.

A theoretical safety concern in the TECARTUS manufacturing process is the generation of RCR. No RCR has been detected in any clinical studies of TECARTUS or YESCARTA, which is manufactured using the same vector.

In vitro characterization included demonstration of CD19-dependent cytotoxicity, cytokine release, and proliferation when co-cultured with tumor cell lines expressing CD19. Additionally, an *in vivo* study conducted using an analogous murine CAR construct recognizing the murine CD19 molecule demonstrated antitumor activity and increased survival in a lymphodepleted syngeneic adoptive transfer mouse model of CD19+ B-cell lymphoma. These studies indicated that the CAR-T cells could target normal B cells; however, no other effects on the overall health of the animals were observed. Traditional *in vitro* and *in vivo* genotoxicity and carcinogenicity/tumorigenicity assessments were not conducted. Published clinical and nonclinical data derived from different CAR-T products supported a relatively low risk for malignant transformation of T cells by retroviral vectors. Additionally, vector integration analysis conducted using a similar product, which used the same retroviral vector and anti-CD19 CAR transgene, found the integration profile consistent with published data for similar vectors. No animal reproductive and developmental toxicity studies were conducted, which is acceptable based on the product characteristics and safety profile.

The product received an accelerated approval and the same warnings and post-marketing requirements.

BREYANZI (lisocabtagene maraleucel) from Juno Therapeutics, Inc., a Bristol-Myers Squibb Company, is a CD19-directed genetically modified autologous T-cell immunotherapy for the treatment of adult patients with relapsed or refractory large B-cell lymphoma after two or more lines of systemic therapy, including DLBCL not otherwise specified (including DLBCL arising from indolent lymphoma), high-grade B-cell lymphoma, primary mediastinal large B-cell lymphoma, and follicular lymphoma grade 3B. The product has a defined composition of CAR-positive viable T cells (consisting of separate CD8 and CD4 DPs). The CAR is comprised of the FMC63 monoclonal antibody-derived single-chain variable fragment (scFv), IgG4 hinge region CD28 transmembrane domain, 4-1BB (CD137) costimulatory domain, and CD3 zeta activation domain. In addition, BREYANZI includes a nonfunctional truncated epidermal growth factor receptor (EGFRt) that is co-expressed on the cell surface with the CD19-specific CAR. Vector integration poses a risk for insertional mutagenesis and through the activation of proto-oncogenes or disruption of tumor suppressor genes has the potential to cause secondary malignancies. To mitigate the risk of insertional mutagenesis, the vector used for BREYANZI manufacturing was designed to remove any known viral enhancer elements (self-inactivating design). Insertion-site analysis did not identify any areas of increased or preferred integration.

In vitro pharmacology studies support the purported MOA of BREYANZI by showing cytokine release, CAR-T-cell expansion, and tumor cell cytotoxicity following exposure to CD19-expressing cancer cells. Additional *in vitro* studies showed that BREYANZI, in combination with various small-molecule drugs demonstrated antitumor activity. Dose-dependent antitumor activity and improved animal survival were demonstrated in immunocompromised rodent models engrafted with CD19-expressing tumor cells following the administration of BREYANZI. Animal studies to assess the long-term safety of BREYANZI were limited because BREYANZI did not survive in immunocompetent rodents and induced GVHD in immunocompromised mice. Studies performed against a panel of normal human tissues showed that on-target/off-tumor and nonspecific recognition against off-target tissues are not a major safety concern. *In vivo* studies in tumor-bearing murine models showed a significant reduction of BREYANZI following the administration of cetuximab; thus, the administration of antibodies targeting the truncated EGFR domain on the surface of BREYANZI may reduce/eliminate the CAR-T cells *in vivo*. The risk of insertional mutagenesis with lentiviral transduction of the T cells, leading to malignant transformation, was studied using unbiased, genome-wide bioinformatics methods. The resulting data demonstrated that the lentivirus used to manufacture BREYANZI did not preferentially integrate at specific genomic sites of concern for oncogenic transformation. In addition, long-term cellular growth assays evaluating the purity and identity profile of BREYANZI suggested that no shift in cellular phenotype due to clonal expansion occurred over time. These data supported the conclusion that any insertional events resulting from lentiviral transduction methods used to generate BREYANZI had a minimal risk for oncogenic transformation. No animal reproductive and developmental toxicity studies were conducted with BREYANZI, which is acceptable based on the product characteristics and safety profile. BREYANZI was approved on February 5, 2021.

ABECMA (idecabtagene vicleucel) from Celgene, a Bristol-Myers Squibb Company, is a B-cell maturation antigen (BCMA)-directed genetically modified (via Lentiviral vector) autologous T-cell immunotherapy indicated for the treatment of adult patients with relapsed or refractory multiple myeloma after four or more prior lines of therapy, including an immunomodulatory agent, a proteasome inhibitor, and an anti-CD38 monoclonal antibody was approved in March 2021. It was approved with similar warnings and post-marketing requirements.

25.11 Special Issues: Case Examples

The section provides cases in retinal diseases to illustrate key points in development in some of the investigational products undergoing development. Although the retinal diseases have different etiologies, the end result is the loss of photoreceptors (PRs). Since currently available treatments, such as the delivery of neurotrophic factors or anti-angiogenic agents, can delay the onset or slow the deterioration of visual impairment, extensive research efforts have focused on the development of novel therapeutic strategies, including cell therapies, that could result in longer duration benefit. The eye is a good target for such an approach because it is easily accessible, small (i.e.,

low volume of cells would be sufficient for therapy), compartmentalized (i.e., permit specific targeting of different ocular tissues) and separated from the rest of the body by the blood-retinal barrier (i.e., ensure ocular immune privilege and minimal systemic dissemination). In addition, the development of high resolution and noninvasive imaging approaches, such as optical coherence tomography and adaptive optics, is of value in evaluating the retinal changes after treatments.

The three main types of cells that are currently being evaluated as potential therapeutics to treat retinal disease are hESCs, human induced pluripotent stem cells (hiPSCs), and adult stem cells. Examples of two cell types are provided below.

25.11.1 Age-Related Macular Degeneration (dry) – hESC-Derived Product

hESCs are being used as a starting point to generate new retinal pigment epithelium on a synthetic scaffold, to replace cells that are lost and lead to vision loss, with clinical trials actively enrolling and implanting patients (Thomas et al. 2016, Kashani et al. 2018, 2019, 2020).

Age-related macular degeneration (AMD) is a degenerative retinal disease associated with aging and the condition affects the macula region of the retina required for sharp central vision. The disease results in a progressive loss of vision in a patient's central visual field and is the leading cause of blindness in older people. The pathophysiology is the damage to the retinal pigment epithelial (RPE) layer, which is a single layer of polarized cells directly beneath the PRs, which are the rods and cones. The RPE layer transports nutrients between choroid blood vessels and PR and plays a key role in the visual cycle. It phagocytoses shed PR membranes every morning powered by light, which is essential for PR renewal. Without RPE, the PR cannot survive or function. Another critical structure in AMD is Bruch's membrane, which separates the choroid vascular bed and RPE. The Bruch's membrane thickens with age, which leads to an accumulation of deposits and drusen, causing breakdown of the membrane. Vision loss in AMD is a secondary effect due to dysfunction /loss of RPE eventually leading to death of PR in the macula. Therapeutic approaches including transplanted cell suspensions may fail to attach to a defective Bruch's membrane, and alternative approaches include the manufacture of an artificial membrane.

In a preclinical rat model in which hESC-derived RPE attached to a parylene substrate was implanted into the eye of a rat, results demonstrated that the cells were nonproliferative; did not migrate and remained at the site of implantation; showed increased neurotrophic growth factor secretion from the apical surface; secreted vascular endothelial growth factor (VEGF) specifically from the basal surface to promote choriocapillaris survival; integrated with PR outer segments, promoting efficient phagocytosis of reactive oxygen species; were more resistant to stress; and had apical and basal domains that promoted appropriate transport functions. A histological cross-section of the orbit from the implanted rat showed the parylene substrate with hESC-RPE interdigitated and the RPE remained localized. An electron micrograph demonstrated that the transplanted RPE were functional in that they phagocytosed the discarded PR outer segments.

Manufacturing processes were locked-in for Phase 1 clinical production and included source of cells with master, working and intermediate cell banks released; reagents that were sourced with no animal sourced reagents; qualification of processes with manufacturing qualification and engineering runs executed, and release testing with critical assays qualified. The hESC-derived RPE had properties of normal healthy RPE, including phenotypic markers of RPE cells; produce pigment; polarize on parylene membrane; produce visual cycle proteins; form tight junctions; do not migrate; secrete pigment epithelium-derived factor (PEDF) from the apical surface to promote PR survival; secrete VEGF from the basal surface to promote choriocapillaris survival, and integrate with PR outer segments to promote an efficient phagocytosis of reactive oxygen species. Parylene membrane support for the cells was designed to mimic the permeability of Bruch's membrane. It provided a healthy substrate for RPE cells to attach and polarize; was fabricated with USP Class VI biocompatible parylene monomer; excellent thermal and mechanical properties; used >30 years in implantables; machined to precise thickness to accommodate required diffusion properties similar to Bruch's membrane; provides flat surface without numerous pores for optimal cell attachment; and allows folding to reduce incision size in sclera and retina, thus increasing safety.

Major IND enabling studies included the efficacy and local toxicity studies; tumorigenicity, systemic toxicity and biodistribution study; pig delivery study; human postmortem eye delivery study, and a CPCB-RPE1 injector loading-unloading study. Results demonstrated improved visual function in Royal College of Surgeons Rats model (an animal model of inherited retinal degeneration); induces PR rescue; performs rod outer segment phagocytosis; does not induce teratomas or tumor formation; has a good toxicity profile; is biocompatible with CPCB-RPE1 insertion forceps; and can be delivered to the pig and human subretinal space safely.

Infrared fundus photography, spectral-domain optical coherence tomography (SD-OCT) imaging, and histology after implantation in the pig subretinal space demonstrated good survival of RPE, proper placement in subretinal space, and no evidence of detachments. In the human cadaveric study, 10/10 human cadaveric eyes underwent successful implantation of CPCB-RPE1, and there was no significant RPE cell loss (<2%) on implant during delivery procedure; surgical delivery of CPCB-RPE1 to the human subretinal space is feasible with custom tool, and known surgical methods and loading and unloading did not increase the number of dead cells on the CPCB-RPE1 implant (Thomas et al. 2016, Kashani et al. 2018, 2019, 2020).

Preclinical data demonstrated the value of two species (rat and pig) for dose extrapolation, the need for tumorigenicity assessment, and the use of large animal as well as human cadaver eyes for the development of the surgical procedure and surgical device tool utilized.

25.11.2 Age-related Macular Degeneration (wet) – iPSC-Derived Product

From Shinya Yamanaka's group in Japan, a clinical study utilizing autologous iPSC-derived RPE cell sheets (generated as a monolayer of cells without any artificial scaffolds) was initiated through Japan's Regenerative Medicine Pathway launched in 2014. In July 2015, the investigator placed the clinical study on hold after one patient had been treated, to evaluate genomic mutation in the cell product from a second patient (Mandai et al. 2017). The investigators subsequently decided not to continue the study.

There had been extensive testing prior to the launch of the clinical trial in 2014 (Kuroda et al. 2012, Assawachanananont et al. 2014, Kamao et al. 2014, Kanemura et al. 2014). The hiPSC-RPE clinical product had been assessed by a range of assessments: assessment of phenotype, i.e., pigmentation, markers of RPE as well as for undifferentiated hiPSCs by qRT-PCR assay that detects 0.002% residual iPSCs (LIN28A), and demonstration of reproducibility with the assessment of gene expression in hiPSC-RPE from 12 patients. Preclinical functional assessment was demonstrated by growth factor secretion, tight junction formation *in vitro*, and efficacy in an animal model of disease (Royal College of Surgeon rats). Safety testing of the hiPSC-derived RPE product to be used in the clinic included studies on immunogenicity and tumorigenicity. The immunogenicity studies included the assessment of MHC I and II (± gamma interferon), mixed lymphocyte reaction, and assessment using implantation in monkeys. The allogeneic implants were rejected (n=3) and an autologous implant persisted for 1 year (n=1). The tumorigenicity studies assessed hiPSCs obtained from six patients and included quality control testing performed on hiPSCs and hiPSC-RPE, and subcutaneous implantation in immunodeficient NOG mice. The investigators tested hiPSC-RPE from three patients, in which they implanted 1×10^6 hiPSC-RPE cells in Matrigel and monitored for tumor formation for up to 64 weeks. In a subretinal implantation (nude rats), they administered $0.8–1.5 \times 10^4$ hiPSC-RPE cells in sheets with hiPSC-RPE from five patients and monitored for tumor formation up to 82 weeks.

Preclinical data demonstrated the morphological properties, *in vitro* and *in vivo* function, gene expression and immunogenicity of authentic RPE, as well as the structural rigidity needed to withstand mechanical stress associated with the transplant procedure.

25.12 FDA Expedited Programs and Interactions

Many of the cell therapies have had success with expedited programs and faster, smoother reviews. The incentive and expedited programs include Orphan product designation and approval (also rare pediatric disease designation and priority review vouchers), priority review, accelerated approval, Fast Track and Breakthrough Therapy Designation (BTD). These programs are available for drug and biologics development; a program unique to regenerative medicine was created in 2016. See Chapter 5 for more on expedited programs.

The 21st Century Cures Act was passed by Congress in December 2016 and included several sections designed to facilitate the development of cell and gene therapies. These included Section 3033 that created a program for the designation of regenerative medicine advanced therapies (RMAT); Section 3034 that mandated guidance regarding devices used in the recovery, isolation, or delivery of regenerative advanced

TABLE 25.3

RMAT Designations between 2017 and March 2021

Fiscal Year	Total Requests Received	Granted	Denied	Withdrawn
2017	31	11	18	2
2018	47	18	27	2
2019	37	17	18	2
2020	34	12	22	0
2021	6	1	2	1

therapies; and Section 3036 focused on efforts to facilitate the development of standards for regenerative medicine therapies.

A drug is eligible for RMAT designation if it is a regenerative medicine therapy that is intended to treat, modify, reverse, or cure a serious or life-threatening disease or condition, and preliminary clinical evidence indicates that it has the potential to address unmet medical needs for such disease or condition. The products within the scope of RMAT includes cell therapies, therapeutic tissue engineering products, human cell and tissue products, combination products associated with the above, and through FDA interpretation by guidance also includes gene therapies, including genetically modified cells that lead to a durable modification of cells or tissues. Potential benefits from RMAT designation include interactions with FDA to expedite development and review of these therapies. The benefits from an RMAT designation are similar to the benefits from a BTD, which can include early discussions with FDA of a proposed potential surrogate or intermediate endpoint to support accelerated approval. The designated products are eligible as appropriate for priority review and accelerated approval, and an expansion of ways to fulfill post-approval requirements under accelerated approval.

The first designation came in 1 day after 21st Century Cures Act was signed into law December 2016. 59 products have been granted designation – 11/31 in 2017, 18/47 in 2018, 17/37 in 2019, 12/34 in 2020, and 1/6 by February 2021. Most are cellular therapy products or cell-based gene therapy products. As of February 2021, there have been 155 RMAT requests and 59 granted designation. Breyanzi is the first RMAT designated product to receive FDA approval. Of note, Breyanzi had also received BTD. Table 25.3 provides the RMAT results over time.

In comparison, as of February 2021, the FDA has approved 201 BTD products, which encompass a broader spectrum of products, and the program had been running since 2012. There have been 1,111 total requests for the designation with 436 designations granted.

An early type of discussion with the FDA is the INitial Targeted Engagement for Regulatory Advice on CBER producTs (INTERACT) meeting (formerly called a pre-pre-IND meeting),[11] frequently encouraged and available for novel cellular and gene therapy approaches, which are reviewed in OTAT. This INTERACT discussion, focused primarily on manufacturing and preclinical issues, and most often conducted by teleconference, is not part of the IND meeting process, i.e., not a PDUFA (User Fee tracked) Type A, B or C meeting. There is a 90-day time frame to schedule these interactions, and this dialogue was created to offer general guidance to sponsors for their IND-enabling preclinical program. An INTERACT meeting does not replace the ability of a sponsor to request a pre-IND meeting with the FDA. An INTERACT meeting provides an opportunity to ask FDA questions and advice on different areas of product development plans, including manufacturing, the range of preclinical studies required to support clinical trials, and high-level clinical trial study design options appropriate for the proposed clinical indication. Approximately 30% of requests for an INTERACT meeting are granted. Meetings are denied either due to the stage of development being premature for discussion, or on the other extent, sufficient progress in development has already been achieved such that a pre-IND meeting is more appropriate.[12]

CBER Advanced Technology Team (CATT) is an interactive mechanism for discussion of advanced technologies or platforms needed for the development of CBER-regulated biologics products; CATT allows access to early and ongoing interactions with CBER before filing of a regulatory submission. The primary focus for CATT is on platforms for manufacturing.[13]

25.12.1 Recent Trends

In 2018, the number of INDs had doubled to 206, and as of 2020 CBER has over 1,000 active cell and gene therapy INDs, a tripling of INDs over the previous 3 years. Former FDA Commissioner Scott Gottlieb and current CBER Center Director Peter Marks in 2019 had noted the potential approval of 10–20 cell and gene therapy products per year starting in 2025, with a prediction of 40–60 product launches and more than 500,000 treated by 2030.[14] It is too soon to predict whether the COVID-19 pandemic and its impact on supply chain manufacturing issues, the work force, and clinical trials implementation and conduct will alter the 2019 modeling predictions.

Clinical Trials[15] facts and figures from 2020 revealed over 1,078 regenerative medicine clinical trials, with the following distribution:

Phase 1 – 394 with 109 in gene therapy, 230 in gene-modified cell therapy, 49 in cell therapy, and 6 in tissue engineering;

---

[11] Very early-type meetings with a follow-up pre-IND meeting initially only readily available in OTAT, are recently now available across CBER, but are much less common in other Centers of the FDA.

[12] Further details on the INTERACT meeting can be found on the FDA website https://www.fda.gov/vaccines-blood-biologics/industry-biologics/interact-meetings-initial-targeted-engagement-regulatory-advice-cber-products.

[13] Further details on CATT can be found on the FDA website https://www.fda.gov/vaccines-blood-biologics/industry-biologics/cber-advanced-technologies-team-catt.

[14] MIT NEWDIGS Research Brief 2018F210-v027-Launches.

[15] Alliance for Regenerative Medicine website 2020.

Phase 2 – 587 with 215 in gene therapy, 225 in gene-modified cell therapy, 125 in cell therapy, and 22 in tissue engineering; and

Phase 3 – 97 with 35 in gene therapy, 16 in gene-modified cell therapy, 30 in cell therapy, and 16 in tissue engineering.

By therapeutic area, 665 (62%) of all current clinical trials are in oncology, including leukemia, lymphoma, and cancers of the brain, breast, bladder, cervix, colon, esophagus, ovaries, pancreas, and others; and 5% (58) are in musculoskeletal disorders, including muscular dystrophies, spinal muscular atrophy, osteoarthritis, degenerative disc disease, bone and cartilage defects, and others.

25.13 Controversies

US House of Representatives on May 22, 2018, passed the Senate's 2017 version of national "right to try" legislation, which was signed by the President of the USA on May 30, 2018. This law, entitled the Trickett Wendler, Frank Mongiello, Jordan McLinn, and Matthew Bellina Right to Try Act of 2017 (s 4788), created a federal framework for patients to access investigational new DPs outside of clinical trials and outside of the US Food and Drug Administration's already-existing expanded access programs. The federal law comes in the wake of a majority of states passing their own right-to-try laws, starting with Arizona in 2014. This was based on the tension between autonomy of choice for patients vs. oversight for the public good. The basic parameters of the federal law include the following:

Anyone "with a life threatening disease or condition…who has exhausted approved treatment options and is unable to participate in a clinical trial"; Eligibility must be "certified" by a treating physician who "will not be compensated directly by the manufacturer for so certifying"…., and "Investigational drugs" that the legislation would make available must have completed a preliminary "phase 1 trial" and must be under active "investigation in a clinical trial that is intended to form the primary basis of a claim of effectiveness in support of approval or licensure."

However, manufacturers are not obligated to provide their investigational products, and insurers are not obligated to pay. To date, it is not clear how many patients or manufacturers will agree to engage in this program, outside of the context of the already-established expanded access program with oversight by the FDA. To date, there is very little public information of the use of access through the Right to Try Act. In July 2020, to facilitate the implementation of the reporting requirements of the Trickett Wendler, Frank Mongiello, Jordan McLinn, and Matthew Bellina Right to Try Act of 2017 (Right to Try Act), the FDA is proposing to establish requirements for the deadline and contents of submission of an annual summary. This proposed rule, if finalized, would implement the statutory requirement under provisions of the Right to Try Act for submission of an annual summary by sponsors and manufacturers who provide an eligible investigational drug for use by an eligible patient.

Stem cell clinics and stem cell tourism of unproven treatments continues. The Institute of Medicine, the International Society for Stem Cell Research, and other professional organizations and regulatory bodies have opined on this issue, including specific examples of risk (Thirabanjasak et al. 2010, Berkowitz et al. 2016, Kuriyan et al. 2017, Marks et al. 2017). Former FDA Commissioner Scott Gottlieb stated new policy steps in August 2017 and enforcement efforts to ensure proper oversight of stem cell therapies and regenerative medicine. To separate promise from unscrupulous hype, he noted stepped up enforcement activity. Incidents included: In California US Marshals Service seized five vials of Vaccinia Virus Vaccine (live) from California Stem Cell Treatment Centers in Rancho Mirage and Beverly Hills – FDA had serious concerns about how StemImmune obtained the product for use as part of an unapproved and potentially dangerous treatment); In Florida the FDA sent a warning letter and inspection to US Stem Cell Clinic) for marketing stem cell products without FDA approval, having significant deviations from cGMP, putting patients at risk (processing adipose tissue into stromal vascular fraction and administering IV or directly into the spinal cord). FDA Guidance documents continue to more clearly describe the rules of the road. In California law (bill SB 512) added section 684 to the Business and Professions Code, signed by Governor Brown October 2, 2017, and required posting in the clinic and a document provided to the patient stating provision of stem cell therapies have not yet been approved by FDA; required Medical Board of California to indicate in its annual report all of the following with regard to licensees who provide stem cell therapies – number of complaints received; any disciplinary actions take, and any administrative actions taken.

The International Society of Stem Cell Research has provided a list of questions and issues to consider for patients considering stem cell treatments, encompassing treatment, scientific evidence and oversight, procedures in place for monitoring safety and mitigating or tackling safety concerns, as well as addressing confidentiality and costs.[16] Responses to these questions can help discriminate the credible resources from those less reputable. In reference to stem cell clinics operating outside of regulatory oversight that provide unproven treatments, they provided the cautionary note that these clinics may state claims that are not supported by a current understanding of science, that patient testimonials and other marketing provided by such clinics may be misleading, and that an experimental treatment offered for sale is not the same as a clinical trial.

25.14 Timeline of Stem Cell Research

The timeline in Table 25.4 provides some of the key scientific and political aspects impacting on the advance of this field.

25.15 Summary and Conclusions

There has been a rapid growth of cell therapy approaches over the past decade, resulting in product approvals providing substantial advancements in the treatments of serious

---

[16] https://www.closerlookatstemcells.org/stem-cells-medicine/stem-cell-treatments-what-to-ask/

TABLE 25.4

Key Scientific and Political Aspects Impacting the Advancement of Stem Cell Research

Year	Noteworthy Event
1961	Till and McCulloch establish foundation for stem cell science
1974	Congress bans federally funded fetal tissue research until National Commission for Protection of Human Subjects of Biomedical and Behavioral Research devises guidelines; in 1975, the Guidelines establish Ethics Advisory Board for fetal and fetal tissue research that originates from abortions
1978	Clinical *in vitro* fertilization for infertile couples is taking place in the U.K, and occurs in the early 1980s for USA
1980	President Reagan does not renew the Ethics Advisory Board, which leads to de facto moratorium halting federal funding of human embryo research
1981	First Embryonic Stem Cells are isolated from mice
1988	Human Fetal Tissue Transplantation Research Panel votes to approve federal funding of embryo research; however, Department of Health and Human Services hears testimony stating embryonic research would lead to an increase in abortions, and the moratorium was extended.
1990	President George H.W. Bush vetoes congressional bill lifting the moratorium
1993	President Clinton signs an executive order removing the moratorium, but in 1994, although NIH human Embryo Research Panel recommends federal government funding, Clinton reverses order based on thousands of letters urging a halt
1995	Embryonic Stem Cells in Primate (Rhesus Monkey)
1997	Congress bans federal funding for research on embryos through Dickey-Wicker amendment, which has passed as a rider on other legislation, every year since 1997, that prohibits HHS/NIH funding for: *creation of a human embryo or embryos for research purposes; or research in which a human embryo or embryos are destroyed, discarded, or knowingly subjected to risk of injury or death...;* i.e., illegal for federal government to fund, but not for private citizens or non-federal funds to carry out research
1997	Dolly the sheep, first artificial animal cloned
1998	Human embryonic stem cells isolated and grown with private/nonfederal funding
1999	President's (Clinton) National Bioethics Advisory Commission again recommended that hESC harvested from embryos discarded after *in vitro* fertilization treatments be eligible for federal funding
1999	Chief Counsel Rabb, Department of Health and Human Services, writes a legal opinion that changes the Clinton Administration opinion and determines US policy; Federal Government cannot fund any destruction of embryos but can fund the research once the stem cells are created; e.g., stem cells do not meet statutory definition of an embryo
2000	NIH Guidelines for Research Using Human Pluripotent Stem Cells go into effect: hESC must be derived with private funds from frozen embryos from fertility clinics; must be created for fertility treatment purposes; must be in excess of the donor's clinical need; and must be obtained with consent of the donor
2001	President (Bush) Similar to Clinton's decision, NIH, could fund research on stem cells after they were created (no funding of embryo destruction); unlike Clinton's decision, these funds were limited to research on the already-established stem cell lines in which: The derivation process was initiated prior to August 9, 2001; must have been derived from embryo that was created for reproductive purposes and was no longer needed and informed consent must have been obtained
2004	California Proposition 71 authorizes the state to fund $3B on stem cell research: other state stem cell focused funding in NY, Maryland, Massachusetts, Connecticut; in November 2020 California Proposition 14 passed to authorize the state to fund $5.5B.
2005	National Academy of Sciences releases Guidelines for Human Embryonic Stem Cell Research, subsequent amendments, for a standard set of requirements for deriving, storing, distributing, and using embryonic stem cell lines.
2005	Fraudulent clones from the research of Woo Suk Hwang of Seoul National University S. Korea. Reported use of technique inspired by the one used to create Dolly the sheep, to create human embryonic stem cells genetically matched to specific people. His work later that year was shown to be false.
2006	International Society for Stem Cell Research releases "Guidelines for the Conduct of Human Embryonic Stem Cell Research," as well as subsequent guidelines for clinical translation
2006	Yamanaka of Kyoto University, Japan, pioneered a way of making embryonic-like cells from adult cells in the mouse, avoiding need to destroy an embryo, and called these new cells "induced pluripotent stem cells " (iPS)
2007	Yamanaka and Thomson independently derive human iPS cells. Utilized skin cells that had four genes inserted into them with viruses, resulting in skin cells acquiring properties similar to embryonic stem cells, and then coaxing them into beating heart cells and nerve cells
2009	President (Obama) issues Executive Order: Removing Barriers to Responsible Scientific Research Involving Human Stem Cells; however, he did not legalize Federal government funding of the creation of new hESC lines
2009	President Obama lifted the Bush restrictions, but also signed an appropriation bill extending the Dickey-Wicker Amendment, thus returning policy to that under the end of the Clinton Administration. In the years between Clinton and Obama, many other stem cell lines were created by private industry or states.
2010	Geron initiates the first clinical trial of hESC-based therapy for patients with spinal cord injury; FDA allows Advanced Cell Technology to test hESC-based therapy for patients with degenerative eye disease
2012	Yamanaka shares Nobel Prize with Gurdon for creating iPS cells
2013	Therapeutic Cloning of hESC from fetal cells by Mitalipov at Oregon National Primate Research Center, the breakthrough falsely claimed by Hwang in 2005
2014	False claims of simple method to rewind adult cell to an embryonic state – Vacanti, Harvard Medical School, and Obokata, Riken Center, Japan
2014	Takahashi at Riken Center, Japan, begins clinical study for first iPSC-based therapy for patients with age-related blindness
2017	First approvals for CAR-Ts in cancer and first approval for gene therapy for rare eye disease

diseases. Much has been learned and continues to evolve with new manufacturing technologies allowing for better defined cell types, and interactions with OTAT can be critical to help address challenges on the development pathway for these products, particularly in the areas of preclinical assessments. The 21st Century Cures Act sought to catalyze development of new medical technologies, including cell therapies, at a unique moment in time when fundamental advances in our understanding of the genetic and protein bases of diseases and advances in medical technology have enabled us to target, arrest, and in some cases have the potential to cure serious and life-threatening, life-disabling diseases.[17]

REFERENCES

Amariglio, N., A. Hirshberg, B. W. Scheithauer, et al. (2009). "Donor-derived brain tumor following neural stem cell transplantation in an ataxia telangiectasia patient." *PLoS Med* **6**(2): e1000029.

Appelbaum, F. R. (2007). "Hematopoietic-cell transplantation at 50." *N Engl J Med* **357**(15): 1472–1475.

Asahara, H. (2019). "Global Focus: Japan's Regenerative Medicine Regulatory Pathways Encouraging Innovation and Patient Access." https://www.fdli.org/2019/02/global-focus-japans-regenerative-medicine-regulatory-pathways-encouraging-innovation-and-patient-access/

Assawachanananont, J., M. Mandai, S. Okamoto, et al. (2014). "Transplantation of embryonic and induced pluripotent stem cell-derived 3D retinal sheets into retinal degenerative mice." *Stem Cell Reports* **2**(5): 662–674.

Berkowitz, A. L., M. B. Miller, S. A. Mir, et al. (2016). "Glioproliferative lesion of the spinal cord as a complication of "Stem-Cell Tourism"." *N Engl J Med* **375**(2): 196–198.

Cavagnaro, J. A. (2008). "Considerations in design of preclinical safety evaluation programs to support human cell-based therapies." *Preclinical Safety Evaluation of Biopharmaceuticals*: 749–781.

FDA (1991). "Points to consider in human somatic cell therapy and gene therapy (1991)." *Hum Gene Ther* **2**(3): 251–256.

FDA (1996). "Guidance on Applications for Products Comprised of Living Autologous Cells Manipulated Ex Vivo and Intended for Structural Repair or Reconstruction." *Federal Register.* https://www.govinfo.gov/content/pkg/FR-1996-05-28/pdf/96-13386

FDA (1997a). "Proposed Approach to Regulation of Cellular and Tissue-Based Products." https://www.fda.gov/regulatory-information/search-fda-guidance-documents/proposed-approach-regulation-cellular-and-tissue-based-products

FDA (1997b). "Proposed Approach to Regulation of Cellular and Tissue-Based Products; Availability and Public Meeting." *Federal Register.* https://www.federalregister.gov/documents/1997/03/04/97-5240/proposed-approach-to-regulation-of-cellular-and-tissue-based-products-availability-and-public

FDA (November 2019). American Society of Cell & Gene Therapy Presentation.

Gatti, R. A., H. J. Meuwissen, H. D. Allen, et al. (1968). "Immunological reconstitution of sex-linked lymphopenic immunological deficiency." *Lancet* **2**(7583): 1366–1369.

Gluckman, E. (2009). "History of cord blood transplantation." *Bone Marrow Transplant* **44**(10): 621–626.

Kamao, H., M. Mandai, S. Okamoto, et al. (2014). "Characterization of human induced pluripotent stem cell-derived retinal pigment epithelium cell sheets aiming for clinical application." *Stem Cell Rep* **2**(2): 205–218.

Kanemura, H., M. J. Go, M. Shikamura, et al. (2014). "Tumorigenicity studies of induced pluripotent stem cell (iPSC)-derived retinal pigment epithelium (RPE) for the treatment of age-related macular degeneration." *PLoS One* **9**(1): e85336.

Kashani, A. H., J. S. Lebkowski, F. M. Rahhal, et al. (2018). "A bioengineered retinal pigment epithelial monolayer for advanced, dry age-related macular degeneration." *Sci Transl Med* **10**(435): eaao4097. doi: 10.1126/scitranslmed.aao4097

Kashani, A. H., A. Martynova, M. Koss, et al. (2019). "Subretinal implantation of a human embryonic stem cell-derived retinal pigment epithelium monolayer in a porcine model." *Adv Exp Med Biol* **1185**: 569–574.

Kashani, A. H., J. Uang, M. Mert, et al. (2020). "Surgical method for implantation of a biosynthetic retinal pigment epithelium monolayer for geographic atrophy: experience from a Phase 1/2a study." *Ophthalmol Retina* **4**(3): 264–273.

Kessler, D. A., J. P. Siegel, P. D. Noguchi, et al. (1993). "Regulation of somatic-cell therapy and gene therapy by the food and drug administration." *N Engl J Med* **329**(16): 1169–1173.

Kochenderfer, J. N., Z. Yu, D. Frasheri, et al. (2010). "Adoptive transfer of syngeneic T cells transduced with a chimeric antigen receptor that recognizes murine CD19 can eradicate lymphoma and normal B cells." *Blood* **116**(19): 3875–3886.

Kuriyan, A. E., T. A. Albini, J. H. Townsend, et al. (2017). "Vision loss after intravitreal injection of autologous "Stem Cells" for AMD." *N Engl J Med* **376**(11): 1047–1053.

Kuroda, T., S. Yasuda, S. Kusakawa, et al. (2012). "Highly sensitive in vitro methods for detection of residual undifferentiated cells in retinal pigment epithelial cells derived from human iPS cells." *PLoS One* **7**(5): e37342.

Mandai, M., A. Watanabe, Y. Kurimoto, et al. (2017). "Autologous induced stem-cell-derived retinal cells for macular degeneration." *N Engl J Med* **376**(11): 1038–1046.

Marks, P. W., C. M. Witten and R. M. Califf (2017). "Clarifying stem-cell therapy's benefits and risks." *N Engl J Med* **376**(11): 1007–1009.

Sato, Y., H. Bando, M. Di Piazza, et al. (2019). "Tumorigenicity assessment of cell therapy products: The need for global consensus and points to consider." *Cytotherapy* **21**(11): 1095–1111.

Sun, C., C. Serra, G. Lee, et al. (2020). "Stem cell-based therapies for Duchenne muscular dystrophy." *Exp Neurol* **323**: 113086.

Thirabanjasak, D., K. Tantiwongse and P. S. Thorner (2010). "Angiomyeloproliferative lesions following autologous stem cell therapy." *J Am Soc Nephrol* **21**(7): 1218–1222.

Thomas, B. B., D. Zhu, L. Zhang, et al. (2016). "Survival and functionality of hESC-derived retinal pigment epithelium cells cultured as a monolayer on polymer substrates transplanted in RCS rats." *Invest Ophthalmol Vis Sci* **57**(6): 2877–2887.

Thomas, E. D., H. L. Lochte, Jr., W. C. Lu, et al. (1957). "Intravenous infusion of bone marrow in patients receiving radiation and chemotherapy." *N Engl J Med* **257**(11): 491–496.

Zakrzewski, W., M. Dobrzynski, M. Szymonowicz, et al. (2019). "Stem cells: Past, present, and future." *Stem Cell Res Ther* **10**(1): 68.

Zhang, Y. M., C. Hartzell, M. Narlow, et al. (2002). "Stem cell-derived cardiomyocytes demonstrate arrhythmic potential." *Circulation* **106**(10): 1294–1299.

---

[17] Paraphrasing remarks from the testimony of former FDA Commissioner Scott Gottlieb before the subcommittee on Health, Energy and Commerce Committee of the US House of Representatives, July 2018

26

Considerations in the Preclinical Development of Gene Therapy Products

Joy A. Cavagnaro
Access BIO, LC

CONTENTS

26.1 Introduction

New discoveries in the field of gene therapy have occurred at an aggressive pace with the hope of not only treating the symptoms of disease but actually providing a "cure" where correction of the defect would persist for the person's lifetime. The types of potential gene therapy products (i.e., product classes) include non-viral vectors (plasmid DNA and mRNA), viral vectors including oncolytic viruses (OV) carrying heterologous transgene(s), bacterial vectors, ex vivo genetically modified cells, and ex vivo and in vivo genome editing. Incorporation of genome editing technology to either correct endogenous disease-causing genes or to specifically target the integration of a therapeutic gene into a defined genetic locus has allowed the advancement of the field beyond gene addition strategies (Chapter 27). The early adverse events with γ-retroviral vectors prompted the shift to use of vectors based on lentivirus which have shown a better preclinical safety profile and more efficient gene delivery to non-dividing cells. Adeno-associated viral (AAV) vectors have gained the widest use as gene therapy vectors due to their non-pathogenic nature, their ability to drive long-term expression in non-dividing cells, and broad tropism of the many serotypes and variants (Flotte and Berns 2005).

The design of the preclinical toxicology studies for gene therapy products incorporates the basic principles used in the preclinical safety evaluation of small molecule (drugs) and large molecule (biologics). Importantly, similar to biologics, the practice of preclinical safety evaluation is based upon a "case-by-case" approach to program design, which takes into consideration not only the indication but also specific attributes of the product (Cavagnaro, 2002, 2008). The perceived challenge and sometimes reluctance to consider a "case-by-case" approach over a prescriptive approach is that since it does not align with a traditional, standardized, or "one-size-fits-all" approach, there is less predictability that a preclinical safety evaluation program will be acceptable to regulatory authorities. Thus, it is imperative to engage regulatory authorities early in planning to better understand the assessments needed for supporting a clinical development program to ensure phase-appropriate manufacturing and appropriate preclinical data to maximize safety and effectiveness of the initial clinical trials.

26.2 Definition of Gene Therapy

The first draft of the human genome sequence was published in 2001, with an estimate of 30,000–40,000 protein-coding sequences (Lander et al., 2001) with about 20–25,000 "haploid" protein-coding genes.

The US Food and Drug Administration (FDA) defines gene therapy as a medical intervention based on the modification of the genetic material of living cells. Cells may be modified ex vivo for subsequent administration to humans or may be altered in vivo by gene therapy given directly to the subject. When the genetic manipulation is performed ex vivo on cells which are then administered to the patient, this is also a form of somatic cell therapy. The genetic manipulation may be intended to have a therapeutic or prophylactic effect or may provide a way of marking cells for later identification. Recombinant DNA materials used to transfer genetic material for such therapy are considered components of gene therapy and as such are subject to regulatory oversight (FDA Guidance for Industry: Guidance for Human Somatic Cell Therapy and Gene Therapy, 1998).

In vivo gene transfer is the direct delivery of the gene therapy product into an animal or human. Direct injection can be *in situ*, i.e., delivered locally into the target tissue (intravitreal, intracerebral, intraarticular, intracardiac etc.), for cancer this may be intratumorally, or via systemic delivery usually intravenous. *Ex vivo* gene transfer is achieved by administering cells that are transduced with vectors that express the desired transgenes or tumor-associated antigens. These genetically modified calls can also be delivered directly to the desired target cell or tissue or delivered systemically.

From 1989 through the first half of 2000, 270 new gene transfer INDs were submitted to the FDA (Zoon, 2000) enrolling more than 4,000 subjects. A search of gene therapy in NIH US Library of Medicine Clinical Trials data base in September of 2020 (search ClinicalTrials.gov) listed over 4,500 ongoing or completed clinical trials. The various studies include but are not limited to gene therapy products intended to treat various genetic disorders, such as diseases due to inborn errors in a single defective gene (e.g., severe combined immunodeficiency (SCID), hemophilia, muscular dystrophy); polygenic diseases (e.g., diabetes mellitus or coronary heart disease); and acquired genetic diseases (e.g., rheumatoid arthritis, cancer). The various strategies include (1) insertion of a normal gene into a non-specific location on the genome to replace a nonfunctional gene, (2) exchanging an abnormal gene for a normal gene, (3) repair of the abnormal gene through selective reverse

mutation that returns the gene to its normal function, and (4) the regulation of a particular gene by turning it "on" or "off") (Serabian and Huang, 2008).

26.3 Historical Background

In a 1972 article in Science entitled "Gene Therapy for Human Disease," Friedmann and Roblin proposed that a sustained effort be made to formulate and develop a complete set of ethicoscientific criteria to guide the development and clinical application of gene therapy techniques. They further stated that such an endeavor could go a long way toward ensuring that gene therapy is used in humans only in those instances where it will prove beneficial, and toward preventing its misuse through premature application (Friedmann and Roblin, 1972).

The first gene therapy clinical trials in the USA began in the late 1980s with the ex vivo transduction of tumor-infiltrating lymphocytes (TIL) with a retroviral vector that carried the marker gene NeoR, administered to melanoma patients. In 1990, ex vivo autologous lymphocytes transduced with a retroviral vector expressing the ADA gene were administered to a child with ADA-SCID (SCID due to adenosine deaminase deficiency). The first trial involving the direct injection of a DNA plasmid occurred in 1992 with the administration of plasmid expressing HLA-B7 into HLA-B7-positive tumors. The first clinical trial using adenovirus (AV) vector occurred in cystic fibrosis patients in 1993 and was extended to the use of AAV vectors in this patient population in 1995. This was followed by an accelerated number of clinical trials with a variety of vectors, peaking in 1999 (Serabian and Huang 2008). However, the field of gene therapy was essentially halted with the death of Jesse Gelsinger, a 17-year-old with an ornithine transcarbamylase (OTC) deficiency, in September of 1999 following the intrahepatic infusion of an adenoviral vector expressing a normal OTC gene.

Following this incident, numerous public meetings were held in the USA to discuss perceived inadequacies in the scientific, ethical, and regulatory oversight of clinical trials involving gene therapy. As a result, regulatory oversight in the USA was increased, as well as wider assurance of public awareness and scientific and ethical discussions regarding this area of medical research through the Recombinant DNA Advisory Committee (RAC) (Serabian and Huang 2008). A key role of the RAC was to advise the NIH Director and the NIH Office of Biotechnology Activities (OBA), which is the NIH locus of oversight for recombinant DNA research.

The first successful administration of autologous ex vivo transduced hematopoietic stem cells for the treatment of children of SCID-XI disease was reported in a clinical trial in France (Cavazzana et al. 2000). Unfortunately, despite the initial reports of efficacy, several children developed a leukemia-like syndrome that was attributed to the combination of the integrating retrovirus and the gene. Again, the field of gene therapy took a pause to reevaluate the safety.

In 2001, as the field was beginning to recover with the potential use of AAV vectors for hemophilia, a clinical trial was halted following an infusion of an AAV vector containing the Factor IX gene into the liver of a patient with hemophilia

B where vector DNA was detected in semen. This result was unexpected since similar studies had been conducted in hemophilic dogs and had shown no evidence of vector DNA in semen. However, because of the risk of germline transmission (the possibility that the vector DNA would be transmitted to the subject's offspring), the field took another pause. In the weeks following the injection, the vector DNA signal in semen DNA gradually diminished and then disappeared, suggesting that the risk was likely short-term (High 2014). Importantly, it was shown that the vector DNA was present in the seminal fluid but not in DNA extracted from motile sperm, providing further reassurance about risks related to germline transmission (Manno et al. 2006).

In hindsight, the enthusiasm to "cure" disease should have more "critically" considered the biological complexity and current unknowns to highlight the increased potential for risks. But perhaps these were necessary events to shift toward better understanding the complexity of gene therapy to allow a refocus on safety.

Thirty-one years after Friedman and Robbins' seminal publication, the first gene therapy product, an adenoviral vector expressing the p53 gene (GENDICINE), was approved in China in 2003 for the treatment of head and neck cancer and a recombinant oncolytic AV (ONCORINE) also for the treatment of head and neck cancer in 2005. At this time these were the only approved gene therapy products globally. As previously mentioned, the 2009 "come-back of gene therapy" was propelled by the early successes in ocular and primary immune deficiency diseases. Three years later, in 2012, the European Medicines Agency (EMA) recommended the approval of GLYBERA (alipogene tiparvovec), an AAV1-based gene therapy as the first validation for a gene therapy treatment in either Europe or the USA. GLYBERA was designed to reverse lipoprotein lipase deficiency (LPLD), a rare inherited disorder that can cause severe pancreatitis. However, failure to gain approval in the USA led to its subsequent withdrawal from the EU market. In 2015, IMLYGIC (talimogene laherparepvec, T-VEC), a genetically modified herpes virus to treat melanoma, was approved in the USA and Europe. In the following year (2016), STRIMVELIS, an autologous CD34+ enriched cell fraction that contains CD34+ cells transduced with retroviral vector that encodes for the human ADA cDNA sequence, was the first ex vivo stem cell gene therapy approved in the EU to treat a rare disease for patients with ADA-SCID. Today only one site in Europe is currently approved for manufacture.

In 2017, KYMRIAH (tisagenlecleucel) became the first gene therapy approval in the USA. This new therapeutic approach of adoptive cell transfer was subsequently approved in the USA and EU in 2018 to treat B-cell acute lymphoblastic leukemia (ALL). Autologous T cells were genetically engineered to make a specific chimeric T-cell receptor ("CAR-T") and an antibody specific to a protein (CD19) that is common on B cells. YESCARTA (axicabtagene ciloleucel), using a similar approach, for large B-cell lymphoma, followed with approvals by FDA and EMA in 2017 and 2018, respectively. LUXTURNA (voretigene neparvovec-rzyl) was approved in the USA in 2017, as the first approval ever for an inherited genetic disease, a rare form of blindness. LUXTERNA is an AAV-2-based treatment delivering the correct copy of the RPE65 gene. ZOLGENSMA (onasemnogene abeparvovec), AAV9-based therapy, was approved in the USA in 2019 as a treatment for spinal muscular atrophy, a severe neuromuscular disorder caused by a mutation in the SMN1 gene. It has been approved for use in children under 2 years of age, with the hope that a single dose will have a lasting effect throughout a patient's lifetime. In 2020, ZOLGENSMA was conditionally approved in Europe.

In August 2018, the NIH and FDA announced a joint proposal to reduce the requirement of joint review to streamline duplicative and burdensome oversight over gene therapy. Because of the changing landscape, NIH refocused the NIH RAC into a role closer to its original mandate, which was to follow and provide advice on safety and ethical issues associated with emerging biotechnologies. Today, these emerging areas of research include, but are not restricted to, technologies surrounding advances in recombinant or synthetic nucleic acid research. Accordingly, the Committee has been renamed the Novel and Exceptional Technology and Research Advisory Committee (*NExTRAC*) to reflect this broader outlook.

Upon receiving the Japan Prize in 2015, Ted Friedmann acknowledged that "We're well past the stage of having to prove the concept of gene therapy and have finally overcome our history of perhaps promising too much too soon. We're at the point where we can truly begin to deliver real treatments to real people."

26.4 Vectors Used in Gene-Based Therapies

The fundamental challenges to generating effective gene therapies are being addressed by selecting vectors that optimize delivery, obtain biologically relevant levels of expression of the transgene, and maintain expression of the transgene without interfering with host gene expression, or effecting gene silencing, for the specific clinical indication. Table 26.1 highlights the fact that gene therapy products are not created equal. While "the principles" in this chapter will address gene-based

TABLE 26.1

All Gene Therapy Products Are Not Created Equal

Product Class	Examples
Non-viral vectors	DNA translated in nucleus; mRNA translated in the cytoplasm
Replication-incompetent viral vectors	Adenovirus, AAV, HSV, lentivirus, viral particles (expressing various transgenes)
Replication-competent viral vectors	Retrovirus, measles, reovirus, adenovirus, VSV, vaccinia, coxsackievirus, New Castle disease virus (may express transgenes)
Gene editing vectors	Transcription activator-like effector Nucleases (TALENs)
	Meganucleases (MNs)
	Zinc finger proteins (ZFPs)
	Clustered regularly interspaced short palindrome repeat (CRISPR)
Genetically engineered microorganisms	Listeria, Salmonella, Clostridium, bacteriophages (expressing various transgenes)
Ex vivo genetically modified cells	Adult stem cells, somatic cells (expressing various transgenes)

therapies in general, since AAV vectors are currently the leading platform for gene delivery used across a variety of diseases, most of "the practices" discussed in the chapter will focus on AAV-based gene therapies.

26.4.1 Non-Viral Vectors

Non-viral vectors are used to transfer nucleic acids. The types of product classes include large DNA molecules (plasmid DNA) and mRNA. Small DNA (oligonucleotides) and related molecules and RNA (e.g., siRNA, miRNA) are regulated as drugs in the USA and EU as they are chemically synthesized and are not functional genetic material that can insert, replicate, be transcribed, or otherwise effect changes in the human genome. Unlike viral vectors which have the natural ability to invade cells, non-viral vectors need to be complexed with delivery vehicles (e.g., chemical carriers, gold nanoparticles, synthetic and natural biodegradable lipids etc.) or subjected to forced entry (e.g., various physical methods). Delivery efficiency is the major hurdle for almost all of the non-viral vectors (Ramamoorth and Narvekar 2015).

26.4.2 Replication-Incompetent Viral Vectors

Replication-incompetent, defective, or deficient mutant viruses are specifically defective for viral functions that are essential for viral genome replication and assembly of progeny virus particles. They are propagated in complementing cell lines that express the missing viral gene product(s) to allow viral replication. AV was the first viral vector developed for gene therapy and was approved for clinical trials in 1990. Since AV vectors allow episomal or stable insertion of therapeutic genes, they carry advantages over vectors that integrate into cellular DNA. AAV, unlike other viruses, requires a few other helper proteins, agents, or viruses such as AV, herpes simplex virus type I/II, pseudorabies virus, cytomegalovirus, genotoxic agents, UV radiation, or hydroxyurea to infect cells and complete replication. The HSV genome carries immediate-early, early, and late genes for replication and allows the creation of replication-competent, replication-incompetent, and helper-dependent vectors, or amplicon vectors. The two most common types of retroviruses are gammaretrovirus and lentivirus, which are derived from murine leukemia virus (MLV) and human immunodeficiency virus (HIV-1), respectively. The advantages of using retroviruses are that they can accommodate a 9–12-kb-large insert size for the gene of interest and produce high titers. The most significant disadvantages are the lack of cell specificity and the possibility of insertional mutagenesis (Goswami et al. 2019, Lundstrom 2018).

26.4.3 Replication-Competent Viral Vectors

In the last two decades, various families of viruses, including both DNA and RNA viruses, have successfully transitioned from preclinical studies into early randomized clinical-phase trials (Eissa et al 2018). The applicability of OV as a therapy for clinical oncology trials is due to their potential selectivity, their ability to kill tumor cells but not normal cells. The current research efforts are focused on increasing efficacy against different cancer types, optimizing delivery as the majority have been delivered intratumorally, enhancing either the innate or adaptive immune response as the immune response can also suppress viral replication, and modifying vectors to reduce impact of pre-existing antibodies which can suppress OV efficacy when administered intravenously. Examples of replication-competent viral vectors include AV, herpes simplex virus, poxvirus including vaccinia virus, vesicular stomatitis virus, reovirus, and measles virus (Lundstrom 2018).

26.4.4 Bacterial Vectors

Bacteria can be used for gene therapy via two strategies – either by the transfection of eukaryotic host cells using bacteria (bactofection) or by "alternative gene therapy" using genetically modified bacteria for direct in situ production of therapeutic molecules. Because the host genome is not affected, it represents an alternative to the standard gene transfer to the nucleus of the target cell. While bactofection is optimal for gene substitution and DNA vaccination, alterative gene therapy is suitable for in situ delivery of proteins. A specific form of a bacteria-mediated gene therapy is transkingdom RNA interference (tkRNAi), which uses bacteria that produce short hairpin RNA, which is further processed by the host cell machinery in the cytoplasm to small interfering RNA which downregulates the expression of specific genes (Celec and Gardlik 2017). Examples of non-pathogenic bacterial vectors being studied include Salmonella, Listeria, Shigella, Escherichia, Lactobacillus, and Clostridium.

26.5 Modifications to Improve Vector Delivery

Important advancements are being made employing various strategies to improve the level of transduction required for therapeutic benefit while minimizing toxicity and immune responses. Researchers are developing novel cell-penetrating peptides, mitochondrial targeting strategies, nano shells, sleeping beauty transposons, and new conjugated polymers to improve non-viral vector delivery (Ramamoothi and Narvekar 2015). There is also notable progress being made in methods to improve transduction for viral vectors. For AAV vectors, these include rational mutagenesis and library-based approaches to create capsids that have increased transfection efficiency for particular cell types as well as decreased tropism for non-target organs in addition to improving barriers within intracellular trafficking pathways. Improvements in transgene design and use of tissue-specific promoters have also improved target-specific gene expression. More recent work has focused on the use of pharmacological agents "transduction enhancing compounds" to improve efficiency. In addition to creating alternative, less immunogenic vectors, strategies to shield viruses through chemical modification or exosome encapsulation, inducing immunologic tolerance, using immunosuppressive agents and plasmapheresis are all being consider in efforts to counteract antiviral immunity to improve therapeutic benefit.

26.6 Preclinical Studies to Support Clinical Trials

Preclinical studies provide the necessary information of the potential activity (proof-of-concept (POC)) and safety (toxicity) which justify the advancement of gene therapies into clinical trials to assess the safety and potential therapeutic to humans. These studies support the initiation of clinical studies and can be conducted in parallel if needed to support later-stage clinical development.

Not unlike protein-based biologicals, the objectives of preclinical studies for gene therapy include the establishment of biological relevance in animal models or species, identification of biologically active dose levels, establishment of feasibility and reasonable safety for the proposed clinical route of administration (ROA), selection of potential starting dose level, and dose escalation schedule and dosing regimen. In addition, preclinical data can be used to support patient eligibility criteria, identify physiological parameters that can guide clinical monitoring, and identify potential health risks, (e.g., to the general public, caregivers, family members, and close contacts) (Table 26.2).

General considerations in animal species selection include comparative physiology and anatomy to humans, permissiveness/susceptibility to infection and replication for a viral vector, immune tolerance to the human transgene, and the ability to use the planned clinical delivery system (device) and procedure. In the latter case, a large animal species may be necessary to more accurately discern the transduction pattern in the desired target and vector spread for optimal translation to humans.

Over the years, the arguments against using animal models for preclinical safety assessment have included their inherent variability, the paucity of robust historical/baseline data, and potential technical limitations based upon physiological and/or anatomical constraints. However, preclinical studies performed in an animal model of disease (AMD) or injury to assess not only efficacy but also safety may provide the best opportunity regarding the relationship of dose (including transduction efficiency) to activity and toxicity as the initial population for therapeutic gene therapy products are patients vs. normal healthy volunteers (Cavagnaro and Silva-Lima 2015).

Existing animal models include spontaneous disease models such as hemophilic dogs, non-spontaneous disease models (chemically, surgically, immunologically induced) such as the N-methyl-4-phenyl-1, 2, 3, 6-tetrahydropyridine (MPTP) non-human primate model of Parkinson's disease, and genetically modified disease models (knock-outs, knock-ins and knock-out/knock-ins, including humanized transgenic mouse models). In cases where there is no AMD and/or in addition to a disease model, patient-derived human cells can be used to support POC.

Key considerations for justifying an AMD or injury include an understanding of the progression of abnormal phenotype; the similarities and differences between the model and human disease, including pathophysiology, molecular and functional changes; the lifespan of the model; the time of administration of the gene therapy relative to disease onset and progression; and the age of the intended clinical population.

If an animal transgene (surrogate) is used due to species specificity, additional characterization of the human product

TABLE 26.2

Specific Preclinical Considerations for Gene Therapy Products

- Determine transduction levels of transgene in the target animal species (in vivo) and/or human (in vitro)
- Use the same assay for vector titer determination for the preclinical lots used in pivotal studies as for the clinical lots
- Provide comprehensive discussion, with accompanying data
  ◦ Biological relevance of model/species to proposed clinical population
  ◦ Show consistency of model
  ◦ Provide gender rationale (one or two)
  ◦ Minimize study bias (e.g., randomization, masked assessment of parameters etc)
  ◦ Describe similarities and differences if using a disease phenotype (e.g., pathophysiology, biochemistry, functional changes etc)
- Consider potential impact of any differences
  ◦ Justify timing for product administration in the model relative to disease status of the proposed clinical population (also consider age)
  ◦ Delivery procedure
- Location of injection, number of injections, total dose volume, volume/area site administered etc.
  ◦ Provide rationale, with supporting data, for the study duration and sacrifice points (consider kinetics of transgene expression)
  ◦ Evaluate vector biodistribution (BD) in blood and selected tissues (multiple sections for tissue targeted delivery). Standard for PCR sensitivity is <50 copes/ug genomic DNA; determine the expression of transgene in tissues that are positive for vector presence
  ◦ Safety endpoints in normal or disease animals including but not limited to clinical observations, body weights, physical examinations, appetite, clinical pathology, immune response, gross pathology, and histopathology
- Evaluate serum antibodies to vector and transgene in serum and if delivery to a specific target area (e.g., ocular, intraarticular, intrathecal etc.)
  ◦ For all unscheduled deaths, provide comprehensive clinical pathology, gross pathology and histopathology and other analyses, as appropriate, to determine the potential cause of death.
- Evaluate two or more dose levels of the intended final clinical product/formulation to justify an Effective Dose (ED)
- Confirm compatibility if delivery device is used
- Optimize dose extrapolation based upon the route of delivery
- Provide complete study reports for studies intended to support safety and the rationale for the clinical trial
- Provide documentation regarding compliance with Good Laboratory Practice
- If study not conducted under GLP consider quality review of the raw data to the final report.

and the animal product is conducted to determine the similarities and differences between the human and animal investigational materials.

For gene-modified cell products, immune-incompetent animals, either genetically immune deficient or chemically immunosuppressed, are used to assess the activity of the human cells. In some cases, syngeneic models are used if an intact immune system is needed.

In all cases when surrogate products are used, an understanding of comparability of the animal specific product to the human product is needed in order to improve extrapolation of the findings to humans.

26.6.1 Proof-of-Concept

POC studies focus on assessing the activity and pharmacologic profile of the gene therapy product in a relevant animal model. The data are used to show the biological feasibility, including the level of expression of the intended therapy. As such, these studies provide the basis for providing information for estimating pharmacologically active dose (PAD) ranges for the clinical trial. It is important therefore to understand dose response to establish a minimally effective dose (MED), an effective dose (ED), and a maximally effective dose or optimal biological dose (OBD). For gene therapy products where subjects often only receive a single dose, the importance for understanding a MED is to provide the justification for the first-in-human dose level to be the ED and the subsequent dose levels to be maximally effective.

26.6.2 Biodistribution

Knowing where a therapeutic product "goes" and how long it "stays" after administration is a key principle for understanding safety. For small molecules, this is achieved through pharmacokinetic (PK) and absorption, disposition, metabolism, and excretion (ADME) assessments (ADME) and PK assessments for protein-based biologicals. While the general scientific principles are the same, the precise practices/specific terms/classical studies (e.g., ADME) either may not apply, or do not currently have widely accepted definitions with respect to use with gene therapy products (US 2013, EU 2018). However, on a case-by-case basis, PK studies may need to be carried out depending on the specific product, e.g., if the gene product is a protein excreted in the blood circulation (EU 2018). These assessments, which are referred to as biodistribution (BD) studies, should focus on the distribution, persistence, clearance, and mobilization of the product and should address the risk of germline transmission. BD relates to the spreading of the vector within the animal model and the patient's body from the site of administration, while shedding is defined as the dissemination of the vector through secretions and/or excreta from the animal model or patients.

Ideally, BD studies are conducted via the intended clinical ROA in species that permit vector transduction and that are biologically responsive to the specific transgene product of interest. BD allows for the determination of vector and expressed transgene to the intended therapeutic site (target site) as well as unintended sites (off-target).

BD is required to be completed prior to the initiation of human clinical trials. Analysis is conducted at the molecular level. The current standard is a quantitative polymerase chain reaction assays (e.g., Q-PCR or ddPCR) that detect the number of vector copies per microgram of genomic DNA. Biological fluids and tissue samples are carefully harvested (to avoid cross-contamination) from control and gene therapy product-injected animals at several time points post-administration (Gonin and Gaillard, 2004). Usually at least a minimal panel of tissues is collected and analyzed, including blood, injection site(s), gonads, brain, liver, kidneys, lung, heart, and spleen. Depending on the vector type and the transgene expressed, as well as the ROA, other tissues may need to be analyzed.

If a significant, persistent positive signal is detected, then a more extensive testing paradigm may be necessary. Further studies to determine the cell type that is positive for vector presence may be needed. In the case of targeted delivery, this assessment is important to understand transduction efficiency, which can help to translate doses for the clinical trials. If the outcome implicates inadvertent germline transfer, then the conduct of reproductive and developmental toxicology studies may be needed in order to assess the potential for vertical transmission of the gene sequences. The presence of a vector sequence in non-target tissues at significant levels may suggest the need for further analysis of the tissue to determine the levels of transgene expressed. These data, coupled with results of other safety endpoints, such as clinical pathology and histopathology evaluation, determine whether vector presence or gene expression is correlated with any detrimental effects on the tissue. The finding that the AAV vector can persist for several years as intact particles in the subretinal space of dogs and non-human primates raised the possibility of low levels of replication, which has never been formally excluded in vivo (Steiger et al, 2017). In vivo persistence of AAV vectors at least for certain serotypes expands the requirement for comprehensive shedding investigations. As mentioned previously, there have been a number of public discussions over the years regarding the potential for vertical transmission. The conclusions from each of these public discussions were that the risk of germline transmission of gene therapies is exceedingly low, and while recommendations of patient monitoring have evolved over time, no advisory committee has determined that the demonstration of vector DNA in gonadal tissue or in patient semen should preclude enrollment in gene therapy trials (MacLachlan et àl. 2013). The risk of dissemination of a viral vector into the environment via excreta (e.g., urine, feces, sweat, saliva, nasopharyngeal fluids, skin, and semen), i.e., shedding from the treated patient, is also a potential safety concern for the environment including contamination of other persons (Schenk-Braat et al. 2007).

The Gene Therapy Discussion Group (GTDG) was established within the International Conference on Harmonisation (ICH) framework in 2000. The goals were to share information and explore harmonizing principles, which resulted in the drafting of three ICH Considerations documents relevant to the GT field, covering germline integration, vector shedding, and OV. In 2009, the GTDG was discontinued due to insufficient resources.

In 2012 global regulators proposed an alternative venue to discuss scientific and clinical advances in the gene therapy GT field. This led to the formation of the Regulators Forum Gene Therapy Discussion Group IPRF GTWG in 2013. In January of 2018, the IPRF was reorganized in the International Pharmaceutical Regulators Programme (IPRP). A reflection paper was composed to communicate the current view of experts from various regions on preclinical BD data and expectations (IPRP 2018). In 2019, a concept paper entitled S12: Nonclinical Biodistribution Considerations for Gene Therapy Products was endorsed by the ICH Management Committee. The guideline which is intended to address areas in which harmonization is needed in order to provide a harmonized approach across regulatory regions reached Step 2b in June of 2021(https://www.ema.europa.eu/en/documents/regulatory-procedural-guideline/ich-guideline-s12-nonclinical-biodistribution-considerations-gene-therapy-products-step-2b_en.pdf)

26.6.3 Gene Expression

In parallel with quantifying BD of vectors after local or systemic administration, the assessment of pharmacologic activity is paramount in verifying the relevance of animal models or species used for preclinical studies. Thus, in addition to profiling where the vectors go and for how long, confirming the pharmacologic activity is a key consideration. For gene therapies, pharmacologic activity is measured as gene transcription and/or protein expression. mRNA can be used to monitor gene expression, but more commonly techniques to monitor for the expression of transgene products are used. These techniques may include enzyme-linked immunosorbent assay (ELISA) and immunohistochemistry (IHC). In the absence of animal models of disease, demonstrating pharmacologic activity in normal animals is important in confirming the relevance of safety data obtained in normal animals.

26.6.4 Integration

Two major challenges gene therapy products are as follows: (1) delivery of vectors to desired tissues and (2) controlling integration into or near to transcriptional units (i.e., reducing concerns of insertional mutagenesis, the potential to randomly integrate into host DNA). Vector systems may be less genotoxic due to their insertional preferences, use of internal promoters, relative enhancer activity, or potential read-through transcription. Vector genome integration has been associated with adverse events: integrating γ-retroviral vectors has been implicated in the clonal expansion of transduced cells in clinical studies.

For ex vivo genetically modified cells using retroviral vectors (e.g., gammaretrovirus, lentivirus and foamy virus vectors), the most important goal for both preclinical and clinical safety assessments of integration site analyses is to rule out the emergence of dominant clones in the sample cell population. However, achieving this goal may not require an ultradeep or comprehensive analysis of the vector site integration. Rather, it is most important to ensure a reliable and unbiased detection of a dominant clone, even at the expense of sensitivity. These preclinical and clinical safety analyses should include the assessment of evidence for patterns of clonal insert site enrichment analyses from in vivo samples compared to in vitro-cultured cells. The expectation is that dominant clones driven by genotoxic insertion should behave as described in the clinical trials with chronic granulomatous disease and Wiskott-Aldrich syndrome, both of which showed a sustained increase of the dominant clone over time at the expense of clonal diversity. In case of recurrent observation in vivo of clonal insertion sites that are skewed from the in vitro pattern and multiple events of clonal dominance, it becomes important to consider the specific subsets of target gene(s) and their oncogenic potential (Kiem et al. 2014).

Although AAV vectors are predominantly non-integrating, it has been shown through direct sequencing that integration can occur. When integration takes place, there is a preference for integrating in regions where DNA breaks occur. These can be regions of endonuclease cleavage, active transcription, cytosine-phosphate-guanosine (CpG) islands, and palindromes. All of these studies describing AAV vector genome integration identified vector integration sites through plasmid rescue of vectors containing bacterial origins of replication. (Hojun et al. 2011). There are multiple variables influencing AAV-mediated insertional mutagenesis and subsequent genotoxicity, including the age of treatment, dose, serotype, enhancer promoter encoded by the vector, and the species genome (Russel 2007, Chandler et al. 2015).

26.6.5 Toxicity Assessments

Toxicity studies are conducted to inform an acceptable risk-benefit ratio for the patients that will receive a particular gene therapy product. The approach or practice of toxicology is similar to that for the safety assessment of biotechnology-derived products, "case-by-case" based upon product attributes (US 2013, EU 2018). Relevant species are used, often the same models used to define POC or pharmacology to also assess safety. The species used should ideally be sensitive not just to infection of the vector but also to the pathological consequences of infection that may be induced by the replication competent virus related to the vector. As previously discussed, in some cases, large animals may be needed to better assess the risks associated with the delivery procedure and/or delivery device.

26.6.5.1 Considerations in Study Design

The toxicology assessment of a gene therapy product should include identification, characterization, and quantification of potential local and systemic toxicities. Outcomes measured are acute/chronic toxicities, reversibility of toxicities, delayed or increased toxicities, and any dose-response effects on these various outcomes. The key safety concerns for gene therapy products are listed in Table 26.3. Based upon the specific product type, the concerns may be higher or lower and the study designs customized based on specific product attributes, e.g., ex vivo vs. in vivo delivery, non-viral vs. viral delivery, direct vs. systemic delivery etc.

TABLE 26.3

Potential Safety Concerns for Gene-Based Therapies

- Vector/virus biodistribution to non-target sites/tissues
- Transduced cell distribution to non-target sites/tissues
- Unregulated level of viral replication; viral persistence, and/or transgene expression in target/non-target tissues
- Undesirable immune response against vector, transgene, or transduced cell
- Insertional mutagenesis; oncogenicity/tumorigenicity
- Germline transmission
- Off-target gene editing
- Viral shedding (transmission to untreated individuals)
- Interactions with concomitant therapies
- Risks of the delivery procedure and/or the anatomic site of delivery

26.6.5.1.1 Ex vivo Transduced Cells

The toxicological assessment of the cellular component of ex vivo transduced cells may include endpoints evaluated for somatic cellular therapies as well as in vivo gene therapies. The intended clinical product may be autologous or allogeneic. Depending on the transduced cell population, the following considerations are incorporated for safety assessments: local environmental influence on cell survival, differentiation/phenotype expression, cell migration, host immune response, local and systemic reactions, and tumorigenicity. Safety evaluations are conducted with normal human cells and intended target cells. In many cases, immune-suppressed animals are needed to support engraftment of the clinical product. As such, graft-vs-host disease is expected and may limit the duration of the study.

26.6.5.1.2 In vivo Administration

Most gene therapy products are intended either as a single administration or as a minimal number of repeat administrations over a limited time interval. The main exceptions to this are e.g., ocular and hearing loss gene therapies where a second administration may be given to the companion eye or ear. As discussed, the ROA of a gene therapy product in animals should mimic the intended clinical scenario as closely as possible.

Adverse effects in animals can be dependent on the vector class and the ROA. For some vectors, there may be a need to consider preexisting antibody levels. Species differences in transduction efficiency can also impact toxicity. As the potential for adverse immune effects (e.g., humoral, cellular, or innate) based on delivering both a non-viral and viral vector, immune assessments are needed in safety assessments.

Neutralizing antibodies can also be formed following administration. These neutralizing antibodies can prevent vector distribution to target tissue, accelerate clearance of the virus, and decrease transgene expression/persistence of expression. Thus, the potential for stimulating an immune response to the nucleic acid, the viral protein, or other parts of the vector construct is important to assess. For some vectors, there may be the need to assess the potential for latency and/or reactivation (e.g., HSV-based vectors).

The safety of the expressed transgene should also be evaluated. In most cases, the same animal species that is biologically sensitive to the vector of interest is also responsive to the translated protein. However, in cases where the transgene is not active, or the expressed protein is highly immunogenic in the animal model, then it is important to assess safety with a surrogate transgene.

While persistent transgene expression may be a desired endpoint for some gene therapy products, toxicity can be an undesired outcome of transgene overexpression and/or a delayed abnormal immune response. Prolonged expression of transgenes may be associated with long-term risks. Therefore, understanding the kinetics of expression is important for designing the duration of the animal study. Multiple time points are generally included in studies to assess early and later effects (e.g., 1, 3, or 6 months). If adverse effects are identified, the addition of a recovery group may be considered not only to evaluate if adverse effects recover but also to evaluate the potential for increased toxicity due to persistence of the transgene.

The safety endpoints are similar to other biological product assessments. These include clinical signs, physical examinations, body weights, food consumption, clinical pathology, immunogenicity assessments to vector and expressed transgene product, ECGs, macroscopic and microscopic pathology. Other endpoints may be specific to vector class (e.g., neuropathology HSV; DRG pathology AAV9 and variant vectors) or to the transgene (e.g., undesired cell proliferation for a growth factor). More specific assessments may be needed based upon the proposed clinical indication (especially if using an AMD) or route of delivery (e.g., ERGs for ocular delivery).

If extensive preclinical or clinical safety data for the same or similar vector type exist, toxicity assessment of the gene therapy product of interest may be less extensive, depending on such factors as the dose levels, ROA, and expression cassette that were previously used. Depending on the extent of the change to a particular vector that has been administered to humans, an in vitro or bridging study may suffice (Huang and Serabian 2008).

Toxicity evaluation allows for an understanding of the relationship between the dose level of the gene therapy product administered and the level and persistence of transgene expression in specific tissues, and any toxicities that are observed should be determined. These data help to inform translation of the initial clinical dose, dose escalation strategy, and appropriate clinical monitoring.

26.6.5.2 Good Laboratory Practices (GLP) Requirements

Translation from scientific insight to product development is dependent of high-quality research, well-designed, reproducible data of the highest integrity. The translation is facilitated by the availability of assay methods and relevant models, the availability of reagents, analysis, and the quality of the data.

Preclinical toxicology studies to support clinical trials are generally conducted in compliance with current good laboratory practices (GLPs) as per the US regulation, 21 CFR part 58. Key elements of a GLP study include: a study protocol, a study director, trained personnel, standard operating procedures (SOPs), adequate facilities (e.g. animal house and calibration and maintenance of equipment), and a quality assurance unit. GLPs are concerned with organization processes and conditions; focused on process, not product; regulation of study procedures; including planning, performance, monitoring, recording, and reporting, for assurance of data quality and integrity.

However, it is important to note that, per US regulation, 21 CFR part 312.23 referring to content and format of INDs "For each nonclinical laboratory study subject to the good laboratory practice regulation under part 58, a statement that the study was conducted in compliance with the good laboratory practice regulation in part 58, or if the study was not conducted in compliance with the regulation, a brief statement of the reason for the noncompliance."

In early 2000 there were congressional hearings to investigate the conduct of gene therapy studies. Concerns were raised that studies were poorly run, there were data discrepancies and delays in reporting. As a result of the deliberations the field was advised to increase attention to overall compliance (e.g. GLPs, GMPs and GCPs) and a requisite description of QA/QC programs.

Preclinical in vitro and in vivo pharmacology studies (i.e., proof of concept) are not expected to be conducted under GLP compliance. However, since in many cases the pharmacology models are also used to assess safety non- GLP studies are generally acceptable as long as they are performed in accordance with a prospectively designed protocol and the data are of sufficient quality and integrity to support the proposed clinical trial. The study report should identify any areas that deviate from the prospectively designed protocol and the potential impact of these deviations on study integrity. As there is a large continuum of rigor for non-GLP studies it is more important to understand how the study was conducted vs just labeling it as non-GLP.

As noted above there is an expectation that pivotal toxicology studies submitted to support a marketing application will be conducted under GLP although some aspects may not be fully compliant especially in cases where the methodology is evolving for specific endpoints. Other areas which fall on the compliance continuum include biochemical and non-animal based in vitro systems, assay systems in support of process change or process development, QC testing for bioactivity and comparability.

26.6.5.3 Late-Stage Product Development

As the gene therapy product development program continues into the later-phase clinical trials and toward the ultimate goal of a marketed product, additional consideration may be needed to inform the product label to communicate associated or perceived risks. These studies may include studies to better understand the mechanism of toxicity if adverse events are noted clinically in order to advance the clinical trial or assessment of potential for reproductive or carcinogenic risks to inform the product label.

26.7 Immunogenicity

While considerable advances in gene-based therapies have been made, the host immune response remains a key challenge that must be overcome to ensure the effective translation of gene therapy products to the clinic. Overall preclinical studies in relevant animal models are critical to the development of immune suppression and gene transfer, but the translation of the results of immunogenicity assessments in preclinical studies may not always be direct. This section focuses on accumulated data with AAV vectors including considerations of preexisting immunity to vector capsid and gene therapy-induced antibodies to vector capsid and antidrug antibodies (ADA) to transgene product.

Experience in the clinic with AAV vectors has highlighted three main issues related to vector immunogenicity: (1) preexisting anti-capsid antibodies able to neutralize the vector in individuals who were already exposed to wild-type AAV, (2) humoral immune responses occurring upon initial vector infusion, and (3) cellular immune responses against vector-transduced cells.

The genetic uniformity of inbred strains and absence of natural infection with AAVs can make it difficult to fully extrapolate outcomes in human studies. It is therefore clear that no single animal model will be able to completely predict human responses. It may also be impossible to model such responses in experimental animal species toward establishing credible expectations when translating these experiments into humans (Lowenstein et al. 2007). For example, the study of cell-mediated responses to the AAV capsid is problematic, as these responses are not easily induced in animal models unless complex immunization protocols are used. Unlike cellular responses, humoral responses to AAV can be robust in animal models (Kuranda et al. 2018). In general, the prevalence and titers are higher in the species from which the virus was isolated, such as AAV2 in humans and AAV8 in macaques, although there is substantial cross-species neutralizing activity. Evaluating the impact of host immune memory to a natural AAV infections on AAV-mediated gene transfer is best performed in a preclinical model in which the wild-type version of the vector is permissive (Wang et al. 2011).

Untoward immune responses to AAV vector in some cases have prevented the achievement of long-lasting efficacy. However, the presence of neutralizing antibodies does not necessarily preclude successful transduction, providing that a critical threshold is not reached or depending on the tissue transduced or the administration route.

Neutralizing antibodies may inhibit the viral entry into non-immune target cells, but immunoglobulin or complement-opsonized virus may be targeted to and taken up by innate immune cells (including antigen-presenting cells (APCs) such as dendritic cells) through Fc receptors and complement receptors. Fc receptor cross-linking or targeting of opsonized virus particles to innate immune cells and the engagement of innate receptors may either induce signal transduction events or facilitate virus entry into these APCs, which can lead to inflammatory responses. Unfortunately, it may not be possible to avoid memory AAV capsid T-cell responses by switching serotypes due to cross-reactive epitopes (Boutin et al. 2010). Of note, anti-AAV nAbs and binding antibodies (bAbs) have been shown to have opposite effects on in vivo liver transduction. Binding antibodies, unlike neutralizing antibodies, are not detrimental to AAV transduction and in some in vitro studies have been shown to enhance transduction efficiency (Fitzpatrick et al. 2018).

Much is being learned about host-vector interactions, such as the role of innate immunity and the activation of T cells and B cells in response to the vector and its transgene product. The impact of preexisting immune to AAV on the outcome of gene transfer in terms of safety and efficacy is also not completely understood. Studies in non-human primates indicate that low levels of capsid-specific neutralizing antibodies can alter the tropism of AAV vector particles directing them to the spleen (Wang et al. 2018). The systemic use of AAV vectors in NHPs with neutralizing antibodies to AAV capsids of titers >1:5 has also failed to permit sufficient vector transduction and transgene expression compared to animals with low or undetectable (Arruda et al. 2009). Experience in human trials also suggests that, above a certain level, nAbs prevent AAV vector transduction and consequently transgene expression (Fitzpatrick et al. 2018).

It has been shown that in human liver non-parenchymal cells, the upregulation of IL1-B and IL-6 expression in response to the AAV capsid depends on TLR2 and its accessory protein CD14. Since blood monocytes express high levels of TLR2 and CD14, similar response can be shown with CD14+ moDCs. moDCs appear to be the main innate responders to the AAV capsid in human peripheral blood. Unlike humans, mice are not natural hosts for AAV, although they readily develop anti-AAV antibodies upon AAV vector injections. Additionally, in mice, the TLR2 expression pattern and regulation are different, and unlike in humans, anti-AAV antibody formation in mice is TLR2 independent (Kuranda et al. 2018).

Tolerance induction or immune suppression are strategies being used to enhance efficacy and the duration of gene expression. The ultimate goal is to achieve the long-term antigen-specific tolerance to the transgene product. Immune suppression strategies that block the activation/proliferation of Tregs or completely deplete them from circulation, however, may hamper tolerance induction, necessitating the long-term use.

Transgene expression restricted to the target tissue by using tissue-specific promoters has also been used to avoid immune responses to transgene. One important strategy to avoid an immune response is to prevent transgene expression within APCs such as dendritic cells, B cells, or macrophages.

Delivering vector to tissues and/or a space considered to be immune-privileged is also a logical option to evade unwanted immune response. However, perturbation of the "immune-privileged sites" by the delivery of the vector may compromise the anatomical integrity of these natural barriers and change local immune responses. Therefore, anti-inflammatory or immunosuppressive therapies may be transiently required (Arruda et al. 2009).

In addition to pharmacological inhibition (immunosuppression) approaches to overcome the inhibition of transduction by neutralizing anti-AAV antibodies, other approaches include but are not limited to the use of alternative serotypes; development of "designer" variants, development of nAb-resistant variants by mutations of the AAV capsid, mutagenesis of known antigenic epitopes, directed evolution for the isolation of nAb-resistant AAV variants, shielding of AAV, e.g., by chemical modification or exosome encapsulation, plasmapheresis, and saline flushing.

Ultimately, humans will likely be the best animal model to study AAV immunity with experience gained from the use of approved AAV biologics and clinical trials. Current questions being asked clinically include: Can testing of PBMC predict CD8+ T-cell responses against AAV capsid and rejection of therapy and how can we better screen patients? Is the immunotoxicity in humans a de novo immune response or a recall response? What is the best immune suppression protocol, agent, and treatment window to prevent capsid-related immunotoxicity? What is the optimal vector dose for each capsid serotype to avoid immunity while providing therapeutic transgene expression? (Martino and Markusic 2020).

26.8 Dose Extrapolation

There is a clinical imperative to deliver not only a safe but an active dose to subjects with disease who may only have the option to receive a single dose. The human equivalent dose (HED) is a dose in humans anticipated to provide the same degree of effect as that observed in animals at a given dose. The PAD is the lowest dose tested in an animal species with the intended pharmacologic activity.

As discussed in the section on BD, the traditional practices of PK (ADME) are not generally applicable to gene therapy products. While it is still important to define a NOAEL in toxicity studies, considerations for defining an active dose is particular important for gene therapy products. However, dose extrapolation can be more complicated than for protein-based biologics based upon the many novel routes of administration to improve target site delivery (e.g., subretinal, intravitreal, intracardiac, intrathecal, intraputamen, intercisternal magna, intracochlear etc.) where comparative area or volume needs to be considered cross-species. Additionally, transduction efficiency across species, in relationship to timing of injection, age of animals, differences in normal vs. disease models, may need to be considered based upon the specific gene therapy product and indication.

Unfortunately, it is difficult to compare vector doses used in different clinical trials because of the wide variations that exist in quantitation of vectors used by different sponsors. For toxicity studies designed within a program, it is important to use the same methods to quantify the vector used preclinically as used clinically to improve dose extrapolation.

26.9 Case Studies

This section provides a few case studies that exemplify the importance of a case-by-case approach to advance gene therapy products into the clinic based on specific product attributes.

Case Studies: Novel Route of Administration

Guidance: *A ROA that mimics the intended clinical route as closely as possible. The delivery device intended for use in the clinical studies should be used to administer the investigational CGT product in the definitive toxicology studies; justification should be provided if the intended clinical delivery device is not used (US 2013).*

Case 1. For a specific gene therapy product, the POC study was determined in a mouse model of disease by a different ROA as the proposed clinical route was not technically feasible. The ROA was technically feasible in pigs but high levels of neutralizing antibodies to the specific vector serotype developed during the time interval after the surgical procedure used to create the model prior to delivery of the vector which is expected to reduce transduction. Non-human primates can be screened for low preexisting antibody titers to vector; however, the ROA is not technically feasible due to anatomical differences, but the delivery device can be used.

Case 2. Direct delivery of gene therapy to an organ requires specialized device(s);

Large AMD exists: single large AMD is injected using human device(s) for safety/BD; Small AMD exists but human devices not feasible; efficacy/safety/BD in small AMD; safety/BD in normal large animal using human devices; no AMD exists: single normal large animal safety and BD study conducted using human device(s); confirm transgene expression.

Case Studies: Number and Types of Studies

Guidance: *The number and type of studies performed will be guided by the biological attributes of the investigational CGT product. Animal species in which the CGT product is biologically active should be used in the toxicology studies. Multiple animal models may be necessary to adequately identify functional aspects and potential toxicities of a single product under study (US 2013).*

Case 3. The clinical construct was used for assessing efficacy and safety in a mouse model of disease; BD and toxicity assessments were conducted in NHPs to assess safety and confirm transduction efficiency.

Case 4. A surrogate construct was developed to assess safety in normal monkeys due to severe immunogenicity of the human construct (clinical candidate); in vitro studies were conducted with clinical candidate to assess POC and safety.

Case 5. The vector efficiency for a particular serotype is known to be much higher in mice than in humans; safety and efficacy were conducted in mice via the intended clinical ROA; the known difference in transduction efficiency was considered in extrapolation of dose.

Case 6. POC and safety studies were conducted in rodent disease models at various ages to justify dosing in earlier pediatric populations.

Case 7. In vitro studies were conducted in patient derived cells due to the lack of availability of an AMD; BD and safety of the clinical candidate were assessed in NHPs; human protein expression confirmed.

Case 8. POC of an OV was demonstrated in immune-suppressed human xenograft models; a transgenic mouse model was developed to provide the human specific receptor to allow the assessment of BD and safety.

Case 9. POC and safety of an OV was determined with a surrogate in a syngeneic tumor model as an intact immune system was required for efficacy. In vitro comparative cytotoxicity was determined for the surrogate and clinical candidate. BD and safety of the clinical candidate were also assessed in mice.

Case 10. For a systemically administered gene editing vector targeting non-human DNA; transgenic rodent model for measuring safety, BD and excision activity; off-target assessment in human cells.

26.10 Regulation of Gene Therapy Products

Successful translation to the clinic, however, is inextricably linked to navigating potential regulatory challenges while taking advantage of regulatory opportunities. The opportunity for expedited regulatory pathways can be challenging as there will be the need to accelerate various processes to synchronize with the pace of these expedited pathways. "Fast Track does not mean the regulators read faster." For example, as potency assays are critical to assess product functional activity, consistency, and stability, developers are being encouraged to evaluate multiple product characteristics that could be used to establish a potency test during initial clinical studies as potency is important for providing evidence of comparability after changes to the manufacturing process.

Different countries or regions have different levels of regulatory oversight and some have limited experience in product regulation. In the USA, the FDA is responsible for the regulation of gene therapies. These products are regulated under the Center for Biologics Evaluation and Research (CBER) in the Office of Tissues and Advanced Therapies (OTAT).

The FDA regulates gene therapy under general drug, biologic, and medical device laws and regulations, as well as specific laws and regulations for human cells, tissues, and cellular and tissue-based products (HCT/Ps). In addition, the FDA generally develops and follows guidance documents that are either applicable to or specifically developed for gene-based therapies (Table 26.4). In 2016 and 2017, respectively, Congress passed into law both the 21st Century Cures Act, and the FDA Reauthorization Act of 2017 (FDARA), respectively. The 21st Century Cures Act contains vital new legislation affecting the CGT fields, such as the Regenerative Medicine Advanced Therapy (RMAT) designation.

Scientific advice is a procedure that can be applied to any one of, or any combination of, quality, preclinical and clinical data relating to the development of a medicinal product, with the principle aim to give advice on scientific information that may be necessary to demonstrate, quality, safety and/or efficacy of the product. Scientific advice is operated by the European Medicines Agency (EMA), the Scientific

TABLE 26.4

Gene Therapy Guidance Documents (US)

Guidance Document	Reference Year[a]
Interpreting Sameness of Gene Therapy Products Under the Orphan Drug Regulations; Draft Guidance for Industry	1/2020
Chemistry, Manufacturing, and Control (CMC) Information for Human Gene Therapy Investigational New Drug Applications (INDs); Guidance for Industry	1/2020
Long Term Follow-up After Administration of Human Gene Therapy Products; Guidance for Industry	1/2020
Testing of Retroviral Vector-Based Human Gene Therapy Products for Replication Competent Retrovirus During Product Manufacture and Patient Follow-up; Guidance for Industry	1/2020
Human Gene Therapy for Hemophilia; Guidance for Industry	1/2020
Human Gene Therapy for Rare Diseases; Guidance for Industry	1/2020
Human Gene Therapy for Retinal Disorders; Guidance for Industry	1/2020
Evaluation of Devices Used with Regenerative Medicine Advanced Therapies; Guidance for Industry	2/2019
Expedited Programs for Regenerative Medicine Therapies for Serious Conditions; Guidance for Industry	2/2019
Regulatory Considerations for Human Cells, Tissues, and Cellular and Tissue-Based Products: Minimal Manipulation and Homologous Use; Guidance for Industry and Food and Drug Administration Staff	Updated: 12/2017
Same Surgical Procedure Exception under 21 CFR 1271.15(b): Questions and Answers Regarding the Scope of the Exception; Guidance for Industry	11/2017
Deviation Reporting for Human Cells, Tissues, and Cellular and Tissue-Based Products Regulated Solely Under Section 361 of the Public Health Service Act and 21 CFR Part 1271; Guidance for Industry	9/2017
Recommendations for Microbial Vectors Used for Gene Therapy; Guidance for Industry	9/2016
Design and Analysis of Shedding Studies for Virus or Bacteria-Based Gene Therapy and Oncolytic Products; Guidance for Industry	8/2015
Considerations for the Design of Early-Phase Clinical Trials of Cellular and Gene Therapy Products; Guidance for Industry	6/2015
Determining the Need for and Content of Environmental Assessments for Gene Therapies, Vectored Vaccines, and Related Recombinant Viral or Microbial Products; Guidance for Industry	3/2015
Guidance for Industry: BLA for Minimally Manipulated, Unrelated Allogeneic Placental/Umbilical Cord Blood Intended for Hematopoietic and Immunologic Reconstitution in Patients with Disorders Affecting the Hematopoietic System (This guidance finalizes the draft guidance of the same title dated June 2013.)	3/2014
IND Applications for Minimally Manipulated, Unrelated Allogeneic Placental/Umbilical Cord Blood Intended for Hematopoietic and Immunologic Reconstitution in Patients with Disorders Affecting the Hematopoietic System - Guidance for Industry and FDA Staff (This guidance finalizes the draft guidance of the same title dated June 2013).	3/2014
Guidance for Industry: Preclinical Assessment of Investigational Cellular and Gene Therapy Products (This guidance finalizes the draft guidance entitled "Guidance for Industry: Preclinical Assessment of Investigational Cellular and Gene Therapy Products" dated November 2012)	11/2013
Guidance for Industry: Preparation of IDEs and INDs for Products Intended to Repair or Replace Knee Cartilage (This guidance finalizes the draft guidance of the same title dated July 2007.)	12/2011
Guidance for Industry: Clinical Considerations for Therapeutic Cancer Vaccines (This guidance finalizes the draft guidance of the same title dated September 2009.)	10/2011
Guidance for Industry: Potency Tests for Cellular and Gene Therapy Products (This guidance finalizes the draft document of the same name, dated October 2008.)	1/2011
Guidance for Industry: Cellular Therapy for Cardiac Disease (This guidance finalizes the draft guidance entitled "Guidance for Industry: Somatic Cell Therapy for Cardiac Disease" dated March 2009)	10/2010
Guidance for Industry: Considerations for Allogeneic Pancreatic Islet Cell Products	9/2009
Guidance for FDA Reviewers and Sponsors: Content and Review of Chemistry, Manufacturing, and Control (CMC) Information for Human Somatic Cell Therapy Investigational New Drug Applications (INDs)	4/2008
Eligibility Determination for Donors of Human Cells, Tissues, and Cellular and Tissue-Based Products; Guidance for Industry	8/2007
Guidance for Industry: Guidance for Human Somatic Cell Therapy and Gene Therapy	3/1998

* https://www.fda.gov/vaccines-blood-biologics/biologics-guidances/cellular-gene-therapy-guidances.

Advice Working Party (SAWP) and the Committee for Human Medicinal Products (CHMP).

Whereas scientific advice procedures are focused on development of a specific medicinal product, the EMA offers the opportunity for early dialogues with developers on product development through its Innovation Task Force. The aim of the EMA Innovation Task force is to foster innovation in relation to early development programs, often where the specific product has yet to be manufactured in a form that could be given to patients.

The PRIME (PRIority MEdicine) scheme exists to facilitate approval of products that target unmet medical need. This is voluntary and open to any type of medicinal product that may address an unmet medical need. Initially, developers form their own view as to why a product meets the definition of a priority medicine: at least, early clinical data are expected.

The Scientific Advice Working Party (SAWP) review applications for PRIME designation taking into account considerations from the Committee for Advanced Therapies (CAT) and where granted there is a Rapporteur appointed who supports development of the product with regular meetings with its developers. In 2012 the European Medicine Agency (EMA) Committee for Advanced Therapies (CAT) assumed the lead role in all aspects concerning the development of advance-therapy medicines in Europe, including developing guidelines, organizing workshops and establishment of ad-hoc groups as and when required to develop specific guidance documents. Guidance documents already developed by the Cell-Based Products Working Party (CPWP) and the Gene Therapy Working Party (GTWP) were transferred to CAT (Table 26.5).

Other European agencies that play a role in the regulation of gene therapy products in member states include the French Agency for the Sanitary Safety of Health Products (AFSSAPS; http://agmed.sante.gouv.fr/), the Gene Therapy Advisory Committee (GTAC) in the United Kingdom (www.doh.gov.uk/ genetics/gtac/index.htm), and the Paul Ehrlich Institute in Germany (www.pei. de/themen/gentherapie/gene_therapy_reg.htm).

Regulatory bodies in Asia that evaluate gene therapy products include the Ministry of Health, Labour and Welfare (MHLW) (www.mhlw.go.jp/english) and the Pharmaceuticals and Medical Devices Agency (www.pmda.go.jp/ index-e.html) in Japan, the Korean Food and Drug Administration (KFDA) in South Korea (www.kfda.go.kr), and the State Food and Drug Administration (SFDA) in China (www.sfda.gov.cn/eng).

Japan's regulatory agency, MHLW, has a special regulatory framework for "regenerative medicinal products" under which gene therapy products are characterized and regulated. "Regenerative medicine" is a separate category defined in the Japanese regulation for academic or clinical research products not seeking marketing approval. The relevant guidance for gene therapy products include the *Regenerative Medicine Promotional Law* (RMP, May 2013), the *Act of Safety of Regenerative Medicine* (RM Act, November 2013), and the *Act on Pharmaceuticals and Medical Devices* (PMD Act, November 2013) (Halioua-Haubold et al 2017).

Ongoing international efforts in Gene Therapy include the IPRP, the ICH, the Asia-Pacific Economic Cooperation (APEC), the Regulatory Harmonization Steering Committee (RHSC); and information exchanges with foreign counterparts, including confidential discussions.

In the USA, additional efforts are being made to accelerate gene therapy programs. A program was initiated by the National Institutes of Health's National Center for Advancing Translational Sciences (NCATS) with the affiliated Cures Acceleration Network Review Board (CANRB). The CANRB is composed of multi-stakeholder representatives, including senior academic scientists, patient advocates, and biopharmaceutical industry leaders who are appointed by the Secretary of the US Department of Health and Human. Services and serve four-year terms. Ex-officio members from NIH, the Office of the Assistant Secretary of Defense for Health Affairs, the Office of the Under Secretary for Health for the Department of Veterans Affairs, the National Science Foundation, and the US FDA also are appointed and serve three-year terms. Their remit is to consider translational sciences solutions that would accelerate progress across the whole field. Issues have been identified that seem to the stakeholder community to be the most urgent and the most amenable to a CANRB/NCATS intervention. The issues that will be addressed include: Development of Standardized Predictive Measures/Assays of Neutralizing or Particle-Clearing Antibodies to Major Serotypes; Immune Response, Suppression, Transduction Attenuation and Re-dosing; Assays for Potency, Biodistribution and Filled-Particle Quantitation; Manufacturing and Dissemination; and Scientific Tools to Inform Clinical Trial Design, Selection of Initial Subjects, Dosing Levels, etc. (Ron Bartek, personal communication).

TABLE 26.5

Gene Therapy Guidance Documents (EU)

Guidance Document	Reference Year[a]
Questions and answers on comparability considerations for advanced therapy medicinal products (ATMP)	EMA/CAT/499821/2019
Guideline on the quality, non-clinical and clinical aspects of gene therapy medicinal products	EMA/CAT/80183/2014
Questions and answers on gene therapy	EMA/CAT/80183/2014
Guideline on scientific requirements for the environmental risk assessment of gene therapy medicinal products	CHMP/GTWP/125491/106
Reflection paper on design modifications of gene therapy medicinal products during development	EMA/CAT/GTWP/44236/2009
Reflection paper on quality, non-clinical and clinical issues relating specifically to recombinant adeno-associated viral vectors	CHMP/GTWP/587488/07
ICH Considerations-Oncolytic Viruses	EMEA/CHMP/ICH/607698/2008
Guideline on quality, non-clinical and clinical aspects of medicinal products containing genetically modified cells	CAT/CHMP/GTWP/671639/2008
Guideline on the non-clinical studies required before first clinical use of gene therapy medicinal products	EMEA/CHMP/ GTWP/125459/2006
Guideline on non-clinical testing for inadvertent germline transmission of the gene transfer vectors	EMEA/273974/2005
Reflection paper on management of clinical risks deriving from insertional mutagenesis	CAT/190186/2012
Guideline on follow-up of patients administered gene therapy medicinal products	EMEA/CHMP/GTWP/60436/2007
Guideline on safety and efficacy follow-up and risk management of advanced therapy medicinal products	EMEA/149995/2008

[a] https://www.ema.europa.eu/en/human-regulatory/research-development/advanced-therapies/guidelines-relevant-advanced-therapy-medicinal-products#genetically.

26.11 Conclusion

Considerable progress has been made in the discovery, pre-clinical and clinical development of a variety of gene therapy products, which has led to product approvals. Gene therapy holds the potential for a "cure" but approaches to ensure safety remain paramount.

Recently, a third subject in a trial of a gene therapy for treating a rare and life-threatening neuromuscular disease died (Carroll 2020). The subject was one of three in the trial who had received the gene therapy at the highest dose tested and begun to demonstrate signs of liver dysfunction within three to four weeks after receiving the dose. The indication includes boys up to the age of 5. All three of the subjects demonstrated signs of preexisting hepatobiliary disease. However, while more than half of the subjects enrolled into the study have shown signs of such disease, the gene therapy was not associated with similar complications including subjects who received the same dose level. For another gene therapy indicated to treat hemophilia, additional data were requested by the regulators based on concerns about the durability of the therapy after factor VIII levels seemed to fall off after 12–18 months, raising the possibility of the need to re-dose to maintain protection against bleeds. And following the initial product approval of ZOLGENSMA in infants and children up to 2 years with a rare genetic condition, possible neurological damage in primates was identified. Additional clinical confirmatory data was recently requested to expand use in older children to confirm adequate risk-benefit although the requested additional study was reportedly not linked to the findings in primates.

While clinical experience suggests that findings in humans may not reliably translate between humans, as preclinical translational scientists we are cognizant that we must continue to optimize our preclinical programs to allow clinical translation. Optimization will most likely be experienced-based. Successful translation will be enabled by the availability, validation, and implementation of new technologies not only for product manufacture, but also for testing and evaluation. We are humbled by the knowledge that for some diseases there may not be a relevant AMD and for some the animal model may not recapitulate key aspects of the human disease. We are excited about the many new technologies that are emerging, including gene-modified cells for non-cancer indications, in vivo delivery of lentiviral vectors, dual vector strategies, editing genes without using DNA breaks, trans-splicing ribozymes, therapeutic interfering particles, sensory switch circuit controls, novel tissue-specific promoters, nanorobotics systems for gene delivery etc.

The translational imperative is to administer both a safe and an active dose to subjects in gene therapy trials. A case-by-case approach is needed because gene therapy products are not created equal. Considerations are based on the various product attributes, including vector, payload, expressed transgene, transduced cell type, ROA, and intended disease indication to optimize dose selection and safety monitoring. The data should determine an adequate assessment of potential risks in order to provide effective means of communication of these risks to the clinicians that oversee the clinical trials and to the individuals consenting to receive these experimental therapies.

It is impossible to summarize the past learnings, current practices, and future hopes for gene therapy in a single chapter. Academia, industry, and regulatory scientists need to consistently share information on more efficient development strategies, methods of assessment, key safety concerns and data expectations to ensure successful clinical development, subsequent approval, and most importantly ultimate availability of gene therapy products for patients.

Acknowledgments

The author wishes to acknowledge the experience gained over the past 30 years from discussions with academic, industry, and regulatory colleagues and the opportunities provided by clients patients, patient advocacy groups, and families in designing and evaluating preclinical safety evaluation programs of gene therapy products that not only have successfully advanced into clinical trials but have also received approval for marketing.

REFERENCES

Arruda V, Favaro P and Finn JD (2009) Strategies to modulate immune responses: a new frontier for gene therapy. *Mol Ther* 17:1492–1503.

Blaese RM, Culver KW, Miller AD et al (1995) T lymphocyte-directed gene therapy for ADA-SCID: initial trial results after 4 years. *Science* 270: 475–80.

Boutin S, V Monteilhet, P Veron et al (2010) Prevalence of serum IgG and neutralizing factors against adeno-associated virus (AAV) types 1, 2, 5, 6, 8 and 9 in the healthy population: Implications for gene therapy using AAV vectors. *Hum Gene Ther* 21: 704–712.

Carroll J (2020) Derailed gene therapy study reports 3rd death as safety and durability issues cloud a booming field. https://endpts.com/derailed-gene-therapy-study-reports-3rd-death-as-safety-and-durability-issues-cloud-a-booming-field/.

Cavagnaro JA (2002) Preclinical safety evaluation of biotechnology-derived pharmaceuticals. *Nature Rev Drug Discov* 1: 469–75.

Cavagnaro JA (2008) The Principles of ICH S6 and the Case-by-Case Approach in *Preclinical Safety Evaluation of Biopharmaceuticals: A Science-based Approach to Facilitating Clinical Trials*, ed. JA Cavagnaro, John Wiley & Sons, Hoboken, NJ. pp 45–65.

Cavagnaro J and Silva-Lima B (2015) Regulatory acceptance of animal models of disease to support clinical trials of medicines and advanced therapy medicinal products. *Eur J Pharm* 752: 51–62.

Cavazzana-Calvo M, Hacein-Bey S, de Saine Basile G et al (2000) Gene therapy of severe combined immunodeficiency (SCID)-X1 disease. *Science* 288: 669–72.

Celic P and R Gardlik (2017) Gene therapy using bacterial vectors. *Fron Biosci* 22, 81–95.

Chandler RJ, MC LaFave, GK Varshey (2015) Vector design influences hepatic genotoxicity after adeno-associated viral gene therapy. *J Clin Invest* 125: 870–80.

Collins M and A Thrasher (2015) Gene therapy: progress and predictions. *Proc R Soc B* 282:20143003. http://dx.doi.org/10.1098/rspb.2014.3003.

Eissa IR, I Bustos-Villalobos, et al. (2018) The current status and future prospects of oncolytic viruses in clinical trials against melanoma, glioma, pancreatic, and breast cancers. *Cancers (Basel).* 2018 Oct; 10(10): 356. Published online 2018 Sep 26. doi: 10.3390/cancers10100356.

EU Guidance on the Quality, Non-clinical and Clinical Aspects of Gene Therapy Medicinal Products (2018).

FDA Guidance for Industry: Guidance for Human Somatic Cell Therapy and Gene Therapy (1998).

FDA Guidance for Industry Preclinical Assessment of Investigational Cellular and Gene Therapy Products (2013).

Fitzpatrick Z, C Leborgne C, E Barbon et al (2018) Influence of pre-existing nti-capsid neutralizing and binding antibodies on AAV vector transduction. *Mol Ther: Methods & Clin Dev* 9: 119–129.

Flotte TR, KI Berns (2005) *Adeno-Associated Viral Vectors for Gene Therapy*, Laboratory Techniques in Biochemistry and Molecular Biology, Volume 31, Elsevier B.V.

Friedmann, T and R Roblin (1972) Gene therapy for human genetic disease? *Science* 175: 949–55.

Gonin P and C Gaillard (2004) Gene transfer vector biodistribution: pivotal safety studies in clinical gene therapy development. *Gen Ther* 11 Suppl 1, S98–S108.

Goswami R, G Subranmanian, L Silayeva et al. (2019) Gene therapy leaves a vicious cycle. *Front Oncol* https://doi.org/10.3389/fonc.2019.00297.

Halioua-Haubold, CL, JG Peyer, JA Smith et al. (2017) Regulatory considerations for gene therapy products in the US, EU and Japan. *Yale J of Bio and Med* 90:683–93.

Herzog, RW, O Cao and A Srivastava (2010) Two decades of clinical gene therapy-success if finally mounting. *Discov Med* 9:105–11.

High K (2014) Gene therapy for hemophilia: The clot thickens. *Hum Gen Ther* 25:915–22.

Hojun L, N Malani, SR Hamilton et al (2011) Assessing the potential for AAV vector genotoxicity in a murine model. *Blood* 117: 3311–19.

IPRP Expectations for Biodistribution (BD) Assessments for Gene Therapy (GT) products (2018) (https://admin.iprp.global/sites/default/files/2018(09/IPRP_GTWG_ReflectionPaper_BD_Final_2018_0713.pdf).

Jeune VL, JA Joergensen, RJ Haijar et al (2013) Pre-existing anti-adeno associated virus antibodies as a challenge in AAV gene therapy. *Hum Gene Ther Methods* 24: 59–67.

Kiem H-P, C Baum, FD Bushman et al (2014) Charting a clear path:The ASCGT standardized pathways conference. *Mol Ther* 22:1235–38.

Kumar SRP, DM Markusic, M Biswas, KA High and RW Herzog (2016) Clinical development of gene therapy: results and lessons from recent successes. *Mol Ther Methods Clin Devel* 3: 16034. doi:10.1038/mtm.2016.34.

Kuranda K, Jean-Alphonse P, Leborgne C (2018) Exposure to wild-type AAV drives distinct capsid immunity profiles in humans. *J Clin Inv* 128: 5267–79.

Lander ES et al (2001) Initial sequencing and analysis of the human genome. *Nature* 409: 860–921. doi:10.1038/35057062.

Lowenstein, PR, RJ Mandel, W-D Xiong et al (2007) Immune responses to adenovirus and adeno-associated vectors used for gene therapy of brain disease: role of immunological synapses in understanding the cell biology of neuroimmune interactions. *Curr Gene Ther.* 7: 347–60.

Lundstrom K (2018) Viral vectors in gene therapy. *Diseases* 6(2):42 Published online 2018 May 21. doi: 10.3390/diseases6020042.

MacLachlan TK, M McIntyre, K Mitrophanous et al (2013) Not reinventing the wheel: applying the 3Rs concepts to viral vector gene therapy biodistribution studies. *Human Gene Ther Part C: Clinical Development* 24:1–4.

Manno C.S., Pierce G.F., Arruda V.R., et al. (2006) Successful transduction of liver in hemophilia by AAV-Factor IX and limitations imposed by the host immune response. *Nat Med* 12: 342–47.

Martino AT, DM Markusic (2020) Immune response mechanisms against AAV vectors in animal models. *Mol Ther: Models Clin Dev* 17:198–208.

Naldini L (2009) Medicine. A Comeback for gene therapy. *Science* 326: 805–6.

Ramamoorth M and A Narvekar (2015) Non-viral vectors in gene therapy-an overview. *J Clin Diagn Res* 9(1): GE01–6. Published online 2015 Jan 1. doi: 10.7860/JCDR/2015/10443.5394.

Russell DW (2007) AAV vectors, insertional mutagenesis and cancer. *Science* 317: 447. doi:1038/sj.mt.6300299.

Schenk-Braat EAM, MMKB van Mierlo, G Wagemaker et al (2007) An inventory of shedding data from clinical gene therapy trials. *J Gene Med* 9:910–21.

Serabian MA and Y Huang (2008) Preclinical safety evaluation in *Preclinical Safety Evaluation of Biopharmaceuticals: A Science-based Approach to Facilitating Clinical Trials*, ed. JA Cavagnaro, John Wiley & Sons, Hoboken, NJ, pp 713–747.

Steiger K, J Schroeder, N Provost et al (2017) Detection of intact rAAV particles up to 6 years after successful gene transfer in the retina of dogs and primates, *Mole Ther* 17: 516–23.

Tang, X, S Xhang, R Fu et al. (2019) Therapeutic Prospects of mRNA-based gene therapy for glioblastoma. *Front Oncol* https://doi.org/10.3389/fonc.2019.01208.

Wang L, Calcedo R, Wang H et al (2011) The pleiotrophic effect of natural AAV infections on liver-directed gene transfer in macaques. *Mol Ther* 18:126–34.

Wang D, Tai, PWL and Gao, G (2019) Adeno-associated virus vectors a platform for gene therapy delivery. *Nature Rev Drug Discov* 18: 358–78.

Yla-Pelto J, L Tripati and P Sushi (2016) Therapeutic use of native and recombinant enteroviruses. *Viruses* 8(3): 57. Published online 2016 Feb 23. doi: 10.3390/v8030057.

Zoon KC. 2000. Approaches to the Regulation of Biotech Products in the USA. 5th Interlaken Conference.

27

Genome Editing Technologies

Kathleen Meyer-Tamaki
Sangamo Therapeutics, Inc.

CONTENTS

27.1 Introduction

Therapeutic application of genome editing with engineered nucleases is one of the most exciting scientific developments in recent years, allowing the investigation of gene function and treatment of genetic, infectious, or acquired diseases. Genome editing technologies are powerful tools for gene therapy because of their ability to inactivate genes, correct mutated genes, or insert intact genes into specific regions of the genome. The engineered nuclease approach has been applied successfully to more than 50 different organisms, including crop plants, livestock, and humans (Carroll 2014). Clinical development of genome editing therapies continues to grow with over 45 ongoing phase 1/2 clinical studies listed in clinicaltrials.gov.

While the genome editing field is rapidly evolving and advancing, key issues remain regarding the specificity, efficiency, and safety of engineered nucleases. Regulatory guidance from the US FDA and EMA focuses on nonclinical aspects of gene therapy development (USFDA 2013, 2020) (EMA 2012, 2018a, 2019); however due to the rapid evolution of the field, guidance on strategies for nonclinical safety aspects of genome editing technologies is not yet available. Fortunately, genome editing products share common features with gene therapy products including nucleic acid delivery methods, assessments of biodistribution, persistence, and transgene expression (Chapter 26). The novel elements for genome editing products are assessment of unintentional nuclease activity at non-target sites within the genome and potential impact of this activity as a long-term or permanent genetic modification of patient cells. Nonclinical programs need to be science-driven, product-focused, and typically are based on a case-by-case assessment due to novelty of genomic medicines and their intended use. Strategies for nonclinical assessment often require creative thinking to address nonclinical safety and risk assessment.

This chapter will discuss advanced genome editing technologies either approaching or being evaluated in clinical studies, and considerations for nonclinical evaluation of these novel genomic medicines. These technologies include zinc finger nucleases (ZFNs), meganucleases, transcription activator-like effector nucleases (TALENs), MegaTALs, and clustered regularly interspaced short palindromic repeats (CRISPR)/CRISPR-associated (Cas) platforms. New editing approaches on the horizon include base editing, which uses components from engineered nuclease systems combined with other enzymes to directly install point mutations into cellular DNA or RNA without making double-strand breaks (DSBs) (Rees and Liu 2018), prime editing, also referred to as "search-and-replace" editing, enables targeted insertions, deletions, and point mutations without requiring DSB or donor templates (Anzalone et al. 2019), peptide nucleic acid (PNA)-based editing, which also relies on a non-enzymatic editing approach to incorporate a permanent site-specific sequence modifications in the genome (Economos et al. 2020), and site-specific recombinases which promote the rearrangement of DNA by breaking and re-joining strands at precisely defined sequence positions (Stark 2014). These exciting approaches are in early preclinical research stages, are not described further in this chapter, but will likely emerge as viable clinical approaches in the future.

Clinical applications are broad and engineered nuclease treatments are administered ex vivo or in vivo to several types of target cells. Scientists in academia and industry continue to improve the specificity and selectivity of these engineered nucleases and find new ways to apply the technology to improve the life of patients. As this field continues to progress, these genomic-based medicines will continue to improve, and new editing products will emerge and advance to the clinic. Knowledge, understanding, and tools to assess these new medicines will also evolve. With the growth and development of these novel genome editing products, the safety evaluation strategies must evolve as well.

27.2 Genome Editing and DNA Repair

The fundamental process common to many genome editing technologies is the use of engineered nucleases to make targeted site-specific DSBs in the genome (Rouet, Smih, and Jasin 1994). The consequences of targeted nuclease activity depend on cellular repair pathways of the DSBs, which are potentially lethal to the cell unless rapidly repaired. Repair of a DSB induced by a nuclease often occurs by one of two potential pathways, including non-homologous end joining (NHEJ) or homology-directed repair (HDR). NHEJ is an error-prone repair pathway that can result in small insertions and deletions of nucleotides at the cut site, referred to as indels, which can disrupt the target gene (or regulatory sequences) by creating frameshift mutations, leading to the expression of a non-functional and/or truncated protein (Cathomen and Joung 2008). NHEJ is regarded as the dominant mechanism for DSB repair in vertebrates, especially in G0, G1, and early S phases of the cell cycle (Lieber et al. 2003).

For the HR repair process, cells use an unbroken sister chromatid or homologous chromosome as a template to copy appropriate information into the break site (Carroll 2014). If an exogenously introduced homologous DNA fragment, referred to as donor DNA, is provided to the cell, this fragment can be incorporated into the break site. Here, the donor DNA is flanked by regions homologous to nucleotides on either side of the cut site to facilitate HR. In the absence of a DSB at the target locus, typically fewer than 1 in 10^5 of targeted cells will contain the desired genetic modification, a frequency too low to be useful for gene therapy (Cathomen and Joung 2008).

The architecture of the donor DNA determines the outcome of the gene targeting event. For example, the donor DNA can be designed to either introduce or correct a mutation in a specific gene locus. Alternatively, the donor DNA can be designed to insert gene-sized fragments, including an entire expression cassette or a corrective DNA fragment of the gene to be corrected. In the latter case, the main benefit of gene addition is that an engineered nuclease combined with a single donor DNA can be used for correcting all mutations located downstream of the DSB in a given gene, while still keeping gene expression under the control of the endogenous promoter (Cathomen and Joung 2008).

The design and exact nature of donor DNA will influence the success of the approach. Successful incorporation of larger DNA inserts requires several hundred homologous base pairs on both sides of the nuclease-induced break. Short single-strand DNA can also be used, but such a template would be limited to applications that require small changes close to the DSB cut site, such as the correction of point mutations (Chen et al. 2011).

Targeted insertion of entire donor expression cassettes is aimed at restoring the cellular phenotype by the integration of a therapeutic expression cassette into an extragenic "safe harbor" such as AAVS1 site or the albumin intron site (Papapetrou and Schambach 2016, Sadelain, Papapetrou, and Bushman 2011, Sharma et al. 2015, DeKelver et al. 2010). Such a "safe harbor" is anticipated to support high, consistent, and sustained transgene expression levels without any signs of genotoxic side effects. Therefore, an engineered nuclease combined with a customized donor DNA could be used for the correction of any given monogenetic inherited disorder that is amendable to genome editing therapy protocols (Lieber et al. 2003). The proof-of-concept was demonstrated in hybrid pharmacology and toxicology studies using ZFNs and cDNA donor inserts for treating hemophilia B, mucopolysaccharidosis (MPS) I, and MPS II (Laoharawee et al. 2018, Li et al. 2012, Ou et al. 2019).

27.3 Genome Editing Technologies

The novel genome editing technologies arising from basic research efforts investigating targeted nucleic acid binding and editing are promising and have brought great potential for new ways to treat disease. A brief summary of each genome editing technology follows.

27.3.1 Zinc Finger Nucleases

ZFNs, the most clinically advanced engineered nuclease platform, are composed of zinc finger-binding proteins fused to a nuclease domain. The zinc finger motif, first identified by Sir Aaron Klug as the DNA-binding region in the transcription factor IIA in *Xenopus laevis*, is one of the most common structural motifs in eukaryote DNA-binding proteins and transcription factors (reviewed in (Carroll 2014, Pabo, Peisach, and Grant 2001). When zinc fingers are fused with a FokI nuclease domain, specific targeting and editing of the genome is achieved (Durai et al. 2005, Li, Wu, and Chandrasegaran 1992).

Nearly 30 years ago, the crystal structure of a zinc finger DNA-binding motif bound to its DNA target was determined, providing the framework for understanding how these transcription factors recognize DNA and suggesting that this motif may provide a useful basis for the design of novel DNA-binding proteins (Pavletich and Pabo 1991). Each zinc finger is comprised of ~30 amino acids that fold into one α-helix and two short β strands (reviewed by (Carroll 2014, Pabo, Peisach, and Grant 2001)) (Figure 27.1). Each finger uses at least six amino acids to bind to ~3 base pairs of DNA, and the α-helix portion of the zinc finger then fits into a region within the major groove. The zinc finger consists of a Cys2-His2 motif, meaning that two cysteine and two histidine residues coordinate with a zinc atom to maintain the structure by holding the α-helix and antiparallel β-sheet together.

Zinc fingers are typically assembled in modules of at least three consecutive fingers to provide adequate binding affinity, where the best three-finger combinations have an equilibrium dissociation constant (Kd) in the low nanomolar range (Carroll 2014, Pabo, Peisach, and Grant 2001). Three to six individual fingers can be linked to enable the construction of arrays that recognize longer sequences of 9–18 base pairs of DNA sequence and can confer specificity within 68 billion base pairs of DNA. Further specificity can be engineered by changing critical residues within the recognition helices. In addition, individual fingers in an array can potentially interact and make base-specific contacts in sequences recognized by adjacent fingers, and optimization of binding can therefore be potentially altered by interactions between individual fingers.

The nuclease domain of the ZFN is derived from the C-terminus of the FokI restriction endonuclease. Chandrasegaran and colleagues found that the FokI recognition and cleavage activities could be separated and demonstrated that cleavage specificity could be altered by linking the nonspecific nuclease domain with the DNA targeting capabilities of zinc fingers (Kim, Cha, and Chandrasegaran 1996). FokI only cuts DNA when it dimerizes, so two sets of zinc fingers are required to induce a DSB, generating a 5′ overhang. These enzymes, however, can be engineered such that within the dimer, one side of the nuclease domain is catalytically active, while its twin is catalytically inactive, which will generate a single-stranded nick rather than a DSB (Corrigan-Curay et al. 2015).

For selective ZFN engineering, there are several regions that can be optimized including the base contacts, space between the ZFN binding sites, length of the linker between the zinc finger and the FokI nuclease, and ZFN residues that make contact with the DNA phosphate backbone (Pabo, Peisach, and Grant 2001, Paschon et al. 2019). Additionally, Miller showed that editing specificity can be enhanced by attenuating DNA cleavage kinetics of FokI, which reduces off-target nuclease activity (Miller et al. 2019). Several groups have attempted to ascertain a zinc finger protein (ZFP)-DNA base recognition code, but the diversity of ZFN side chain-base interactions precludes the deciphering of a simple code. Thus, as with monoclonal antibody engineering, ZFN engineering requires knowledge, experience, plus empirical testing to generate optimal ZFNs.

ZFPs can also be engineered to function as transcriptional regulators. In vitro and in vivo preclinical studies evaluated allele-selective zinc fingers protein-transcription factors (ZFP-TFs) targeting the mutant form of the huntingtin gene, repressing its transcription and selectively lowering the production of the human huntingtin protein (Zeitler et al. 2019). The ZFP-TFs lack the FokI nuclease motif, and instead, the ZFPs are tethered to a transcriptional repression domain.

Clinical studies evaluating ZFN technology are summarized in Table 27.1. The first clinical study to evaluate ex vivo

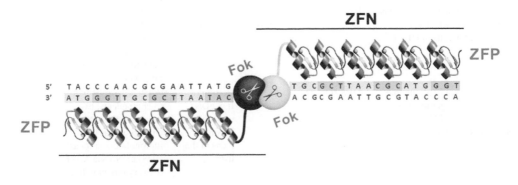

FIGURE 27.1 Zinc finger nuclease.

TABLE 27.1

Summary of Ongoing Clinical Studies with Genome Editing Technologies (as of September 2020; clinicaltrials.gov)

Nuclease Type	Study Title	Disease	Route	Target/ Modification	Delivery	Clinical Stage	ClinicalTrials. gov Identifier
ZFN	Study of molecular-targeted therapy using zinc finger nuclease in cervical precancerous lesions	CIN	In vivo	HPV E6 and E7 disruption	In situ delivery of plasmid ZFN DNA (ZFN-603 and ZFN-758) via suppository formulation	Phase 1	NCT02800369
ZFN	A phase 1 study of T cells genetically modified at the CCR5 gene by zinc finger nucleases SB-729mR in HIV-infected patients	HIV	Ex vivo	CCR5 disruption	SB-728mR ZFNs (mRNA electroporation) to autologous CD4+ T cells	Phase 1	NCT02388594
ZFN	Ascending dose study of genome editing by zinc finger nuclease therapeutic SB-FIX in subjects with severe hemophilia B	Hemophilia B	In vivo	Insertion of FIX cDNA into albumin intron 1 locus in liver	IV delivery of SB-FIX (3 components; two separate ZFN cDNAs and promoterless FIX cDNA) via AAV6 delivery targeting liver	Phase 1	NCT02695160
ZFN	CCR5-modified T cells for HIV infection	HIV	Ex vivo	CCR5 disruption	SB-728-T ZFNs (adenovirus transduction) to autologous CD4+ T cells	Phase 1	NCT03666871
ZFN	Autologous T cells genetically modified at the CCR5 gene by zinc finger nucleases SB-728 for HIV	HIV	Ex vivo	CCR5 disruption	SB-728-T ZFNs (adenovirus transduction) to autologous CD4+ T cells	Phase 1	NCT00842634
ZFN	Study of autologous T cells genetically modified at the CCR5 gene by zinc finger nucleases in HIV-infected subjects	HIV	Ex vivo	CCR5 disruption	SB-728-T ZFNs (adenovirus transduction) to autologous CD4+ T cells	Phase 1	NCT01252641
ZFN	Ascending dose study of genome editing by the zinc finger nuclease (ZFN) therapeutic SB-318 in subjects with MPS I	MPS I	In vivo	Insertion of IDUA cDNA into albumin intron 1 locus in liver	IV delivery of SB-318 (3 components; two separate ZFN cDNAs and promoterless IDUA cDNA via AAV6 delivery targeting liver	Phase 1	NCT02702115
ZFN	Phase 1 dose escalation study of autologous T cells genetically modified at the CCR5 gene by zinc finger nucleases in HIV-infected patients	HIV	Ex vivo	CCR5 disruption	SB-728mR-HSPC ZFNs (mRNA electroporation) to autologous hematopoietic stem/ progenitor cells	Phase 1	NCT01044654
ZFN	Safety study of zinc finger nuclease CCR5-modified hematopoietic stem/progenitor cells in HIV-1 infected patients	HIV	Ex vivo	CCR5 disruption	SB-728mR-HSPC ZFNs (mRNA electroporation) to autologous hematopoietic stem/ progenitor cells	Phase 1	NCT02500849
ZFN	Ascending dose study of genome editing by zinc finger nuclease (ZFN) therapeutic SB-913 in subjects with MPS II	MPS II	In vivo	Insertion of IDS cDNA into albumin intron 1 locus in the liver	IV delivery of SB-913 (3 components; two separate ZFN cDNAs and a promoterless iduronidate-2-sulfatase (IDS) cDNA via AAV6 delivery targeting liver	Phase 1	NCT03041324

(Continued)

TABLE 27.1 (*Continued*)

Summary of Ongoing Clinical Studies with Genome Editing Technologies (as of September 2020; clinicaltrials.gov)

Nuclease Type	Study Title	Disease	Route	Target/ Modification	Delivery	Clinical Stage	ClinicalTrials. gov Identifier
ZFN	Repeat doses of SB-728mR-T after cyclophosphamide conditioning in HIV-infected subjects on HAART	HIV	Ex vivo	CCR5 disruption	SB-728mR-T ZFNs (mRNA electroporation) to autologous CD4+ T cells	Phase I	NCT02225665
ZFN	CD4 CAR+ ZFN-modified T cells in HIV therapy	HIV	Ex vivo	CCR5 disruption	SB-728mR ZFNs (mRNA electroporation) and CD4 CAR+ autologous T cells	Pilot	NCT03617198
ZFN	Long-term follow-up of HIV subjects exposed to SB-728-T or SB-728mR-T	HIV-1	Ex vivo	CCR5 disruption	SB-728-T ZFNs (adenovirus transduction) or SB-728mR-T (mRNA electroporation) to autologous CD4+ T cells	Phase 1	NCT04201782
ZFN	A study to assess the safety, tolerability, and efficacy of ST-400 for the treatment of transfusion-dependent beta-thalassemia (TDT)	Transfusion-dependent beta-thalassemia	Ex vivo	BCL11A enhancer disruption	ST-400 ZFNs (mRNA electroporation) to autologous CD34+ hematopoietic stem/progenitor cells	Phase 1	NCT03432364
ZFN	A study to assess the safety, tolerability, and efficacy of BIVV003 for autologous hematopoietic stem cell transplantation in patients with severe sickle cell disease	Severe sickle cell disease	Ex vivo	BCL11A enhancer disruption	BIVV003 ZFNs (mRNA electroporation) to autologous hematopoietic stem/progenitor cells	Phase 1	NCT03653247
Homing Endonuclease	Dose-escalation study of safety of PBCAR0191 in patients with r/r NHL and r/r B-cell ALL	Relapsed/refractory (r/r) B cell precursor ALL; r/r NHL	Ex vivo	TCR disruption	Engineered homing endonuclease (mRNA electroporation) to knock out the T-cell receptor to produce allogeneic anti-CD19 CAR T cells	Phase 1/2	NCT03666000
Homing Endonuclease	Dose escalation study of safety of PBCAR20A in subjects with r/r NHL or r/r CLL/SLL	r/r NHL; r/r CLL or SLL	Ex vivo	TCR disruption	Engineered homing endonuclease (mRNA electroporation) to knock out the T-cell receptor and produce allogeneic anti-CD20 CAR T-cell therapy	Phase 1/2	NCT04030195
Homing Endonuclease	A dose escalation study to evaluate the safety and clinical activity of PBCAR269A in study participants with relapsed/refractory multiple myeloma	Multiple myeloma	Ex vivo	TCR disruption	Engineered homing endonuclease (mRNA electroporation) to knock out the T-cell receptor and produce allogeneic anti-BCMA CAR T-cell therapy	Phase 1/2a	NCT04171843
TALEN	Study of targeted therapy using transcription activator-like effector nucleases in cervical precancerous lesions	HPV persistency and HPV16-positive CIN	In vivo	HPV16 oncoproteins E6 and E7 disruption	In situ delivery of plasmid DNA encoding TALEs (T27 and T512) via suppository formulation targeting HPV16 oncoproteins E6 and E7, respectively	Phase 1	NCT03226470

(*Continued*)

TABLE 27.1 (*Continued*)

Summary of Ongoing Clinical Studies with Genome Editing Technologies (as of September 2020; clinicaltrials.gov)

Nuclease Type	Study Title	Disease	Route	Target/ Modification	Delivery	Clinical Stage	ClinicalTrials. gov Identifier
TALEN and CRISPR	A safety and efficacy study of TALE and CRISPR/Cas9 in the treatment of HPV-related cervical intraepithelial neoplasia	HPV persistency and HPV16- and HPV18- positive CIN	In vivo	HPV16 and HPV18 oncoproteins E6 and E7 disruption	In situ delivery of plasmid DNA via suppository formulation of TALEN or CRISPR/Cas 9 plasmids targeting HPV16 and HVP18 oncoproteins E6 and E7	Phase 1	NCT03057912
TALEN	Study evaluating safety and efficacy of UCART targeting CS1 in patients with relapsed/refractory multiple myeloma	Multiple myeloma	Ex vivo	TRAC and CD52 disruption	TALENs (mRNA electroporation) to knock out the T-cell receptor alpha chain and CD52 and produce allogeneic anti-CS1 CAR T cells, alemtuzumab	Phase 1	NCT04142619
TALEN	Phase 1 study of UCART22 in patients with relapsed or refractory CD22+ B-cell acute lymphoblastic leukemia (BALLI-01)	B-cell ALL	Ex vivo	TRAC and CD52 disruption	TALENs (mRNA electroporation) to knock out the T-cell receptor alpha chain and CD52 and produce allogeneic anti-CD22 CAR T cells	Phase 1	NCT04150497
TALEN	Study evaluating safety and efficacy of UCART123 in patients with relapsed/refractory acute myeloid leukemia	Acute myeloid leukemia	Ex vivo	TRAC and CD52 disruption	TALENs (mRNA electroporation) to knock out the T-cell receptor alpha chain and CD52 and produce allogeneic anti-CD123 CAR T cells	Phase 1	NCT03190278
CRISPR/ Cas9	A study of metastatic gastrointestinal cancers treated with tumor-infiltrating lymphocytes in which the gene encoding the intracellular immune checkpoint CISH is inhibited using CRISPR genetic engineering	Gastro-intestinal cancers	Ex vivo	CISH disruption	CRISPR/Cas9 (mRNA electroporation) targeting the CISH gene in autologous tumor-infiltrating lymphocytes	Phase 1	NCT04426669
CRISPR/ Cas9	Safety of transplantation of CRISPR CCR5-modified CD34+ cells in HIV-infected subjects with hematological malignancies	HIV-infected subjects	Ex vivo	CCR5 disruption	CRISPR/Cas9 (mRNA electroporation) targeting the CCR5 gene in autologous CD34+ cells	Phase 1	NCT03164135
CRISPR/ Cas9	NY-ESO-1-redirected CRISPR (TCRendo and PD1) edited T cells (NYCE T cells)	Multiple myeloma, melanoma, synovial sarcoma, myxoid/round cell liposarcoma	Ex vivo	PD-1 and TCR disruption	CRISPR/Cas9 (mRNA electroporation) targeting the PD-1 and endogenous TCR genes in autologous T cells to target NY-ESO-1 expressing neoplasia	Phase 1	NCT03399448
CRISPR/ Cas9	Study of CRISPR-Cas9-mediated PD-1 and TCR gene-knocked-out mesothelin-directed CAR-T cells in patients with mesothelin-positive solid tumors	Multiple mesothelin-positive neoplasias	Ex vivo	PD-1 TCR	CRISPR/Cas9 (mRNA delivery not specified) targeting PD-1 and TCR genes to produce allogeneic mesothelin-directed CAR-T cells	Phase 1	NCT03545815

(*Continued*)

TABLE 27.1 (*Continued*)

Summary of Ongoing Clinical Studies with Genome Editing Technologies (as of September 2020; clinicaltrials.gov)

Nuclease Type	Study Title	Disease	Route	Target/ Modification	Delivery	Clinical Stage	ClinicalTrials. gov Identifier
CRISPR/ Cas9	CRISPR (HPK1)-edited CD19-specific CAR-T cells (XYF19 CAR-T cells) for CD19+ leukemia or lymphoma	CD19+ leukemia or lymphoma	Ex vivo	HPK1	CRISPR/Cas9 (mRNA delivery not specified) targeting the HPK1 gene to produce anti-CD19 CAR-T cells	Phase 1	NCT04037566
CRISPR/ Cas9	A safety and efficacy study evaluating CTX120 in subjects with relapsed or refractory multiple myeloma	r/r multiple myeloma	Ex vivo	TRAC and B2M disruption	CRISPR/Cas9 (mRNA electroporation) targeting TRAC and B2M to generate allogeneic BCMA-directed CAR T cells	Phase 1	NCT04244656
CRISPR/ Cas9	A safety and efficacy study evaluating CTX001 in subjects with transfusion-dependent beta-thalassemia	Transfusion-dependent beta-thalassemia	Ex vivo	BCL11A enhancer	CRISPR/Cas9 (mRNA electroporation) targeting BCL11A enhancer in autologous CD34+ hematopoietic stem and progenitor cells	Phase 1	NCT03655678
CRISPR/ Cas9	A safety and efficacy study evaluating CTX130 in subjects with relapsed or refractory renal cell carcinoma	r/r renal cell carcinoma	Ex vivo	TRAC and B2M disruption	CRISPR/Cas9 (mRNA electroporation) targeting TRAC and B2M to generate allogeneic CD70-directed CAR T cells	Phase 1	NCT04438083
CRISPR/ Cas9	A safety and efficacy study evaluating CTX130 in subjects with relapsed or refractory T- or B-cell malignancies	r/r T or B cell malignancies	Ex vivo	TRAC and B2M disruption	CRISPR/Cas9 (mRNA electroporation) targeting TRAC and B2M to generate allogeneic CD70-directed CAR T cells	Phase 1	NCT04502446
CRISPR/ Cas9	A safety and efficacy study evaluating CTX110 in subjects with relapsed or refractory B-cell malignancies	r/r B cell malignancies	Ex vivo	TRAC and B2M disruption	CRISPR/Cas9 (mRNA electroporation) targeting TRAC and B2M to generate allogeneic CD19-directed CAR T cells	Phase 1	NCT04035434
CRISPR/ Cas9	A safety and efficacy study evaluating CTX001 in subjects with severe sickle cell disease	Sickle cell disease	Ex vivo	BCL11A enhancer disruption	CRISPR/Cas9 (mRNA electroporation) targeting BCL11A enhancer in autologous CD34+ hematopoietic stem and progenitor cells	Phase 1	NCT03745287
CRISPR/ Cas9	iHSCs with the gene correction of HBB intervent subjects with beta-thalassemia mutations	Beta-thalassemia	Ex vivo	HBB gene correction	CRISPR/Cas9 (delivery not specified) HBB gene correction of autologous iHSCs administered to beta-thalassemia patients	Phase 1	NCT03728322
CRISPR/ Cas9	Study of PD-1 gene-knocked-out mesothelin-directed CAR-T cells with the conditioning of PC in mesothelin-positive multiple solid tumors	Mesothelin positive multiple solid tumors	Ex vivo	PD-1 disruption	CRISPR/Cas9 (delivery not specified) PD-1 disruption in autologous CAR-T cells	Phase 1	NCT03747965

(Continued)

TABLE 27.1 (*Continued*)

Summary of Ongoing Clinical Studies with Genome Editing Technologies (as of September 2020; clinicaltrials.gov)

Nuclease Type	Study Title	Disease	Route	Target/ Modification	Delivery	Clinical Stage	ClinicalTrials. gov Identifier
CRISPR/ Cas9	A study evaluating UCART-19 in patients with relapsed or refractory CD19+ leukemia and lymphoma	r/r CD19+ leukemia and lymphoma	Ex vivo	TCR and B2M disruption	CRISPR/Cas9 (mRNA electroporation) TCR and B2M disruption to generate allogeneic anti-CD19 CAR T cells	Phase 1	NCT03166878
CRISPR/ Cas9	A long-term follow-up study in subjects who received CTX001	Beta-thalassemia SCD	Ex vivo	BCL11A enhancer disruption	CRISPR/Cas9 (mRNA electroporation) targeting BCL11A enhancer in autologous CD34+ hematopoietic stem and progenitor cells	Phase 1	NCT04208529
CRISPR/ Cas9	PD-1-knockout engineered T cells for advanced esophageal cancer	Advanced esophageal cancer	Ex vivo	PD-1 disruption	CRISPR/Cas9 (delivery not specified) targeting PD-1 in autologous T cells	Phase 1	NCT03081715
CRISPR/ Cas9	A feasibility and safety study of universal dual specificity CD19 and CD20 or CD22 CAR-T cell immunotherapy for relapsed or refractory leukemia and lymphoma	r/r B-cell leukemia and lymphoma	Ex vivo	TCR and B2M disruption	TCR and B2M disruption (delivery not specified) to generate allogeneic CAR T cells	Phase 1	NCT03398967
CRISPR/ Cas9	TACE combined with PD-1-knockout engineered T cells in advanced hepatocellular carcinoma	Hepato-cellular carcinoma	Ex vivo	PD-1 disruption	PD-1 knockout (delivery not specified) in autologous T cells	Phase 1	NCT04417764
CRISPR/ Cas9	Cell therapy for high-risk T-cell malignancies using CD7-specific CAR expressed on autologous T cells	T-cell leukemia or lymphoma	Ex vivo	CD7 disruption	CD7-knockout (delivery not specified) in autologous T cells	Phase 1	NCT03690011
CRISPR/ Cas9	PD-1-knockout engineered T cells for muscle-invasive bladder cancer	Bladder cancer	Ex vivo	PD-1 disruption	PD-1-knockout (delivery not specified) in autologous T cells	Phase 1	NCT02863913
CRISPR/ Cas9	PD-1-knockout engineered T cells for castration-resistant prostate cancer	Prostate cancer	Ex vivo	PD-1 disruption	PD-1-knockout (delivery not specified) in autologous T cells	Phase 1	NCT02867345
CRISPR/ Cas9	PD-1-knockout engineered T cells for metastatic renal cell carcinoma	Renal cell carcinoma	Ex vivo	PD-1 disruption	PD-1-knockout (delivery not specified) in autologous T cells	Phase 1	NCT02867332
CRISPR/ Cas9	PD-1-knockout engineered T cells for metastatic non-small-cell lung cancer	Non-small-cell lung cancer	Ex vivo	PD-1 disruption	PD-1-knockout (delivery not specified) in autologous T cells	Phase 1	NCT02793856
CRISPR/ Cas9	PD-1-knockout EBV-CTLs for advanced state EBV associated malignancies	EBV+ malignancies	Ex vivo	PD-1 disruption	PD-1-knockout (delivery not specified) in autologous T cells	Phase 1	NCT03044743
CRISPR/ Cas9	Single ascending dose study in participants with LCA10	Leber congenital amaurosis 10	In vivo	IVS26 mutation in CEP290 gene	Subretinal injection of EDIT-101 (AAV5 delivery) targeting specific mutation of CEP290 gene	Phase 1	NCT03872479
CRISPR/ Cas9	Study to evaluate safety, tolerability, pharmacokinetics, and pharmacodynamics of NTLA-2001 in patients with hereditary transthyretin amyloidosis with polyneuropathy	AATR amyloidosis	In vivo	Transthyretin (TTR) disruption	TTR knock out and delivery via lipid nanoparticles	Phase 1	NCT0460151

AAV, adeno-associated virus; ALL, acute lymphoblastic leukemia; BCMA, B-cell maturation antigen; CIN, cervical intraepithelial neoplasia; CLL, chronic lymphocytic leukemia; EBV, Epstein-Barr virus; HAART, highly active antiretroviral therapy; HBB, hemoglobin subunit beta; iHSC, induced hematopoietic stem cells; IV, intravenous; IDUA, iduronidase; IDS, iduronidate-2-sulfatase; NHL, non-Hodgkin's lymphoma; r/r, relapsed or refractory; PC, paclitaxel and cyclophosphamide; SCD, sickle cell disease; SLL, small lymphocytic lymphoma, TCR, T-cell receptor; TRAC, T-cell receptor alpha chain.

genome engineered cells used ZFNs targeting the CCR5 locus in autologous CD4+ T cells and experiences in T-cell adoptive transfer (reviewed in (Wang and Cannon 2016)). The initial study in HIV-1-positive subjects employed ex vivo adenoviral delivery of ZFNs to autologous T cells, and following early demonstration of clinical safety, subsequent studies were designed to further optimize treatment, including cell input and switching from adenoviral delivery of ZFNs to using mRNA electroporation. Engineering CD34+ hematopoietic stem and progenitor cells (HSPCs) instead of CD4+ T cells provided the potential to provide a long-lasting source of modified cells and to additionally protect CD4+ myeloid cells that are susceptible to HIV-1.

Additional ongoing studies are evaluating ZFNs targeting the BCL11A enhancer for the treatment of beta thalassemia and sickle cell disease. As in the HIV-1 study, ZFNs are delivered to autologous CD34+ HSPCs ex vivo and engineered cells are infused back into the donor subject.

Other investigators used ZFNs targeting the human papillomavirus (HPV)-type 18 oncoprotein E7, delivered as plasmid DNA formulated as a suppository, with potential antineoplastic activity for the treatment of cervical intraepithelial neoplasia.

Three clinical studies used in vivo AAV6 delivery of ZFNs and a corrective cDNA donor gene for the treatment of hemophilia B, MPS I, and MPS II (Clinicaltrials.gov). These were the first *in vivo* editing studies in human subjects (GEN 2017, Marchione 2017). Here the ZFN and cDNA donor genes were delivered in separate AAV6 vectors by intravenous infusion. The vectors target the liver, and ZFN expression is driven by a liver-specific promoter. The ZFNs are expressed and induce a DSB at the albumin intron 1 locus, and the cDNA donor is inserted into the cut site with transgene (e.g., Factor IX, iduronidase, and iduronate-2-sulfatase, respectively, for hemophilia B, MPS I, and MPS II) expression driven by the albumin promoter. The primary focus of these early phase 1/2 studies was safety, and further work is ongoing to optimize ZFN architecture and delivery.

27.3.2 Meganucleases

Meganucleases, also known as homing endonucleases, were first described by Bolotin and colleagues (Bolotin et al. 1971) and are microbial DNA-cleaving enzymes that mobilize their own reading frames by generating DSB at specific genomic invasion sites, where their open reading frames are then specifically duplicated into recipient alleles of a host gene

(Stoddard 2011). Homing endonucleases are considered selfish genetic elements that use host DNA repair mechanisms and homologous recombination to insert and multiply their genetic material without damaging the host.

An excellent review is provided by Stoddard (2011). These nucleases are found in microbes, yeast, phage, viruses, and some plants, but with no reports of homing endonuclease genes within genomes of more complex organisms. There are five families of homing endonucleases, with the most widespread and well-known LAGLIDADG family primarily used for genome editing applications. These exist as homodimers (two identical protein subunits – 160–200 residues in size) and a monomeric protein (100–120 residues in size) where tandem repeats of two domains are connected by a peptide linker. These nucleases generate a DSB with a four-base 3′ overhang.

These natural proteins recognize long stretches of DNA sequences (typically 20–30 base pairs) with high specificity but do not have distinct DNA binding and enzymatic cleavage domains; thus, engineering a meganuclease to modify DNA binding specificity frequently results in reduced nuclease activity (Figure 27.2). These challenges to engineering have hampered the preclinical development of homing endonucleases for therapeutic use. These nucleases, however, are small and can be easily packaged in commonly used vectors. They offer potentially high binding specificity, but challenges with their engineering and lack of customizable reagents pose a high hurdle for developing agents for clinical applications (Silva et al. 2011). To overcome this challenge, researchers shifted focus to the FokI nuclease, which has two separate domains for DNA recognition and cleavage (Kim and Chandrasegaran 1994, Li, Wu, and Chandrasegaran 1992) paving the way for the development of zinc finger and TALE nucleases.

There are three phase 1/2 clinical studies (as of September 2020; Clintrials.gov) using engineered homing endonuclease editing to generate allogeneic CAR T cells by inserting the CAR gene into the cut site at the T-cell receptor (TCR) (Table 27.1). The edited anti-CD19 CAR T cells are being evaluated in adult patients with relapsed/refractory B-cell precursor acute lymphoblastic leukemia and relapsed/refractory non-Hodgkin's lymphoma (NHL); edited anti-CD20 CAR T cells for the treatment of relapsed/refractory NHL, relapsed/refractory chronic lymphocytic leukemia, or relapsed/refractory small lymphocytic lymphoma; and edited anti-BCMA CAR T cells for the treatment of patients with multiple myeloma.

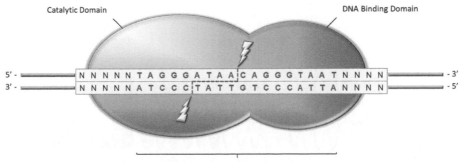

FIGURE 27.2 Meganuclease (Adapted from Jantz and J. 2012).

27.3.3 TALENs

TALENS are clinical-stage TALE DNA-binding proteins fused to a FokI nuclease domain. TALEs were first described in 2009 by Boch and Moscous and Bogdanove (2009). The genomes of some plant-pathogenic bacteria (*Xanthomonas* and related genera) encode proteins that are imported into the host cell nucleus and activate genes to promote infection (Carroll 2014). The TALE proteins have DNA-binding domain modules made up of tandem repeats of ~34 amino acids (Figure 27.3). These modules are unique structures and not related to other DNA-recognition motifs. The framework is highly conserved among modules, but residues in positions 12 and 13, termed repeat variable di-residues (RVDs), vary in concert with individual base pairs in the target DNA sequence. The structures of TALE repeats binding to DNA show a helical staircase-like form, with consecutive modules closely opposed to each other. The RVD of each repeat is on a loop that is directed into the major groove. Only residue 13 makes contact with DNA, while the residue 12 side chain folds back and makes stabilizing contacts with other residues in the module.

Table 27.2 shows the accepted code for DNA recognition by TALEs, along with alternative RVDs that may be useful. The standard RVD for G is NN (asparagine in positions 12 and 13),

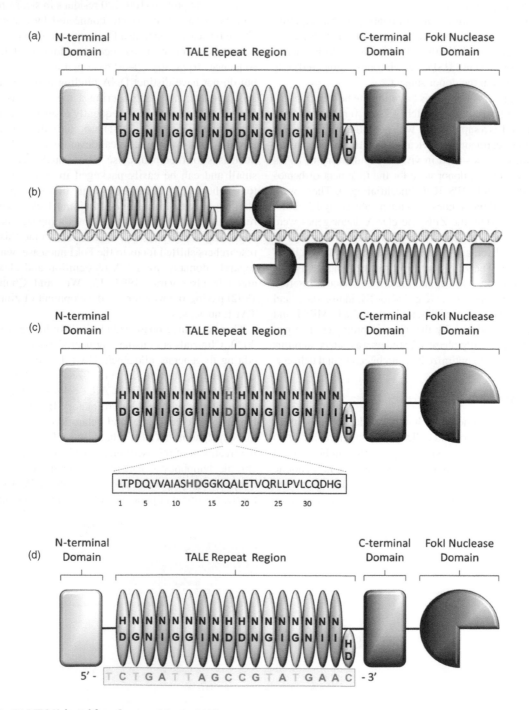

FIGURE 27.3 TALEN (Adapted from Joung and Sander 2013).

TABLE 27.2

TALE Modules Used in DNA Recognition

Base Pair	Canonical Module[a,b]	Alternatives
A:T	NI	-
C:G	HD	N[*c]
G:C	NN	NK, NH[d]
T:A	NG	-

Source: From Carroll (2014).

[a] Modules are identified by the amino acid positions 12 and 13 of the TALE repeat, using one-letter codes: D, aspartic acid; G, glycine; H, histidine; I, isoleucine; K, lysine; N, asparagine. The asterisk indicates no residue.

[b] Modules HD and NN, for C:G and G:C base pairs, respectively, are considered strong in terms of binding affinity.

[c] This module alleviates inhibition by methylation on position 5 of cytosine and binds more weakly than HD.

[d] These alternatives are more specific for G:C but have weaker affinity than NN.

but it recognizes A in some contexts. NK and NH have greater specificity for G but bind in a weaker manner. To engineer DNA-binding specificity, individual TALE repeats are assembled into an array that is designed to recognize the target DNA sequence of about 13–20 base pairs. Numerous schemes for assembling new combinations of TALE modules for new targets have been published, and most of the building blocks have been made publicly available (Carroll 2014).

Once the TALE recognition code was identified and tested, the parallel to ZFN recognition became obvious, and it was not long before fusions with the FokI cleavage domain were produced (reviewed in (Carroll 2014)). Although the FokI nuclease domain is the same for TALENs and ZFNs, in contrast to ZFNs and for reasons that are not yet understood, TALENs cannot be manipulated to create nicks rather than DSBs.

There are several ongoing clinical studies using TALENs to edit hematopoietic cells (Table 27.1) (Clinicaltrials.gov). The first clinical use of TALENs involved compassionate use of allogeneic (universal) gene-modified chimeric antigen receptor (CAR) T cells to successfully treat two infants with refractory relapsed B-cell acute lymphoblastic leukemia (B-ALL) (Qasim et al. 2017). Allogeneic cells were obtained from healthy volunteers and edited to disable specific gene(s) to mitigate host recognition of the foreign cell as well as gene(s) involved in the donor cells mounting an immune response against the host. Here the T-cell receptor alpha chain constant (TRAC) region was disrupted to prevent TCR-mediated recognition of the patient's HLA antibodies and the CD52 loci was disrupted to permit alemtuzumab use in lymphodepletion. These allogeneic anti-CD19 CAR T cells also expressed the RQR8 CD20 mimotope safety switch allowing targeted elimination of RQR8+ cells by rituximab, which can halt runaway responses associated with CAR T treatment. These cells, using a different manufacturing process, are also being evaluated in patients with relapsed/refractory NHL and relapsed/refractory multiple myeloma. The same investigators are evaluating allogeneic CAR T cells targeting the CS1 antigen on plasma cells for the treatment of patients with multiple myeloma. Other studies using TALEN-edited TRAC and CD52 T cells include anti-CD22 CAR T cells for relapsed refractory B-ALL

and anti-CD123 CAR T cells for relapsed/refractory B acute myeloid leukemia and CD123 expressing hematopoietic malignancies such as blastic plasmacytoid dendritic cell neoplasm (BPDCN) and acute myeloid leukemia.

TALENs are also being evaluated for the treatment of infectious disease using polymer-coated plasmids (formulated as suppositories) encoding TALENs targeting HPV oncoproteins E6 and E7 for the treatment of cervical intraepithelial neoplasia (Hu et al. 2015).

27.3.4 CRISPR/Cas9

In 2012, Jennifer Doudna and Emmanuelle Charpentier discovered a bacterial defense system called clustered regularly interspaced short palindromic repeats (CRISPR)/CRISPR-associated (Cas) that protects organisms from invading virus and plasmids (Jinek et al. 2012) and has subsequently been used as a specific genome editing tool. This platform, derived from a bacterial innate immune system, has rapidly progressed on its development and captured considerable attention due to the relative ease of engineering its RNA-based targeting component. Within a year of discovery, four groups applied these reagents to genomic targets in human cells (Cho et al. 2013, Cong et al. 2013, Jinek et al. 2013, Mali et al. 2013).

CRISPR/Cas9 is distinct from previous engineered nucleases as an RNA guide is used to re-direct the Cas9 nuclease for site-specific genome editing. In bacteria and archaea, type II CRISPR systems process foreign sequences from invading bacteriophages or plasmids into small segments that are then introduced into a CRISPR array. These fragments of foreign DNA become templates for 20-nucleotide sequence of CRISPR RNA (crRNA), which now contains a variable sequence from the invading DNA. This crRNA then hybridizes with a trans-activating RNA (tracrRNA), and the RNAs form complexes with the Cas9 nuclease protein (Jinek et al. 2012). The next time this foreign sequence is detected, it is cleaved and degraded, thereby combating the intrusion.

The crRNA and tracrRNA can be combined into a single RNA molecule known as a guide RNA (gRNA) that can still engage the Cas9 protein (Figure 27.4). The gRNA should have a 20-nucleotide guide sequence corresponding to the desired target followed by 80 nucleotides of hybrid crRNA/tracRNA (Jinek et al. 2012). Similar to ZFNs, it is possible to make a nick rather than a DSB with this system. However, unlike ZFNs and TALEs, the DSB cut made by CRISPR/Cas9 leaves mostly blunt ends.

Another feature of this system, the Cas9 nuclease, is directed to cleave the complementary target DNA sequence if it is adjacent to a short sequence known as the protospacer adjacent motif (PAM). This PAM sequence commonly used from *Streptococcus pyogenes* has the sequence 5′-[N]GG, although 5′-[N]AG can also be used. Many bacteria have the Cas9 system, but not all possess the PAM sequences, providing some additional variability. The first crystal structures of Cas9 protein alone and in complex show how the protein domains are arranged and how recognition and cleavage is accomplished. These structures provide the basis for engineering Cas9 to have enhanced specificity and altered PAM recognition, among other valuable features (Carroll 2014).

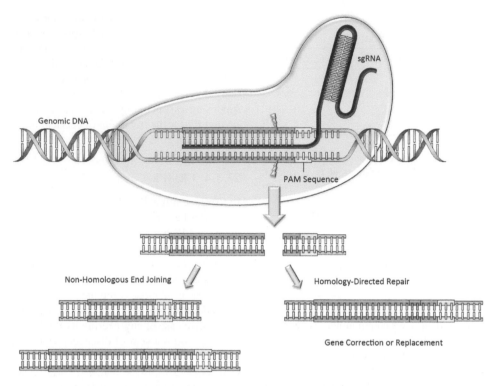

FIGURE 27.4 CRISPR/Cas System (Adapted from Tu et al. 2015).

Some researchers have made Cas9 hybrid cleavage reagents using meganucleases, ZFNs, or TALE domains to make recognition more flexible, and fusion to recombinases has been completed (Carroll 2014). Additionally, nuclease-inactivated versions of Cas9 protein linked to RNA binding domain can serve as an RNA-guided transcription factor (Carroll 2014).

There are currently over 23 ongoing phase 1/2 clinical studies using CRISPR/Cas9 technology as of November 30, 2020 (Clinicaltrials.gov), primarily focused on editing hematopoietic cells (e.g., HSPC, T cells, and CAR T cells) as well as a few studies evaluating the treatment of ocular disease or solid tumors (Table 27.1).

Many investigators are using CRISPR/Cas9 to edit autologous hematopoietic cells. Here, the target cells are collected from a patient, modified ex vivo via transient expression of CRISPR/Cas9 to inactivate target gene(s), and then returned to the same patient. This autologous cell strategy is being used to inactivate the CCR5 locus in CD34+ HSPC for the treatment of HIV-1-infected subjects, the erythroid-specific BCL11A enhancer locus in CD34+ HSPC for the treatment of beta thalassemia and sickle cell disease. Autologous T cells have been edited with CRISPR/Cas9 targeting the TRAC and PD-1 genes for the treatment of hematopoietic cell cancer and induced hematopoietic stem cells (iHSC) edited at the hemoglobin B gene for the treatment of patients with beta thalassemia. Autologous T cells were also engineered to express a cancer-testis antigen NY-ESO-1-directed TCR and edited to inactivate the PD-1 and redirect the endogenous TCR genes for the treatment of NY-ESO-1-expressing neoplasia. Other investigators have used CRISPR/Cas9 to disrupt the expression of TCR α and β chains and PD-1 for the treatment of

multiple myeloma, to disrupt the PD-1 gene for CAR T cells directed to cancer cells expressing mesothelin or the HPK1 gene in CD19 CAR T cells for the treatment of leukemia and lymphoma. CRISPR/Cas9 is also being used to inactivate the intracellular immune checkpoint CISH in autologous tumor-infiltrating lymphocytes (TILs) for the treatment of gastrointestinal cancer.

Allogeneic (universal) CAR T cells are being developed to rapidly provide immune therapy with off-the-shelf cell products that have been edited to mitigate the risk of GVHD. Several researchers have accomplished this by using CRISPR/Cas9 editing to eliminate the TRAC and major histocompatibility I (MHC I) beta-2 microglobulin (β2M) genes in T cells. These edited allogeneic T cells are then transduced to express CARs targeting validated tumor targets, including the BCMA antigen-expressed B cells for the treatment of multiple myeloma, the CD70 antigen expressed on both hematologic cancers and solid tumors including relapsed remitting renal cell carcinoma, the CS1 antigen for multiple myeloma, or dual anti-CD20 and anti-CD22 CAR T cells for the treatment of lymphocytic leukemia. The same group developing allogeneic anti-CD19 CAR T cells using TALEN editing is also exploring CRISPR/Cas9 editing for the treatment of leukemia and lymphoma.

CRISPR/Cas9 therapy is also being evaluated in patients with Leber congenital amaurosis 10 (LCA 10), by targeting a specific mutation of the gene CEP290 in the retina. This is the first in vivo editing clinical study using CRISPR/Cas9 (Ledford 2020) and is based on a strategy of delivering AAV vectors encoding two gRNAs targeting the CEP290 gene to photoreceptors by a subretinal injection. Nuclease expression results in a cut to excise the mutation-containing region and restoration of normal function to the gene. CRISPR/Cas9 mRNA components encapsulated in lipid nanoparticles is being evaluated in patients with hereditary ATTR amyloidosis (Gillmore et al. 2021).

27.3.5 Hybrid Nucleases

Hybrid versions of endonucleases have been developed by combining various DNA- or RNA-binding motifs with different nuclease domains. Boissel and colleagues describe the combination of the DNA-binding region of TALE with a site-specific meganuclease, and this technology is currently in preclinical studies targeting the CCR5 locus in human CD4+ cells for HIV treatment (Boissel et al. 2014). Additionally, the mRNA-based megaTAL platform is in the preclinical stages of development and approaching clinical development.

27.4 Delivery of Genome Editing Technologies for Therapeutic Use

One of the key challenges for successful therapy with engineered nucleases relies on the ability to deliver all components efficiently, effectively, and safely to target cells in culture or within the body. This challenge is especially true for systemic delivery in vivo and likely explains the plethora of ex vivo hematopoietic cell-targeted therapies in clinical trials. For HSPCs, T cells, or CAR T cells, engineered nucleases can be delivered via transfection or electroporation with synthetic mRNA. These methods result in transient exposure to nucleases. For in vivo delivery, DNA-coding sequences are generally delivered via recombinant AAV vectors, with some investigators exploring the use of lipid nanoparticle delivery of mRNA-encoding engineered nucleases in preclinical studies. Much work is ongoing to understand the most safe and effective ways to effectively deliver engineered nucleases to various body compartments (e.g., eye, synovium), systemically to various tissues (e.g., liver, skeletal muscle, brain), or into the CNS compartment (e.g., intracerebroventricular, intrathecal). Designs for AAV vector constructs, DNA expression constructs including choice of tissue-specific promotors, other regulatory motifs, and/or mRNA are also critical for the development of successful genomic medicines yet are beyond the scope of this chapter.

27.5 Nonclincial Evaluation of Engineered Nucleases

Genome editing technologies continue to evolve, making progress towards improving engineered nuclease activity, specificity, and sensitivity. More genome editing programs are transitioning from laboratory bench to clinical studies, targeting a diverse collection of human diseases. Regulatory guidance and nonclinical development strategies for these novel compounds are evolving as well. For a toxicologist new to the field of genome editing and responsible for designing a nonclinical program for an engineered nuclease, it is important to partner with molecular biologist colleagues in the research group and gain a deep understanding of the editing technology and tools at hand.

The underlying pharmacology and toxicology philosophy guiding the development of small molecules and biologics provides the foundation for safety assessment of these novel editing therapies, yet due to the unique nature of engineered nuclease products and their intended indications, new types of investigations and tools are necessary to add to the nonclinical assessment toolbox.

27.5.1 Nonclinical Program Objectives and Strategy

The objective of the nonclinical program for genome editing medicines is to provide sufficient information for a risk/benefit assessment for use of the investigational product in humans, based on the assessment of product pharmacology, biodistribution/pharmacokinetics, and toxicology profiles. Many aspects guiding nonclinical development of engineered nucleases are shared with gene therapy products including the assessment of potential effects of the vector backbone (e.g., viral, bacterial, plasma-derived sequences), expressed transgene, medical delivery device used, or excipients (EMA) (Chapter 26). Features unique to engineered nucleases include the assessment of on- and off-target editing, functional consequences of editing, and associated safety risk.

The nature and extent of the nonclinical program depends on the intended use of the engineered nuclease (ex vivo or in vivo editing), targeted cell type(s), availability of relevant animal models, intended route of administration, study population, and treatment regimen in clinical studies. A case-by-case approach to nonclinical development is customary due to the novelty of the technology and anticipated use in the clinic.

The US FDA summarizes key objectives for a successful nonclinical program for gene therapy medicines (USFDA 2013), which are also applicable to engineered nucleases, including:

1. Establishment of biological plausibility.
2. Identification of biologically active dose levels.
3. Selection of potential starting dose level, dose-escalation schedule, and dosing regimen for clinical trials.
4. Establishment of feasibility and reasonable safety of the investigational product's proposed clinical route of administration.
5. Support of patient eligibility criteria.
6. Identification of physiologic parameters that can guide clinical monitoring.
7. Identification of potential public health risks (e.g., to the general public, caregivers, family members, close contacts (for example, co-workers), and intimate contacts).

The data from the nonclinical program should thus guide the design of early-stage clinical studies, as well as provide the foundation for the conduct of future nonclinical studies supporting the product development.

27.5.2 Pharmacology

The pharmacology evaluation of genome editing products focuses on assessing the expression profile of the engineered nuclease, intended editing activity (defined as % insertions and deletions [% indels]) at the target site, persistence over time in target tissue, subsequent pharmacologic activity related to either disabling a specific gene element, or if the edits result in incorporation of a donor cDNA encoding a therapeutic protein, the functional consequences of the donor transgene expression. Pharmacology studies can also characterize the lack of expression and activity in non-target tissues.

Selection of relevant species for pharmacological assessment is critical to the success of the nonclinical program, and this may pose an additional challenge when species-specific sequence differences are present within the target genomic site or if no relevant animal models are available. For the former case, surrogate engineered nucleases will likely be needed. A combined hybrid pharmacology and toxicology study is recommended for genome editing therapies since most are intended for rare monogenic diseases and animal disease models are necessary to establish proof-of-concept and build confidence that the editing technology can work and have a positive impact on disease (Cavagnaro and Silva Lima 2015).

For ex vivo nuclease editing of immune cells (e.g., edited HSPC, T cells, or CAR T cells), % indels and editing persistence can be evaluated in human cells prepared with the clinically representative manufacturing process. Demonstrating functional activity will likely require an animal model, if feasible. The edited human immune cell product should ideally be pharmacologically active in the animal model, although often animal models lack the human target antigen and/or necessary human cytokines and/or growth factors to allow the long-term assessment. There are also challenges associated with xenoreactivity of human hematopoietic cells in immunodeficient mice and generation of graft-versus-host disease (GvHD), which limits study duration.

27.5.2.1 On-Target Nuclease Activity Assessment

Assessment of on-target nuclease activity is typically conducted via next-generation sequencing (NGS; also referred to as deep sequencing or massive parallel sequencing) of the target region of DNA within the genome. This high-throughput and cost-effective technology has evolved over the last 10 years and will continue to revolutionize genetic analysis. The primary NGS read-out for effectiveness of engineered nuclease activity is percentage of polymerase chain reaction (PCR) products/alleles/genes with insertions and deletions (% indels) at the target site.

NGS enables the interrogation of hundreds to thousands of genes at one time in multiple samples, as well as discovery and analysis of different types of genomic features in a single sequencing run, from single nucleotide variants, to copy number and structural variants, and even RNA fusions (ThermoFisher 2020).

NGS sequencing involves DNA extraction, library preparation, target enrichment, and sequencing (Goodwin, McPherson, and McCombie 2016, Slatko, Gardner, and Ausubel 2018,

Yohe and Thyagarajan 2017). Library preparation refers to the process of preparing DNA for use on a sequencer, and involves extraction, the locus of interest directly amplified with primers that have additional primer or bar-coded sequences directly encoded in them. Target enrichment can be performed by hybridization to complementary sequences or by PCR. Clinical and preclinical sequencing is generally performed with specialized instruments such as Illumina sequencers (HiSeq, MiSeq, and NexSeq) or Ion Torrent sequencers (IonPGM, IonProton, and IonS5).

27.5.2.2 In Vitro Pharmacology Studies

In vitro pharmacology studies for genome editing products should characterize the nuclease expression and activity (% indels) in target cells/tissue and subsequent functional activity related to the inactivation of the target gene or expression of an inserted gene. For ex vivo editing programs, human cells most reflective of the final clinical manufactured cell product are recommended for the study. For in vivo editing programs, the target cell type (e.g., primary human hepatocytes and/or hepatocyte cell lines) is recommended for characterization. Additionally, cell lines or primary cells derived from animal species used in pharmacology and toxicology studies should be used to characterize the nuclease activity, if necessary, and will often require species-specific surrogate engineered nucleases for in vivo investigation due to species sequence differences at the nuclease cut site. On- and off-target nuclease activity of species-specific surrogate nucleases will need characterization, and a discussion of any notable differences should be provided with regulatory submissions.

27.5.2.3 In Vivo Pharmacology Studies

The primary objective of vivo pharmacology studies for genome editing products is to understand the pharmacologic dose-response relationship (e.g., vector dose, % indels, pharmacological impact of editing) and justify dose selection for testing in clinical studies. These studies should use the most appropriate pharmacologically relevant animal models available, or an explanation of why the available models are not relevant or available.

Considerations for species selection include the presence of appropriate receptors for the uptake of virus/bacteria into cells, vector construct and regulatory elements driving tissue-specific expression of engineered nuclease, specificity of engineered nuclease binding to nucleic acid target, and expression level (and activity) of donor transgene or lack of expression of disrupted gene. If no relevant animal models are available, in vitro models representative of the disease state (collected from patient donors) can likely be used.

A hybrid pharmacology/toxicology approach is recommended for in vivo editing as well as gene therapy programs, allowing assessment in the same model, reduction in animal use, and an understanding of the pharmacology and toxicology profile in the presence of a disease state (USFDA 2013). The disease model can be used to characterize the levels of nuclease expression, degree of gene modification, persistence of edited cells over time, as well as the expression of inserted donor genes and the relationship to pharmacodynamic response in the disease model. Evaluating the safety of engineered nuclease administration and any potential adverse effects in the disease model is also helpful.

For ex vivo edited immune cells, demonstrating functional activity will likely require an animal model, if feasible. Efficiency and persistence of ZFN-mediated disabling of the CCR5 gene in T cells and HSPC was assessed in human edited cells, and these cells were then administered to an immunodeficient NOG mouse model to evaluate efficacy to HIV challenge (Cannon and June 2011, Perez et al. 2008, DiGuisto et al. 2016). TALENs were used to disrupt both the TRAC region to reduce the risk of GvHD and the CD52 gene to evade the depletion effects of alemtuzumab (anti-CD52 monoclonal antibody) to generate allogeneic anti-CD19 CAR T cells. This CRISPR/Cas9-edited cell product was evaluated for antitumor effects in a lymphoma model using NSG mice (Poirot et al. 2015). CRISPR/Cas9 was also used to disrupt the TRAC and CD52 loci for the production of allogeneic anti-CD19 CAR T cells, which were evaluated for anti-leukemic effects in NSG-immunodeficient mice (Georgiadis et al. 2018).

Although it is possible to evaluate pharmacologic activity of edited human HSPC, T cells, or CAR T cells in short-term studies in immunodeficient animals, characteristics of the model preclude long-term studies. Human T cells can induce a GvHD response in normal and immunodeficient animals leading to animal mortality, and mice lack cross-reactive cytokines or growth factors needed to support the growth and differentiation of human hematopoietic cells. Both of these aspects create challenges to product evaluation in longer-term studies.

Animal pharmacology studies are generally not used to select clinical doses for ex vivo modified cell therapy, as these cell dose determinations often follow the clinical use of hematopoietic cells used for transplantation (e.g., HSPC, T cells), or other more relevant estimations of cell dose. Dose extrapolation for in vivo genome editing programs generally utilizes data from gene modification assessment (% indels) and transgene expression, collected from mouse (hybrid pharmacology toxicology and wildtype) and NHP studies.

27.5.3 Safety Pharmacology

The necessity of including safety pharmacology assessments (e.g., CNS, cardiovascular and respiratory) as part of the pharmacology/toxicology studies for genome editing therapeutics is determined on a case-by-case basis, driven by biodistribution of the product in relation to exposure in the therapeutic range and intended pharmacological activity of expressed transgene (EMA 2018a). Early discussion with regulatory authorities is recommended to ensure alignment.

27.5.4 Pharmacokinetics, Biodistribution, and Shedding

The traditional absorption, distribution, metabolism, and excretion (ADME) studies necessary for the development of small molecule therapeutics are not feasible for genome editing or gene therapy products; however, it is still necessary to characterize the pharmacokinetics, biodistribution,

persistence, and clearance of delivery vector and/or modified cell. For biodistribution studies for AAV-delivered nucleases, the AAV vector is typically measured in plasma and tissues using a validated qPCR method (limit of quantification ≤ 50 copies/μg genomic DNA, so the assay can detect this limit with 95% confidence), including blood, injection site, brain, heart, liver, lung, kidney, spleen, gonads, and other relevant tissues depending on the product (USFDA 2020). Biodistribution of ex vivo edited hematopoietic cells in blood and tissues can be assessed by flow cytometry.

Understanding vector copy levels or cell number in plasma and target tissue is valuable when assessing the transgene expression and any toxicity findings, and interim necropsies allow understanding the distribution profile over time. A set of tissue samples can be collected at interim and final necropsy times, with only key tissues from the high dose group initially evaluated for vector copy number. In addition, if using the same AAV platform for multiple programs, it may be possible to bridge the full biodistribution package from one program to a second program that assesses a limited list of tissues (MacLachlan et al. 2013). The remainder can be held for possible future analysis. Obtaining regulatory feedback on a reduced scope for biodistribution analysis is recommended.

Viral vector shedding evaluation in bodily fluids (e.g., saliva, plasma, urine, semen [typically only mice due to sexually mature status], and feces) in animals is also necessary to communicate potential risk to patients, family, or caregivers.

27.5.5 Toxicology Evaluation

Based on the novel nature of genome editing technologies, the exponential growth as a consequence of basic research, and varied therapeutic targets and uses for these genomic medicines, toxicologists need to consider safety evaluation programs tailored to the genomic medicine and use in patients. Early and ongoing communication with regulators is highly recommended for a successful nonclinical safety evaluation program.

Although there are no dedicated international regulatory guidance documents for assessing the safety of genome editing medicines, the US FDA and EMA do address some considerations for nonclinical safety assessment for genome editing compounds, and current gene therapy guidance documents do provide a high-level roadmap of considerations that are also relevant for these novel medicines (EMA 2018b, 2019, USFDA 2020). A US FDA guidance draft document for nonclinical assessment of genome editing medicines is anticipated in 2021-2022. Each safety evaluation program needs to be science-based and designed on a case-by-case basis to support clinical studies and product development.

As summarized in the US FDA long-term follow-up guidance document (USFDA 2020), preclinical safety evaluation of genome editing products should consider (1) the technology used to edit the genome, (2) the target cell types that are modified, (3) the genomic sites that are modified, (4) the vector used to deliver the genome-editing components; and (5) the clinical route of administration. Preclinical studies evaluating these factors can inform the scope of the clinical long-term follow-up observations.

Genome editing, whether ex vivo or in vivo, introduces the risk for delayed adverse effects, due to (1) the permanent nature of change; (2) the potential for off-target genome modifications that can lead to aberrant gene expression, chromosomal translocation, induce malignancies, etc.; (3) the risk for insertional mutagenesis when integrating or non-integrating vectors are used to deliver the genome editing components, and the associated risk of tumorigenicity; and/or (4) the possibility of an immune response to the genome editing components or the expressed transgene (USFDA 2020).

For studies where animal models of disease can be used to establish the proof-of-concept, hybrid pharmacology/toxicology studies provide understanding of the relationship between dose, protein expression levels, their impact on the disease under study, and potential toxicity from protein overexpression in the disease model.

For ex vivo therapies, unique aspects of edited immune cells need to be considered in designing the safety assessment plan. CAR T and TCR-modified immune cells have the potential for on-target/off-tumor toxicity that needs to be addressed, as feasible, either in appropriate animal model or by an alternative approach using a combination of in silico and in vitro analyses. Additionally, human T cells can induce a GvHD response and subsequent toxicity can confound safety evaluation.

27.5.5.1 Off-Target Nuclease Activity Assessment

Although current scientific knowledge is far from fully understanding the interpretation of off-target findings, an important part of safety assessment of engineered nucleases is evaluating the unintended binding and cleavage of off-target genomic sites that share sequence homology with the on-target site. Off-target nuclease activity can result in indel formation following NHEJ-mediated DNA repair that can lead to frameshift changes resulting in gene inactivation or truncation (Cathomen and Joung 2008).

The methods for off-target assessment continue to evolve and fall into two categories: biased and unbiased assessment. Earlier methods used bioinformatics to search the genome for homologous off-target binding sites followed by the evaluation of indels at these prespecified sites, thus the term "biased assessment." This method is useful when designing and screening engineered nucleases; however, software tools do not take into account accessibility of a potential off-target site in vivo, which can be affected by the dynamic epigenetic status of the locus, thus reducing predictive power (Yee 2016).

Newer unbiased genome wide methods are designed to tag each region where a DSB occurs followed by tag-specific amplification and sequencing the captured off-target site. This strategy designed to map DSBs includes the following methods, integration-defective lentiviral vector (IDLV), GUIDE-Seq, high-throughput, genome-wide, translocation sequencing (HTGTS) and breaks labeling, enrichment and next-generation sequencing (BLESS) (reviewed in (EMA 2018b, Yee 2016)). The most sensitive and commonly used methods are IDLV (0.5-1% indels) and GUIDE-Seq (~0.1% indels) (Tsai et al. 2015, Wang et al. 2015, Yee 2016). New orthogonal methods also include CIRCLE-Seq (Tsai et al. 2017), which is an in vitro method for selective sequencing of nuclease cleaved genomic DNA fragments (EMA 2018b), and CHANGE-Seq, which is another new type of unbiased tagging and sequencing method (Lazzarotto et al. 2020).

Once a list of potential off-target sites is determined, the genes at each site can be curated and a risk assessment performed based on the location of the cut site (falling in a coding or non-coding region), expression of the edited gene in the target tissue, cut site location relative to an oncogene or tumor suppressor gene, or if editing is anticipated to result in a truncated or chimeric protein. This assessment is conducted for both ex vivo and in vivo engineered nuclease products.

For ex vivo edited HSPC, T cell, or CAR T-cell products where cells can be cultured and expanded, the next step after determining the potential off-target sites is conducting a molecular translocation analysis. Bioinformatics are used to assess all possible translocations that can occur between cutting at on- and off-target sites, then probes are designed to search for these translocations in the edited cells (Ando and Meyer 2017). A risk assessment is done in parallel to evaluate possible outcomes of the identified translocations and health risk.

27.5.5.2 Genotoxicity Studies

Due to the nature of engineered nucleases, the nonclinical assessment of genotoxicity is much different than that found for small molecule therapeutics. Small molecule compounds can be directly administered in vitro or in vivo and assessed using the traditional, well-validated standard battery of genotoxicity tests (e.g., Ames test, mouse micronucleus test), whereas engineered nucleases are delivered as DNA or RNA via different methods/vectors (e.g., electroporation, adeno-associated viral vectors, lipid nanoparticles) and require cellular expression of the nuclease before any genotoxicity assessment can ensue. Thus, new ways of testing have been needed, using several orthogonal methods to assess genotoxicity risk.

The intended use of ex vivo or in vivo nuclease-modified cells will guide which methods are most relevant for safety assessment. Standard genotoxicity assays may be required, however, if there is a concern about an impurity or a component of the delivery system (e.g., nucleic acid complexing material) (EMA 2019). The field continues to evolve as more is learned about the use of these methods and ability to translate results to the clinic.

There is no prescribed way to assess genotoxicity risk of engineered nucleases due to the diverse target cells and intended clinical use of these novel medicines. There are many tools to choose from and it is recommended to design a plan and discuss with regulators early on. These tools will continue to evolve as more understanding of genome editing ensues.

For cells that undergo ex vivo editing, such as HSPC or universal CAR T cells, the edited target cells can be studied in ways not possible when delivering engineered nucleases in vivo to target cells in the body. Potential genotoxicity of ex vivo ZFN-modified HSPCs targeting the CCR5 locus was assessed using off-target analysis, karyotyping evaluating structural and numerical aberrations, and the 53BP1 DSB assay (Ando and Meyer 2017), and cells evaluated should be prepared using the clinical-scale manufacturing process. Karyotype analysis is a traditional way of assessing structural and numerical chromosome aberrations in genome-modified cells by a trained cytogeneticist and can be conducted in compliance with Good Laboratory Practices (GLP) or Good Manufacturing Practices (GMP). The 53BP1 assay assesses the presence of DSBs over time in clinically relevant cells. Induction of a DSB triggers the recruitment of cellular factors involved in DNA repair to the site of the break. One such protein, 53BP1, is recruited (within 24 hours) to the sites of DSBs (Rappold et al. 2001, Schultz et al. 2000), and sites can be visualized as distinct foci within the nucleus using immunofluorescence microscopy with antibodies that recognize 53BP1. The number of 53BP1 foci per nucleus is an accurate measure of the number of DSBs that occurred in the cell.

The risk of insertional mutagenesis of AAV vector-delivered genome editing medicines needs to be considered as part of the genotoxicity assessment and long-term follow-up risk of adverse effects, considering the delivery vector and characteristics of the engineered nuclease. AAV vectors do not have a propensity to integrate or reactivate and generally present a low risk of delayed adverse events (USFDA 2013); however, a vector integration study may be necessary. The presence of a promoter/enhancer may be the main driver for risk potential (Chandler, Sands, and Venditti 2017). If vector integration studies are not conducted, a discussion on why the study was not performed and evidence supporting the assessment of risk of delayed adverse events posed by the product is expected.

27.5.5.3 In Vitro Tumorigenicity

Studies evaluating the in vitro tumorigenicity risk of engineered nuclease off-target activity include the soft agar colony transformation assay. The soft agar colony formation assay is a well-established method for characterizing the ability of transformed cells to acquire anchorage-independent growth on a solid surface and is a stringent test for malignant transformation in cells (Ando and Meyer 2017, Borowicz et al. 2014). As tumor growth and invasion represent a complex multistep process involving anchorage-independent growth, motility, and proteolytic degradation of extracellular matrix, aspects of these processes can be assessed by measuring the ability of a cell to grow independently of substrate adhesion and to form colonies in a soft agar matrix. Thus, transformed cells can be easily differentiated from normal cells in vitro since the growth of normal cells is anchorage dependent (Ando and Meyer 2017, Puck, Marcus, and Cieciura 1956). The soft agar transformation assay can be conducted as GLP compliant.

As dysregulation of IL-2 production can lead to spontaneous T-cell transformation in vitro, assessing the potential risk for oncogenic transformation of edited T-cell products cultured in the absence of IL-2 is necessary (Nagarkatti et al. 1994). IL-2 is a major T-cell growth factor and T cells in culture have been shown to undergo spontaneous transformation resulting from continuous production of and responsiveness to autocrine IL-2. Edited T cells are assessed for viability and growth and monitored over time to see if cells acquire tumorigenic properties.

Taken together, the off-target assessment and results from selected in vitro genotoxicity and tumorigenicity studies make up the overall genotoxicity risk assessment.

27.5.5.4 In Vivo Toxicology Studies

In vivo safety assessment of engineered nuclease products is considered on a case-by-case basis depending on the type of modified cell and whether ex vivo or in vivo genome editing was used. For ex vivo delivery to cells in culture, the engineered nucleases are typically delivered by mRNA electroporation and are transiently expressed. For in vivo delivery to target cells by AAV vectors, the engineered nucleases are anticipated to be episomal with chronic long-lasting expression, thus necessitating the long-term evaluation in animals. Long-term follow-up for clinical trial subjects is also necessary to characterize the safety profile of these products.

Typically, two species are recommended for safety evaluation of in vivo delivered engineered nucleases, though it may be possible on a case-by-case basis to justify testing in one species. A combined hybrid pharmacology and toxicology study using the animal disease model is recommended for genome editing therapies since most editing and gene addition products are intended for rare monogenic diseases and animal disease models are necessary to establish the proof-of-concept. Pharmacology and toxicology evaluations can be combined in the animal disease model, which can result in reduction of animal use in safety assessment. For mouse studies, larger group sizes can be used to evaluate the safety of editing, whereas for nonhuman primates, expected to more closely approximate the clinical situation and be more relevant for dose selection, can use smaller group sizes.

For in vivo delivered nuclease components, biopsy/necropsy target tissues can be assessed for nuclease mRNA and protein levels, on- and off-target gene modification (% indels), and correlated with any safety findings. The persistence of engineered nuclease and therapeutic transgene expression can be evaluated over time, triggering additional investigation if expression of either is lost. These studies allow the assessment of unwanted consequences of biodistribution and persistence of delivery vector, its transduction, expression and biologic activity of vector genes and engineered nucleases as well as expression and activity of therapeutic gene, if a donor gene is used as part of the therapy. Assessing the risk of inadvertent editing of gonad cells is of ultimate importance; thus, demonstrating the lack of engineered nuclease expression and the lack of genome editing in ovaries and testes is critical. Assessment of local tolerance and immunogenicity to the delivery vector, expressed nuclease, and/or therapeutic transgene or any unanticipated pharmacological effects is also possible. For in vivo administered editing products, animal toxicology studies should include standard toxicology assessments (clinical observations, body weight, clinical, macroscopic, and microscopic pathology evaluations) in addition to the assessment specific to the engineered nuclease and expressed therapeutic transgene, and the GLP study duration should be at least 6 months and negotiated with regulators based on overall risk assessment of product.

The standard types of toxicology studies are generally not relevant to ex vivo delivered nuclease programs involving T cell- and CAR T cell-based products that lack the human target in normal or immunodeficient animals, GvHD response to the human cells in immunodeficient animals, and the relatively short survival time of human cells in animal models due to the lack of human cytokine/growth factor milieu. Generally, toxicology assessments can be added to the short-term (~ 2-month duration) pharmacology efficacy and biodistribution studies conducted to evaluate T-cell fate and distribution.

The toxicology studies are expected to be conducted in compliance with GLP (21CFR Part 58); however, some assessments may not be fully compliant with GLP regulations. For example, some hybrid pharmacology and toxicology studies can only be conducted at academic institutions with sole access to the disease model and benefit of strong scientific and husbandry experience with specific models. To mitigate the lack of GLP oversight, having an independent Quality Assurance unit/person provide an oversight function with respect to the conduct of the toxicology study and final study report is recommended (USFDA 2013). For studies conducted at GLP-compliant laboratories, some of the endpoint analyses may not be available at the facility, such as NGS analysis of insertions and deletions, vector biodistribution, cell fate, transgene expression, or specific immunological evaluations. If the study or some of the endpoint analyses are not conducted in compliance with GLPs, a brief statement of the reason for the noncompliance needs to be submitted in the final study report. This explanation should include the areas of deviation and whether the deviation(s) impacted study outcome.

Safety margins can be generated by both toxicology species and used to support the clinical starting dose and dose escalation range for in vivo genome editing programs. For ex vivo programs, the human cell dose is not based on animal study data but rather on clinical results showing the number of human HSPCs needed for successful transplantation or number of CAR T cells shown to be efficacious in other clinical programs.

27.5.5.5 Tumorigenicity Risk Evaluation

Standard lifetime carcinogenicity studies in rodents are not generally required for safety evaluation of engineered nuclease agents; however, the oncogenic and tumorigenic potential is expected to be investigated in relevant nonclinical models for neoplasm signals, oncogene activation, or cell proliferation index. The decision to proceed should follow a weight of evidence approach that is based on knowledge of the engineered nuclease target cell type and molecular target, off-target profile, and genotoxicity risk assessment.

The risk for potential tumorigenicity due to genome editing can be evaluated with in vitro assays such as the fibroblast soft agar assay or IL-2 clonality assay for assessing T cells, as described earlier. For in vivo genome editing programs, potential tumorigenicity can also be assessed histologically in the toxicology studies, although the duration is shorter than traditional two-year cancer bioassays. For example, with liver targeted programs, histopathology assessment of multiple liver tissue sections from all treated animals can be used to identify any findings of hepatocellular hyperplasia or neoplasia risk.

For edited HSPC cells, immunodeficient NSG transgenic mice have been used to evaluate the engraftment of edited cells, persistence, biodistribution, and potential tumorigenesis

(Ando and Meyer 2017). NSG mice lack a functional common IL-2 receptor (R) γ-chain and functional T and B cells, natural killer cells and also have impaired dendritic cell function, so that they are able to accept transplantations of human hematopoietic cells and to establish longer-lived grafts of human HSPC and their progeny. These studies typically deliver a full human HSPC dose split among many animals to determine if any human hematopoietic cell tumors arise from the edited cells. A new NSG-variant, the NBSGW mouse strain, is similar to NSG but with a mutation in the *Kit* gene that promotes the engraftment of donor cells without myeloablative irradiation (McIntosh et al. 2015), allowing the tumorigenicity study to be conducted at traditional GLP contract laboratory organization sites without access to a radiation source. Obtaining regulatory feedback on study design is highly recommended before embarking on a tumorigenicity study in immunodeficient mouse models.

Tumorigenicity studies are not considered appropriate for edited CAR T cells or T cells, as the human target (e.g., CD19 or CD22) is generally absent in normal or immunodeficient mice, and there is no activation or proliferation of T cells following administration in these species. Additionally, human T-cell engraftment in immunodeficient animal models is limited by a xenograft versus host disease generally occurring about 2 months following the administration of T cells (Ehx et al. 2018). This short lifespan of human T cells in the mouse consequently limits the ability to investigate the potential adverse effects and tumorigenicity of edited T cells or CAR T cells in these mouse models (Wen et al. 2019).

27.5.5.6 Reproductive/Developmental Risk Evaluation

The potential for a genome editing product to cause reproductive or developmental toxicity will depend on the product type, mechanism of action, biodistribution and shedding profile, and target patient population (EMA 2018a). The risk of inadvertent germline transmission can be assessed by AAV vector biodistribution in gonads, and by demonstrating both lack of nuclease expression and activity in the gonads. If necessary, sperm fractionation studies can be conducted to demonstrate the absence of transduction of spermatozoa (Roehl et al. 2000). Breeding studies may be required if the risks cannot be unequivocally determined. Embryo-fetal development studies should be considered for gene therapy products unless otherwise justified on basis of the edited cell and reproductive/developmental risk assessment.

27.6 Summary and Conclusion

Nonclinical development of genome editing products is challenging as the technologies and tools evaluating activity and safety continue to evolve. The safety evaluation toxicologist needs to think creatively and design a program fit for the product, intended target cell, duration of nuclease expression, on-/off-target editing profile, mechanism of action, and patient population. Much of the available regulatory guidance for gene therapy serves as a foundation for the nonclinical program and is combined with specific evaluations for genome editing products and subsequent risk/benefit assessment. Communication early and often with regulators is recommended to develop a successful case-by-case approach tailored to the editing product. Developing engineered nuclease products is rewarding as these novel genomic medicines offer great promise for treating serious rare genetic, acquired, or infectious diseases in patients.

Acknowledgment

Special thanks to Michael C. Holmes and Gregory Davis for review of the manuscript, in particular, the genome editing sections, and Melanie Butler-Gauthier for designing the meganuclease, TALEN, and CRISPR/Cas figures.

LIST OF GENOME EDITING- AND GENE THERAPY-RELATED ABBREVIATIONS

AAV	Adeno-associated virus
B2M	Beta-2-microglobulin
cDNA	Complementary deoxyribonucleic acid
CAR	Chimeric antigen receptor
CAR	T-cell Chimeric antigen receptor T cell
CRISPR/Cas9	Clustered regularly interspaced short palindromic repeats (CRISPR)/CRISPR-associated (Cas) platforms
DSB	Double-strand break
DNA	Deoxyribonucleotide
HDR	Homology-directed repair
HSPC	Hematopoietic stem and progenitor cell
MegaTAL	Engineered nuclease composed of a meganuclease and TALE binding region
NHEJ	Non-homologous end joining
mRNA	Messenger ribonucleic acid
NGS	Next-generation sequencing
RVD	Repeat variable diresidue
TALE	Transcription activator-like effectors
TALEN	Transcription activator-like effectors nuclease
TCR	T-cell receptor
TRAC	T-cell receptor alpha chain constant region
PAM	Protospacer adjacent motif
PCR	Polymerase chain reaction
vg	Vector genome(s)
ZFN	Zinc finger nuclease
ZFP	Zinc finger protein

REFERENCES

Ando, D., and K. Meyer. 2017. "Gene editing: Regulatory and translation to clinic." *Hematol Oncol Clin North Am* 31 (5):797–808. doi: 10.1016/j.hoc.2017.06.002.

Anzalone, A. V., P. B. Randolph, J. R. Davis, A. A. Sousa, L. W. Koblan, J. M. Levy, P. J. Chen, C. Wilson, G. A. Newby, A. Raguram, and D. R. Liu. 2019. "Search-and-replace genome editing without double-stgrand breaks or donor DNA." *Nature* 576 (7785):149–157.

Boch, J., H. Scholze, S. Schornack, A. Landgraf, S. Hahn, S. Kay, T. Lahaye, A. Nickstadt, and U. Bonas. 2009. "Breaking the code of DNA binding specificity of TAL-type III effectors." *Science* 326 (5959):1509–1512. doi: 10.1126/science.1178811.

Boissel, S., J. Jarjour, A. Astrakhan, A. Adey, A. Gouble, P. Duchateau, J. Shendure, B. L. Stoddard, M. T. Certo, D. Baker, and A. M. Scharenberg. 2014. "megaTALs: A rare-cleaving nuclease architecture for therapeutic genome engineering." *Nucleic Acids Res* 42 (4):2591–2601. doi: 10.1093/nar/gkt1224.

Bolotin, M, D. Coen, J. Deutsch, B. Dujon, P. Netter, E. Petrochilo, and Slonimski P. P. 1971. "La recombinaison des mitochondries chez *Saccharomyces cerevisiae*." *Bull Inst Pasteur* 69:215–239.

Borowicz, S., M. Van Scoyk, S. Avasarala, M. K. Karuppusamy Rathinam, J. Tauler, R. K. Bikkavilli, and R. A. Winn. 2014. "The soft agar colony formation assay." *J Vis Exp* (92):e51998. doi: 10.3791/51998.

Cannon, P., and C. June. 2011. "CCR5 knockout strategies." *Curr Opin HIV AIDs* 6 (1):74–79.

Carroll, D. 2014. "Genome engineering with targetable nucleases." *Annu Rev Biochem* 83: 409–439 doi: 10.1146/annurev-biochem-060713-035418.

Cathomen, T., and J. K. Joung. 2008. "Zinc-finger nucleases: the next generation emerges." *Mol Ther* 16 (7):1200–1207. doi: 10.1038/mt.2008.114.

Cavagnaro, J., and B. Silva Lima. 2015. "Regulatory acceptance of animal models of disease to support clinical trials of medicines and advanced therapy medicinal products." *Eur J Pharmacol* 759:51–62 doi: 10.1016/j.ejphar.2015.03.048.

Chandler, R. J., M. S. Sands, and C. P. Venditti. 2017. "Recombinant adeno-associated viral integration and genotoxicity: Insights from animal models." *Human Gene Ther* 28 (4):314–322.

Chen, F., S. M. Pruett-Miller, Y. Huang, M. Gjoka, K. Duda, J. Taunton, T. N. Collingwood, M. Frodin, and G. D. Davis. 2011. "High-frequency genome editing using ssDNA oligonucleotides with zinc-finger nucleases." *Nat Methods* 8 (9):753–755.

Cho, S. W., S. Kim, J. M. Kim, and J. S. Kim. 2013. "Targeted genome engineering in human cells with the Cas9 RNA-guided endonuclease." *Nat Biotechnol* 31 (3):230–232. doi: 10.1038/nbt.2507.

Clinicaltrials.gov.

Cong, L., F.A. Ran, D. Cox, S. Lin, R. Barretto, N. Habib, P. Hsu, X. Wu, W. Jiang, L.A. Marraffini, and F. Zhang. 2013. "Multiplex genome engineering usign CRISPR/Cas systems." *Science* 339:819–823.

Corrigan-Curay, J., M. O'Reilly, D. B. Kohn, P. M. Cannon, G. Bao, F. D. Bushman, D. Carroll, T. Cathomen, J. K. Joung, D. Roth, M. Sadelain, A. M. Scharenberg, C. von Kalle, F. Zhang, R. Jambou, E. Rosenthal, M. Hassani, A. Singh, and M. H. Porteus. 2015. "Genome editing technologies: Defining a path to clinic." *Mol Ther* 23 (5):796–806. doi: 10.1038/mt.2015.54.

DeKelver, R. C., V. M. Choi, E. A. Moehle, D. E. Paschon, D. Hockemeyer, S. H. Meijsing, Y. Sancak, X. Cui, E. J. Steine, J. C. Miller, P. Tam, V. V. Bartsevich, X. Meng, I. Rupniewski, S. M. Gopalan, H. C. Sun, K. J. Pitz, J. M. Rock, L. Zhang, G. D. Davis, E. J. Rebar, I. M. Cheeseman,

K. R. Yamamoto, D. M. Sabatini, R. Jaenisch, P. D. Gregory, and F. D. Urnov. 2010. "Functional genomics, proteomics, and regulatory DNA analysis in isogenic settings using zinc finger nuclease-driven transgenesis into a safe harbor locus in the human genome." *Genome Res* 20 (8):1133–1142.

DiGuisto, D. L., P. M. Cannon, M. C. Holmes, L. Li, A. Rao, J. Wang, G. Lee, P. D. Gregory, K. A. Kim, S. B. Hayward, K. Meyer, C. Exline, E. Lopez, J. Henley, N. Gonzalez, V. Bedell, R. Stan, and J. A. Zaia. 2016. "Preclinical development and qualification of ZFN-mediated CCD5 disruption in human hematopoietic stem/progenitor cells." *Mol Ther Methods Clin Dev* 3 (January 1):1–12.

Durai, S., M. Mani, K. Kandavelou, J. Wu, M. H. Porteus, and S. Chandrasegaran. 2005. "Zinc finger nucleases: custom-designed molecular scissors for genome engineering of plant and mammalian cells." *Nucleic Acids Res* 33 (18):5978–5990. doi: 10.1093/nar/gki912.

Economos, N. G., S. Oyaghire, E. Quijano, A. S. Ricciardi, W. M. Saltzman, and P. M. Glazer. 2020. "Peptide nucleic acids and gene editing: perspectives on structure and repair." *Molecules* 25 (3):735–755.

Ehx, G., J. Somja, H. J. Warnatz, C. Ritacco, M. Hannon, L. Delens, G. Fransolet, P. Delvenne, J. Muller, Y. Beguin, H. Lehrach, L. Belle, S. Humblet-Baron, and F. Baron. 2018. "Xenogeneic Graft-Versus-Host Disease in Humanized NSG and NSG-HLA-A2/HHD Mice." *Front Immunol* 9:1943. doi: 10.3389/fimmu.2018.01943.

EMA. 2012. Guideline of quality, non-clinical and clinical aspects of medicinal products containing genetically modified cells. edited by Committee for Advanced Therapies European Medicines Agency.

EMA. 2018a. Guideline on the quality, non-clinical and clinical aspects of gene therapy medicinal products. edited by Committee for Advanced Therapies European Medicines Agency.

EMA. 2018b. Report of the EMA expert meeting on genome editing technologies used in medicinal product development. edited by Human Medicines Research and Development Support Division European Medicines Agency and Human Medicines Inspections, Pharmacovigilance and Committees Division.

EMA. 2019. Draft Guideline on quality, non-clinical and clinical requirements for investigational advanced therapy medicinal products in clinical trials. edited by Committee for Advanced Therapies European Medicines Agency.

GEN. 2017. "Sangamo genome editing trial, assessing MPS II candidate, treats first patient." *Genetic Engineering & Biotechnology News*.

Georgiadis, C., R. Preece, L. Nickolay, A. Etuk, A. Petrova, D. Ladon, A. Danyi, N. Humphryes-Kirilov, A. Ajetunmobi, D. Kim, J. S. Kim, and W. Qasim. 2018. "Long Terminal Repeat CRISPR-CAR-Coupled "Universal" T Cells Mediate Potent Anti-leukemic Effects." *Mol Ther* 26 (5):1215–1227. doi: 10.1016/j.ymthe.2018.02.025.

Gillmore, J. D. et al. 2021. "CRISPR-Cas9 In Vivo Gene Editing for Transthyretin Amyloidosis." *N. Engl. J. Med.* https://www.nejm.org/doi/full/10.1056/NEJMoa2107454

Goodwin, S., J. D. McPherson, and W. R. McCombie. 2016. "Coming of age: Ten years of next-generation sequencing technologies." *Nat Rev Genet* 17:333–351.

Hu, Z., W. Ding, D. Zhu, L. Yu, X. Jiang, X. Wang, C. Zhang, L. Wang, T. Ji, D. Liu, D. He, X. Xia, T. Zhu, J. Wei, P. Wu, C. Wang, L. Xi, Q. Gao, G. Chen, R. Liu, K. Li, S. Li, S. Wang, J. Zhou, D. Ma, and H. Wang. 2015. "TALEN-mediated targeting of HPV oncogenes ameliorates HPV-related cervical malignancy." *J Clin Invest* 125 (1):425–36. doi: 10.1172/JCI78206.

Jantz, D., and Jefferson-Smith J. 2012. Rationally-designed meganuclease variants of lig-34 and I-crei for maize genome engineering.

Jinek, M., K. Chylinski, I. Fonfara, M. Hauer, J. A. Doudna, and E. Charpentier. 2012. "A programmable dual-RNA-guided DNA endonuclease in adaptive bacterial immunity." *Science* 337 (6096):816–21. doi: 10.1126/science.1225829.

Jinek, M., A. East, A. Cheng, S. Lin, E. Ma, and J. A. Doudna. 2013. "RNA-programmed genome editing in human cells." *Elife* 2:e00471.

Joung, J. K., and J. D. Sander. 2013. "TALENs: A widely applicable technology for targeted genome editing". *Nat Rev Mol Cell Biol* 14 (1):49–55.

Kim, Y. G., J. Cha, and S. Chandrasegaran. 1996. "Hybrid restriction enzymes: Zinc finger fusions to Fok I cleavage domain." *Proc Natl Acad Sci U S A* 93 (3):1156–1160. doi: 10.1073/pnas.93.3.1156.

Kim, Y. G., and S. Chandrasegaran. 1994. "Chimeric restriction endonuclease." *Proc Natl Acad Sci U S A* 91 (3):883–887. doi: 10.1073/pnas.91.3.883.

Laoharawee, K., R. C. DeKelver, K. M. Podetz-Pedersen, M. Rohde, S. Sproul, H. O. Nguyen, T. Nguyen, S. J. St Martin, L. Ou, S. Tom, R. Radeke, K. E. Meyer, M. C. Holmes, C. B. Whitley, T. Wechsler, and R. S. McIvor. 2018. "Dose-dependent prevention of metabolic and neurologic disease in murine MPS II by ZFN-mediated in vivo genome editing." *Mol Ther* 26 (4):1127–1136. doi: 10.1016/j.ymthe.2018.03.002.

Lazzarotto, C. R., N. L. Malinin, Y. Li, R. Zhang, Y. Yang, G. Lee, E. Cowley, Y. He, X. Lan, K. Jividen, V. Katta, N. G. Kolmakova, C. T. Petersen, Q. Qi, E. Strelcov, S. Maragh, G. Krenciute, J. Ma, Y. Cheng, and S. Q. Tsai. 2020. "CHANGE-seq reveals genetic and epigenetic effects on CRISPR-Cas9 genome-wide activity." *Nat Biotechnol.* doi: 10.1038/s41587-020-0555-7.

Ledford, H. 2020. "CRISPR treatment inserted directly into body for first time." *Nature* 579 (12 March):185.

Li, H, V. Haurigot, Y. Doyan, T. Li, S. Y. Wong, A. S. Bhagwat, N. Malani, X. M. Anguela, R. Sharma, L. Ivanciu, S. L. Murphy, J. D. Finn, F. R. Khazi, S. Zhou, D. E. Paschon, E. J. Rebar, F. D. Bushman, P. D. Gregory, and M. C. Holmes. 2012. "In vivo genome editing restores hemostasis in a mouse model of hemophilia." *Nature* 475 (7355):217–221.

Li, L., L. P. Wu, and S. Chandrasegaran. 1992. "Functional domains in Fok I restriction endonuclease." *Proc Natl Acad Sci U S A* 89 (10):4275–4279. doi: 10.1073/pnas.89.10.4275.

Lieber, M. R., Y. Ma, U. Pannicke, and K. Schwarz. 2003. "Mechanism and regulation of human non-homologous DNA end-joining." *Nat Rev Mol Cell Biol* 4 (9):712–720. doi: 10.1038/nrm1202.

MacLachlan, T., M. McIntyre, K. Mitrophanous, D. J. Miskin, D. J. Jolly, and J. A. Cavagnaro. 2013. "Not reinventing the wheel: Applying the 3Rs concepts to viral vector gene therapy biodistribution studies". *Human Gene Ther Clin Dev* 24 (1):1–4.

Mali, P., L. Yang, K. M. Esvelt, J. Aach, M. Guell, J. E. DiCarlo, J. E. Norville, and G. M. Church. 2013. "RNA-guided human genome engineering via Cas9." *Science* 339 (6121):823–826. doi: 10.1126/science.1232033.

Marchione, M. 2017. "US scientists try 1st gene editing in the body." *Associated Press News.* https://apnews.com/4ae98919b52e43d8a8960e0e260feb0a/AP-Exclusive:-US-scientists-try-1st-gene-editing-in-the-body.

McIntosh, B. E., M. E. Brown, B. M. Duffin, J. P. Maufort, D. T. Vereide, Slukvin, II, and J. A. Thomson. 2015. "Nonirradiated NOD,B6.SCID Il2rgamma-/- Kit(W41/W41) (NBSGW) mice support multilineage engraftment of human hematopoietic cells." *Stem Cell Reports* 4 (2):171–180. doi: 10.1016/j.stemcr.2014.12.005.

Miller, J. C., D. P. Patil, D. F. Xia, C. B. Paine, F. Fauser, H. W. Richards, D. A. Shivak, Y. R. Bendana, S. J. Hinkley, N. A. Scarlott, S. C. Lam, A. Reik, Y. Zhou, D. E. Paschon, P. Li, T. Wangzor, G. Lee, L. Zhang, and E. J. Rebar. 2019. "Enhancing gene editing specificity by attenuating DNA cleavage kinetics." *Nat Biotechnol* 37 (8):945–952. doi: 10.1038/s41587-019-0186-z.

Moscou, M. J., and A. J. Bogdanove. 2009. "A simple cipher governs DNA recognition by TAL effectors." *Science* 326 (5959):1501. doi: 10.1126/science.1178817.

Nagarkatti, M., M. Hassuneh, A. Seth, K Manickasundari, and P. Nagarkatti. 1994. "Constituitive activation of the interleukin 2 gene in the induction of spontaneous in vitro transformation and tumorigenicity of T cells." *Proc Natl Acad Sci U S A* 91:7638–7642.

Ou, L., R. C. DeKelver, M. Rohde, S. Tom, R. Radeke, S. J. St Martin, Y. Santiago, S. Sproul, M. J. Przybilla, B. L. Koniar, K. M. Podetz-Pedersen, K. Laoharawee, R. D. Cooksley, K. E. Meyer, M. C. Holmes, R. S. McIvor, T. Wechsler, and C. B. Whitley. 2019. "ZFN-mediated in vivo genome editing corrects murine hurler syndrome." *Mol Ther* 27 (1):178–187. doi: 10.1016/j.ymthe.2018.10.018.

Pabo, C. O., E. Peisach, and R. A. Grant. 2001. "Design and selection of novel Cys2His2 zinc finger proteins." *Annu Rev Biochem* 70:313–40 doi: 10.1146/annurev.biochem.70.1.313.

Papapetrou, E. P., and A. Schambach. 2016. "Gene insertion into genomic safe harbors for human gene therapy." *Mol Ther* 24 (4):678–684.

Paschon, D. E., S. Lussier, T. Wangzor, D. F. Xia, P. W. Li, S. J. Hinkley, N. A. Scarlott, S. C. Lam, A. J. Waite, L. N. Truong, N. Gandhi, B. N. Kadam, D. P. Patil, D. A. Shivak, G. K. Lee, M. C. Holmes, L. Zhang, J. C. Miller, and E. J. Rebar. 2019. "Diversifying the structure of zinc finger nucleases for high-precision genome editing." *Nat Commun* 10 (1):1133. doi: 10.1038/s41467-019-08867-x.

Pavletich, N. P., and C. O. Pabo. 1991. "Zinc finger-DNA recognition: Crystal structure of a Zif268-DNA complex at 2.1 A." *Science* 252 (5007):809–17. doi: 10.1126/science.2028256.

Perez, E. E., J. Wang, J. C. Miller, Y. Jouvenot, K. A. Kim, O. Liu, N. Wang, G. Lee, V. V.v Bartsevich, Y. Lee, D. Y. Guschin, I. Rupniewski, A. J. Waite, C. Carpenito, R. G. Carroll, J. S. Orange, F. D. Urnov, E. J. Rebar, D. Ando, P. D. Gregory, J. L. Riley, M. C. Holmes, and C. H. June. 2008. "Establishment of HIV-1 resistence in CD4+ T cells by genome editing using zinc finger nucleases." *Nat Biotechnol* 26 (7):808–816.

Poirot, L., B. Philip, C. Schiffer-Mannioui, D. Le Clerre, I. Chion-Sotinel, S. Derniame, P. Potrel, C. Bas, L. Lemaire, R. Galetto, C. Lebuhotel, J. Eyquem, G. W. Cheung, A. Duclert, A. Gouble, S. Arnould, K. Peggs, M. Pule, A. M. Scharenberg, and J. Smith. 2015. "Multiplex genome-edited T-cell manufacturing platform for "Off-the-Shelf" adoptive T-cell immunotherapies." *Cancer Res* 75 (18):3853–3864. doi: 10.1158/0008-5472.CAN-14-3321.

Puck, T. T., P. I. Marcus, and S. J. Cieciura. 1956. "Clonal growth of mammalian cells in vitro; growth characteristics of colonies from single HeLa cells with and without a feeder layer." *J Exp Med* 103 (2):273–283. doi: 10.1084/jem.103.2.273.

Qasim, W., H. Zhan, S. Samarasinghe, S. Adams, P. Amrolia, S. Stafford, K. Butler, C. Rivat, G. Wright, K. Somana, S. Ghorashian, D. Pinner, G. Ahsan, K. Gilmour, G. Lucchini, S. Inglott, W. Mifsud, R. Chiesa, K. S. Peggs, L. Chan, F. Farzeneh, A. J. Thrasher, A. Vora, M. Pule, and P. Veys. 2017. "Molecular remission of infant B-ALL after infusion of universal TALEN gene-edited CAR T cells." *Sci Transl Med* 9 (374). doi: 10.1126/scitranslmed.aaj2013.

Rappold, I., K. Iwabuchi, T Date, and J. Chen. 2001. "Tumor suppressor p53 binding protein 1 (53BP1) is involved in DNA damage-signaling pathways." *J Cell Biol* 153 (3):613–620.

Rees, H. A., and D. R. Liu. 2018. "Base editing: Precision chemistry on the genome and transcriptome of living cells." *Nat Rev Genetics* 19 (12):770–788.

Roehl, H. H., M. E. Leibbrandt, J. S. Greengard, E. Kamantigue, W. G. Glass, M. Giedlin, K. Boekelheide, D. E. Johnson, D. J. Jolly, and N. C. Sajjadi. 2000. "Analysis of testes and semen from rabbits treated by intravenous injection with a retroviral vector encoding the human factor VIII gene: No evidence of germ line transduction." *Hum Gene Ther* 11 (18):2529–2540. doi: 10.1089/10430340050208000.

Rouet, P., F. Smih, and M. Jasin. 1994. "Expression of a site-specific endonuclease stimulates homologous recombination in mammalian cells." *Proc Natl Acad Sci U S A* 91 (13):6064–6068. doi: 10.1073/pnas.91.13.6064.

Sadelain, M., E. P. Papapetrou, and F. D. Bushman. 2011. "Safe harbours for the integration of new DNA in the human genome." *Nat Rev Cancer* 12 (1):51–58. doi: 10.1038/nrc3179.

Schultz, LB, N. H. Chehab, A. Malikzay, and T. D. Halazonetis. 2000. "p53 binding protein (53BP1) is an early participant in the cellular response to DNA double-strand breaks." *J Cell Biol* 151 (7):1381–1390.

Sharma, R., X. M. Anguela, Y. Doyon, T. Wechsler, R. C. DeKelver, S. Sproul, D. E. Paschon, J. C. Miller, R. J. Davidson, D. Shivak, S. Zhou, J. Rieders, P. D. Gregory, M. C. Holmes, E. J. Rebar, and K. A. High. 2015. "In vivo genome editing of the albumin locus as a platform for protein replacement therapy." *Blood* 126 (15):1777–1784. doi: 10.1182/blood-2014-12-615492.

Silva, G., L. Poirot, R. Galetto, J. Smith, G. Montoya, P. Duchateau, and F. Paques. 2011. "Meganucleases and other tools for targeted genome engineering: Perspectives and challenges for gene therapy." *Curr Gene Ther* 11 (1):11–27. doi: 10.2174/156652311794520111.

Slatko, B. E., A. F. Gardner, and F. M. Ausubel. 2018. "Overview of next-generation sequencing technologies." *Curr Protoc Mol Biol* 122 (1):e59. doi: 10.1002/cpmb.59.

Stark, W. M. 2014. "The serine recombinases." *Microbiol Spectr* 2 (6). doi: 10.1128/microbiolspec.MDNA3-0046-2014.

Stoddard, B. L. 2011. "Homing endonucleases: From microbial genetic invaders to reagents for targeted DNA modification." *Structure* 19 (1):7–15. doi: 10.1016/j.str.2010.12.003.

ThermoFisher. 2020. "What is next generation sequencing."

Tsai, S. Q., Z. Zheng, N. T. Nguyen, M. Liebers, V. V. Topkar, V. Thapar, N. Wyvekens, C. Khayter, A. J. Iafrate, L. P. Le, M. J. Aryee, and J. K. Joung. 2015. "GUIDE-seq enables genome-wide profiling of off-target cleavage by CRISPR-Cas nucleases." *Nat Biotechnol* 33 (2):187–197. doi: 10.1038/nbt.3117.

Tsai, S., N. T. Nguyen, J. Malagon-Lopex, V. V. Topkar, M. J. Aryee, and J. K. Joung. 2017. "CIRCLE-seq: a highly senstive in vitro screen for genome-wide CRISPR-Cas9 nuclease off-targets." *Nat Methods* 14:607–614.

Tu, Z., W. Yang, S. Yan, X. Guo, and X. J. Li. 2015. "CRISPR/Cas9: A powerful genetic engineering tool for establishing large animal models of neurodegenerative diseases." *Mol Neurodegener* 10:35. doi: 10.1186/s13024-015-0031-x.

USFDA. 2013. Guidance for Industry - Preclinical Assessment of Investigational Cellular and Gene Therapy Products. edited by Center for Biologics Evaluation and Research US Food and Drug Administration.

USFDA. 2020. Guidance for Industry - Long Term Follow-up After Administration of Human Gene Therapy Products. edited by Center for Biologics Evaluation and Research US Food and Drug Administration.

Wang, C. X., and P. M. Cannon. 2016. "The clinical applications of genome editing in HIV." *Blood* 127 (21):2546–2552. doi: 10.1182/blood-2016-01-678144.

Wang, X, Y. Wang, X. Wu, J. Wang, Z. Qiu, T. Chang, H. Huang, R. Lin, and J-K. Yee. 2015. "Unbiased detection of off-target cleavage by CRISPR-Cas9 and TALENs using integrase-defective lentiviral vectors." *Nat Biotechnol* 33:175–178.

Wen, H., Z. Qu, Y. Yan, C. Pu, C. Wang, H. Jiang, T. Hou, and Y. Huo. 2019. "Preclinical safety evaluation of chimeric antigen receptor-modified T cells against CD19 in NSG mice." *Ann Transl Med* 7 (23):735. doi: 10.21037/atm.2019.12.03.

Yee, J. K. 2016. "Off-target effects of engineered nucleases." *FEBS J* 283 (17):3239–3248. doi: 10.1111/febs.13760.

Yohe, S., and B. Thyagarajan. 2017. "Review of clinical next-generation sequencing." *Arch Pathol Lab Med* 141 (11):1544–1557. doi: 10.5858/arpa.2016-0501-RA.

Zeitler, B., S. Froelich, K. Marlen, D. A. Shivak, Q. Yu, D. Li, J. R. Pearl, J. C. Miller, L. Zhang, D. E. Paschon, S. J. Hinkley, I. Ankoudinova, S. Lam, D. Guschin, L. Kopan, J. M. Cherone, H. B. Nguyen, G. Qiao, Y. Ataei, M. C. Mendel, R. Amora, R. Surosky, J. Laganiere, B. J. Vu, A. Narayanan, Y. Sedaghat, K. Tillack, C. Thiede, A. Gartner, S. Kwak, J. Bard, L. Mrzljak, L. Park, T. Heikkinen, K. K. Lehtimaki, M. M. Svedberg, J. Haggkvist, L. Tari, M. Toth, A. Varrone, C. Halldin, A. E. Kudwa, S. Ramboz, M. Day, J. Kondapalli, D. J. Surmeier, F. D. Urnov, P. D. Gregory, E. J. Rebar, I. Munoz-Sanjuan, and H. S. Zhang. 2019. "Allele-selective transcriptional repression of mutant HTT for the treatment of Huntington's disease." *Nat Med* 25 (7):1131–1142. doi: 10.1038/s41591-019-0478-3.

Part IV

Practical Applications

28

Nonclinical Development of Anticancer Biotherapeutics

Marque Todd
Renaissance Consulting

Cris Kamperschroer
Labcorp

Rafael Ponce
Shape Therapeutics

Timothy MacLachlan
Novartis Institutes for Biomedical Research

Jonathan Heyen
Pfizer

CONTENTS

28.1 Introduction

There has been continuous advancement in the number and diversity of biotechnology-derived therapeutics (biotherapeutics) used to treat multiple diseases including cancer.

Biotherapeutics are usually highly selective due to their specificity for a given target. More traditional biotherapeutics like proteins, monoclonal antibodies and their derivatives, and recombinant wild-type and modified cytokines are used frequently in clinical trials and in oncology clinical practice. Due

DOI: 10.1201/9781003124542-32

to the success of conventional biotherapeutic approaches as well as some of their limitations, there is a push to develop novel variations of these modalities as well as new modalities to target cancer with its diverse mechanisms of growth and treatment resistance.

The understanding of the underlying mechanisms of cancer has also advanced significantly, resulting in an explosion of more complex biological modalities designed to do more than directly target antigens on the cancer cell surface or its supporting vasculature. The newest area of anticancer research aims to modulate the immune system by taking the breaks off of immune checkpoints, using complex molecules that recognize the cancer cell and at the same time engage and activate cells of the immune system, taking advantage of the oncolytic properties of some viruses, and designing vaccines that target cancer cells. Other complex modalities like antibody-drug conjugates (ADCs) aim to take advantage of traditional cytotoxic agents by linking them to antibodies that directly target tumor cells.

In the wake of this plethora of new modalities, health authorities have started to create comprehensive regulatory guidelines that specifically address the safety aspects of some of these newer modalities and the different risk/benefit considerations for patients with late-stage cancer. The aim of many of these guidelines is to deliver safe therapies to cancer patients while taking into consideration the need for more rapid advancement of anticancer drug development programs due to the serious life-threatening nature of the disease and the lack of other treatment options.

28.2 Nonclinical Regulatory Considerations for the Development of Anticancer Biotherapeutics

28.2.1 Protein-Based Biotherapeutics

This section will specifically focus on the guidelines most applicable to the development of protein-based biotherapeutics for oncology, including the International Committee of Harmonization (ICH) guidelines: ICH S6(R1): *Preclinical Safety Evaluation of Biotechnology-Derived Pharmaceuticals*; ICH S9: *Nonclinical Evaluations for Anticancer Pharmaceuticals,* and ICH S9 Q&A: *Nonclinical Evaluations for Anticancer Pharmaceuticals Questions and Answers* (collectively called ICH S9). Many of the general principles that apply to the nonclinical development of all biotherapeutics and outlined in ICH S6(R1) can be applied to biotherapeutics for anticancer indications (e.g., selection of pharmacologically relevant species, immunogenicity testing). However, a tremendous amount of effort has gone into developing a specific regulatory framework for the nonclinical development of anticancer drugs (including small molecules and biotherapeutics) by health authorities and industry through the creation of specific guidelines including ICH S9 and its associated question and answer document (ICH S9 Q&A). ICH S9 describes the principles and special considerations for the nonclinical development of anticancer drugs, including biotherapeutics, and was finalized in 2009. The follow-up guideline ICH S9 Q&A was finalized in 2018 to clarify and/ or update specific areas of the original ICH S9 document. ICH

S6(R1), ICH S9, and ICH S9 Q&A thus provide the framework for the nonclinical development of protein-based anticancer biotherapeutics. ICH S6(R1) outlines the general principles, and the ICH S9 guidelines give specific recommendations for the nonclinical development of anticancer drugs, and in some instances touches upon special considerations for biotherapeutics (e.g., ADCs, non-human primate [NHP] developmental toxicity studies). In general, all protein biotherapeutics, including those being developed for oncology indications, fall under the scope of ICH S6(R1) with additional considerations as highlighted in ICH S9 and the associated Q&A document. However, some other types of modalities are specifically excluded from the scope of ICH S6(R1), including vaccines (DNA and viral), gene therapies, and cell therapies, and the ICH S9 guidelines are generally silent on non-protein-based biotherapeutics. Non-protein-based anticancer biotherapeutics with a few exceptions are generally covered by the same guidelines as for other noncancer indications with some special considerations for cancer indications based on the different risk-benefit considerations in this therapeutic area (see Section 28.2.2 for regulatory considerations for non-protein-based anticancer biotherapeutics).

Many clinical studies often involve cancer patients whose disease condition is progressive and fatal, and many existing anticancer drugs have limited effectiveness. Thus, it was recognized that the risk/benefit factors used to determine the appropriate nonclinical and clinical studies and study endpoints, as well as the timing of those studies, are different from other indications. For these reasons, flexibility is needed in designing a program of nonclinical studies for new anticancer therapies. The ICH S9 guidelines were written to ensure that drugs being developed for late-stage cancer indications could be provided to patients as expeditiously as possible while still protecting patient safety. One key difference for anticancer drugs versus drug for other indications is that the clinically efficacious exposure level in patients is often near to or even exceeds the observed adverse effect levels in the animal toxicity studies. More safety risk is tolerated for anticancer drugs, because patients with late-stage cancer have limited time and treatment options for their disease. The possible benefit to these patients outweighs the potentially greater risk that these drugs may pose during early clinical investigation. Because of the increased safety risk and also the opportunity for benefit, most of the initial clinical trials conducted with anticancer drugs occur in patients with late-stage cancer rather than in healthy volunteers. For all these reasons, there is a greater sense of urgency, which requires a more flexible, and somewhat less conservative approach to the development of anticancer drugs. This approach does not mean that patient safety is compromised or downplayed but that physicians and patients are willing to assume a greater amount of risk because of the severity and seriousness of their illness. It does mean that the nonclinical development program under ICH S9 guidance can enhance the speed at which critical drugs can be delivered to patients in a number of ways: (1) decrease the number of required animal toxicity studies; (2) streamline the endpoints or numbers of animals required on studies; (3) delay some studies until later in development; and/or (4) using different toxicity criteria (i.e., the highest non-severely toxic dose [HNSTD] in non-rodents and the severely toxic dose in 10% or less of the animals [STD_{10}]) to determine the starting dose in first-in-human (FIH) clinical trials.

The scope of ICH S9 was originally defined as providing guidance on nonclinical development programs for drugs that are intended to "treat cancer in patients with serious and life-threatening malignancies" (i.e., advanced and/or late-stage cancer). ICH S9 Q&A further clarifies that ICH S9 pertains to development programs in both adults and children "whose disease is resistant and refractory to available therapy." A clarification in the ICH S9 Q&A guideline on scope states that if the cancer is not resistant and refractory, then ICH S9 can be used as a starting point but other guidelines may need to be used as appropriate (e.g., ICH M3[R2] titled *Guidance on nonclinical safety studies for the conduct of human clinical trials and marketing authorization for pharmaceuticals and S6[R1]*) and additional studies may be warranted. For example, follow-on clinical trials in adjuvant and neoadjuvant settings are covered by ICH S9 even when there is a lack of detectable residual disease. Nonclinical and clinical data generated in patients with late-stage cancer can be considered, and may be used, to abbreviate any additional nonclinical studies for follow on cancer indications. The guideline further defines that in cases where there is a high cure rate and/or a low or long delay in recurrence rate, then further studies (e.g., developmental and reproductive studies [DART]) will likely be needed prior to registration for those indications. In contrast, if recurrence is high and/or rapid, the need for additional studies can be addressed on a case-by-case basis taking into account the totality of nonclinical and clinical safety data, cure rate, and expected time to recurrence. However, if the initial development program is in the adjuvant or neoadjuvant setting, additional nonclinical studies may be needed, including longer-term general toxicity studies (i.e., a 6-month repeat-dose toxicity study for a biotherapeutic). ICH S9 does not apply to all cancer-related indications, for example, biotherapeutics designed as supportive care drugs in the oncology setting (e.g., erythropoietin for cancer drug-related anemia).

The ICH S9 guidelines discuss when the nonclinical development program can diverge from that described in other more general guidelines such as ICH M3(R2) or ICH S6(R1) or when these guidelines should still be followed. When determining which guideline to follow first, in most cases the more specific guideline should be followed first, and where it is silent on a topic, the next specific guideline should be consulted. For anticancer biotherapeutics, this means that ICH S9 and S9 Q&A would be consulted first, and if the information that is being sought is not in these guidelines, then ICH S6(R1) would be consulted next, and finally the more general guidelines on specific topics such specialty toxicity studies (e.g., ICH S5(R3) *Detection of toxicity to reproduction for medicinal products & toxicity to male fertility* for DART studies and ICH M3(R3) on timing of the studies).

Several important considerations are highlighted in the ICH S9 guidelines that influence the conduct and timing of nonclinical studies to specifically support a late-stage anticancer drug development program. Table 28.1 highlights the similarities and major differences in the requirements for the nonclinical toxicity testing of late-stage anticancer biotherapeutics based on the ICH S9 guidelines (and where applicable the ICH S6(R1) guideline) versus for non-oncology indications.

A more detailed discussion of these considerations is presented in Section 28.3.

28.2.1.1 Safety Margin Considerations and Starting Dose Selection for FIH Clinical Trials

Identifying a no observable adverse effect level (NOAEL) is not critical nor required under ICH S9 to support clinical use of an anticancer biopharmaceutic, and this should be taken into consideration when selecting doses for the general toxicity studies. Although safety and tolerability are still the primary endpoints in a FIH clinical trial with an anticancer biotherapeutic, based on ethical considerations (i.e., ensuring patients can possibly gain some benefit from the new biotherapeutic), all dose levels tested in patients should provide a minimal level of pharmacological activity. Safety margins to support the starting dose in an FIH clinical trial with a biotherapeutic can be calculated using a variety of approaches, including NOAEL, STD_{10}, HNSTD, or minimal anticipated biological effect level (MABEL). Whichever approach is used to set the clinical starting dose, it should be scientifically justified using all available nonclinical data (i.e., efficacy, pharmacokinetics, pharmacodynamics, and toxicity) and also deliver the highest pharmacologically active dose (PAD) possible while still protecting patient safety.

Since a different level of safety risk is acceptable for anticancer drugs that will be used in FIH clinical trials, different approaches beyond using a NOAEL can and should be considered when defining toxic dose levels and subsequent safety margins in general toxicity studies. Besides NOAEL, ICH S9 encourages the use of the STD_{10} for rodent studies (i.e., mice and rats) and the HNSTD for non-rodent studies (i.e., dogs and monkeys) as first defined by (DeGeorge et al. 1998). ICH S9 Q&A further clarifies that the use of these endpoints can be acceptable for biotherapeutics as well as small molecules. The STD_{10} is a dose level that is severely toxic to ≤10% of the animals. Severely toxic is usually defined as mortality, life-threatening toxicity, or observation of toxicities that are not reversible during a recovery period and would substantively diminish organ function. The highest non-severely toxic dose (HNSTD) is defined as the dose where severe toxicity including mortality and the other parameters mentioned above is not observed but there may still be adverse findings. Usually, the clinical starting dose in a FIH clinical trial is calculated using data from the most sensitive species based on the extent and types of toxicity and associated exposure levels. If the rodent is the most relevant species, then 1/10th the STD_{10} is considered to be an appropriate starting dose in patients, whereas if the non-rodent species is the most relevant species, then 1/6th the HNSTD is considered most appropriate. Depending on the type of toxicities observed (e.g., cardiovascular toxicity) and/or how steep the dose-toxicity response curve is, an additional safety factor (e.g., 5–10X) may be added to lower the starting dose further while still ensuring an active dose. In some cases, depending on the half-life of the biotherapeutic, the duration of toxicological effects, and/or the steepness of the dose-toxicity response curve, it may be more appropriate to use the NOAEL to define safety margins and set dose levels for FIH clinical trials.

Some classes of anticancer drugs are considered to have a higher risk of causing adverse events (e.g., agonistic

TABLE 28.1

General Considerations for the Nonclinical Testing Strategy Supporting Late-Stage Anticancer Biotherapeutics in Comparison to Non-oncology Indications

Area of Consideration	Late-Stage Anticancer Indication	Other Indications
Species selection	• If two pharmacologically relevant species identified (one rodent and one non-rodent), testing is required in both species • If one pharmacologically relevant species identified; testing is required in one species • If no pharmacologically relevant species identified; no in vivo studies may be required (use of surrogates is discouraged) and safety endpoints in in vivo pharmacology models and in vitro studies supporting safety may suffice	• If two pharmacologically relevant species identified (one rodent and one non-rodent), testing is required in both species • If one pharmacologically relevant species identified, testing is required in one species • If no pharmacologically relevant species identified, in vivo studies using a homologous protein (i.e., surrogate) or transgenic animal model may be used
General toxicity studies	• 13-week study longest required duration needed to support late-stage clinical development and marketing authorization • Identification of a NOAEL is not required; identification of a HNSTD in non-rodents and a STD_{10} in rodents is sufficient • Assessment of recovery should be conducted in at least one study • TK assessments should be incorporated • ADA assessment incorporated to meet recommendations in ICH S6(R1)	• 26-week study longest duration needed to support late-stage clinical development and marketing authorization • Identification of a NOAEL is generally required • Assessment of recovery should be conducted in at least one study • TK assessments should be incorporated • ADA assessment incorporated to meet recommendations in ICH S6(R1)
Safety pharmacology assessments	• Can be incorporated into non-rodent and rodent (if relevant) general toxicity studies	• Can be incorporated into non-rodent and rodent (if relevant) general toxicity studies
Tissue cross-reactivity studies (IHC) or alternative methods to assess target binding/ site distribution	• Not required except when no pharmacologically relevant species has been identified • May be useful for molecules where on-target or off-target binding in normal non-tumor tissues can cause severe toxicity (e.g., CAR T cells, CD3 bispecifics, ADCs)	• Required for all biotherapeutics containing a CDR
DART studies	• EFD study in one pharmacologically relevant species is sufficient • If biotherapeutic belongs to a class of drugs that has been well characterized, then EFD study may not be needed and risk is communicated in the label • If monkey is the only relevant species, strong consideration will be given to not conducting an EFD study and risk is communicated in the label • Fertility and PPND studies not required; not required to use sexually mature animals on 13-week monkey toxicity study if only relevant species	• EFD studies generally conducted in two pharmacologically relevant species (or in one species if only one pharmacologically relevant species) • Rare that EFD study (or equivalent) requirement is waived • If monkey is the only relevant species, an EFD study or equivalent (EFD study with surrogate or evaluation in enhanced PPND study) is generally required • Fertility (or assessment of reproductive organs in mature animals on 26-week monkey study) and PPND studies are generally required
Genotoxicity and carcinogenicity studies	• Not required	• Genotoxicity studies not required for biotherapeutics • Assessment of carcinogenic potential may be needed
Juvenile toxicity studies	• Generally not required	• May be required on a case-by-case basis based on intended clinical population
Combination studies	• Generally not required if the toxicity of each drug has been well characterized individually • When the toxicity profile of one of the drugs has not been well characterized, limited safety endpoints from a supportive pharmacology study, such as mortality, clinical signs and body weight, may suffice	• May be needed on a case-by-case basis

ADA = antidrug antibodies; ADC = antibody-drug conjugate; CAR = chimeric antigen receptor; CDR = complementarity-determining region; DART = developmental and reproductive toxicity; EFD = embryo-fetal development; HNSTD = highest non-severely toxic dose; NOAEL = no observable effect level; PPND = pre- and postnatal development; STD_{10} = severely toxic dose in 10% of the animals; TK = toxicokinetics.

immunomodulating drugs) and require a more conservative approach to selecting the appropriate starting dose in cancer patients. The importance of understanding the in vitro and in vivo pharmacology versus relying solely on in vivo toxicity data for these types of agonist immunomodulators was highlighted by the FIH clinical trial with an anti-CD28 super-agonist monoclonal antibody (Tegenero TGN1412) that resulted in severe adverse effects in healthy volunteers (Suntharalingam et al. 2006). More recently, severe adverse effects in clinical trials with chimeric antigen receptor T cells (CAR-T) have also been reported (Anand et al. 2019). The Committee for Medicinal Products for Human Use (CHMP) of the European Medicines Agency (EMA) published and then revised a guideline designed to mitigate risks when initiating clinical trials and for clinical starting dose selection for these types of molecules including the use of MABEL or PAD (pharmacologically active dose) (EMA 2017) approaches as alternative methods for determining the safe clinical starting dose for FIH clinical trials with anticancer drugs. Factors such as the affinity of the biopharmaceutical for the target and across species (i.e., potency), understanding of the receptor-occupancy-response relationships and the potential for "on-off" switch mechanisms (i.e., steep dose response relationships), and in vitro/in vivo mechanistic pharmacology/toxicity (e.g., cell killing and cytokine release) should be considered for these molecules when selecting a clinical starting dose (Leach et al. 2020). There is still the expectation even for these higher-risk drugs that the starting dose will provide the potential for efficacy in patients with advanced cancer.

Saber et al. from the FDA Office of Hematology and Oncology Products produced three informative papers (Saber and Leighton 2015; Saber et al. 2016, 2017) that highlight the variety of approaches used in selecting the FIH clinical trial starting dose and subsequent impact on duration of the clinical trials and on how quickly doses were reached where adverse events are observed. Saber and Leighton (2015) analyzed nonclinical toxicity study data including selection of the HNSTD and/or STD10, the methods used to calculate the clinical starting dose, and FIH clinical trial outcomes for several ADCs (see Chapter 22). The analyses concluded that 1/6th the HNSTD in cynomolgus monkeys or 1/10th the STD_{10} in rodents using a body surface area (BSA) scaling approach to convert from animal to human doses appeared to result in the most acceptable balance between safety and efficacy during the dose escalation phase (Saber and Leighton 2015). Other acceptable approaches included 1/10th the HNSTD in monkeys using BSA scaling or using 1/10th the NOAEL in rodents or monkeys using body weight scaling. The same group analyzed data on immune system antagonist antibodies and the use of the MABEL approach for FIH clinical trial starting dose selection (Saber et al. 2016). Analyses of the data showed that for approximately half of the antibodies examined, the selected starting dose based on a MABEL approach was too low and required many dose escalations to reach the maximally tolerated dose (MTD) in patients. This is not considered an optimum scenario for clinical trials enrolling patients with late-stage cancer where there is an expectation that patients will receive doses of drug that are pharmacologically active. On the other hand, using 1/6th of the HNSTD or 1/10th of the NOAEL resulted in unsafe starting doses. In the third publication (Saber et al. 2017), the use of different approaches for the selection of FIH clinical trial starting doses for a subset of immune activating products, CD3 bispecific molecules, was explored. Those analyses showed that FIH clinical dose selection approaches based on in vitro receptor occupancy assays or on the NHSTD or NOAEL dose level derived from monkey toxicity studies were not acceptable approaches, because these doses were at, or exceeded, the MTD in patients. A MABEL/PAD approach using an FIH starting dose corresponded to 10%–30% activity in in vitro pharmacology assays (e.g., T-cell activation, cytotoxicity, and

effector function assays) gave more acceptable results; in most cases, using 50% pharmacological activity was also acceptable. These three publications highlight the complexities of setting the FIH clinical trial starting dose with considerations as to the type of modality, the pharmacological mechanism of action, and the types of in vitro and in vivo data collected all influencing which approach will be most appropriate.

28.2.1.2 Other Regulatory Considerations to Support Clinical Trials

The ICH S9 guideline also advises on dose escalation, the highest dose that can be used in clinical trials based on dose levels tested in the nonclinical studies, as well as on the duration and dosing schedule of toxicity studies to support initial clinical trials.

In general, the highest dose/exposure tested in the repeat-dose toxicity studies does not limit the dose escalation or highest dose that can be investigated in the clinical trials. However, if a steep dose- or exposure-toxicity response curve has been observed or if a severe, non-monitorable toxicity has been identified in nonclinical studies, then smaller-than-usual dose increments should be considered in the clinical trial. Clinical trials can continue beyond the highest dose and duration of completed toxicity studies based on individual patient responses.

The dosing intervals selected for the toxicity studies should be chosen based on the pharmacokinetic profile of the test article and to allow for flexibility of dosing schedules in the clinic and may also be based on test article tolerability. It is not expected that the exact clinical schedule be followed in the toxicity studies, but that drug exposure and toxicity data be sufficient to support the clinical dose and schedule and to identify potential target organ toxicities. This is particularly important for protein-derived pharmaceuticals where more protracted dose intervals have the potential for increased immunogenicity in animals. Examples of potential nonclinical and clinical dosing schedules include daily, weekly, or once every 3-week dosing.

The nonclinical data used to support Phase 1 clinical trials in conjunction with Phase 1 clinical data are normally sufficient to support entry into Phase 2 clinical trials. Three-month repeat-dose toxicity studies are required under ICH S9 to initiate the registrational clinical trials for a late-stage cancer indication. Recently, many registrational clinical trials for late-stage cancer are Phase 2 trials, and repeat-dose toxicity studies of 3 months in duration are still required to initiate these clinical trials (i.e., what is important to consider is if the clinical trial is registration-enabling, and not the designated phase of the clinical trial [Phase 2 or Phase 3]).

28.2.2 Regulatory Considerations for Non-protein-Based Biotherapeutics

There are a plethora of non-protein-based biotherapeutic modalities including cell therapies (some with gene modifications), oncolytic viruses (some with gene modifications), and anticancer vaccines that are being developed for use in late-stage cancer indications. Each modality has its own set of nonclinical development regulatory considerations. As with standard protein-based biotherapeutics, the nonclinical development programs for these modalities will be considered on a case-by-case basis by health authorities. The development programs may be based on similar guidelines as used for non-oncology indications for the same type of modality and/or take these guidelines into consideration but with modifications due to the program supporting a late-stage cancer indication. Toxicity assessments need to be considered on a case-by-case basis depending on the modality and the risks presented and may involve in vivo or in vitro assessments, or a mix of both. For non-protein-based biotherapeutics, the process of choosing an animal model for toxicity studies, or even whether to use an animal model is complex. In addition, the length of any animal studies may be different from more standard biotherapeutics considering that in some cases the therapy is permanent after only one administration or in other cases the biotherapeutic may be administered multiple times and have variable persistence in blood and/or tissues. Finally, some concerns of health authorities are very specific to the type of modality or intended indication. Based on all these considerations, it is strongly recommended that a pre-IND meeting with the FDA or the equivalent for other countries is planned to discuss the overall nonclinical development strategy with the relevant health authorities. In addition, FDA CBER offers the INTERACT meeting, which is an even earlier opportunity to receive feedback on the nonclinical development of novel biotherapeutics (see Chapter 6 for detailed information on interactions with worldwide health authorities). Table 28.2 gives an overview of some general regulatory considerations for non-protein-based cancer biotherapeutics (with reference to later sections of this chapter or other chapters in the book that give more details based on the type of modality).

TABLE 28.2

Nonclinical Regulatory Considerations for the Toxicity Testing of Non-protein-Based Biotherapeutics for Oncology

Modality (Other Reference Sections/Chapters)	Regulatory Considerations
Cell therapies (see Section 28.4.1.3; also see Chapter 25)	• There may be no relevant animal model if the therapy uses autologous cells and/or the mechanism of action is human cell-specific (e.g., T-cell immunotherapies); in the case where there is no relevant animal model, in vitro efficacy and safety studies may be used to support a FIH clinical trial • Toxicity studies may be conducted in pharmacologically relevant normal animals, in murine tumor models including syngeneic models and/or in immunosuppressed mice if human cells are used; these studies should only be conducted if the animal models are pharmacologically relevant • The required duration, dosing regimen, and route of administration of any animal toxicity studies will be based on the clinical trial duration, dosing regimen, and route of administration, and also allow for full characterization of biodistribution • Biodistribution and persistence studies may be required • In vitro and/or in vivo tumorigenicity studies may be required to evaluate the potential of a stem cell therapy or genetically modified cells to form a tumor • If the cell therapy includes any added or modified genes, a genomic integration assessment may be required
Oncolytic viruses (see Section 28.4.5)	• Selection of the animal model should take into consideration viral tropism, infectivity, replication ability, and cytopathic potential; if the virus contains a transgene, it is important that the animal model be pharmacologically responsive to any expressed proteins • Mechanisms for oncolytic specificity/risk to normal tissue should be addressed • Animal toxicity studies may be conducted in normal animals and/or murine tumor models; tumor models may be more relevant • A toxicity study in immunosuppressed mice may be required as a "worst-case scenario" if the virus will be given to immunocompromised patients • Biodistribution, persistence, and latency/reactivation studies will likely be required, based on the known attributes of the virus • If the virus can integrate into the host genome, then a genomic integration assessment will likely be required • Intended and unintended biodistribution assessments are required to understand the tropism and persistence of the virus in tissues and the peripheral blood, and based on the anticipated route of administration • Viral shedding will need to be evaluated in animal studies to understand how the virus may be shed in bodily fluids and/or feces and for how long after dose administration • Safety of any expressed transgene products should be established using predicted exposure levels in patients • An embryo-fetal development study may be required (dependent on patient population) • Risks of recombination with wild-type viruses, and environmental transfer to animal species should be considered
Cancer vaccines (see Section 28.4.6; and Chapter 23)	• Need to select a pharmacologically relevant species (e.g., transgenic mice or non-human primate) based on target antigen homology and tissue distribution between species • Cancer vaccine toxicity studies are generally similar in design and duration to infectious disease vaccine toxicity studies (e.g., route of administration, dose, and number of doses administered) • Measurement of antigen-specific humoral (i.e., antibody generation) and/or cellular immune responses as well as duration of the response depending on the vaccine's mechanism of action will typically be required • Novel adjuvants or combinations with immunostimulating therapies may need to be tested in stand-alone toxicity studies • If the vaccine contains nucleic acids and/or is delivered via a viral or bacterial, biodistribution and persistence, and shedding studies may be required • An embryo-fetal development study may be required

28.3 Special Considerations for Toxicology Programs Supporting Protein-Based Biotherapeutics

This section applies to most protein-based biotherapeutics such as monoclonal antibodies and their derivatives, fusion proteins, and recombinant proteins such as wild-type and modified cytokines that target cancer cell antigens. These modalities, except for some that specifically target the immune system, will not be discussed in further detail beyond what is provided in this section. This is because any other details of the nonclinical development programs beyond those outlined below are similar to non-oncology indications, and other chapters of this book go into greater detail for those considerations (see Chapters 20, 29, and 30). The considerations below are for biotherapeutics where the initial indication is for the treatment of advanced, late-stage cancer (disease is resistant and refractory) in accordance with ICH S9. For other initial development programs and for follow-on indications in cancer that are not resistant and refractory, aspects of ICH S9 and S9 Q&A may apply and should be used as a starting point with other nonclinical studies being added as appropriate with reference to ICH M3(R2) and S6(R1).

28.3.1 General Toxicity Studies

The approach for general toxicity study conducted to support protein-based anticancer biotherapeutics is outlined in ICH S9 and ICH S9 Q&A. As is the case in the development of most biotherapeutics, each molecule should be considered on a case-by-case basis as the target, modality, species selectivity, and other factors will influence the overall strategy for designing the toxicity studies. Many of the principles that apply to general toxicity studies to support non-oncology indications apply to anticancer biotherapeutics. However, the use of homologous proteins (i.e., surrogate molecules) is generally discouraged for indications supported by ICH S9; however, in some cases, they have been used particularly for novel modalities where there is no clinical experience.

As has been discussed previously in this chapter, identifying a NOAEL or NOEL is not considered essential to aid in selecting the starting dose for a FIH clinical trial for a late-stage cancer drug. More relevant endpoints for oncology include the HNSTD in non-rodents and the STD_{10} in rodents and taking into account binding affinity differences between animals and humans. Dose levels for the repeat-dose toxicity studies are selected similarly to those supporting non-oncology indications. However, an important exception is that the highest dose level/exposure tested in the toxicity studies does not limit the dose escalation or highest dose that can be investigated in clinical trials. In addition, clinical trials can continue beyond the highest dose and duration of completed toxicity studies based on patient responses.

The dosing intervals selected for the toxicity studies should be chosen based on the pharmacokinetic profile of the test article and to allow for flexibility of dosing schedules in the clinic and may also be based on drug tolerability for more toxic biotherapeutics (e.g., ADCs). It is not expected that the exact clinical schedule be followed in the toxicity studies, but that drug exposure and toxicity data are sufficient to support the clinical dose and schedule and to identify potential target organ toxicities.

Three-month repeat-dose toxicity studies following the intended clinical schedule (or a more intensive schedule) must be available prior to initiation of the pivotal clinical trial that will support registration of the biotherapeutic (i.e., registrational clinical trials can be Phase 2 or Phase 3 clinical studies) for a late-stage cancer indication. In addition, general toxicity studies longer than 3 months in duration in rodents and non-rodents do not have to be conducted for follow-on anticancer indications including in adjuvant and neoadjuvant settings.

Anticancer biotherapeutics may be inherently more toxic based on their targets and/or mechanisms of action. Study design changes may be implemented to align with the 3 R's (replacement, reduction, and refinement) and ensure quality data is obtained from the study. Staggered dosing designs can be employed where either (1) one animal in a dose group is administered the drug and monitored for clinical signs and/or changes in clinical pathology parameters indicative of tolerability before giving the drug to the rest of the animals in the dose group, or (2) all animals in a dose group are administered the drug and monitored for toxicity during the full dosing duration before the next group of animals are given the drug. These approaches minimize the number of animals exposed to concentrations of drug that could result in severe toxicity and/or mortality, and also allows for flexibility to increase or decrease the next dose level based on data from the previous dose levels. Other strategies that can be employed include intra-animal dose escalation or priming and maintenance regimens; these approaches can also minimize the number of animals needed to identify severe toxicity.

28.3.2 Developmental and Reproductive Toxicity (DART) Studies

An assessment of DART risk is not considered essential to support clinical trials in patients with late-stage cancer but is needed to support product registration (also see Chapter 12). If there is sufficient information on the target or drug class, literature, specifics of the patient population, limited relevant exposure, and/or other relevant information to sufficiently inform the human risk assessment (e.g., product label), then that weight of evidence should be proposed in lieu of an in vivo developmental toxicity study (Bowman and Chapin 2016; Rocca et al. 2018).

Particularly when the monkey is the only relevant species for an anticancer biotherapeutic, a weight-of-evidence assessment of reproductive risk should be provided to health authorities. As stated in ICH S9 Q&A, a monkey study to assess developmental toxicity should not be considered the default approach. If the weight of evidence clearly indicates a risk, an embryo-fetal development (EFD) study in monkey is not needed and the risk can be communicated in the product label.

If a weight-of-evidence evaluation of developmental toxicity risk is considered insufficient by a health authority, in vivo experimental evidence of developmental toxicity in at least one pharmacological relevant species is considered sufficient to support late-stage cancer product registration. If embryo-fetal lethality or malformations are identified in a dose-range finding EFD study, then a definitive study is generally not warranted and the dose-range finding study can support product registration. If no developmental toxicity is observed in the dose-range finding study, then a definitive EFD study should be conducted.

Fertility and early embryonic studies are generally not warranted to support late-stage cancer indications. Information available from general toxicology studies of the effects on reproductive organs can be used as a basis for the assessment of fertility. The use of mature monkeys in repeat-dose studies is not necessary for the assessment of the reproductive organs for late-stage cancer indications. Pre- and post-natal toxicity studies are also generally not warranted for late-stage cancer indications. In addition, lactation or placental transfer studies are not needed. However, if follow-on indications move away from late-stage cancer (e.g., indications with longer patient life expectancy or non-oncology indications), additional DART studies may be needed.

Juvenile animal toxicity studies are generally not needed to support advanced cancer indications. Potential toxicities that could occur in pediatric patients are generally understood from the known biology of the drug and from the nonclinical and clinical studies that have already been conducted where toxicity/safety has been evaluated (Leighton et al. 2016). In addition, dosing and clinical monitoring for young patients is typically done in a hospital setting, which decreases the risk (Leighton et al. 2016).

28.3.3 Tissue Cross-Reactivity Studies

In accordance with ICH S9 Q&A, tissue cross-reactivity studies are not generally needed for anticancer biotherapeutics with complementarity-determining regions (CDR) (e.g., antibody- or Fab-containing modalities) unless there is a specific cause for concern (see Chapter 11).

Certain modalities may have greater cause for concern because on-target or off-target binding in normal tissues carries a much greater risk for serious toxicity; examples include CD3-bispecifics, CAR T cells, and ADCs. In these cases, a more rigorous characterization of where the target is expressed may be warranted. These assessments do not need to be conducted in a regulated tissue cross-reactivity study and in fact, better reagents/methods may be available for this purpose than those used for regulated tissue cross-reactivity studies.

If there is no pharmacologically relevant species and in vivo toxicity studies cannot be conducted, a human tissue cross-reactivity study will be required to support the first clinical trial (ICH S9 Q&A).

28.3.4 Genotoxicity and Carcinogenicity Studies

As for other biotherapeutics, genotoxicity studies are generally not needed. Carcinogenicity studies are not warranted to support registration of late-stage cancer biotherapeutics (ICH S9). However, if less life-threatening follow-on indications are pursued, a carcinogenicity assessment, and potentially a carcinogenicity study (if there is a pharmacologically relevant rodent species), may be needed.

28.3.5 Phototoxicity Studies

Phototoxicity studies are generally not needed for biotherapeutics used in advanced cancer indications. One exception may be when the biotherapeutic contains a small molecule such as an ADC or a nanoparticle. In these cases, the assessment should be restricted to the small-molecule portion of the biotherapeutic.

28.3.6 Combination Studies

ICH S9 clearly states that, "In general, toxicology studies investigating the safety of combinations of pharmaceuticals intended to treat patients with advance cancer are not warranted." The ICH S9 and S9 Q&A guidelines further clarify the position by stating (1) any therapeutic intended for use in combination should be well studied individually (i.e., the toxicological evaluation is sufficient to support clinical studies of the individual drug alone); (2) if there is no, or very limited, human safety data for one of the drugs in the combination, then a study to support the clinical use of the combination is needed. The provided pharmacology study should show increased pharmacologic activity in the absence of a substantial increase in toxicity. Toxicity assessment in the combination pharmacology study can be based on limited endpoints, including mortality, clinical signs, and body weight. If the available clinical and nonclinical data are insufficient to determine a safe clinical starting dose for the combination, a combination toxicity study specifically designed to establish a safe starting dose should be considered.

This guidance is helpful particularly for biotherapeutics where combinations of biotherapeutics or combinations of biotherapeutics and small molecules can be challenging due to concerns over immunogenicity in the first case and differences in pharmacologically active species in the latter case. See Chapter 14 for more discussion on combinations.

28.3.7 Considerations for Programs with No Pharmacologically Relevant Species

There are several examples of pharmacologic targets and therapeutic modalities for which a suitable animal model for pharmacology and/or toxicity testing may not be available. The initiation of clinical trials is still feasible in these cases. An in vitro assay-based safety strategy can be successfully implemented to assess efficacy and safety, to highlight potential safety risks for patients, and to help set a safe clinical starting dose. Examples of such programs include biotherapeutics that exclusively bind the human target antigen and do not bind the target antigen nor have pharmacological activity in standard species used in toxicity testing (e.g., mouse, rat, rabbit, dog, and cynomolgus and rhesus monkeys). This approach has been accepted by health authorities based on the risk/benefit of anticancer therapeutics for late-stage cancer patient populations. It should be stressed that although this is a viable approach, the nonclinical program strategy if using only in vitro assays should be presented in advance of filing an IND or CTA to the appropriate health authorities to ensure acceptability of the approach.

Typically, in vitro only programs will still attempt to address as many aspects of safety as possible in lieu of having data from animal toxicity studies. Potential assays to characterize the safety of the biotherapeutic can include a thorough evaluation of target expression in tissues, cytotoxicity assays and/or activated cell killing assays in normal human and tissue-matched tumor cells, Fc function assays (i.e., antibody-dependent cellular cytotoxicity [ADCC] and complement-dependent cytotoxicity [CDC] assays), receptor occupancy assays, CRA, and/or a human tissue cross-reactivity study. The types of in vitro assays used, and their specific format and output, will be wholly dependent on the target, mechanism of action, and type of modality. In addition, it is not uncommon that an in vivo single-dose PK study is also conducted in rodents or non-rodents to characterize the pharmacokinetics of the biotherapeutic even in the absence of target binding or pharmacologic activity in that species. It should also be recognized that the clinical starting dose will be selected based on a MABEL or PAD approach in the absence of animal toxicity data (Leach et al. 2020), meaning that a lower clinical starting dose may be needed.

If a pharmacologically relevant animal model can be identified, this is still the best approach to fully characterize the safety of a new biotherapeutic. This approach has the advantage of potentially giving additional useful information including in vivo pharmacokinetics, and characterization of pharmacodynamic effects and their relationship to pharmacokinetics and toxicity. These additional data can be used to (1) understand potential exposure in patients; (2) aid in selecting the clinical starting dose; (3) characterize potential clinical pharmacodynamic markers; and (4) better understand the relationships between biotherapeutic exposure, pharmacodynamics, and any observed toxicity. Another advantage in assessing potential toxicity in a pharmacologically relevant species if possible is that the proposed clinical starting dose may be higher than that obtained using a MABEL or PAD approach based solely on in vitro data and the dose escalation strategy may be more aggressive.

28.3.8 Toxicity Evaluation When Targeting the Immune System

With the clinical success of immunotherapies targeting checkpoint inhibitors including cell death receptor or ligand (i.e., the PD1/PDL1 axis) and cytotoxic T-lymphocyte associated protein 4 (CTLA4) in a number of cancer indications, there has been a renewed interest in harnessing the immune system as a viable treatment for tumors (Ribas and Wolchok 2018). Broadly speaking, immunomodulatory therapies for cancer can be classified as either antagonists or agonists of targeted pathways. On the one hand, immune system antagonists can act by abrogating an inhibitory signaling pathway that would normally lead to downregulation of the immune system's ability to detect and/or respond to tumor cells. For example, PD1

antagonists promote antitumor activity of T cells by removing a signal meant to downregulate the T-cell response (Ribas and Wolchok 2018). On the other hand, immune system agonists typically act by stimulating or activating pathways known to increase antitumor activities such as cytolysis. Recent examples include tumor necrosis factor alpha (TNF-α) superfamily members CD134 and CD137, and stimulator of interferon genes (STING) agonists (Chester et al. 2018; Buchan, Rogel, and Al-Shamkhani 2018; Villanueva 2019). Immune agonists are considered to have a higher risk for cytokine release syndrome (CRS) and other acute immune-related adverse reactions. Immune agonists are specifically highlighted in ICH S9 with respect to understanding the immune activation properties of the molecule and ensuring the proper assessments and adjustments to calculate the clinical starting dose (i.e., consideration of MABEL).

Each immunomodulatory biotherapeutic should be considered case-by-case with mechanism of action and the pharmacologic and pharmacodynamic profile influencing the in vitro and in vivo toxicity testing strategy. There is an expectation by health authorities that there is a thorough evaluation of immune system endpoints for both immune antagonists and immune agonists used as anticancer therapies. Typical evaluations in rodent and/or non-rodent toxicity studies can include standard hematology parameters, evaluation of immune system organs (e.g., lymph nodes, spleen, thymus, bone marrow, and gut-associated lymphoid tissue) including organ weights and microscopic evaluations, immunophenotyping of peripheral blood or tissues to further characterize subsets of immune cells and/or activation of specific types of immune cells, and cytokine levels. The T-cell-dependent antigen response (TDAR) assay is more commonly used to broadly assess immune system function, typically for immune system antagonists. There is limited experience with using this assay for immune-stimulating cancer therapies and little data available to support its utility. Additionally, in vitro human CRAs are generally used to assess the potential for an immunomodulatory biotherapeutic to induce cytokine release.

28.3.8.1 Cytokine Release and Potential for Cytokine Storm

Many immuno-oncology therapies induce cytokine release as part of their expected mechanism of action and pharmacological activity, and the cytokine release may or may not contribute to antitumor efficacy. While cytokine release can represent a safety concern and is important to characterize, the hazard may have already been identified in pharmacology studies. In such cases, a separate in vitro CRA to confirm cytokine release may not be needed. In situations where cytokine release is expected, it is useful to distinguish between using cytokine measurements as a pharmacologic readout versus using the CRAs to identify safety risk. In certain situations (e.g., CD3-bispecific molecules), cytokine release data may be used as a measure of pharmacology to aid in the determination of the clinical starting dose (i.e., as part of a MABEL approach). However, in vitro CRAs conducted as part of the safety evaluation are only considered useful for hazard identification, and not generally for quantitative risk assessment (Vidal et al. 2010; Finco et al. 2014).

Assessments of cytokine production can also be added to rodent or non-rodent toxicity studies and may add to understanding the potential relationship between pharmacodynamic activity and toxicity. The details of measuring cytokine endpoints on toxicity studies, such as the timing of sample collection and the panel of cytokines evaluated, should be carefully considered in the context of the study goals. In general, the assessment of cytokines can be limited to a subset of pharmacologically meaningful cytokines (e.g., 3–5 cytokines) that are sufficiently sensitive, are relevant to the biologic pathways of interest, and/or are related to toxicity concerns. The assessment of large and broad panels of cytokines is normally unnecessary and does not provide additional value. Additional consideration should be given to the species where the cytokines will be measured. In general, rodents (i.e., mice and rats) may tolerate higher and more prolonged circulating levels of cytokines without showing clinical signs of toxicity or other adverse sequelae related to cytokine production as compared to primates (cynomolgus and human). Thus, the use of a rodent model may suggest a lesser risk for cytokine production-related toxicity that may not be relevant to patients in clinical trials. The evaluation of in vivo cytokine production can also be correlated with clinical signs or other endpoints, including changes in body temperature, increased heart rate, decreased blood pressure, and/or emesis, depending upon the species.

Overall, CRAs are considered of value for identifying the potential hazard of cytokine release and can be used in conjunction with cytokine data generated in vivo. The impact of cytokine data on a given therapeutic program and the decisions made in response to the data are determined on a case-by-case basis. The decisions are influenced by multiple factors including the biological pathway being targeted, whether cytokine production is considered to be part of the pharmacologic mechanism of action, the results from nonclinical in vitro and in vivo studies, the patient population being treated, and information available from literature.

28.3.8.2 *Immunophenotyping in Peripheral Blood or Tissues*

Immunophenotyping by flow cytometry is commonly added to rodent and/or monkey toxicity studies to evaluate the presence and/or activity of immune cell populations in the peripheral blood and/or tissues after the administration of immuno-oncology biotherapeutics. There are currently only limited immune cell markers available for the dog; therefore, immunophenotyping options are limited in this species.

Flow cytometry-based immunophenotyping assays using whole blood and/or tissues can be used to characterize CD4+ and CD8+ T cells, central and effector memory T cells, regulatory T cells, B-cell subsets, natural killer (NK) cells, monocytes/macrophages, and dendritic cell subsets (Wang and Lebrec 2017). In addition, many of the same immune cell biomarkers can be used in animal pharmacology and clinical studies allowing for an understanding of nonclinical

to clinical translation of efficacy and/or potential toxicity. Immunophenotyping typically includes counts and percentage of CD4+ and CD8+ T cells, CD20+ B cells, and NK cells. This panel can be easily expanded to understand activation and/or proliferation of individual cell populations. In addition, monocytic and dendritic cell markers are also available and can be assessed if the mechanism of action may be related to these cellular subsets. Other cellular subsets (e.g., subsets of FoxP3+ regulatory T cells) can be evaluated to further delineate the potential impact of immuno-oncology biotherapeutics on the immune system.

Consideration must be given to the understanding of the mechanism of action and primary pharmacology of the molecule to inform of any potential species or translation differences that may impact data interpretation. Care should be given to the interpretation of immunophenotyping in studies which employ a low number of animals as a high degree of inter-animal variability may be observed. The use of baseline assessments can be useful in establishing individual animal profiles and may be used in conjunction with historical control and published data aid in the interpretation of potential effects following treatment.

28.4 Nonclinical Development of Novel Cancer Biotherapeutics

A wide array of biotherapeutic modalities are used in the treatment of cancer and are selected based on their ability to enhance specific biological mechanisms that specifically target cancer cells while attempting to reduce toxicity in healthy cells and tissues. The landscape of modalities is continuously changing in oncology as more is learned about each modality's strengths and weaknesses in different cancer indications and as more is understood about the biology of cancer. Because of the numerous types of modalities and their diverse mechanisms of action, a standardized approach to nonclinical development and toxicity testing is not always feasible. Any approach must take into account the specific modality and generic mechanism of action of that modality, the specific biological pathways that are being targeted, and any specific regulatory requirements that pertain to that modality (e.g., ADCs) or class of drugs (i.e., immuno-oncology biotherapeutics).

This section will specifically focus on anticancer modalities where there has been at least one product brought to market, thus paving the way for the development programs that follow and allowing for a more thorough discussion of the nonclinical safety program considerations as well as any safety information derived from clinical experience. For the most part, the modalities in this section fall into a broad class of drugs specifically being developed to target the immune response to cancer, including checkpoint inhibitors, CD3 bispecifics, T-cell immunotherapies, and oncolytic viruses, and cancer vaccines. In addition, ADCs will be addressed because of their complex nonclinical development programs and to give overall context to the breadth of molecules being developed for oncology indications.

28.4.1 Overview of Immuno-Oncology Biotherapeutics

A role for the immune system in host defense against cancer was first proposed by Ehrlich in the beginning of the 20th century (Ehrlich 1909). These findings were contemporaneously supported by the surgeon William Coley who had identified a number of case reports of spontaneous tumor regression following streptococcal erysipelas skin infection, and led Coley to investigate the use of various bacterial preparations as a cancer treatment (Coley 1891, 1991). Over a 40-year period of clinical experimentation, Coley treated over 1,000 patients, achieved cures in approximately 10% of patients, and had tumor regressions in as many as half of these patients (Nauts and McLaren 1990; Wiemann and Starnes 1994). However, a number of factors challenged widespread acceptance of his approach, including the absence of a theoretical framework for understanding how the immune system could distinguish tumor cells from healthy cells (Parish 2003; McCarthy 2006; Wiemann and Starnes 1994); difficulties in establishing long-term benefit due to poor patient follow-up; and inconsistent preparation and administration of the toxins, which created variability in the outcome and made it difficult for other clinicians to obtain similar results. Additionally, the patients experienced a range of severe, potentially life-threatening adverse effects (Parish 2003; McCarthy 2006; Wiemann and Starnes 1994).

Since these humble beginnings, a wealth of emergent data support a role for specific components of innate and adaptive immunity in host defense against cancer, including epidemiologic studies of congenital (primary) immunodeficiencies (Salavoura et al. 2008; Mueller 1995; Filipovich et al. 1994), therapeutically induced immunodeficiencies (Penn 1998; Kasiske et al. 2004; Penn 2000), and acquired immunodeficiencies (Boshoff and Weiss 2002; Engels et al. 2008; Grulich et al. 2007). Conversely, increased cancer risk is also associated with chronic immune system activation, including increased cancer rates in patients with chronic infections or autoimmunity (Yoshida et al. 2014; Ponce et al. 2014; Chiesa Fuxench et al. 2016). Taken together, these data indicate that immunosuppression and inflammation are both associated with increased cancer risk, and in the case of immunosuppression, an increased risk is identified for both cancers associated with a viral etiology and others for which no such viral etiology has been identified.

In addition to these epidemiology data, emerging clinical data that characterize the immune composition and distribution in the tumor microenvironment as a predictor of survival outcomes in cancer patients is providing important insights into the nature of immune- and tumor-associated factors that influence tumor rejection and survival outcomes. Galon et al. (2006) indicated that the location and density of T-cell infiltrates (e.g., CD4+helper T cells, CD8+ cytotoxic T cells, CD45RO memory T cells) in the tumor microenvironment, and expression of effector molecules (e.g., granzymes, interferon-gamma [IFN-γ], T-bet, interferon regulatory factor 1 [IRF1], interleukin 12 [IL-12] were a potentially stronger predictor of long-term patient survival when compared to traditional histopathological scoring of colorectal tumors; these data have since been reaffirmed (Tosolini et al. 2011). A number of studies have subsequently evaluated the "immune contexture" of tumors as a predictor of patient survival outcomes. A recent meta-analysis of 23 clinical studies reported that hepatocellular carcinoma patients with high levels of CD8+ and CD3+ tumor-infiltrating lymphocytes (TILs) had better overall survival and disease-free survival (along with CD4+ T cells) compared to those with low levels of these TILs, and conversely high levels of FoxP3+ regulatory TILs had poor prognosis (Yao et al. 2017). Similar findings regarding the importance of a T helper type 1 (TH1)-associated TIL phenotype on patient outcomes are available for a number of other cancer types, including oral cancer (Feng et al. 2017), ovarian cancer (Feng et al. 2017; Zhang et al. 2003; Sato et al. 2005), breast cancer (Al-Saleh et al. 2017), and esophageal cancer (Jesinghaus et al. 2017). These data were supported by interventional data with therapeutic immunomodulators that provide direct insight into the control and elimination of various cancers. Biologic immunomodulators with a clinically validated impact on host defense towards cancer, excluding monoclonal antibodies targeting cancer antigens, are summarized in Table 28.3.

The observed epidemiological and clinical data in patients are supported by a wealth of experimental and mechanistic data, which have culminated in the articulation of the immunoediting model of cancer by Schreiber and colleagues (Dunn et al. 2005; Vesely et al. 2011). This mechanistic model serves an important role in integrating the disparate in vitro and on vivo experimental observations that characterize the role of different components of immunity in protecting or subverting host defense against cancer, and the continuous co-evolution of the tumor under the selective pressure of the host immune response.

Taken as a whole, the emergent observational, interventional, and mechanistic data provide the current framework for guiding design of novel strategies and combinatorial approaches for treating cancer. Such approaches are exemplified below.

28.4.1.1 Monoclonal Antibodies Directed Against Immune Activation "Checkpoints"

The human immune system is highly regulated to ensure it does not target endogenous cells or allow overstimulation in response to minor insults (Topalian, Drake, and Pardoll 2015). Pathways that aid in regulating the immune system are referred to as "checkpoints"; checkpoint receptors and/or ligands can be present on normal cells as well as T cells. Some cancer cells have taken advantage of these pathways to escape detection by the immune system by upregulating checkpoint receptor and/or ligands on their cell surface. An intensive evaluation of a number inhibitory checkpoint pathways has been undertaken to develop biotherapeutics that can impact checkpoint pathways through the inhibition of either receptors or ligands, thus allowing the immune system to recognize tumor cells (Lenschow, Walunas, and Bluestone 1996). The first two checkpoint receptors to be discovered, CTLA-4 and PD-1, ultimately led to the first generation of immuno-oncology biotherapeutics. CTLA-4, discovered in 1987, was found to impact T-cell activation primarily by competing for the CD80 and

TABLE 28.3

US FDA-Approved Immunomodulatory Late-Stage Cancer Biotherapeutics (to 2020)

Class	Agent	Cancer Type
Checkpoint modulator	Bavencio (avelumab, anti-PD-L1)	Merkel cell carcinoma; bladder cancer
	Imfinzi (durvalumab, anti-PD-L1)	Bladder cancer
	Keytruda (pembrolizumab, anti-PD-1)	NSCLC, melanoma, squamous cell head and neck cancer, Hodgkin lymphoma, bladder cancer, any unresectable/metastatic solid tumor with certain genetic markers
	Opdivo (nivolumab, anti-PD-1)	NSCLC, melanoma, renal cell carcinoma, Hodgkin lymphoma, squamous cell head and neck cancer, bladder cancer
	Libtayo (cemiplimab, anti-PD-1)	Metastatic cutaneous squamous cell carcinoma (CSCC)
	Tecentriq (atezolizumab, anti-PD-L1)	Bladder cancer, NSCLC
	Yervoy (ipilimumab, anti-CTLA-4)	Melanoma
Oncolytic virus	Imlygic (talimogene laherparepvec, modified HSV-1 virus)	Melanoma
Bispecific T-cell engager (BiTE)	Blinatumomab (blinatumomab, CD19-directed CD3 T-cell engager antibody)	B-cell precursor acute lymphoblastic leukemia
Chimeric antigen receptor (CAR) T cell	Yescarta (axicabtagene ciloleucel, anti-CD19)	Large B-cell lymphoma (including diffuse large B-cell lymphoma (DLBCL) not otherwise specified, primary mediastinal large B-cell lymphoma, high grade B-cell lymphoma, and DLBCL arising from follicular lymphoma)
	Kymriah (tisagenlecleucel, anti-CD19)	B-cell acute lymphoblastic leukemia; diffuse large B-cell lymphoma (DLBCL), high-grade B-cell lymphoma and DLBCL arising from follicular lymphoma
Cytokine	Proleukin (aldesleukin, IL-2)	Metastatic melanoma and renal cell carcinoma
	Pegintron (peginterferon alfa-2b, IFN-α)	Melanoma
	Roferon-A (hIFN-α2a)	Hairy cell leukemia, chronic myelogenous leukemia, Kaposi's sarcoma, melanoma
	Intron A (hIFN-α2b)	Renal cell cancer, melanoma
Dendritic cell	Provenge (sipuleucel-T, GM-CSF, and prostatic acid phosphatase-primed cells)	Prostate cancer

CD86 ligands on antigen-presenting cells (Brunet et al. 1987). Normally, these ligands would engage CD28, a receptor critical for the activation of T cells; however, CTLA-4 has a much higher affinity for CD80/CD86. The centrality of CTLA-4 to this process has been shown in animals by pharmacologic inhibition or knockout of the gene, either leading to rampant systemic inflammation (Leach, Krummel, and Allison 1996). In addition to interaction with CD80/CD86, CTLA-4 is also present on regulatory T cells, and depletion of these cells by checkpoint inhibitors likely adds to the unwanted proinflammatory effects observed in patients treated with these therapies (Selby et al. 2013).

Another checkpoint pathway involving the receptor PD-1 and the ligand PD-L1 is also key in inhibiting the activation of T cells (Ahmadzadeh et al. 2009; Sfanos et al. 2009). In contrast to CTLA-4, PD-1 receptors respond to a significant overexpression of the PD-L1 ligand on tumor cells, making this event highly local to the tumor microenvironment (Ahmadzadeh et al. 2009; Sfanos et al. 2009). This has been demonstrated by differences observed between PD-1-knockout mice, which display a more muted response, and CTLA-4-knockout mice, which show late-onset organ specific inflammation that is made more apparent when crossed with other immune activating phenotypes (Parry et al. 2005). This more limited activation appears to lead to a more targeted response against the tumor. The PD-L1 ligand is expressed in many human cancers, whereas the receptor is also highly expressed except on TILs (Dong et al. 2002), thus lending additional proof to this hypothesis.

Currently, five checkpoint inhibitor monoclonal antibodies are on the market and all of them target either the CTLA-4 or PD-1/PD-L1 pathways (Table 28.3). There are many other checkpoint inhibitor monoclonal antibodies in nonclinical and clinical development targeting other proteins involved with tumor immune surveillance. These include, but are not limited to, TIM-3, LAG-3, GITR, OX40, TIGIT, B7-H3, VISTA, and others.

Nonclinical safety studies for most of these agents have largely been performed in the NHP due to a lack of cross-reactivity to the target antigen in rabbits and rodents. It should also be noted that these targets, which are active and, in some cases, highly expressed in tumors, are present at much more moderate levels in healthy individuals, including in the animal models used for safety assessment, making the translatability of the nonclinical data to the clinic more challenging.

In the nonclinical toxicology program for ipilimumab, administration of 10 mg/kg on various dosing schedules was well tolerated in 1- and 6-month repeat-dose monkey toxicity studies (FDA 2011). A more recent monkey study evaluating 50 mg/kg/week for 1 month was associated with widespread inflammation in tissues such as the GI track and kidney (Selby et al. 2016). In investigative studies, treatment with ipilimumab was associated with colitis in a small number of animals (Selby et al. 2013). Clinically, patients experience an array of inflammatory conditions; most notably colitis and dermatitis occurred in 12% and 15% of subjects, respectively, in the pivotal clinical trial (Di Giacomo, Biagioli, and Maio 2010). Also observed were incidences of hepatitis, neuropathies, and endocrinopathies and other immune-related adverse events. In the nonclinical evaluations for the PD-1 targeting antibodies nivolumab and pembrolizumab, no adverse findings were observed in any of the monkey studies conducted with either biotherapeutic. The primary finding was the observation of inflammatory cell infiltrates in multiple tissues, which in some instances could have been attributed to normal background findings (Herzyk and Haggerty 2018). Clinically, and similar to ipilimumab, colitis was observed for both nivolumab and pembrolizumab in addition to other inflammatory conditions such as hepatitis and pneumonitis. The nonclinical program for atezolizumab was unique in that the antibody also cross-reacts with rodent PD-L1, and as a result, toxicity studies were conducted in both monkeys and mice. Again, minimal non-adverse inflammatory infiltrates were observed in both species (Mease, Kimzey, and Lansita 2017). Finally, checkpoint inhibitors have the potential to break down the self/non-self immune recognition tolerance during pregnancy, and this can lead to early abortions (Prell, Halpern, and Rao 2016).

The current clinical direction for these types of therapies is to combine two or more checkpoint inhibitors, in an attempt to further immune system responses to tumor cells, while not exacerbating the existing clinical adverse event profile. Because of the potential for potent activation of the immune system and suprapharmacologic effects that could substantively increase toxicity, some of these combinations have been investigated in nonclinical toxicity studies prior to entering the clinic, an approach not typically required for anticancer therapeutics in accordance with the ICH S9 guideline. Combination toxicity studies in monkeys have been described for anti-LAG3 and nivolumab, and ipilimumab and nivolumab (Selby et al. 2016). In both combination studies, increased inflammation in tissues was observed and manifested as epididymitis, central nervous system (CNS) vasculitis, and gastrointestinal inflammation. However, these findings were not replicated in the clinic besides showing that immune system-related effects and inflammation are enhanced in general.

It is clear that the healthy animals used in evaluating checkpoint inhibitors have been of limited value in identifying risks for patients other than generalized inflammation, which was already known based on their mechanism of action. Single-agent toxicity studies in normal animals are still required for initiation and continuation of clinical trials with new checkpoint inhibitors. Clinical studies with combinations of checkpoint inhibitors are now largely supported with nonclinical efficacy data that serves as the rationale for the proposed clinical trial, with additional in vitro safety studies such as CRAs completing the nonclinical package. Alternative animal models are currently under investigation for their utility in providing more insight into potential autoimmune risk for these therapeutics. Data using different variants of transgenic mice with a humanized immune system after the administration of checkpoint inhibitors have been presented at scientific meetings, some showing inflammation in various organs of greater severity than that observed in normal animals. Much

more work needs to be done prior to using these models in lieu of normal animal studies or to support the nonclinical safety evaluation of new checkpoint inhibitors. See Chapter 20 for more discussion on monoclonal antibodies as a modality.

28.4.1.2 CD3 Bispecifics

T cells are critical for protection against emerging cancers in the body, yet cancers develop at least in part because T cells specific for the tumor cells either are not initially generated against the tumor cells, or they are ineffective because they cannot gain access to the tumor microenvironment or are suppressed (or die) once they enter the tumor microenvironment. One promising approach to overcome at least some of these hurdles is the development of CD3-bispecific molecules. These molecules bind to CD3 on T cells and simultaneously to an antigen target on the tumor cells. This trimolecular interaction not only forms a "bridge," bringing the T cell and the tumor cell into close contact, but also binds to and stimulates the CD3 signaling complex, activating the T cell to respond against and ultimately kill the tumor cell expressing the target antigen. A major advantage to this approach is that by directly engaging CD3, the bispecific molecule bypasses the antigen specificity of the T cell that it binds to, and thus can theoretically recruit any T cell to respond against the tumor.

The approach was first proposed over 30 years ago (Staerz and Bevan 1986), but it has taken decades of engineering and development to turn the idea into effective anticancer biotherapeutics. The first approved CD3 bispecific was catumaxomab (it was approved in the European Union and has since been withdrawn). The only currently approved CD3 bispecific is blinatumomab, which targets CD19 on B-cell lymphomas (Benjamin and Stein 2016). Blinatumomab is a bispecific T-cell engager (BiTE) (Einsele et al. 2020) comprising two linked scFv regions derived from antibodies recognizing CD3 and CD19. The impressive efficacy of blinatumomab in B-cell acute lymphoblastic leukemia (Topp et al. 2015; Kantarjian et al. 2017) has led to a resurgence of interest in the CD3-bispecific approach. Currently, there are dozens of other bispecific molecule formats in development (Wang et al. 2019), each with its own advantages and disadvantages in terms of exposure half-life, tumor penetration, stability, manufacturability, and tumor selectivity. There have also been more recent modifications, including altering the CD3 binding domain to reduce cytokine release (Trinklein et al. 2019; Hernandez-Hoyos et al. 2016) or "masking" binding sites to minimize target recognition on normal (non-tumor) cells (Geiger et al. 2020; Panchal et al. 2020). Additionally, there are CD3 bispecifics that target tumor-associated major histocompatibility complex (MHC)-peptide complexes instead of native cell surface tumor antigens (He et al. 2019; Høydahl et al. 2019). Finally, there are bispecific antibodies in development that engage other immune cells such as NK cells (e.g., through CD16), although those will not be addressed in this chapter.

The development of bispecific molecules raises new challenges for nonclinical development and safety assessment, including expanded nonclinical species justification (e.g., to evaluate species-specific interactions on both target binding arms), assay development (e.g., whether it is necessary to characterize antidrug antibodies against both arms), study design, interpretation, and dose selection. Because mass-balance relationships between drug and target (that define free vs bound ratios) can differ across individuals and species based on target selection (e.g., soluble vs cell bound), target regulation (e.g., total target expression, target internalization and production), drug clearance and binding affinity, the relative distribution of free and bound drug between two targets can differ markedly between species and over time. These principles can help explain the pharmacodynamic, pharmacokinetic, and toxicological profile, and understanding these factors can aid nonclinical dose selection and study interpretation, and can help justify the initial clinical dose and dose escalation strategy.

There are two primary safety concerns with CD3 bispecifics: cytokine release and damage to normal cells expressing the target antigen. The release of cytokines, including (but not limited to) interleukin 6 (IL-6), TNF-α, IFN- γ, interleukin 2 (IL-2), interleukin 10 (IL-10), and granulocyte-macrophage colony-stimulating factor (GM-CSF), generally occurs rapidly, within hours of dosing in both monkeys and humans. In monkeys, CD3 bispecifics generally induce cytokine release that is accompanied by clinical signs, including emesis, hunched posture, and reduced activity, and can be life-threatening depending on the magnitude of the cytokine release. In humans, flu-like symptoms (pyrexia, chills) accompany mild cytokine release, but CRS is associated with higher cytokine concentrations and is often characterized by hypotension, tachycardia, dyspnea, and hypoxia, and can progress to life-threatening hypovolemic shock and multiorgan failure. There are established guidelines for the grading of clinical CRS (Lee et al. 2019), but no such criteria exist for nonclinical evaluation of cytokine release symptoms in monkeys. Many of the parameters measured in humans (e.g., blood pressure, heart rate, oxygen saturation) are not routinely monitored in monkey toxicity studies, which could at least partly contribute to the perception that sensitivity of monkeys to cytokine release is different from humans. Typically, cytokine release in monkeys is qualitatively predictive of cytokine release in humans, although quantitatively they do often tend to be less sensitive.

Overall, the monkey appears to be an appropriate animal model for evaluating toxicities related to T-cell activation, cytokine release, and other downstream toxicities induced by CD3 bispecifics. Recent nonclinical evidence suggests that TNF-α and GM-CSF produced by T cells are key activators of macrophage production of cytokines (e.g., interleukin 1 [IL-1], IL-6) that drive the clinical signs associated with CRS (Li et al. 2019; Sterner et al. 2019). Cytokine release has commonly been evaluated with in vitro CRAs, and multiple CRA formats may be employed with or without target tumor cells added. However, current CRAs are appropriate for hazard identification only (Grimaldi et al. 2016), and cytokine release is a well-established hazard with CD3 bispecifics. It has therefore recently been suggested that stand-alone in vitro CRAs are not warranted for CD3 bispecifics (Kamperschroer et al. 2020), assuming that cytokine release has been confirmed (i.e., in in vitro assays or in in vivo pharmacology or toxicity studies).

Damage to normal cells is an expected on-target toxicity in cases where normal cells express the target antigen of the bispecific. Because any target-expressing cell is susceptible to T cell-mediated killing, a thorough evaluation of target expression is a key initial step towards understanding the potential toxicity profile of any given bispecific. Tissue target expression can be evaluated by standard immunohistochemistry (IHC) or in situ hybridization (ISH) or (less frequently) polymerase chain reaction (PCR) approaches. The evaluation is not always straightforward, because activated T cells are highly sensitive to low amounts of antigen. A small number of target molecules expressed on a cell can be sufficient to trigger the T cell to attack, particularly if the interaction between the target on the cells and the bispecific are of high affinity. In some cases, the method to detect target expression on a cell may be less sensitive than the functional responses of T cells against a cell expressing the target, and this must be taken into consideration when measuring target antigen expression on cells.

An approach to evaluating the potential for toxicity to normal tissues after the administration of a bispecific is to assess cell killing in vitro. Experiments can be conducted in parallel with tumor cells of the same tissue type or in different tissues to aid in understanding if there is a differential sensitivity of tumor cells versus normal cells. However, a number of cell types cannot be cultured in vitro, or change phenotype and possibly antigen expression in culture, so this approach is not always feasible. The potential for damage to normal tissues can also be evaluated in monkey toxicity studies, assuming the monkey is a relevant species and that the expression profile of the target antigen in monkeys is similar to that of human. Data from in vivo toxicity studies generally carry the most weight for safety-related decision making. The nonclinical in vivo pharmacology and toxicity studies can also be used to evaluate potential biomarkers of toxicity for clinical use, depending on what tissues are targeted and what biomarkers are available to evaluate specific toxicities.

In addition to cytokine release and targeting of normal cells, neurotoxicity has been associated with blinatumomab and other T cell-directed therapies (e.g., CAR-T) that target B cells through antigens such as CD19. The neurotoxicity is associated with symptoms such as tremors, encephalopathy (i.e., disorientation or confusion), cerebellar symptoms, speech impairment, and convulsions (Topp et al. 2015). The mechanism of the neurotoxicity has been best studied with CAR-T therapies, and the current understanding of mechanism is that T-cell activation and T-cell-derived cytokines (e.g., GM-CSF and TNF- α) (Sterner et al. 2019) stimulate macrophage activation and further production of cytokines that activate the endothelium, increased vascular permeability, loss of blood-brain barrier integrity, and CNS inflammation following access of cytokines and immune cells into the CNS (Chou and Turtle 2019). Interleukin 1 may be a key cytokine driving neurotoxicity (Norelli et al. 2018; Giavridis et al. 2018), and certain parameters reflecting endothelial activation like Ang1/Ang2 ratios have been proposed as risk biomarkers (Gust et al. 2017; Chou and Turtle 2019); however, the details of the mechanism of neurotoxicity is still being elucidated. An important point is that CNS neurotoxicity as described above has not been reported for CD3 bispecifics targeting non-B-cell antigens, so it does not appear to be a toxicity common to all CD3 bispecifics and it may be dependent on the target antigen.

A challenge to the nonclinical development of first generation CD3 bispecifics (e.g., catumaxomab, blinatumomab, carcinoembryonic [CEA] BiTE) was the lack of cross-reactivity of the anti-CD3 domain with any standard nonclinical species. Different early development programs used different approaches to overcome this problem: by conducting studies in non-relevant species (e.g., catumaxomab); by using a surrogate molecule (e.g., blinatumomab); or by evaluating safety in in vitro studies only (e.g., CEA BiTE) and selecting a more conservative clinical starting dose based on a MABEL approach (Prell, Halpern, and Rao 2016). Conducting toxicity studies in non-pharmacologically relevant species is strongly discouraged by health authorities. The majority of CD3 bispecifics currently in development contain a CD3 binding domain that cross-reacts with monkey CD3, allowing for toxicity studies in this species as long as the other target binding domain of the bispecific can bind to the monkey target antigen and the pharmacologic activity in monkeys is comparable to what would be expected in humans. However, there will continue to be cases where a relevant species cannot be identified. For example, CD3 bispecifics targeting MHC-peptide complexes will not cross-react with monkeys because even if the target peptide is identical between monkey and human, the monkey does not express the human MHC molecule that presents the peptide to T cells. For these cases, there are limited options to assess toxicity in in vivo studies. While mice expressing human MHC molecules as transgenes have been explored, they are not commonly used, in part because even if the target peptide were conserved in mice, it is often not generated by the proteolytic machinery in mouse cells or it is not efficiently expressed on mouse cells. These and other challenges have limited the use of humanized transgenic mouse models. In most cases, CD3 bispecifics targeting MHC-peptide complexes have relied on a combination of in silico and in vitro studies for nonclinical evaluation of the potential for cross-reactivity and other safety concerns (He et al. 2019).

When evaluating monkey as a relevant species, it is important to confirm not just binding to the monkey target antigen and monkey CD3, but also to demonstrate pharmacologic activity with both "arms" of the CD3 bispecific. This can be confirmed in vitro using CTL assays showing that monkey T cells can kill target antigen-expressing cells. Once species relevance has been clearly demonstrated, there is still much to consider in the design of nonclinical toxicity studies in monkeys supporting bispecific programs. Due to the difficulty in predicting tolerable dose levels in the initial exploratory toxicity study, small "lead-in" groups of 1–2 animals per cohort may be used prior to administering the bispecific to the rest of the study animals in order to minimize the impact of doses that are not tolerated. Also, intra-animal dose escalations may be performed in exploratory studies in order to explore a wider dose range in the same number of animals and/or to better characterize tissue-related toxicity if cytokine release-related toxicities limit the ability to dose higher. Intra-animal dose escalations are generally not performed in definitive toxicity studies because determining how any observed toxicity relates to specific doses/exposures becomes complicated. It is useful to measure cytokine release because CRS is a key safety concern common to CD3 bispecifics. As indicated earlier in this section, a wide range of cytokines can be induced by CD3 bispecifics, but a limited subset of cytokines (e.g., IL-6, IFN-γ, IL-2, and IL-10) and time points (0, 3, and 6–7 hours relative to dose administration) are generally sufficient to evaluate cytokine release. The acute-phase marker C-reactive protein (CRP) is also a simple and sensitive indicator downstream of cytokine release and can be added to standard clinical chemistry panels. Immunophenotyping is also useful for confirming the expected pharmacologic effects on T cells, including activation (e.g., CD69 and CD25 markers) and proliferation (e.g., Ki-67 marker). As another indicator of T-cell activation, soluble CD25 (IL-2 receptor alpha) can also be measured. Soluble CD25 has the advantage of being a simple ELISA-based measurement that can be used with frozen serum samples. Transient lymphocyte decreases are a hallmark of CD3 bispecific-mediated T-cell stimulation, occur within hours of dose administration, are readily detected 24 hours after dosing, and progressively return to baseline values over the next few days. In early exploratory studies, pharmacologic activity can be confirmed by measuring lymphocyte decreases and CRP. More extensive pharmacologic activity assessments in the definitive toxicity studies where larger numbers of animals are available can be useful for understanding PK/PD relationships where the exposure of the CD3 bispecific in relationship to T-cell responses can be modeled and help to predict responses in patients. Significant levels of antidrug antibodies are commonly observed with CD3 bispecifics in monkeys and often lead to the loss of exposure of the CD3 bispecific. In longer term (e.g., 3-month) studies, ADA-induced loss of exposure can present challenges or may even invalidate a toxicity study if most or all animals are affected. These and other considerations regarding nonclinical evaluation of CD3 bispecifics have been addressed and presented along with case studies in a recent publication (Kamperschroer et al. 2020).

Another major challenge with CD3 bispecifics is to determine a starting dose in patients that is low enough to be safe, but high enough so as few patients as possible are exposed to subtherapeutic doses that will not provide any clinical benefit. Clinical starting doses based on data from in vivo toxicity studies (e.g., using the HNSTD) generally are not considered appropriate so most sponsors have used a MABEL approach to determine the clinical starting dose. However, this approach has led to prolonged Phase 1 dose escalations where large numbers of patients are treated with subtherapeutic doses (Saber et al. 2017). MABEL calculations in these cases relied heavily on in vitro assays with human cells to determine concentration responses to the CD3 bispecific. These assays appear to overestimate the potency of the CD3 bispecific and drive very low starting doses. This may be due to inappropriately high effector to target ratios, use of cell lines with high antigen density, use of purified T cells, or other parameters that may not reflect the in vivo situation, and more work is needed to understand what conditions are most appropriate. After analyzing nonclinical and clinical data from 17 CD3 bispecific programs, Saber et al (2017) concluded that selecting the clinical starting dose based on receptor occupancy, HNSTD, or NOAEL was not acceptable as it resulted in doses too close to the MTD in patients. The authors recommended that using a PAD approach with pharmacologic activity from in vitro assays in the 10%–30% range was an acceptable approach to select the clinical starting dose. In all but one case, using 50% pharmacologic activity would have also been acceptable. With the development of more sophisticated modeling approaches (Betts et al. 2019) and refinements to the in vitro assays, the hope is to arrive at an approach that more often leads to clinical starting doses that are safe yet provide clinical benefit for as many patients as possible.

28.4.1.3 T-Cell Immunotherapies

While all the aforementioned therapeutic strategies involve approaches to jump start T-cell activity towards a cancer cell by one means or another, one group of cancer immunologists have spent the last few decades utilizing T cell themselves as the modality (Rosenberg and Restifo 2015; Sadelain, Rivière, and Riddell 2017). Commonly referred to as T-cell immunotherapy, this strategy involves removing a patient's T cells, placing them in culture and genetically modifying them to specifically target a particular cancer antigen, and then finally infusing them back into the patient in hopes that these armed T cells will attack the tumor. Since this treatment involves the patient's own cells, it is a form of autologous immunotherapy, whereas some T-cell immunotherapies are allogeneic and involve using T cells from a single source, genetically engineering those cells, and then use them in several different patients.

The main two modifications that have been used in the clinic are genetically engineered T cells that express either (1) an optimized T-cell receptor (TCR) that can recognize a peptide/MHC complex specific to the cancer; or (2) a CAR that combines a target binding portion of a monoclonal antibody (scFv) that is specific to the cancer antigen and expressed on the extracellular side of the T cell, and a variety of T-cell signaling domains that are expressed on the intracellular side of the T cell (Weber, Maus, and Mackall 2020). Thus, T-cell immunotherapies are a cross between a classic gene and cell therapy. A lentiviral vector is typically used to introduce and integrate the gene expressing the TCR or CAR into the genome of the T cells ex vivo, and then the cells are cultured and administered to the patient as an autologous immunotherapy. Both approaches have their advantages and disadvantages, but in general a key differentiator is that optimized TCRs will be able to recognize intracellular cancer antigens (as long as they are presented by MHC) and CARs recognize proteins that are at least in part displayed on the surface of cells, such as growth factor receptors.

While the field has spent many years investigating TCR-based therapies targeting melanoma among other cancers, widespread success was found with a handful of sponsors using CARs targeting CD19 in leukemia, lymphoma, and other B-cell-driven malignancies. Initial publications of these clinical trials described dramatic responses in a limited number of pediatric and adult patients who had become resistant to more standard therapies against B cells, essentially curing them (Kochenderfer et al. 2010). Two T-cell immunotherapies have progressed to market, tisagenlecleucel and axicabtagene ciloleucel approved for leukemia and lymphoma indications, respectively (FDA 2017a, 2017b) (Table 28.3). Safety concerns with these and other liquid tumor targets not surprisingly

very much mirror that of the CD3 bispecific programs outlined above, with substantial cytokine release during the period shortly after dosing while the T cells are expanding in response to antigen recognition, as well as varying incidence and severity of neurotoxicity (Neelapu et al. 2018). Treatment of the cytokine syndrome in the clinic can be complicated, as cytokines are required for the activity of the modified T cells and a blunt tool like steroids used to dampen this response can eliminate any hope for efficacy. More directed mitigation steps have been used to target specific cytokines such as IL-6 to reduce rather than shut down T-cell activity in this phase.

As these programs have ventured outside of blood-borne cancers, the potential for reactivity of the TCR or CAR with endogenous antigens has increased (Rafiq, Hackett, and Brentjens 2020). In clinical trials with these T cells, several instances of adverse events have occurred that are the result of either on- or off-target activity. Some of the first T-cell immunotherapy products were designed against melanoma antigens including MART-1 (Johnson et al. 2009). While highly expressed in melanoma cells, this antigen is also expressed in normal melanocytes in the skin, eye, and ear, which led to significant toxicity in these organs. In another example, a clinical trial with a TCR targeting MAGE-A3, another antigen commonly found in melanoma, led to lethal cardiac toxicity in two patients (Cameron et al. 2013). This unexpected result was linked to the ability of the TCR to not only bind to the MAGE-A3 peptide in MHC, but also an antigen in heart muscle (i.e., titin), which caused massive cardiac inflammation and ultimately heart failure. CARs are thought to have better selectivity to their target, as many candidate scFvs can be screened for high affinity and selective binding to their target. Still, as liver toxicity in a trial using a CAIX-targeting CAR and pulmonary safety issues with a CAR binding Her2 have shown, "on-target, off-tumor" toxicities are still observed with this modality.

Thus, it is clear that while significant promise lies with this new and growing modality, major safety liabilities exist. Given the autologous cell therapy nature of the vast majority of these approaches, there are significant challenges in evaluating these products in a nonclinical setting. One in particular is the availability of an animal model that (1) is responsive to tumor targeting TCRs or CARs; (2) possesses an intact immune system providing support for expansion of the T cells after target engagement; and (3) allows the engraftment of human T cells without subsequent graft-versus-host (GvH) issues. Certainly the "distribution" of these cells in models where GvH exists as a potential outcome can be very complicated and highly irrelevant to what would be expected in humans.

Efficacy studies are typically performed in immune-compromised mice engrafted with human tumors; however, these systems have limitations in that they cannot assess "off-tumor" targeting, notably in the lack of binding of either a TCR or CAR to the mouse target antigen. Human TCRs on T-cell immunotherapies are unable to recognize the mouse MHC alleles, let alone the homologous expressed peptide, which may or may not be processed in the same way as it is in human cells.

CARs suffer the same challenges as more standard monoclonal antibody programs, containing scFvs that rarely cross-react to target antigens in species lower than NHPs. Tool CARs can be prepared that do cross-react in mice; however, this approach involves a significant amount of work to generate a product solely to understand off-tumor safety liabilities and should probably only be pursued if such risks are particularly high. Additionally, these mouse models lack a fully functional immune system, which may contribute to the overall activity of the autologous T cells administered to patients. This could not only hamper the evaluation of tissue targeting but may also minimize any safety issue such as cytokine release.

More recently, attempts have been made to generate CAR-T cells in NHPs, using monkey T cells and CARs that cross-react to the endogenous target antigen in animals with fully intact immune systems. Some progress has been made, with groups reporting expected pharmacology and even neurological signs secondary to significant cytokine release. These approaches are laborious, with requirements for several new reagents to create monkey CAR-Ts, the manufacturing of a T-cell product for each individual animal, and so on. Nevertheless, there may be new opportunities in the in vivo nonclinical space to answer key safety-related questions and to more finely tune these products to reduce the risk of adverse events for patients.

An additional consideration for T-cell immunotherapies is the means by which these cells have the tumor-targeting entity added to the genome. Since part of the lifecycle of this modality is to have the cells expand significantly and ultimately overwhelm the tumor, the introduced gene needs to be anchored to the genome rather than be episomally expressed; otherwise, the gene would be lost in a matter of a few cell divisions. This is accomplished with the use of retroviruses, and more recently lentiviruses, which in general randomly integrate their genetic information into the host genome. Historically, another subset of retroviruses, gamma-retroviruses, which preferentially integrate near growth-promoting genes caused several incidences of leukemia in some non-oncology clinical trials. While gamma retroviruses were initially used for T-cell immunotherapies, currently third-generation lentiviruses are the preferred vector. There have been some reports of integration and disruption of tumor suppressor genes such as TET2, which have led to growth advantages to subsets of the T-cell preparations, but no secondary malignancies have been observed in patients. As such, there may be a need to evaluate the genomic integration profile of a T-cell preparation when initially characterizing the product. However, these data are largely uninformative in the absence of a clinical event, suggesting growth advantage or clonality. Sponsors have also utilized in vitro growth kinetic experiments for these preparations, in particular the IL-2-independent growth assay. Importantly, data from these assays have not detected any dangerous uncontrolled growth.

In large part, current nonclinical safety evaluation of these T-cell immunotherapies involves thoroughly evaluating the specificity of target antigen tissue expression. With TCRs, a full evaluation of other similar peptides that may be presented in MHC is usually performed, while with CARs, some sponsors are testing the scFv for potential to bind other targets through either protein interaction arrays, IHC, or specific assessment of the binding of proteins with similar sequences. Thus, nonclinical packages supporting these programs have typically employed efficacy assessments in immune-compromised animals without any direct safety evaluations

and an in vitro assessment of tumor targeting receptor specificity. Considering the late-stage cancer indications these products have been used for, these approaches have largely been accepted worldwide. However, as T-cell immunotherapies become more "front line" therapies, more investment will need to be made on identifying better in vivo models to assess safety. A case-by-case approach is necessary to allow maturation of this field while balancing safety concerns.

28.4.1.4 Oncolytic Viruses

Case reports of spontaneous cancer regressions, particularly hematological malignancies, following viral infections date back to the mid-1800s (Kelly and Russell 2007). These data supported contemporaneous observations by Coley and others regarding spontaneous cancer regressions following bacterial infections. These observations began to inform a role for host immunity in the defense against cancer, which culminated in the current cancer immunoediting model (described in Section 28.4.1, above). However, these data also began to inform a potential therapeutic role for using viruses as direct oncolytic agents. Early therapeutic strategies administered sera or tissues from virus-infected patients, including hepatitis virus, West Nile virus, and others (Hoster, Zanes, and Von Haam 1949).

In the intervening years, numerous viruses, both wild-type and engineered, were evaluated in model systems (and in some patients), with mixed success. Engineered, replication incompetent viruses, which could deliver transgenes to drive tumor growth inhibition or destruction, while safe, were generally insufficiently potent to treat large tumor masses. Thus, in the 1990s, Martuza and colleagues engineered replication competent herpes simplex virus type 1 (HSV-1) for the treatment of malignant glioma (Martuza et al. 1991). These pioneering efforts led to a renewed interest and investment, which culminated in the Chinese approval of the first oncolytic virus (Garber 2006), and the US approval of talimogene laherparepvec in 2015.

Oncolytic viruses can be wild-type or naturally attenuated strains of viruses that are generally genetically modified to selectively replicate and lyse cancer cells. These modifications can include (1) the mutation of the viral-coding genes that are critical for viral replication in normal cells, (2) the control of early gene expression by using tumor-specific promoters, (3) a change in the viral tissue tropism and/or cell entry process, and (4) the incorporation of transgenes into the viral genome to modify the immune response or the immune environment.

In 2009, ICH released a "Considerations" document addressing this modality, including guidance on nonclinical studies [Oncolytic viruses (ICH 2009b)]. Three main topics are central to evaluating these viruses: use of an animal model that will support replication, distribution of the virus within the organism, and shedding of the virus outside the organism. In addition, when an oncolytic virus contains a transgene, it is important that the animal species be pharmacologically responsive to the expressed protein and that evidence of the pharmacologic activity of the expressed transgene be determined. If the expressed transgene is inactive in the animal species (e.g., human GM-CSF is inactive in mice), the oncolytic virus can be engineered to express the analogous species-specific transgene and used in nonclinical studies to assess both activity and safety. In these instances, characterization of the oncolytic virus administered to animals should be performed to assess the extent of comparability to the clinical candidate (e.g., level of transgene expression).

Selection of the animal species should take into consideration viral tropism, infectivity, replication ability, cytopathic potential, and antitumor effect of the oncolytic virus. The permissiveness of the animal species to the virus needs to be considered. Standard animal species routinely used for nonclinical testing might not be appropriate; therefore, other animal species (e.g., cotton rats, Syrian hamsters) may need to be considered. The species used should ideally be sensitive not just to infection by the virus, but also to the pathological consequences of infection that can be induced by the virus. Both non-tumor-bearing animal species and tumor-bearing xenograft or syngeneic animal models are useful for nonclinical toxicity testing. Tumor-bearing mouse models can be used to assess efficacy, pharmacodynamics, viral shedding, and safety. Ideally, a xenograft or syngeneic model should represent the tumor biology and pathology of the target clinical population to the extent that efficacy observed in the animal model will be an indication of clinical outcome. This desired effect should be considered when evaluating the safety of the oncolytic virus, as the level of viral presence and the extent of persistence in various biological samples of a tumor-bearing model can be significantly different than in a non-tumor-bearing animal. There are limitations to these models however, as the lack of an intact immune system and inability of the virus to infect mouse cells in some cases may limit the ability to study safety. As the intent of the virus is to replicate, an evaluation in one or more of these models on where the virus distributes is critical. And like any viral replication scenario, how the virus may leave the body and through what route (i.e., viral shedding) is another part of the pharmacokinetics of the virus that will need to be understood.

Imlygic (talimogene laherparepvec, T-VEC, Onco-VEX^{GM-CSF}) was approved for the treatment of late-stage metastatic melanoma by the FDA in 2015 as the first US-approved oncolytic virus. This approval represented the culmination of scientific and clinical effort that began with the case reports in the mid-1800s of cancer remissions in patients following viral infection, which led to clinical trials in the 1940s to 1950s, which yielded some promising results, although with toxicity (Kelly and Russell 2007).

Imlygic was based on a novel primary isolate (named JS-1) of HSV-1 virus, which demonstrated superior in vitro cell lysis over common laboratory passaged strains. Subsequent engineering of JS-1 virus was conducted to remove the primary HSV-1 neurovirulence factor ICP34.5, which also conferred tumor-selective replication. Further modifications included elimination of ICP47, immediate early expression of US11, and the introduction of two copies of the huGM-CSF gene in place of ICP34.5. These modifications were collectively designed to limit viral pathogenesis in normal tissues, while allowing selective replication in tumor tissues and enhancing the immunogenicity of infected tumor cells. The replacement of both copies of ICP34.5 by huGM-CSF was designed to minimize the likelihood that a recombination event could restore wild-type ICP34.5 in the genetically modified virus. The engineering and pharmacological activity, including mechanistic support for the genetic modifications to Imlygic, its tumor-selective replication, and the induction of both direct tumor cell lysis and the development of a systemic adaptive immune response, have been previously reported (Liu et al. 2003; Hughes et al. 2014; Moesta et al. 2017).

As a replication competent, genetically engineered virus, Imlygic, posed unique challenges during nonclinical development as compared to traditional biologic or gene therapeutics. Extant guidance documents by ICH [Oncolytic viruses (ICH 2009b)] and FDA [Preclinical Assessment of Investigational Cellular and Gene Therapy Products (FDA 2013); Considerations for the Design of Early-Phase Clinical Trials of Cellular and Gene Therapy Products (FDA 2015)] provide critical insights into the breadth of considerations for developing a product like Imlygic and serve to guide early nonclinical safety testing.

The mouse served as a useful model for evaluating the nonclinical safety of Imlygic as it is a well-characterized model species for understanding HSV-1 virology and phenocopies characteristic of human HSV-1 infection and neurovirulence; however, it is not a strong model for testing reactivation following latency. Direct CNS infection confirmed an approximately 10,000-fold reduction in neurovirulence of Imlygic (attributable to ICP34.5 elimination) as compared to wild-type HSV-1, consistent with prior publications (Bolovan, Sawtell, and Thompson 1994).

Mechanistic pharmacology studies demonstrated that intratumoral injection was associated with expanding tumor cell lysis concomitant with logarithmic viral replication in infected tumors, whereas adjacent normal tissue could be infected with virus without overt pathology. The mechanisms underlying tumor-selective replication of an ICP34.5-deficient HSV-1 virus are not fully understood, but are attributed to deficient innate, Type 1 IFN-mediated antiviral responses in many tumors, rendering them susceptible to HSV-1 infection even with ICP34.5 attenuation (Liu et al. 2003).

Several unique considerations for the development of Imlygic included dose scaling (allometry), the assessment of viremia risk with immune suppression (or immune deficiency), protection of secondary contacts and healthcare providers from inadvertent exposure (either through viral shedding or through a needle stick during dosing), and the risk of maternal-fetal transfer during pregnancy/birthing.

There is no established allometric method for scaling HSV-1 dosing in animals to humans. This translational scaling is challenging because of the absence of traditional nonclinical safety data in animal models that allow traditional allometric relationships to be established. Fundamental questions about the suitability of using traditional allometry (used to establish dose equivalency from animals to humans) for viruses, and the complication that a replicating virus will likely behave fundamentally differently in experimental animal tumor models as compared to humans also need to be considered. Moreover, the viral drug product is replication-competent, and the exposure will increase in the patient following intratumoral dosing as the virus undergoes oncolytic expansion in the patient's tumor. In the absence of available allometric methods for scaling dose and in recognition of the patient-specific factors that drive the pharmacokinetics (i.e., expansion and clearance) of the drug, initial clinical experience using low, titrated doses guided dose setting. In practice, subsequent interspecies dose scaling was conducted on the basis of viral potency units (i.e., plaque-forming units) per kg body weight.

In vitro testing was conducted to ensure that Imlygic remained susceptible to treatment with the standard anti-HSV-1 therapy, acyclovir (Vere Hodge and Field 2013). Specifically, in vitro testing over a range of concentrations demonstrated comparable antiviral potency of acyclovir towards Imlygic and wild-type HSV-1, and supported the use of acyclovir in clinical staff who could inadvertently be exposed to Imlygic upon needle sticks during clinical testing.

In vivo pharmacology studies evaluated the antitumor activity of Imlygic towards syngeneic mouse tumors (in an immune competent mouse) and human tumor xenografts in immuno-compromised mice. These studies were conducted to assess the induction of a systemic antitumor immune response following tumor oncolysis. However, these studies revealed susceptibility of immune-deficient (SCID and nude) mice to systemic viremia upon dosing with Imlygic. These studies demonstrated that whereas the normal antiviral host response is sufficient to protect immune-competent animals from systemic infection by Imlygic, severe immunodeficiency could pose a risk. As a result, Imlygic acquired a label warning about the risks of use in patients with compromised immunity.

Extensive biodistribution and shedding studies were conducted in mice (and subsequently in patients) to characterize the persistence and clearance of Imlygic, and to identify the likely shedding routes. The biodistribution of Imlygic following intratumoral injection was predominantly restricted to the tumor and blood, and to tissues likely associated with immune-mediated viral clearance (spleen, lymph node, liver). The absence of viral DNA in the lachrymal glands, nasal mucosa, or feces indicated a low likelihood of secondary exposure (i.e., shedding) of viral DNA from tears, mucous, or feces. Viral DNA found in the brains of two virus-injected mice was not associated with adverse effects in these animals. These data were challenging to interpret as no contemporaneous assessment of viral replication was conducted on these samples, so whether the detected virus represented intact virus was not established.

Separate studies were conducted to characterize potential risks to reproduction and development in mice, and the potential for maternal-fetal viral transfer following maternal dosing. These studies used a "worst-case" assumption of viral exposure based on IV dosing of the pregnant dams. No overt adverse effect was seen on reproduction and development. Nevertheless, because HSV-1 can infect neonates following maternal viral shedding during birthing, potentially leading to systemic viremia, encephalitis, or death (Straface et al. 2012), FDA required a warning label around the risk to pregnancy from Imlygic.

During global regulatory discussions, certain countries were especially concerned with the environmental risks, including risks of infection to household pets and the risk of generating novel strains via recombination with wild-type herpes viruses.

These risks were generally addressed by a combination of literature data and careful explanation of the design of the viral vector and an explanation of the role of each engineering modification to HSV-1 fitness and function, and the intentional design to minimize the likelihood that recombination events could produce a novel strain with unique properties.

28.4.1.5 Cancer Vaccines

The concept of treating cancer with a vaccine has been an aspiration of scientists for some time and is closely linked with the recent resurgence of immuno-oncology. The goal of a cancer vaccine approach is to create a response to tumors that have become refractory to conventional treatments by utilizing tumor-specific antigens that can leverage the host immune system to target the lesions. In this way, the response should be specific to the tumor and sparing of normal tissues and allow for the long-term control of the cancer. There have been multiple challenges to developing safe and effective cancer vaccines with limited clinical success thus far. Vaccines secondarily relevant to cancer include the two prophylactic vaccines for hepatitis B virus and human papillomavirus, both viruses have clear links to the development of cancer. These more traditional approaches along with use of Bacillus Calmette-Guerin (BCG), which is used to treat certain forms of bladder cancer, are some of the few success stories to date (Morales, Eidinger, and Bruce 1976). However, these efforts fall short of the idea of treating refractory cancers with the host immune system. Sipuleucel-T (Provenge), an immune cell-based vaccine, is a first-in-class-approved cancer vaccine with a demonstrated increased overall survival in hormone-refractory prostate cancer patients (Cheever and Higano 2011). There are currently a number of vaccines in development and in clinical trials for the treatment of cancer.

The challenge of developing additional effective cancer vaccines remains (Schreiber, Old, and Smyth 2011; Zhou and Levitsky 2012), and to that end, many different scientific approaches are being evaluated. The cancer vaccine field remains very active in the nonclinical and clinical space, and can be subdivided into several major categories of vaccine modalities; each modality brings its own unique challenges and considerations in regard to developing a nonclinical safety testing strategy. Cell vaccines (tumor or immune cell), protein/peptide vaccines, and genetic (DNA, RNA, and viral) vaccines are all being actively pursued as potential solutions to the cancer vaccine challenge. Table 28.4 outlines the key aspects of different approaches and their pros and cons, as well as outlines general nonclinical safety strategy considerations. As would be expected, the broad range of modalities and materials making up the modalities (i.e., proteins, cells, and/or genes) translates to a case-by-case approach when determining the nonclinical toxicity testing strategy for any given therapeutic cancer vaccine. These strategies can range from an in vitro approach to safety evaluation due to the lack of an available animal model to what may be considered a more standard nonclinical safety package that more closely follows ICH S6(R1) and/or the ICH S9 guidelines. The most appropriate regulatory guidelines to follow will be specific to the type of vaccine being developed, and in some cases, specific guidelines are not

TABLE 28.4

Overview of Cancer Vaccine Approaches and Nonclinical Development Considerations

Vaccine Type	Key Aspects	Pros and Cons	Nonclinical Considerations	Examples of Development Programs
Protein/ peptide-based	Typically based on mutated or tumor-associated antigens or peptides including neoantigens	Pros: • Ease of manufacture • Low toxicity potential Cons: • HLA restriction • Low immunogenic potential	• Monkey is often but not always the most relevant species • Expression pattern of the protein/peptide in normal tissue will guide species selection	• Ras mutations • NY-ESO1 (testis antigens)
Cell-based	Use engineered antigen-presenting cells to prime T cells for antitumor response	Pros: • High immunogenic potential particularly cellular responses • Specificity of antigen response Cons: • Vascular toxicity potential	• Appropriate animal models may not exist • Potential for cytokine release may need to be evaluated • An evaluation of product tumorigenicity may be needed	• Provenge (DC) • GVAX (tumor cell based)
Gene-based (RNA and DNA-based approaches)	Multiple tumor antigen sequences are encoded to be expressed and recognized by the immune system	Pros: • Multiple antigens can be targeted • Designed to induce both cellular and humoral immune responses • Not HLA-restricted Cons: • Low immunogenic potential • Cold storage requirements and other supply chain considerations may limit availability	• Monkeys have been used to support toxicity assessment • Species tropism is an important consideration in species selection • Consideration of genetic toxicity potential, insertional mutagenesis • Understanding of vaccine distribution and tissues and organs that uptake and express antigens	• INO-5401 • VGX-3100 • GX-188E
Viral/ bacterial-based	Use of pathogens to deliver tumor antigen sequences	Pros: • Historical evidence of high immunogenic potential (humoral and cellular) • Ease of manufacture Cons: • Potential for increased toxicity • Infection potential dependent upon vector • May be only single use if immunogenicity against the vector develops or there are preexisting antibodies	• Two species assessment (rodent and non-rodent) typically needed • Biodistribution study should be considered to understand viral/bacterial tropism, persistence, shedding • Potential for immunotoxicity and infection should be thoroughly evaluated and understood	• TroVax • TG4010 • Lm-LLO-E7

available and a case-by-case approach based on several guidelines may be need. See Chapter 23 on Vaccines.

For many cancer vaccines, it is especially important to establish the pharmacological and thus toxicological relevance of the chosen animal model and/or species. In the case where the target of a cancer vaccine immune response is a self-antigen, it is important to understand both the homology of the antigen(s) and the distribution of the target between humans and the nonclinical species. The use of monkeys has dominated the cancer vaccine field based on similarities between NHP and human immune systems. However, in vitro and in vivo assessments should be completed to support species selection and confirm relevant pharmacology. The use of rodents has also proven to be valuable for some approaches. For these programs, it is not uncommon that safety data are acquired from studies that evaluate both efficacy and safety aspects rather than having dedicated studies for each assessment. These studies also typically support pharmacologic relevance and safety of the clinical route, aid in selecting the clinical starting dose and dosing regimen based on pharmacodynamic effects and duration of responses. When conducting in vivo animal studies, particularly for vaccines targeting self-antigens, general

considerations for dose, dose volume, and number of doses are similar to those for infectious disease vaccines.

For many cancer vaccines, the primary mechanism of action is to elicit a cellular immune response. Evidence of a cellular immune response can be measured in the nonclinical species as a measure of pharmacologic activity; however, it is important to note that the cellular immune response may not correlate with clinical efficacy. If the vaccine contains nucleic acids and is delivered via a viral or bacterial vector, a biodistribution study should be considered to understand vector tropism, persistence, and shedding. If an established viral or bacterial platform is used, a biodistribution study may not be required.

Lastly, to overcome some of the early limitations of the cancer vaccine approaches, different delivery systems and ways to boost the immune response (e.g., viral or bacterial, nanoparticles, adjuvants, co-administration of other immunomodulatory agents) have been developed. The safety of each individual component should be considered as part of the nonclinical assessment as well as the safety of the overall cancer vaccine that includes all the components. Combination pharmacology/toxicity studies with all the vaccine components and co-stimulating agents (e.g., checkpoint inhibitors) should be

TABLE 28.5

Currently Approved Antibody-Drug Conjugates

Generic Name (Brand Name)	Target/Payload	Approval Date	Approved Treatment(s)[a]
Gemtuzumab ozogamicin (Mylotarg)	CD33/N-acetyl-γ-calicheamicin dimethylhydrazide	2001 2017[b]	Relapsed acute myelogenous leukemia
Brentuximab vedotin (Adcetris)	CD30/monomethyl auristatin E (MMAE)	2011	Relapsed Hodgkin's lymphoma and relapsed systemic anaplastic large cell lymphoma
Trastuzumab emtansine (Kadcyla)	HER2/emtansine (DM1)	2013	HER2-positive metastatic breast cancer
Inotuzumab ozogamicin (Besponsa)	CD22/N-acetyl-γ-calicheamicin dimethylhydrazide	2017	Relapsed or refractory CD22-positive acute lymphoblastic leukemia
Polatuzumab vedotin (Polivy)	CD79b/monomethyl auristatin E (MMAE)	2019	Relapsed or refractory diffuse large B-cell lymphoma
Enfortumab vedotin (Padcev)	Nectin-4/monomethyl auristatin E (MMAE)	2019	Locally advanced or metastatic urothelial cancer
Trastuzumab deruxtecan (Enhertu)	HER2/MAAA-1181a (derivative of exatecan)	2019	Unresectable or metastatic HER2-postitive breast cancer
Sacituzumab govitecan (Trodelvy)	Trop-2/SN-38 (active metabolite of irinotecan)	2020	Metastatic triple-negative breast cancer
Belantamab mafodotin (Blenrep)	BCMA/auristatin F	2020	Relapsed or refractory multiple myeloma

[a] See labels for specific details on approved treatments.

[b] After a request from the US FDA, Mylotarg was withdrawn from the US market in June 2010; it remained on the market in Japan. It was re-introduced into the US market in 2017 and also authorized for use in the EU.

considered as appropriate to support the identification of key risks of the total vaccine package in early clinical trials. The use of reagents and components that have existing safety information can be supportive in understanding potential risk and reduce the need for novel combination studies. The inclusion of genotoxicity and DART studies may be needed for some but not all vaccine modalities and should be considered on a case-by-case basis. Patient population and tumor characteristics will also inform the overall risk assessment and support the final nonclinical strategy and approach.

28.4.2 Antibody-Drug Conjugates

This section will provide a brief introduction to ADCs in the context of other biotherapeutics/modalities used in late-stage cancer. For a comprehensive overview of ADCs and nonclinical development strategies, see Chapter 20. ADCs are complex molecules comprising a monoclonal antibody linked to a small-molecule drug through an organic linker. The small-molecule portion of the ADC is typically a potent cytotoxic drug (also known as the payload), and each ADC has a range in the number of payload molecules per each antibody (also known as the antibody-drug ratio or DAR; i.e., 2–4 or 3–5, etc.). In addition to the targeting antibody and the cytotoxic payload, a key design feature of ADCs resides in the chemical nature of the linker connecting the antibody and the cytotoxic agent. Two general classes of linkers exist: cleavable linkers that are susceptible to chemical or enzymatic degradation and non-cleavable linkers that contain no sites for such degradation in biological systems. All three components of an ADC can contribute to its toxicity profile, thus making the nonclinical toxicology strategy for the assessment of this modality complex.

ADCs were initially developed for hematologic malignancies. This was due in part to the large size of the intact ADC and relatively less distribution into tissues, including solid tumors, from the peripheral circulation. There have been recent breakthroughs with newer ADCs that show activity in solid tumors. The currently approved ADCs are shown in Table 28.5.

The original promise of ADCs was that by targeting only cells that express the target antigen there would be less toxicity than that observed by directly administering a potent cytotoxic agent alone (Chari 2008). Although the original hypothesis was shown to be true in some respects, most ADCs still show steep dose-toxicity response curves, small safety margins, and serious and sometimes life-threatening toxicities in patients. The toxicity profile (i.e., target organs or underlying pathology in target organs) of the full ADC may be different from the toxicity profile of the payload alone in animals and humans. In addition, the toxicity observed after a single dose may not fully represent the toxicity profile observed after multiple doses due to observed cumulative toxicity even with less-intensive dosing schedules (e.g., doses given every 2 or 3 weeks).

Any cell expressing the target antigen/epitope may be a target for the ADC and subjected to the toxicity of the payload, including normal cells with low levels of target expression. In addition to target-dependent toxicity (i.e., that is associated with binding to the target), target-independent toxicity unrelated to binding of the antibody to the intended target can be observed. Target independent toxicity can be observed with the release of free payload from cells back into the peripheral circulation or can be due to the non-specific uptake of an ADC into highly perfused organs like the liver or lungs. Target-independent toxicity due to non-specific uptake was not well understood in the early days of ADC development and became better appreciated as development programs matured. Mylotarg (gemtuzumab ozogamicin) is an example where the non-specific uptake of the ADC by liver cells causes liver toxicity and associated acute thrombocytopenia in both cynomolgus monkeys and humans (Guffroy et al. 2017). These effects, although associated with non-specific uptake, are also payload dependent with calicheamicin-based ADCs showing greater hepatotoxicity versus mitotic inhibitor-based ADCs.

In addition to the toxicity associated with some of the specific distribution characteristics of ADCs, the physiochemical properties of the ADC may also contribute to the toxicity profile. The number of payload molecules associated with each antibody (the DAR), the type of linker used (i.e., cleavable or non-cleavable), as well as the mechanism of action and associated toxicity of the payload can all contribute to the toxicity of an ADC. For example, the toxicity of ADCs using various linkers and cytotoxic agents was tested in rats where an anti-CD22-based ADC did not cross-react with rodent CD22. Only the cleavable linkers yielding membrane-permeable payloads were associated with hepatic and hematological toxicities. Similar types of studies have shown the relationship between increasing the DAR and increased toxicity, even when a concomitant increase in efficacy is not always observed (Hamblett et al. 2004). There have been recent efforts to re-evaluate the use of cleavable linkers in ADCs to enhance the potential for a bystander effect. The bystander effect occurs once antigen-positive cells in a heterogeneous tumor process the ADC and the payload diffuses out of the cells and into neighboring antigen negative cells and induces cytotoxicity (Singh, Sharma, and Shah 2016).

Taking into consideration that an ADC is comprised of three components (i.e., antibody, linker, and payload), the nonclinical testing strategy has to address not only the toxicity of the full ADC but also each individual component. From a regulatory perspective, the ICH S9 Q&A guideline makes several recommendations specifically for ADCs that were not covered in the original ICH S9 guideline. The ADC topics in ICH S9 Q&A include: when characterization of the individual components of an ADC (antibody, linker and payload) are required, what toxicokinetic analyses to perform on the total ADC and the components, plasma stability in the toxicology species and humans, recommendations for setting clinical starting dose, supporting clinical trial dosing regimens, and species selection. In addition, ICH S6(R1) directly addresses the testing strategy for novel payloads versus well-characterized payloads where literature on toxicity of the payload is available and/or previous studies with the payload only have been conducted (ICH S6(R1) 2011, Note 2). Table 28.6 outlines some general considerations for the nonclinical testing strategy for ADCs taking into consideration the recommendations in applicable ICH guidelines.

28.5 Future Directions for an Ever-Expanding Array of Novel Modalities

There is no shortage of creativity and diversity in advancing the field of anticancer biotherapeutics. Multiple novel approaches are currently in the early stages of discovery and development with the hope of becoming the next generation of biotherapeutics for the treatment of cancer. These approaches use a wide variety of modalities and encompass a broad range of design and engineering and in some cases combinations of modalities. The nonclinical safety strategy may not have been fully established for many of these modalities, but as always, past experience can provide valuable insight into the design of the nonclinical toxicity program for new biotherapeutics.

Engineered antibodies continue to evolve particularly in the field of oncology to enhance treatment options for patients.

In addition to bispecific approaches discussed in this chapter, there are currently many additional modalities and approaches in early- and late-stage clinical development. Some examples include engineered cytokines to bias for receptor binding, cytokine payloads, and other modifications (Conlon, Miljkovic, and Waldmann 2019; Mizui 2019). The intent of the new modifications is to improve risk/benefit by improving safety and efficacy. The nonclinical strategy for engineered cytokines aligns well with existing ICH S6(R1)/S9 guidance with emphasis on the potential for immunotoxicity.

The field of cellular therapies continues to advance with enhanced design and engineering intended to provide greater efficacy and safety. In addition to T-cell immunotherapies, NK cells, monocytes, and other immune cell subtypes are currently being explored for their potential to treat various tumor types (Chu et al. 2020; Moyes et al. 2017). Additionally, the ability to genetically manipulate mesenchymal stem cells and other cell types in an ex vivo environment makes them an attractive delivery system option for oncolytic viruses and gene therapies. Stem cells can be modulated to express proteins of interest, carry oncolytic viruses, and exosomes and have many other potential applications. The nonclinical safety evaluation of these new modalities will need to consider multiple factors and proceed using a case-by-case approach. Existing nonclinical strategies for cellular therapies can be used as a starting point.

Another exciting area of research is using biotherapeutics to access intracellular proteins and cancer neoantigens. Neoantigens are aberrantly expressed proteins that are presented on the surface of cancer cells by MHC proteins (i.e., human leukocyte antigens [HLAs]), with the intent of having T cells recognize the neoantigen peptide, become activated, and kill the transformed cell. However, T cells are often impaired in their ability to identify these cells as abnormal. Monoclonal antibodies that are designed to behave like a TCR, termed "T-cell receptor mimics," can bind the neoantigens in the context of the HLA, thus allowing access to unique intracellular cancer cell targets (Trenevska, Li, and Banham 2017). Such an approach can harnesses the whole Fc receptor expressing compartment of the immune system to assist T-cell recognition of the neoantigen. Viable therapeutic candidates against novel cancer antigens such as WT1 and PRAME have been described in the literature with promising results in nonclinical studies (Chang et al. 2017; Dubrovsky et al. 2014). Additionally, investigators have sought to take a combined TCR mimic/CD3 bispecific approach in an attempt to amplify the response against these antigens (Dao et al. 2015).

A key challenge in obtaining relevant nonclinical safety information for TCR mimics is identifying an animal model where the antibody is able to recognize the targeted human MHC in an animal model. Transgenic mice are available commercially that express some MHC proteins (e.g., HLA-A2). These mice could be used to understand if any safety liabilities exist if the novel cancer antigen is unexpectedly expressed in normal tissues. However, more work needs to be done to evaluate the expression levels and locations of HLA-A2 in these mice. Alternatives to a more classic in vivo safety program will likely include in vitro analyses of primary human cells where the antigen is known to be expressed as well as a thorough examination of the specificity of the antibody to the HLA-antigen complex. Comparative binding to other similar antigen sequences can be evaluated as

TABLE 28.6

Nonclinical Test Strategy for ADCs and Their Components

Study Type	ADC[a]	Well-Characterized Payload[b]	Novel Payload
General toxicity studies	• Studies need to be conducted in rodent and non-rodent species if pharmacologically active in both • If only pharmacologically active in one species, then studies are conducted in that species only • If there are no pharmacologically active species, a short-term multiple-dose toxicity study still needs to be conducted in one species • Single-dose PK studies (with tolerability assessments) are useful but not required • Multiple-dose range-finding toxicity studies • Multiple-dose definitive toxicity studies with recovery and immunogenicity assessment	• No additional testing need	• Consider including a payload only arm on studies with the ADC or conduct stand-alone studies in a rodent species (definitive study can be short duration [i.e., 2–4 weeks] and non-GLP)
hERG assay	• Not required	• Not required	• Required
In vivo safety pharmacology studies	• Endpoints incorporated into definitive repeat-dose non-rodent toxicity study	• Not required	• May be needed if only conducting stand-alone rodent studies
Tissue cross-reactivity studies	• Human tissue cross-reactivity study only required if no relevant species for toxicity testing • Recommend using full ADC and not just antibody portion	• Not applicable	• Not applicable
DART studies	• If rodent and/or rabbit are relevant species, then an EFD study in one species • If monkey is the only relevant species, then a WOE approach may be sufficient • Evaluation of male and female reproductive organs on the definitive repeat-dose toxicity study (mature animals not required) • No other DART studies are required	• Not required	• EFD should be considered if monkey is the only relevant species for the full ADC • Evaluation of male and female reproductive organs in any definitive repeat-dose toxicity studies • No other DART studies are required
Genotoxicity studies	• Not required	• Not Required	• Full battery of genotoxicity assays required for BLA submission
Carcinogenicity studies	• Not required	• Not required	• Not required

ADC = antibody-drug conjugate; BLA = biologics license application; DART = developmental and reproductive toxicity; EFD = embryo-fetal development; GLP = Good Laboratory Practice; PK = pharmacokinetic; WOE = weight of evidence.

[a] Assessment of the antibody only or linker only is not required in accordance with ICH S9 Q&A.

[b] Well-characterized means that toxicity studies have already been conducted with the payload on a previous program, that the payload has been extensively used clinically including in marketed products, and/or there is extensive publicly available literature supporting characterizing the safety of the payload.

well as any potential for cross-reactivity to other extracellular proteins unrelated to MHC/HLA complexes.

The general term "nanoparticle" encompasses several different modalities (polymeric, liposomal, and magnetic nanoparticles; liposomes; carbon nanotubes; quantum dots; dendrimers; metallic nanoparticles, etc.) that are currently being tried in new anticancer therapies. A nanoparticle typically consists of several components, including the nanomaterial, a payload (the pharmacologically active moiety), and a targeting ligand (often a biotherapeutic). The targeting ligand

may consist of monoclonal antibodies or peptides intended to drive tissue-specific uptake of the nanoparticle. The payload can consist of any number of modalities, for example, small molecules, oncolytic viruses, and RNA/DNA. The nanoparticle approach was traditionally used to increase the safety or efficacy of older anticancer agents through new or targeted delivery systems (Fornaguera and García-Celma 2017; Shi et al. 2017). Similar to other novel modalities, the nonclinical safety strategy of nanoparticles will need to encompass the assessment of multiple components to ensure the potential contributions of each to the overall toxicity profile. Two key considerations in the toxicity assessment of nanoparticles is an understanding of the pharmacokinetics/tissue distribution of the nanoparticle and the release of the payload into the blood and tissue compartments. Understanding both of these factors is critical to understanding potential human safety risks.

The discovery and development of novel biotherapeutics for the treatment of cancer remains an active and exciting field of research. With each advancement comes unknown potential risks, which can be investigated and characterized with a knowledge of previous development programs and a well-thought-out nonclinical safety strategy. Using the deep pool of knowledge of biotherapeutic safety testing already available and a rigorous scientific case-by-case approach will continue to be needed to ensure the successful development of new novel biotherapeutics for cancer patients.

REFERENCES

Ahmadzadeh, M., L. A. Johnson, B. Heemskerk, J. R. Wunderlich, M. E. Dudley, D. E. White, and S. A. Rosenberg. 2009. "Tumor antigen-specific CD8 T cells infiltrating the tumor express high levels of PD-1 and are functionally impaired." *Blood* 114 (8): 1537–1544. https://doi.org/10.1182/blood-2008-12-195792.

Al-Saleh, K., N. A. El-Aziz, A. Ali, W. Abozeed, A. A. El-Warith, A. Ibraheem, J. Ansari, A. Al-Rikabi, S. Husain, and J.-M. Nabholtz. 2017. "Predictive and prognostic significance of CD8(+) tumor-infiltrating lymphocytes in patients with luminal B/HER 2 negative breast cancer treated with neo-adjuvant chemotherapy." *Oncol Lett* 14 (1): 337–344. https://doi.org/10.3892/ol.2017.6144. https://pubmed.ncbi.nlm.nih.gov/28693173.

Anand, K., E. Burns, D. Sano, S. R. Pingali, J. Westin, L. J. Nastoupil, H. J. Lee, F. Samaniego, S. Parmar, M. Wang, M. Hawkins, S. Adkins, L. Fayad, R. Steiner, R. Nair, S. Ahmed, N. H. Fowler, S. S. Neelapu, and S. P. Iyer. 2019. "Comprehensive report of anti-CD19 chimeric antigen receptor T cells (CAR-T) associated non-relapse mortality (CART-NRM) from FAERS." *J Clin Oncol* 37 (15_suppl): 2540–2540. https://ascopubs.org/doi/abs/10.1200/JCO.2019.37.15_suppl.2540.

Benjamin, J. E., and A. S. Stein. 2016. "The role of blinatumomab in patients with relapsed/refractory acute lymphoblastic leukemia." *Ther Adv Hematol* 7 (3): 142–156. https://doi.org/10.1177/2040620716640422.

Betts, A., N. Haddish-Berhane, D. K. Shah, P. H. van der Graaf, F. Barletta, L. King, T. Clark, C. Kamperschroer, A. Root, A. Hooper, and X. Chen. 2019. "A translational quantitative systems pharmacology model for CD3 bispecific molecules: application to quantify T cell-mediated tumor cell killing by P-Cadherin LP DART(®)." *Aaps J* 21 (4): 66. https://doi.org/10.1208/s12248-019-0332-z.

Bolovan, C. A., N. M. Sawtell, and R. L. Thompson. 1994. "ICP34.5 mutants of herpes simplex virus type 1 strain 17syn+ are attenuated for neurovirulence in mice and for replication in confluent primary mouse embryo cell cultures." *J Virol* 68 (1): 48–55. https://doi.org/10.1128/jvi.68.1.48-55.1994.

Boshoff, C., and R. Weiss. 2002. "AIDS-related malignancies." *Nat Rev Cancer* 2 (5): 373–382. https://doi.org/10.1038/nrc797.

Bowman, C. J., and R. E. Chapin. 2016. "'Goldilocks' determination of what new in vivo data are "Just Right" for different common drug development scenarios, part 1." *Birth Defects Res B Dev Reprod Toxicol* 107 (4–5): 185–194. https://doi.org/10.1002/bdrb.21184.

Brunet, J. F., F. Denizot, M. F. Luciani, M. Roux-Dosseto, M. Suzan, M. G. Mattei, and P. Golstein. 1987. "A new member of the immunoglobulin superfamily – CTLA-4." *Nature* 328 (6127): 267–270. https://doi.org/10.1038/328267a0.

Buchan, S. L., A. Rogel, and A. Al-Shamkhani. 2018. "The immunobiology of CD27 and OX40 and their potential as targets for cancer immunotherapy." *Blood* 131 (1): 39–48. https://doi.org/10.1182/blood-2017-07-741025.

Cameron, B. J., A. B. Gerry, J. Dukes, J. V. Harper, V. Kannan, F. C. Bianchi, F. Grand, J. E. Brewer, M. Gupta, G. Plesa, G. Bossi, A. Vuidepot, A. S. Powlesland, A. Legg, K. J. Adams, A. D. Bennett, N. J. Pumphrey, D. D. Williams, G. Binder-Scholl, I. Kulikovskaya, B. L. Levine, J. L. Riley, A. Varela-Rohena, E. A. Stadtmauer, A. P. Rapoport, G. P. Linette, C. H. June, N. J. Hassan, M. Kalos, and B. K. Jakobsen. 2013. "Identification of a Titin-derived HLA-A1-presented peptide as a cross-reactive target for engineered MAGE A3-directed T cells." *Sci Trans Med* 5 (197): 197ra103–197ra103. https://pubmed.ncbi.nlm.nih.gov/23926201.

Chang, A. Y., T. Dao, R. S. Gejman, C. A. Jarvis, A. Scott, L. Dubrovsky, M. D. Mathias, T. Korontsvit, V. Zakhaleva, M. Curcio, R. C. Hendrickson, C. Liu, and D. A. Scheinberg. 2017. "A therapeutic T cell receptor mimic antibody targets tumor-associated PRAME peptide/HLA-I antigens." *J Clin Invest* 127 (7): 2705–2718. https://doi.org/10.1172/jci92335.

Chari, R. V. 2008. "Targeted cancer therapy: conferring specificity to cytotoxic drugs." *Acc Chem Res* 41 (1): 98–107. https://doi.org/10.1021/ar700108g.

Cheever, M. A., and C. S. Higano. 2011. "PROVENGE (Sipuleucel-T) in prostate cancer: the first FDA-approved therapeutic cancer vaccine." *Clin Cancer Res* 17 (11): 3520–3526. https://doi.org/10.1158/1078-0432.Ccr-10-3126.

Chester, C., M. F. Sanmamed, J. Wang, and I. Melero. 2018. "Immunotherapy targeting 4-1BB: mechanistic rationale, clinical results, and future strategies." *Blood* 131 (1): 49–57. https://doi.org/10.1182/blood-2017-06-741041.

Chiesa Fuxench, Z. C., D. B. Shin, A. Ogdie Beatty, and J. M. Gelfand. 2016. "The risk of cancer in patients with psoriasis: a population-based cohort study in the health improvement network." *JAMA Dermatol* 152 (3): 282–290. https://doi.org/10.1001/jamadermatol.2015.4847.

Chou, C. K., and C. J. Turtle. 2019. "Insight into mechanisms associated with cytokine release syndrome and neurotoxicity after CD19 CAR-T cell immunotherapy." *Bone Marrow Transplant* 54 (Suppl 2): 780–784. https://doi.org/10.1038/s41409-019-0602-5.

Chu, D. T., T. T. Nguyen, N. L. B. Tien, D. K. Tran, J. H. Jeong, P. G. Anh, V. V. Thanh, D. T. Truong, and T. C. Dinh. 2020. "Recent progress of stem cell therapy in cancer treatment: molecular mechanisms and potential applications." *Cells* 9 (3). https://doi.org/10.3390/cells9030563.

Coley, W. B. 1891. "II. Contribution to the knowledge of sarcoma." *Annals Surg* 14 (3): 199–220. https://doi.org/10.1097/00000658-189112000-00015.

Coley, W. B. 1991. "The treatment of malignant tumors by repeated inoculations of erysipelas. With a report of ten original cases. 1893." *Clin Orthop Relat Res* (262): 3–11.

Conlon, K. C., M. D. Miljkovic, and T. A. Waldmann. 2019. "Cytokines in the treatment of cancer." *J Interferon Cytokine Res* 39 (1): 6–21. https://doi.org/10.1089/jir.2018.0019.

Dao, T., D. Pankov, A. Scott, T. Korontsvit, V. Zakhaleva, Y. Xu, J. Xiang, S. Yan, M. D. de Morais Guerreiro, N. Veomett, L. Dubrovsky, M. Curcio, E. Doubrovina, V. Ponomarev, C. Liu, R. J. O'Reilly, and D. A. Scheinberg. 2015. "Therapeutic bispecific T-cell engager antibody targeting the intracellular oncoprotein WT1." *Nat Biotechnol* 33 (10): 1079–1086. https://doi.org/10.1038/nbt.3349.

DeGeorge, J. J., C. H. Ahn, P. A. Andrews, M. E. Brower, D. W. Giorgio, M. A. Goheer, D. Y. Lee-Ham, W. D. McGuinn, W. Schmidt, C. J. Sun, and S. C. Tripathi. 1998. "Regulatory considerations for preclinical development of anticancer drugs." *Cancer Chemother Pharmacol* 41 (3): 173–185. https://doi.org/10.1007/s002800050726.

Di Giacomo, A. M., M. Biagioli, and M. Maio. 2010. "The emerging toxicity profiles of anti-CTLA-4 antibodies across clinical indications." *Semin Oncol* 37 (5): 499–507. https://doi.org/10.1053/j.seminoncol.2010.09.007.

Dong, H., S. E. Strome, D. R. Salomao, H. Tamura, F. Hirano, D. B. Flies, P. C. Roche, J. Lu, G. Zhu, K. Tamada, V. A. Lennon, E. Celis, and L. Chen. 2002. "Tumor-associated B7-H1 promotes T-cell apoptosis: a potential mechanism of immune evasion." *Nat Med* 8 (8): 793–800. https://doi.org/10.1038/nm730.

Dubrovsky, L., D. Pankov, E. J. Brea, T. Dao, A. Scott, S. Yan, R. J. O'Reilly, C. Liu, and D. A. Scheinberg. 2014. "A TCR-mimic antibody to WT1 bypasses tyrosine kinase inhibitor resistance in human BCR-ABL+ leukemias." *Blood* 123 (21): 3296–3304. https://doi.org/10.1182/blood-2014-01-549022.

Dunn, G. P., H. Ikeda, A. T. Bruce, C. Koebel, R. Uppaluri, J. Bui, R. Chan, M. Diamond, J. M. White, K. C. Sheehan, and R. D. Schreiber. 2005. "Interferon-gamma and cancer immunoediting." *Immunol Res* 32 (1–3): 231–245. https://doi.org/10.1385/ir:32:1-3:231.

Ehrlich. 1909. "Ueber den jetzigen stand der Karzinomforschung." *Ned Tijdschr Geneeskd* 5: 273–290.

Einsele, H., H. Borghaei, R. Z. Orlowski, M. Subklewe, G. J. Roboz, G. Zugmaier, P. Kufer, K. Iskander, and H. M. Kantarjian. 2020. "The BiTE (bispecific T-cell engager) platform: development and future potential of a targeted immuno-oncology therapy across tumor types." *Cancer* 126 (14): 3192–3201. https://doi.org/10.1002/cncr.32909.

EMA. 2017. "Guideline on strategies to identify and mitigate risks for first-in-human and early clinical trials with investigational medicinal products." Committee for Medicinal Products for Human Use.

Engels, E. A., R. J. Biggar, H. I. Hall, H. Cross, A. Crutchfield, J. L. Finch, R. Grigg, T. Hylton, K. S. Pawlish, T. S. McNeel, and J. J. Goedert. 2008. "Cancer risk in people infected with human immunodeficiency virus in the United States." *Int J Cancer* 123 (1): 187–194. https://doi.org/10.1002/ijc.23487.

FDA. 2011. "Yervoy (ipilimumab) Summary Basis of Approval: Pharmacology Review." Accessed February 15, 2020. http://www.accessdata.fda.gov/drugsatfda_docs/nda/2011/125377Orig1s000PharmR.pdf.

FDA. 2013. "Preclinical Assessment of Investigational Cellular and Gene Therapy Products." FDA Guidance for Industry.

FDA. 2015. "Considerations for the Design of Early-Phase Clinical Trials of Cellular and Gene Therapy Products." FDA Guidance for Industry.

FDA. 2017a. "FDA Approves Tisagenlecleucel for B-cell ALL and Tocilizumab for Cytokine Release Syndrome." Accessed February 15, 2020. https://www.fda.gov/drugs/resources-information-approved-drugs/fda-approves-tisagenlecleucel-b-cell-all-and-tocilizumab-cytokine-release-syndrome.

FDA. 2017b. "FDA Approves Axicabtagene Ciloleucel for Large B-cell Lymphoma." Accessed February 15, 2020. https://www.fda.gov/drugs/resources-information-approved-drugs/fda-approves-axicabtagene-ciloleucel-large-b-cell-lymphoma.

Feng, Z., D. Bethmann, M. Kappler, C. Ballesteros-Merino, A. Eckert, R. B. Bell, A. Cheng, T. Bui, R. Leidner, W. J. Urba, K. Johnson, C. Hoyt, C. B. Bifulco, J. Bukur, C. Wickenhauser, B. Seliger, and B. A. Fox. 2017. "Multiparametric immune profiling in HPV- oral squamous cell cancer." *JCI insight* 2 (14): e93652. https://doi.org/10.1172/jci.insight.93652.

Filipovich, A. H., A. Mathur, D. Kamat, J. H. Kersey, and R. S. Shapiro. 1994. "Lymphoproliferative disorders and other tumors complicating immunodeficiencies." *Immunodeficiency* 5 (2): 91–112.

Finco, D., C. Grimaldi, M. Fort, M. Walker, A. Kiessling, B. Wolf, T. Salcedo, R. Faggioni, A. Schneider, A. Ibraghimov, S. Scesney, D. Serna, R. Prell, R. Stebbings, and P. K. Narayanan. 2014. "Cytokine release assays: current practices and future directions." *Cytokine* 66 (2): 143–155. https://doi.org/10.1016/j.cyto.2013.12.009.

Fornaguera, C., and M. J. García-Celma. 2017. "Personalized nanomedicine: a revolution at the nanoscale." *J Pers Med* 7 (4). https://doi.org/10.3390/jpm7040012.

Galon, J., A. Costes, F. Sanchez-Cabo, A. Kirilovsky, B. Mlecnik, C. Lagorce-Pagès, M. Tosolini, M. Camus, A. Berger, P. Wind, F. Zinzindohoué, P. Bruneval, P. H. Cugnenc, Z. Trajanoski, W. H. Fridman, and F. Pagès. 2006. "Type, density, and location of immune cells within human colorectal tumors predict clinical outcome." *Science* 313 (5795): 1960–1964. https://doi.org/10.1126/science.1129139.

Garber, K. 2006. "China approves world's first oncolytic virus therapy for cancer treatment." *JNCI J Natl Cancer Inst* 98 (5): 298–300. https://doi.org/10.1093/jnci/djj111.

Geiger, M., K. G. Stubenrauch, J. Sam, W. F. Richter, G. Jordan, J. Eckmann, C. Hage, V. Nicolini, A. Freimoser-Grundschober, M. Ritter, M. E. Lauer, H. Stahlberg, P. Ringler, J. Patel, E. Sullivan, S. Grau-Richards, S. Endres, S. Kobold, P. Umaña, P. Brünker, and C. Klein. 2020. "Protease-activation using anti-idiotypic masks enables tumor specificity of a folate receptor 1-T cell bispecific antibody." *Nat Commun* 11 (1): 3196. https://doi.org/10.1038/s41467-020-16838-w.

Giavridis, T., S. J. C. van der Stegen, J. Eyquem, M. Hamieh, A. Piersigilli, and M. Sadelain. 2018. "CAR T cell-induced cytokine release syndrome is mediated by macrophages and abated by IL-1 blockade." *Nat Med* 24 (6): 731–738. https://doi.org/10.1038/s41591-018-0041-7.

Grimaldi, C., D. Finco, M. M. Fort, D. Gliddon, K. Harper, W. S. Helms, J. A. Mitchell, R. O'Lone, S. T. Parish, M. S. Piche, D. M. Reed, G. Reichmann, P. C. Ryan, R. Stebbings, and M. Walker. 2016. "Cytokine release: a workshop proceedings on the state-of-the-science, current challenges and future directions." *Cytokine* 85: 101–108. https://doi.org/10.1016/j.cyto.2016.06.006.

Grulich, A. E., M. T. van Leeuwen, M. O. Falster, and C. M. Vajdic. 2007. "Incidence of cancers in people with HIV/AIDS compared with immunosuppressed transplant recipients: a meta-analysis." *Lancet* 370 (9581): 59–67. https://doi.org/10.1016/s0140-6736(07)61050-2.

Guffroy, M., H. Falahatpisheh, K. Biddle, J. Kreeger, L. Obert, K. Walters, R. Goldstein, G. Boucher, T. Coskran, W. Reagan, D. Sullivan, C. Huang, S. Sokolowski, R. Giovanelli, H. P. Gerber, M. Finkelstein, and N. Khan. 2017. "Liver microvascular injury and thrombocytopenia of antibody-calicheamicin conjugates in cynomolgus monkeys-mechanism and monitoring." *Clin Cancer Res* 23 (7): 1760–1770. https://doi.org/10.1158/1078-0432.Ccr-16-0939.

Gust, J., K. A. Hay, L. A. Hanafi, D. Li, D. Myerson, L. F. Gonzalez-Cuyar, C. Yeung, W. C. Liles, M. Wurfel, J. A. Lopez, J. Chen, D. Chung, S. Harju-Baker, T. Özpolat, K. R. Fink, S. R. Riddell, D. G. Maloney, and C. J. Turtle. 2017. "Endothelial activation and blood-brain barrier disruption in neurotoxicity after adoptive immunotherapy with CD19 CAR-T cells." *Cancer Discov* 7 (12): 1404–1419. https://doi.org/10.1158/2159-8290.Cd-17-0698.

Hamblett, K. J., P. D. Senter, D. F. Chace, M. M. Sun, J. Lenox, C. G. Cerveny, K. M. Kissler, S. X. Bernhardt, A. K. Kopcha, R. F. Zabinski, D. L. Meyer, and J. A. Francisco. 2004. "Effects of drug loading on the antitumor activity of a monoclonal antibody drug conjugate." *Clin Cancer Res* 10 (20): 7063–7070. https://doi.org/10.1158/1078-0432.Ccr-04-0789.

He, Q., X. Jiang, X. Zhou, and J. Weng. 2019. "Targeting cancers through TCR-peptide/MHC interactions." *J Hematol Oncol* 12 (1): 139. https://doi.org/10.1186/s13045-019-0812-8.

Hernandez-Hoyos, G., T. Sewell, R. Bader, J. Bannink, R. A. Chenault, M. Daugherty, M. Dasovich, H. Fang, R. Gottschalk, J. Kumer, R. E. Miller, P. Ravikumar, J. Wiens, P. A. Algate, D. Bienvenue, C. J. McMahan, S. K. Natarajan, J. A. Gross, and J. W. Blankenship. 2016. "MOR209/ES414, a novel bispecific antibody targeting PSMA for the treatment of metastatic castration-resistant prostate cancer." *Mol Cancer Ther* 15 (9): 2155–2165. https://doi.org/10.1158/1535-7163.Mct-15-0242.

Herzyk, D. J., and H. G. Haggerty. 2018. "Cancer immunotherapy: factors important for the evaluation of safety in non-clinical studies." *AAPS J* 20 (2): 28. https://doi.org/10.1208/s12248-017-0184-3.

Hoster, H. A., R. P. Zanes, Jr., and E. Von Haam. 1949. "Studies in Hodgkin's syndrome; the association of viral hepatitis and Hodgkin's disease; a preliminary report." *Cancer Res* 9 (8): 473–480.

Høydahl, L. S., R. Frick, I. Sandlie, and GÅ Løset. 2019. "Targeting the MHC ligandome by use of TCR-like antibodies." *Antibodies (Basel)* 8 (2). https://doi.org/10.3390/antib8020032.

Hughes, T., R.S. Coffin, C. E. Lilley, R. Ponce, and H. L. Kaufman. 2014. "Critical analysis of an oncolytic herpesvirus encoding granulocyte-macrophage colony stimulating factor for the treatment of malignant melanoma." *Oncolytic Virother* 3: 11–20. https://doi.org/10.2147/OV.S36701.

ICH. 2009a. "ICH S9: Nonclinical Evaluation for Anticancer Pharmaceuticals." International Conference on Harmonisation of Technical Requirements for Registration of Pharmaceuticals for Human Use.

ICH. 2009b. "Oncolytic Viruses." International Conference on Harmonisation of Technical Requirements for Registration of Pharmaceuticals for Human Use.

ICH. 2011. "ICH S6(R1): Preclinical Safety Evaluation of Biotechnology-Derived Pharmaceuticals." International Conference on Harmonisation of Technical Requirements for Registration of Pharmaceuticals for Human Use.

ICH. 2018. "ICH S9: Nonclinical Evaluations for Anticancer Pharmaceuticals Questions and Answers." International Conference on Harmonisation of Technical Requirements for Registration of Pharmaceuticals for Human Use.

Jesinghaus, M., K. Steiger, J. Slotta-Huspenina, E. Drecoll, N. Pfarr, P. Meyer, B. Konukiewitz, M. Bettstetter, K. Wieczorek, K. Ott, M. Feith, R. Langer, W. Weichert, K. Specht, and M. Boxberg. 2017. "Increased intraepithelial CD3+ T-lymphocytes and high PD-L1 expression on tumor cells are associated with a favorable prognosis in esophageal squamous cell carcinoma and allow prognostic immunogenic subgrouping." *Oncotarget* 8 (29): 46756–46768. https://doi.org/10.18632/oncotarget.18606.

Johnson, L. A., R. A. Morgan, M. E. Dudley, L. Cassard, J. C. Yang, M. S. Hughes, U. S. Kammula, R. E. Royal, R. M. Sherry, J. R. Wunderlich, C.-C. R. Lee, N. P. Restifo, S. L. Schwarz, A. P. Cogdill, R. J. Bishop, H. Kim, C. C. Brewer, S. F. Rudy, C. VanWaes, J. L. Davis, A. Mathur, R. T. Ripley, D. A. Nathan, C. M. Laurencot, and S. A. Rosenberg. 2009. "Gene therapy with human and mouse T-cell receptors mediates cancer regression and targets normal tissues expressing cognate antigen." *Blood* 114 (3): 535–546. https://doi.org/10.1182/blood-2009-03-211714.

Kamperschroer, C., J. Shenton, H. Lebrec, J. K. Leighton, P. A. Moore, and O. Thomas. 2020. "Summary of a workshop on preclinical and translational safety assessment of CD3 bispecifics." *J Immunotoxicol* 17 (1): 67–85. https://doi.org/10.1080/1547691x.2020.1729902.

Kantarjian, H., A. Stein, N. Gökbuget, A. K. Fielding, A. C. Schuh, J. M. Ribera, A. Wei, H. Dombret, R. Foà, R. Bassan, Ö Arslan, M. A. Sanz, J. Bergeron, F. Demirkan, E. Lech-Maranda, A. Rambaldi, X. Thomas, H. A. Horst, M. Brüggemann, W. Klapper, B. L. Wood, A. Fleishman, D. Nagorsen, C. Holland, Z. Zimmerman, and M. S. Topp. 2017. "Blinatumomab versus chemotherapy for advanced acute lymphoblastic leukemia." *N Engl J Med* 376 (9): 836–847. https://doi.org/10.1056/NEJMoa1609783.

Kasiske, B. L., J. J. Snyder, D. T. Gilbertson, and C. Wang. 2004. "Cancer after kidney transplantation in the United States." *Am J Transplant* 4 (6): 905–913. https://doi.org/10.1111/j.1600-6143.2004.00450.x.

Kelly, E., and S. J. Russell. 2007. "History of oncolytic viruses: genesis to genetic engineering." *Mol Ther* 15 (4): 651–659. https://doi.org/10.1038/sj.mt.6300108.

Kochenderfer, J. N., W. H. Wilson, J. E. Janik, M. E. Dudley, M. Stetler-Stevenson, S. A. Feldman, I. Maric, M. Raffeld, D. A. Nathan, B. J. Lanier, R. A. Morgan, and S. A. Rosenberg. 2010. "Eradication of B-lineage cells and regression of lymphoma in a patient treated with autologous T cells genetically engineered to recognize CD19." *Blood* 116 (20): 4099–4102. https://doi.org/10.1182/blood-2010-04-281931.

Leach, D., M. Krummel, and J. Allison. 1996. "Enhancement of antitumor immunity by CTLA-4 blockade." *Science* 271: 1734–1736.

Leach, M. W., O. Clarke D, S. Dudal, C. Han, C. Li, Z. Yang, F. R. Brennan, W. J. Bailey, Y. Chen, A. Deslandes, L. I. Loberg, K. Mayawala, M. C. Rogge, M. Todd, and N. V. Chemuturi. 2020. "Strategies and recommendations for using a data-driven and risk-based approach in the selection of first-in-human starting dose: an international consortium for innovation and quality in pharmaceutical development (IQ) assessment." *Clin Pharmacol Ther*. https://doi.org/10.1002/cpt.2009.

Lee, D. W., B. D. Santomasso, F. L. Locke, A. Ghobadi, C. J. Turtle, J. N. Brudno, M. V. Maus, J. H. Park, E. Mead, S. Pavletic, W. Y. Go, L. Eldjerou, R. A. Gardner, N. Frey, K. J. Curran, K. Peggs, M. Pasquini, J. F. DiPersio, M. R. M. van den Brink, K. V. Komanduri, S. A. Grupp, and S. S. Neelapu. 2019. "ASTCT consensus grading for cytokine release syndrome and neurologic toxicity associated with immune effector cells." *Biol Blood Marrow Transplant* 25 (4): 625–638. https://doi.org/10.1016/j.bbmt.2018.12.758.

Leighton, J. K., H. Saber, G. Reaman, and R. Pazdur. 2016. "An FDA oncology view of juvenile animal studies in support of initial pediatric trials for anticancer drugs." *Regul Toxicol Pharmacol* 79: 142–143. https://doi.org/10.1016/j.yrtph.2016.03.001.

Lenschow, D. J., T. L. Walunas, and J. A. Bluestone. 1996. "CD28/B7 system of T cell costimulation." *Annu Rev Immunol* 14: 233–258. https://doi.org/10.1146/annurev.immunol.14.1.233.

Li, J., R. Piskol, R. Ybarra, Y. J. Chen, J. Li, D. Slaga, M. Hristopoulos, R. Clark, K. Modrusan, K. Totpal, M. R. Junttila, and T. T. Junttila. 2019. "CD3 bispecific antibody-induced cytokine release is dispensable for cytotoxic T cell activity." *Sci Transl Med* 11 (508). https://doi.org/10.1126/scitranslmed.aax8861.

Liu, B. L., M. Robinson, Z. Q. Han, R. H. Branston, C. English, P. Reay, Y. McGrath, S. K. Thomas, M. Thornton, P. Bullock, C. A. Love, and R. S. Coffin. 2003. "ICP34.5 deleted herpes simplex virus with enhanced oncolytic, immune stimulating, and anti-tumour properties." *Gene Ther* 10 (4): 292–303. https://doi.org/10.1038/sj.gt.3301885.

Martuza, R. L., A. Malick, J. M. Markert, K. L. Ruffner, and D. M. Coen. 1991. "Experimental therapy of human glioma by means of a genetically engineered virus mutant." *Science* 252 (5007): 854–856. https://doi.org/10.1126/science.1851332.

McCarthy, E. F. 2006. "The toxins of William B. Coley and the treatment of bone and soft-tissue sarcomas." *Iowa Orthop J* 26: 154–158.

Mease, K. M., A. L. Kimzey, and J. A. Lansita. 2017. "Biomarkers for nonclinical infusion reactions in marketed biotherapeutics and considerations for study design." *Curr Opin Toxicol* 4: 1–15. https://doi.org/10.1016/j.cotox.2017.03.005.

Mizui, M. 2019. "Natural and modified IL-2 for the treatment of cancer and autoimmune diseases." *Clin Immunol* 206: 63–70. https://doi.org/10.1016/j.clim.2018.11.002.

Moesta, A. K., K. Cooke, J. Piasecki, P. Mitchell, J. B. Rottman, K. Fitzgerald, J. Zhan, B. Yang, T. Le, B. Belmontes, O. F. Ikotun, K. Merriam, C. Glaus, K. Ganley, D. H. Cordover, A. M. Boden, R. Ponce, C. Beers, and P. J. Beltran. 2017. "Local delivery of OncoVEX(mGM-CSF) generates systemic antitumor immune responses enhanced by cytotoxic T-lymphocyte-associated protein blockade." *Clin Cancer Res* 23 (20): 6190–6202. https://doi.org/10.1158/1078-0432.Ccr-17-0681.

Morales, A., D. Eidinger, and A. W. Bruce. 1976. "Intracavitary Bacillus Calmette-Guerin in the treatment of superficial bladder tumors." *J Urol* 116 (2): 180–183. https://doi.org/10.1016/s0022-5347(17)58737-6.

Moyes, K. W., N. A. Lieberman, S. A. Kreuser, H. Chinn, C. Winter, G. Deutsch, V. Hoglund, R. Watson, and C. A. Crane. 2017. "Genetically engineered macrophages: a potential platform for cancer immunotherapy." *Hum Gene Ther* 28 (2): 200–215. https://doi.org/10.1089/hum.2016.060.

Mueller, N. 1995. "Overview: viral agents and cancer." *Environ Health Perspect* 103 (Suppl 8): 259–261. https://doi.org/10.1289/ehp.95103s8259.

Nauts, H. C., and J. R. McLaren. 1990. "Coley toxins – the first century." *Adv Exp Med Biol* 267: 483–500. https://doi.org/10.1007/978-1-4684-5766-7_52.

Neelapu, S. S., S. Tummala, P. Kebriaei, W. Wierda, C. Gutierrez, F. L. Locke, K. V. Komanduri, Y. Lin, N. Jain, N. Daver, J. Westin, A. M. Gulbis, M. E. Loghin, J. F. de Groot, S. Adkins, S. E. Davis, K. Rezvani, P. Hwu, and E. J. Shpall. 2018. "Chimeric antigen receptor T-cell therapy - assessment and management of toxicities." *Nat Rev Clin Oncol* 15 (1): 47–62. https://doi.org/10.1038/nrclinonc.2017.148.

Norelli, M., B. Camisa, G. Barbiera, L. Falcone, A. Purevdorj, M. Genua, F. Sanvito, M. Ponzoni, C. Doglioni, P. Cristofori, C. Traversari, C. Bordignon, F. Ciceri, R. Ostuni, C. Bonini, M. Casucci, and A. Bondanza. 2018. "Monocyte-derived IL-1 and IL-6 are differentially required for cytokine-release syndrome and neurotoxicity due to CAR T cells." *Nat Med* 24 (6): 739–748. https://doi.org/10.1038/s41591-018-0036-4.

Panchal, A., P. Seto, R. Wall, B. J. Hillier, Y. Zhu, J. Krakow, A. Datt, E. Pongo, A. Bagheri, T. T. Chen, J. D. Degenhardt, P. A. Culp, D. E. Dettling, M. V. Vinogradova, C. May, and R. B. DuBridge. 2020. "COBRA™: a highly potent conditionally active T cell engager engineered for the treatment of solid tumors." *MAbs* 12 (1): 1792130. https://doi.org/10.1080/19420862.2020.1792130.

Parish, C. R. 2003. "Cancer immunotherapy: the past, the present and the future." *Immunol Cell Biol* 81 (2): 106–113. https://doi.org/10.1046/j.0818-9641.2003.01151.x.

Parry, R. V., J. M. Chemnitz, K. A. Frauwirth, A. R. Lanfranco, I. Braunstein, S. V. Kobayashi, P. S. Linsley, C. B. Thompson, and J. L. Riley. 2005. "CTLA-4 and PD-1 receptors inhibit T-cell activation by distinct mechanisms." *Mol Cell Biol* 25 (21): 9543–9553. https://doi.org/10.1128/mcb.25.21.9543-9553.2005.

Penn, I. 1998. "Occurrence of cancers in immunosuppressed organ transplant recipients." *Clin Transpl* 147–158.

Penn, I. 2000. "Post-transplant malignancy: the role of immunosuppression." *Drug Saf* 23 (2): 101–113. https://doi.org/10.2165/00002018-200023020-00002.

Ponce, R. A., T. Gelzleichter, H. G. Haggerty, S. Heidel, M. S. Holdren, H. Lebrec, R. D. Mellon, and M. Pallardy. 2014. "Immunomodulation and lymphoma in humans." *J Immunotoxicol* 11 (1): 1–12. https://doi.org/10.3109/1547691X.2013.798388.

Prell, R. A., W. G. Halpern, and G. K. Rao. 2016. "Perspective on a modified developmental and reproductive toxicity testing dtrategy for vancer immunotherapy." *Int J Toxicol* 35 (3): 263–273. https://doi.org/10.1177/1091581815625596.

Rafiq, S., C. S. Hackett, and R. J. Brentjens. 2020. "Engineering strategies to overcome the current roadblocks in CAR T cell therapy." *Nat Rev Clin Oncol* 17 (3): 147–167. https://doi.org/10.1038/s41571-019-0297-y.

Ribas, A., and J. D. Wolchok. 2018. "Cancer immunotherapy using checkpoint blockade." *Science* 359 (6382): 1350–1355. https://doi.org/10.1126/science.aar4060.

Rocca, M., L. L. Morford, D. L. Blanset, W. G. Halpern, J. Cavagnaro, and C. J. Bowman. 2018. "Applying a weight of evidence approach to the evaluation of developmental toxicity of biopharmaceuticals." *Regul Toxicol Pharmacol* 98: 69–79. https://doi.org/10.1016/j.yrtph.2018.07.006.

Rosenberg, S. A., and N. P. Restifo. 2015. "Adoptive cell transfer as personalized immunotherapy for human cancer." *Science* 348 (6230): 62–68. https://doi.org/10.1126/science.aaa4967.

Saber, H., P. Del Valle, T. K. Ricks, and J. K. Leighton. 2017. "An FDA oncology analysis of CD3 bispecific constructs and first-in-human dose selection." *Regul Toxicol Pharmacol* 90: 144–152. https://doi.org/10.1016/j.yrtph.2017.09.001.

Saber, H., R. Gudi, M. Manning, E. Wearne, and J. K. Leighton. 2016. "An FDA oncology analysis of immune activating products and first-in-human dose selection." *Regul Toxicol Pharmacol* 81: 448–456. https://doi.org/10.1016/j.yrtph.2016.10.002.

Saber, H., and Leighton. 2015. "An FDA oncology analysis of antibody-drug conjugates." *Reg Toxicol Pharmacol* 71 (3): 444–452. https://doi.org/10.1016/j.yrtph.2015.01.014.

Sadelain, M., I. Rivière, and S. Riddell. 2017. "Therapeutic T cell engineering." *Nature* 545 (7655): 423–431. https://doi.org/10.1038/nature22395.

Salavoura, K., A. Kolialexi, G. Tsangaris, and A. Mavrou. 2008. "Development of cancer in patients with primary immunodeficiencies." *Anticancer Res* 28 (2b): 1263–1269.

Sato, E., S. H. Olson, J. Ahn, B. Bundy, H. Nishikawa, F. Qian, A. A. Jungbluth, D. Frosina, S. Gnjatic, C. Ambrosone, J. Kepner, T. Odunsi, G. Ritter, S. Lele, Y. T. Chen, H. Ohtani, L. J. Old, and K. Odunsi. 2005. "Intraepithelial CD8+ tumor-infiltrating lymphocytes and a high CD8+/regulatory T cell ratio are associated with favorable prognosis in ovarian cancer." *Proc Natl Acad Sci U S A* 102 (51): 18538–43. https://doi.org/10.1073/pnas.0509182102.

Schreiber, R. D., L. J. Old, and M. J. Smyth. 2011. "Cancer immunoediting: integrating immunity's roles in cancer suppression and promotion." *Science* 331 (6024): 1565–1570. https://doi.org/10.1126/science.1203486.

Selby, M. J., J. J. Engelhardt, R. J. Johnston, L. S. Lu, M. Han, K. Thudium, D. Yao, M. Quigley, J. Valle, C. Wang, B. Chen, P. M. Cardarelli, D. Blanset, and A. J. Korman. 2016. "Preclinical development of ipilimumab and nivolumab combination immunotherapy: mouse tumor models, in vitro functional studies, and cynomolgus macaque toxicology." *PLoS One* 11 (9): e0161779. https://doi.org/10.1371/journal.pone.0161779.

Selby, M. J., J. J. Engelhardt, M. Quigley, K. A. Henning, T. Chen, M. Srinivasan, and A. J. Korman. 2013. "Anti-CTLA-4 antibodies of IgG2a isotype enhance antitumor activity through reduction of intratumoral regulatory T cells." *Cancer Immunol Res* 1 (1): 32–42. https://doi.org/10.1158/2326-6066.Cir-13-0013.

Sfanos, K. S., T. C. Bruno, A. K. Meeker, A. M. De Marzo, W. B. Isaacs, and C. G. Drake. 2009. "Human prostate-infiltrating CD8+ T lymphocytes are oligoclonal and PD-1+." *Prostate* 69 (15): 1694–703. https://doi.org/10.1002/pros.21020.

Shi, J., P. W. Kantoff, R. Wooster, and O. C. Farokhzad. 2017. "Cancer nanomedicine: progress, challenges and opportunities." *Nat Rev Cancer* 17 (1): 20–37. https://doi.org/10.1038/nrc.2016.108.

Singh, A. P., S. Sharma, and D. K. Shah. 2016. "Quantitative characterization of in vitro bystander effect of antibody-drug conjugates." *J Pharmacokinet Pharmacodyn* 43 (6): 567–582. https://doi.org/10.1007/s10928-016-9495-8.

Staerz, U. D., and M. J. Bevan. 1986. "Hybrid hybridoma producing a bispecific monoclonal antibody that can focus effector T-cell activity." *Proc Natl Acad Sci U S A* 83 (5): 1453–1457. https://doi.org/10.1073/pnas.83.5.1453. https://pubmed.ncbi.nlm.nih.gov/2869486.

Sterner, R. M., R. Sakemura, M. J. Cox, N. Yang, R. H. Khadka, C. L. Forsman, M. J. Hansen, F. Jin, K. Ayasoufi, M. Hefazi, K. J. Schick, D. K. Walters, O. Ahmed, D. Chappell, T. Sahmoud, C. Durrant, W. K. Nevala, M. M. Patnaik, L. R. Pease, K. E. Hedin, N. E. Kay, A. J. Johnson, and S. S. Kenderian. 2019. "GM-CSF inhibition reduces cytokine release syndrome and neuroinflammation but enhances CAR-T cell function in xenografts." *Blood* 133 (7): 697–709. https://doi.org/10.1182/blood-2018-10-881722.

Straface, G., A. Selmin, V. Zanardo, M. De Santis, A. Ercoli, and G. Scambia. 2012. "Herpes simplex virus infection in pregnancy." *Infect Dis Obstet Gynecol* 2012: 385697. https://doi.org/10.1155/2012/385697.

Suntharalingam, G., M. R. Perry, S. Ward, S. J. Brett, A. Castello-Cortes, M. D. Brunner, and N. Panoskaltsis. 2006. "Cytokine storm in a phase 1 trial of the anti-CD28 monoclonal antibody TGN1412." *N Engl J Med* 355 (10): 1018–1028. https://doi.org/10.1056/NEJMoa063842.

Topalian, S. L., C. G. Drake, and D. M. Pardoll. 2015. "Immune checkpoint blockade: a common denominator approach to cancer therapy." *Cancer Cell* 27 (4): 450–461. https://doi.org/10.1016/j.ccell.2015.03.001.

Topp, M. S., N. Gökbuget, A. S. Stein, G. Zugmaier, S. O'Brien, R. C. Bargou, H. Dombret, A. K. Fielding, L. Heffner, R. A. Larson, S. Neumann, R. Foà, M. Litzow, J. M. Ribera, A. Rambaldi, G. Schiller, M. Brüggemann, H. A. Horst, C. Holland, C. Jia, T. Maniar, B. Huber, D. Nagorsen, S. J. Forman, and H. M. Kantarjian. 2015. "Safety and activity of blinatumomab for adult patients with relapsed or refractory B-precursor acute lymphoblastic leukaemia: a multicentre, single-arm, phase 2 study." *Lancet Oncol* 16 (1): 57–66. https://doi.org/10.1016/s1470-2045(14)71170-2.

Tosolini, M., A. Kirilovsky, B. Mlecnik, T. Fredriksen, S. Mauger, G. Bindea, A. Berger, P. Bruneval, W. H. Fridman, F. Pagès, and J. Galon. 2011. "Clinical impact of different classes of infiltrating T cytotoxic and helper cells (Th1, th2, treg, th17) in patients with colorectal cancer." *Cancer Res* 71 (4): 1263–1271. https://doi.org/10.1158/0008-5472.Can-10-2907.

Trenevska, I., D. Li, and A. H. Banham. 2017. "Therapeutic antibodies against intracellular tumor antigens." *Front Immunol* 8: 1001. https://doi.org/10.3389/fimmu.2017.01001.

Trinklein, N. D., D. Pham, U. Schellenberger, B. Buelow, A. Boudreau, P. Choudhry, S. C. Clarke, K. Dang, K. E. Harris, S. Iyer, B. Jorgensen, P. P. Pratap, U. S. Rangaswamy, H. S. Ugamraj, O. Vafa, A. P. Wiita, W. van Schooten, R. Buelow, and S. Force Aldred. 2019. "Efficient tumor killing and minimal cytokine release with novel T-cell agonist bispecific antibodies." *MAbs* 11 (4): 639–652. https://doi.org/10.1080/19420862.2019.1574521.

Vere Hodge, R. A., and H. J. Field. 2013. "Antiviral agents for herpes simplex virus." *Adv Pharmacol* 67: 1–38. https://doi.org/10.1016/b978-0-12-405880-4.00001-9.

Vesely, M. D., M. H. Kershaw, R. D. Schreiber, and M. J. Smyth. 2011. "Natural innate and adaptive immunity to cancer." *Annu Rev Immunol* 29: 235–271. https://doi.org/10.1146/annurev-immunol-031210-101324.

Vidal, J. M., T. T. Kawabata, R. Thorpe, B. Silva-Lima, K. Cederbrant, S. Poole, J. Mueller-Berghaus, M. Pallardy, and J. W. Van der Laan. 2010. "In vitro cytokine release assays for predicting cytokine release syndrome: the current state-of-the-science. Report of a European Medicines Agency Workshop." *Cytokine* 51 (2): 213–215. https://doi.org/10.1016/j.cyto.2010.04.008.

Villanueva, M. T. 2019. "STINGing systemically." *Nat Rev Drug Discov* 18 (1): 15. https://doi.org/10.1038/nrd.2018.236.

Wang, and H. Lebrec. 2017. "Immunophenotyping: application to safety assessment." *Toxicol Pathol* 45 (7): 1004–1011. https://doi.org/10.1177/0192623317736742.

Wang, Q., Y. Chen, J. Park, X. Liu, Y. Hu, T. Wang, K. McFarland, and M. J. Betenbaugh. 2019. "Design and production of bispecific antibodies." *Antibodies (Basel, Switzerland)* 8 (3): 43. https://doi.org/10.3390/antib8030043. https://pubmed.ncbi.nlm.nih.gov/31544849.

Weber, E. W., M. V. Maus, and C. L. Mackall. 2020. "The emerging landscape of immune cell therapies." *Cell* 181 (1): 46–62. https://doi.org/10.1016/j.cell.2020.03.001.

Wiemann, B., and C. O. Starnes. 1994. "Coley's toxins, tumor necrosis factor and cancer research: a historical perspective." *Pharmacol Ther* 64 (3): 529–564. https://doi.org/10.1016/0163-7258(94)90023-x.

Yao, W., J. C. He, Y. Yang, J. M. Wang, Y. W. Qian, T. Yang, and L. Ji. 2017. "The prognostic value of tumor-infiltrating lymphocytes in hepatocellular carcinoma: a systematic review and meta-analysis." *Sci Rep* 7 (1): 7525. https://doi.org/10.1038/s41598-017-08128-1.

Yoshida, T., J. Kato, I. Inoue, N. Yoshimura, H. Deguchi, C. Mukoubayashi, M. Oka, M. Watanabe, S. Enomoto, T. Niwa, T. Maekita, M. Iguchi, H. Tamai, H. Utsunomiya, N. Yamamichi, M. Fujishiro, M. Iwane, T. Takeshita, T. Ushijima, and M. Ichinose. 2014. "Cancer development based on chronic active gastritis and resulting gastric atrophy as assessed by serum levels of pepsinogen and *Helicobacter pylori* antibody titer." *Int J Cancer* 134 (6): 1445–1457. https://doi.org/10.1002/ijc.28470.

Zhang, L., J. R. Conejo-Garcia, D. Katsaros, P. A. Gimotty, M. Massobrio, G. Regnani, A. Makrigiannakis, H. Gray, K. Schlienger, M. N. Liebman, S. C. Rubin, and G. Coukos. 2003. "Intratumoral T cells, recurrence, and survival in epithelial ovarian cancer." *N Engl J Med* 348 (3): 203–213. https://doi.org/10.1056/NEJMoa020177.

Zhou, G., and H. Levitsky. 2012. "Towards curative cancer immunotherapy: overcoming posttherapy tumor escape." *Clin Dev Immunol* 2012: 124187–124187. https://doi.org/10.1155/2012/124187.

29

Non-Clinical Safety Evaluation of Immunomodulatory Biological Therapeutics for the Treatment of Immune-Mediated Diseases

Frank R. Brennan
Novartis Institute of BioMedical Research

CONTENTS

29.1 Introduction

Chronic inflammatory, autoimmune and allergic diseases and transplant rejection are diseases driven by a dysregulated immune system. The aim of an effective therapeutic for these immune-mediated diseases is to suppress or modify the immune system to dampen the inflammation. As of January 2020, there are approximately 42 innovator biological drugs (monoclonal antibodies (mAbs) and immunoglobulin (Ig)G Fc-fusion proteins) and 6 biosimilars approved for treatment of chronic human inflammatory, autoimmune and allergic diseases and organ transplantation (henceforth referred to as immune-mediated diseases), including rheumatoid arthritis (RA), ankylosing spondylitis (AS), psoriatic arthritis (PsA),

psoriasis (Ps), multiple sclerosis (MS), systemic lupus erythematosus (SLE), Crohn's disease (CrD), ulcerative colitis (UC), atopic dermatitis (AD) and asthma (Table 29.1) [1]. Many more are in late-stage clinical development for these and other diseases such as uveitis, type-1 diabetes (T1D), type-2 diabetes (T2D), autoantibody-driven autoimmune diseases, idiopathic pulmonary fibrosis (IPF) and chronic obstructive pulmonary disease (COPD) [2,3]. The vast majority of drugs indicated for the treatment of these diseases are generally designed to dampen the activity of soluble mediators (cytokines, growth factors, complement, pathogenic immunoglobulins, etc.), inhibit the function of cell surface receptors or deplete cells that are driving disease pathogenesis with resulting immunosuppression [2–5]. The clinical success of some of these mAbs/fusions proteins, such as the tumor necrosis

DOI: 10.1201/9781003124542-33

TABLE 29.1

mAbs and Fc-Fusion Proteins Approved by FDA and/or EMA for Inflammatory/Autoimmune Disease Indications (Excludes Biosimilars)

INN Name	Trade Name	Company	Species/Isotype	Target	Inflammatory Indication(s)	MoA
Alefacept	Amevive®	Astellas	Human LFA-3-FcIgG1	CD2	Ps	Inhibition of T cell function (binds CD2 on T cells blocking interaction with LFA-3 on APC)
Muromonab	Orthoclone-OKT3®	Janssen-Cilag	Mouse IgG2a	CD3	Organ rejection (renal, heart, liver)	Inhibits T cell function
Efalizumab	#Raptiva®	Genentech, Merck Serono	Humanized IgG1	CD11a (LFA-1)	Ps	Blocks inflammatory T cell migration
Daclizumab	#Zenapax®	Roche	Humanized IgG1	CD25 (IL-2R)	Organ rejection (renal)	Inhibits T cell function
Basilixumab	Simulect®	Novartis	Chimeric IgG1	CD25	Organ rejection (renal)	Inhibits T cell function
Natalizumab	Tysabri®	Biogen IDEC, Elan	Humanized IgG4	CD49d (VLA-4)	MS, CrD	Blocks inflammatory T cell migration
Vedolizumab	Entyvio®	Takeda-Millennium	Humanized IgG1	α4β7	UC, CrD	Inhibits cellular adhesion interactions between α4β7 and MAdCAM-1 and fibronectin, thus inhibiting lymphocyte migration to gut
Abatacept	Orencia®	Bristol-Myers Squibb	Human CTLA4-FcIgG1	CD80, CD86	RA, JIA	Inhibition of T cell function (binds to CD80 and CD86 on APCs leading to blocking of CD28 interaction and T cell activation)
Belatacept	Nulojix®	Bristol-Myers Squibb	Human CTLA-4-IgG Fc-IgG4	CD80, CD86	Organ rejection (renal)	Inhibition of T cell function (binds to CD80 and CD86 on APCs leading to blocking of CD28 interactions and T cell activation)
Rituximab	Rituxan®, Mabthera™	Biogen-IDEC, Roche	Chimeric IgG1	CD20	RA*	B cell depletion by ADCC, CDC and apoptosis
Ocrelizumab	Ocrevus®	Roche	Humanized IgG1	CD20	MS	Induce B cell depletion by ADCC, CDC and apoptosis induction
Belimumab	Benlysta® Lymphostat B	Human Genome Sciences	Human IgG1	BLyS (BAFF)	SLE	B cell depletion by apoptosis (block BLyS binding to BCMA, BAFFR and TACI required for B cell maturation/survival)
Alemtuzumab	Campath®	Genzyme, Bayer	Humanized IgG1	CD52	RA, MS	Depletes leukocytes (T and B cells monocytes, macrophages) by ADCC
Infliximab	Remicade®	Johnson & Johnson	Chimeric IgG1	TNFα	RA, CrD, UC, AS, Ps, PsA	Blocks TNFα-mediated leukocyte migration, inhibition of apoptosis, macrophage, osteoclast, and EC activation
Etanercept	Enbrel®	Amgen, Pfizer	Human TNFR-FcIgG1	TNFα	RA, Ps, CrD	Blocks TNFα-activity
Adalimumab	Humira®/ Trudexa®	Abbott	Human IgG1	TNFα	RA, CrD, AS, Ps, PsA, JIA	Blocks TNFα-activity
Certolizumab pegol	Cimzia®	UCB	Humanized Fab-PEG	TNFα	CrD	Blocks TNFα activity
Golimumab	Simponi®	Johnson & Johnson	Human IgG1	TNFα	RA, AS, PsA	Blocks TNFα activity
Anakinra	Kineret	Biovitrum	IL-1RA (modified)	IL-1	RA. AOSD	Blocks IL-1β-mediated leukocyte migration, macrophage and osteoclast activation, DC activation, Th17 differentiation
Rilonacept	Arcalyst®	Regeneron	IL1R1-IL-1RAcP-IgG1-Fc-fusion protein (soluble decoy receptor)	IL-1	CAPS	Blocks IL-1β-mediated leukocyte migration, macrophage and osteoclast activation, DC activation, Th17 differentiation; binds IL-1α and IL-1 receptor antagonist (IL-1ra) with reduced affinity
Canakinumab	Ilaris®	Novartis	Human IgG1	IL-1β	CAPS	Blocks IL-1β-mediated leukocyte migration, macrophage and osteoclast activation, DC activation, Th17 differentiation

(Continued)

TABLE 29.1 (*Continued*)

mAbs and Fc-Fusion Proteins Approved by FDA and/or EMA for Inflammatory/Autoimmune Disease Indications (Excludes Biosimilars)

INN Name	Trade Name	Company	Species/Isotype	Target	Inflammatory Indication(s)	MoA
Dupilumab	Dupixent®	Regeneron, Sanofi	Human IgG4	IL-4Rα	Asthma (eosinophilic), AD	Blocking IL-4Rα with dupilumab inhibits IL-4 and IL-13 cytokine-induced responses, including the release of proinflammatory cytokines, chemokines and IgE
Mepolizumab	Nucala®	GlaxoSmithkline	Humanized IgG1	IL-5	Asthma (eosinophilic)	Inhibits IL-5-mediated eosinophil maturation, activation and migration (binds IL-5, thereby blocking binding to IL-5R on eosinophils).
Reslizumab	Cinqair®	Teva (Ception Therapeutics)	Humanized IgG4	IL-5	Asthma (eosinophilic)	Inhibits IL-5 activity
Benralizumab	Fasenra®	AZ-MedImmune	Humanized IgG1 (afucosylated)	IL-5Rα	Asthma (eosinophilic)	Inhibits IL-5 activity
Tocilizumab	Actemra® RoActemra®	Roche/Chugai	Humanized IgG1	IL-6R	RA, JIA	Binds soluble and membrane-bound IL-6 receptors, hindering IL-6 induced inflammation. Blocks IL-6-mediated B/T cell and osteoclast activation, inhibition of T cell apoptosis, Th17 differentiation
Sarilumab	Kevzara®	Sanofi (from Regeneron)	Human IgG1	IL-6Rα	RA	Inhibits IL-6 activity
Siltuximab	Sylvant®	Janssen	Chimeric IgG1	IL-6	Castleman's Disease	Inhibits IL-6 activity
Ustekinumab	Stelara®	Janssen, Johnson & Johnson	Human IgG1	IL-12, IL-23 (p40)	Ps	Binds to the p-40 subunit of both IL-12 and IL-23, blocking T-cell activation and inflammatory responses. Blocks IL-12-mediated TH1/NK cell activation and TNFα/IFN-γ release; blocks IL-23-mediated TH17 cell expansion and IL-17/IL-22 release
Secukinumab	Cosentyx®	Novartis	Human IgG1	IL-17A	Ps, RA/PsA, AS	Blocks IL-17A-mediated proinflammatory cytokine/chemokine production, granulocyte and monocyte mobilization, TNFα/IL-1b production, ICAM-1 expression, DC maturation, EC and osteoclast activation
Ixekizumab	Talz®	Eli Lilly	Humanized IgG4	IL-17A	Ps, PsA, RA	Blocks IL-17A activity
Brodalumab	Siliq®/ Kyntheum®	Valeant Pharma	Human IgG2	IL-17RA	Ps	Inhibits IL-17A receptor (blocks activity of IL-17A, C, E (IL-25), F and A/F); IL-17RA is found on a variety of cells including fibroblasts, epithelial cells and monocytes
Guselkumab	Tremfya®	J&J-Janssen	Human IgG1	IL-23 (p19)	Ps, RA	Blocks IL-23-mediated activation of IL-17-producing cells
Tildrakizumab	Ilumya®/ Ilumetri	Sun Pharma	Humanized IgG1	IL-23 (p19)	Ps	Blocks IL-23-mediated activation of IL-17-producing cells
Risankizumab	Skyrizi™	BI/AbbVie	Humanized IgG4	IL-23 (p19)	Ps	Blocks IL-23-mediated activation of IL-17-producing cells
Emapalumab	Gamifant®	NovImmune	Human	IFN-γ	HLH	Blocks IL-IFN-γ activity
Omalizumab	Xolair®	Genentech, Roche, Novartis	Humanized IgG1	IgE	Allergic Asthma	Blocks IgE binding to, and cross-linking of FcεRI, mast cells
Eculizumab	Soliris®	Alexion	Humanized IgG2/4	C5	PNH	Blocks complement C5, inhibiting its cleavage to C5a and C5b and generation of membrane attack complex C5b-C9
Ravulizumab	Ultomiris™	Alexion	Humanized	C5	PNH, aHUS	Blocks complement C5, inhibiting its cleavage to C5a and C5b and generation of membrane attack complex C5b-C9

#Products now withdrawn; *also approved in non-Hodgkin's lymphoma.

AD, atopic dermatitis; ADCC, antibody-dependent cellular cytotoxicity; aHUS. Atypical hemolytic uremic syndrome; AOSD, adult-onset Still's disease; APC, antigen-presenting cell; AS, ankylosing spondylitis; BAFF, B cell-activating factor; BCMA, B cell maturation antigen; CAPS, cryopyrin-associated period syndromes; CDC, complement-dependent cytotoxicity; CrD, Crohn's disease; CTLA-4, cytotoxic T lymphocyte antigen-4; C5, complement C 5; DC, dendritic cell; EC, endothelial cell; HLH, hemophagocytic lymphohistiocytosis; IFN-γ. Interferon-gamma; IL, Interleukin; INN, International Non-Proprietary Name, JIA, juvenile idiopathic arthritis; LFA-1/3, leukocyte function antigen-1/3; MS, multiple sclerosis; NK, natural killer; PNH, paroxysmal nocturnal hemoglobinuria; Ps, psoriasis; PsA, psoriatic arthritis; RA, rheumatoid arthritis; SLE; systemic lupus erythematosus; TACI, transmembrane activator and calcium modulator and cyclophilin ligand interactor; Th, T helper; TNFα, tumor necrosis factor-α; UC, ulcerative colitis; VLA-4, very late antigen-4.

factor (TNF) and IL-17 blockers, has served unmet medical needs and greatly improved the lives of many patients. Accordingly, the development and approval of biologics have grown steadily over the past 10 years and many more are expected to be approved, encouraged by the desire to improve on the clinical efficacy achieved by the first-generation products and the growing understanding of the mechanism of action (MoA) of protein-based therapeutics and disease etiologies that might realize the potential for disease modification, immune tolerance, immune reset, tissue repair and ultimately to disease resolution [6,7]. The high specificity of biological drugs, in combination with their multifunctional properties, high potency, long half-life (permitting intermittent dosing and prolonged pharmacological effects) and general lack of off-target toxicity, makes them ideal therapeutics, with the potential to intervene early in at-risk populations and prevent tissue damage. In parallel, there is the continuing development of bioengineering technologies to both optimize and overcome existing biophysical, functional and immunogenic limitations of biologics, and to develop molecules with new specificities and functions and optimized pharmacokinetic (PK)/pharmacodynamic (PD) properties.

Dosing with mAbs/proteins for these severe and debilitating but often non-life-threatening diseases is usually prolonged, for several months (mos) or years, and affects not only adults, including sensitive populations such as women of child-bearing potential (WoCBP) and the elderly, but also children. Immunosuppression is usually a therapeutic goal of these mAbs and when administered to patients whose treatment program often involves other immunosuppressive therapies, there is an inherent risk for frank immunosuppression and reduced host defense, which when prolonged, increases the risk of infection and cancer. In addition, when mAbs and other biologics interact with the immune system, they can induce other adverse immune-mediated drug reactions such as infusion reactions, cytokine release syndrome, anaphylaxis, immune-complex-mediated pathology and autoimmunity.

This chapter provides a brief overview of the pathogenesis of the major immune-mediated diseases, the classes of drugs being developed to treat these diseases and their MoAs. Specific emphasis is placed on mAbs (and mAb-related constructs) and Fc-fusion proteins since these represent all of the approved products (Table 29.1). Other classes of biologics in preclinical and early clinical development, such as tolerogenic peptides and dendritic cells (DCs), stem cells and T regulatory cells (T regs)-based therapies [6,8], gene editing-based therapies [9] and oligonucleotide-based therapies [10], may be more antigen-specific, but harboring the same safety concerns regarding prolonged immunosuppression/immunomodulation, albeit potentially reduced. Hence, they will only be briefly discussed since the modality-specific safety concerns associated with these therapies will be covered in separate chapters. The non-clinical safety assessment and risk mitigation strategies utilized to characterize these immunosuppressive biologics is reviewed, with case studies to highlight some of the key challenges. These include the design of studies to qualify animal species for toxicology studies, early studies to investigate the safety and define PK/PD relationships, general toxicity studies, immunotoxicity, developmental, reproductive and juvenile toxicity studies, assessing the potential for immunosuppression and reduced host defense against infection and cancer and first-in-human (FIH) dose setting.

29.2 Overview of the Immune System and Key Immunological Pathways Driving Inflammatory, Autoimmune and Allergic Diseases

The immune system is composed of a complex array of diverse immunocompetent cells (predominantly leukocytes such as T and B lymphocytes, monocytes/macrophages, granulocytes, mast cells and DCs), and proinflammatory and anti-inflammatory mediators (cytokines, chemokines, growth factors and complement components) that coexist in regulated networks (Figures 29.1 and 29.2; refer also to the Glossary of Immunological Terms in Appendix 1). These components interact through cascades and utilize positive and negative feedback loops to maintain normal inflammation (e.g., during wound healing) and immunosurveillance against invading pathogens. However, during autoimmune and allergic diseases, a foreign or self (auto)-antigen or allergen might trigger the dysregulation of these networks leading to altered immunity, persistent inflammation and ultimately pathologic sequelae [11,12]. Indeed, there is a considerable body of data demonstrating that various components of the immune system including leukocytes and proinflammatory cytokines are dysregulated in a number of immunological diseases. These diseases can be broadly categorized into those inflammatory/autoimmune diseases that exhibit an immunological profile characterized by a T helper cell (Th) 1/Th17 response (e.g., RA, Ps, MS, and inflammatory bowel disease (IBD)) versus allergic diseases (e.g., asthma and AD) with a predominantly Th2 cell profile although it is accepted that certain diseases, and indeed, subsets of patients within a disease do not fit this simplistic classification. The initiation of an adaptive cell-mediated immune response (to both foreign and self-antigen) begins with the production of proinflammatory cytokines from innate immune cells (myeloid cells such as DCs, monocytes/macrophages and granulocytes), as well as from tissue cells such as fibroblasts, smooth muscle cells and epithelial and endothelial cells) in response to an induction stimulus (e.g., infection, injury, and allergen exposure) that drives the activation of naive CD4$^+$ T cells and their differentiation into specific Th cell subsets with distinct effector functions (Figure 29.1). Autocrine production of interferon-γ (IFN-γ) (driven by IL-12 and IL-18), interleukin-4 (IL-4) and IL-21 promotes the differentiation of Th1, Th2 and T follicular helper (TFH) cells, respectively, while IL-6, IL-23, IL-1 and transforming growth factor-β (TGF-β)) produced by non-T cells create an environment that favors Th17 development. IFN-γ and TNFα secreted by Th1 cells activate macrophages and DCs to generate, e.g., reactive oxygen and nitrogen species, and recruited neutrophils, all of which are pivotal in mediating host defense against microbial species but also can induce collateral tissue damage. In addition, Th1 memory

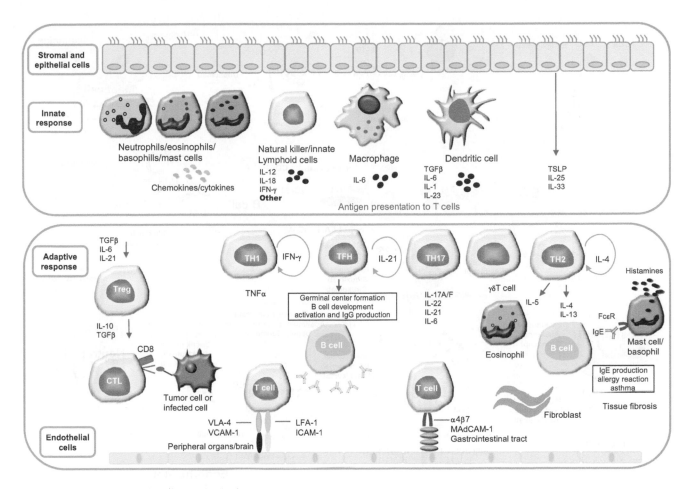

FIGURE 29.1 Overview of innate and adaptive immune responses

cells are key for the survival and function of memory CD8+ T cells. IL-21 secreted by TFH cells promotes germinal center formation and B cell development, activation and immuno-globulin production. Cytokines such as IL-4 and IFN-γ pro-mote immunoglobulin class switching. IL-17A, IL-17F and IL-22 produced by Th17 cells and γδ T cells mediate an anti-bacterial activity at epithelial barriers by promoting recruit-ment and activation of neutrophils and macrophages (type-1 effector) and epithelial cells.

However, dysregulated Th17 cells can also drive organ-specific autoimmunity, e.g., RA, Ps, IBD via secretion of IL-17A/F. IL-1, IL-6, IL-12, IL-18 and colony-stimulating fac-tor (CSF)2 (granulocyte/monocyte (GM-CSF)) from macro-phages, DCs and other cells promote these autoinflammatory Th1 and Th17 responses. TH2 cells protect against chronic nematode infection but are also responsible for allergy, asthma and tissue fibrosis by the secretion of IL-4, IL-5 and IL-13. Cytokines such as thymic stromal lymphopoietin (TSLP), IL-25 and IL-33 produced by stromal cells and other T cells induce the production of these cytokines and serve to induce and amplify this Th2 cell allergic environment. IL-5 is key for eosinophilic inflammation, whereas IL-4 and IL-13 pro-mote B cell immunoglobulin E (IgE) production (that binds FcεR and drives mast cell activation following cross-linking by an allergen), goblet cell mucus secretion, fibrosis and alternative activation of macrophages (type-2 macrophages). Tregs (e.g., natural CD4+/CD25+FoxP3+ cells and induced IL-10-secreting cells) interacting with specific tolerogenic DC subsets can efficiently control effector T cells response to self- and non-self-antigens through the expression of anti-inflammatory molecules such as IL-10, TGF-β and IL-35 and/or inhibitory receptors such as CTLA-4, LAG-3, GITR, CD39 and CD73 [13]. These T regs and DCs are frequently dysregulated during inflammatory diseases. In view of their pivotal role in autoimmune and allergic disease development, maintenance and chronicity, T and B cells, cytokines, che-mokines and other soluble mediators as well as cell surface receptors that promote the recruitment, activation, regula-tion and survival of these and other leukocytes represent the major targets of mAbs for immunological disease therapy (see Tables 29.1 and 29.2 and Figure 29.2). Other cell types such as macrophage subsets, granulocytes, NK-T cell and inate lymphoid cells (ILCs), MAIT cells and fibroblasts are also targets for reducing and resolving inflammation and promot-ing tissue repair [5]. However, since many of the immune cells and pathways are involved in combating infections by bacte-ria, viruses, fungi and parasites as well as involved in tumor immunosurveillance, and biologic therapies aim to suppress/modulate these responses, efficacy/benefit has to be finely bal-anced with the increased infection and cancer risk.

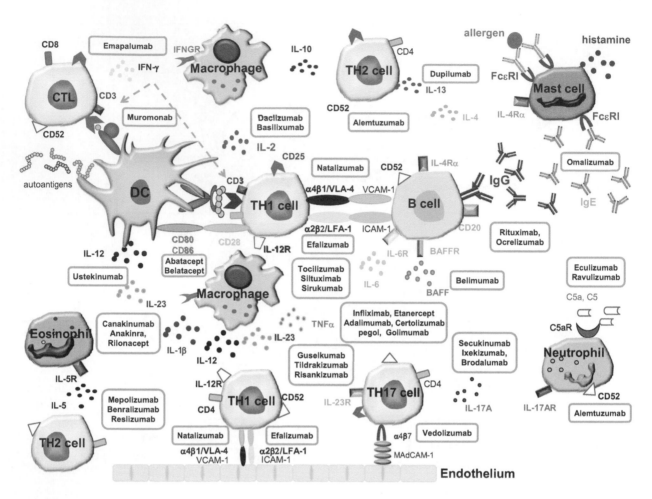

FIGURE 29.2 Overview of approved mAbs and Fc-fusion proteins and their immune targets

TABLE 29.2

Toxicology Studies Performed for FDA-/EMEA-Approved mAbs/Fusion Proteins for Inflammatory/Autoimmune Disease Indications

INN Name	Target	Toxicology Species	Key Toxicology Studies	Findings
Alefacept	CD2	Cyno, baboon	44–47-wk tox. and EFD-PPND studies in cynos; 3-mo study in baboons	↓T cells in blood and lymphoid organs; mild↓TDAR to KLH but not HSA; lymphoma in 1 animal after 28 wks
Muromonab	CD3	Rhesus macaque	2-wk tox. study with 10-mo observation period	↑number and size of germinal centers in spleen and LNs
Efalizumab	CD11a (LFA-1)	Mouse (surrogate)	26-wk nonterminal chimpanzee study; 4-wk mouse tox., fertility, EFD and PPND (with surrogate); 6-mo carcinogenicity study in p53 KO mice	↓humoral response, ↑WBC, ↓LN cellularity; ↓DTH a and TDAR responses
Daclizumab	CD2 (IL-2R)	Cynomolgus macaque (cyno)	SD mouse and rabbit tox. 4-wk cyno tox.	None
Basilixumab	CD25	Rhesus, cyno	4-wk rhesus tox., cyno EFD	None
Vedolizumab	α4β7	Cyno, rabbit	13-wk rabbit and cyno tox., 26-wk cyno tox; rabbit EFD, cyno ePPND; rhesus EAE model	↓lymphocytes in GI tract. No impact on TDAR/NK cells Lymphoplasmacytic gastritis at all doses in 26- wk cyno (NOAEL not identified) ADA-related lymphoid hyperplasia No ↓CNS immunosurveillance in rhesus EAE model; no reprotox.

(Continued)

TABLE 29.2 (*Continued*)

Toxicology Studies Performed for FDA-/EMEA-Approved mAbs/Fusion Proteins for Inflammatory/Autoimmune Disease Indications

INN Name	Target	Toxicology Species	Key Toxicology Studies	Findings
Natalizumab	CD49d (VLA-4)	Cyno, rhesus, guinea pig, mouse	2-wk tox. mouse 26-wk tox. and EFD cyno 26-wk juvenile tox. cyno Fertility, EFD and PPND guinea pig; 4-wk combination tox. with Avonex (IFN-β) rhesus Effects on VLA-4-expressing tumor growth in SCID and nude mice	(↑WBC, ↑reticulocytes, ↑spleen weight and follicular hypertrophy, ↓liver and thymus weight (neonates only), lymphoplasmacytic inflammation of the colon; ↓female fertility; glomerulonephritis in cynos related to immunogenicity; anaphylaxis in guinea pigs related to immunogenicity
Abatacept	CD80, CD86	Cyno, mouse rat, rabbit	4-, 26- and 52-wk tox. cyno; 26-wk tox. mouse, rat fertility, EFD and PPND; rabbit EFD; 84–88-wk mouse carcinogenicity study	↓serum IgG, ↓T and B cell activation, ↓splenic B cells in adults, ↑TDAR and thyroid inflammation in neonates; ↑lymphoma and mammary gland tumors
Belatacept	CD80, CD86	Cyno, rat, rabbit	4-wk tox. cyno; fertility, EFD and PPND studies in rat; EFD study in rabbit	↓serum IgG, ↓germinal centers in spleen and LN, low-level infection in pregnant dams, ↑TDAR and thyroid inflammation in female neonates
Rituximab	CD20	Cyno	8-wk tox., EFD and PPND cyno	↓B cells in blood and lymphoid organs of mothers and infants
Ocrelizumab	CD20	Cyno	4- and 20-wk tox., EFD and ePPND cyno	Reversible dose-related ↓B cells, lymphocytes, RBC, ↑reticulocytes; histopath: lymphoid follicular atrophy in lymph nodes and spleen; erythroid cell hypercellularity of bone marrow Perinatal mortality: both affected neonates had bacterial infections
Belimumab	BLyS (BAFF)	Cyno	4- and 26-wk tox. and EFD-PPND cyno	↓B cells in blood and lymphoid organs of mother and infants; ↓IgG, IgM and IgE; interstitial and germinal cell hyperplasia in ovaries; hyperplasia in stomach, vasculitis in heart and arterial hyperplasia in kidney at high dose; slight ↑fetal death
Alemtuzumab	CD52	Cyno	30-day cyno tox. (ADA restricted dosing duration)	↓WBCs, lymphopenia, neutropenia, ↓serum total protein and albumin
Infliximab	TNFα	Chimp, mouse (surrogate)	5-day nonterminal chimp study; 26- wk tox. EFD and PPND mouse (with surrogate)	No significant effects (possibly slight ↓male fertility, bilateral crystalline deposits in lens capsule of males of unknown relevance. No reprotox.
Etanercept	TNFα	Cyno, rat, rabbit	28-day and 26-wk cyno tox. 12-wk immunogenicity studies in mice, rats and rabbits; rat EFD and PPND; rabbit EFD	No significant effects (mild ↑eosinophil and lymphocytes at injection site) No reprotox.
Adalimumab	TNFα	Cyno	4- and 39-wk tox. and EFD-PPND cyno	↓thymus weight and involution, ↓splenic follicular centers and DCs; ↓T cells in thymus and B cells in spleen (males only) No reprotox.
Certolizumab pegol	TNFα	Cyno, mouse (surrogate)	28-day, 13-, 26- and 52-wk cyno tox; 52- wk cyno juvenile tox.; rat FEED, EFD & PPND (with surrogate)	↓hemoglobin, RBC and PCV, ↑WBC, histiocytic vacuolation (foamy macrophages) at high dose at injection sites, lymphoid organs, choroid plexus and other organs, ↑aPTT (all in cynos) No reprotox.
Golimumab	TNFα	Cyno	1-mo, 25- and 26-wk tox, EFD and PPND cyno; supporting data from mouse FEED, EFD and PPND studies with surrogate mAb used to support infliximab approval	Mild ↓TDAR in 25-wk IV study but not in 26-wk SC study, mild reversible ↑B cells No reprotox.
Anakinra	IL-1	Rhesus, rats, rabbits	2-and 4-wk rhesus tox. 2-wk and 6-mo rat tox.; rat and rabbit EFD, rat FEED	No significant effects (injection site reactions) No reprotox.
Rilonacept	IL-1	Cyno, mouse (surrogate)	3-, 6- (non-GLP) and 26-wk tox. and EFD cyno Mouse FEED and EFD (with surrogate)	ADA-related tox. in multiple organs at the low and mid doses. Mineralization of ovaries, mononuclear cell infiltration of ovaries and uterus, ↓estrogen, ↓ossification of growth plate; atrophy of thymus and lymph nodes

(*Continued*)

TABLE 29.2 (*Continued*)

Toxicology Studies Performed for FDA-/EMEA-Approved mAbs/Fusion Proteins for Inflammatory/Autoimmune Disease Indications

INN Name	Target	Toxicology Species	Key Toxicology Studies	Findings
Canakinumab	IL-1β	Marmoset, mouse (surrogate)	4-, 13- and 26-wk tox. and EFD marmoset; mouse FEED, EFD, PPND and juvenile tox. with surrogate mAb	No effect in 26-wk study but minimal-slight lymphoid hyperplasia in spleen in 13-wk study; slight developmental delay, incomplete bone ossification in mice and marmoset F1, slight ↑bent tail in marmoset F1, slight ↓reproductive performance in mice; slight ↑histiocytosis in lymph nodes in F1 mice; deaths related to immunogenicity of surrogate in mice
Dupilumab	IL-4α	Cyno, mouse (surrogate)	13- and 26-wk cyno tox.; Cyno EFD/PPND; mouse FEED (with surrogate)	No effects except ↓ IgE levels in 13- wk study No reprotox.
Mepolizumab	IL-5	Cyno, mouse (surrogate)	1- and 6-mo tox. cyno ePPND cyno, mouse FEED/EFD (with surrogate)	Significantly↓ circulating eosinophils and blocked blood eosinophilia after hIL-2 administration No reprotox.
Reslizumab	IL-5	Cyno, mouse	1- and 6-mo tox. cyno and mouse Mouse and rabbit EFD, mouse PPND and juvenile tox., cyno 1-mo juvenile bridging tox.	Significantly↓ circulating eosinophils No reprotox. or juvenile tox.
Benralizumab	IL-5Rα	Cyno	39-wk cyno tox. and ePPND cyno	1 animal with reversible postdose reaction (bruising/reddening).↓eosinophils in blood, bone marrow and bronchoalveolar lavage fluid of cynos; transient reduction in neutrophils. No reprotox., ↓eosinophils at birth that ↑ postnatally
Tocilizumab	IL-6R	Cyno, mouse (surrogate)	26-wk tox. and EFD in cyno; 4- wk rat tox. FEED and EFD; rabbit EFD (rat and rabbit not pharmacologically relevant); mouse FEED and PPND study (with surrogate; FDA request)	Liver granulomas and skeletal muscle degeneration in adult cynos, slight ↑abortion and fetal death in cynos; slight ↓in leukocytes but no effect on TDAR on newborn mice administered surrogate
Sarilumab	IL-6Rα	Cyno, mouse (surrogate)	3- and 6-mo tox and ePPND cyno, mouse FEED and juvenile tox. (with surrogate)	Injection site inflammation, ↑neutrophils, fibrinogen and/or CRP, ↓TDAR
Siltuximab	IL-6	Cyno, mouse (surrogate)	3-mo and 6-mo tox, EFD and ePPND cyno; mouse fertility (with surrogate)	Slight ↓TDAR No reprotox.
Ustekinumab	IL-12/23 (p40)	Cyno, mouse (surrogate)	1 and 6-mo tox., EFD, EFD-PPND and male fertility cyno; female mouse FEED (with surrogate)	1 monkey in 26- wk study had bacterial enteritis; neonatal deaths in the ePPND (1 in each treated group)
Secukinumab	IL-17A	Cyno, mouse (surrogate)	4- and 26- tox, EFD cyno; mouse EFD and PPND (with surrogate), *M. tuberculosis* acute infection model (with surrogate)	Slight ↓ CD4+ T cells, ↑ NK cells, ↓TDAR, ↓NK function; skin lesions and immunotox. in 1 high-dose animal in 26-wk study. No reprotox. No impact on *M. tuberculosis* infection
Ixekizumab	IL-17A	Cyno	8-wk and 9-mo tox., 13-wk fertility, EFD and ePPND cyno	Severe injection site reaction in 1 animal in 9-mo study No effects on IPT, NK cells or TDAR No reprotox. effects
Brodalumab	IL-17RA	Cyno	1-, 3- and 6-mo tox; ePPND cyno; rabbit local tolerance	Muco-cutaneous inflammation/mild skin changes and histopath, ↑neutrophils, ↓albumin/ globulin ratios. No effects on IPT or TDAR Moderate to severe edema at injection site in rabbits No reprotox.
Guselkumab	IL-23 (p19)	Cyno, guinea pig	5-wk and 24-wk tox. and ePPND cyno; guinea pig FEED	No effects on lymphoid organs or TDAR Possibly slight ↑neonatal death rate in cynos
Tildrakizumab	IL-23 (p19)	Cyno	13- and 39-wk tox., EFD and ePPND cyno	No effects on lymphoid organs or TDAR; slight ↑ neonatal deaths; (2 high-dose deaths attributable to viral infection)
Risankizumab	IL-23 (p19)	Cyno	4-wk and 26- wk tox; 26- wk fertility and ePPND cyno	No effects on immune-histopathological T- and B-cell evaluation of the lymphoid tissues nor in TDAR Slight ↑ fetal/infant loss

(Continued)

TABLE 29.2 (*Continued*)

Toxicology Studies Performed for FDA-/EMEA-Approved mAbs/Fusion Proteins for Inflammatory/Autoimmune Disease Indications

INN Name	Target	Toxicology Species	Key Toxicology Studies	Findings
Emapalumab	IFN-γ	Cyno, mouse (surrogate)	8- and 13-wk cyno tox.; mouse EFD (with surrogate)	Diarrhea, dehydration, ↓body weigh;↓ body temp. subdued behavior, ↑ WBCs, PMNs, histopath changes, mortality due to GI infections (also seen predosing) in 13- wk study No effects in follow-up 8-wk study except ↓ primary TDAR Slight ↑ postimplantation loss
Omalizumab	IgE	Cyno	26-wk tox., fertility (mating), EFD-PPND and juvenile tox. cyno	↓Platelets in adult cynos, TCP in juvenile cynos
Eculizumab	C5	Mouse (surrogate)	26-wk mouse tox., fertility, FEED, EFD and PPND (with surrogate)	None
Ravulizumab	C5	Mouse (surrogate)	None. Leveraged tox. data with surrogate used to support Eculizumab approval	None

↑ increased; ↓decreased; AEs, adverse effects; aPTT, activated partial thromboplastin time; CRP, C-reactive protein; DR, dose-related; DTH, delayed-type hypersensitivity; EAE, experimental autoimmune leukoencephalopathy; EFD, embryofetal development; FEED, fertility and early embryonic development; HSA, human serum albumin; IPT, immunophenotyping; KLH, keyhole limpet hemocyanin; LN, lymph nodes; mo, month; NK, natural killer; PCV, packed cell volume; PML, progressive multifocal leukoencephalopathy; PPND, pre/postnatal development; RBC, red blood cell; SD, single dose; TDAR, T cell-dependent antibody response; WBC, white blood cells; wk, week.

29.3 Overview of the Major Classes of Biologics Targeting Immune-Mediated Diseases

29.3.1 Monoclonal Antibodies/IgG-Fc-Fusion Proteins

The vast majority of all mAb therapeutics are based on IgG due to its long half-life and Fc effector function. The antigen-binding fragment (Fab) domains bind the intended target, and the Fc region binds both the neonatal Fc receptor (FcRn), giving it a long half-life, and IgG Fc gamma receptors (FcγR) on immune cells. The majority of new mAbs in clinical development have been rationally designed to increase potency, optimize desirable pharmacology, enhance PK and minimize potential immunogenicity, while avoiding undesirable effects that could increase safety concerns. Most mAbs currently in development are fully human or humanized (95% human) proteins to reduce the potential for immunogenicity. IgGs can be functionally optimized in both their Fab and Fc domains to improve efficacy and minimize safety concerns. Different approaches can be applied such as increasing the affinity of IgGs to give low picomolar affinity for their specific targets or by using the modular nature of antibody to produce new highly potent and sometimes multimeric mAb constructs. A wide range of structures has been explored, including whole IgGs and related fragments such as F(ab)₂, Fabs, scFvs and single domains. Antibody domains can also be combined with multivalent or multispecific molecules (with increased avidity and the ability to bind two (bi-specific) or more different targets, to bind two epitopes on the same target (bi-paratopic) or to cotarget other functional domains [14]. Antibodies derived from other species, e.g., camel (nanobodies), or shark (IgNAR), with favorable physicochemical properties, as well as alternative protein scaffolds (lipocalins, ankyrin, fibronectin, etc.) are also being developed [15–17].

The primary MoA of most anti-inflammatory mAbs and Fc-fusion proteins is to directly or indirectly modulate one or more aspects of the immune system (humoral, cell-mediated and innate immunity), with the potential to induce immunosuppression or immunomodulation. They are often designed to bind directly to receptors on immune cells, e.g., T cells, B cells, granulocytes, monocytes, dendritic cells (DCs) in order to deplete these cells (e.g., rituximab, alemtuzumab, ofatumumab, ocrelizumab), downregulate and/or block activation receptors to suppress their function (e.g., efalizumab, omalizumab, epratuzumab, abatacept) or prevent their homing to lymphoid organs and inflammatory sites (e.g., natalizumab, efalizumab, vedolizumab). Others are designed to neutralize pleiotropic mediators such as cytokines, chemokines or growth factors that have multiple contributions to inflammatory disease pathogenesis (e.g., infliximab and the other TNF blockers, canakinumab, ustekinumab, belimumab). Many of the immunomodulatory effects of mAbs are desirable, intended immunopharmacology required to suppress the etiologies of inflammatory disease required for clinical efficacy. However, activation or suppression/depletion of nontarget immune cells and mediators, or permanent non-reversible changes to immune target cells/pathways, or any unintended effects of the intended pharmacology, e.g., severe infusion reactions, cell and tissue injury, inflammation, "cytokine storms", infection and cancer would constitute immunotoxicity.

It is important that mAbs for inflammatory disease do not unnecessarily activate immune effector cells (NK cells, phagocytes and DCs) for antibody-dependent cellular cytotoxicity (ADCC) and complement-dependent cytotoxicity (CDC) or induce cytokines via FcγR interaction on these cells. Hence, many of these anti-inflammatory mAbs that are designed to inhibit immune function (rather than deplete immune cells) are of the IgG₁ isotypes that have been preselected for low/

no Fc effector function (Table 29.1), although a few are IgG_2 or IgG_4 isotypes (with lower natural effector function) [18]. Loss of effector function can also be achieved through structural changes including mutations in the CH2 domain to completely prevent FcγR interaction [19,20] and mAb aglycosylation to completely remove effector function [21]. However, immunogenicity of any non-natural mutation or structure needs to be considered. Avoidance of effector function can also be achieved through the use of non-Fc-bearing antibody fragments such as Fabs, diabodies, scFvs, single domains and alternative scaffolds [14,17]. Monovalent antibody fragments might also be used to block receptors while avoiding receptor cross-linking. When these non-Fc-containing fragments are intended for chronic dosing, the half-life can be extended by strategies such as conjugation to polyethylene glycol (PEG), fusion to human serum albumin (HSA; which binds FcRn) and incorporating anti-HSA binding domains to name but a few strategies [22]. However, for molecules such as PEG, the potential formation of PEG-containing vacuoles in cells and the formation of anti-PEG antibodies observed with some pegylated molecules need to be considered [23].

mAbs primarily indicated for hemopoietic cancers are now showing promise in autoimmune disease indications such as RA, SLE and MS through their ability to deplete B and T cells and thereby inhibit the antigen-presenting and autoantibody-producing function of B cells (rituximab, belimumab, ocrelizumab, alemtuzumab) [24] and autoimmune T cell activity (alemtuzumab) [25]. Other mAbs are designed to deplete eosinophils in allergic diseases (e.g., benralizumab) [26]. However, these mAbs are of the IgG_1 isotype with high FcγR binding, which can be further optimized by Fc engineering and glycoengineering (e.g., afucosylation) [26,27] to promote increased FcγR binding and enhanced killing of (proinflammatory) immune cells by triggering of Fc-mediated immune effector mechanism such as ADCC by NK cells and CDC. This activity of ADCC and CDC leads to the unwanted (but unavoidable) release of proinflammatory cytokines, e.g., TNFα, IFN-γ, IL-6 and complement activation. Alternative routes of administration are also being used to improve efficacy and mitigate against safety risks. Local delivery of IgG and antibody fragments, e.g., by intraocular (IVT), intrajoint, and inhalation administration, seek to maximize mAb delivery to the intended site of action in the inflamed tissue while minimizing systemic pharmacology (not required for efficacy) and safety concerns and decreasing immunogenicity.

29.4 Next-Generation Experimental Therapies beyond mAbs and Proteins

All approved therapies for immune-mediated diseases are mAb/proteins that mainly induce immunosuppression to reduce inflammation and must be administered for extended periods of time (e.g., they are treatments, not cures), some have serious side effects, and considerable numbers of patients do not respond. In an effort to address these deficiencies, there are a number of next-generation therapies in early development with the aim of not only resolving the inflammation but also achieving genetic correction, immune tolerance, disease modification and tissue repair with the hope for, in some cases, disease cure (Table 29.3) [7]. The following section provides a brief overview of these technologies. The reader is referred to recent comprehensive reviews [6,8–10]. Modality-specific safety considerations for cell and gene therapies, gene editing and oligonucleotides are covered in other chapters. However, the intended pharmacological effects of these novel therapies for treating immune-mediated diseases, i.e., immune suppression, will present some of the same safety concerns described later for mAbs and proteins.

Tolerogenic Vaccines: In many immune-mediated diseases, immune homeostasis and self-tolerance are impaired. T cells are often driving this autoreactive response, promoting B cells and other immune cells to induce tissue damage [6]. If the self-protein recognized by these autoreactive T cells is known, then it can be used to induce antigen-specific self-tolerance. Short peptides representing key sequences of autoantigens or allergens are delivered intradermally (or mucosally) in the absence of adjuvant, with the aim of directly binding to **major histocompatibility complex** (MHC) molecules on immature DCs and being recognized by T cells without costimulation.

TABLE 29.3

New (Non-mAb/Protein-Based) Therapies for Immune-Mediated Diseases

Modality	Therapeutic Aim(s)	Antigen-Specific	Immune Diseases
Gene-edited **HSPCs**	Genetic correction	No	Inherited poly inflammatory disease
Gene-edited **iPSCs** (e.g., to express cytokine inhibitors	Inhibit inflammation, tissue repair	No	Broad applicability
Mesenchymal stem cells (MSCs)	Inhibit inflammation, tissue repair	No	Broad applicability
Tolerogenic Vaccines (autoantigenic peptides, altered peptide ligands administered intradermally, ±immature DCs, liposomes containing rapamycin, TGF-β, IL-10)	Autoantigen-specific self-tolerance; disease modification	Yes	Immune-mediated disease for which the autoantigens are known (IDDM, MS, etc.)
Tregs (in vitro expanded, in vivo modulated, e.g., low-dose IL-2)	Non-autoantigen-specific tolerance, disease modification	No	Broad applicability, e.g., RA, IIDM, GvHD
Gene-edited T regs (chimeric autoantigen receptor T regs; **CAR-Tregs**; T cell receptor T regs (**TCR-Tregs**)	Autoantigen-specific self-tolerance, disease modification	Yes	Immune-mediated disease for which the autoantigens are known (IDDM, MS, etc.)
Oligonucleotides (antisense, siRNA)	Resolution of inflammation, immune reset	Yes	Broad applicability

This leads to antigen-specific T cell anergy/tolerance to the peptides and induction of autoantigen-specific T regs [28,29]. Such immune tolerance approaches have the potential to induce drug-free remission in patients with diseases but also to be used prophylactically to prevent disease in patients at risk of developing autoimmunity. Antigen-specific tolerance is achieved without the generalized immunosuppression seen with immunosuppressive drugs, nor the non-antigen-specific T reg induction induced by non-activating anti-CD3 mAbs [30,31]. Peptide-based therapies are under investigation in T1D (e.g., proinsulin, insulin, GAD65 and islet cell antigen (ICA) peptides) [29,32], MS (e.g., myelin basic protein (MBP), proteolipid protein (PLP) and myelin oligodendrocyte glyco-protein (MOG) peptides) [28], celiac disease (gluten peptides) [33], RA (e.g., HSP70) [34] and allergy (e.g., cat dander and grass pollen peptides) [35,36]. Therapeutic dose levels are low (range of 1–100 µg of peptide) and mixtures of peptides across more than 1 autoantigen, as well as encapsulation in nanoparti-cles or liposomes (with or without rapamycin, TGF-β or IL-10), are being used to enhance the power and breadth of effect [6,32,37,38]. Tolerance-promoting peptides can also be loaded onto the MHC class II of immature DCs and these tolerogenic DCs reinfused back into the patient to induce antigen-specific T regs [39]. Tolerogenic peptides are also being expressed in the liver using adeno-associated virus (AAV) and lentivirus (LV) vectors, where sinusoidal endothelial cells and DCs can promote antigen-specific T reg induction [38,40,41].

Gene Editing-Based Therapies: The development of pre-cise and robust gene editing technologies to insert or modify effector protein expression, structure or function has generated interest in using targeted genetic modifications for inflamma-tory disease therapies. Applications include the correction of monogenic autoinflammatory syndromes with genetically edited hematopoietic stem and progenitor cells, modification of induced pluripotent stem cells (iPSCs) for controlled cyto-kine delivery and tissue regeneration, targeting of specific cellular subsets necessary for disease or disrupting traffick-ing to affected tissues, ex vivo expansion and modification of T regs, and the production of chimeric antigen receptor T cell (CAR-T cell) therapy for autoantigen-specific targeting and suppression of pathologic B or T cell clones [9,42]. As with vaccines, these targeted therapies might avoid generalized immunosuppression. Genetic modification tools include zinc finger nuclease (ZFNs), Transcription activator-like effector nucleases (TALENS) and CRISPR/Cas9, base editing, ribo-nucleic acid (RNA) editing, targeted activators and repressors of transcription and targeted epigenetic modifiers [43–45]. Gene editing facilitates efficient and accurate modification of deoxyribonucleic acid (DNA) at a specific locus or loci by the generation of a double-stranded break (DSB). DSBs are then modified by endogenous cellular machinery that mediates either homologous recombination (homology-directed repair [HDR]) or non-homologous end joining (NHEJ). HDR can use an exogenous DNA repair template to perform precise knock-in of a desired alteration of the genomic DNA, while NHEJ is error-prone and induces disruptive insertions and/or dele-tions of varying sizes (termed indels) at the target (repair) site, which can mutate the protein coding sequence in a negative fashion. The editing machinery must successfully enter the nucleus of targeted cells in order to facilitate transcription and eventually translation. Nuclear delivery of plasmids encoding proteins required for genome editing can be greatly enhanced by the use of viral vectors (retrovirus (RV)/ lentivirus (LV), adenovirus (AV) and AAV), non-viral vectors (nanoparticles, cationic carriers lipofectamine and polymeric) and nonvector methods (electroporation and mechanical deformation with microfluidic devices) [9]. Gene editing can also be performed on cells ex vivo and the modified cells reinfused back in to the patient (see below).

Cell Therapies: Stem Cells. There is considerable inter-est in genetically modifying stem cells for the treatment of immune-mediated diseases. **Hematopoietic stem cells (HSCs)** can be treated with RVs or LV expressing the wild-type gene to correct monogenic inflammatory diseases and immunodeficiencies [46,47]. **iPSCs** have broader applicability and exhibit in vivo durability can differentiate into multiple tissue types affected by chronic inflammatory diseases, and abundant quantities can be produced without using embryos/ products of conception. iPSCs can be gene-edited to be inflam-mation-resistant with the aim of utilizing the engineered cells for regenerative medicine in a hostile, inflammatory microen-vironment (e.g., in the RA or OA joint). When gene editing was used to delete the IL-1 receptor type-1 gene, and specific dif-ferentiating factors used to generate cartilage from the edited iPSC clones, the resulting genetically modified cartilage was resistant to cytokine-mediated tissue degradation [48]. iPSCs can be gene-edited to express anticytokine molecules (e.g., IL-1Ra, sTNFR1) only upon inflammatory stimuli for con-trolled delivery [49], avoiding the repeated dosing and side effects of mAbs as a result of loss of cytokine function in all tissues. **Mesenchymal stem cells (MSCs)**, isolated from adult bone marrow and adipose tissues and neonatal umbilical cord and placenta, show an extensive proliferation ability and mul-tipotency, are genetically stable and are poorly immunogenic (due to low MHC class II and costimulatory molecule expres-sion). Moreover, MSCs have trophic, homing/migration and immunosuppression functions [50]. MSCs can also serve as bioreactors of soluble factors that will promote tissue regener-ation from the damaged tissue cellular progenitors. A number of clinical trials are using MSCs for therapeutic interventions CrD and graft-versus host disease (GvHD), alone or in combi-nation with other drugs. MSCs interfere with different path-ways of the immune response by means of direct cell-to-cell interactions and soluble factor secretion. In vitro, MSCs inhibit T cells, B cells, NK cells and DC proliferation, cytokine secre-tion and cytotoxicity of T and NK cells; B cell maturation and antibody secretion; DC maturation and activation, as well as antigen presentation. MSCs need to be activated to exert their immunomodulatory effects, facilitated by an inflammatory disease environment. MSCs recruit T regs to inflammatory sites and the production of prostaglandin E2, TGF-β, IL-10, HLA-G5, matrix metalloproteinases, indoleamine-2,3-dioxy-genase and nitric oxide likely drive their immunosuppressive effects. Promising preclinical data in animal models of trans-plantation, GvHD, lung injury, MS, RA, T1D and SLE have led to human clinical trials in some of these diseases [51].

Cell Therapies: Tregs. Tregs (CD4+CD25+- FOXP3+ cells) are naturally occurring Th cells with immunoregulatory functions including the suppression of antigen-specific T cells and maintenance of peripheral tolerance [13]. Mutations in the FoxP3 gene impair Treg function, causing severe autoimmunity in mice and humans [52], promoting interest in using Tregs for therapy. Tregs exert their suppressive function in both contact-independent and contact-dependent manners, including the release of inhibitory cytokines (e.g., TGF-β), disruption of metabolic pathways, suppression of antigen-presenting cells (APCs), and cytotoxic mechanisms. Tregs inhibit allograft rejection and autoimmunity in animal models, while **polyclonal Tregs** have shown promising disease-modifying effects in clinical trials of GvHD, T1D and SLE without AEs [53]. However, the large amounts of cells needed for infusions and the risk of nonspecific immunosuppression (viral reactivation has been observed) are major drawbacks, potentially overcome by using antigen-specific Tregs, which require fewer cells to exert more localized and targeted suppression. Antigen-specific Tregs are generated by expanding Tregs with APCs and specific antigens. However, CD4+ T cells can also be genetically engineered to express FoxP3 (**iFoxp3 Tregs**) that promotes differentiation into a large population of Tregs [54]. T cell receptor (TCR) gene transfer/editing to direct polyclonal Tregs to express a specific TCR gene and thus redirect specificity toward a single (auto)antigenic epitope (**TCR-Tregs**) can also be done [55]. iFoxP3Tregs and TCR-Tregs have shown efficacy in murine models of transplantation and arthritis and in human T cells for islet cell targeting [54–56]. However, TCR-Tregs are still MHC-restricted, limiting the modular application to individual patients. An MHC-independent strategy is to engineer Tregs with genes encoding chimeric antigen receptors (CARs) (**CAR-Tregs**) specific for targets driving immune-mediated diseases [8]. CARs typically consist of a single-chain variable fragment (scFv) that mediates target binding, an extracellular hinge, a transmembrane region and intracellular signaling domains [57]. CAR-T effector cells are mainly used in oncology; however, this technology has been extended to Treg therapies using CARs specific for autoantigens or autoantigen receptors on autoreactive T cell and autoantibody-producing B cells, to direct T regs to sites of inflammation for targeted immunosuppression [55,58,59]. CAR-Tregs have shown potential for treating IBD, MS, RA, T1D, asthma and transplant rejection [60–64].

Oligonucleotide Therapies: Antisense oligonucleotides (ASOs) are short, single-stranded deoxynucleotides that interfere with gene expression by binding to the complementary target mRNA directly within the nucleus or cytoplasm. Most ASOs induce RNase H endonuclease activity that cleaves the RNA–DNA heteroduplex (others inhibit 5′ cap formation, alter splicing or sterically hinder ribosomal activity), resulting in a significant reduction of target gene translation and reduced intracellular and extracellular target levels [10,65,66]. Sequence specificity of ASOs is key, since only 6–7 base pairs between the ASO and nontarget mRNA can initiate RNase activity, leading to cleavage of the wrong target. Most ASOs are phosphorothioated [67], which facilitates ASO binding to plasma proteins, thereby reducing their renal loss and improving organ uptake. However, phosphorothioate ASOs containing CpG motifs can bind Toll-like receptor (TLR) 9 and trigger innate immune responses, circumvented by selecting ASOs containing no CpG or replacing the

C with 5methylC. Increased ASO binding affinity and biostability are achieved with ribose modifications and locked nucleic acid (LNA)] technology that reduces conformational plasticity [68]. **Small Interfering RNA (siRNA)** are double-stranded RNA molecules, consisting of two short-stranded RNA molecules, a passenger sense strand and a guide (antisense) strand that is complementary to the target mRNA. The siRNA duplex is separated by an enzyme called DICER and the guide antisense strand is loaded onto the RNA-induced silencing complex (RISC), which leads to sequence-specific gene silencing by catalytic cleavage and degradation of the targeted mRNA [69]. The single antisense strand/ RISC complex is highly stable; hence, multiple mRNA transcripts can be catalytically degraded. As with ASOs, siRNAs must be modified to prevent degradation by endonucleases. Both ASOs and siRNAs can be complexed with nanoparticles and coupled with cell-targeting moieties, e.g., N-acetylgalactosamine (GalNAc) to enhance asialoglycoprotein receptor (ASGR)-mediated uptake into liver hepatocytes for enhanced bioavailability and target cell penetration [70–72]. However, nanoparticles can increase the toxicity of the compound or alter the PK and biodistribution of the oligonucleotides. A number of ASOs and one siRNA (Patisiran) are FDA-approved for noninflammatory disease indications [73–75]. ASOs targeting ICAM-1, NF-kB, Smad7, *GATA3 transcription factor and carbohydrate sulfotransferase 15 (CHST15)* are being developed to treat IBD and other inflammatory diseases [76–80], with some evidence of efficacy in humans [81,82]. A siRNA targeting CHST15 is in clinical development for IBD [83].

29.5 General Safety Considerations for Biologics Targeting Immune-Mediated Diseases

Therapeutic mAbs and Fc-fusion proteins for inflammatory diseases have shown to be generally well-tolerated, with any toxicity primarily due to exaggerated pharmacology as a result of inhibiting or enhancing the activities of the target antigen on target cells in blood and tissues. This is often predictable based on an understanding of the pharmacology and data from non-clinical studies in pharmacologically responsive species.

A potential risk for all chronically administered immunosuppressive biologics is the increased risk of infection and cancer. Prolonged and pronounced inhibition of one or more arms of the immune system by mAbs and other immunosuppressive therapies, coupled with the concomitant administration of other immunosuppressive drugs (e.g., methotrexate, corticosteroids, cyclosporin, cyclophosphamide, azathioprine, 6-mercaptopurine) increases the patient risk for opportunistic bacterial, fungal or parasitic infections, chronic viral infection (e.g., EBV and CMV), or virally induced cancers (e.g., lymphoma, skin cancer, Kaposi's sarcoma and hepatocellular carcinoma). RA patients treated chronically with anti-TNFα biologics (e.g., infliximab, adalimumab or etanercept) are at increased risk of nasopharyngitis and upper respiratory tract infections, opportunistic infections and intracellular granulomatous infections such as tuberculosis (especially reactivation of latent tuberculosis hence, patients are prescreened via tuberculin skin test prior to treatment), histoplasmosis, listeriosis and pneumocytosis. These class effects are seen with all anti-TNF therapies [84,85]. Frequent infections are also observed in patients treated with alemtuzumab [86] and rituximab [87]. Chronic treatment of MS and CrD patients with natalizumab (anti-VLA-4 mAb), either alone or in combination with IFN-β may increase the risk of progressive multifocal leukoencephalopathy (PML), a rare, but potentially lethal, brain disorder caused by reactivation of latent polyoma virus, i.e., John Cunningham (JC) virus, infection [88]. Natalizumab is designed to inhibit inflammatory T cell migration to the brain, and the increased incidence of PML is thought to be due to reduced homing of virus clearing Th and T cytotoxic cells (cytotoxic T lymphocytes; CTLs) to the brain [89]. Natalizumab was initially withdrawn from the market, but the FDA subsequently approved its return as a monotherapy, subject to a special restricted distribution program following a comprehensive review of a large number of patients. PML has also been observed in a small number of Ps patients treated with efalizumab (anti-CD11a (LFA-1), a mAb which also affects lymphocyte recirculation, and this has led to market withdrawal due to an unfavorable risk:benefit profile [90]. PML has also been observed with rituximab [91], belimumab [92], belatacept (anti-CD80) [93], ofatumumab (anti-CD20) [94] and tocilizumab (anti-IL6R) [95]. Boxed warnings for an increased risk of infections and/or PML are seen for several of the immunomodulatory mAbs, as these rare events are often only observed once substantial clinical data are available and a low increased risk in treated patients becomes evident. It is recommended not to administer live vaccines during immunosuppressive mAb therapy. The risk of infection, PML and cancer are poorly/not predicted by non-clinical studies, although animal models are being developed [96], and hence, risk mitigation for these effects will also rely on a weight-of-evidence approach to benefit:risk assessment and careful clinical risk management based on the unique characteristics of the product, the target and patient population to be treated.

The likelihood of unintended toxicity is dependent on the pharmacological effect of target binding, the degree of target antigen expression, the role of the target in normal physiologic processes and the potential of the mAb Fc domain to interact with immune effector cells and/or complement. For highly characterized targets whose biology and tissue distribution are well-defined, potential target organs for unwanted toxicity can often be identified and predicted. Anti-GM-CSFR (CSF2R) mavrilimumab causes pulmonary alveolar proteinosis (PAP) at high dose levels in cynomolgus monkeys [97] due to the inhibition of the known role of GM-CSF in pulmonary surfactant homeostasis [98]. This was not unexpected since GM-CSF KO mice have impaired alveolar macrophage function and develop PAP, which is also observed in patients with anti-CSF2 autoantibodies (**see Case Study 2**).

For less well-characterized targets, although toxicity can often be hypothesized based on likely organ expression profiles and target function, a more exploratory investigation is likely to be required. A mAb specific for a target antigen that is not only expressed on inflammatory cells but also highly expressed on normal cells and involved in normal cell function is likely to have greater potential toxicity, possibly involving both disease-targeted organs and non-disease-targeted organs, than a mAb against an antigen that has a restricted tissue expression or function or is only expressed in the diseased state. Nontarget-related (off-target) toxicity of mAbs are rare but not unheard of.

Unintended immune activation by mAbs could lead to infusion and hypersensitivity reactions, generic terms describing a set of related clinical and laboratory findings that can be caused by several immune-mediated mechanisms, including allergic reactions, pseudoallergic reactions and cytokine release syndrome (CRS) [99,100]. Therapeutic mAbs and Fc-fusion proteins have the potential to trigger systemic CRS in humans, either by cross-linking and clustering of the antigen target on immune cells by the Fab arms, by the interaction of the Fc region with Fc gamma receptors (FcγR) on NK cells and neutrophils, or by a combination of both [101,102]. An example is shown in **Case Study 1**. True allergic reactions mediated by antidrug IgE require prior exposure to the mAb, e.g., as with infliximab [99] and hence do not occur on the first infusion, except in rare cases where patients have preexisting antibodies that cross-react with the drug [103]. Severe allergic reactions with anaphylaxis are exceedingly rare. Pseudoallergic/anaphylactoid reactions (IgE-independent reactions mediated possibly by direct immune cell and complement activation) and CRS both occur primarily on the first infusion of drug, although they can also occur on subsequent administrations. Antidrug antibody (ADA, not IgE) has also been shown to induce infusion reactions, e.g., in infliximab- and adalimumab-treated patients that often precludes further treatment since the ADA leads to loss of efficacy [104,105]. The symptoms of all three types of immunologically mediated infusion reactions overlap, but they can often be discriminated by their scope, duration, severity and response to therapy. Some approved mAbs, including rituximab, alemtuzumab, belimumab and muromonab, carry a "Black Box" warning for infusion reactions, and sometimes CRS, which is associated with systemic increases in proinflammatory cytokines TNFα, IFN-γ and IL-6 although others such as IL-2, IL-8 and IL-10 may also be present. The systemic and local presence of these molecules and the associated inflammation and hemodynamic effects damage tissues and organs and can result in disseminated intravascular coagulation, organ failure and death if untreated. In vitro and in vivo studies to assess the potential of mAbs for cytokine release have been reviewed [102,106–108].

CRS as a consequence of mAb infusion may be related to the intended immunopharmacological activity of the mAb and mediated by target-specific binding that either triggers cellular activation, leading to cytokine release, e.g., muromonab or TGN1412, or, when associated with Fc-mediated effector functions (see **Case Study 2**) such as ADCC and CDC, leads to cellular lysis and cytokine release, e.g., rituximab and alemtuzumab. The cytokine release induction by rituximab and alemtuzumab is reduced in RA and MS patients compared to oncology patients where the high tumor burden promotes higher levels of cytokine release following tumor cell killing. CRS can be mild to life-threatening and characterized by fever, chills, nausea, rash, myalgia, flushing, vascular leak, shortness of breath and/or hypotension [100]. Immune activation can in rare cases also lead to the undesirable activation of autopathogenic cells and the development of autoimmunity as observed in a small number of patients treated with alemtuzumab [109] and anti-TNFα biologics [110].

29.6 General Approaches to Initial Biologics Safety Testing

In order to maximize the chances of identifying immunomodulatory mAbs with the potential for adverse effects in humans, non-clinical safety testing programs supporting early clinical trials, including FIH, must be rationally designed with a strong scientific understanding of the product, including its method of manufacture, purity, sequence, structure, class/isotype, pharmacological and immunological effects, the biology of the target and intended clinical use (e.g., indication, patient population and dosing regimen). In silico, in vitro and in vivo studies to assess the safety of immunomodulatory biologics have been reviewed in detail previously [101,102,111–113]. Here, we will illustrate the utility of such studies using case studies. There is no specific guidance relating to the safety assessment of autoimmune/inflammatory disease therapies as there is for oncology. Hence, ICHM3 (R2) [114], ICHS6 and ICHS(R1) (R1) [115,116] are the key documents. ICHS8 (immunotoxicity) [117] is also important.

29.7 In Silico and In Vitro Studies with Biologics for Immune-Mediated Diseases

From target proposal through to lead candidate selection, in silico studies are performed to confirm the knowledge of the expression, cellular localization and function of the target protein, as well as the clinical immunopharmacology, pharmacogenetic and safety data from individuals with genetic disorders lacking the target or populations with modified levels of the target (if available). These data can be informative, especially when correlated with corresponding data generated in knockout, transgenic or other animal models (**see Case Study 3**). Once candidate molecules are identified, in vitro studies to characterize the immunopharmacological and potential immunotoxicological effects, as well as to understand the risk of some types of MoA-driven immunotoxicity may be performed. The relative cell/antigen specificity of mAb binding to the immune system in humans and animals should be determined using methods such as flow cytometry, cell-based assays or competitive immunoassays. In addition, the binding to human and animal tissues can be determined using immunohistochemical (IHC) techniques (TCR studies) or alternative techniques (e.g., mammalian cell surface display (Retrogenix, Integral Molecular), in situ hybridization (ISH)). The relative affinity and immunopharmacological activity of the lead candidate mAb for the immune-based target in humans and animal species used for toxicology studies should be determined using clinically relevant in vitro/ex vivo assays (e.g., to assess cell depletion, suppression, activation and cytokine production). The full dose–response curve should be thoroughly characterized in humans and animals in vitro by exploring immunological effects at both the low and high ends of the curve using clinically relevant cell-based assays (if available). Potential unwanted immunological or other effects should be assessed in these assays (e.g., to demonstrate lack of agonism of an antagonist mAb or lack of cell depletion of a receptor blocking mAb, or lack of unwanted on-target toxicity (**see Case Studies 2 and 4**). Data from these studies should provide an understanding of whether (or not) complete human-relevant immunopharmacology can be elicited in the toxicology species and how predictive the toxicology species are likely to be for human immunotoxicity. These studies should also identify whether there are any potential immunotoxicity in humans that will not be predicted in animals and will require an assessment within in vitro studies with human cells or within early clinical trials and whether there are any immunological effects in human cells that might preclude clinical development (**Case Study 2**).

29.8 In Vivo Studies

29.8.1 Species Selection

Toxicology species selection should ideally consider target sequence homology, target expression and distribution, structural homology, relative target binding affinity, ligand occupancy and kinetics and functional equivalence of PD effects (e.g., relative IC_{50} or IC_{90} between humans and the toxicology species, including (when relevant) for mAb-based products Fc-mediated effects [115,116] and, if relevant, genotypic difference between strains. A relevant species is one in which complete inhibition of the target for the duration of each dosing interval can be achieved, which can often be predicted by combining concentration/biological effect data with simple exposure predictions of human IgG in animals and/or with PK/PD modeling. Historically, many immunomodulatory mAbs/proteins have been tested in only one species, mainly non-human primates (NHP) because only one relevant species could be identified (see Table 29.2). If binding and relevant pharmacology is seen in NHP and rodents, then studies in both NHP and rodents should be performed, as was done for natalizumab, etanercept and abatacept (Table 29.2), **and Case Study 2**, but the potentially higher levels of neutralizing antibodies in lower species impacting exposure and PD should be considered. If there is no pharmacologically relevant species, then the use of surrogate mAbs/proteins and human transgenic models should be considered [113,118–120] as done for infliximab [121], efalizumab [122] and eculizumab [123]; as well as for reproductive toxicity and efficacy studies for certolizumab pegol, ustekinumab and canakinumab. It may be possible to support clinical studies with a wholly in vitro package as done for oncology; however, such packages have rarely been done for mAbs/proteins for non-life-threatening inflammatory diseases.

29.9 In Vivo Studies Supporting First-in-Human Studies

Study design and dose selection for PK/PD and toxicology studies with mAbs/proteins have been described in detail previously

[113,124]. These studies are supported by a range of bioanalytical assays for the detection of the dosed mAb (PK), PD parameters and antidrug (mAb) antibody (ADA) which are not discussed herein and have been extensively reviewed elsewhere [125–129]. By nature of the intended pharmacological effects of modulating the immune system (most induce immune suppression and/or modulation and many mAbs have low Fc effector function), the majority of biologics for autoimmune/inflammatory disease do not have overt adverse events in toxicology studies which are performed in normal animals, often with a low expression of the immune target compared to the inflammatory disease situation (see Table 29.1). This often makes PK/PD assessment challenging due to the lack of PD markers.

29.10 Pharmacokinetic (PK)/ Pharmacodynamic (PD) Studies

A single- or multiple-dose PK/PD study may be performed in one more species to better understand exposure and proposed dose regimen. An example is shown in **Case Study 1**. The PK and PD data generated in these studies allow a preliminary determination of the PK/PD relationship and these simple exposure–response relationships or more complex modeling and simulation approaches can be used to confirm the relevance of the toxicology species (e.g., target saturation can be achieved throughout the study) and guide the choice of dose levels, dosing regimen and length of the recovery period for the subsequent FIH-enabling study. PD parameters related to mAb binding to the target antigen and/or downstream pharmacological activity can be assessed (if available) to provide evidence of target engagement (TE; binding to target and resulting in a functional effect) and pharmacologic effect. The data from these studies might also help to build a human PK/PD model for FIH study dose selection and allow optimal translation of drug effects into the clinic and refinement of clinical biomarker assays and strategies.

Case Study 1: PK/PD Study to Inform Dose Selection for the Toxicology and FIH Studies

Rozanolixizumab is an anti-FcRn mAb in Phase 3 for autoimmune disease indications, designed to promote the degradation of IgG, including IgG autoantibodies [130]. Rozanolixizumab binds and inhibits the function of human and cynomolgus monkey FcRn with comparable affinity and potency. The PK/PD of rozanolixizumab was characterized in cynomolgus monkeys (n=3–4/group) using a wide range of dose levels (5–30 mg/kg), with several single and repeated dosing regimens, and by both the IV and SC routes. The PK was characterized by complex PK/PD behavior driven by a combination of target-mediated drug disposition (TMDD) related to high-affinity binding to abundant cell surface FcRn and the intended pharmacologic effect of rozanolixizumab that inhibits FcRn, thus accelerating the clearance of rozanolixizumab and endogenous IgG (measured using standard clinical chemistry measurements of cyno IgG). As a result, the PK of rozanolixizumab was not dose proportional, exhibiting more rapid elimination at lower doses. The rapid elimination of rozanolixizumab was also evident at doses as high as 30 mg/kg, where after a single IV dose, no detectable drug was observed after 5 days, demonstrating much faster elimination compared to other mAbs [131] in NHPs. Intermittent or daily dosing of rozanolixizumab showed that the PK was consistent over time, with no unexpected accumulation or diminution in an exposure. However, there was evidence of ADA to rozanolixizumab that substantially reduced exposure with repeated dosing. These data informed the subsequent repeat-dose good laboratory practice (GLP)-compliant toxicology study to use dose levels of 30–150 mg/kg rozanolixizumab every 3 days [130]. A PK/PD model was developed to characterize the relationship between UCB7665 PK and IgG levels. The PK/PD data were analyzed by nonlinear mixed-effects modeling. System- and drug-related parameters were translated from cyno to human using a combination of literature, in vivo and in vitro data. Uncertainty in the translation was included in the simulations of possible FIH scenarios. A two-compartment PK/PD model with TMDD in the central compartment [132] and an indirect-effect model where the free drug stimulates IgG catabolism characterized the PK–IgG relationship in cynos. Simulations from the cyno-to-human translated model were used to optimize the FIH design. A range of doses between a starting dose corresponding to a minimal effect (<10% IgG reduction) and a maximum dose providing a −70% mean change from baseline IgG were chosen for the FIH study. The model adequately described the FIH data.

29.11 Preliminary Toxicology Studies

For novel (first-in-class) biologics with a higher perceived risk of toxicity (e.g., based on target expression/pharmacology and in vitro studies), a non-GLP dose-range finding (DRF) toxicity may be performed, prior to the conduct of the first GLP-compliant study supporting FIH dosing. DRF studies are typically conducted in a relatively small number of animals, usually cynomolgus monkeys but also rodents if a relevant species. The general design of such studies has been described in detail [113].

Case Study 2: DRF NHP Study and In Vitro Studies Identify Human Safety Risks Leading to Candidate Termination

This case study is an example of biologic that did have a high perceived acute safety risk and for which multiple in vitro studies and a DRF toxicity study were performed. The DRF study was able to identify a potentially human translatable toxicity in addition to the safety risks identified from in vitro studies, leading to candidate termination.

The molecule is a multimeric antibody-related molecule designed to bind to and block the activation of FcγRs by pathogenic autoantibodies in autoimmune diseases [133]. There are known differences in the target receptor expression, distribution, and functions between rodents and primates (including humans); however, the NHP has the greater pharmacological similarity to human compared to rodents. Since FcγRs are expressed on leukocytes and platelets and the molecule had the potential for complement activation, in vitro human cellular studies of cytokine release, platelet and complement activation, as well as studies to assess potency (immunomodulation of disease-relevant immune cells), were conducted to optimize the safety and efficacy of the candidate series. Additionally, in vivo mouse studies were conducted with the understanding that there might be differences in pharmacologic activity based on receptor disposition or functionality. In mice, there were highly variable strain-dependent safety effects, including anaphylactoid reactions, observed with all candidates, despite favorable in vitro safety profiles with human cells. Based on the human in vitro studies, three optimized lead candidates modified to reduce/remove the safety risk but retaining varying degrees of potency (TE and inhibition) were selected for in vivo assessment in a DRF study in NHPs in a small number of animals (n=3/candidate, with intra-animal dose escalation, starting with the candidate with the lowest potency [134]. After the first dose, the least potent candidate showed no AEs while the second (more potent) candidate caused bruising in the absence of clinical signs; both candidates were administered to monkeys at higher dose levels without additional findings. The final and most potent candidate, however, induced severe anaphylactoid reactions and bruising in all animals after the first low dose. Despite the different clinical signs, all three candidates induced high serum levels of C-reactive protein (CRP) and serum amyloid A (SAA), with little-to-no changes in complement activation and only a slight increase in serum IL-6. Animals were redosed with the third candidate, with or without a platelet-activating factor (PAF) blocker which markedly reduced adverse symptoms, suggesting that PAF was mediating the anaphylactoid reactions, with PAF-mediated platelet activation potentially also involved. The third candidate was subsequently shown to stimulate PAF release from human blood cells in vitro, raising the concern that the adverse events observed in monkeys could translate to humans. Neither the acute-phase response, platelet activation nor anaphylactoid reactions were anticipated by in vitro studies with human cells. The mouse was also not a good translatable model since even the safest candidates that had good in vitro human safety profiles and which induced no clinical symptoms in NHPs, induced anaphylactoid reactions in mice. The acute-phase response in NHPs was observed at low doses of even the least potent candidate meaning that it would be very difficult to avoid such effects in humans with this series. Such proinflammatory responses would be unacceptable in autoimmune disease patients with an already activated immune system. Since the safety margins were considered unacceptable, all candidates were terminated before clinical trials and alternative drug formats were considered.

29.12 Pivotal Repeat-Dose Toxicology Studies

A GLP-compliant toxicology study is performed to support the FIH study. In many cases, the FIH study for a biologic for a chronic inflammatory disease indication is a single ascending dose (SAD) study either in healthy volunteers or sometimes in patients. However, the SAD phase is often followed by a rapid transition to a multiple ascending dose phase (MAD) in patients with treatment for up to 3 mos in order to define an active dose. Hence, it is common for the first GLP toxicity study (or studies) to be of a 13-week (wk) duration. An off-dose recovery period might be included to assess reversibility of any pharmacological and toxicological effects. The clinical route of administration is used, often IV for an FIH/Phase 1 safety study but sometimes a subcutaneous (SC) formulation (the preferred route intended for marketing of many mAbs/proteins for inflammatory diseases) has been developed and can be tested within this study. Dose selection may be informed by the PK/PD study and aims to identify a dose that gives the maximum intended pharmacological effect for the entire study duration as well as a dose achieving a ten-fold exposure multiple over the maximum predicted human exposure, corrected for potency differences between the toxicology species and humans. Standard in-life toxicology investigations and safety pharmacology parameters, as well as additional endpoints, including a range of immunological parameters, including immune function testing depending on the MoA of the target and an extended histopathology assessment of the lymphoid organs [135] are generally included.

Many mAbs/proteins and other biologics for inflammatory disease therapy will be indicated for chronic use hence a 26-wk repeat-dose toxicity study will normally be required. If a mAb has a comparable safety profile in the earlier 4- or 13-wk toxicity studies in NHPs and rodents, or the findings are understood from the MoA of the mAb, then longer term general toxicity studies in one species (preferably rodent; [136]) are considered sufficient [115,116]. The design of this study will follow very closely that described for the FIH-enabling study in that species but if NHPs are used, then the study may include sexually mature NHPs to assess effects on fertility. The clinical route of administration is used (usually SC). Dose levels will generally be the same as those used for the earlier studies unless toxicity was noted and/or the updated PK/PD model recommends alternative dose levels. A recovery period may be included, however, if there is little notable toxicity observed in the shorter toxicity studies, or recovery has been previously observed, then recovery groups may not be required [137]. Additional parameters might include further immunology assessments not included in the 13- wk study, including a close assessment for signs of infection, male and female fertility assessments and, depending on the target, an assessment of whether the mAb/protein can promote cell growth and proliferation, including lymphoproliferative disease that might point to an increased risk of tumor development (see Immunotoxicity Assessment section). Frequent PK and PD monitoring (where possible) is performed throughout the dosing and recovery period of these toxicity studies and the data can be used to update the PK/PD model. ADA is measured if there is evidence of altered PD activity, unexpected changes in the PK profile or evidence of immune-mediated reactions. For many mAbs for inflammatory diseases, there will be no unexpected on-target toxicity in repeat-dose studies (the case for the anti-FcRn mAb in **Case Study 1**). However,

Case Studies 3 and 4 below describe mAbs with undesirable on-target/off-therapeutic toxicity in NHPs, but the repeat-dose toxicology studies coupled with in vitro studies with human cells were able to support clinical entry and progression of the candidates.

Case Study 3: Undesirable On-Target/ Off-Therapeutic Toxicity: GLP Toxicology Studies Identify Safe Human Exposures

Mavrilimumab is an antigranulocyte-macrophage colony-stimulating factor receptor (GM-CSFRα) mAb that blocks the activity of GM-CSF and is currently in clinical development for RA (RA) [138]. It inhibits GM-CSF signaling and is intended to decrease the number of activated inflammatory macrophages and granulocytes at inflammatory sites. However, GM-CSF is also known to serve a role in pulmonary surfactant homeostasis. GM-CSF KO mice [139] accumulate phospholipids and proteins in the lung. PAP is a rare restrictive human lung disorder that is caused either by GM-CSFα mutations or by anti-GM-CSF autoantibodies [98,140]. Patients can manifest lung surfactant and protein accumulation and, in severe cases, respiratory failure. Mavrilimumab was tested in several repeat-dose toxicity studies in cynomolgus monkeys [97], the only pharmacologically relevant species based on similar binding affinity and potency in functional assays using human and cynomolgus monkey granulocytes [141]. Foamy alveolar macrophages in lungs due to intracellular accumulation of neutral lipids were seen on the studies of 11 wks or longer, but not in the studies of 4-wk duration and was deemed "non-adverse" as it reflected the normal clearance function of macrophages without necrosis or impact on lung structure or function. In a 26-wk study, foamy macrophages were observed, but there was also a buildup of foreign material, cholesterol clefts and granulomatous inflammation, deemed "adverse" because the normal functions of macrophages were impaired, leading to accumulated debris and inflammation; this resembled human PAP. These latter findings occurred at high multiples of clinical exposure. At lower multiples of clinical exposure, no such effects were observed in animals that maintained exposure despite ADA generation. Thus, the toxicity studies correlated exposure with a response and showed that the GM-CSFRa could be targeted safely with a mAb, without triggering an adverse impact on lung or respiratory function. Clinical trials proceeded with doses that were approximately 3–5 times below the exposures associated with NHP foamy macrophages [97,138].

Case Study 4: Undesirable On-Target/Off-Therapeutic Toxicity: GLP Toxicology Study and In Vitro Safety Studies Support Lack of Human Safety Risk and Candidate Progression

Dapirolizumab pegol (DZP or Dapimab)is an antibody Fab' fragment directed against CD40 ligand (CD40L or CD154) and conjugated to PEG. CD40L is primarily expressed on activated T cells and, through interactions with its receptor CD40, plays an important role in regulating interactions between T cells and other immune cells, notably B cells and APCs, and thus affects several important functional events thought to be involved in autoimmune disease [142]. CD40L can also be found on other cell types including macrophages, B cells, platelets and non-hematopoietic cells. The biology of CD40L appears to be similar in humans, NHPs and rodents, and there is no evidence for differences in functions or modes of inhibition across these species. Blockade of CD40L is efficacious in treating inflammatory and autoimmune conditions in a range of animal models. In CD40 or CD40L KO mice, there is little Ig class switching or germinal center formation, and immune responses are severely inhibited, while human CD40L deficiency results in an inability to undergo Ig class switching and is associated with hyper-IgM syndrome [143]. CD40L inhibition has also shown similar effects on other pharmacological endpoints in both mice and NHPs. The development of Dapimab was guided by previous clinical experience with the humanized anti-CD40L IgG1mAb, hu5c8 (BG9588, ruplizumab). This whole IgG mAb was studied in a series of Phases 1 and 2 clinical trials in numerous indications [144]. A related full IgG drug was studied in similar trials by IDEC (IDEC-131; toralizumab) [145]. Although promising activity trends were noted, eight patients suffered a thromboembolic event (TE) presenting with either myocardial infarction, pulmonary embolism, or stroke, which was fatal in one patient [144]. Development of both hu5c8 and IDEC-131 was terminated. Prior to this, hu5c8 had shown no unexpected adverse events in toxicology studies in cynomolgus monkeys. However, a subsequent safety evaluation of hu5c8 in rhesus monkeys revealed pulmonary vascular thrombi with pulmonary arterial and arteriolar thrombosis with intimal hyperplasia. In vitro studies with human, cynomolgus and rhesus platelets showed aggregation/activation of both human and rhesus platelets with hu5c8 but not cynomolgus platelets pointing to a translatable link between platelet activation in vitro and TE in vivo in humans and rhesus, but not cynomolgus, monkeys. Hence, in vitro platelet studies and in vivo rhesus toxicity studies could be used as key risk assessment tools for TE prior to undertaking clinical studies with anti-CD40L mAbs. A program was undertaken to design a new, safer drug that did not cause platelet aggregation. One hypothesis for mAb-induced aggregation was that the Fc portion of the mAb might be responsible for activating platelets via binding to CD32 (FcγRIIa) on the platelet surface [146] . To test the hypothesis, Dapimab was developed, a PEGylated anti-CD40L Fab' fragment which lacks an Fc region and cannot bind CD32 [147]. Dapimab, like hu5c8, has equivalent binding and potency for human, cynomolgus and rhesus CD40L but does not bind to rodent CD40L. Dapimab, as well as an aglycosyl version of hu5c8 that lacks FcγR binding activity, showed no evidence of human or rhesus platelet activation in vitro and no TE or vasculopathy in vivo in 3-mo rhesus toxicology studies at high multiples of the clinical exposure (whereas hu5c8 tested in parallel showed clear platelet activation in vitro and TE events in vivo) [147]. The only observed effects were expected modulation of lymphocytes and dose-responsive reversible decreases in antigen-specific antibody responses following immunization. This PK/PD relationship was used to model pharmacologically active dosing regimens in patients. The intensively reviewed pathology in the rhesus monkey studies as well as in vitro investigations on platelets provided assurance for human trial safety. To date, Dapimab has shown no evidence of TE events or other adverse events in humans.

29.13 Immunotoxicity Assessment

Extensive immunotoxicity assessment, including immune function testing, is common for many anti-inflammatory biologics since they are designed to directly modulate the immune sytems. Both immune status and immune function can be assessed in toxicity studies [117] and are designed to detect expected (primary pharmacology-driven), significant direct effects on specific cell type, e.g., B cell depletion or activation of a major T cell population, but should be comprehensive and careful enough to detect subtle, minor, downstream effects that may be unanticipated effects related to the primary pharmacology. Importantly, recovery of the immune system to normal on cessation of dosing and an absence of long-lasting or irreversible effects on immune function or toxicological or pathological effects resulting from the immune modification should be demonstrated. At present, there is no agreement on the level of histopathological change (number of endpoints altered or severity of lesion) that constitutes a biologically significant immune effect [148,149]. The correlation between histopathologic effects and other immune assays such as immunophenotyping and immune function is also not well established, although in some cases correlations between histopathologic findings and other immune tests have been observed, e.g., thymic cortex effects and cell-mediated host resistance [150].

If mAb-/protein-mediated histopathologic changes are observed, immunophenotyping of the affected tissues by IHC to identify the affected cell types can be considered. Immunophenotyping (absolute and relative cell counts) of lymphocytes, e.g., T, B and NK cells, from both blood and lymphoid organs can be done by flow cytometry including an evaluation of specific cell subsets (Th, T cytotoxic, T naïve, T effector, T memory and Tregs and a range of B cell subsets) and activation status. Multiple sampling of biologics-treated and control groups prior to dosing will enhance the chances of detecting a biologics-related change and can be useful to compare each animal to its own predose values to assess for drug-related changes. As with histopathology, it is unclear how small/large a change is necessary to predict a biologically significant consequence/clinical concern and what relationship exists between immunophenotypic change and effects on immune function. Abatacept (CTLA-4-Ig) is immunosuppressive and inhibits a T cell-dependent antibody response (TDAR) in monkeys and rodents, and even ADA production in rodents; however, it had no effects on the numbers of T or B cells in either species [151]. Conversely, alefacept (LFA3-Ig) causes T cell depletion in blood and tissues of monkeys and yet has no effect on the TDAR responses to HSA and only a minimal effect on the keyhole limpet hemocyanin (KLH) response

[152]. Efalizumab (anti-CD11a) depletes T cells and has also significant effects on the TDAR response in chimpanzees, as does the surrogate anti-mouse CD11a mAb in mice [153].

Evaluation of other target-relevant immune parameters should be considered on a case-by-case basis, depending on the MoA, e.g., serum cytokines (for mAbs, such as IgG1, that bind to the surface of immune cells and with strong effector function), acute phase proteins, serum immunoglobulins, complement components, clotting factors, ex vivo lymphocyte Stat-6 activation, ex vivo T cell proliferation, receptor occupancy (RO). If considered relevant, ECGs can be timed to coincide with cytokine release sampling to assess whether any observed increased cytokine levels correlate with CV effects. For mAbs that target the immune system, secondary tests (immune function tests) may be included within the GLP toxicology studies in the primary species, even if no effects are observed in the primary screens described above. Ideally, the functional assays should reflect the cells/pathways targeted by the mAb (T, B, NK, macrophage, etc.) and the MoA (immunosuppression or activation). Assessment of the effects of a mAb on the TDAR to KLH or tetanus toxoid (TT) in cynomolgus monkeys, or sheep red blood cells (SRBC)/KLH in rodents, is a common functional endpoint. Both the primary (IgM, IgG) and secondary (IgG) responses to antigen(s) administered during dosing and recovery can be determined to assess the effect of the mAb on immune priming and boosting (immune memory) and recovery from any effects. An effect on the TDAR means possible effects on APCs, B cells and T cells; hence, positive effects in the TDAR could be followed up with other functional tests to further define the target cells/mechanism, such as specific assessment of T/B cell or APC function, e.g., delayed-type hypersensitivity (DTH) responses, proliferation in response to B and T cell mitogens, e.g., conA, PHA, anti-CD3, lipopolysaccharide (LPS), or antigen, cytokines/ Ig responses to stimuli (antigens, infective agents), in vitro APC function, etc. If the TDAR is not relevant, other functional assays can be considered depending on the target and MoA, e.g., macrophage/neutrophil function assessments such as phagocytosis and chemotaxis assessment by flow cytometry. As with the other tests, there is limited understanding of the extent of reduced immune function required to have a significant biological effect, e.g., increased risk of infection and tumor development in humans. A weight-of-evidence approach where all immunotoxicity data are considered as a whole (and in consideration of the MoA of the mAb, the predicted extent and duration of human exposure, the clinical population, disease status, concomitant medication, etc.) is recommended when interpreting the findings of immunotoxicity assays and in considering the risk of clinically significant immunotoxicity occurring in humans.

If in the initial toxicity studies, immunosuppression is associated with infections that deleteriously affect the health of the animals and their ability to remain on study, subsequent studies might include prophylactic or therapeutic treatment with antibiotics prior to mAb/protein dosing, especially in cases where the animal species is oversensitive to infection with specific organisms of limited relevance to humans [154]. This might allow a wider range of dose levels and longer durations of dosing and hence a more thorough safety assessment.

If severe immunosuppressive effects are observed, detailed histopathology/IHC assessment (e.g., Ki67, PCNA staining) to look for early signs of lymphoproliferative disease and possible increased risk of tumors could be included in the chronic toxicity studies if there is sufficient concern. Monitoring for the effects of the mAb on titers of endogenous tumor-promoting viruses, e.g., lymphocryptovirus (LCV; a gamma-herpes virus similar to human Epstein-Barr virus (EBV)) in monkeys could also be considered as a measure of the impact of the mAb on immunosurveillance to an oncogenic virus, as has been done previously for alefacept and abatacept [151,152]; however, the relevance of any observed effects for humans is unknown. LCV and other tumor-promoting viruses induce polymorphic B cell hyperplasia or plasmacytoid hyperplasia that could result in lymphoproliferative changes and potentially to lymphoma [155]. Indicators of viral load (viral DNA/gene products) could be monitored during chronic toxicity studies (in addition to any clinical manifestations of viral infection) to determine whether they are increased following treatment with an immunosuppressive mAb. Increased titers of LCV were observed after chronic treatment of monkeys with alefacept, and lymphoma was observed in a single monkey although the relevance of this finding for humans is not clear (no mAb-induced lymphomas have been reported with alefacept to date in humans) [152]. With abatacept, no change in viral infection status was observed in a 52-wk NHP study, whereas virus-induced tumors were observed in a 2-year mouse carcinogenicity study [151]. It is not known whether an effect on tumor-promoting viruses and/or occurrence of lymphoma in animals within a chronic toxicity study in any way predicts effects on human tumor-promoting viruses and the risk of human lymphoma and other neoplasms. Human lymphoma is caused by human viruses (HVs) (e.g., EBV, HTLV-1, HHV-8 and HPV), which are different from the animal viruses. The endogenous levels of these HVs are also expected to be different from the animal viruses present in normal toxicology species. The immunological status of human patients and viral control mechanisms are also likely to differ from normal toxicology animals. In addition, it may be that lymphoma will only be observed in humans after longer exposure to an immunosuppressive mAb (years) that is not detected in a 26- wk toxicity study. However, viral monitoring in animals might add to the overall weight of evidence for immunosuppression and decreased host resistance.

29.14 Studies of Host Defense in Animal Disease Models (Host Resistance Assays)

Host resistance assays, i.e., effect of biologics on growth and pathogenesis/mortality following challenge with bacteria, viruses, fungi, parasites or tumors should be considered on a case-by-case basis for mAbs with broad-spectrum immunosuppressive activity and/or having shown suppressive effects on the TDAR and/or other immune function tests. Host resistance assays might potentially be useful in determining if the immune system is compromised to the point of ineffectiveness in providing protection from specific organisms, in determining the length of reduced resistance and relationship with the PK/PD and might confirm the affected cell population from immune function tests by decreasing resistance to organism controlled by certain cell types [156]. Host resistance assays might also help to rank/benchmark a reduced host defense effect versus an immunosuppressive agent with clinical experience and might help to avoid the requirement for clinical infection studies. If such studies are deemed useful, then the choice of host resistance model is dependent on the MoA, i.e., the particular immune cells/pathways targeted by the mAb. For example, for a mAb that affects neutrophil/phagocyte function, models of extracellular bacterial infection such as *Streptococcus pneumoniae* controlled by neutrophils should be considered. For a mAb that affects cell-mediated immunity or macrophage function, then a challenge with a facultative intracellular parasite such as *Listeria* might be relevant. However, host resistance assays are not routinely performed within the industry since their predictive value for humans is unproven, although rodent models of infection with influenza virus, Candida albicans (fungus), Mycobacterium tuberculosis and other pathogens have been used with some mAbs [156,157], including secukinumab (Table 29.2).

Host resistance assays are rarely performed in the NHP due to lack of qualified models, low animal numbers, high inter-animal variation and lack of specific pathogen-free (SPF) animals, and variable pathogen profiles between NHPs. Testing in rodent models usually requires the use of a surrogate mAb and is both time-consuming and expensive. These assays also require specialized external CRO expertise and, due to overlapping and compensatory immune pathways, the effects on immune function may not result in decreased host resistance unless multiple host resistance models (a combination of bacterial, viral and tumor models) and immune function tests are utilized to increase the weight of evidence [150]. The susceptibility to infection in animals is dependent on both the degree of immunosuppression and the number of challenge organisms. The productivity of such models for humans, where the degree of immunosuppression may be variable in the out-bred population and the number/nature of challenge organisms cannot be controlled, is further questioned. Infection in humans occurs on a background of concomitant medication and underlying disease, e.g., RA, Ps, variables not tested in host resistance models. The available host resistance database is limited to a small number of usually high immunosuppressive (NCE) drugs, and hence, the question remains as to whether these models can detect the effect of a mild/moderate immunosuppressant on host defense. Hence, even if a mAb shows no effects in a range of host resistance assays, one cannot conclude that no such effects will occur in humans. One should first consider whether the target is involved in mediating defense against particular organisms that might be a risk in humans and if existing "class effect" data are known in animals and/or humans or whether infectious agent/tumor challenge data exist from animals treated with a mAb against the same target or from target knockout mice. In these cases host resistance studies may be of little value since a negative result in a challenge model(s) would not negate the existing data and a general label of potential increased risk of infection and cancer is likely. This was the case with ustekinumab

[158] (see Carcinogenicity Studies section) not]. In such cases, many investigators choose to address the potential impaired resistance to microbial pathogens/tumors in clinical trials and in the subsequent clinical risk management and pharmacovigilance plans. Alternatively, in vitro assays with human immune cells may have value in answering specific questions relating to infection risk. For the anti-IL-17 mAb secukinumab, an in vitro study was performed to assess the effect of anti-TNFα adalimumab and secukinumab on dormant *M. tuberculosis* H37Rv in a novel human 3-D microgranuloma model [159]. Anti-TNFα, but not secukinumab, treatment showed evidence of mycobacterial reactivation.

29.15 Reproductive Toxicity Studies

MAbs for inflammatory disease therapy are frequently indicated for chronic administration to WoCBP and to fertile men. Many of these patients are often taking disease-modifying and/or immunosuppressive drugs that are contraindicated in pregnancy and known to have teratogenic effects. Woman participating in clinical trials must practice highly effective methods of contraception. Since very low numbers of pregnancies still occur and to also identify any potential of a mAb to effect reproduction and development of the offspring (the outcome of which may help to inform the physician and the pregnant mother on whether to continue her accidental pregnancy), reproductive toxicity studies are usually required to support license application of mAbs (see Table 29.2).

Immunomodulatory mAbs used for inflammatory disease therapy, by impacting immune cells and their produced mediators, have the potential to affect different aspects of pregnancy. Ovulation, implantation, placentation, fetal growth and parturition each require a unique immune environment [160]. T cells, NK and macrophages produce various cytokines, chemokines and growth factors (e.g., TNFα, IFN-γ, IL-6, IL-8) that affect ovarian folliculogenesis and ovulation [161]. In the first trimester of pregnancy, a proinflammatory Th1 environment promotes blastocyst/trophoblast implantation and embryo uterine attachment. Uterine NK cells are involved in angiogenesis, vascular transformation and trophoblast infiltration [162]. In the second trimester, there is a switch to a more anti-inflammatory immunosuppressive Th2 milieu that is necessary for fetal growth [163,164]. In women with healthy pregnancies, there is a prevalence of CD4+ Th2 cells (producing IL-4 and IL-10) and CD4+CD25+Foxp3+ T reg cells (producing IL-10 and TGF-β), that, together with immune checkpoints and the programmed cell death system, serve to inhibit proinflammatory IFN-γ production, and to enhance tolerance to the fetal allograft. Tregs also control the activity of Th17 that protects the maternal-fetal interface from microbial infection [165]. In women with recurrent abortions, the protective Th2 environment during the fetal growth stage is compromised and there is an increase in decidual Th1 cells producing IFN-γ and TNFα, Th17 (producing IL-17 only), Th17/Th1 (producing IL-17 and IFN-γ) and Th22 cells (producing IL-22 only), as well as increases in NK and NK-T cells producing IFN-γ [166–168]. Toward parturition, the protective Th2 immune response shifts toward a proinflammatory Th1 response in which IL-6, IL-1β, and TNFα, produced by T cells, NK cells, macrophages and neutrophils, play an important role in parturition and delivery, driving NF-kB signaling and increasing prostaglandins that stimulate cervical ripening and contraction of the myometrium [164,167]. Hence, effects on cellular immune function affecting these different cell subsets (and impacting the Th1/Th2/Th17/Treg and IL-4/IFN-γ balance) and direct neutralization of key cytokines by a mAb/other biologics could, in theory, affect these diverse processes and impact pregnancy.

The fetal and neonatal immune systems are vitally important in protection against infection and uncontrolled inflammation. However, humans are born with an immature immune system with regard to antigen experience and immune memory, and the neonate already has an increased risk of infection compared to adults, relying in part on innate immune responses and maternal IgG antibodies transferred across the placenta and secretory IgA (sIgA) via breast milk. If the fetus and neonate are exposed to immunomodulatory mAbs/Fc-fusion proteins through placental transfer, then there is the potential to adversely impact the developing immune system in the fetus and the maturing immune system in the infant leading to neonatal immunosuppression [169]. Potential short-term effects could be increased risk of infections or dissemination of live attenuated vaccines. Potential longer term effects might be severe infections, atopy, allergies and malignancies, especially lymphoid cancers. However, in a recent study of infants born to mothers with IBD treated with TNF inhibitors, when assessed at 1 year of age, birth outcomes, growth, infection rate, allergies, eczema and adverse reactions to vaccines in the newborn of mothers treated for IBD appear to be unaffected by TNFα inhibitor treatment, whether stopped before the third trimester (to minimize placental transfer) or continued [170]. However, a tragic case of neonatal death due to disseminated Bacillus Calmette-Guérin (BCG) infection occurred after BCG vaccination in an infant born to a mother treated with infliximab throughout pregnancy [171]. Hence, administration of live vaccines should be avoided in newborns exposed to TNFα inhibitors, for at least 6 mos postpartum [170,172]. Biologics that do not cross the placenta will avoid immune modulation of the fetus/neonate.

The NHP is often the only relevant species for mAbs/proteins and is most similar to humans in reproductive physiology, endocrine control and placental transport, as well as having a more morphologically and functionally mature immune system at birth (compared to other species where considerable postnatal immune maturation). The enhanced pre-/postnatal development PPND (ePPND) study in cynomolgus monkeys as advocated in ICHS6 [115,116] and outlined in comprehensive reviews [173,174] is widely performed to generate both embryofetal development (EFD) and pre-/postnatal development (PPND) data with mAbs, as was done for Ustekinumab [158], and all the approved mAbs post-2010 (see Table 29.2 and **Case Study 5**). Pregnant females are dosed from GD20 onward (once pregnancy is confirmed; hence it will not assess impact on implantation or placentation) until the end of gestation to achieve human-relevant levels of fetal exposure. Plasma levels in the infant at birth are usually comparable to those of the mother and the long half-life of most mAbs ensures the exposure of the infant for several mos at pharmacological levels. For immunomodulatory mAbs/proteins, important critical immunological development windows in the NHP are the development of the lymphoid organs (thymus, spleen, lymph nodes and mucosal-associated lymphoid tissues) and their population by immune cells (T cells, B cells, APCs and macrophages), predominantly in the second trimester between GD50 to GD100 [175]. CD3+ T cells and double-positive CD4+CD8+ T cells are present in the thymus from GD60 and GD80, respectively. In the spleen, B cells appear around GD65 and by GD80, the red and white pulps (T and B cells areas) and demarcated [175,176]. The development of B cell follicles/germinal centers and the generation of antibody-producing cells in the spleen and LNs occurs later in the third trimester and continues postnatally. Immune endpoints can also be assessed postnatally. If an impact on immune function is anticipated, then the timing should allow for the development of immune competence to be completed. Developmental immunotoxicity (DIT) measurements such as lymphocyte immunophenotyping (from 1 mo after birth), TDAR (from 3 to 6 mos after birth) and other immune function tests can be included in postnatal assessments within the ePPND study in NHPs or rodents depending on the MoA of the mAb. Infant lymphoid organ weights and histopathology can be performed at termination. The developing immune system may be more susceptible to immune perturbation than the adult immune system and critical windows of DIT that differ from the adult immune system and could be adversely affected by immunomodulatory drugs have been described [177]. Although there is some evidence in animals with xenobiotic NCEs to support this [177,178], there is little evidence to suggest that this is also the case with highly specific mAbs. This might be because mAbs get transferred mainly in the late second and third trimesters when the lymphoid organs will have formed and hence, any impact would be on immune system maturation which may be more difficult to detect.

If rodents and/or rabbits are also relevant species for the mAb/biologic, then these should be used for reproductive toxicity studies rather than the NHP [115]. These rat FEED and rat/rabbit EFD study designs would generally follow those commonly performed for NCEs and have been reviewed previously [113]. IgG crosses the yolk sac in rodents/rabbits via FcRn and exposure begins during the late organogenesis and continues throughout gestation [179]. However, this transfer is lower in rodents than the placental transfer of IgG in humans, NHPs and rabbits, with the majority being transferred postnatally in milk. Thus, the fetal rat has lower exposure during organ maturation compared to humans [179], and since the period of organogenesis is longer in rats and rabbits, the likelihood of placental transfer during organogenesis is higher compared to NHPs and humans and so could overestimate the risk of developmental effects. Abatacept was tested in mice, rat and rabbit, and etanercept was tested in rats and rabbits (Table 29.2). For infliximab, efalizumab, eculizumab and canakinumab, surrogates were used for reproductive toxicity studies in rats/rabbits. The relevance of the surrogate approach for assessing at least some aspects of reproductive toxicity is questioned in light of the observed increase in pregnancy

loss with a sIL-4R in cynomolgus monkeys which was not observed with the mouse sIL-4R surrogate in rodents [180] (see also **Case Study 5**).

There are few instances of mAbs/Fc-fusion proteins for inflammatory disease having reprotoxic effects in animals, despite theoretically impacting immune homeostasis at the materno-fetal interface, high placental transfer and hence potential impacts on the developing immune system of the fetus/neonate (Table 29.2) [181]. Teratogenic effects are also rare due to the MoA of most mAbs/Fc-fusion proteins not impacting development but also due to the lack of placental transfer during organogenesis in NHPs. TNF inhibitors show no reprotoxicity in animals or humans. In humans, register-based cohort studies, case–control studies and meta-analyses in patients with RA, IBD, AS, and Ps suggest that these agents do not pose a significant clinical risk to conception, teratogenicity and congenital malformations, intrauterine death, or increase the risk of adverse outcomes or the risk of infection of the neonate or infant when dosed at all stages of pregnancy [182,183]. Hence, TNFα inhibitors can be used in the preconception period and during the first and second trimesters and even in the third trimester [182,183] to control active disease and flares in certain patients where the risk:benefit is justified (since active RA/IBD disease negatively impacts pregnancy). The anti-IL-4Ra mAb (blocking IL-4 and IL-13) dupilumab (Tables 29.1 and 29.2), which should reduce allo-protective Th2 responses, had no impact on successful pregnancy in an NHP ePPND study [184]. This probably reflects the redundancy in cytokine networks. However, as mentioned above, a sIL-4R protein did increase abortion/embryofetal death in an EFD study monkeys [180].

The anti-IL-6 mAb, olokizumab, is a notable exception where severe effects or parturition were observed (see **Case Study 5**). Another IL-6 inhibitory mAb tocilizumab (anti-IL-6R) [185] caused a slight increase in abortion rate and fetal death in cynomolgus monkeys (despite only being dosed from gestation days 20–50). With other anti-IL-6 mAbs dosed throughout gestation, sirukumab caused an increased incidence of embryofetal loss, while siltuximab and sarilumab had no adverse effects on the fetus nor parturition [186,187]). Belimumab (anti-BLyS) caused a slight increase in abortion rate and fetal death in cynomolgus monkeys [188]. Each of the anti-IL-23 mAbs guselkumab, tildrakizumab and risankizumab induced slight increased incidence of fetal/neonatal death [189–191]. Canakinumab induced incomplete bone ossification in F1 marmosets and mice (with surrogate) and bent tail in F1 marmosets [192]. Hematologic changes were observed in cynomolgus monkey fetuses exposed to natalizumb (decreased platelets in guinea pigs also) [193] as well as in fetuses and offspring exposed to rituximab (decreased B cells and total serum IgG but only small (nonsignificant) effects on immune function (TDAR to KLH and TT) [194]. Immunological effects were also noted in mice treated with the efalizumab (anti-CD11a) surrogate (increased circulating lymphocytes, increased spleen weight and decreased cellularity of the lymph nodes) or rats treated with abatacept (increased TDAR, thyroid inflammation)(see Table 29.2) [153]. In each case, these effects were most likely related to the MoA of the mAb, observed in adult animals, mild (compared to the phenotype of target KO mice, e.g., in the case of natalizumab, α4 integrin KO mice have cardiac effects not observed in mAb-treated animals probably due to no/low mAb exposure during organogenesis) and reversible.

Case Study 5: mAb Causing Human-Relevant Reproductive Toxicity in NHPs But Not Rodents

The molecule is an anti-IL-6 mAb (IgG4) used in the development of inflammatory diseases [195]. The cynomolgus monkey was the only pharmacologically relevant species for safety assessment, based on in vitro potency on downstream signaling comparable to human, in vivo efficacy in a disease model and literature about similar distribution and function of the target. KO mouse studies and mice dosed with a homolog mAb did not reveal any adverse findings. General toxicity studies conducted in the adult healthy monkey with the clinical lead mAb were uneventful. Since the treated population would include WoCBP and young infants, it was necessary to assess toxicity during pregnancy. In an ePPND study, pregnant monkeys were treated from gestation day 20 to parturition and infants were monitored for 9 mos. mAb treatment was well tolerated during pregnancy and did not increase the normal incidence of abortions. However, in all treated pregnant animals, the duration of gestation was significantly increased, and mortality was seen in some animals at delivery without prior signs of distress. Pathologic findings suggested that the difficult deliveries (dystocia) were caused by placental retention and, in some cases, associated with significant genital blood loss. Infant losses were also seen and judged secondary to dystocia. Infants who survived the difficult parturition developed normally, including their immune systems. None of the findings of this ePPND study were observed in KO mice nor in pregnant mice treated with an anti-mouse cytokine receptor mAb, as a consequence of a difference in the physiology of parturition between rodents and higher mammals. Based on these findings, a deeper review of parturition literature suggested that the target could be one of many factors involved in labor-associated inflammation, cervical ripening, and the digestion of the interface between placenta and uterus in human and higher mammals; in fact, the cytokine was shown to be indispensable for normal parturition. This study showed for the first time that this factor was more critical than previously appreciated in primate parturition and that pregnant women might also be at risk of dystocia, hemorrhage and infant loss if undergoing treatment with the mAb. In conclusion, the only appropriate species for assessing reproductive and developmental toxicity was the cynomolgus monkey. Conducting the study identified a life-threatening hazard for women and infants during the latter stages of pregnancy, one that was not predicted from prior literature, nor from mice (KO or mAb-treated). As a result of the ePPND study in monkeys, the mAb continued development in patients with autoimmune diseases without unexpected safety findings, but labeling specifically warns against use in pregnancy and instructs that women who become pregnant while receiving the mAb must stop treatment immediately.

29.16 Juvenile Toxicity Studies

The mAbs/proteins targeting immune-mediated diseases are frequently indicated for diseases that affect children and adolescents. The need for a toxicity study in juvenile animals will depend on the age of children to be included in trials, the risk:benefit to the intended juvenile patients, the duration of dosing, the MoA and expression of the target in adults compared to juveniles, existing pharmacology/toxicology data in animals and humans (including data from target KO mice if available) and the timing of the trials during development [196,197]. The human and NHP immune systems are anatomically developed and functional at birth; however, there is a considerable postnatal immune functional maturation, coupled with increasing exposure to antigens and allergens and the development of immune memory (not adult equivalent until aged 15), that continues through the neonatal period and childhood [175,176]. For example, at birth and during the early neonatal period, IgG levels are low (mainly coming from the mother) and innate immune function, cytokine production and NK cell and T cell function is low at birth. However, by 1–2 years, there are effective T and B cell responses and cytokine responses and the complement system is fully developed, although B cells do not produce adult levels of IgG and IgA at 5 and 12 years, respectively. In assessing the need for a juvenile toxicity study. consider if the effects on the immune system in juvenile animals are likely to be different from those observed in studies in older adult/adolescent animals used in general toxicology studies. Frequently, cynomolgus monkeys aged 2–3 years (8–12-year-old human equivalent) are used to support adult clinical trials and hence may be used to support dosing of children/juveniles. It might also be possible to gather data from the postnatal phase of an ePPND study, whereby the neonates are exposed to a mAb through maternal transfer. High exposure couple with the long half-life can often ensure sustained exposure of the neonates for several wk s or mos after birth, which could cover the equivalent human neonatal period. Hence, the key question then is whether the gap in immune system exposure between the end of the exposure in the ePPND study and the start of dosing/exposure in the general toxicity study in adolescents is important for the drug in question with regard to the long-term impact on the human immune system and so needs to be assessed by dosing of juvenile animals. In most of the cases, no such study is required as any potential effects are likely to be observed in adult animals and juvenile-specific effects on the maturing immune system are likely reversible.

However, if clinical studies in children and infants below the age of 2 are planned, and there are no/insufficient supporting data from the ePPND and toxicology studies, and the MoA highlights a risk, then a juvenile toxicity study may be required. The age of the animals for postnatal dosing and the duration of dosing should take into account both the age of the infants/children to be treated, any species differences in the timing and duration of target organ system development between animals and humans and the duration of clinical dosing. Preferably, rats are used if it is a pharmacologically responsive species. However, the considerable postnatal immune system development in rodents compared to humans and monkeys needs to be considered in the study design and dosing interval. Abatacept was tested in juvenile rats [151]. If the only pharmacologically responsive species for a mAb is the NHP, then studies in juvenile NHPs can be performed. Both natalizumab [193] and omalizumab [198] were tested in juvenile NHPs (1.5–2.5 years old and 6–15 mos old, respectively), with studies of up to 6-mo duration (Table 29.2). Certolizumab pegol (Cimzia) was recently tested in a 52-wk juvenile toxicity study in NHPs, primarily to confirm that the safety profile of the attached PEG moiety and associated cellular vacuolation was no different in juvenile animals compared to adults [199]. Another option is to evaluate effects in juvenile rodents using a surrogate molecule as was done for canakinumab [192]. Adalimumab [200] was tested in a transgenic mouse RA model with dosing from day 10 postpartum through 10 wk s of age.

29.17 Carcinogenicity

Many therapeutic mAbs/proteins targeting immune-mediated diseases are administered chronically and so a carcinogenicity assessment is needed prior to market application [201]. The risk for these molecules is not through direct mutagenicity or promotion of new or existing tumors but rather the potential to adversely impact the host's defense against tumors. This can be through interfering with the process of immunoediting (a dynamic process wherein the tumor evolves under the selective pressure of the immune response, while the immune system continues to adapt to the evolving tumor [202]) or by altering immunosurveillance of oncogenic viruses (e.g., Kaposi's sarcoma virus (HHV-8), EBV or HPV). Immune components such as NK cells, dendritic cells, CTLs and NKT cells can directly kill tumor cells and suppress or clear virus/virally infected cells, produce proinflammatory cytokines (e.g., interleukin [IL]-12, IL-18, IFN-γ and IL-6, TNFα) and promote the cellular production of IFN-α, which both directly interferes with viral replication and promotes antiviral immunity [203].

Traditional tools such as lifetime (2-year) studies in rodents and alternative ras-H2 transgenic and P53 KO models are not relevant for these molecules [204,205] since there is no tumor directing immune editing, and when tumors have been observed as a result of endogenous animal oncogenic viruses (e.g., with alefacept in NHPs and with abatacept in mice) [151,152,204], they have not been observed in humans. Other options include rodent initiation-promotion models, e.g., chemical, radiation, UV skin carcinogenesis and viral carcinogenesis models (reviewed in Ref. [206]), which have been used to assess the tumor-promotion potential of cyclosporine and azathioprine, and to assess the cancer risk of mAbs against, e.g., TNFα, IL-12 and IL-17 [207,208]. Also, implanted tumor cell host resistance assays, e.g., B16 melanoma model, used to assess the effect of an anti-CD4 mAb in human transgenic mice [209] or PDV squamous cell carcinoma model used to assess an anti-IL-12/23 mAb [210] can be used to assess the potential of a mAb to suppress host defense against experimental lung metastases. Tumor immunization models can be used to assess the effects of a mAb on tumor-specific immune responses [211]. Bugelski et al. [212] proposed to use these models, together with knowledge of the MoA, to evaluate the relative hazard for decrease immunosurveillance of tumors by mAbs. While these approaches may be helped in demonstrating the relative immunosuppressant potency of a mAb (compared with drugs with clinical experience of immunosuppression and cancer development) and may contribute to the overall weight of evidence for or against carcinogenic risk, they are fraught with difficulties in interpretation and relevance for human risk assessment [206]. Many express irrelevant tumor types for an immunomodulatory mAb, i.e., they may not use virus-induced lymphomas or other tumor types observed following immunosuppression in humans. The murine viruses and other initiators used may not be relevant to humans and they lack proper validation and background data. Models such as EBV infection and resultant lymphoma in human immune system transgenic mice are being developed and might have utility in the carcinogenicity assessment of immunosuppressive mAbs and other drugs [213]. Age, race, genetics, underlying diseases, concomitant medication and immune status are likely to be highly variable in patients. Hence, the balance of immunosuppression versus antitumor effects is likely to be quite different in animals and humans.

For the vast majority of immunosuppressive biologics, a weight-of-evidence approach is taken in determining the relative risk of target neutralization by an immunosuppressive/immunomodulatory biologic on tumor promotion and in devising a carcinogenicity testing plan [214]. This is documented in a Carcinogenicity Assessment Document (CAD) that will ultimately be used to communicate risk and provide input to the risk management plan, labeling proposals, clinical monitoring and postmarketing surveillance. In assessing carcinogenic risk of a therapeutic mAb, understanding the biology of the target and the potential downstream effects following chronic modulation through a detailed review of the literature is key. Consider the level and kinetics of target expression on tumor cells and the mechanisms that may be related to the tumor-promoting processes. Data from humans with genetic deficiency of the target, genetically modified animals (KO/KI mice), animals treated with drugs that modulate the pathway and xenograft models evaluating the effect of treatment on the growth of nascent or implanted tumor cells [209,210] can be informative. Since the main potential for increased tumor growth for the majority of anti-inflammatory mAbs relates to reduced cancer immunosurveillance, one must consider carefully the immunopharmacology and immunotoxicity data. Does neutralization of the target by the mAb affect key immune parameters, including immune function, in target KO mice (if data available), in toxicology studies, and in early clinical studies? A lack of general immunosuppression by target neutralization (e.g., no effect on immunophenotyping, histopathology of lymphoid organs, TDAR or NK cell function, no signs of lymphoproliferative disease/preneoplastic changes or increase in markers of proliferation (Ki67, PCNA), following long-term assessment in KO mice or following administration of the mAb at high doses for 6 mos to animals) would provide strong evidence of a lack of generalized immunosuppression. One might expect highly specific mAbs designed to neutralize, e.g., individual cytokines/pathways or the function of specific cell types should provide more targeted therapies for inflammatory diseases with potentially a reduced risk of tumor development than broad-spectrum and strong immunosuppressants such as azathioprine and cyclosporine that induce frank immunosuppression. If the mAb does effect immune function at clinically relevant dose levels, then further consideration of the MoA will be required, especially if it affects, or is likely to affect, the generation of a Th1 cell-type response (and associated IFN-γ and IL-12 secretion), or to generate, activate or influence tumor penetration by CTLs or NK cell responses in vitro, and/or in animal models of cancer and infection (especially viral infection) [203,210,215]. These are all potent antitumor immune response mechanisms and inhibition could impair host immunosurveillance of viruses/tumors, although the considerable redundancy in the immune system is recognized. However, one must consider that the inhibition of some of these immune mechanisms is desirable immunopharmacology required for efficacy. It is also important to evaluate any potential effect of the disease state on cancer incidence in the targeted patient population. Patients treated with anti-TNF biologics have an approximately two to three-fold higher rate of lymphoma in RA patients [216], although these patients are already at a higher risk of lymphoma and lung cancer than the general population [217] and thus it is not clear whether this is a real increase in the cancer incidence. More recent studies have not identified such an increased cancer risk with TNF inhibitors compared to untreated RA patients [218].

For immunomodulatory mAbs, consider if further preclinical studies will influence risk assessment or impact labeling. A conservative approach is usually taken by Health Authorities whereby any mAb with an immunosuppressive MoA will have a label that states that there is a risk of decreased immunosurveillance and a potential for carcinogenicity irrespective of results observed in non-clinical studies. Indeed, this is the case for muromonab, ustekinumab, belimumab infliximab, abatacept, alefacept and belatacept; therefore, there may be no value in performing non-clinical studies and it may be simpler to accept the label. This was the approach taken for ustekinumab [158]. A literature review revealed that systemic administration of IL-12 exhibits an antitumor effect in mice [219] and inhibition of IL-12/IL-23 expression with a murine mAb and IL-12/23 KO mice have enhanced tumor formation/growth in mice [206,209]. It was concluded that "there is sufficient non-clinical data in the literature indicating an increased carcinogenic risk with inhibition of IL-12/IL-23 expression to justify inclusion in the labeling of this animal data to inform prescribers about the potential carcinogenic risk from ustekinumab use". Further studies would not affect the risk assessment of the mAb. Indeed, for many immunomodulatory biologics, the Weight-Of-Evidence (WoE) will reveal an extensive and often conflicting literature for the potential effects of target neutralization on tumor promotion such that performing further non-clinical studies with the clinical candidate would not inform human risk assessment. Hence, a waiver of standard lifetime carcinogenicity studies and other non-clinical studies would be requested and carcinogenic potential is assessed through clinical pharmacovigilance for malignancies as outlined in **Case Study 6**.

Case Study 6

CAD summary for an anti-IL-17 mAb. mAbX is a selective cytokine inhibitor blocking IL-17, acting mainly on muco-epidermal immunity [220]). Hence, it is not a broad-spectrum immunosuppressant that is expected to greatly reduce the key functions of effector memory CTLs, NK and NKT cells that contribute to oncogenic virus and tumor immune- surveillance. Overall, data generated with the approved anti-IL-17 mAbs Cosentyx™, Taltz™, Siliq™ or Stelara™ do not suggest an increased risk of tumorigenicity for the different pathological conditions considered. The carcinogenic risk of mAbX is not expected to be significantly different from these approved mAbs. IL-17 can promote tumors by 1/ increasing angiogenesis, 2/ attracting myeloid-derived suppressor cells (MDSCs) to the tumor and promoting their development, 3/ decreasing apoptosis and 4/ attracting neutrophils to the tumor, contributing to the maintenance of inflammation. Therefore, mAbX, by neutralizing IL-17, could be protective against tumors. This is supported by the correlation of IL-17 (and Th17) and tumor progression in many cancer types, the evidence of increased growth of IL-17-transfected tumor cells, as compared to their wild-type counterparts, and the protection against tumor development in IL-17/IL-23 KO mice or upon anti-IL-17 mAb treatment in several models. However, conversely, IL-17 might also inhibit tumors through its role in tumor immune surveillance, and hence, mAbX might have a deleterious effect by reducing immune surveillance. For example, IL-17KO mice show greater metastasis than wildtype mice in a colon carcinoma model and there are examples of human tumors regressing upon IL-17 treatment. A positive correlation between the levels of IL-17 in ascites and survival has also been reported in some solid tumor types. The effects of IL-17 may depend on the specific tumor microenvironment and tumor/immune cell phenotype in each individual. It is also possible that the role of Th17 cells varies according to cancer cause, type, location and stage of the disease. However, no strong impact on immune function/status was observed in toxicity studies with the mAb. The risk for the mAb is not expected to be different from other IL-17 and IL-23 blockers. A waiver for 2-year bioassays and mouse transgenic models is proposed based on the lack of cross-reactivity of the mAb with rodent IL-17, the lack of availability of a surrogate reagent and post importantly the fact that any additional non-clinical study data will not alter the already conflicting database. Hence, immunosurveillance of tumors will be included in the Clinical Risk Management Plan.

29.18 Combination Toxicology Studies

In an effort to improve on clinical efficacy achieved with individual mAbs, one or more mAbs may be combined with other mAbs, biologics or NCEs. Guidelines for combination toxicology studies have been published [221,222]. Combination toxicity studies are rarely performed for mAbs/proteins for immune-mediated diseases as the perceived safety risks of the combinations are usually perceived to be low. Non-clinical combination studies are generally not required to support the administration of an immunomodulatory mAb as an adjunctive/concomitant therapy with standard-of-care drugs such as methotrexate. No such studies were performed for the approved TNFα inhibitors. A combination study might be considered if there is cause for concern around the combined PD activity of the two drugs, although this information may well be obtained from in vitro studies with human cells and/or in efficacy/pharmacology studies rather than from a dedicated toxicology study. Non-clinical safety studies were conducted to evaluate the safety and PD effects (decreased blood and tissue B cell and serum Ig) of atacicept (TACI-Ig, blocks BLyS and APRIL-mediated survival of B cells) combined with mycophenolate mofetil (MMF) in mice and with atacicept combined with rituximab in cynomolgus monkeys [223]. Combining two immunosuppressive drugs likely brings an increased risk of infection. However, it should be noted that the potential increased risk of infection when combining two immunosuppressive biologics (e.g., increased infections with Enbrel (anti-TNFα) and Kineret (IL-1ra) [224]; PML observed with natalizumab (anti-α4-integrin mAb) and Avonex (IFN-β1a) [225] would not be detected in a non-clinical combination study.

29.19 Limitations to the Predictive Value of Non-Clinical Testing of mAbs for Immune-Mediated Diseases

The main adverse events observed with mAbs/proteins for immune-mediated disease, namely hypersensitivity (including anaphylaxis), infusion reactions, CRS, PML, autoimmunity, allergy and decreased immune surveillance leading to infection are often of low incidence in patients and are poorly predicted from non-clinical studies with mAbs. The overall concordance of non-clinical and clinical data is low; however, the direct and/or exaggerated immunopharmacology of mAbs/proteins is modeled well in non-clinical studies [134], whereas indirect outcomes of immunomodulation (e.g., infection, PML) and CRS are not [226,227]. This may be partly dues to patient-specific factors (age, race and patient genetics (MHC), underlying disease, concomitant medication, immune status), which are likely to be highly variable in patient's population, as well as to species differences in the expression profile and function of immune targets/pathways between animals and humans [101]. Hence, there is a need to develop sensitive and robust assays/endpoints in both animals and humans to assess immunological activities beyond immunosuppression and the standard tier immunotoxicity tests (flow cytometry, TDAR, histopathology of lymphoid organs), such as effects on key functions of T regs, Th1-Th2 cells, CTLs, dendritic cells, NK cell, macrophage subsets and mast cells. The use of techniques such as IHC, genomics, proteomics and humanized/transgenic/KO animals should be promoted to try and detect more sensitive markers of immunotoxicity.

29.20 Selection of a Safe Starting Dose in Humans

The selection of a safe starting dose for a mAb/protein should utilize all relevant biological and pharmacological information and has been extensively reviewed [124,132,228–230]. Key considerations include (1) the MoA (nature and duration of the pharmacological effect(s) (e.g., is it an antagonist or does it have agonist activity with strong immune cell activation and cytokine release potential), (2) novelty of the agent (standard IgG or multivalent and/or highly engineered construct) and (3) the availability of in vitro human systems and in vivo animal models to assess/predict the safety of the pharmacological effect of the biologic (dependent on relative target binding and in some cases FcγR binding, target distribution and expression level and pharmacological activity between animals and humans). The presence of these real or perceived risk factors will determine whether the biologic is considered a high-risk molecule for which a more conservative starting dose might be justified (e.g., based on a minimum anticipated biological effect level (MABEL), theoretically maximizing safety for clinical trial subjects [228–233] or low risk where a higher degree of pharmacological activity of the starting dose might be acceptable (e.g., pharmacologically active dose (PAD), anticipated therapeutic dose (ATD)) [233].

Generally, for most drugs, the FIH starting dose is selected based on consideration of both toxicology data (NOAEL) and pharmacology data (MABEL, PAD and ATD). The use of the NOAEL to determine the FIH starting dose is described in the 2005 FDA guidance [231]. The NOAEL in the most appropriate animal species is determined and then converted to a HED (direct mg/kg animal to human for mAbs) to which a safety factor is applied to provide the Maximum Recommended Starting Dose (MRSD). However, for the vast majority of highly specific immunomodulatory mAbs designed to inhibit the function and/or deplete immune cells, there will be no or little acute and/or severe safety concerns. The NOAEL within the toxicity studies is often the highest dose tested, e.g., 100–200 mg/kg, and hence, the Human Equivalent Dose (HED) based on toxicity data would be 10-20 mg/kg which is too high a starting dose, hence rarely do the toxicology data drive the starting dose for immunosuppressive biologics, which is mainly derived from the pharmacology data (see **Case Study 7**). Pharmacology data-based methods include in vitro or in vivo data (e.g., target occupancy (TO; binding to target but not necessarily resulting in a functional effect), TE and pharmacological activity/efficacy data (pathways downstream of TE, including effects on disease in a non-clinical model) that defines the exposure–response curve from which a PAD in humans can be estimated. Differences in pharmacological activity and relative potency between humans and the chosen toxicology species should be accounted for when extrapolating the in vitro and in vivo toxicological and pharmacological responses observed in animals to those predicted in humans [233]. Data from one or several of these assays (perhaps the most sensitive of the assays, the assay considered to be the most biologically relevant, a combination of relevant assays or an average of multiple assays) are used to estimate the pharmacological responses in humans across a range of dose levels. In recent years, empirical calculation methods have been replaced by state-of-the-art PK/PD and physiologically based PK (PBPK) modeling to guide dose selection that describes exposure–response relationships based on a mixture of data and estimated parameters (**Case Study 7**). PK/PD modeling can be used to integrate mAb concentrations in blood and tissue with in vitro and in vivo TO, pharmacological activity and toxicological data in animals, enabling the prediction of PD effects in humans over time at different dose levels, based upon adjusted animal parameters [234]. They are considered more holistic in the way they incorporate multiple parameters such as binding affinity to target (KD), mechanism, drug disposition, and the relationship of the drug to the target.

Since the majority of mAbs/proteins for immune-mediated diseases discussed herein are not designated as a high risk, a MABEL-based starting dose would rarely be appropriate and a less conservative approach could be considered (with scientific justification), with the starting dose producing a higher level of TO /pharmacological activity (PAD and ATD). In this way, a therapeutic dose (e.g., recommended Phase 2 dose) will be reached within fewer cohorts, thereby both safeguarding healthy volunteers and patients from adverse events but also minimizing the number of patients exposed to sub-therapeutic doses. Indeed, the European Medicines Agency (EMA) 2017 guidance recommends that for patients, the starting dose should consider the disease and should not be substantially lower than the expected pharmacological dose. In the less frequent cases where a molecule would be considered high risk, e.g., a first-in-class molecule for which acute responses might be anticipated (e.g., cytokine release or rapid cell depletion, potential for unintended immune cell activation (**Case Study 8**), then a MABEL approach may be justified, based on low TO or TE levels (e.g., 10%), or a low effective concentration (EC) or inhibitory concentration (IC) from the in vitro assays (e.g., EC10 and EC20) or the lowest dose providing exposures predicted to show a trend toward a biological effect in the PK/PD model.

Case Study 7: Lower risk, Antagonist mAb, MABEL Not Used

The molecule is a novel multivalent mAb-based construct designed to inhibit the pharmacological activity of three soluble inflammatory cytokines in autoimmune diseases. The expression and function of all three targets are well characterized and there is considerable clinical experience with monotherapy mAbs targeting the individual cytokines. There is no risk for acute toxicity. The main risk for humans is the potential to increase the risk of infection after long-term dosing due to inhibition of innate immunity (the case for many such immunosuppressive mAbs targeting cytokines). The molecule neutralizes the pharmacological of the three cynomolgus monkey cytokines to a similar extent as to the human cytokines but does not inhibit the cytokines from lower species. The molecule was well tolerated in NHPs, although a NOAEL could not be assigned due to the presence of adverse skin findings due to bacterial outgrowth. These findings are not directly translatable to humans. Hence, based on the antagonist MoA, the existing knowledge of the targets, the availability of

pharmacologically relevant in vitro and in vivo models and the clinical safety experience with the monotherapy, it was considered low risk, and hence, a MABEL-based starting dose was not proposed. A model-based approach [235] was taken. The human PK in plasma was expected to be linear and was predicted using an allometric scaling of the PK model based on NHP data. Prediction of the PK in the target tissue was made assuming a partition of approximately 0.25. The binding model included the plasma and target tissue compartments, with expression and turnover of the three cytokines in each compartment. Values for target expression and turnover were obtained from in-house in vitro experiments, tissue expression data and literature values. Since the FIH study was in patients with mild inflammatory disease, very low TO was to be avoided in order to minimize the number of patients receiving sub-therapeutic exposures. At the proposed starting dose, the model predicted target binding of 20%, 10% and 95% for the three cytokines in the target tissue. While the degrees of target binding for two of the cytokines were predicted to be low, binding to the third cytokine would result in a pharmacological effect at the starting dose. Given the extensive experience with neutralizing this cytokine, the risk of significant AEs was considered low. Target binding to all three cytokines in blood was predicted to be greater than 95%.

Case Study 8: High-Risk Molecule with Immune-Activating Potential, MABEL Defined Using In Vitro Pharmacology Data

This case study is a theoretical case study based on the novel Fc multimer constructs described in Case Study 1, but for which an alternative format was developed with a favorable safety profile, allowing potential progression to the clinic. A starting dose based on MABEL was proposed due to the potential high safety risk of complement and platelet activation, cytokine release and acute immunotoxicity seen with other molecules within the class. Pharmacologically relevant in vitro and in vivo assays were available and confirmed the favorable safety profile of the alternative format Fc multimer. However, translation was uncertain due to the differences in expression and activities of FcγRs in humans and NHPs. In addition, the Fc multimer showed complex PK and extremely short serum half-life in vivo due to rapid TMDD, making it difficult to relate exposure to the degree of RO and PD effect/safety biomarker in NHPs and to model this in humans. A dose predicted to achieve a max plasma concentration (Cmax) equating to the mean EC$_{10}$ for CR or platelet-activating factor release (whichever was lowest) in vitro with human cells, with a safety factor applied (to account for the biological difference between humans and NHPs), would be selected for the FIH dose in HVs.

29.21 Conclusions

Immune-mediated diseases are chronic, generally incurable diseases that have been mainly managed to date through the use of broad-spectrum immunosuppressant small molecule drugs as well as more targeted biological therapies, many of which have gained regulatory approval. At an earlier stage of development are a number of more highly focused antigen- and cell-specific therapies, based on tolerogenic peptide identification, gene editing and gene and cell therapy technologies with the potential to achieve disease modification, immune tolerance, immune reset, tissue repair and ultimately to disease resolution. However, each of the immunomodulatory therapies has a risk of immunotoxicity, frequently driven by exaggerated immunopharmacology. A combination of *in vitro* and *in vivo* immunosafety studies in pharmacologically relevant species is required to try and predict adverse immune effects and select safe dose levels for patients. However, although these models are able to predict the intended pharmacological effects of these mAbs in humans, they are not very good at predicting immunotoxicity such as hypersensitivity (including anaphylaxis), infusion reactions, CRS, PML, autoimmunity and risk of infection and cancer. Efforts must be made to developing new and/or optimized animal models, assays and biomarkers as well as clinical safety assays to predict the potential for immunotoxicity. However, some of these events are relatively rare and can never realistically be assessed in non-clinical studies with small numbers of animals or human cells. Risk mitigation for these effects will rely on a weight-of-evidence approach to benefit: risk assessment and careful clinical risk management based on the unique characteristics of the product, the target and the patient population to be treated.

APPENDIX—GLOSSARY OF IMMUNOLOGICAL TERMS

Adaptive (acquired) immunity: Antigen-specific, lymphocyte-mediated immune defense mechanisms that take several days to become protective and are designed to remove the specific antigen.

ADCC (antibody-dependent cell cytotoxicity): is the killing of an antibody-coated target cell by a cytotoxic effector (e.g., NK cell) cell following binding to its FcγR resulting in the release of cytotoxic granules or cell death-inducing molecules.

ADCP (antibody-dependent cell phagocytosis): phagocytosis of antibody-coated target cells by phagocytes expressing FcgRIIa (primarily).

Allergy: Hypersensitivity caused by exposure to an exogenous antigen (allergen) resulting in a marked increase in reactivity and responsiveness to that antigen on subsequent exposure, resulting in adverse health effects.

Anaphylaxis: A type of immune-mediated hypersensitivity reaction. Anaphylactic (type I) or immediate hypersensitivity reactions involve specific IgE antibodies.

Antibody (Ab): Immunoglobulin molecule produced by B lymphocytes (B cells) in response to immunization/sensitization with a specific antigen that specifically reacts with that antigen.

Antigen-presenting cell (APC): A cell that presents antigen to lymphocytes, enabling its specific recognition by receptors on the cell surface. In a more restricted way, this term is used to describe MHC class II-positive (accessory) cells that are able to present (processed) antigenic peptides complexed with MHC class II molecules to T helper (Th) cells. These cells include macrophage populations (in particular Langerhans cells, and dendritic or interdigitating cells), B cells, activated T lymphocytes (T cells), certain epithelial and endothelial cells (after MHC class II antigen induction by, e.g., interferon-γ).

Autoantibodies: Immunoglobulins (antibodies) that are directed against endogenous molecules of the host. They circulate in the serum but may be also detectable in other body fluids or bound in target tissue structures. Autoantibodies may occur as a part of the natural immunoglobulin repertoire (natural antibodies) or are induced by different mechanisms (non-natural or pathological autoantibodies). A number of non-natural autoantibodies are diagnostic markers of defined autoimmune diseases regardless of their pathogenetic activity. They may be directed against conserved non-organ-specific autoantigens, organ-specific autoantigens or cell-specific autoantigens.

Autoantigens: Self-constituents (antigens) of the organism, which may be targets of autoimmune responses mediated by autoreactive B cells (*see* Autoantibodies) or T cells; they include proteins, glycoproteins, nucleic acids, phospholipids and glycosphingolipids.

Autoimmune disease: Disease caused by antibodies or T cells targeting self-antigens.

Autoimmunity: A state of immune reactivity toward self-constituents (*see* Autoantigens) that may be either destructive or nondestructive. Destructive autoimmunity is associated with the development of autoimmune diseases.

B lymphocyte/cells: Lymphocytes expressing immunoglobulin (antibody) surface receptors (on naive B cells IgM and IgD) that recognize nominal antigen and after activation, proliferate and differentiate into antibody-producing plasma cells. During a T cell-dependent process, there is an immunoglobulin class switch (from IgM to IgG, IgA, IgD or IgE) with the maintenance of the antigen binding domain. For T cell-independent antigens, cells differentiate only to IgM-producing plasma cells.

Basophils: White blood cells (granulocytes) with granules that stain with basic dyes and which have a function similar to mast cells (*see* Mast cell).

Biologicals: Proteins, poly- or monoclonal antibodies and fusion proteins generated by recombinant DNA technology.

CD: Cluster of differentiation, e.g., CD4 and CD8. This is a standard naming system for cell surface proteins of the immune system. For example, CD4 and CD8 identify different subsets of T cells, and CD69 is a cell surface protein induced upon short-term activation of T cells.

CD4+: T helper cells recognize antigenic peptides in association with MHC class II molecules. They mediate their effector functions by enhancing the persistence of antigen-stimulated T cells or through the secretion of effector cytokines.

CD8⁺: T cytotoxic cells or Cytotoxic T lymphocytes (CTLs) recognize antigenic peptides in association with MHC class I molecules and mediate their effector functions by killing the cells presenting the relevant antigenic peptides or secreting effector cytokines.

Cell-mediated immunity: Immunological reactivity mediated by T cells.

Complement-dependent cytotoxicity (CDC): The immune process involving complement by which the antibody–antigen complex activates a cascade of proteolytic enzymes that ultimately result in the formation of a terminal lytic complex that is inserted into a cell membrane, resulting in lysis and cell death.

Complement system: Series of proteolytic enzymes in blood, capable of lysing microbes and enhancing the uptake of microbes by phagocytes.

Cytokines: Proteins secreted by activated immunocompetent cells that act as intercellular mediators regulating cellular differentiation and activation, particularly within the immune system. They are produced by a number of tissue or cell types rather than by specialized glands and generally act locally in a paracrine or autocrine manner often with overlapping or synergistic actions.

Dendritic cells (DC): Leukocytes in tissue that show elongations/protrusions of cytoplasm in the parenchyma, representing a specialized type of antigen-presenting cell derived from lymphocytes or monocytes.

Effector T cells: T cells that perform immune functions, i.e., T helper cells and cytotoxic T cells (CTLs).

Eosinophils: Granular leukocytes stained by eosin that contains a typically bi-lobed nucleus and large specific granules. The eosinophils reside predominantly in submucosal tissue and normally low in blood. The cells participate in phagocytosis and inflammatory responses.

Fab region: Region of an antibody that contains the antigen-binding site.

Fc receptor: Cell surface receptor on phagocytes and other (mostly immune) cells, e.g., NK cells involved in the recognition of Fc regions of Ig. Fc receptor triggering in phagocytes can trigger various effector functions, including phagocytosis, degranulation and intracellular (oxidative) killing.

Fc region: Region of an antibody responsible for binding to Fc receptors and the C1q component of complement.

HLA: *see* Major histocompatibility complex

Humoral immunity: Immunological reactivity mediated by antibodies.

Hypersensitivity: Abnormally increased, immunologically mediated response to a stimulus. Sometimes used loosely for any increased response or to describe allergy. The reaction can be mimicked by non-immunological mechanisms (e.g., chemical stimulation of mast cell degranulation).

Immune system: A system including all aspects of host defense mechanisms against xenobiotics and pathogens that are encoded in the genes of the host. It includes barrier mechanisms, all organs of immunity, the innate (immediate, nonspecific) immune response effectors (proteins, bioactive molecules and cells—mainly phagocytes) and the adaptive (delayed, specific) immune response effectors (T and B cells and their products). The two responses (specific and nonspecific) act synergistically for a fully effective immune response.

Immunoglobulin: Immunoglobulins (Ig) are synthesized by plasma cells. The basic subunit consists of two identical heavy chains (about 500 amino acid residues, organized into four homologous domains; for μ chain in IgM about 600 amino acid residues, organized in five homology domains) and two identical light chains (about 250 amino acid residues organized into two homologous domains), each consisting of a variable domain and 1–3 constant domains (in the μ chain four constant domains). The antigen-binding fragment (Fab) consists of variable domains of heavy and light chains (two per basic subunit). Five classes of immunoglobulins exist, which differ according to heavy chain type (constant domains): IgG (major Ig in blood), IgM (pentamer consisting of five basic units), IgA (major Ig in secretions, here present mainly as a dimeric Ig molecule), IgD (major function as receptor on B lymphocytes) and IgE. Effector functions after antigen binding are mediated by constant domains of the heavy chain (Fc part of the molecule) and include complement activation (IgG, IgM), binding to phagocytic cells (IgG), sensitization and antibody-dependent cell-mediated cytotoxicity (IgG), adherence to platelets (IgG) and sensitization and degranulation of mast cells and basophils (IgE). IgA lacks these effector functions and acts mainly in immune exclusion (prevention of entry into the body) at secretory surfaces.

Immunomodulation: Immunomodulation is directed toward either enhancement or suppression of host immunological mechanisms, such as phagocytosis and bactericidal activity, cytokine production, lymphocyte proliferation, antibody response and cellular immunity.

Immunosuppression: Defects in one or more components of the nonspecific/innate or specific/adaptive immune system, resulting in inability to eliminate or neutralize non-self-antigens. Congenital or primary immunodeficiencies are genetic or due to developmental disorders. Acquired or secondary immunodeficiencies develop as a consequence of immunosuppressive compounds, malnutrition, malignancies, radiation or infection. This may result in decreased resistance to infection, the development of certain types of tumors or immune dysregulation and stimulation, thereby promoting allergy or autoimmunity.

Inflammation: A complex biological and biochemical process involving cells of the immune system and a plethora of biological mediators (particularly cytokines); it may be defined as the normal response of living tissue to mechanical injury, chemical toxins, invasion by microorganisms or hypersensitivity reactions.

Excessive or chronic inflammation can lead to disease/pathology.

Inflammatory cytokines: Cytokines that primarily contribute to inflammatory reactions, including interferon-γ, interleukins, tumor necrosis factor-a (TNFα) and chemokines.

Innate immune system/innate (nonspecific) immunity: Non-adaptive, non-antigen-specific host defense system against pathogens and injurious stimuli, present at birth and consisting of phagocytes (macrophages, neutrophils), natural killer (NK) cells and other innate lymphocyte populations and the complement system.

Leukocytes: Also called white blood cells, comprising granulocytes (polymorphonuclear neutrophilic granulocytes, eosinophilic granulocytes and basophilic granulocytes), monocytes and lymphocytes.

Lymphocytes: Cells belonging to the lymphoid lineage of bone marrow-derived hematopoietic cells. A more restricted designation is that of a small resting or recirculating mononuclear cell in blood or lymphoid tissue that measures about 7–8 μm and has a round nucleus containing densely aggregated chromatin and little cytoplasm. Lymphocytes play a key role in immune reactions through specific recognition of antigens.

Lymphoid organ: It is an organ in which cells of the immune system, mainly lymphocytes, are lodged in an organized microenvironment, either in a resting stage or in a stage of activation/differentiation/proliferation. Lymphoid organs include bone marrow, thymus, lymph nodes, spleen and mucosal-associated lymphoid tissue. Central (primary) lymphoid organs are those in which T and B cells develop and mature (bone marrow, thymus); peripheral (secondary) lymphoid organs are those where immunocompetent lymphocytes recognize antigen and subsequently initiate immunological reactions and produce effector elements of these reactions.

Macrophages: Large 12–20-μm mononuclear phagocytic and antigen-presenting cells are present in tissues, constituting the mononuclear phagocytic system that includes monocytes, macrophages, dendritic cells (in lymphoid organs), Langerhans cells (in skin) and Kupffer cells (in liver).

Major histocompatibility complex (MHC): Set of genes that code for tissue compatibility markers, called HLA (human leukocyte antigens, which are targets in the rejection of an allograft (matched grafted tissue or organ from a different individual) and hence determine the fate of allografts, also play a central role in the control of cellular interactions (e.g., T cells) during immunological reactions. Tissue compatibility is coded by class I and class II gene loci.

Mast cell: Tissue (mainly skin and mucosa)-associated cell activated by antigen/allergen bridging of surface-bound IgE antibodies, releasing enzymes and vasoactive mediators, especially histamine: a key driver of allergic reactions.

Monoclonal antibodies (mAbs): Identical copies of antibody with the same antigen specificity consist of one heavy chain class and one light chain type.

Monocytes: Large 10–15-μm non-differentiated mononuclear cell, present in blood and lymphatics, comprising the circulating component of the mononuclear phagocyte system.

Natural killer (NK) cells: Lymphocyte-like cells of the innate immune system capable of killing virus-infected and tumor-transformed cells in an antigen-independent manner.

Neutrophils: Highly specialized white blood cells characterized by a multilobed nucleus (polymorphonuclear) and a granular cytoplasm that is "neutral" to histological staining under the light microscope. Specialized constituents of the neutrophil membrane, cytoplasmic granules and cytosol together mediate ingestion and killing of bacteria; after attachment and internalization of the microorganism into the phagocytic vacuole (phagosome), its destruction is mediated by the release of an array of antimicrobial polypeptides and reactive oxidant species.

Phagocytosis: Process by which phagocytes bind and engulf material > 1 μm (e.g., microbes) in an Fc receptor-dependent manner, with accessory help of complement receptors. Phagocytosis occurs *via* a "zipper" mechanism, whereby the particle, opsonized (coated) with antibody or complement, becomes enclosed by the cell membrane of the phagocyte. The particle is then incorporated into a vacuole (phagosome) where it is degraded by proteases and an NADPH oxidase-mediated oxidative burst with the formation of superoxide anion, peroxide anion and hydroxyl radicals.

T cell: Thymus-derived lymphocytes that induce, regulate and effect specific immunological reactions stimulated by antigen, mostly in the form of processed antigen complexed with MHC on an antigen-presenting cell. Subsets include T helper (Th), T cytotoxic (Tc/CTL) and T regulatory (Treg) cells.

T cell receptor (TCR): Heterodimeric molecule on the surface of the T cell that recognizes antigens. The polypeptide chains have a variable and a constant part and can be an α, β or γ chain. The αβT cell receptor occurs on most T cells and recognizes antigenic peptides in combination with the polymorphic determinant of MHC molecules (self-MHC restricted). The γδT cell receptor occurs on a small subpopulation, e.g., in mucosal epithelium, and can recognize antigen in a non-MHC-restricted manner. The T cell receptor occurs exclusively in association with the CD3 molecule that mediates transmembrane signaling.

T cytotoxic (Tc) cell/CTL: Functional subset of predominantly CD8+ T cells that differentiate from precursor to effector cytotoxic cells and subsequently kill target cells. CD8+ CTLs recognize antigenic peptides in association with MHC class I molecules. CD8+ T cells mediate their effector functions by killing the cells presenting the relevant antigenic peptides, or secreting effector cytokines. CD4[+] T helper cells recognize antigenic peptides in association with MHC class II molecules. They mediate their effector functions by enhancing the persistence of antigen-stimulated T cells or through secretion of effector cytokines.

T helper (Th) cells: Functional subset of predominantly CD4[+] T cells that can help to generate cytotoxic T cells (CTLs) and cooperates with B cells in the production of antibody. Th1, Th2 and Th17 subpopulations exist: Th1 cells produce interleukin (IL)-2, interferon (IFN)-γ, tumor necrosis factor (TNF)α and tumor necrosis factor (TNF)β, granulocyte/macrophage colony-stimulating factor (GM-CSF), function in the induction of delayed-type hypersensitivity (DTH), macrophage activation and IgG1 synthesis. Th2 cells produce IL-3, -4, -5, TNFα and GM-CSF; function in the induction of IgG4, IgA and IgE synthesis, and induction of eosinophilic granulocytes; and drive allergic responses. Th17 cells produce IL-17 that drive proinflammatory T cell and neutrophil responses and are important in muco-epidermal immunity and skin inflammation.

T regulatory cells (Tregs): Functional subset of T cells that regulate the activity and function of other T cells and immune cells through the production of mediators such as IL-10 and TGF-β.

Tolerance: A state of unresponsiveness to antigenic stimulation, due to the absence of responding elements or the loss of capacity of existing elements to mount a reaction; synonym for anergy.

REFERENCES

1. Kaplon H, Reichert JM. Antibodies to watch in 2019. *mAbs* 2019;11:219–38.
2. Brennan FR. Monoclonal antibodies in Phase 1 and 2 clinical studies for immunological disorders. In: Dubel S, Reichert J, editors. *Handbook of Therapeutic Antibodies.* John Wiley & Sons Inc; 2014. Chapter 30; pp. 927–67.
3. Ward P, Bodmer M, Sloan V. Monoclonal antibodies in Phase III clinical studies for immunological disorders. In: Dubel S, Reichert J, editors. *Handbook of Therapeutic Antibodies.* John Wiley & Sons Inc; 2014. Chapter 29; pp. 851–925.
4. Wolfe RM, Ang DC. Biologic therapies for autoimmune and connective tissue diseases. *Immunol Allergy Clin North Am* 2017;37:283–99.
5. Schett G, Neurath MF. Resolution of chronic inflammatory disease: Universal and tissue-specific concepts. *Nat Commun* 2018;9:3261.
6. Rayner F, Isaacs JD. Therapeutic tolerance in autoimmune disease. *Semin Arthritis Rheum* 2018;48:558–62.
7. Schett G. Resolution of inflammation in arthritis. *Semin Immunopathol* 2019;41:675–79.
8. Zhang Q, Lu W, Liang CL, Chen Y, Liu H, Qiu F, Dai Z.Chimeric antigen receptor (CAR) Treg: A promising approach to inducing immunological tolerance. *Front Immunol* 2018;9:2359.
9. Ewart D, Peterson EJ, Steer CJ. A new era of genetic engineering for autoimmune and inflammatory diseases. *Semin Arthritis Rheum* 2019;49:e1–e7.
10. Di Fusco D, Dinallo V, Marafini I, Figliuzzi MM, Romano B, Monteleone G. Antisense oligonucleotide: Basic concepts and therapeutic application in inflammatory bowel disease. *Front Pharmacol* 2019;10:305.
11. Kopf M, Bachmann MF, Marsland BJ. Averting inflammation by targeting the cytokine environment. *Nat Rev Drug Discov* 2010;9:703–18.
12. McInnes IB, Buckley CD, Isaacs JD. Cytokines in rheumatoid arthritis - shaping the immunological landscape. *Nat Rev Rheumatol* 2016;12:63–8.
13. Shevach EM, Thornton AM. tTregs, pTregs, and iTregs: Similarities and differences. *Immunol Rev* 2014;259:88–102.
14. Brinkmann U, Kontermann RE. The making of bispecific antibodies. *mAbs* 2017;9:182–212.
15. Siontorou CG. Nanobodies as novel agents for disease diagnosis and therapy. *Int J Nanomedicine* 2013;8:4215–27.
16. Kovaleva M, Ferguson L, Steven J, Porter A, Barelle C. Shark variable new antigen receptor biologics - a novel technology platform for therapeutic drug development. *Expert Opin Biol Ther* 2014;14:1527–39.
17. Hober S, Lindbo S, Nilvebrant J. Bispecific applications of non-immunoglobulin scaffold binders. *Methods* 2019;154:143–52.
18. Brezski RJ, Georgiou G. Immunoglobulin isotype knowledge and application to Fc engineering. *Curr Opin Immunol* 2016;40:62–9.
19. Schlothauer T, Herter S, Koller CF, Grau-Richards S, Steinhart V, Spick C, Kubbies M, Klein C, Umaña P, Mössner E. Novel human IgG1 and IgG4 Fc-engineered antibodies with completely abolished immune effector functions. *Protein Eng Des Sel* 2016;29:457–66.
20. Wang X, Mathieu M, Brezski RJ. IgG Fc engineering to modulate antibody effector functions. *Protein Cell* 2018;9:63–73.
21. Jefferis R. Glyco-engineering of human IgG-Fc to modulate biologic activities. *Curr Pharm Biotechnol* 2016;17:1333–47.
22. Kontermann RE. Half-life extended biotherapeutics. *Expert Opin Biol Ther* 2016;16:903–15.
23. Zhang P, Sun F, Liu S, Jiang S. Anti-PEG antibodies in the clinic: Current issues and beyond PEGylation. *J Control Release* 2016;244(Pt B):184–93.
24. Reddy V, Dahal LN, Cragg MS, Leandro M. Optimising B-cell depletion in autoimmune disease: Is obinutuzumab the answer? *Drug Discov Today* 2016 Aug;21(8):1330–38.
25. Willis MD, Robertson NP. Alemtuzumab for multiple sclerosis. *Curr Neurol Neurosci Rep* 2016 Sep;16(9):84.
26. Matucci A, Maggi E, Vultaggio A. Eosinophils, the IL-5/IL-5Rα axis, and the biologic effects of benralizumab in severe asthma. *Respir Med* 2019 Nov 11;160:105819.
27. Pereira NA, Chan KF, Lin PC, Song Z. The "less-is-more" in therapeutic antibodies: Afucosylated anti-cancer antibodies with enhanced antibody-dependent cellular cytotoxicity. *mAbs* 2018 Jul;10(5):693–711.
28. Chataway J, Martin K, Barrell K, Sharrack B, Stolt P, Wraith DC. ATX-MS1467 Study Group. Effects of ATX-MS-1467 immunotherapy over 16 weeks in relapsing multiple sclerosis. *Neurology* 2018;90:e955–e962.

29. Roep BO, Wheeler DCS, Peakman M. Antigen-based immune modulation therapy for type 1 diabetes: The era of precision medicine. *Lancet Diabetes Endocrinol* 2019;7:65–74.

30. Vlasakakis G, Napolitano A, Barnard R, Brown K, Bullman J, Inman D, Keymeulen B, Lanham D, Leirens Q, MacDonald A, et al. Target engagement and cellular fate of **otelixizumab**: A repeat dose escalation study of an anti-CD3ε mAb in new-onset type 1 diabetes mellitus patients. *Br J Clin Pharmacol* 2019;85:704–14.

31. Herold KC, Bundy BN, Long SA, Bluestone JA, DiMeglio LA, Dufort MJ, Gitelman SE, Gottlieb PA, Krischer JP, Linsley PS, et al. An anti-CD3 antibody, teplizumab, in relatives at risk for type 1 diabetes. *N Engl J Med* 2019;381:603–61.

32. Smith EL, Peakman M. Peptide immunotherapy for type 1 diabetes-clinical advances. *Front Immunol* 2018;9:392.

33. Di Sabatino A, Lenti MV, Corazza GR, Gianfrani C. Vaccine immunotherapy for celiac disease. *Front Med (Lausanne)* 2018 Jun 26;5:187.

34. van Eden W, Jansen MAA, Ludwig IS, Leufkens P, van der Goes MC, van Laar JM, Broere F. Heat shock proteins can be surrogate autoantigens for induction of antigen specific therapeutic tolerance in rheumatoid arthritis. *Front Immunol* 2019 Feb 22;10:279.

35. Hoffmann HJ, Valovirta E, Pfaar O, Moingeon P, Schmid JM, Skaarup SH, Cardell LO, Simonsen K, Larché M, Durham SR, et al. Novel approaches and perspectives in allergen immunotherapy. *Allergy* 2017;72:1022–34.

36. Satitsuksanoa P, Głobińska A, Jansen K, van de Veen W, Akdis M. Modified allergens for immunotherapy. *Curr Allergy Asthma Rep* 2018;18:9.

37. Pearson RM, Casey LM, Hughes KR, Miller SD, Shea LD. In vivo reprogramming of immune cells: Technologies for induction of antigen-specific tolerance. *Adv Drug Deliv Rev* 2017;114:240–55.

38. Carambia A, Freund B, Schwinge D, Bruns OT, Salmen SC, Ittrich H, Reimer R, Heine M, Huber S, Waurisch C, et al. Nanoparticle-based autoantigen delivery to Treg-inducing liver sinusoidal endothelial cells enables control of autoimmunity in mice. *J Hepatol* 2015;62:1349–56.

39. Benham H, Nel HJ, Law SC, Mehdi AM, Street S, Ramnoruth N, Pahau H, Lee BT, Ng J, Brunck ME, et al. Citrullinated peptide dendritic cell immunotherapy in HLA risk genotype-positive rheumatoid arthritis patients. *Sci Transl Med* 2015;7:290ra87.

40. Akbarpour M, Goudy KS, Cantore A, Russo F, Sanvito F, Naldini L, Annoni A, Roncarolo MG. Insulin B chain 9-23 gene transfer to hepatocytes protects from type 1 diabetes by inducing Ag-specific FoxP3+ Tregs. *Sci Transl Med* 2015;7:289ra81.

41. Keeler GD, Kumar S, Palaschak B, Silverberg EL, Markusic DM, Jones NT, Hoffman BE. Gene therapy-induced antigen-specific Tregs inhibit neuro-inflammation and reverse disease in a mouse model of multiple sclerosis. *Mol Ther* 2018;6:173–83.

42. Singh DD, Hawkins RD, Lahesmaa R, Tripathi SK. CRISPR/Cas9 guided genome and epigenome engineering and its therapeutic applications in immune mediated diseases. *Semin Cell Dev Biol* 2019;96:32–43.

43. Porteus MH. Towards a new era in medicine: Therapeutic genome editing. *Genome Biol* 2015;16:286.

44. Maeder ML, Gersbach CA. Genome-editing technologies for gene and cell therapy. *Mol Ther* 2016;24:430–46.

45. Kotagama OW, Jayasinghe CD, Abeysinghe T. Era of genomic medicine: A narrative review on CRISPR technology as a potential therapeutic tool for human diseases. *Biomed Res Int* 2019;2019:1369682.

46. Hacein-Bey Abina S, Gaspar HB, Blondeau J, Caccavelli L, Charrier S, Buckland K, Picard C, Six E, Himoudi N, Gilmour K, et al. Outcomes following gene therapy in patients with severe Wiskott-Aldrich syndrome. *JAMA* 2015;313:1550–63.

47. Cavazzana M, Ribeil JA, Lagresle-Peyrou C, André-Schmutz I. Gene therapy with hematopoietic stem cells: The diseased bone marrow's point of view. *Stem Cells Dev* 2017;26:71–6.

48. Brunger JM, Zutshi A, Willard VP, Gersbach CA, Guilak F. CRISPR/Cas9 editing of murine induced pluripotent stem cells for engineering inflammation-resistant tissues. *Arthritis Rheumatol* 2017;69:1111–21.

49. Brunger JM, Zutshi A, Willard VP, Gersbach CA, Guilak F. Genome engineering of stem cells for autonomously regulated, closed-loop delivery of biologic drugs. *Stem Cell Rep* 2017;8:1202–13.

50. De Miguel MP, Fuentes-Julián S, Blázquez-Martínez A, Pascual CY, Aller MA, Arias J, Arnalich-Montiel F. Immunosuppressive properties of mesenchymal stem cells: Advances and applications. *Curr Mol Med* 2012;12:574–91.

51. Wang LT, Ting CH, Yen ML, Liu KJ, Sytwu HK, Wu KK, Yen BL. Human mesenchymal stem cells (MSCs) for treatment towards immune- and inflammation-mediated diseases: Review of current clinical trials. *J Biomed Sci* 2016;23:76.

52. Sakaguchi S, Sakaguchi N, Asano M, Itoh M, Toda M. Immunologic self-tolerance maintained by activated T cells expressing IL-2 receptor α-chains (CD25): Breakdown of a single mechanism of self-tolerance causes various autoimmune diseases. *J Immunol* 1995;155:1151–64.

53. Duggleby R, Danby RD, Madrigal JA, Saudemont A. Clinical grade regulatory CD4+ T cells (Tregs): Moving toward cellular-based immunomodulatory therapies. *Front Immunol* 2018;9:252.

54. Jaeckel E, von Boehmer H, Manns MP. Antigen-specific FoxP3-transduced T-cells can control established type 1 diabetes. *Diabetes* 2005;54:306–10.

55. Adair PR, Kim YC, Zhang AH, Yoon J, Scott DW. Human Tregs made antigen specific by gene modification: The power to treat autoimmunity and antidrug antibodies with precision. *Front Immunol* 2017;8:1117.

56. Zavvar M, Abdolmaleki M, Farajifard H, Noorbakhsh F, Azadmanesh K, Vojgani M, Nikcnam MH. Collagen II-primed Foxp3 transduced T cells ameliorate collagen-induced arthritis in rats: The effect of antigenic priming on t regulatory cell function. *Iran J Allergy Asthma Immunol* 2018;17:361–71.

57. Charrot S, Hallam S. CAR-T cells: Future perspectives. *Hemasphere* 2019;3:e188.

58. Scott DW. From IgG fusion proteins to engineered-specific human regulatory T cells: A life of tolerance. *Front Immunol* 2017;8:1576.

59. Koristka S, Kegler A, Bergmann R, Arndt C, Feldmann A, Albert S, Cartellieri M, Ehninger A, Ehninger G, Middeke JM, et al. Engrafting human regulatory T cells with a flexible modular chimeric antigen receptor technology. *J Autoimmun* 2018;90:116–31.

60. Elinav E, Adam N, Waks T, Eshhar Z. Amelioration of colitis by genetically engineered murine regulatory T cells redirected by antigen-specific chimeric receptor. *Gastroenterology* 2009;136:1721–31.

61. Lee JC, Hayman E, Pegram HJ, Santos E, Heller G, Sadelain M, Brentjens R. In vivo inhibition of human CD19-targeted effector T cells by natural T regulatory cells in a xeno-transplant murine model of B cell malignancy. *Cancer Res* 2011;71:2871–81.

62. Fransson M, Piras E, Burman J, Nilsson B, Essand M, Lu B, Harris RA, Magnusson PU, Brittebo E, Loskog AS. CAR/FoxP3-engineered T regulatory cells target the CNS and suppress EAE upon intranasal delivery. *J Neuroinflammation* 2012;9:112.

63. Skuljec J, Chmielewski M, Happle C, Habener A, Busse M, Abken H, Hansen G. Chimeric antigen receptor-redirected regulatory T cells suppress experimental allergic airway inflammation, a model of asthma. *Front Immunol* 2017;8:1125.

64. Sicard A, Levings MK, Scott DW. Engineering therapeutic T cells to suppress alloimmune responses using TCRs, CARs, or BARs. *Am J Transplant* 2018;18:1305–11.

65. Bennett CF, Baker BF, Pham N, Swayze E, Geary RS. Pharmacology of antisense drugs. *Annu Rev Pharmacol Toxicol* 2017;57:81–105.

66. Crooke ST. Molecular mechanisms of antisense oligonucleotides. *Nucleic Acid Ther* 2017;27:70–7.

67. Eckstein F. Phosphorothioates, essential components of therapeutic oligonucleotides. *Nucleic Acid Ther* 2014;24: 374–87.

68. Hagedorn PH, Persson R, Funder ED, Albæk N, Diemer SL, Hansen DJ, Møller MR, Papargyri N, Christiansen H, Hansen BR, et al. Locked nucleic acid: Modality, diversity, and drug discovery. *Drug Discov Today* 2018;23:101–14.

69. Li Z, Rana TM. Molecular mechanisms of RNA-triggered gene silencing machineries. *Acc Chem Res* 2012;45:1122–31.

70. Nair JK, Willoughby JL, Chan A, Charisse K, Alam MR, Wang Q, Hoekstra M, Kandasamy P, Kel'in AV, Milstein S, et al. Multivalent N-acetylgalactosamine-conjugated siRNA localizes in hepatocytes and elicits robust RNAi-mediated gene silencing. *J Am Chem Soc* 2014;136:16958–61.

71. Tatiparti K, Sau S, Kashaw SK, Iyer AK. siRNA delivery strategies: A comprehensive review of recent developments. *Nanomaterials (Basel)* 2017;7:E77.

72. Xue XY, Mao XG, Zhou Y, Chen Z, Hu Y, Hou Z, Li MK, Meng JR, Luo XX. Advances in the delivery of antisense oligonucleotides for combating bacterial infectious diseases. *Nanomedicine* 2018;14:745–58.

73. Stein CA, Castanotto D. FDA-approved oligonucleotide therapies in 2017. *Mol Ther* 2017;25:1069–75.

74. Adams D, Gonzalez-Duarte A, O'Riordan WD, Yang CC, Ueda M, Kristen AV, Tournev I, Schmidt HH, Coelho T, Berk JL, et al. Patisiran, an RNAi therapeutic, for hereditary transthyretin amyloidosis. *N Engl J Med* 2018;379:11–21.

75. Rüger J, Ioannou S, Castanotto D, Stein CA. Oligonucleotides to the (Gene) rescue: FDA approvals 2017–2019. *Trends Pharmacol Sci* 2019;pii: S0165-6147(19)30249-4.

76. Bennett CF, Kornbrust D, Henry S, Stecker K, Howard R, Cooper S, Dutson S, Hall W, Jacoby HI. An ICAM-1 anti-sense oligonucleotide prevents and reverses dextran sulfate sodium-induced colitis in mice. *J Pharmacol Exp Ther* 1997;280:988–1000.

77. Stepkowski SM, Wang ME, Amante A, Kalinin D, Qu X, Blasdel T, Condon T, Kahan BD, Bennett CF. Antisense ICAM-1 oligonucleotides block allograft rejection in rats. *Transplant Proc* 1997;29:1285.

78. Murano M, Maemura K, Hirata I, Toshina K, Nishikawa T, Hamamoto N, Sasaki S, Saitoh O, Katsu K. Therapeutic effect of intracolonically administered nuclear factor kappa B (p65) antisense oligonucleotide on mouse dextran sulphate sodium (DSS)-induced colitis. *Clin Exp Immunol* 2000;120:51–8.

79. Laudisi F, Dinallo V, Di Fusco D, Monteleone G. Smad7 and its potential as therapeutic target in inflammatory bowel diseases. *Curr Drug Metab* 2016;17:303–6.

80. Scarozza P, Schmitt H, Monteleone G, Neurath MF, Atreya R. Oligonucleotides-A novel promising therapeutic option for IBD. *Front Pharmacol* 2019;10:314.

81. Greuter T, Vavricka SR, Biedermann L, Pilz J, Borovicka J, Seibold F, Sauter B, Rogler G. Alicaforsen, an antisense inhibitor of intercellular adhesion molecule-1, in the treatment for left-sided ulcerative colitis and ulcerative proctitis. *Dig Dis* 2018;36:123–9.

82. Feagan BG, Sands BE, Rossiter G, Li X, Usiskin K, Zhan X, Colombel JF. Effects of mongersen (GED-0301) on endoscopic and clinical outcomes in patients with active Crohn's disease. *Gastroenterology* 2018;154:61–4.e6.

83. Suzuki K, Yokoyama J, Kawauchi Y, Honda Y, Sato H, Aoyagi Y, Terai S, Okazaki K, Suzuki Y, Sameshima Y, et al. Phase 1 clinical study of siRNA targeting carbohydrate sulphotransferase 15 in Crohn's disease patients with active mucosal lesions. *J Crohns Colitis* 2017;11:221–8.

84. Hindryckx P, Novak G, Bonovas S, Peyrin-Biroulet L, Danese S. Infection risk with biologic therapy in patients with inflammatory bowel disease. *Clin Pharmacol Ther* 2017;102:633–41.

85. Fernández-Ruiz M, Aguado JM. Risk of infection associated with anti-TNF-α therapy. *Expert Rev Anti Infect Ther* 2018;16:939–56.

86. Buonomo AR, Zappulo E, Viceconte G, Scotto R, Borgia G, Gentile I. Risk of opportunistic infections in patients treated with alemtuzumab for multiple sclerosis. *Expert Opin Drug Saf* 2018;17:709–17.

87. Grøn KL, Glintborg B, Nørgaard M, Mehnert F, Østergaard M, Dreyer L, Krogh NS, Hetland ML. Overall infection risk in rheumatoid arthritis during treatment with abatacept, rituximab and tocilizumab; an observational cohort study. *Rheumatology (Oxford)* 2019;pii:kez530.

88. Berger JR. Classifying PML risk with disease modifying therapies. *Mult Scler Relat Disord* 2017;12:59–63.

89. Iannetta M, Zingaropoli MA, Bellizzi A, Morreale M, Pontecorvo S, D'Abramo A, Oliva A, Anzivino E, Lo Menzo S, D'Agostino C, et al. Natalizumab affects T-cell phenotype in multiple sclerosis: Implications for JCV reactivation. *PLoS One* 2016;11:e0160277.

90. Schwab N, Ulzheimer JC, Fox RJ, Schneider-Hohendorf T, Kieseier BC, Monoranu CM, Staugaitis SM, Welch W, Jilek S, Du Pasquier RA, et al. Fatal PML associated with efalizumab therapy: Insights into integrin αLβ2 in JC virus control. *Neurology* 2012;78:458–67.

91. Berger JR, Malik V, Lacey S, Brunetta P, Lehane PB. Progressive multifocal leukoencephalopathy in rituximab-treated rheumatic diseases: A rare event. *J Neurovirol* 2018;24:323–31.

92. Fredericks CA, Kvam KA, Bear J, Crabtree GS, Josephson SA. A case of progressive multifocal leukoencephalopathy in a lupus patient treated with belimumab. *Lupus* 2014;23:711–3.

93. Dekeyser M, de Goër de Herve MG, Hendel-Chavez H, Labeyrie C, Adams D, Nasser GA, Gasnault J, Durrbach A, Taoufik Y. Refractory T-cell anergy and rapidly fatal progressive multifocal leukoencephalopathy after prolonged CTLA4 therapy. *Open Forum Infect Dis* 2017;4:ofx100.

94. Focosi D, Tuccori M, Maggi F. Progressive multifocal leukoencephalopathy and anti-CD20 monoclonal antibodies: What do we know after 20 years of rituximab. *Rev Med Virol* 2019;29:e2077.

95. Kobayashi K, Okamoto Y, Inoue H, Usui T, Ihara M, Kawamata J, Miki Y, Mimori T, Tomimoto H, Takahashi R. Leukoencephalopathy with cognitive impairment following tocilizumab for the treatment of rheumatoid arthritis (RA). *Intern Med* 2009;48:1307–9.

96. White MK, Gordon J, Berger JR, Khalili K. Animal models for progressive multifocal leukoencephalopathy. *J Cell Physiol* 2015;230:2869–74

97. Ryan PC, Sleeman MA, Rebelatto M, Wang B, Lu H, Chen X, Wu CY, Hinrichs MJ, Roskos L, Towers H, et al. Nonclinical safety of mavrilimumab, an anti-GMCSF receptor alpha monoclonal antibody, in cynomolgus monkeys: Relevance for human safety. *Toxicol Appl Pharmacol* 2014;279:230–9.

98. Carey B, Trapnell BC. The molecular basis of pulmonary alveolar proteinosis. *Clin Immunol* 2010;135:223–35.

99. Matucci A, Nencini F, Maggi E, Vultaggio A. Hypersensitivity reactions to biologics used in rheumatology. *Expert Rev Clin Immunol* 2019;15:1263–71.

100. Gupta KK, Khan MA, Singh SK. Constitutive inflammatory cytokine storm: Major threat to human health. *J Interferon Cytokine Res* 2019;doi: 10.1089/jir.2019.0085.

101. Brennan FR, Kiessling A.Translational immunotoxicology of immunomodulatory monoclonal antibodies. *Drug Discov Today Technol* 21–22:85–93.

102. Brennan FR, Kiessling A. In vitro Assays supporting the safety assessment of immunomodulatory monoclonal antibodies. *Toxicol In Vitro* 2017;45(Pt 3):296–308.

103. Chung CH, Mirakhur B, Chan E, Le QT, Berlin J, Morse M, Murphy BA, Satinover SM, Hosen J, Mauro D, et al. Cetuximab-induced anaphylaxis and IgE specific for galactose-α-1,3-galactose. *N Engl J Med* 2008;358:1109–17.

104. Murdaca G, Spanò F, Contatore M, Guastalla A, Penza E, Magnani O, Puppo F. Immunogenicity of infliximab and adalimumab: What is its role in hypersensitivity and modulation of therapeutic efficacy and safety? *Expert Opin Drug Saf* 2016;15:43–52.

105. Liau MM, Oon HH. Therapeutic drug monitoring of biologics in psoriasis. *Biologics* 2019;13:127–32.

106. Walker M, Makropoulos D, Achuthanandam R, Bugelski P. Recent advances in the understanding of drug-mediated infusion reactions and cytokine release syndrome. *Curr Opin Drug Discov Dev* 13:124–35.

107. Finco D, Grimaldi C, Fort M, Walker M, Kiessling A, Wolf B, Salcedo T, Faggioni R, Schneider A, Ibraghimov A, et al. Cytokine release assays: Current practices and future directions. *Cytokine* 2014 Apr;66(2):143–55.

108. Grimaldi C, Finco D, Fort MM, Gliddon D, Harper K, Helms WS, Mitchell JA, O'Lone R, Parish ST, Piche MS, et al. Cytokine release: A workshop proceedings on the state-of-the-science, current challenges and future directions. *Cytokine* 2016;85:101–8.

109. Devonshire V, Phillips R, Wass H, Da Roza G, Senior P. Monitoring and management of autoimmunity in multiple sclerosis patients treated with alemtuzumab: Practical recommendations. *J Neurol* 2018;265:2494–505.

110. Atzeni F, Talotta R, Salaffi F, Cassinotti A, Varisco V, Battellino M, Ardizzone S, Pace F, Sarzi-Puttini P. Immunogenicity and autoimmunity during anti-TNF therapy. *Autoimmun Rev* 2013;12:703–8.

111. Lynch CM, Hart BW, Grewal IS. Practical considerations for nonclinical safety evaluation of therapeutic monoclonal antibodies. *mAbs* 2009 Jan–Feb;1(1):2–11. Review.

112. Brennan FR, Dill Morton L, Spindeldreher S, Kiessling A, Allenspach A, Hey A, Muller PY, Frings W, Sims J. Safety and immunotoxicity testing of immunomodulatory monoclonal antibodies. *mAbs* 2010;2:233–55.

113. Brennan FR, Cauvin, A, Tibbitts J, Wolfreys A. Optimized nonclinical safety assessment strategies supporting clinical development of therapeutic monoclonal antibodies targeting inflammatory diseases. *Drug Dev Res* 2014;75:115–61.

114. ICHM3(R2). Nonclinical safety studies for the conduct of human clinical trials with pharmaceuticals. 2009; Available at: http://www.ema.europa.eu/pdfs/human/ich/ 028695en. pdf

115. ICH S6. Preclinical safety evaluation of biotechnology-derived pharmaceuticals. 1997; Available at: http://www. ich.org

116. ICHS6 (R1). Preclinical safety evaluation of biotechnology-derived pharmaceuticals. 2011; Step 2 Addendum. Available at: http://www.ich.org/LOB/media/ MEDIA5784.pdf

117. ICHS8. Notes for guidance on immunotoxicity testing of human pharmaceuticals. 2004; Available at: http://www. ema.europa.eu /pdfs/human/ich /16723504en.pdf

118. Bugelski PJ, Herzyk DJ, Rehm S, Harmsen AG, Gore EV, Williams DM, Maleeff BE, Badger AM, Truneh A, O'Brien SR, et al. Preclinical development of keliximab, a primatized anti-CD4 monoclonal antibody, in human CD4 transgenic mice: Characterization of the model and safety studies. *Hum Exp Toxicol* 2000;19:230–43.

119. Bussiere JL, Martin P, Morner M, Couch J, Flaherty M, Andrews L, Beyer J, Horvath C. Alternative strategies for toxicity testing of species-specific biopharmaceuticals. *Int J Toxicol* 2009;28:230–53.

120. Flaherty MM, MacLachlan TK, Troutt M, Magee T, Tuaillon N, Johnson S, Stein KE, Bonvini E, Garman R, Andrews L. Nonclinical evaluation of GMA161--an antihuman CD16 (FcγRIII) monoclonal antibody for treatment of autoimmune disorders in CD16 transgenic mice. *Toxicol Sci* 2012;125:299–309.

121. Treacy G. Using an analogous monoclonal antibody to evaluate the reproductive and chronic toxicity potential for a humanized anti-TNF-α monoclonal antibody. *Hum Exp Toxicol* 2000;19:226–9.

122. Clarke J, Leach W, Pippig S, Joshi A, Wu B, House R, Beyer J. Evaluation of a surrogate antibody for preclinical safety testing of an anti-CD11a monoclonal antibody. *Regul Toxicol Pharmacol* 2004;40:219–26.

123. Soliris. Pharmacology review. 2007; Available at: https://www.accessdata.fda.gov/drugsatfda_docs/nda/2007/125166s0000_PharmR.pdf

124. Muller PY, Brennan FR. Safety assessment and dose selection for first-in-human clinical trials with immuno-modulatory monoclonal antibodies. *Clin Pharmacol Ther* 2009;85:247–58.

125. Gupta S, Devanarayan V, Finco D, Gunn GR 3rd, Kirshner S, Richards S, Rup B, Song A, Subramanyam M. Recommendations for the validation of cell-based assays used for the detection of neutralizing antibody immune responses elicited against biological therapeutics. *J Pharm Biomed Anal* 2011;55:878–88.

126. Wadhwa M, Knezevic I, Kang HN, Thorpe R. Immunogenicity assessment of biotherapeutic products: An overview of assays and their utility. *Biologicals* 2015;43: 298–306.

127. EMA. Guideline on immunogenicity assessment of therapeutic proteins. 2017; Available at: https://www.ema.europa.eu/en/documents/ scientific -guideline/guideline-immunogenicity-assessment-therapeutic-proteins-revision-1_en.pdf

128. FDA. Bioanalytical method validation. Guidance for industry. 2018; Available at: https://www.fda.gov/files/drugs/published/Bioanalytical-Method-Validation-Guidance-for-Industry.pdf

129. FDA. Immunogenicity testing of therapeutic proteins-Developing and validating assays for anti-drug antibody detection. 2019; Available at: https://www.fda.gov/media/119788/download

130. Kiessling P, Lledo-Garcia R, Watanabe K, Langdon G, Tran D, Bari M, Christodoulou L, Jones E, Price G, Smith B, et al. The FcRn inhibitor Rozanolixizumab reduces human serum IgG concentration: A randomized Phase I study. *Science Translational Med* 2017;9(414). pii: eaan1208.

131. Deng R, Iyer S, Theil F-P, Mortensen DL, Fielder PJ, Prabhu S. Projecting human pharmacokinetics of therapeutic antibodies from nonclinical data: What have we learned? *mAbs* 2011;3:61–6.

132. Lowe PJ, Tannenbaum S, Wu K, Lloyd P, Sims J. On setting the first dose in man: Quantitating biotherapeutic drug-target binding through pharmacokinetic and pharmacodynamic models. *Basic Clin Pharmacol Toxicol* 2010;106:195–209.

133. Rowley TF, Peters SJ, Aylott M, Griffin R, Davies NL, Healy LJ, Cutler RM, Eddleston A, Pither TL, Sopp JM, et al. Engineered hexavalent Fc proteins with enhanced Fc-gamma receptor avidity provide insights into immune-complex interactions. *Commun Biol* 2018;1:146.

134. Brennan FR, Cavagnaro J, McKeever K, Ryan PC Schutten M, Vahle J, Weinbauer G, Marrer-Berger E, Black LE. Safety testing of monoclonal antibodies in non-human primates: Case studies highlighting their important impact on risk assessment for humans. *mAbs* 2018;10:1–17.

135. Haley PJ. The role of histopathology in the identification of immunotoxicity. *J Immunotoxicol* 2005;2:181–3.

136. Prior H, Baldrick P, de Hann L, Downes N, Jones K, Mortimer-Cassen E, Kimber I. Reviewing the utility of two species in general toxicology related to drug development. *Int J Toxicol* 2018;37:121–4.

137. Perry R, Farris G, Bienvenu JG, Dean C Jr, Foley G, Mahrt C, Short B; Society of Toxicologic Pathology. Society of Toxicologic Pathology position paper on best practices on recovery studies: The role of the anatomic pathologist. *Toxicol Pathol* 2013;41:1159–69.

138. Burmester GR, McInnes IB, Kremer J, Miranda P, Korkosz M, Vencovsky J, Rubbert-Roth A, Mysler E, Sleeman MA, Godwood A, et al. A randomised phase IIb study of mavrilimumab, a novel GM-CSF receptor alpha monoclonal antibody, in the treatment of rheumatoid arthritis. *Ann Rheum Dis* 2017;76:1020–30.

139. Stanley E, Lieschke GJ, Grail D, Metcalf D, Hodgson G, Gall JA, Maher DW, Cebon J, Sinickas V, Dunn AR. Granulocyte/macrophage colony-stimulating factor-deficient mice show no major perturbation of hematopoiesis but develop a characteristic pulmonary pathology. *Proc Natl Acad Sci U S A* 1994;91:5592–6.

140. Sakagami T, Beck D, Uchida K, Suzuki T, Carey BC, Nakata K, Keller G, Wood RE, Wert SE, Ikegami M, et al. Patient-derived granulocyte/macrophage colony-stimulating factor autoantibodies reproduce pulmonary alveolar proteinosis in nonhuman primates. *Am J Respir Crit Care Med* 2010;182:49–61.

141. Minter RR, Cohen ES, Wang B, Liang M, Vainshtein I, Rees G, Eghobamien L, Harrison P, Sims DA, Matthews C, et al. Protein engineering and preclinical development of a GM-CSF receptor antibody for the treatment of rheumatoid arthritis. *Br J Pharmacol* 2013;168:200–11.

142. Gommerman JL, Summers DeLuca L. LTbR and CD40: Working together in dendritic cells to optimize immune responses. *Immunol Rev* 2011;244:85–98.

143. Xu J, Foy TM, Laman JD, Elliott EA, Dunn JJ, Waldschmidt TJ, Elsemore J, Noelle RJ, Flavell RA. Mice deficient for the CD40 ligand. *Immunity* 1994;1:423–31.

144. Boumpas DT, Furie R, Manzi S, Illei GG, Wallace DJ, Balow JE, Vaishnaw A; BG9588 Lupus Nephritis Trial Group. BG9588 Lupus Nephritis Trial Group. A short course of BG9588 (anti-CD40 ligand antibody) improves serologic activity and decreases hematuria in patients with proliferative lupus glomerulonephritis. *Arthritis Rheum* 2003;48:719–27.

145. Kuwana M, Nomura S, Fujimura K, Nagasawa T, Muto Y, Kurata Y, Tanaka S, Ikeda Y. Effect of a single injection of humanized anti-CD154 monoclonal antibody on the platelet-specific autoimmune response in patients with immune thrombocytopenic purpura. *Blood* 2004;103:1229–36.

146. Langer F, Ingersoll SB, Amirkhosravi A, Meyer T, Siddiqui FA, Ahmad S, Walker JM, Amaya M, Desai H, Francis JL. The role of CD40 in CD40L- and antibody-mediated platelet activation. *Thromb Haemost* 2005;93:1137–46.

147. Shock A, Burkly L, Wakefield I, Peters C, Garber E, Ferrant J, Taylor FR, Su L, Hsu YM, Hutto D, et al. CDP7657, an anti-CD40L antibody lacking an Fc domain, inhibits CD40L-dependent immune responses without thrombotic complications: An in vivo study. *Arthritis Res Ther* 2015;17:234.

148. Germolec DR, Kashon M, Nyska A, Kuper CF, Portier C, Kommineni C, Johnson KA, Luster MI. The accuracy of extended histopathology to detect immunotoxic chemicals. *Toxicol Sci* 2004;82:504–14

149. DeWitt JC, Germolec DR, Luebke RW, Johnson VJ. Associating changes in the immune system with clinical diseases for interpretation in risk assessment. *Curr Protoc Toxicol* 2016; 67:18.1.1–22.

150. Luster MI, Portier C, Pait DG, Rosenthal GJ, Germolec DR, Corsini E, Blaylock BL, Pollock P, Kouchi Y, Craig W, et al. Risk assessment in immunotoxicology. II. Relationships between immune and host resistance tests. *Fundam Appl Toxicol* 1993;21:71–82.

151. Orencia. European public assessment report; Scientific discussion, EMEA. 2007; Available at: http://www.ema.europa. eu /humandocs/ PDFs /EPAR/orencia/H-701-en6.pdf

152. Amevive. BLA review, pharmacology and toxicology assessment, FDA. 2002; Available at: http://www.fda.gov/ downloads/Drugs/DevelopmentApprovalProcess/How DrugsareDevelopedandApproved/ApprovalApplications/ TherapeuticBiologic Applications/ucm086014.pdf

153. Raptiva. European public assessment report, scientific discussion, EMEA. 2004; Available at: http://www.ema.europa. eu/ humandocs/PDFs/EPAR/raptiva/ 6565604en6.pdf

154. Price KD. Bacterial infections in cynomolgus monkeys given small molecule immunomodulatory antagonists. *J Immunotoxicol* 2010;7(2):128–37.

155. McInnes EF, Jarrett RF, Langford G, Atkinson C, Horsley J, Goddard MJ, Cozzi E, Schuurman HJ. Posttransplant lymphoproliferative disorder associated with primate gamma-herpesvirus in cynomolgus monkeys used in pig-to-primate renal xenotransplantation and primate renal allotransplantation. *Transplantation* 2002;73:44–52.

156. Burleson SCM, Freebern WJ, Burleson FG, Burleson GR, Johnson VJ, Luebke RW. Host resistance assays. *Methods Mol Biol* 2018;1803:117–45.

157. Park H, Solis NV, Louie JS, Spellberg B, Rodriguez N, Filler SG. Different tumor necrosis factor α antagonists have different effects on host susceptibility to disseminated and oropharyngeal candidiasis in mice. *Virulence* 2014;5:625–9.

158. Stelara. FDA nonclinical pharmacology review. 2007; Available here: https://www.accessdata.fda.gov/drugsatfda_ docs/nda/2016/761044Orig1s000PharmR.pdf

159. Kammüller M, Tsai TF, Griffiths CE, Kapoor N, Kolattukudy PE, Brees D, Chibout SD, Safi J Jr, Fox T. Inhibition of IL-17A by secukinumab shows no evidence of increased *Mycobacterium tuberculosis* infections. *Clin Transl Immunol* 2017;6:e152.

160. Mor G, Abrahams VM. *Immunology of Pregnancy in Creasy and Resnik's Maternal-Fetal Medicine: Principles and Practice.* In: Resnik R, Lockwood CJ, Moore TR, Greene MF, Copel JA, Silver RM, editors, 8th edition, Elsevier Inc; Philadelphia, PA, 2019. Chapter 8; pp. 127–40.

161. Vinatier DP, Dufour N, Tordjeman-Rizzi JF, Prolongeau S, Depret-Moser, Monnier JC. Immunological aspects of ovarian function: Role of the cytokines. *Eur J Obstet Gynecol Reprod Biol* 1995;63:155–68.

162. Boots CE, Jungheim ES. Inflammation and human ovarian follicular dynamics. *Semin Reprod Med* 2015;33:270–5.

163. Mor G, Aldo P, Alvero AB. The unique immunological and microbial aspects of pregnancy. *Nat Rev Immunol* 2017;17:469–82.

164. Ander SE, Diamond MS, Coyne CB. Immune responses at the maternal-fetal interface. *Sci Immunol* 2019;4. pii: eaat6114.

165. Salvany-Celades M, van der Zwan A, Benner M, Setrajcic-Dragos V, Bougleux Gomes HA, Iyer V, Norwitz ER, Strominger JL, Tilburgs T. Three types of functional regulatory T cells control T cell responses at the human maternal-fetal interface. *Cell Rep* 2019;27:2537–47.

166. Yuan J, Li J, Huang SY, Sun X. Characterization of the subsets of human NKT-like cells and the expression of Th1/Th2 cytokines in patients with unexplained recurrent spontaneous abortion. *J Reprod Immunol* 2015 Aug;110:81–8.

167. Yang F, Zheng Q, Jin L. Dynamic function and composition changes of immune cells during normal and pathological pregnancy at the maternal-fetal interface. *Front Immunol* 2019;10:2317.

168. Logiodice F, Lombardelli L, Kullolli O, Haller H, Maggi E, Rukavina D, Piccinni MP. Decidual interleukin-22-producing CD4+ T cells (Th17/Th0/IL-22+ and Th17/Th2/IL-22+, Th2/IL-22+, Th0/IL-22+), which also produce IL-4, are involved in the success of pregnancy. *Int J Mol Sci* 2019;20. pii: E428.

169. Arsenescu R, Arsenescu V, de Villiers WJ. (2011). TNF-α and the development of the neonatal immune system: Implications for inhibitor use in pregnancy. *Am J Gastroenterol* 2011 Apr;106(4):559–62.

170. Luu M, Benzenine E, Doret M, Michiels C, Barkun A, Degand T, Quantin C, Bardou M. Continuous anti-TNFα use throughout pregnancy: Possible complications for the mother but not for the fetus. A Retrospective Cohort on the French National Health Insurance Database (EVASION). *Am J Gastroenterol* 2018;113:1669–77.

171. Cheent K, Nolan J, Shariq S, Kiho L, Pal A, Arnold J. Case report: Fatal case of disseminated BCG infection in an infant born to a mother taking infliximab for Crohn's disease. *J Crohns Colitis* 2010;4:603–5.

172. Julsgaard M, Christensen LA, Gibson PR, Gearry RB, Fallingborg J, Hvas CL, Bibby BM, Uldbjerg N, Connell WR, Rosella O, et al. Concentrations of adalimumab and infliximab in mothers and newborns, and effects on infection. *Gastroenterology* 2016;151:110–9.

173. Stewart J. Developmental toxicity testing of monoclonal antibodies: An enhanced pre- and post-natal study design option. *Reproductive Toxicol* 2009;28:220–5.

174. Weinbauer GF, Luft J, Fuchs A. The enhanced pre- and postnatal development study for monoclonal antibodies. *Methods Mol Biol* 2013;947:185–200.

175. Skaggs H, Chellman GJ, Collinge M, Enright B, Fuller CL, Krayer J, Sivaraman L, Weinbauer GF. Comparison of immune system development in nonclinical species and humans: Closing information gaps for immunotoxicity testing and human translatability. *Reprod Toxicol* 2019;89:178–88.

176. Kuper CF, van Bilsen J, Cnossen H, Houben G, Garthoff J, Wolterbeek A. Development of immune organs and functioning in humans and test animals: Implications for immune intervention studies. *Reprod Toxicol* 2016;64:180–90.

177. Dietert RR. Developmental Immunotoxicology (DIT): Windows of vulnerability, immune dysfunction and safety assessment. *J Immunotoxicol* 2008;5:401–12.

178. Burns-Naas LA, Hastings KL, Ladics GS, Makris SL, Parker GA, Holsapple MP. What's so special about the developing immune system? *Int J Toxicol* 2008;27:223–54.

179. Bowman CJ, Breslin WJ, Connor AV, Martin PL, Moffat GJ, Sivaraman L, Tornesi MB, Chivers S. Placental transfer of Fc-containing biopharmaceuticals across species, an industry survey analysis. *Birth Defects Res B Dev Reprod Toxicol* 2013;98:459–85.

180. Carlock LL, Cowan LA, Oneda S, Hoberman A, Wang DD, Hanna R, Bussiere JL. A comparison of effects on reproduction and neonatal development in cynomolgus monkeys given human soluble IL-4R and mice given murine soluble IL-4R. *Regul Toxicol Pharmacol* 53:226–34.

181. Ishihara-Hattori K, Barrow P. Review of embryo-fetal developmental toxicity studies performed for recent FDA-approved pharmaceuticals. *Reprod Toxicol* 2016;64:98–104.

182. Chambers CD, Johnson DL, Xu R, Luo Y, Lopez-Jimenez J, Adam MP, Braddock SR, Robinson LK, Vaux K, Lyons Jones K, et al. Birth outcomes in women who have taken adalimumab in pregnancy: A prospective cohort study. *PLoS One* 2019;14:e0223603.

183. Huang V, Leung Y, Nguyen GC, Seow CH. Management of inflammatory bowel disease in pregnancy: A practical approach to new guidelines. *Can J Gastroenterol Hepatol* 2016;2016:9513742.

184. Dupixent. Pharmacology review. 2017; Available at: https://www.accessdata.fda.gov/drugsatfda_ocs/nda/2017/761055Orig1s000PharmR.pdf

185. Actemra. Pharmacology review. 2010; Available at: https://www.accessdata.fda.gov/drugsatfda_docs/nda/2010/125276s000PharmR.pdf

186. Sylvant. Pharmacology review. 2014; Available at: https://www.accessdata.fda.gov/drugsatfda_docs/nda/2014/125496Orig1s000PharmR.pdf

187. Kevzara. Pharmacology review. 2018; Available at: https://www.accessdata.fda.gov/drugsatfda_docs/nda/2017/761037Orig1s000PharmR.pdf

188. Benlysta. Pharmacology review. 2010; Available at: https://www.accessdata.fda.gov/drugsatfda_docs/nda/2011/125370Orig1s000PharmR.pdf

189. Tremfya. Multi-Disciplinary review. 2017; Available at: https://www.accessdata.fda.gov/ drugsatfda_ docs/nda/2017/761061Orig1s000MultidisciplineR.pdf

190. Ilumya. Multi-disciplinary review. 2018; Available at: https://www.accessdata.fda.gov/drugsatfda_ docs/nda/2018/761067Orig1s000MultdisciplineR.pdf

191. Skyrizi. Pharmacology review. 2019; Available at: https://www.accessdata.fda.gov/drugsatfda_ docs/nda/2019/761105Orig1s000MultidisciplineR.pdf

192. Ilaris. Pharmacology review. 2009; Available at: https://www.accessdata.fda.gov/drugsatfda_ docs/nda/2009/125319s000_PharmR_P2.pdf

193. Tysabri. Pharmacology review. 2004; Available at: https://www.accessdata.fda.gov/drugsatfda_ docs/nda/2004/125104s000_Natalizumab_Pharmr_P3.pdf

194. Vaidyanathan A, McKeever K, Anand B, Eppler S, Weinbauer GF, Beyer JC. Developmental imunotoxicology assessment of rituximab in cynomolgus monkeys. *Toxicol Sci* 2010;119:116–25.

195. Cauvin A, Peters C, Brennan FR. Advantages and limitations of commonly used nonhuman primate species in research and development of biopharmaceuticals. In: Bluemel J, Korte S, Schenck E, Weinbauer G, editors. *The Non-Human Primate in Nonclinical Drug Development and Safety Assessment*. Academic Press. Elsevier, 125 London Wall, London, EC2Y 5AS, UK; 2015. Chapter 19; pp. 379–95.

196. FDA. Guidance for industry: Non-clinical safety evaluation of pediatric drug products. 2006; Available at: http://www.fda.gov/downloads/Drugs/GuidanceCompliance RegulatoryInformation/ Guidances /ucm079247.pdf

197. EMEA. Guideline on the need for non-clinical testing in juvenile animals of pharmaceuticals for paediatric indications. 2008; Available at: http://www.ema.europa.eu/docs/en_GB/ document_library/ Scientific_ guideline/ 2009/09/WC500003305.pdf

198. Xolair. EMA. European public assessment report scientific discussion. 2005; Available at: http://www.ema.europa.eu/docs/en_GB/document_library/EPAR_-_Scientific_Discussion/human/000606/WC500057295.pdf

199. Depelchin BO. 52-week juvenile toxicity study in cynomolgus monkeys with certolizumab-pegol to assess impact of PEG on choroid plexus function. *Presented at the Biosafe General Membership Meeting*, May 2–4, 2017. https://www.bio.org/sites/default/files/legacy/bioorg/docs/2017%20BioSafe%20GMM%20v.2.pdf

200. Adalimumab. Pharmacology review. 2002; Available here: https://www.accessdata.fda.gov /drugsatfda_docs/nda/2002/BLA_125057_S000_HUMIRA_PHARMR.PDF

201. ICHS1A.The need for long-term rodent carcinogenicity studies of pharmaceuticals. 1996; Available at: http://www.ema.europa.eu/docs/en_GB/document_library/Scientific_guideline/2009/09/ WC500002699.pdf

202. Mittal D, Gubin MM, Schreiber RD, Smyth MJ. New insights into cancer immunoediting and its three component phases--elimination, equilibrium and escape. *Curr Opin Immunol* 2014;27:16–25.

203. Ponce RA, Gelzleichter T, Haggerty HG, Heidel S, Holdren MS, Lebrec H, Mellon RD, Pallardy M. Immunomodulation and lymphoma in humans. *J Immunotoxicol* 2014;11:1–12.

204. Vahle JL, Finch GL, Heidel SM, Hovland DN Jr, Ivens I, Parker S, Ponce RA, Sachs C, Steigerwalt R, Short B, et al. Carcinogenicity assessment of biotechnology-derived pharmaceuticals: A review of approved molecules and best practice recommendations. *Toxicol Pathol* 2010;38:522–53.

205. Cavagnaro JA. Preclinical evaluation of cancer hazard and risk of biopharmaceuticals. In: Cavagnaro JA, editor. *Preclinical Safety Evaluation of Biopharmaceuticals*. John Wiley & Son, Hoboken, NJ, 2008; pp. 209–40.

206. Bugelski, PJ, Volk, A, Walker, MR, Krayer, JH, Martin, P, Descotes, J. Critical review of preclinical approaches to evaluate the potential of immunosuppressive drugs to influence human neoplasia. *Int J Toxicol* 2010;29:435–66.

207. Maeda A, Schneider SW, Kojima M, Beiddert S, Schwarz T, Schwarz A. Enhanced photocarcinogenesis in interleukin-12-deficient mice. *Cancer Res* 2006;66:2962–9.

208. Xiao M, Wang C, Zhang J, Li Z, Zhao X, Qin Z. IFNγ promotes papilloma development by up-regulating Th17-associated inflammation. *Cancer Res* 2009;69:2010–7.

209. Herzyk DJ, Gore ER, Polsky R, Nadwodny KL, Maier CC, Liu S, Hart TK, Harmsen AG, Bugelski PJ. Immunomodulatory effects of anti-CD4 antibody in host resistance against infections and tumors in human CD4 transgenic mice. *Infect Immun* 2001;69:1032–43.

210. Langowski JL, Zhang X, Wu L, Mattson JD, Chen T, Smith K, Basham B, McClanahan T, Kastelein RA, Oft M. IL-23 promotes tumor incidence and growth. *Nature* 2006;442:461–5.

211. Mahnke YD, Schirrmacher V. Characteristics of a potent tumor vaccine-induced secondary anti-tumor T cell response. *Int J Oncol* 2004;24:1427–34.

212. Bugelski PJ, Sachs C, Cornacoff J, Martin P, Treacy G. Immunomodulatory biopharmaceuticals and risk of neoplasia. In: Cavagnaro JA, editor. *Preclinical Safety Evaluation of Biopharmaceuticals.* John Wiley & Son, Hoboken, NJ; 2008; pp. 601–32.

213. Strowig, T, Gurer C, Ploss A, Liu Y-F, Arrey F, Sashihara J, Koo G, Rice CM, Young JW, Chadburn A, et al. Priming of protective T cell responses against virus-induced tumors in mice with human immune system components. *J Exp Med* 206:1423–34.

214. Lebrec H, Brennan FR, Haggerty H, Herzyk D, Kamperschroer C, Maier CC, Ponce R, Preston BD, Weinstock D, Mellon RD. HESI/FDA workshop on immunomodulators and cancer risk assessment: Building blocks for a weight-of-evidence approach. *Regul Toxicol Pharmacol* 2016;75:72–80.

215. Kryczek I, Wei S, Zou L, Szeliga W, Vatan L, Zou W. Endogenous IL-17 contributes to reduced tumor growth and metastasis. *Blood* 2009;114:357–9.

216. Keystone EC. Does anti-tumor necrosis factor-α therapy affect risk of serious infection and cancer in patients with rheumatoid arthritis? A review of long-term data. *J Rheumatol* 2011;38:1552–62.

217. Simon TA, Thompson A, Gandhi KK, Hochberg M, Suissa S. Incidence of malignancy in adult patients with rheumatoid arthritis: A meta-analysis. *Arthritis Res Ther* 2015;17:212.

218. Harrold LR, Griffith J, Zueger P, Litman HJ, Gershenson B, Islam SS, Barr CJ, Guo D, Fay J, Greenberg JD. Long-term, real-world safety of adalimumab in rheumatoid arthritis: Analysis of a prospective US-based registry. *J Rheumatol* 2020;47:959–967.

219. Brunda MJ, Luistro L, Warrier RR, Wright RB, Hubbard BR, Murphy M, Wolf SF, Gately MK. Antitumor and anti-metastatic activity of interleukin 12 against murine tumors. *J Exp Med* 1993;78:1223–30.

220. Li X, Bechara R, Zhao J, McGeachy MJ, Gaffen SL. IL-17 receptor-based signaling and implications for disease. *Nat Immunol* 2019;20:1594–602.

221. EMA. Guideline on the non-clinical development of fixed combinations of medicinal products. 2008; Available at: http://www.ema.europa.eu/docs/en_GB/document_library/Scientific _guideline /2009/10/WC500003976.pdf

222. FDA. Guidance for industry: Nonclinical safety evaluation of drug or biologic combinations. 2006; Available at: http://www.fda.gov/downloads/Drugs/GuidanceCompliance RegulatoryInformation/ Guidances/ucm079243.pdf

223. Ponce R. Preclinical support for combination therapy in the treatment of autoimmunity with atacicept. *Toxicol Pathol* 2009;37:89–99.

224. Genovese MC, Cohen S, Moreland L, Lium D, Robbins S, Newmark R, Bekker P; 20000223 Study Group. Combination therapy with etanercept and anakinra in the treatment of patients with rheumatoid arthritis who have been treated unsuccessfully with methotrexate. *Arthritis Rheum* 2004;50:1412–9.

225. Kleinschmidt-DeMasters BK, Tyler KL. Progressive multifocal leukoencephalopathy complicating treatment with natalizumab and interferon beta-1a for multiple sclerosis. *N Engl J Med* 2005;353:369–74.

226. Bugelski PJ, Martin PL. Concordance of preclinical and clinical pharmacology and toxicology of therapeutic monoclonal antibodies and fusion proteins: Cell surface targets. *Br J Pharmacol* 2012;166:823–46.

227. Martin PL, Bugelski PJ. Concordance of preclinical and clinical pharmacology and toxicology of monoclonal antibodies and fusion proteins: Soluble targets. *Br J Pharmacol* 2012;166:806–22.

228. Muller PY, Milton M, Lloyd P, Sims J, Brennan FR. The Minimum Anticipated Biological Effect Level (MABEL) for selection of first human dose in clinical trials with monoclonal antibodies. *Curr Opin Biotechnol* 2009;20:1–8.

229. Tibbitts J, Cavagnaro JA, Haller CA, Marafino B, Andrews PA, Sullivan JT. Practical approaches to dose selection for first-in-human clinical trials with novel biopharmaceuticals. *Regul Toxicol Pharmacol* 2010;58:243–51.

230. Leach M, Clarke O, Dudal S, Han C, Li C, Yang Z, Brennan FR, Bailey WJ, Chen Y, Deslandes A, et al. Strategies and recommendations for using a data-driven and risk-based approach in the selection of first-in-human starting dose: An International Consortium for Innovation and Quality in Pharmaceutical Development (IQ) Assessment. *Clin Pharmacol Ther* 2021;109:1395–1415..

231. FDA. Guidance for industry estimating the maximum safe starting dose in initial clinical trials for therapeutics in adult healthy volunteers. 2005; Available at: http://www.fda.gov/downloads/Drugs/GuidanceCompliance RegulatoryInformation/Guidances/ ucm078932.pdf

232. EMEA. Guideline on strategies to identify and mitigate risks for first-in-human clinical trials with investigational medicinal products. 2007; Available at: http://www.ema.europa.eu/docs/en_ GB/ document_ library/ Scientific_ guideline/2009/09/WC500002988.pdf

233. EMA. Guideline on strategies to identify and mitigate risks for first-in-human and early clinical trials with investigational medicinal products. 2017; Available at: https://www.ema.europa.eu/en/documents/ scientific-guideline/guideline-strategies-identify-mitigate-risks-first-human-early-clinical-trials-investigational_en.pdf

234. Yang Z, Wang H, Salcedo TW, Suchard SJ, Xie JH, Schneeweis LA, Fleener CA, Calore JD, Shi R, Zhang SX, et al. Integrated pharmacokinetic/pharmacodynamic analysis for determining the minimal anticipated biological effect level of a novel anti-CD28 receptor antagonist BMS-931699. *J Pharmacol Exp Ther* 2015;355:506–15.

235. Davda JP, Hansen RJ. Properties of a general PK/PD model of antibody-ligand interactions for therapeutic antibodies that bind to soluble endogenous targets. *mAbs* 2010;2:576–88.

30

Nonclinical Safety Program Considerations for Biologic Therapeutics for Neurodegenerative Conditions

D.N. Hovland, Jr.
Eledon Pharmaceuticals, Inc.

B.B. Smith
Vir Biotechnology

C.W. Chen
Tox and Text Solutions, LLC

CONTENTS

30.1 Introduction and Background

Neurodegenerative disorders, such as Alzheimer's disease (AD), Parkinson's disease (PD), amyotrophic lateral sclerosis (ALS), Huntington's disease (HD), and multiple sclerosis (MS), are conditions associated with progressive degeneration of specific populations of neurons in the central or peripheral nervous system (Hebert et al. 2013, Mehta et al. 2018, N.O.R.D. 2020, Parkinson's Foundation 2020, Robertson and Moreo 2016, Trapp and Nave 2008). Neurodegenerative disorders are associated with debilitating manifestations in affected individuals that can include cognitive and motor function deficits, disability, and death. Neurodegenerative conditions are devastating for those affected, but also to families and caregivers supporting individuals with the diseases (Caga et al. 2019, Cheng 2017, Maguire and Maguire 2020, Tan et al. 2020).

While these disorders have unique and varied etiology, mechanisms, and prognoses, they share critical fundamental traits. Neurodegenerative diseases are typically progressive, meaning that the associated damage proceeds along a pathway of increasing severity. The neuronal loss common to neurodegenerative disorders is, in most cases, considered irreversible. Therefore, damage done cannot be repaired or reversed. There are relatively few pharmacological therapies available for patients with these diseases, and existing treatments primarily focus on management of signs and symptoms. Consequently, there is a large unmet medical need for neurodegenerative disease treatments that are effective and safe and can be used early in the disease lifecycle to prevent the progression of irreversible damage. Therapies that modify disease progression are a major goal of therapeutic intervention.

DOI: 10.1201/9781003124542-34

Biologic therapeutics (e.g., biotechnology-derived pharmaceuticals, gene therapies, and cellular therapies) possess unique attributes (e.g., high degree of specificity and prolonged residence time) that offer potential benefits as treatments for neurodegenerative conditions. This chapter discusses considerations for the design of appropriate nonclinical safety programs to support the clinical development of biologic therapeutics for these conditions. Design of informative and efficient nonclinical safety programs requires a case-by-case, science-based approach that appropriately considers the nature and progression of the specific neurodegenerative condition, the characteristics of the affected population, the treatment paradigm, and the biologic therapeutic modality's properties.

30.2 Health Authority Perspective

30.2.1 Treatment Options for Neurodegenerative Conditions Are Limited

Global health authorities (e.g., United States Food and Drug Administration (US FDA), European Medicines Agency (EMA), and Health Canada) responsible for oversight of the development and registration of pharmaceuticals consider many neurodegenerative diseases, such as AD, ALS, HD, PD, and MS, as serious, life-threatening, and/or severely debilitating conditions (EMA 2018a, Health Canada 2008, 2016, US FDA 2014, 2019a). Health authority acknowledgment that a new product shows potential promise as a treatment for these conditions may facilitate consideration of opportunities for expedited development and registration.

Formal programs for expedited development of promising therapies are in place with major global health authorities (Hwang, Darrow, and Kesselheim 2017, Khera 2020, Nagai 2019). These programs include Breakthrough, Fast Track, Accelerated Approval, and Priority Review in the United States (US FDA 2014); Priority Review or Notice of Compliance with Conditions (NOC/c) in Canada (Health Canada 2008, 2016); accelerated assessment, adaptive pathways, conditional marketing authorization, and PRIME in Europe (EMA 2018a, 2016a, 2016b, 2016c); and priority review, conditional early approval system, and Sakigake designation in Japan (Nagai 2019). In addition, many neurodegenerative disorders may qualify as rare or orphan conditions (US FDA 2019b). These programs recognize the need for new therapies for serious conditions and are intended to facilitate efficient development of therapies offering a potential benefit for these conditions, providing additional opportunities for health authority engagement during development, conditional approval based on surrogate endpoints, and shorter review timelines for marketing applications.

Health authority acknowledgment of the value of new therapies for serious conditions without adequate therapies, like neurodegenerative diseases, also translates to their perspective on the scope of appropriate nonclinical safety programs, reflected in key guidance documents.

30.2.2 Unmet Medical Need Impact on Nonclinical Safety Programs

Nonclinical development programs supporting the clinical development of pharmaceutical treatments should be designed in full consideration of the disease/condition to be treated, the characteristics of the patient population to be treated, the intended duration of treatment, and the scope of proposed clinical trials. To facilitate the development of appropriate nonclinical programs, guidance documents on nonclinical development programs to support clinical development and registration of pharmaceuticals have been published by national (e.g., country-specific) and regional health authorities (e.g., European Union). In addition, globally applicable guidance documents followed by the majority of national and regional health authorities (e.g., US FDA, EMA, Health Canada, and Japan's Pharmaceutical and Medical Device Agency) have been published by the International Conference on Harmonisation (ICH) of Technical Requirements for Registration of Pharmaceuticals for Human Use.

Many of the available guidance documents provide nonclinical study type-specific information (e.g., for assessment of reproductive/developmental toxicity, genotoxicity, or carcinogenicity). However, selected guidance documents provide information supporting the design of nonclinical safety *programs*, presenting considerations for sponsors developing an appropriate complement of nonclinical studies to support clinical development and registration of pharmaceuticals.

A key program-level ICH nonclinical guidance document is ICH M3, Nonclinical Safety Studies for the Conduct of Human Clinical Trials and Marketing Authorization for Pharmaceuticals (ICH 2009a). ICH M3 provides details on the appropriate type and duration of nonclinical safety studies, and the appropriate timing of such studies, to support the conduct of clinical trials and ultimate marketing authorization for pharmaceuticals. The majority of the study-specific guidance (e.g., study type and duration) in ICH M3 is not directly relevant to biologic therapeutics. This information is more appropriately addressed in other guidance documents, such as ICH S6, described below (ICH 2011). However, ICH M3's general pharmacology/toxicology principles, its perspective on serious/life-threatening conditions, and its study timing considerations in alignment with clinical development stage can be applied to biologic therapeutics.

ICH M3 states that for pharmaceutical treatments for life-threatening or serious diseases without current effective therapy, a case-by-case approach is warranted to optimize and expedite development (ICH 2009a). In these cases, which could include the development of treatments for neurodegenerative disorders, the full complement of typical nonclinical studies may not be required to support clinical development and registration; "particular studies can be abbreviated, deferred, omitted, or added" (ICH 2009a). This brief statement in ICH M3 is notable; however, there is limited, specific health authority guidance detailing appropriate nonclinical development programs for therapeutics for serious or life-threatening conditions outside of the oncology or rare disease (US FDA

2019b, Prescott et al. 2017). ICH S9, Nonclinical Evaluation for Anticancer Pharmaceuticals (ICH 2009b), describes a case-by-case, flexible approach for the design of nonclinical development programs for small molecule and biotechnology-derived pharmaceuticals for advanced cancer directed at expediting the availability of new treatments where the death rate is high and existing therapies have limited effectiveness. Given the progressive and irreversible disability, reduced life expectancy, adversely affected quality of life, and unmet medical need of neurodegenerative disorders, the concepts described in ICH S9 for the design of appropriate nonclinical development programs for advanced cancer therapeutics may also be applicable to pharmaceutical treatments for these conditions (Prescott et al. 2017).

Variation from the standard nonclinical study paradigm for treatment for neurodegenerative conditions would appropriately consider the disease characteristics and affected patient population, facilitating prioritized interest in certain studies while identifying those studies that may be less informative in the interest of expediting the availability of new treatments. For example, as the typically affected patient population for PD and AD is typically ≥60 years of age, nonclinical studies evaluating reproductive and developmental toxicity may not provide meaningful information regarding human risk. Therefore, omission or abbreviation of typical reproductive/developmental toxicity studies may be acceptable. Specifically, the patient populations for PD and AD do not typically include women of childbearing potential. Therefore, developmental toxicity studies would not be informative and should not be included in nonclinical safety programs of therapeutics for these conditions (Rocca et al. 2018). Another example could be applied to carcinogenicity studies of therapies intended for these conditions. Given the advanced age of patients and the irreversible progression of PD and AD, delaying registration of new therapies for these conditions to allow for completion of standard 2-year rodent carcinogenicity would not be warranted. Furthermore, while expediting the progression of novel therapies through clinical development, the elimination of noncritical studies also reduces animal use. Note that the study value determination examples mentioned above may not be applicable to early-onset variations of PD and AD, emphasizing the need for case-by-case evaluation by sponsors.

30.2.3 Health Authority Perspective on Nonclinical Safety Programs for Biologic, Cellular, and Gene Therapies

While high-level guidance in ICH M3 regarding appropriate timing for the conduct of key nonclinical studies, with respect to the clinical development stage, is generally applicable to biologic therapeutics, the source and diverse nature of biotechnology-derived pharmaceuticals (biologics) require special consideration when designing informative nonclinical development programs. Health authority perspective on this special consideration is detailed in ICH S6, Preclinical Safety Evaluation of Biotechnology-Derived Pharmaceuticals (ICH 2011), which describes key principles for the design of

appropriate nonclinical programs supporting the development of biologic pharmaceutical therapeutics for human use.

The unique properties of biotechnology-derived pharmaceuticals require flexibility to achieve appropriate characterization of safety. Given the diversity of modalities and intended function, a flexible, case-by-case, science-based approach to nonclinical safety evaluation is required. Health authority guidance notes challenges for biologic pharmaceuticals, relative to typical small molecules, that include their exceptionally high degree of species-specific activity (e.g., not always active in rodents; often limited to large animal species such as nonhuman primates), more invasive nature of delivery (e.g., injection instead of oral administration), and potential for antidrug immunogenicity (e.g., antibodies developed against human-specific molecule).

These challenges lead to recommendations against defaulting to a standard list of nonclinical studies. A sponsor should consider each of the nonclinical study categories listed in S6, in the context of the intended patient population and their specific biological pharmaceutical's properties. Major health authorities also acknowledge the need for flexibility in nonclinical safety programs for gene and cellular therapies. Guidance documents have been published by the US FDA and EMA that discuss nonclinical safety programs for these unique products.

As per the US FDA's Guidance for Industry, Preclinical Assessment of Investigational Cellular and Gene Therapy Products (US FDA 2013), the basic testing principles in ICH S6 may be a useful reference for the nonclinical evaluation of cellular and gene therapies (US FDA 2013). In addition, recommendations as to the timing of reproduction/developmental toxicity studies in ICH M3 may be useful to consider for cellular and gene therapy products. The US FDA's cellular/gene therapy product guidance reiterates a flexible, science-driven review process to address safety issues in a context that considers both the biology of the product and the intended clinical indication (US FDA 2013).

The high degree of specificity and potential for the extended activity of cellular and gene therapy products may provide meaningful benefits for the treatment of neurodegenerative conditions. However, these traits must be considered when designing informative nonclinical programs. Prolonged activity may impact definitive study duration and dosing paradigms; specificity of activity may limit the scope of available species/models and the potential for immunogenicity; and the requirement for parenteral, potentially invasive administration routes may confound study results. As with biological pharmaceuticals, studies in irrelevant species are discouraged to avoid the generation of noninformative data and to reduce animal use.

Unique gene therapy features impacting the requirements for nonclinical development include the potential in vivo effects of the transgene or other recombinant nucleic acid sequences and the vector backbone (i.e., viral, bacterial, or plasmid-derived sequences) (EMA 2018b). Key to nonclinical safety evaluation of gene therapy products is characterization of biodistribution, evaluation of persistence, and potential for integration (intended or unintended) into the host genome (Chapter 26). Given the specificity of these therapies, as with biologic pharmaceuticals

TABLE 30.1

Neurodegenerative Disorders: Onset, Prevalence, and Genetic Therapeutic Targets

Disorder	Age of Onset	Prevalence in US	Genetic Therapeutic Targets
Spinal muscular atrophy[a]	Birth–6 months	1–2 per 100,000	SMN1, non-5qSMA
Batten disease[b]	6 months–10 years	2–4 per 100,000	CLN genes
Friedreich's ataxia[c]	1.5–30 years	2 per 100,000	FXN
Multiple sclerosis[d]	20–50 years	913,925	HLA-DRB1
Early-onset Alzheimer's disease[e]	30–65 years	200,000	APP, PSEN1, PSEN2
Huntington's disease[f]	30–50 years	30,000	HTT
Prion disease[g]	45–75 years	1.2 per 1 million annually	PRPN
Frontotemporal dementia[h]	50–60 years	50,000–60,000	C9orf72, MAPT (tau), GRN (progranulin)
Amyotrophic lateral sclerosis[i]	55–75 years	5 per 100,000	SOD1, C9orf72
Parkinson's disease[j]	~60 years	930,000 (est. 2020)	LRRK2, PARK7, PINK1, PRKN, SNCA (α-synuclein)
Alzheimer's disease[e]	~ 65 years old	5.6 million	Aβ, APP, PSEN1, PSEN2, APOE-ε4

APOE: apolipoprotein E; C9orf72: chromosome 9 open reading frame 72; CLN: ceroid lipofuscinosis, neuronal; FXN: frataxin; HTT: huntingtin; LLRK: leucine-rich repeat kinase; PARK: parkinsonism-associated deglycase; PINK: PTEN-induced kinase; PRKN: Parkin RBR E3 ubiquitin ligase; PRPN: prion protein gene; PSEN: presenilin; SMN: survival motor neuron; SOD1: superoxide dismutase 1.

[a] Verhaart et al. (2017)
[b] N.I.N.D.S. (2020)
[c] Bidichandani and Delatycki (2017)
[d] Wallin et al. (2019)
[e] Hebert et al. (2013)
[f] N.O.R.D. (2020)
[g] Maddox et al. (2020)
[h] Knopman and Roberts (2011)
[i] Mehta et al. (2018)
[j] Parkinson's Foundation (2020)

(ICH 2011), a single species may be sufficient for toxicity studies (EMA 2018b) including the assessment of safety within an animal model of disease. Likewise, the potential for immunogenicity should be considered. For gene therapies, the potential for immunogenicity may need to be considered against both the vector and the transgene product (EMA 2018b).

30.3 Neurodegenerative Disorder Considerations

Neurodegenerative disorders have a devastating effect on not only the patient, but their support system as well. While AD and PD are typically associated with the aged population, several neurodegenerative disorders are diagnosed in childhood or young adulthood, such as Friedreich's ataxia, spinal muscular atrophy (SMA), and MS. Age of onset for prion disease, ALS, and HD falls in the middle, typically between the ages of 40 and 75. The ideal age for intervention in these conditions will vary and be largely dependent upon early diagnosis prior to irreversible neuronal damage. When designing the nonclinical program, some topics to consider discussing with health authorities include acceptable margins of safety, appropriate benefit-to-risk relationship (e.g., does the therapeutic treat symptoms or modify disease), age of onset, and anticipated life expectancy of the patient. For instance, most treatments today are palliative in nature; however, more latitude may be warranted if the therapeutic represents the first disease-modifying therapeutic and the patient can anticipate a significantly longer life span as a result. The molecular basis of the disorders, including the pathology of the conditions, has been gradually

linked to the genetic causes, paving the way toward the identification of transformative therapies (Martin 1999). Some neurodegenerative disorders have hereditary components, whereas many are sporadic, but regardless of the underlying cause of genetic change, diagnoses based on genetic screening could enable early treatment with a potentially disease-modifying therapeutic (Pihlstrom, Wiethoff, and Houlden 2017). Table 30.1 demonstrates some of the genetic linkages to a representative list of neurodegenerative disorders, along with the age of onset.

30.4 Challenges and Opportunities for Design of Informative and Efficient Nonclinical Safety Programs for Biologic Therapeutics

The high degree of specificity of biologic therapeutics for disease-related targets and their potential for prolonged effect provide promise as treatments for complex neurodegenerative conditions. However, their diverse nature and unique properties create challenges for the design of appropriate nonclinical safety programs and may impact their utility for patients.

30.4.1 Species Specificity

Species specificity is a primary consideration in the nonclinical development of biologic therapeutics that is largely inconsequential when developing small molecule drugs. Studies in non-relevant species are discouraged; specifically, studies in species in which the biological pharmaceutical is not active are not informative. Avoiding non-relevant nonclinical studies of biologics increases the efficiency of development programs and reduces animal use. If the mechanism of the therapeutic and etiology of the disease is well understood, an initial assessment of which species share that mechanism is paramount. The relevance of a species should correlate to how translatable findings will be to humans. This is of particular importance for gene and cell-based therapies where both safety and efficacy can be simultaneously assessed to provide evidence for direct benefits in conditions where the initial population may be in children.

Species selection should prepare for potential immunogenic responses if the therapeutic modality is human specific. Considering the likely chronic administration for neurodegenerative diseases, potential development of an immunogenic response should be monitored. Choosing the appropriate preclinical species can help anticipate prolonged biological activity. While animal studies may not accurately predict potential immunogenicity of a product in humans designed for a unique human target, a properly designed surrogate product or animal model of disease could be helpful in anticipating clinical responses. Note that the use of surrogate molecules to characterize safety requires careful consideration and should only be relied upon if unable to evaluate the clinical therapeutic in a single species (Bussiere et al. 2009). Some notable limitations of surrogate monoclonal antibodies are technical limitations of providing a close enough species-specific epitope match to the clinical candidate and potentially varying impurity profiles (Lynch, Hart, and Grewal 2009). As with all surrogate approaches, the clinical candidate is not being tested, and therefore, while it does not offer an ideal strategy to understand potential risks, it has shown to be helpful in specialty toxicology studies such as reproduction and development (Bussiere 2008).

A similar approach is undertaken for cellular and gene therapy products. If the clinical therapeutic is directed toward a uniquely human target, analogous products aimed at the equivalent animal target or the utilization of animal models of disease may be preferable to healthy animals (US FDA 2013). Disease models are also important for helping to evaluate potential adverse effects as the first subjects in these trials typically are patients and not healthy volunteers. There is an expectation that animal studies will guide the design of the clinical studies and that there should be a demonstrated biological response to the investigational product in the preclinical species (ICH 2011). Dose scaling between animals and humans may require more effort due to species specificity. For example, relative brain (Bartus et al. 2011) or cerebrospinal fluid (CSF) volumes between animals and humans, coordinates for stereotaxic injection to the appropriate region of the brain, relative target concentrations, whether the biochemical feature of the targeted disease condition exists to the same degree in the animals, and immunogenicity should all be taken into consideration when extrapolating safe and efficacious doses.

30.4.2 Blood–Brain Barrier

Targets for neurodegenerative disorders are typically located in the central nervous system (CNS); as such, there will be the added challenge of finding a way to overcome the protective blood–brain barrier (BBB) (Pardridge 2019). Monoclonal antibodies are too large to readily pass, and bivalent binding of the antibody to a receptor can lead to it being trapped in the brain endothelial cells such that the fraction getting through to the target may be subefficacious.

Direct routes such as intracerebroventricular (ICV) (Nutt et al. 2003, Zhang et al. 1997), intraparenchymal (Hovland et al. 2007, Lang et al. 2006), and intrathecal (IT) (Hinderer, Bell, et al. 2018) have risks associated with invasive administration and do not guarantee access to specific anatomical targets in the CNS (Vuillemenot et al. 2016). One product that successfully uses ICV infusion is cerliponase alfa (Brineura®), the first approved enzyme replacement therapy by ICV infusion for the treatment of Batten disease (de Los Reyes et al. 2020). Some cellular and gene therapy options may require direct stereotaxic delivery into specific regions of the brain. In these cases, nonhuman primate animal models will be preferable due to anatomic similarity to humans which may better allow for the use of the clinically intended delivery device. Consequently, the benefit–risk profile for local delivery methods may not be acceptable for clinical studies in healthy volunteers. While initiating clinical trials with more severe or advanced disease patients may appear to help mitigate this risk, selecting patients who have less advanced neurodegeneration would be anticipated to have a higher likelihood of demonstrating a neuroprotective effect than someone who has little function left to measure. Patients earlier in the time course of disease may also be less likely to have concomitant therapeutics or co-morbidities, enabling a more focused assessment of safety. Anticipated equipment or delivery devices for administering the product in the clinical setting should then be adapted for use in nonclinical animal models. However, invasive routes of administration in laboratory animals can pose risks of infection that exceed clinical incidence simply due to grooming behaviors; therefore, additional considerations of wound care for animal welfare should be well defined.

Some recommendations have been published regarding the development of gene therapies for the treatment of neurodegenerative disorders. Use of adeno-associated virus (AAV) vectors with high permeability of the BBB is a potential route for gene therapy approaches (Choong, Baba, and Mochizuki 2016). AAV2 has been identified as a vector of choice due to high specificity for neurons (Axelsen and Woldbye 2018, Fiandaca, Bankiewicz, and Federoff 2012) while largely avoiding transducing antigen-presenting cells (APCs). However, AAV2 transduction of human neural cells has not proven very efficient and has an associated downside of preexisting human seropositivity in up to 30% of adults (Cearley et al. 2008, Halbert et al. 2006, Mijanovic et al. 2020). This can lead to a higher likelihood of neutralizing antibodies that diminish the therapeutic benefit of the gene therapy. The AAV9 vector has also been recently used due to identified specificity toward transduction of astrocytes and neurons following systemic intravenous (IV) administration, albeit at an apparently lower transduction efficiency (Foust et al. 2009, Manfredsson, Rising, and Mandel 2009, Merkel et al. 2017). Nevertheless, this provides an attractive advantage of avoiding the BBB without invasive direct injection. Other potential AAV serotypes applicable for neurodegenerative diseases have been recently reviewed (Hocquemiller et al. 2016). Delivery methods that optimize distribution such as convection-enhanced delivery (CED) can deliver higher doses to a larger area than diffusion-based delivery. Optimization of cannula placement and use of reflux-resistant cannulas along with real-time imaging are other options (Fiandaca, Bankiewicz, and Federoff 2012). Lastly, having a target-specific vector with high transduction efficiency along with optimized tissue affinity of the formulation should also increase the probability of reaching the desired target within the brain.

Delivery of neurotrophic factors via AAV vectors was attempted with CERE-120, an AAV2 encoding human neurturin. After bilateral stereotactic injections to rhesus monkeys to multiple sites within both the caudate and putamen, expression was observed after a year and no safety concerns were raised (Bartus et al. 2011). While studies in animal models suggested axonal retrograde transport from cell terminals to cell bodies efficiently protected degenerating dopaminergic (DA) neurons, later hypotheses suggested that the lack of notable improvement in clinical trials may have been due to limited retrograde transport in subjects with PD (Warren Olanow et al. 2015). Alternative variants of neurturin were developed by another group with the goal of improving diffusion by limiting heparin-binding potential (Runeberg-Roos et al. 2016). Unfortunately, only limited effects were observed with CERE-120 in Phase 2a and 2b trials and the program was discontinued.

Onasemnogene abeparvovec-xioi (Zolgensma®), an AAV9 vector encoding the survival motor neuron (SMN) gene designed to have high ubiquitous expression especially in the nervous system (Gray et al. 2011, Zincarelli et al. 2008), was administered as an IT dose to monkeys. The monkeys developed inflammation in dorsal root ganglia (DRG), sometimes with degeneration or necrosis. However, this effect was not observed in earlier nonclinical animal studies conducted to support IV onasemnogene abeparvovec-xioi administration, including a non-GLP single-dose IV study in monkeys, likely because the dose tested, 6.7×10^{13} vg/kg, was too low (Novartis 2019, EMA 2020). The results prompted the US FDA to place a partial clinical hold on clinical trials for IT administration (Novartis 2019); no adverse effects related to DRG inflammation were observed at low or mid-doses (6×10^{13} and 1.2×10^{14} vg, respectively) in Phase 1. However, similar DRG lesions have been noted after intracisternal injection with AAV9 vectors being tested for neurodegenerative diseases, e.g., at approximately 3 months after injection with $\geq 10^{12}$ genome copies of an AAV9 vector carrying the transgene for α-L-iduronidase, which encodes a lysosomal enzyme deficient in Hurler syndrome (Hordeaux et al. 2018). Given the current data, inflammation and degeneration of the DRG noted after AAV9 gene therapy vector dosing are potentially dose- and timing-related (EMA 2020).

Receptor-mediated transcytosis and exosomes were initially thought to hinder CNS drug delivery; however, researchers are finding ways to harness these mechanisms to facilitate delivery. In general, the challenge of overcoming the BBB can be addressed by increasing the dose of the therapeutic to saturate the potential uptake (Bevan et al. 2011) or use of BBB-crossing biotherapeutics as a "Trojan horse" (Stanimirovic, Sandhu, and Costain 2018, Freskgard, Niewoehner, and Urich 2017).

To circumvent the BBB, but reach CNS targets at efficacious concentrations, sometimes researchers will administer a high systemic dose, an approach that may lead to adverse systemic effects. A high IV dose (2×10^{14} vg/kg) of AAV9 vector carrying a human SMN transgene was administered to juvenile monkeys and piglets to examine motor neuron transduction efficiency (Hinderer, Katz, et al. 2018). The IV administration led to extensive transduction of the spinal motor neurons; nonetheless, marked toxicity was observed in the liver (in monkeys only) and DRG. Ironically, DRG toxicity was also noted after IT AAV9 vector (onasemnogene abeparvovec-xioi) administration to monkeys, as mentioned earlier; this illustrates the challenge of delivering AAV vectors that demonstrate high distribution to the NS without incurring toxicity, regardless of the route.

Using antibodies targeting the insulin receptor (IR) or transferrin receptor (TfR), biologic payloads can be transported across the BBB (Pardridge 2015). However, translation to humans has not been ideal as there have been noted species differences as well as safety concerns considering the distribution of these receptors beyond the BBB (Couch et al. 2013). The manner in which the carrier and transporting receptor interact is important to understand, as Fc effector functionality and receptor dimerization can prove problematic (Freskgard, Niewoehner, and Urich 2017).

As described above, there are clearly challenges to safely and effectively breaching the BBB to deliver gene therapies. Direct routes of administration or utilizing a Trojan horse technique to bypass the BBB may appear ideal but have demonstrated limited effectiveness thus far. Research suggests modulating the neuroinflammatory response to AAV-based gene therapies for CNS diseases may be possible by considering vector design, pre-immunity or immunomodulation, route of administration, transgene overexpression or expression in nontarget tissues, postdose immunomodulation, and CSF biomarker selection for postdose monitoring (Perez et al. 2020).

30.4.3 Models of Disease

If a preclinical model of the neurodegenerative disease exists, or can be reliably developed, a simultaneous assessment of safety and efficacy can be undertaken. This is an acceptable approach for gene and cell-based therapies; however, for protein-based therapies, disease-specific models have not been routinely accepted for the assessment of safety. Many models of neurodegenerative diseases appear to mimic pathology or symptoms, yet have fallen short to recapitulate the progressive nature of these conditions (Dawson, Golde, and Lagier-Tourenne 2018). For instance, the traditional neurotoxin-induced rodent models of PD utilizing 6-hydroxydopamine (6-OHDA) or 1-methyl-4-phenyl-1,2,3,6-tetrahydropyridine (MPTP) are more useful as models of symptomatology of PD than disease modification (Kin et al. 2019, Tieu 2011). These lesion models do not necessarily capture the degenerative course of the disease, instead offering visibility to a static time point within the disease. Models capturing earlier phases or the full scope of the disease are gaining more visibility (Grandi, Di Giovanni, and Galati 2018).

If the target does not exist in animal species, there may be significant value in evaluating knock-in or knockout strains or transgenic species expressing the human target (humanized). Several transgenic mouse models exist those phenotypically reproduce aspects of Alzheimer's pathology, modeling Aβ or tau pathology, either independently or simultaneously (Nair et al. 2019). Yet behavioral alterations (such as loss of function, impaired cognition, and altered mood) in these models fail to correlate with AD in humans and to date, promising therapeutics in these transgenic strains have not proven successful in clinical trials. DJ-1, Parkin, and PTEN-induced putative kinase 1 (PINK1) have been linked to familial forms of PD in humans (Sarkar, Raymick, and Imam 2016). Even though genetic variations account for a small percentage of all cases, models incorporating the variations can help identify therapeutics that may alter disease progression (Barker and Bjorklund 2020, Grandi, Di Giovanni, and Galati 2018).

The ability to model the human disease in a preclinical animal species is paramount to understanding the translatability of therapeutic effects to humans. Special attention should be given as to understanding whether the model utilized will have the ability to demonstrate potential disease-modifying action or relief of symptoms. Alignment between the stage of the disease being modeled in animals and the clinical intent of treatment timing is critical. Different patients with the same disease may have different genotypes that may warrant additional steps in genetically screening patients for a more uniform population. An example of this may be edaravone, which demonstrated an attenuation of symptom progression and motor neuron degeneration in G93A mutant SOD1 transgenic mice (Ito et al. 2008). However, a Phase 3 study did not demonstrate a significant difference in the Revised ALS Functional Rating Scale when compared to placebo. Post hoc analysis demonstrated that in a subset of the patient population defined as early stage, edaravone had a greater magnitude of effect in modifying the progression of the disease (Writing Group and Edaravone A.L.S. Study Group 2017). Additionally, including safety endpoints in pharmacology studies in preclinical models of disease may better characterize anticipated adverse events in patients (Chapter 2).

Dawson et al. (2018) propose that future models of neurodegenerative diseases should aim to demonstrate the progressive degeneration of all cell types, not just neurons, and that perhaps multiple pathways will need simultaneous targeting. Neurodegenerative diseases appear to be multifactorial. Success in a single-disease model should lead to further preclinical investigations in other models as opposed to premature conduct of expensive human clinical studies. Several recent reviews of animal models of neurodegenerative diseases have been published that discuss the strengths and limitations of each model (Barker and Bjorklund 2020, Dawson, Golde, and Lagier-Tourenne 2018, Fisher and Bannerman 2019, JPND Action Group 2014, Ransohoff 2018).

One example of disease models being used for safety evaluation is the nonclinical development program for cerliponase alfa that incorporated safety pharmacology endpoints into general toxicity studies performed in a model of Batten disease. Neurological examinations, CNS biodistribution, magnetic resonance imaging, and cardiovascular endpoints were included within the repeat-dose studies in TPP1-null juvenile dachshund dogs. Three of these repeat-dose studies were between 9 and 10 months in duration and perhaps due to the uniqueness of the animal model; none of the studies in dachshunds were performed GLP, and there were no other species tested for repeat-dose toxicity. The US FDA's perspective on nonclinical development programs for enzyme replacement products is summarized in the 2019 Guidance for Industry, Investigational Enzyme Replacement Therapy Products: Nonclinical Assessment (US FDA 2019c).

Another example of using an animal model of disease within the nonclinical safety package can be demonstrated with gantenerumab, a human monoclonal antibody directed against Aβ for the treatment of AD. While the patient population affected by typical AD is generally aged beyond childbearing years (Table 30.1), gantenerumab was also being considered for potential future use in the prevention of AD, treating the condition early to slow or stop its irreversible disease progression (Barrow et al. 2017). This would require clinical trials in younger patients, of reproductive age. Therefore, a full complement of nonclinical developmental/reproductive toxicity studies (e.g., fertility, embryo-fetal development, and pre- and postnatal development (PPND)) was deemed necessary. However, health authorities agreed that these studies did not need to be completed prior to clinical trials with gantenerumab given the low number of non-elderly patients in the initial clinical development program and the requirement for contraception in premenopausal women. Instead, the studies needed to be completed before the submission of a marketing application. In addition, the studies were conducted in transgenic mice (PS2APP model), as gantenerumab's target is aggregated forms of Aβ that are not present in healthy animal models more commonly used for pharmaceutical developmental/reproductive toxicity studies (Barrow et al. 2017).

Additionally, while there are no stem cell therapies currently approved for neurodegenerative diseases in the US, animal models of disease have been used to explore safety and efficacy challenges. Historically, tumorigenicity had been an issue when transplanting pluripotent stem cells (Liu et al. 2016). Researchers sorted human-induced pluripotent stem cells (iPSCs; somatic cells that have been transduced with exogenous genes to induce pluripotency) with a cell surface marker often co-located with DA progenitor neurons before transplanting into the PD model of 6-OHDA lesioned rats. The transplanted iPSCs differentiated into midbrain DA neurons and resulted in significant improvement of motor behavior, and notably, at up to 4 months after the transplantation of the sorted iPSCs, no tumors were noted (Doi et al. 2014). Mesenchymal stem cells were also tested in the 6-OHDA rat model and demonstrated that cells that were engineered to express both tyrosine hydroxylase (TH; a differentiation marker for DA neurons) and glial cell line-derived neurotrophic factor (GDNF) were able to perform significantly better in behavioral tests and express significantly more DA and GDNF than any of the other treatment groups including either MSCs expressing TH or GDNF alone (Shi et al. 2011).

30.5 Nonclinical Safety Programs for Biologic Therapeutics for Neurodegenerative Disorders

Given the substantial unmet medical need for effective therapies for serious neurodegenerative diseases, there is an opportunity to take an approach that is science-based and agency-interactive to efficiently develop novel biopharmaceuticals. Below, key features of nonclinical safety programs for US FDA-approved biologic therapeutics for neurodegenerative conditions are described; these programs are targeted, with focused scope based on active consideration of the condition to be treated, the patient population, and the specific properties of the modality and therapeutic target but maintain a science-based approach that appropriately addresses traditional toxicological principles. Table 30.2 summarizes the nonclinical programs for a select list of biopharmaceuticals approved in the US.

30.5.1 Safety Pharmacology

Considering targets within the CNS, safety pharmacology evaluations of CNS safety may be particularly helpful in identifying exaggerated pharmacology or off-target effects, and per ICH S6, endpoints can be incorporated into general toxicology studies. There were no stand-alone safety pharmacology studies conducted in support of the MS therapies daclizumab (Zinbryta®) or ocrelizumab (Ocrevus®), or the SMA gene therapy onasemnogene abeparvovec-xioi (US FDA 2016d, 2017e, 2019e). However, for daclizumab, the sponsor did conduct neurobehavioral assessments in a 2-week neurotoxicity study as a follow-up to histopathological findings from chronic toxicology studies, as a targeted assessment to understand the mechanism of toxicity as opposed to fulfill the need for a stand-alone safety pharmacology study (US FDA 2016d).

Regarding cardiovascular safety pharmacology evaluation, ICH S6 and industry working groups have recommended against conducting dedicated safety pharmacology studies to support biopharmaceutical development, instead recommending inclusion of ECG evaluations in large animal studies (Berman et al. 2014, ICH 2011, Vargas et al. 2008). It has been noted that the ICH guidelines are not clear on safety pharmacology recommendations for antisense oligonucleotides (ASOs), as they appear to exist in a gray area between small molecules and biologics (Kim et al. 2014). Stand-alone cardiovascular and respiratory safety assessments were conducted for nusinersen. However, results from these studies demonstrate that stand-alone safety pharmacology assays for ASOs have low utility and that incorporation of endpoints within general toxicity studies should be sufficient.

The general toxicity program for onasemnogene abeparvovec-xioi mainly consisted of a definitive extended single-dose toxicity study in one species, neonatal mice, and included clinical pathology, histopathology, and biodistribution. A non-GLP extended single-dose toxicity study was also conducted in infant monkeys, and the pharmacologic effect was investigated in an SMA disease model in juvenile piglets (US FDA 2019e). This nonclinical program supported use in the targeted population of patients <2 years old.

30.5.2 Safety Margins

In light of the unmet medical need and serious life-threatening conditions that can exist with neurodegenerative disorders, health authorities may be willing to consider biologic therapeutics that are efficacious, even if safety margins are low. There is precedent for limited safety margins supporting the approval of biopharmaceuticals for neurodegenerative diseases. For daclizumab (US FDA 2016d), in repeat-dose subcutaneous toxicity studies in monkeys up to 9 months, the main drug-related adverse effects consisted of skin and CNS findings that persisted in monkeys at the highest dose following recovery. There was no NOAEL (No Observed Adverse Effect Level) for the dermal histopathology findings. The safety margin for the microglial aggregates was approximately nine times the anticipated human exposure. Although a nonclinical pharmacology reviewer recommended against the approval of the drug, the supervisor memo determined that the microglial aggregate lesions do not prevent the approval of daclizumab since there was a NOAEL, an exposure margin, and lesions were minimal. Subsequently, the approval was based on the balance of efficacy and safety findings noted in subjects (US FDA 2016d). While daclizumab was approved in 2016, it was withdrawn from the market in 2018 due to shifting and complex safety issues, including CNS inflammation that was noted preclinically with a much lower severity (AbbVie 2018, US FDA 2016d, 2018) and the small number of patients dosed as a consequence of being considered a third-line therapy. This example illustrates the need for both regulators and industry to continually re-evaluate the benefit–risk profile in developing and marketing biopharmaceuticals for neurodegenerative diseases.

Another example of low or no margins of safety to the clinical dose can be found in the approval of nusinersen (Spinraza®; US FDA 2016b), an ASO for the treatment of SMA. In the repeat-dose IT toxicity studies in juvenile monkeys, slight to minimal histological findings in the CNS were noted at the mid- and high doses; lesions remained after the recovery period. The NOAEL for the CNS histopathology was similar to the proposed clinical maintenance dose and was associated with exposure margins of safety that were <1 (US FDA 2016b).

For onasemnogene abeparvovec-xioi (US FDA 2019e), a gene therapy for SMA described earlier, a safety margin could not be calculated. Serum chemistry and cardiac findings were observed at all doses in neonatal mice and a NOAEL was unable to be defined. The lowest dose tested in the toxicity studies was lower than the recommended clinical IV infusion dose for onasemnogene abeparvovec-xioi (US FDA 2019e).

30.5.3 Genotoxicity and Carcinogenicity

Standard genotoxicity studies are typically not necessary for biologic therapeutics (ICH S6). They were performed for nusinersen (US FDA 2016b), as ASOs are generally regulated more like small molecules than as biologics. For gene therapies, some vectors have a potential for insertional mutagenesis and integration. In the case of onasemnogene abeparvovec-xioi, lack of genotoxicity was supported by citing low frequency for random integration of recombinant AAV vectors (AAV9

TABLE 30.2

Summary of Nonclinical Safety Evaluation Programs for Selected US FDA-Approved Biologic Therapeutics for Neurodegenerative Disorders

Product/Description	US FDA Approval Date, Route, and Indication	Approval Notes	Key Nonclinical Safety Program Aspects	References
Ocrelizumab (Ocrevus®) Humanized IgG1 mAb directed against CD20-expressing B-cells	28 Mar 2017 IV infusion Treatment of relapsing or primary progressive forms of MS in adults	BLA Fast Track, Breakthrough Therapy, and Priority Review designation	• Tissue cross-reactivity conducted • No dedicated safety pharmacology studies • No single-dose toxicity studies • Single relevant species for repeat-dose toxicity • No genotoxicity or carcinogenicity studies • Additional expanded PPND study (containing TDAR) conducted as PMR	(US FDA 2017e)
Daclizumab (Zinbryta®) Humanized mAb directed against α-subunit of interleukin 2 receptor (IL-2Rα/CD25)	27 May 2016 SC injection Treatment of relapsing forms of MS in adults	BLA Review period extended by 3 months for major amendment; Withdrawn from the market in 2018 by sponsor	• Tissue cross-reactivity conducted • No dedicated safety pharmacology studies • No genotoxicity or carcinogenicity studies • No juvenile toxicity studies[a] • Low safety margin for unmonitorable CNS lesions • Neurotoxicity study conducted for further evaluation of histopathology lesions and neurobehavioral effects[b]	(US FDA 2016d, AbbVie 2018)
Alemtuzumab (Lemtrada®) Humanized IgG1 kappa mAb directed against the cell surface glycoprotein, CD52	14 Nov 2014 IV infusion Treatment of relapsing forms of MS in adults	BLA Approved for MS as a supplement to the 2001 accelerated approval for patients with B-cell CLL; available for MS only through a restricted access program under a REMS	• Tissue cross-reactivity conducted • Dedicated safety pharmacology studies conducted for initial CLL indication • No genotoxicity or carcinogenicity studies • PPND study conducted as a PMR	(US FDA 2001, EMA 2013, Genzyme Corporation 2020)
Natalizumab (Tysabri®) Humanized IgG4 kappa mAb that binds to α4-integrin	23 Nov 2004 IV infusion Treatment of relapsing forms of MS in adults	BLA Accelerated Approval	• Tissue cross-reactivity conducted • No carcinogenicity studies • Tumor promotion potential explored by in vitro and in vivo studies • Final report for PPND study submitted as PMR	(US FDA 2004b)

(Continued)

TABLE 30.2 (Continued)

Summary of Nonclinical Safety Evaluation Programs for Selected US FDA-Approved Biologic Therapeutics for Neurodegenerative Disorders

Product/Description	US FDA Approval Date, Route, and Indication	Approval Notes	Key Nonclinical Safety Program Aspects	References
Onasemnogene abeparvovec-xioi (Zolgensma®) AAV9 vector-based gene therapy containing a transgene for human SMN	24 May 2019 IV infusion Treatment of SMA with bi-allelic mutations in the survival motor neuron 1 (SMN1) gene in pediatric patients <2 years of age	BLA Fast Track, Breakthrough Therapy, Priority Review, and Orphan Drug designation	• No safety pharmacology studies or endpoints evaluated • Single-dose toxicity study in juvenile mice • No repeat-dose toxicity studies • Limited safety margin • No genotoxicity or carcinogenicity studies • No reproductive toxicity studies	(US FDA 2019e)
Nusinersen (Spinraza®) Antisense oligonucleotide that binds to a specific sequence in the intron downstream of exon 7 of the SMN2 transcript	23 Dec 2016 IT injection Treatment of SMA in pediatric and adult patients	NDA Fast Track, Priority Review, and Orphan Drug designation	• Dedicated safety pharmacology studies conducted • Limited safety margin • Genotoxicity studies conducted • Carcinogenicity study conducted as PMR • PPND completed as PMR	(US FDA 2016b)
Cerliponase alfa (Brineura®) Recombinant human tripeptidyl peptidase-1 (rhTPP1)	27 Apr 2017 ICV infusion Treatment to slow the loss of ambulation in symptomatic pediatric patients ≥3 years of age with late infantile neuronal CLN2, also known as TPP1 deficiency	BLA Breakthrough Therapy, Priority Review, and Orphan Drug designation	• No dedicated safety pharmacology studies • No genotoxicity or carcinogenicity studies • Non-GLP, single species for repeat-dose toxicity[c] • No reproductive toxicity studies	(US FDA 2017b)

α: alpha; AAV: adeno-associated virus; BLA: biologics license application; CD: cluster of differentiation; CLL: chronic lymphocytic leukemia; CLN2: ceroid lipofuscinosis type 2; CNS: central nervous system; EMA: European Medicines Agency; FDA: Food and Drug Administration; ICV: intracerebroventricular; IgG: immunoglobulin G; IL-2Rα: interleukin-2 receptor; IT: intrathecal; IV: intravenous; κ: kappa; mAb: monoclonal antibody; MS: multiple sclerosis; NDA: new drug application; N/A: not applicable; PMR: postmarketing requirement; PMS: primary multiple sclerosis; PPND: pre- and postnatal development; REMS: risk evaluation and mitigation strategy; SC: subcutaneous; SMA: spinal muscular atrophy; SMN: survival motor neuron; TDAR: T-cell-dependent antibody response.

[a] Due to toxicity, sponsor did not intend to treat juvenile patients with drug.

[b] A 2-week neurotoxicity study was conducted to follow up on histological changes in the chronic studies; this study included neurobehavioral assessments.

[c] Non-GLP, chronic, repeat-dose toxicity studies were conducted in a disease model of dogs.

vectors) and absence of hepatic genotoxicity in recombinant AAV genomic integration in liver samples from monkeys and humans (Chandler, Sands, and Venditti 2017, Gil-Farina et al. 2016, Nowrouzi et al. 2012, US FDA 2019e).

As per health authority guidance, standard rodent carcinogenicity studies are not typically conducted for biologic (ICH 2011, Vahle et al. 2010) or gene and cellular therapies (US FDA 2013). However, for biologics, there is the expectation of an assessment of carcinogenic risk based upon the understanding of the target, mechanism of action, results of general toxicity studies, and alternative methods to assess tumorigenicity. For example, in vitro tumor cell growth assays and xenograft studies were performed for natalizumab (Tysabri®) for relapsing MS (US FDA 2004b). Completion of a 2-year carcinogenicity study in a single rodent species (mice) was a postmarketing requirement for nusinersen, an ASO for the treatment of SMA (US FDA 2016b). However, as stated above for genotoxicity studies, ASOs are regulated more as small molecules than as biologics. For cellular therapies, especially those derived from embryonic stem cells and iPSCs, it is important to assess tumorigenicity prior to initial clinical trials. For the development of biopharmaceuticals for neurodegenerative diseases, it may be important to also consider the patient population, severity of disease, and expected prognosis in formulating a carcinogenicity plan.

30.5.4 Reproduction and Developmental Toxicity

Studies investigating effects on reproduction and development are dependent upon the age of the population and anticipated outcome (Rocca et al. 2018). Advanced age in AD and PD may negate the need for evaluating potential reproductive risk. However, both conditions can have an earlier onset in a subset of patients. As mentioned earlier, developmental and reproductive toxicity studies in PS2APP transgenic mice were conducted for the investigational monoclonal antibody gantenerumab, targeting Aβ in AD (Barrow et al. 2017). But even for childhood-onset conditions, if the treatment is not anticipated to alter the course of the disease, the patient may be expected to die well before reaching reproductive potential. Accordingly, no reproductive toxicity studies were conducted for cerliponase alfa, a treatment for Batten disease (US FDA 2017b). For onasemnogene abeparvovec-xioi, the gene therapy product approved for SMA, reproductive toxicity studies were not conducted. This approach was justified based on low vector DNA in the gonads within general toxicology studies and the fact that patients will likely be less than 1 year old at the time of treatment, many years from reaching reproductive maturity (US FDA 2019e).

Based upon the specific product, indication, and scientific rationale, animal studies might be delayed until after a product is approved by gaining agreement with health agencies on postponing requirements to the postmarketing phase. This option has been applied for the PPND studies supporting several biopharmaceutical reproductive development programs. To support alemtuzumab (Lemtrada®), a humanized immunoglobulin G (IgG)4 monoclonal antibody against α4β1 integrin for the treatment of patients with relapsing MS, a PPND study was conducted in a transgenic mouse expressing human

cluster of differentiation (CD)52 during postmarketing (US FDA 2001). For natalizumab, a humanized IgG1 κ monoclonal antibody against CD52 also for the treatment of patients with relapsing forms of MS, the final report for a PPND study was submitted to the US FDA during postmarketing (US FDA 2004b). For nusinersen, an ASO for the treatment of SMA, a PPND study ongoing at the time of approval was completed as a postmarketing requirement (US FDA 2016b).

30.5.5 Abuse Liability

Given the intended CNS activity of therapeutics for neurodegenerative disorders, abuse potential should be considered in alignment with appropriate health authority expectations (Gauvin, Zimmermann, and Baird 2019, de Zafra et al. 2018), such as the US FDA's Guidance for Industry, Assessment of Abuse Potential of Drugs (US FDA 2017c). The scope of this guidance includes biologic pharmaceuticals regulated by the US FDA's Center for Drug Evaluation and Research (CDER) but does not cover gene and cellular therapies regulated by the Center for Biologics Evaluation and Research (CBER). Therapeutics with high abuse potential may require special abuse-related nonclinical or clinical studies. Nonclinical data contributing to the characterization of abuse potential could include behavior evaluations from safety pharmacology studies, drug-discrimination studies, self-administration studies, or physical dependence studies (US FDA 2017c). While CNS activity would be an expected goal of most treatments for neurodegenerative disorders, sponsors should consider the specific molecular target and intended mechanism of action of their therapeutic to assess whether there would be a particular concern for abuse (e.g., treatment produces euphoria, hallucinations, or effects consistent with CNS depression or stimulation). Due to their required administration by a health care provider, biologic therapeutics may have a reduced potential for abuse, relative to small molecules. In addition, if the nonclinical characterization of abuse potential is warranted, the properties and specificity of biologic therapeutics must be considered in designing appropriate investigations; typical animal models may not be relevant. For the biologic therapeutic products summarized in Table 30.2, the US FDA's medical reviews identified no concerns for abuse associated with the therapeutics' mechanisms of action, and there were no observations in clinical studies suggestive of abuse potential. Consequently, no specific abuse-related nonclinical or clinical studies were conducted to support approval (US FDA 1996, 2004a, 2016a, 2016c, 2017a, 2017d, 2019d).

30.6 Conclusions and Recommendations

Given the progressive, degenerative, and irreversible nature of degenerative disorders of the CNS, and the limited number of available therapies, there remains a significant unmet medical need for novel pharmacological interventions. Global health authorities responsible for regulating pharmaceuticals recognize this need and have provided guidance for sponsors to reference in the design of appropriate and efficient clinical and nonclinical development programs to facilitate the rapid availability of new treatments to patients.

The examples of US FDA-approved biologic therapeutics provided in this chapter provide a framework for sponsors that emphasizes the importance of a case-by-case approach based upon product attributes for nonclinical development programs for biotherapeutics intended to treat neurodegenerative disorders.

The patient populations for neurodegenerative disorders are demographically diverse, with unique prevalence and etiology across many factors, including age and sex. Therefore, certain nonclinical studies may not be informative for the evaluation of human risk. When designing nonclinical safety programs for biopharmaceuticals for neurodegenerative conditions, sponsors must take a case-by-case, science-based approach that thoughtfully considers the specific condition, the characteristics of the affected population, the treatment approach, and the properties of the therapeutic modality. Special consideration should be given to the appropriate approach to manage the BBB and engage the target. Importantly, the collection of safety endpoints in animal models of disease may be critical in understanding translatability to the clinic.

While health authority guidance and approved precedent provide solid reference for sponsors to use when developing informative nonclinical safety programs for biotherapeutics for neurodegenerative disorders, early and frequent engagement (e.g., meetings, written correspondence) with health authorities is strongly recommended. Notably, health authority guidance encourages these opportunities (US FDA 2013, 2014, 2020, EMA 2018a, US FDA 2019b) to discuss novel development programs. Health authority engagement allows validation of the program design considerations being applied by the sponsor and can facilitate a collaborative working partnership directed at the shared goal of providing novel, effective therapies to patients with neurodegenerative disorders in the most efficient way possible.

REFERENCES

AbbVie. 2018. "Biogen and AbbVie Announce the Voluntary Worldwide Withdrawal of Marketing Authorizations for ZINBRYTA® (daclizumab) for Relapsing Multiple Sclerosis." https://news.abbvie.com/news/press-releases/biogen-and-abbvie-announce-voluntary-worldwide-withdrawal-marketing-authorizations-for-zinbryta-daclizumab-for-relapsing-multiple-sclerosis.htm. 02 Mar 2020 (Accessed 19 Aug 2020).

Axelsen, T. M., and D. P. D. Woldbye. 2018. "Gene therapy for Parkinson's disease, an update." *J Parkinsons Dis* 8 (2):195–215. doi: 10.3233/JPD-181331.

Barker, R. A., and A. Bjorklund. 2020. "Animal models of Parkinson's disease: are they useful or not?" *J Parkinsons Dis*. doi: 10.3233/JPD-202200.

Barrow, P., L. Villabruna, A. Hoberman, B. Bohrmann, W. F. Richter, and C. Schubert. 2017. "Reproductive and developmental toxicology studies with gantenerumab in PS2APP transgenic mice." *Reprod Toxicol* 73:362–371. doi: 10.1016/j.reprotox.2017.07.014.

Bartus, R. T., L. Brown, A. Wilson, B. Kruegel, J. Siffert, E. M. Johnson, Jr., J. H. Kordower, and C. D. Herzog. 2011. "Properly scaled and targeted AAV2-NRTN (neurturin) to

the substantia nigra is safe, effective and causes no weight loss: support for nigral targeting in Parkinson's disease." *Neurobiol Dis* 44 (1):38–52. doi: 10.1016/j.nbd.2011.05.026.

Berman, C. L., K. Cannon, Y. Cui, D. J. Kornbrust, A. Lagrutta, S. Z. Sun, J. Tepper, G. Waldron, and H. S. Younis. 2014. "Recommendations for safety pharmacology evaluations of oligonucleotide-based therapeutics." *Nucleic Acid Ther* 24 (4):291–301. doi: 10.1089/nat.2013.0477.

Bevan, A. K., S. Duque, K. D. Foust, P. R. Morales, L. Braun, L. Schmelzer, C. M. Chan, M. McCrate, L. G. Chicoine, B. D. Coley, P. N. Porensky, S. J. Kolb, J. R. Mendell, A. H. Burghes, and B. K. Kaspar. 2011. "Systemic gene delivery in large species for targeting spinal cord, brain, and peripheral tissues for pediatric disorders." *Mol Ther* 19 (11):1971–80. doi: 10.1038/mt.2011.157.

Bidichandani, S. I., and M. B. Delatycki. 2017. "Friedreich Ataxia. 1998 Dec 18 [Updated 2017 Jun 1]." In *GeneReviews [Internet]*, edited by M. P. Adam, H. H. Ardinger and R. A. Pagon. Seattle, WA: University of Washington, Seattle; 1993–2020. Available from: https://www.ncbi.nlm.nih.gov/books/NBK1281/.

Bussiere, J. L. 2008. "Species selection considerations for preclinical toxicology studies for biotherapeutics." *Expert Opin Drug Metab Toxicol* 4 (7):871–877. doi: 10.1517/17425255.4.7.871.

Bussiere, J. L., P. Martin, M. Horner, J. Couch, M. Flaherty, L. Andrews, J. Beyer, and C. Horvath. 2009. "Alternative strategies for toxicity testing of species-specific biopharmaceuticals." *Int J Toxicol* 28 (3):230–253. doi: 10.1177/1091581809337262.

Caga, J., S. Hsieh, P. Lillo, K. Dudley, and E. Mioshi. 2019. "The impact of cognitive and behavioral symptoms on ALS patients and their caregivers." Front Neurol 10 (192):1–7. doi: 10.3389/fneur.2019.00192.

Cearley, C. N., L. H. Vandenberghe, M. K. Parente, E. R. Carnish, J. M. Wilson, and J. H. Wolfe. 2008. "Expanded repertoire of AAV vector serotypes mediate unique patterns of transduction in mouse brain." Mol Ther 16 (10):1710–1718. doi: 10.1038/mt.2008.166.

Chandler, R. J., M. S. Sands, and C. P. Venditti. 2017. "Recombinant Adeno-Associated Viral Integration and Genotoxicity: Insights from Animal Models." Hum Gene Ther 28 (4):314–322. doi: 10.1089/hum.2017.009.

Cheng, S. T. 2017. "Dementia caregiver burden: A research update and critical analysis." Curr Psychiatry Rep 19:64. doi: 10.1007/s11920-017-0818-2.

Choong, C. J., K. Baba, and H. Mochizuki. 2016. "Gene therapy for neurological disorders." Expert Opin Biol Ther 16 (2):143–59. doi: 10.1517/14712598.2016.1114096.

Couch, J. A., Y. J. Yu, Y. Zhang, J. M. Tarrant, R. N. Fuji, W. J. Meilandt, H. Solanoy, R. K. Tong, K. Hoyte, W. Luk, Y. Lu, K. Gadkar, S. Prabhu, B. A. Ordonia, Q. Nguyen, Y. Lin, Z. Lin, M. Balazs, K. Scearce-Levie, J. A. Ernst, M. S. Dennis, and R. J. Watts. 2013. "Addressing safety liabilities of TfR bispecific antibodies that cross the blood-brain barrier." Sci Transl Med 5 (183):183ra57, 1–12. doi: 10.1126/scitranslmed.3005338.

Dawson, T. M., T. E. Golde, and C. Lagier-Tourenne. 2018. "Animal models of neurodegenerative diseases." Nat Neurosci 21 (10):1370–1379. doi: 10.1038/s41593-018-0236-8.

de Los Reyes, E., L. Lehwald, E. F. Augustine, E. Berry-Kravis, K. Butler, N. Cormier, S. Demarest, S. Lu, J. Madden, J. Olaya, S. See, A. Vierhile, J. W. Wheless, A. Yang, J. Cohen-Pfeffer, D. Chu, F. Leal-Pardinas, and R. Y. Wang. 2020. "Intracerebroventricular Cerliponase Alfa for Neuronal Ceroid Lipofuscinosis Type 2 Disease: Clinical Practice Considerations From US Clinics." Pediatr Neurol 110:64–70. doi: 10.1016/j.pediatrneurol.2020.04.018.

de Zafra, C. L. Z., C. G. Markgraf, D. R. Compton, and T. J. Hudzik. 2018. "Abuse liability assessment for biologic drugs - All molecules are not created equal." Regul Toxicol Pharmacol 92:165–172. doi: 10.1016/j.yrtph.2017.11.019.

Doi, D., B. Samata, M. Katsukawa, T. Kikuchi, A. Morizane, Y. Ono, K. Sekiguchi, M. Nakagawa, M. Parmar, and J. Takahashi. 2014. "Isolation of human induced pluripotent stem cell-derived dopaminergic progenitors by cell sorting for successful transplantation." *Stem Cell Reports* 2 (3):337–350. doi: 10.1016/j.stemcr.2014.01.013.

EMA. 2013. "Lemtrada (alemtuzumab) Public Assessment Report. 27 Jun 2013. Procedure No. EMEA/H/C/003718/0000." European Medicines Agency. https://www.ema.europa.eu/en/documents/assessment-report/lemtrada-epar-public-assessment-report_en.pdf.

EMA. 2016a. "Guidance for Companies Considering the Adaptive Pathways Approach." EMA/527726/2016.

EMA. 2016b. "Guideline on the Scientific Application and the Practical Arrangements Necessary to Implement Commission Regulation (EC) No 507/2006 on the Conditional Marketing Authorisation for Medicinal Products for Human Use Falling within the Scope of Regulation (EC) No 726/2004." Committee for Medicinal Products for Human Use. EMA/CHMP/509951/2006, Rev. 1.

EMA. 2016c. "Guideline on the Scientific Application and the Practical Arrangements Necessary to Implement the Procedure for Accelerated Assessment Pursuant to Article 14(9) of Regulation (EC) No 726/2004." Human Medicines Evaluation Division. EMA/CHMP/671361/2015 Rev. 1.

EMA. 2018a. "Enhanced Early Dialogue to Facilitate Accelerated Enhancement of PRIority Medicines (PRIME)." Committee for Medicinal Products for Human Use. EMA/CHMP/57760/2015, Rev. 1.

EMA. 2018b. "Guideline on the Quality, Non-clinical and Clinical Aspects of Gene Therapy Medicinal Products." Committee for Advanced Therapies. EMA/CAT/80183/2014.

EMA. 2020. "Zolgensma (onasemnogene abeparvovec) Assessment Report. 26 Mar 2020. Procedure No. EMEA/H/C/004750/0000." European Medicines Agency. https://www.ema.europa.eu/en/documents/assessment-report/zolgensma-epar-public-assessment-report_en.pdf.

Fiandaca, M. S., K. S. Bankiewicz, and H. J. Federoff. 2012. "Gene therapy for the treatment of Parkinson's disease: the nature of the biologics expands the future indications." *Pharmaceuticals (Basel)* 5 (6):553–590. doi: 10.3390/ph5060553.

Fisher, E. M. C., and D. M. Bannerman. 2019. "Mouse models of neurodegeneration: know your question, know your mouse." *Sci Transl Med* 11 (493). doi: 10.1126/scitranslmed.aaq1818.

Foust, K. D., E. Nurre, C. L. Montgomery, A. Hernandez, C. M. Chan, and B. K. Kaspar. 2009. "Intravascular AAV9 preferentially targets neonatal neurons and adult astrocytes." *Nat Biotechnol* 27 (1):59–65. doi: 10.1038/nbt.1515.

Freskgard, P. O., J. Niewoehner, and E. Urich. 2017. "Time to open the blood–brain barrier gate for biologics?." *Fut Neurol* 9 (3):243–245.

Gauvin, D. V., Z. J. Zimmermann, and T. J. Baird. 2019. "In further defense of nonclinical abuse liability testing of biologics." *Regul Toxicol Pharmacol* 101:103–120. doi: 10.1016/j.yrtph.2018.11.009.

Genzyme Corporation. 2020. "Lemtrada (alemtuzumab injection, solution, concentrate) prescribing information. Version June 2020." Daily Med. U.S. National Library of Medicine. Retrieved 18 Aug 2020. https://dailymed.nlm.nih.gov/dailymed/drugInfo.cfm?setid=6236b0bc-82e9-4447-9a78-f57d94770269.

Gil-Farina, I., R. Fronza, C. Kaeppel, E. Lopez-Franco, V. Ferreira, D. D'Avola, A. Benito, J. Prieto, H. Petry, G. Gonzalez-Aseguinolaza, and M. Schmidt. 2016. "Recombinant AAV integration is not associated with hepatic genotoxicity in nonhuman primates and patients." *Mol Ther* 24 (6):1100–1105. doi: 10.1038/mt.2016.52.

Grandi, L. C., G. Di Giovanni, and S. Galati. 2018. "Animal models of early-stage Parkinson's disease and acute dopamine deficiency to study compensatory neurodegenerative mechanisms." *J Neurosci Methods* 308:205–218. doi: 10.1016/j.jneumeth.2018.08.012.

Gray, S. J., S. B. Foti, J. W. Schwartz, L. Bachaboina, B. Taylor-Blake, J. Coleman, M. D. Ehlers, M. J. Zylka, T. J. McCown, and R. J. Samulski. 2011. "Optimizing promoters for recombinant adeno-associated virus-mediated gene expression in the peripheral and central nervous system using self-complementary vectors." *Hum Gene Ther* 22 (9):1143–1153. doi: 10.1089/hum.2010.245.

Halbert, C. L., A. D. Miller, S. McNamara, J. Emerson, R. L. Gibson, B. Ramsey, and M. L. Aitken. 2006. "Prevalence of neutralizing antibodies against adeno-associated virus (AAV) types 2, 5, and 6 in cystic fibrosis and normal populations: Implications for gene therapy using AAV vectors." *Hum Gene Ther* 17 (4):440–447. doi: 10.1089/hum.2006.17.440.

Health Canada. 2008. "Guidance for Industry: Priority Review of Drug Submissions." Health Products and Food Branch. Minister of Health.

Health Canada. 2016. "Guidance Document: Notice of Compliance with conditions (NOC/c)." Health Products and Food Branch. Minister of Health.

Hebert, L. E., J. Weuve, P. A. Scherr, and D. A. Evans. 2013. "Alzheimer disease in the United States (2010–2050) estimated using the 2010 census." *Neurology* 80 (19):1778–1783. doi: 10.1212/WNL.0b013e31828726f5.

Hinderer, C., P. Bell, N. Katz, C. H. Vite, J. P. Louboutin, E. Bote, H. Yu, Y. Zhu, M. L. Casal, J. Bagel, P. O'Donnell, P. Wang, M. E. Haskins, T. Goode, and J. M. Wilson. 2018. "Evaluation of intrathecal routes of administration for adeno-associated viral vectors in large animals." *Hum Gene Ther* 29 (1):15–24. doi: 10.1089/hum.2017.026.

Hinderer, C., N. Katz, E. L. Buza, C. Dyer, T. Goode, P. Bell, L. K. Richman, and J. M. Wilson. 2018. "Severe toxicity in nonhuman primates and piglets following high-dose intravenous administration of an adeno-associated virus vector expressing human SMN." *Hum Gene Ther* 29 (3):285–298. doi: 10.1089/hum.2018.015.

Hocquemiller, M., L. Giersch, M. Audrain, S. Parker, and N. Cartier. 2016. "Adeno-associated virus-based gene therapy for CNS diseases." *Hum Gene Ther* 27 (7):478–496. doi: 10.1089/hum.2016.087.

Hordeaux, J., C. Hinderer, T. Goode, N. Katz, E. L. Buza, P. Bell, R. Calcedo, L. K. Richman, and J. M. Wilson. 2018. "Toxicology study of intra-cisterna magna adeno-associated virus 9 expressing human alpha-L-iduronidase in rhesus macaques." *Mol Ther Methods Clin Dev* 10:79–88. doi: 10.1016/j.omtm.2018.06.003.

Hovland, D. N., Jr., R. B. Boyd, M. T. Butt, J. A. Engelhardt, M. S. Moxness, M. H. Ma, M. G. Emery, N. B. Ernst, R. P. Reed, J. R. Zeller, D. M. Gash, D. M. Masterman, B. M. Potter, M. E. Cosenza, and R. M. Lightfoot. 2007. "Six-month continuous intraputamenal infusion toxicity study of recombinant methionyl human glial cell line-derived neurotrophic factor (r-metHuGDNF in rhesus monkeys." *Toxicol Pathol* 35 (7):1013–1029. doi: 10.1177/01926230701481899.

Hwang, T. J., J. J. Darrow, and A. S. Kesselheim. 2017. "The FDA's expedited programs and clinical development times for novel therapeutics, 2012–2016." *JAMA* 318 (21):2137–2138. doi: 10.1001/jama.2017.14896.

ICH. 2009a. "Guidance on Nonclinical Safety Studies for the Conduct of Human Clinical Trials and Marketing Authorization for Pharmaceuticals M3(R2)." International Conference on Harmonisation of Technical Requirements for Registration of Pharmaceuticals for Human Use.

ICH. 2009b. "Nonclinical Evaluation for Anticancer Pharmaceuticals (S9)." International Conference on Harmonisation of Technical Requirements for Registration of Pharmaceuticals for Human Use.

ICH. 2011. "Preclinical Safety Evaluation of Biotechnology-Derived Pharmaceuticals S6(R1)." International Conference on Harmonisation of Technical Requirements for Registration of Pharmaceuticals for Human Use.

Ito, H., R. Wate, J. Zhang, S. Ohnishi, S. Kaneko, H. Ito, S. Nakano, and H. Kusaka. 2008. "Treatment with edaravone, initiated at symptom onset, slows motor decline and decreases SOD1 deposition in ALS mice." *Exp Neurol* 213 (2):448–455. doi: 10.1016/j.expneurol.2008.07.017.

JPND Action Group. 2014. "Experimental Models for Neurodegenerative Diseases." Report of the JPND Action Group. EU Joint Programme – Neurodegenerative Disease Research. https://www.neurodegenerationresearch.eu/uploads/media/JPND_Exp_Models_Final_report_Jan_2014_-_DM.pdf.

Khera, A. 2020. "Expediting drug development regulatory pathways globally." *Clin Res* 34 (3):18-28.

Kim, T. W., K. S. Kim, J. W. Seo, S. Y. Park, and S. P. Henry. 2014. "Antisense oligonucleotides on neurobehavior, respiratory, and cardiovascular function, and hERG channel current studies." *J Pharmacol Toxicol Methods* 69 (1):49–60. doi: 10.1016/j.vascn.2013.10.005.

Kin, K., T. Yasuhara, M. Kameda, and I. Date. 2019. "Animal models for Parkinson's disease research: trends in the 2000s." *Int J Mol Sci* 20 (21). doi: 10.3390/ijms20215402.

Knopman, D. S., and R. O. Roberts. 2011. "Estimating the number of persons with frontotemporal lobar degeneration in the US population." *J Mol Neurosci* 45 (3):330–335. doi: 10.1007/s12031-011-9538-y.

Lang, A. E., S. Gill, N. K. Patel, A. Lozano, J. G. Nutt, R. Penn, D. J. Brooks, G. Hotton, E. Moro, P. Heywood, M. A. Brodsky, K. Burchiel, P. Kelly, A. Dalvi, B. Scott, M. Stacy, D. Turner, V. G. Wooten, W. J. Elias, E. R. Laws, V. Dhawan, A. J. Stoessl, J. Matcham, R. J. Coffey, and M. Traub. 2006. "Randomized controlled trial of intraputamenal glial cell line-derived neurotrophic factor infusion in Parkinson disease." *Ann Neurol* 59 (3):459–466. doi: 10.1002/ana.20737.

Liu, C. C., D. L. Ma, T. D. Yan, X. Fan, Z. Poon, L. F. Poon, S. A. Goh, S. G. Rozen, W. Y. Hwang, V. Tergaonkar, P. Tan, S. Ghosh, D. M. Virshup, E. L. Goh, and S. Li. 2016. "Distinct responses of stem cells to telomere uncapping-A potential strategy to improve the safety of cell therapy." *Stem Cells* 34 (10):2471–2484. doi: 10.1002/stem.2431.

Lynch, C. M., B. W. Hart, and I. S. Grewal. 2009. "Practical considerations for nonclinical safety evaluation of therapeutic monoclonal antibodies." *MAbs* 1 (1):2–11. doi: 10.4161/mabs.1.1.7377.

Maddox, R. A., M. K. Person, J. E. Blevins, J. Y. Abrams, B. S. Appleby, L. B. Schonberger, and E. D. Belay. 2020. "Prion disease incidence in the United States: 2003–2015." *Neurology* 94 (2):e153-e157. doi: 10.1212/WNL.0000000000008680.

Maguire, R., and P. Maguire. 2020. "Caregiver burden in multiple sclerosis: recent trends and future directions." *Curr Neurol Neurosci Rep* 20 (7):18. doi: 10.1007/s11910-020-01043-5.

Manfredsson, F. P., A. C. Rising, and R. J. Mandel. 2009. "AAV9: a potential blood-brain barrier buster." *Mol Ther* 17 (3):403–405. doi: 10.1038/mt.2009.15.

Martin, J. B. 1999. "Molecular basis of the neurodegenerative disorders." *N Engl J Med* 340 (25):1970–1980. doi: 10.1056/NEJM199906243402507.

Mehta, P., W. Kaye, J. Raymond, R. Punjani, T. Larson, J. Cohen, O. Muravov, and K. Horton. 2018. "Prevalence of amyotrophic lateral sclerosis - United States, 2015." *MMWR Morb Mortal Wkly Rep* 67 (46):1285–1289. doi: 10.15585/mmwr.mm6746a1.

Merkel, S. F., A. M. Andrews, E. M. Lutton, D. Mu, E. Hudry, B. T. Hyman, C. A. Maguire, and S. H. Ramirez. 2017. "Trafficking of adeno-associated virus vectors across a model of the blood-brain barrier; a comparative study of transcytosis and transduction using primary human brain endothelial cells." *J Neurochem* 140 (2):216–230. doi: 10.1111/jnc.13861.

Mijanovic, O., A. Brankovic, A. Borovjagin, D. V. Butnaru, E. A. Bezrukov, R. B. Sukhanov, A. Shpichka, P. Timashev, and I. Ulasov. 2020. "Battling neurodegenerative diseases with adeno-associated virus-based approaches." *Viruses* 12 (4). doi: 10.3390/v12040460.

N.I.N.D.S. 2020. "Batten Disease Fact Sheet." National Institute of Neurological Disorders and Stroke (N.I.N.D.S). https://www.ninds.nih.gov/Disorders/Patient-Caregiver-Education/Fact-Sheets/Batten-Disease-Fact-Sheet#:~:text=It%20is%20not%20known%20how,children%20in%20the%20United%20States (Accessed 17 Aug 2020).

N.O.R.D. 2020. "Huntington's Disease." National Organization for Rare Disorders. Rare Disease Database. https://rarediseases.org/rare-diseases/huntingtons-disease/ (Accessed 17 Aug 2020).

Nagai, S. 2019. "Flexible and expedited regulatory review processes for innovative medicines and regenerative medical products in the US, the EU, and Japan." *Int J Mol Sci* 20 (15). doi: 10.3390/ijms20153801.

Nair, R. R., S. Corrochano, S. Gasco, C. Tibbit, D. Thompson, C. Maduro, Z. Ali, P. Fratta, A. A. Arozena, T. J. Cunningham, and E. M. C. Fisher. 2019. "Uses for humanised mouse models in precision medicine for neurodegenerative disease." *Mamm Genome* 30 (7–8):173–191. doi: 10.1007/s00335-019-09807-2.

Novartis. 2019. "Novartis announces AVXS-101 intrathecal study update." 30 Oct 2019 Press Release. https://www.novartis.com/news/media-releases/novartis-announces-avxs-101-intrathecal-study-update.

Nowrouzi, A., M. Penaud-Budloo, C. Kaeppel, U. Appelt, C. Le Guiner, P. Moullier, C. von Kalle, R. O. Snyder, and M. Schmidt. 2012. "Integration frequency and intermolecular recombination of rAAV vectors in non-human primate skeletal muscle and liver." *Mol Ther* 20 (6):1177–1186. doi: 10.1038/mt.2012.47.

Nutt, J. G., K. J. Burchiel, C. L. Comella, J. Jankovic, A. E. Lang, E. R. Laws, Jr., A. M. Lozano, R. D. Penn, R. K. Simpson, Jr., M. Stacy, G. F. Wooten, and ICV GDNF Study Group. Implanted intracerebroventricular. Glial cell line-derived neurotrophic factor. 2003. "Randomized, double-blind trial of glial cell line-derived neurotrophic factor (GDNF) in PD." *Neurology* 60 (1):69–73. doi: 10.1212/wnl.60.1.69.

Pardridge, W. M. 2015. "Blood-brain barrier drug delivery of IgG fusion proteins with a transferrin receptor monoclonal antibody." *Expert Opin Drug Deliv* 12 (2):207–222. doi: 10.1517/17425247.2014.952627.

Pardridge, W. M. 2019. "Blood-brain barrier and delivery of protein and gene therapeutics to brain." *Front Aging Neurosci* 11:373. doi: 10.3389/fnagi.2019.00373.

Parkinson's Foundation. 2020. "Prevalence Project." https://www.parkinson.org/understanding-parkinsons/statistics/Prevalence-Project (Accessed 17 Aug 2020).

Perez, B. A., A. Shutterly, Y. K. Chan, B. J. Byrne, and M. Corti. 2020. "Management of neuroinflammatory responses to AAV-mediated gene therapies for neurodegenerative diseases." *Brain Sci* 10 (2). doi: 10.3390/brainsci10020119.

Pihlstrom, L., S. Wiethoff, and H. Houlden. 2017. "Genetics of neurodegenerative diseases: an overview." *Handb Clin Neurol* 145:309–323. doi: 10.1016/B978-0-12-802395-2.00022-5.

Prescott, J. S., P. A. Andrews, R. W. Baker, M. S. Bogdanffy, F. O. Fields, D. A. Keller, D. M. Lapadula, N. M. Mahoney, D. E. Paul, S. J. Platz, D. M. Reese, S. A. Stoch, and J. J. DeGeorge. 2017. "Evaluation of therapeutics for advanced-stage heart failure and other severely-debilitating or life-threatening diseases." *Clin Pharmacol Ther* 102 (2):219–227. doi: 10.1002/cpt.730.

Ransohoff, R. M. 2018. "All (animal) models (of neurodegeneration) are wrong. Are they also useful?" *J Exp Med* 215 (12):2955–2958. doi: 10.1084/jem.20182042.

Robertson, D., and N. Moreo. 2016. "Disease-modifying therapies in multiple sclerosis: overview and treatment considerations." *Fed Pract* 33 (6):28–34.

Rocca, M., L. L. Morford, D. L. Blanset, W. G. Halpern, J. Cavagnaro, and C. J. Bowman. 2018. "Applying a weight of evidence approach to the evaluation of developmental toxicity of biopharmaceuticals." *Regul Toxicol Pharmacol* 98:69–79. doi: 10.1016/j.yrtph.2018.07.006.

Runeberg-Roos, P., E. Piccinini, A. M. Penttinen, K. Matlik, H. Heikkinen, S. Kuure, M. M. Bespalov, J. Peranen, E. Garea-Rodriguez, E. Fuchs, M. Airavaara, N. Kalkkinen, R. Penn, and M. Saarma. 2016. "Developing therapeutically more efficient Neurturin variants for treatment of Parkinson's disease." *Neurobiol Dis* 96: 335–345. doi: 10.1016/j.nbd.2016.07.008.

Sarkar, S., J. Raymick, and S. Imam. 2016. "Neuroprotective and therapeutic strategies against Parkinson's disease: recent perspectives." *Int J Mol Sci* 17 (6). doi: 10.3390/ijms17060904.

Shi, D., G. Chen, L. Lv, L. Li, D. Wei, P. Gu, J. Gao, Y. Miao, and W. Hu. 2011. "The effect of lentivirus-mediated TH and GDNF genetic engineering mesenchymal stem cells on Parkinson's disease rat model." *Neurol Sci* 32 (1):41–51. doi: 10.1007/s10072-010-0385-3.

Stanimirovic, D. B., J. K. Sandhu, and W. J. Costain. 2018. "Emerging technologies for delivery of biotherapeutics and gene therapy across the blood-brain barrier." *BioDrugs* 32 (6):547–559. doi: 10.1007/s40259-018-0309-y.

Tan, S. B., A. F. Williams, E. K. Tan, R. B. Clark, and M. E. Morris. 2020. "Parkinson's disease caregiver strain in Singapore." *Front Neurol* 11:455. doi: 10.3389/fneur.2020.00455.

Tieu, K. 2011. "A guide to neurotoxic animal models of Parkinson's disease." *Cold Spring Harb Perspect Med* 1 (1):a009316. doi: 10.1101/cshperspect.a009316.

Trapp, B. D., and K. A. Nave. 2008. "Multiple sclerosis: an immune or neurodegenerative disorder?" *Annu Rev Neurosci* 31:247–269. doi: 10.1146/annurev.neuro.30.051606.094313.

US FDA. 1996. "Copaxone (glatiramer acetate) Review. Application No. 020622. Approved 20 Dec 1996." https://www.accessdata.fda.gov/drugsatfda_docs/nda/pre96/020622Orig1s000rev.pdf.

US FDA. 2001. "Campath (alemtuzumab) Pharmacology Review. Application No. 125104. Approved 07 May 2001." https://www.accessdata.fda.gov/drugsatfda_docs/nda/2000/103948s000_CampathTOC.cfm.

US FDA. 2004a. "Tysabri (natalizumab) Medical Review. Application No. 125104. Approved 23 Nov 2004." https://www.accessdata.fda.gov/drugsatfda_docs/nda/2004/125104s000_Natalizumab.cfm.

US FDA. 2004b. "Tysabri (natalizumab) Pharmacology Review. Application No. 125104. Approved 23 Nov 2004." https://www.accessdata.fda.gov/drugsatfda_docs/nda/2004/125104s000_Natalizumab.cfm.

US FDA. 2013. "Guidance for Industry: Preclinical Assessment of Investigational Cellular and Gene Therapy Products." Center for Biologics Evaluation and Research (CBER). U.S. Department of Health and Human Services.

US FDA. 2014. "Guidance for Industry: Expedited Programs for Serious Conditions — Drugs and Biologics." Center for Drug Evaluation and Research (CDER). Center for Biologics Evaluation and Research (CBER). U.S. Department of Health and Human Services.

US FDA. 2016a. "Spinraza (nusinersen) Medical Review. Application No. 209531. Approved 23 Dec 2016." https://www.accessdata.fda.gov/drugsatfda_docs/nda/2016/209531Orig1s000TOC.cfm.

US FDA. 2016b. "Spinraza (nusinersen) Pharmacology Review. Application No. 209531. Approved 23 Dec 2016." https://www.accessdata.fda.gov/drugsatfda_docs/nda/2016/209531Orig1s000TOC.cfm.

US FDA. 2016c. "Zynbryta (daclizumab) Medical Review. Application No. 761029. Approved 27 May 2016." https://www.accessdata.fda.gov/drugsatfda_docs/nda/2016/761029Orig1s000TOC.cfm.

US FDA. 2016d. "Zynbryta (daclizumab) Pharmacology Review. Application No. 761029. Approved 27 May 2016." https://www.accessdata.fda.gov/drugsatfda_docs/nda/2016/761029Orig1s000TOC.cfm.

US FDA. 2017a. "Brineura (cerliponase alfa) Medical Review. Application No. 761053. Approved 27 Apr 2017." https://www.accessdata.fda.gov/drugsatfda_docs/nda/2017/761052Orig1s000MedR.pdf.

US FDA. 2017b. "Brineura (cerliponase alfa) Pharmacology Review. Application No. 761053. Approved 27 Apr 2017." https://www.accessdata.fda.gov/drugsatfda_docs/nda/2017/761052Orig1s000PharmR.pdf.

US FDA. 2017c. "Guidance for Industry: Assessment of Abuse Potential of Drugs." Center for Drug Evaluation and Research (CDER). U.S. Department of Health and Human Services.

US FDA. 2017d. "Ocrevus (ocrelizumab) Medical Review. Application No. 761053. Approved 28 Mar 2017." https://www.accessdata.fda.gov/drugsatfda_docs/nda/2017/761053Orig1s000TOC.cfm.

US FDA. 2017e. "Ocrevus (ocrelizumab) Pharmacology Review. Application No. 761053. Approved 28 Mar 2017." https://www.accessdata.fda.gov/drugsatfda_docs/nda/2017/761053Orig1s000TOC.cfm.

US FDA. 2018. "FDA working with manufacturers to withdraw Zinbryta from the market in the United States." https://www.fda.gov/drugs/drug-safety-and-availability/fda-working-manufacturers-withdraw-zinbryta-market-united-states. Content current as of 14 Mar 2018 (Accessed 19 Aug 2020).

US FDA. 2019a. "CDER Breakthrough Therapy Designation Approvals." Center for Drug Evaluation and Research (CDER). U.S. Department of Health and Human Services.

US FDA. 2019b. "DRAFT Guidance for Industry: Rare Diseases: Common Issues in Drug Development." Center for Drug Evaluation and Research (CDER). Center for Biologics Evaluation and Research (CBER). U.S. Department of Health and Human Services. https://www.fda.gov/media/119757/download.

US FDA. 2019c. "Guidance for Industry: Investigational Enzyme Replacement Therapy Products: Nonclinical Assessment." Center for Drug Evaluation and Research (CDER). U.S. Department of Health and Human Services. https://www.fda.gov/media/131295/download.

US FDA. 2019d. "Zolgensma (onasemnogene abeparvovec-xioi) Clinical Review Memo. Application No. 125694. Approved 24 May 2019." https://www.fda.gov/vaccines-blood-biologics/zolgensma.

US FDA. 2019e. "Zolgensma (onasemnogene abeparvovec-xioi) Pharmacology-Toxicology Review. Application No. 125694. Approved 24 May 2019." https://www.fda.gov/vaccines-blood-biologics/zolgensma.

US FDA. 2020. "SOPP 8214: INTERACT Meetings with Sponsors for Drugs and Biological Products. Version 2. Effective Date 12 Jun 2020." Center for Biologics Evaluation and Research (CBER). U.S. Department of Health and Human Services. https://www.fda.gov/media/124044/download.

Vahle, J. L., G. L. Finch, S. M. Heidel, D. N. Hovland, Jr., I. Ivens, S. Parker, R. A. Ponce, C. Sachs, R. Steigerwalt, B. Short, and M. D. Todd. 2010. "Carcinogenicity assessments of biotechnology-derived pharmaceuticals: a review of approved molecules and best practice recommendations." *Toxicol Pathol* 38 (4):522–553. doi: 10.1177/0192623310368984.

Vargas, H. M., A. S. Bass, A. Breidenbach, H. S. Feldman, G. A. Gintant, A. R. Harmer, B. Heath, P. Hoffmann, A. Lagrutta, D. Leishman, N. McMahon, S. Mittelstadt, L. Polonchuk, M. K. Pugsley, J. J. Salata, and J. P. Valentin. 2008. "Scientific review and recommendations on preclinical cardiovascular safety evaluation of biologics." *J Pharmacol Toxicol Methods* 58 (2):72–76. doi: 10.1016/j.vascn.2008.04.001.

Verhaart, I. E. C., A. Robertson, I. J. Wilson, A. Aartsma-Rus, S. Cameron, C. C. Jones, S. F. Cook, and H. Lochmuller. 2017. "Prevalence, incidence and carrier frequency of 5q-linked spinal muscular atrophy - a literature review." *Orphanet J Rare Dis* 12 (1):124. doi: 10.1186/s13023-017-0671-8.

Vuillemenot, B. R., S. Korte, T. L. Wright, E. L. Adams, R. B. Boyd, and M. T. Butt. 2016. "Safety evaluation of CNS administered biologics-study design, data interpretation, and translation to the clinic." *Toxicol Sci* 152 (1):3–9. doi: 10.1093/toxsci/kfw072.

Wallin, M. T., W. J. Culpepper, J. D. Campbell, L. M. Nelson, A. Langer-Gould, R. A. Marrie, G. R. Cutter, W. E. Kaye, L. Wagner, H. Tremlett, S. L. Buka, P. Dilokthornsakul, B. Topol, L. H. Chen, N. G. LaRocca, and U. S. Multiple Sclerosis Prevalence Workgroup. 2019. "The prevalence of MS in the United States: a population-based estimate using health claims data." *Neurology* 92 (10):e1029–e1040. doi: 10.1212/WNL.0000000000007035.

Warren Olanow, C., R. T. Bartus, T. L. Baumann, S. Factor, N. Boulis, M. Stacy, D. A. Turner, W. Marks, P. Larson, P. A. Starr, J. Jankovic, R. Simpson, R. Watts, B. Guthrie, K. Poston, J. M. Henderson, M. Stern, G. Baltuch, C. G. Goetz, C. Herzog, J. H. Kordower, R. Alterman, A. M. Lozano, and A. E. Lang. 2015. "Gene delivery of neurturin to putamen and substantia nigra in Parkinson disease: a double-blind, randomized, controlled trial." *Ann Neurol* 78 (2):248–257. doi: 10.1002/ana.24436.

Writing Group, and Edaravone A.L.S. Study Group. 2017. "Safety and efficacy of edaravone in well defined patients with amyotrophic lateral sclerosis: a randomised, double-blind, placebo-controlled trial." *Lancet Neurol* 16 (7):505–512. doi: 10.1016/S1474-4422(17)30115-1.

Zhang, Z., Y. Miyoshi, P. A. Lapchak, F. Collins, D. Hilt, C. Lebel, R. Kryscio, and D. M. Gash. 1997. "Dose response to intraventricular glial cell line-derived neurotrophic factor administration in parkinsonian monkeys." *J Pharmacol Exp Ther* 282 (3):1396–1401.

Zincarelli, C., S. Soltys, G. Rengo, and J. E. Rabinowitz. 2008. "Analysis of AAV serotypes 1–9 mediated gene expression and tropism in mice after systemic injection." *Mol Ther* 16 (6):1073–1080. doi: 10.1038/mt.2008.76.

31

Nonclinical Development of Biologics for Infectious Diseases

B.B. Smith
Vir Biotechnology

CONTENTS

31.1 Introduction and Background

Long before the world seemingly screeched to a halt in early 2020 with the introduction and rapid spread of coronavirus disease 2019 (COVID-19), biologics had been in active development to address a variety of infectious diseases within the population. Whether it is vaccines to prevent infection or monoclonal antibodies to treat infection, scientists for hundreds of years have sought to optimize our immune system in defense of pestilence. The ability to safely grow viruses in a laboratory opened the door to many advancements and innovations. Common childhood ailments such as polio, smallpox, measles, mumps, and rubella became a reduced burden on society with the development of vaccines. And in parallel, the safety of such products came under heightened scrutiny along with an alarming rise of conspiracy theories and the anti-vaccination movement. While this chapter will focus on viral infectious diseases, similar applications can be considered for bacterial, fungal, or parasitic infectious diseases. An in-depth chapter specific to vaccines can be found in Chapter 23.

Many viral infectious diseases do not require treatment and are self-limiting, resolving without medical intervention. Others such as human immunodeficiency virus (HIV), herpes simplex, herpes zoster, varicella, and influenza have historically been treated with small molecule antiviral drugs unfortunately often with only modest success (Razonable 2011). Success as an antiviral medication relies on completely blocking the virus life cycle, via inactivation of the virus prior to entry, blocking attachment to host cells, or prevention of viral genome replication, synthesis of the viral protein or release of the new virions. However, disrupting the virus life cycle risks disrupting the host cell as well, causing toxicity. Ineffective inhibition of the virus can lead to the virus learning how to avoid inactivation, also known as escape mutants. One highly publicized example of escape mutants was the variants of the severe acute respiratory syndrome coronavirus-2 (SARS-CoV-2) that made headlines in late 2020 and early 2021, with speculation as to the continued efficacy of the monoclonal antibody (mAb) cocktails and messenger ribonucleic acid (mRNA) vaccines that had received Early Use Authorization by the Food and Drug Administration (FDA). Another limitation of small molecule antiretroviral treatment is that some viruses such as HIV and hepatitis B virus (HBV) manage to maintain a hidden stockpile of proviruses that can lead to viral rebound following a course of therapy. Researchers continue to look for novel ways either to neutralize the stockpile (sterilizing cure) or optimize the immune system independent of antiviral therapeutic treatment (functional cure) (Halper-Stromberg et al. 2016).

Until more recently, biologics for infectious diseases have primarily focused on vaccines, with fewer approved biologic therapies (Table 31.1). The benefits of biologic therapeutics would include reduced treatment burden due to extended pharmacokinetics and increased specificity to avoid potentially severe adverse off-target effects. Development of mAb therapies has historically been time-consuming; however, new proposals to use clonal pools in Investigational New Drug application (IND)-enabling toxicology studies as opposed to waiting for the single cell clone can provide opportunities for rapid development in the face of emerging health crises (Kelley 2020; Bolisetty 2020). Escape mutants may be better addressed through the usage of broad neutralizing antibodies that target more consistent, conserved regions of the virus. In HIV, however, rapid viral resistance has been observed following broadly neutralizing antibodies, as a consequence of the high mutation rate of HIV (Awi and Teow 2018).

TABLE 31.1

Selected Viruses and Status of Biologic Treatments or Vaccines

Virus	Existing Biologic Treatment	Existing Vaccine
HAV	None	Havrix™, Vaqta®
CHB	Intron® A, Roferon® A, HBIg	Engerix™ B, Recombivax HB®
CHC	Intron® A, Roferon® A	None
HIV	Trogarzo™	In development
TB	Remicade®	BCG vaccine
EVD	Inmazeb™, Ebanga™	Ervebo®
COVID-19	Monoclonal antibodies	mRNA and adenovector vaccines
Influenza	Antibody therapies in development	Inactive, inactivated, live-attenuated, and egg-free
RSV	Synagis®	In development
Rotavirus	None	Rotarix®, RotaTeq®
VZV	Antibody therapies in development	Live attenuated, Shingrix® (recombinant), Zostavax® (live)

BCV = Bacillus of Calmette and Guerin; HAV = hepatitis A virus; CHB = chronic hepatitis B; HBIg = hepatitis B immune globulin; CHC = chronic hepatitis C; HIV = human immunodeficiency virus; TB = tuberculosis; EVD = Ebola virus disease; COVID-19 = coronavirus disease 2019; RSV = respiratory syncytial virus; VZV = varicella-zoster virus

The nonclinical development of biologics for infectious diseases holds some unique considerations. The typical scope of nonclinical studies is significantly narrowed as many study types are not considered relevant. While treatment of diseases may vary in duration, from chronic such as HIV, hepatitis B, or hepatitis C, to acute such as respiratory infections, the duration of repeat-dose toxicity studies is less variable. This chapter will discuss which nonclinical safety studies should be anticipated when developing biologics for treatment and prevention of infectious diseases.

31.2 Viral Immunology

Both the innate and adaptive immune systems are critical to defend against infectious diseases. The innate immune system provides the initial defenses with the help of interferon and other cytokines. The adaptive immune system is recruited if the task is too much for the innate response, bringing in antibodies tailored to neutralizing the virus and T-cells to eliminate the infected cells. Novel approaches to improve upon our natural immune responses have included, for example, the recent mRNA vaccine technology for COVID-19 (Sandbrink and Shattock 2020; Batty et al. 2021; Ho et al. 2021) and utilization of cytomegalovirus vectors to maximize prophylactic or therapeutic vaccine potency (Früh and Picker 2017).

Passive immune therapy via infusion of convalescent plasma, or plasma collected from disease survivors, has been used for over a century (Keller and Stiehm 2000). Convalescent plasma is an early treatment option in the face of emerging infectious diseases, as was observed for Ebola and more recently with COVID-19 (Winkler 2015; Katz 2021). Evaluating the polyclonal antibody response in convalescent plasma and selecting the most active B-cell clones to create recombinant monoclonal antibodies effectively bypasses the typical lag time for a patient's own adaptive immune response (Sparrow et al. 2017). Early recombinant monoclonal antibodies targeting different epitopes may also be grouped together as a cocktail in hopes to improve virus neutralization.

Effector functions are also an important aspect of the immune response to foreign invaders (Wang 2020). Effector functions are a result of Fcγ receptors (FcγR) engaging the Fc domain of an antibody, while the Fab domain binds to the viral epitopes to neutralize the virus. While the predominant mAb isotype for infectious diseases is IgG, IgA monoclonal antibodies have also been evaluated for potent effector functions in some bacterial and viral infection settings (Davis et al. 2020). The variable affinity and specificity for an antibody's Fc domain to bind to the different activating and/or inhibiting FcγRs on a variety of leukocyte subsets control the flavor of immune response. The end result can include antibody-dependent cellular cytotoxicity (ADCC) and/or antibody-dependent cellular phagocytosis (ADCP) that each helps to clear infected host cells, reducing viral load and propagation (Bournazos et al. 2020). Antibody-mediated complement activation can also lead to complement-dependent cytotoxicity (CDC). While these effector functions are necessary for a healthy immune response to many viral infections (van Erp et al. 2019; Huang et al. 2019), they raise the theoretical possibility of antibody-dependent enhancement (ADE) if the phagocytic cell does not inactivate the virus.

31.2.1 Antibody-Dependent Enhancement and Vaccine-Associated Enhanced Disease

Antibody-dependent enhancement (ADE) of disease is defined as the worsening of an infection directly related to the antibodies produced through either previous exposure, vaccine administration, or passive transfer (Arvin et al. 2020; Bournazos et al. 2020). A related and rarely observed condition called vaccine-associated enhanced disease (VAED) is defined as an immune response to a vaccine that increases the severity of the infection compared to those who have not been vaccinated (Haynes et al. 2020). However, it is challenging to differentiate ADE or VAED from severe disease resulting from the pathogen alone. Several hypotheses have been raised about how antibodies could enhance disease, including suboptimal neutralization due to low titers, incomplete neutralization by cross-reactive antibodies from infection by a related virus and antibodies that bind but have little or no neutralizing function. Two antibody-mediated outcomes with the theoretical potential to enhance disease are uptake of the virus by phagocytic cells followed by the production of progeny virus instead of inactivation or the formation of immune complexes that are deposited in tissues and trigger complement activation and inflammation. Observations of ADE/VAED have occurred in cross-reactive serotypes of dengue fever and an early formalin-inactivated RSV vaccine, but fortunately the evidence of widespread risk of ADE is low (Arvin et al. 2020; Rao 2019; Taylor et al. 2015). Potential mechanisms also differ depending on the virus; for example, dengue targets phagocytic cells for infection, whereas uptake of other viruses by antibody mechanisms results in inactivation, as shown with coronaviruses. Importantly, there have been no advancements in clinical differentiation between severe viral infection and one exacerbated by immune dysfunction. Although there are investigative models for select diseases as discussed below, there are no validated in vitro or in vivo nonclinical models for determining the potential for ADE. In vitro assays can help to identify how the antibody impacts viral fusion, etc. but the translation to in vivo ADE is lacking. In vivo limitations include lack of models (of human disease or predictive of enhanced disease), variability between FcγRs in animals versus humans, and the anti-human antibody responses within the animal that fails to recapitulate the potential human immune response. A thorough review of VAED in the setting of coronavirus concluded there was currently no evidence of a higher potential for VAED for COVID-19 vaccines and that nonclinical models have failed to demonstrate translation to humans (Haynes et al. 2020). As for any virus, there is a theoretical risk of ADE of disease in coronavirus; however, large studies of convalescent plasma and clinical trials of mAb therapeutics have not shown a safety signal in treated patients (Arvin et al. 2020). The most relevant manner to screen for potential ADE/VAED is placebo-controlled trials designed to detect any increase in disease severity among subjects who received the intervention. While it is common to expect animal models to help translate anticipated findings in advance of clinical studies, the development of an animal model of ADE/VAED prior to having knowledge of specific immune enhancement in people would require guessing potential mechanisms, and a lack of effect in such studies could be interpreted either as a lack of ADE/VAED signal or as an inadvertent selection of a nonrelevant mechanism. Regardless of the challenges and the lack of current formal guidance, regulatory agencies will likely continue to request nonclinical data to inform on the potential for producing clinical ADE/VAED and, therefore, an acceptable proposal will need regulatory concurrence.

31.3 Therapeutics for Infectious Diseases

The typical emphasis of conducting toxicity studies in a pharmacologically relevant species shifts when your product is directed at a foreign, exogenous target such as viruses (ICH 2011;). The ICH S6 guideline briefly touches on monoclonal antibodies for viral targets in the Addendum, "…a short-term safety study … in one species (choice of species to be justified by the sponsor) can be considered; no additional toxicity studies, including reproductive toxicity studies, are appropriate." Efforts to use the lowest phylogenetic species, to align with the principles of animal use refinement, are encouraged. An alternative is also mentioned, to incorporate a safety assessment within a proof-of-concept pharmacology study when conducted in an animal model of disease to help identify target-associated toxicities.

However, animal models of disease can be challenging to develop if the virus is only known to occur/infect humans or when novel viruses are initially discovered. The ability of the virus to invade the species, the nature of immune response, as well as the ramifications of infection all help to identify potential models. The cotton rat has been used to create a model of various virus infections such as RSV, influenza, measles, herpes simplex virus, and VZV. SARS-CoV-2 has been studied in the Syrian hamster model, rhesus monkeys, and others (Muñoz-Fontela et al. 2020; Hewitt et al. 2020). It may be necessary to develop surrogates of the virus, such as the simian immunodeficiency virus (SHIV) nonhuman primate (NHP) model of HIV, a virus that combines the simian and human genomes of the immunodeficiency virus, or the simian varicella virus (SVV) in rhesus monkeys that closely resembles both primary and reactivated varicella-zoster infections, also known as chicken pox and shingles, respectively (Mahalingam et al. 2019). Another alternative to study pharmacology in animal models is to modify the candidate antibody to better align with species-specific variations in immune response, such as FcγRs, or modify the virus to recognize the animal's viral entry receptors. An example of the latter is the novel mouse-adapted model of SARS-CoV-2 that remodeled the SARS-CoV-2 spike receptor-binding domain at the mouse angiotensin-converting enzyme receptor-2 (mACE2) binding interface to allow for infection (Dinnon et al. 2020, 2021; Schäfer et al. 2021).

Tissue cross-reactivity (TCR) studies are commonly performed to help identify potential off-target tissues (Leach et al. 2010; Bussiere et al. 2011). The study is particularly important for exogenous targets as it provides the justification for safety assessment in the lowest phylogenetic species. The guidance also allows for alternatives such as validated in vitro protein arrays (ICH 2011; MacLachlan 2021). However, when monoclonal antibodies are selected from the plasma of recovered patients, cross-reactivity may not be anticipated as they would have been subject to immune negative selection mechanisms that eliminate autoreactive antibodies. While not explicitly discussed in guidelines, human fetal TCR studies are also currently recommended by regulators in lieu of reproductive animal studies seemingly to provide additional "comfort" prior to treating pregnant women clinically. However, the collection of these tissues for studies raises ethical questions, and the appropriate interpretation of positive specific reactivity in light of limited tissue panels or singular donors supports that acceptable alternatives should be investigated by both industry and regulatory agencies.

Two recently approved biologic therapeutics, Inmazeb and Ebanga, for *Zaire ebolavirus* illustrate the nonclinical safety program that may be expected for a biologic product targeting an infectious disease. Inmazeb is cocktail of three monoclonal

TABLE 31.2

Comparison of Two Antibody Therapeutics for Ebola

Inmazeb	Ebanga
3-week IV rat	4-week IV rhesus monkey
• Each antibody was studied independently at a single dose, and the combination was administered at three dose levels, up to a high dose of 65 mg/kg each, once weekly for three administrations	• Antibody was dosed either weekly at 50 or 500 mg/kg or 50 mg/kg three times per week
• 10-week recovery	• Tissue distribution and Ebola glycoprotein binding included
• CNS and CV safety pharmacology endpoints included	• 8-week recovery
	• CNS, CV, and respiratory safety pharmacology endpoints included
TCR in adult human and rat tissues	TCR in adult human tissues
TCR in fetal human tissues	Postmarketing commitment to perform TCR in fetal human tissues

antibodies (1:1:1) intended to be administered as a single intravenous (IV) infusion of 50 mg/kg of each component. Ebanga, approved approximately 2 months later, is a single mAb also administered as a single IV infusion of 50 mg/kg (Table 31.2).

Antidrug antibodies (ADAs) were not evaluated in the toxicology study for Inmazeb nor in the nonhuman primate pharmacokinetic (NHP PK) study, citing that ADAs in preclinical species are not predictive of immunogenicity in humans. Instead, a visual inspection of concentration–time profiles from the PK study was performed and animals exhibiting a "sudden precipitous decline" were considered ADA positive and excluded from pharmacokinetic mean analysis (FDA 2019: Inmazeb). Later in development, ADA assays were developed for clinical use and samples from the NHP PK study were used to confirm the accuracy of the assay. ADAs were evaluated for Ebanga in the NHP PK study and are typically considered helpful in the interpretation of toxicity findings, and critical if you want to attribute morbidity/unscheduled deaths to ADAs. While the ICH S6 Addendum is not explicit as to the need for inclusion of safety pharmacology endpoints within the toxicity evaluation, the lack of relevant species or anticipated tissue cross-reactivity due to an exogenous target would suggest these endpoints may not bring value. In the TCR studies with Inmazeb, unexpected membrane staining prompted a follow-up competition TCR study which suggested the observed membrane staining was the result of nonspecific binding. Genetic toxicity, carcinogenicity, and reproductive toxicity studies were absent from both programs consistent with current guidance.

31.4 Vaccine Development for Infectious Diseases

The concepts discussed below are expanded upon in the chapter on Vaccines and Adjuvants authored by Klas and Novicki. Guidelines have been established by the World Health Organization (WHO) for the nonclinical evaluation of vaccines (WHO Annex 1 2005; WHO Annex 2 2014). Nonclinical immunization studies are useful for providing efficacy proof of concept as well as the nature of the intended immune

response following vaccination and subsequent challenge with the antigen. However, it is acknowledged that again, there are limitations in the animal models either failing to recapitulate the disease in humans or failing to predict efficacy due to species variation in immune response.

The World Health Organization (WHO) recommendations for toxicology studies in support of vaccines largely follow recommended ICH guidelines (ICH 2011), emphasizing relevant animal species, dosing schedule, route of administration, and options to include toxicity endpoints into animal efficacy studies. The animal species should develop an immune response to the vaccine antigen and a single species is usually sufficient. The dose studied should provide a maximal immune response in the animal and is often the highest anticipated clinical dose, as opposed to a dose–response evaluation, and the number of administered doses should be equal to or greater than the number proposed in humans. Studies often include one administration more than proposed clinically to allow for flexibility in clinical trial design should another dose be warranted. As with other biologics, a shorter dosing interval between doses may be used, particularly if driven by the kinetics of the anticipated immune response. Local tolerability or inflammatory reactions to treatment are important to monitor, along with the evaluation of draining lymph nodes, systemic toxicity, and immune system effects (antigen-specific antibody titers, seroconversion rates, activation of cytokine-secreting cells, and/or measures of cell-mediated immune responses) (FDA 2007). Specific and helpful recommendations regarding the timing of endpoint collections are provided in the WHO guidelines. As with all biologics, inappropriate and unintended immune reactions from early studies could prompt specialized immunotoxicity studies to further investigate mechanisms, such as potential to induce cytokine storm or cytokine release syndrome. Autoimmune diseases such as systemic lupus erythematosus, multiple sclerosis, and Guillain–Barré syndrome have also been observed following vaccination against various infectious diseases, potentially a result of adjuvants, cross-reactive epitopes on endogenous proteins (molecular mimicry), or background genetic susceptibility to autoimmune disorders; however, there is currently inadequate evidence of causality to vaccines (Vadalà et al. 2017). Nonclinical models to evaluate the potential to cause autoimmune disease are discussed in Chapter 23.

Developmental toxicity studies are indicated if the vaccine is intended for administration to pregnant women or women of childbearing potential and should be performed in animals that demonstrate an immune response to the vaccine (WHO Annex 1 2005; WHO Annex 2 2014; FDA 2006). Typically, peri/postnatal and embryofetal development studies are necessary, and dosing is tailored to maximize the immune response during critical phases of reproduction (Stages C through E, ICH S5[R3] (ICH 2020)). Maternal antibody transfer is assessed by measuring cord or fetal blood antibody levels. Developmental toxicity studies may not be considered necessary if sufficient data already exist for vaccines within a similar product class (FDA 2006).

Novel adjuvants or additives such as excipients or preservatives were initially recommended to be characterized independently with a full toxicology battery of studies, as would be expected of any new chemical entity, including genotoxicity and carcinogenicity assessments (WHO Annex 1 2005). However, Annex 2 revised the recommendation and proposed that inclusion of a study arm receiving adjuvant alone in general toxicology studies may be sufficient and that while genotoxicity testing is still recommended, previous experience suggests that carcinogenicity studies for new adjuvants are not necessary (WHO Annex 2 2014). Pharmacokinetic studies are also normally not needed; however, distribution studies may hold value for new routes of administration or novel adjuvants.

An example of a nonclinical development package for vaccines can be found in the summary basis for regulatory action for the recently approved live vaccine for *Zaire ebolavirus*, ERVEBO (https://www.fda.gov/vaccines-blood-biologics/ervebo). The vaccine was supported by two repeat-dose toxicity studies administering two intramuscular injections of two concentrations, 2 weeks apart in mice and cynomolgus monkeys, followed by 4-week recovery periods. A reproductive and developmental toxicity study in rats was supported by exploratory immunogenicity/viremia data, and dosing was optimized to provide maximal immune response during critical developmental stages. Only a single dose level was evaluated; the initial dose occurred 28 days prior to mating, and the study was taken until postnatal Day 21. Antibody analysis confirmed active delivery of the vaccine and the presence of maternal antibodies in the pups. Several challenge models in multiple species supported the preclinical proof of concept. A biodistribution study in cynomolgus monkeys established persistence of vaccine virus RNA in lymphoid tissues and a low potential for viral shedding. An additional study in cynomolgus monkeys evaluated the potential for neurovirulence after intrathalamic brain inoculation.

31.5 Animal Rule

Raxibacumab and obiltoxaximab received FDA approvals in 2012 and 2016, respectively, for the treatment of inhaled anthrax, a bacterial infection caused by Bacillus anthracis, in an assessment driven by the "Animal Rule" (Pelfrene et al. 2019). Under the FDA Animal Rule guidance, approval of drugs or biologics may be based on animal studies when human efficacy studies are not considered ethical or feasible (FDA 2002, 2015). While this guideline focuses on animal efficacy and pharmacokinetic/pharmacodynamic (PK/PD) assessments to extrapolate to proposed human doses, toxicology studies are not addressed. Insight can be gained by the Summary Basis of Approval documents; raxibacumab incorporated gross and histopathologic evaluation into the good laboratory practice (GLP), anthrax-challenged rabbit efficacy study, with emphasis on selected organs including the central nervous system (CNS), as a result of CNS findings observed in earlier rabbit and monkey toxicology studies in healthy animals. TCR studies were performed in human, monkey, and rabbit tissues. A single embryofetal development study was also performed in rabbits. For obiltoxaximab, a single-dose cardiovascular and toxicity study in monkeys was performed along with repeat-dose studies up to 14 days in rats and embryofetal development evaluation in rabbits. As with raxibacumab, obiltoxaximab also had TCR studies performed using human, rat, and monkey tissues and a targeted neuropathology assessment from treated infected monkeys and treated infected and noninfected rabbits.

31.6 Accelerated Approval Pathways and Specific Regulatory Guidance

COVID-19 has elevated the visibility to regulatory acceleration mechanisms in place to improve the availability of vaccines and therapeutics for emerging serious health crises (Grobler et al. 2020). Pre-IND meeting requests with the FDA were streamlined specifically for COVID-19 (FDA 2020a). Fast Track and Breakthrough Therapy designations with the FDA can be applied for by sponsors to allow for rolling submissions and opportunities to expedite development and review (Kepplinger 2015). Emergency Use Authorizations (EUAs) are a mechanism employed by FDA to enable the use of medical products with limited data to help rapidly address public health emergencies and, in October 2020, released a guideline specifically for COVID-19 vaccine EUAs (FDA 2020b). Health Canada has a similar process termed an Interim Order and the European Medicines Agency (EMA) has the authority to grant conditional marketing authorizations (Pelfrene et al. 2019). The FDA also has several Guidance for Industry documents specific to indications such as influenza (April 2011), respiratory syncytial virus (October 2017, draft), and hepatitis B (November 2018, draft). In October 2016, FDA provided guidance on priority review vouchers to sponsor's applications for the prevention or treatment of a "tropical disease." Priority review vouchers help to incentivize development for rare diseases and can be granted by the FDA or purchased from another company that was granted a voucher that they have decided not to utilize for their own development. As the name implies, the priority review voucher will reduce FDA review of the application to 6 months from the typical 10-month time frame of a standard review, allowing for potentially more rapid financial recuperation of development costs. In summary, regulatory agencies are keen to help developers understand expectations unique to infectious diseases and expedite development in times of need.

31.7 Conclusion

The COVID-19 pandemic has brought worldwide attention to the significant need for a rapid development of new therapeutics and vaccines for infectious diseases. The extent of nonclinical safety evaluation is targeted based on the specific attributes of the product and, as such, may not be as extensive as for other biologics. The utility of TCR studies for exogenous targets or the development of animal studies to identify potential for clinical ADE/VAED prior to evidence of immune enhancement in people will require special attention. As with all biologics, robust scientific justification in discussions with regulatory authorities is encouraged to ensure successful translation to the clinic.

REFERENCES
Arvin AM, Fink K, Schmid MA, Cathcart A, Spreafico R, Havenar-Daughton C, Lanzavecchia A, Corti D, Virgin HW. A perspective on potential antibody-dependent enhancement of

SARS-CoV-2. *Nature.* 2020 Aug;584(7821):353–363. doi: 10.1038/s41586-020-2538-8. Epub 2020 Jul 13. PMID: 32659783.

Awi NJ, Teow SY. Antibody-mediated therapy against HIV/AIDS: where are we standing now? *J Pathog.* 2018 Jun 3;2018: 8724549. doi: 10.1155/2018/8724549. PMID: 29973995; PMCID: PMC6009031.

Batty CJ, Heise MT, Bachelder EM, Ainslie KM. Vaccine formulations in clinical development for the prevention of severe acute respiratory syndrome coronavirus 2 infection. *Adv Drug Deliv Rev.* 2021 Feb;169:168–189. doi: 10.1016/j. addr.2020.12.006. Epub 2020 Dec 13. PMID: 33316346; PMCID: PMC7733686.

Bolisetty P, Tremml G, Xu S, Khetan A. Enabling speed to clinic for monoclonal antibody programs using a pool of clones for IND-enabling toxicity studies, MAbs. 2020 Jan–Dec;12(1):1763727.

Bournazos S, Gupta A, Ravetch JV. The role of IgG Fc receptors in antibody-dependent enhancement. *Nat Rev Immunol.* 2020 Oct;20(10):633–643. doi: 10.1038/s41577-020-00410-0. Epub 2020 Aug 11. PMID: 32782358; PMCID: PMC7418887.

Bussiere JL, Leach MW, Price KD, Mounho BJ, Lightfoot-Dunn R. Survey results on the use of the tissue cross-reactivity immunohistochemistry assay. *Regul Toxicol Pharmacol.* 2011 Apr;59(3):493–502. doi: 10.1016/j.yrtph.2010.09.017. Epub 2010 Oct 14. PMID: 20951178.

Davis SK, Selva KJ, Kent SJ, Chung AW. Serum IgA Fc effector functions in infectious disease and cancer. *Immunol Cell Biol.* 2020 Apr;98(4):276–286. doi: 10.1111/ imcb.12306. Epub 2020 Jan 19. PMID: 31785006; PMCID: PMC7217208.

Dinnon KH 3rd, Leist SR, Schäfer A, Edwards CE, Martinez DR, Montgomery SA, West A, Yount BL Jr, Hou YJ, Adams LE, Gully KL, Brown AJ, Huang E, Bryant MD, Choong IC, Glenn JS, Gralinski LE, Sheahan TP, Baric RS. A mouse-adapted model of SARS-CoV-2 to test COVID-19 countermeasures. *Nature.* 2020 Oct;586(7830):560–566. doi: 10.1038/s41586-020-2708-8. Epub 2020 Aug 27. Erratum in: *Nature.* 2021 Jan 19; PMID: 32854108.

Dinnon KH 3rd, Leist SR, Schäfer A, Edwards CE, Martinez DR, Montgomery SA, West A, Yount BL Jr, Hou YJ, Adams LE, Gully KL, Brown AJ, Huang E, Bryant MD, Choong IC, Glenn JS, Gralinski LE, Sheahan TP, Baric RS. Publisher correction: a mouse-adapted model of SARS-CoV-2 to test COVID-19 countermeasures. *Nature.* 2021 Jan 19. doi: 10.1038/s41586-020-03107-5. Epub ahead of print. Erratum for: *Nature.* 2020 Oct;586(7830):560–566. PMID: 33469219.

Früh K, Picker L. CD8+ T cell programming by cytomegalovirus vectors: applications in prophylactic and therapeutic vaccination. *Curr Opin Immunol.* 2017 Aug;47:52–56. doi: 10.1016/j.coi.2017.06.010. Epub 2017 Jul 19. PMID: 28734175; PMCID: PMC5626601.

FDA. Final Rule, New Drug and Biological Drug Products: Evidence Needed to Demonstrate Effectiveness of New Drugs When Efficacy Studies are Not Ethical or Feasible, 67 FR 37988, May 31, 2002.

FDA. Guidance for Industry: Considerations for Developmental Toxicity Studies for Preventive and Therapeutic Vaccines for Infectious Disease Indications, February 2006.

FDA. Guidance for Industry: Considerations for Plasmid DNA Vaccines for Infectious Disease Indications, November 2007.

FDA. Guidance for Industry, Influenza: Developing Drugs for Treatment and/or Prophylaxis, April 2011.

FDA. Guidance for Industry, Product Development Under the Animal Rule, October 2015.

FDA. Guidance for Industry, Respiratory Syncytial Virus Infection: Developing Antiviral Drugs for Prophylaxis and Treatment, October 2017 draft.

FDA. Guidance for Industry, Chronic Hepatitis B Virus Infection: Developing Drugs for Treatment, November 2018 draft.

FDA. Inmazeb (atoltivimab, maftivimab, and odesivimab-ebgn) Multi-Discipline Review, 2019. Application No. 761169. Approved 14 Oct 2020.

FDA. Guidance for Industry and Investigators, COVID-19 Public Health Emergency: General Considerations for Pre-IND Meeting Requests for COVID-19 Related Drugs and Biological Products, May 2020a.

FDA. Guidance for Industry, Emergency Use Authorization for Vaccines to Prevent COVID-19, October 2020b.

Grobler JA, Anderson AS, Fernandes P, Diamond MS, Colvis CM, Menetski JP, Alvarez RM, Young JAT, Carter KL. Accelerated preclinical paths to support rapid development of COVID-19 therapeutics. *Cell Host Microbe.* 2020 Nov 11;28(5):638–645. doi: 10.1016/j.chom.2020.09.017. Epub 2020 Oct 1. PMID: 33152278; PMCID: PMC7528945.

Halper-Stromberg A, Nussenzweig MC. Towards HIV-1 remission: potential roles for broadly neutralizing antibodies. *J Clin Invest.* 2016 Feb;126(2):415–23. doi: 10.1172/JCI80561. Epub 2016 Jan 11. PMID: 26752643; PMCID: PMC4731188.

Haynes BF, Corey L, Fernandes P, Gilbert PB, Hotez PJ, Rao S, Santos MR, Schuitemaker H, Watson M, Arvin A. Prospects for a safe COVID-19 vaccine. *Sci Transl Med.* 2020 Nov 4;12(568):eabe0948. doi: 10.1126/scitranslmed. abe0948. Epub 2020 Oct 19. PMID: 33077678.

Hewitt JA, Lutz C, Florence WC, Pitt MLM, Rao S, Rappaport J, Haigwood NL. ACTIVating Resources for the COVID-19 pandemic: in vivo models for vaccines and therapeutics. *Cell Host Microbe.* 2020 Nov 11;28(5):646–659. doi: 10.1016/j.chom.2020.09.016. Epub 2020 Oct 1. PMID: 33152279; PMCID: PMC7528903.

Ho W, Gao M, Li F, Li Z, Zhang XQ, Xu X. Next-generation vaccines: nanoparticle-mediated DNA and mRNA delivery. *Adv Healthc Mater.* 2021 Jan 18;e2001812. doi: 10.1002/ adhm.202001812. Epub ahead of print. PMID: 33458958.

Huang Y, Dai H, Ke R. Principles of effective and robust innate immune response to viral infections: a multiplex network analysis. *Front Immunol.* 2019 Jul 24;10:1736. doi: 10.3389/fimmu.2019.01736. PMID: 31396233; PMCID: PMC6667926.

ICH. 2011. "Preclinical Safety Evaluation of Biotechnology-Derived Pharmaceuticals S6(R1)." International Conference on Harmonisation of Technical Requirements for Registration of Pharmaceuticals for Human Use.

ICH. 2020. "Detection of Reproductive and Developmental Toxicity for Human Pharmaceuticals S5(R3)." International Conference on Harmonisation of Technical Requirements for Registration of Pharmaceuticals for Human Use.

Katz LM. (A Little) Clarity on convalescent plasma for Covid-19. *N Engl J Med Editor.* 2021 Jan 13; at NEJM.org

Keller MA, Stiehm ER. Passive immunity in prevention and treatment of infectious diseases. *Clin Microbiol Rev.* 2000 Oct;13(4):602–14. doi: 10.1128/cmr.13.4.602–614.2000. PMID: 11023960; PMCID: PMC88952.

Kelley, B. Developing therapeutic monoclonal antibodies at pandemic pace. *Nat Biotechnol.* 2020;38:540–545. https://doi.org/10.1038/s41587-020-0512-5

Kepplinger EE. FDA's expedited approval mechanisms for new drug products. *Biotechnol Law Rep.* 2015 Feb 1;34(1):15–37. doi: 10.1089/blr.2015.9999. PMID: 25713472; PMCID: PMC4326266.

Leach MW, Halpern WG, Johnson CW, Rojko JL, MacLachlan TK, Chan CM, Galbreath EJ, Ndifor AM, Blanset DL, Polack E, Cavagnaro JA. Use of tissue cross-reactivity studies in the development of antibody-based biopharmaceuticals: history, experience, methodology, and future directions. *Toxicol Pathol.* 2010 Dec;38(7):1138–1166. doi: 10.1177/0192623310382559. Epub 2010 Oct 6. PMID: 20926828.

MacLachlan TK, Price S, Cavagnaro J, Andrews L, Blanset D, Cosenza ME, Dempster M, Galbreath E, Giusti AM, Heinz-Taheny KM, Fleurance R, Sutter E, Leach MW, Classic and evolving approaches to evaluating cross reactivity of mAb and mAb-like molecules – A survey of industry 2008–2019, Regul Toxicol Pharmacol. 2021 Apr;121:104872.

Mahalingam R, Gershon A, Gershon M, Cohen JI, Arvin A, Zerboni L, Zhu H, Gray W, Messaoudi I, Traina-Dorge V. Current in vivo models of varicella-zoster virus neurotropism. *Viruses.* 2019 May 31;11(6):502. doi: 10.3390/v11060502. PMID: 31159224; PMCID: PMC6631480.

Muñoz-Fontela C, Dowling WE, Funnell SGP, Gsell PS, Riveros-Balta AX, Albrecht RA, Andersen H, Baric RS, Carroll MW, Cavaleri M, Qin C, Crozier I, Dallmeier K, de Waal L, de Wit E, Delang L, Dohm E, Duprex WP, Falzarano D, Finch CL, Frieman MB, Graham BS, Gralinski LE, Guilfoyle K, Haagmans BL, Hamilton GA, Hartman AL, Herfst S, Kaptein SJF, Klimstra WB, Knezevic I, Krause PR, Kuhn JH, Le Grand R, Lewis MG, Liu WC, Maisonnasse P, McElroy AK, Munster V, Oreshkova N, Rasmussen AL, Rocha-Pereira J, Rockx B, Rodríguez E, Rogers TF, Salguero FJ, Schotsaert M, Stittelaar KJ, Thibaut HJ, Tseng CT, Vergara-Alert J, Beer M, Brasel T, Chan JFW, García-Sastre A, Neyts J, Perlman S, Reed DS, Richt JA, Roy CJ, Segalés J, Vasan SS, Henao-Restrepo AM, Barouch DH. Animal models for COVID-19. *Nature.* 2020 Oct;586(7830):509–515. doi: 10.1038/s41586-020-2787-6. Epub 2020 Sep 23. PMID: 32967005.

Pelfrene E, Mura M, Cavaleiro Sanches A, Cavaleri M. Monoclonal antibodies as anti-infective products: a promising future? *Clin Microbiol Infect.* 2019 Jan;25(1):60–64. doi: 10.1016/j.cmi.2018.04.024. Epub 2018 Apr 30. PMID: 29715552; PMCID: PMC7128139.

Rao GK, Prell RA, Laing ST, Burleson SCM, Nguyen A, McBride JM, Zhang C, Sheinson D, Halpern WG, *In Vivo* assessment of antibody-dependent enhancement of influenza B infection. *Toxicol Sci.* 2019 June;169(2):409–421. https://doi.org/10.1093/toxsci/kfz053

Razonable RR, Antiviral drugs for viruses other than human immunodeficiency virus. Mayo Clin Proc. 2011; 86(10):1009–1026.

Sandbrink JB, Shattock RJ. RNA vaccines: a suitable platform for tackling emerging pandemics? *Front Immunol.* 2020 Dec 22;11:608460. doi: 10.3389/fimmu.2020.608460. PMID: 33414790; PMCID: PMC7783390.

Schäfer A, Muecksch F, Lorenzi JCC, Leist SR, Cipolla M, Bournazos S, Schmidt F, Maison RM, Gazumyan A, Martinez DR, Baric RS, Robbiani DF, Hatziioannou T, Ravetch JV, Bieniasz PD, Bowen RA, Nussenzweig MC, Sheahan TP. Antibody potency, effector function, and combinations in protection and therapy for SARS-CoV-2 infection in vivo. *J Exp Med.* 2021 Mar 1;218(3):e20201993. doi: 10.1084/jem.20201993. PMID: 33211088; PMCID: PMC7673958.

Sparrow E, Friede M, Sheikh M, Torvaldsen S. Therapeutic antibodies for infectious diseases. *Bull World Health Organ.* 2017 Mar 1;95(3):235–237. doi: 10.2471/BLT.16.178061. Epub 2017 Feb 2. PMID: 28250538; PMCID: PMC 5328111.

Taylor A, Foo SS, Bruzzone R, Dinh LV, King NJ, Mahalingam S. Fc receptors in antibody-dependent enhancement of viral infections. *Immunol Rev.* 2015 Nov;268(1):340–364. doi: 10.1111/imr.12367. PMID: 26497532; PMCID: PMC7165974.

Vadalà M, Poddighe D, Laurino C, Palmieri B. Vaccination and autoimmune diseases: is prevention of adverse health effects on the horizon? *EPMA J.* 2017 Jul 20;8(3):295–311. doi: 10.1007/s13167-017-0101-y. PMID: 29021840; PMCID: PMC5607155.

van Erp EA, Luytjes W, Ferwerda G, van Kasteren PB. Fc-mediated antibody effector functions during respiratory syncytial virus infection and disease. *Front Immunol.* 2019 Mar 22;10:548. doi: 10.3389/fimmu.2019.00548. PMID: 30967872; PMCID: PMC6438959.

Wang P, Gajjar MR, Yu J, Padte NN, Gettie A, Blanchard JL, Russell-Lodrique K, Liao LE, Perelson AS, Huang Y, Ho DD, Quantifying the contribution of Fc-mediated effector functions to the antiviral activity of anti-HIV-1 IgG1 antibodies in vivo. PNAS. 2020 Jul 28;117(30):18002–18009.

Winkler AM, Koepsell SA, The use of convalescent plasma to treat emerging infectious diseases: focus on Ebola virus disease. Curr Opin Hematol. 2015; 22:521–526.

World Health Organization. WHO guidelines on nonclinical evaluation of vaccines. Annex 1. WHO Technical Report Series. 2005;927:31–63.

World Health Organization. WHO guidelines on nonclinical evaluation of vaccines. Annex 2. WHO Technical Report Series. 2014;987:59–100.

Index

Note: **Bold** page numbers refer to tables and *italic* page numbers refer to figures.

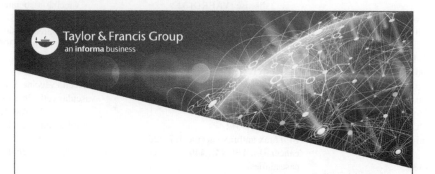